Cardiovascular Medicine

Cardiovascular Medicine
Practice and management

Edited by

Richard C Becker MD
Professor of Medicine, University of Massachusetts
Medical School, Worcester, Massachusetts, USA

and

Joseph S Alpert MD
Professor of Medicine, University of Arizona School of
Medicine, Tucson, Arizona, USA

ARNOLD

A member of the Hodder Headline Group
LONDON   NEW YORK   NEW DELHI

First published in Great Britain in 2001 by
Arnold, a member of the Hodder Headline Group,
338 Euston Road, London NW1 3BH

http://www.arnoldpublishers.com

Distributed in the United States of America by
Oxford University Press Inc.,
198 Madison Avenue, New York, NY 10016
Oxford is a registered trademark of Oxford University Press

Whilst the advice and information in this book are believed to be
true and accurate at the date of going to press, neither the authors
nor the publisher can accept any legal responsibility or liability for
any errors or omissions that may be made. In particular (but without
limiting the generality of the preceding disclaimer) every effort has
been made to check drug dosages; however it is still possible that
errors have been missed. Furthermore, dosage schedules are
constantly being revised and new side-effects recognized. For these
reasons the reader is strongly urged to consult the drug companies'
printed instructions before administering any of the drugs
recommended in this book.

British Library Cataloguing in Publication Data
A catalogue record for this book is available from the British Library

Library of Congress Cataloging-in-Publication Data
A catalog record for this book is available from the Library of
Congress

ISBN 0 340 76286 1

1 2 3 4 5 6 7 8 9 10

Commissioning Editor: Joanna Koster
Project Editor: Sarah de Souza
Production Editor: Rada Radojicic
Production Controller: Bryan Eccleshall
Cover design: Terry Griffiths

Typeset in 10/12 pt Minion by Phoenix Photosetting, Chatham, Kent
Printed and bound in Italy by Giunti Industrie Grafiche

Dedicated to clinicians around the world who are devoted to the management and optimal care of patients with cardiovascular disease.

Dedicated to our families in recognition of their support and inspiration.

Contents

Contributors

Rami Alharethi MD
Resident in Internal Medicine, St Joseph Hospital, Chicago, IL, USA

Joseph S Alpert MD
Professor of Medicine, University of Arizona School of Medicine, Tucson, AZ, USA

Ezra A Amsterdam MD
Professor of Medicine, Director, Coronary Care Unit, University of California – Davis, Sacramento, CA, USA

Jack E Ansell MD
Vice Chair of Medicine for Clinical Affairs, Boston University, Boston, MA, USA

Jill Auger PharmD
St Vincent Hospital – Worcester Medical Center, Worcester, MA, USA

Richard C Becker MD
Professor of Medicine, Division of Cardiology, Department of Medicine, University of Massachusetts Medical School, Worcester, MA, USA

Edward Bessman MD
Director, Department of Emergency Medicine, Johns Hopkins Bayview Medical Center, Baltimore, MD, USA

Marie Bosak MS, RN, CS
Acute Care Practitioner, Beth Israel-Deaconess Medical Center, Boston, MA, USA

Maureen M Burns MD
Cardiology Internist, Health Alliance Leominster, Leominster, MA, USA

Christopher P Cannon MD
Assistant Professor of Medicine, Harvard Medical School, Cardiovascular Division, Brigham and Women's Hospital, Boston, MA, USA

Eugene S Chung MD
Assistant Professor of Medicine, University of Cincinnati College of Medicine, Cincinnati, OH, USA

David M Clive MD
Associate Professor of Medicine, Renal Medicine/Dialysis, UMass-Memorial Medical Center, Worcester, MA, USA

Jeanne Corrao MS, RN, CS, ACNP
Division of Cardiovascular Medicine, UMass-Memorial Medical Center Associate Faculty, Graduate School of Nursing, Worcester, MA, USA

Jay Cyr RN, MS, CCRN
Medical Cardiovascular Patient Care, UMass-Memorial Medical Center, Worcester, MA, USA

Kim A Eagle MD
Albion Walter Hewlett Professor of Internal Medicine, Interim Chief, Division of Cardiology, Chief, Clinical Cardiology, University of Michigan Health System, Ann Arbor, MI, USA

Cara B Ebbeling PhD
Childrens Hospital, Division of Endocrinology, Boston, MA, USA

Jean Einerson MS
Preventive Cardiology, University of Wisconsin Hospital and Clinics, Madison, WI, USA

Mindy Fain MD
Assistant Professor of Clinical Medicine, University of Arizona College of Medicine, Tucson, AZ, USA

Pang-Yen Fan MD
Associate Professor of Clinical Medicine, Renal Medicine, UMass-Memorial Medical Center, Worcester, MA, USA

John Foley MD
Cardiology Associates, Norwich, CT, USA

James S Forrester MD
George Burns and Gracie Allen Professor of Cardiology, Cedars-Sinai Medical Center, Los Angeles, CA, Professor of Medicine, UCLA, Division of Cardiology, Los Angeles, CA, USA

William H Gaasch MD
Professor of Medicine, University of Massachusetts Medical School, Worcester, MA, and Lahey Clinic, Burlington, MA, USA

Pritesh J Gandhi PharmD
Assistant Professor of Clinical Pharmacy, Massachusetts College of Pharmacy and Health Sciences, Cardiovascular Pharmacotherapy Specialist, UMass-Memorial Medical Center, Worcester, MA, USA

Edward P Gerstenfeld MS, MD
Division of Cardiology, Department of Medicine, Hospital of the University of Pennsylvania, Philadelphia, PA, USA

Gary B Green MD, MPH
Associate Professor of Emergency Medicine, Johns Hopkins University School of Medicine, Baltimore, MD, USA

Peter Hagan MD
Clinical Assistant Professor, Division of Cardiology, Department of Internal Medicine, University of Michigan Health System, Ann Arbor, MI, USA

Marguerite A Hawley MD
Assistant Professor of Medicine, Renal Medicine, UMass-Memorial Medical Center, Worcester, MA, USA

James R Hebert PhD
Professor and Chairman, Norman J Arnold School of Public Health, Department of Epidemiology and Biostatistics, University of South Carolina, Charlston, SC, USA

Russell D Hull MD
Thrombosis Research Unit, University of Calgary, Foothills Hospital, Calgary, Alberta, Canada

Karen B James MD
Department of Cardiology, Cleveland Clinic Foundation, Cleveland, OH, USA

Glenn R Kershaw MD
Associate Professor of Clinical Medicine, Department of Medicine, Division of Renal Medicine, UMass-Memorial Medical Center, Worcester, MA, USA

Costas T Lambrew MD
Maine Medical Center, Division of Cardiovascular Medicine, Portland, ME, USA

Jeffrey I Leavitt MD
Assistant Professor of Medicine, Brown University School of Medicine, Cardiology Division, Memorial Hospital of Rhode Island, Pawtucket, RI, USA

Wendy A Leong PharmD
Consultant in Health Care Research and Education, Clinical Research Coordinator and Investigator, Clinical Assistant Professor of Pharmacy, University of British Columbia, Vancouver, BC, Canada

William R Lewis MD
Associate Professor of Medicine, Director, Echocardiography and Exercise Testing Laboratories, University of California-Davis Medical Center, Sacramento, CA, USA

Farrell J Lloyd MD, MPH
Clinical Assistant Professor of Medicine, University of Arizona Health Sciences Center, Tucson, AZ, USA

Yungsheng Ma MD, MPH
Department of Behavior Medicine, UMass-Memorial Medical Center, Worcester, MA, USA

Theresa Mazzarelli MS, RN, ACNP, CCRN
Division of Cardiovascular Medicine, UMass-Memorial Medical Center Associate Faculty, Graduate School of Nursing, Worcester, MA, USA

Patrick McBride MD, MPH
Professor, Department of Medicine and Family Medicine, University of Wisconsin Medical School, Madison, WI, USA

Christopher A McGrew MD
Associate Professor, Division of Sports Medicine, University of New Mexico Health Sciences Center, Albuquerque, NM, USA

Kevin M McIntyre MD
Associate Clinical Professor of Medicine, Harvard Medical School, Boston, MA, USA

Theo E Meyer MD
Professor of Medicine, Director, Heart Failure Clinic and Heart Failure Wellness Center, Department of Cardiovascular Medicine, UMass-Memorial Medical Center, MA, USA

Robert S Mittleman MD
Section of Electrophysiology and Pacing, Cardiovascular Medicine, UMass-Memorial Medical Center, Worcester, MA, USA

Boris A Murillo MD
Department of Medicine, Berkshire Medical Center, Pittsfield, MA, USA

Patrick T O'Gara MD
Associate Professor of Medicine, Harvard Medical School, Director, Clinical Service, Cardiovascular Division, Department of Medicine, Brigham and Women's Hospital, Boston, MA, USA

Ira S Ockene MD
Professor of Medicine, Division of Cardiovascular Medicine, UMass-Memorial Medical Center, Worcester, MA, USA

Judith K Ockene PhD
Director, Division of Preventive and Behavioral Medicine, UMass-Memorial Medical Center, Worcester, MA, USA

Lynn B Oertel MS, ANP
Coordinator, Anticoagulation Therapy Research, Departments of Medicine and Neurology, Massachusetts General Hospital, Boston, MA, USA

John A Paraskos MD
Professor of Medicine, Division of Cardiovascular Disease, UMass-Memorial Medical Center, Worcester, MA, USA

Liberto Pechet MD
Professor of Medicine Emeritus, Division of Hematology and Laboratory Medicine, UMass-Memorial Medical Center, Worcester, MA, USA

Graham F Pineo MD
Thrombosis Research Unit, University of Calgary, Foothills Hospital, Calgary, Alberta, Canada

Susan J Rehm MD
Division of Infectious Disease, Cleveland Clinic Foundation, Cleveland, OH, USA

Tammy B Retalic MS, RN
Nursing Director for In-patient Medical/Surgical and Out-patient Pain and Oncology Services at UMass Memorial-Marlborough Hospital, Marlborough, MA, USA

Valerie F Reyna PhD
Professor and Director, Informatics and Decision-Making Laboratory, Departments of Surgery and Medicine, University of Arizona Health Sciences Center, Tucson, AZ, USA

David N Rubin MD
The Heart Group, Ravenna, OH, USA

Nicholas A Smyrnios MD
Associate Professor of Medicine, Director, Medical Intensive Care Unit, Division of Pulmonary, Allergy, and Critical Care Medicine, University of Massachusetts Medical School, Worcester, MA, USA

Frederick A Spencer MD
Assistant Professor of Medicine, Cardiovascular Medicine, UMass-Memorial Medical Center, Worcester, MA, USA

Alan J Taege MD
Division of Infectious Disease, Cleveland Clinic Foundation, Cleveland, OH, USA

Eric J Topol MD
Chairman, Department of Cardiology, Cleveland Clinic Foundation, Cleveland, OH, USA

Stephen J Voyce MD
Allegheny University – Hahnemann MCP School of Medicine, Scranton, PA, USA

Ann Ward PhD
Department of Kinesiology, University of Wisconsin – Madison, Madison, WI, USA

Sylvan Lee-Weinberg MD
4555 Southern Boulevard, Dayton, OH, USA

Foreword

Cardiovascular medicine has been filled with innovations in practice methods over the past decade. Randomized controlled clinical trials have produced evidence that continually modify our practice on an almost monthly basis. The need for a textbook to assimilate all of this data into principles for improved patient management is obvious. Drs Becker and Alpert have done a masterful job of organizing the various aspects of cardiovascular management and solicited input from expert authors to create a textbook which can be used both by students as well as a reference by all. The text is timely and includes psychological and treatment differences between genders. The sections on emergency, critical care, laboratory testing and post-hospital management logically follow.

There has never been any greater awareness by clinicians of the importance of acute cardiovascular emergencies because of our new technologies. The treatment of myocardial infarction has changed from quiet observation to the routine use of thrombolytic agents or emergent angiography and angioplasty and coronary interventions when necessary. New biological markers are present to help stratify the risk of patients with unstable coronary syndromes so that they might be better selected for the use of low molecular weight heparins and glycoprotein IIb/IIIa receptor antagonists. Teams of cardiologists and emergency physicians work in new observation units to help stratify patients with chest pain who are at low risk for coronary events and better manage these patients and resources. Quality improvement programs permeate the practice of medicine throughout the cardiovascular units and have been sophisticated with identification of the problems, design, measurement and improvements.

This book brings together many important sources of information which will become useful on a regular basis by both trainees and specialists in cardiovascular and critical care medicine.

W. Douglas Weaver MD

Preface

Medicine, when considered broadly and mechanistically, is a discipline that intricately links the fundamentals of biology, chemistry, anatomy and physiology with the complexities of psychology and sociology. While medicine could be viewed simply as the marriage of art and science, perhaps a more honest interpretation places the latter within the original foundation and defines the former as a vehicle that provides a structured means for science to serve mankind. In keeping with this philosophy, the practice of medicine is, in essence, the golden thread that joins careful observation, scientific fact, applied knowledge, and compassion – four vital components of patient care.

Cardiovascular Medicine: Practice and management was developed and written by experienced clinicians for clinicians with a specific goal of providing clear, concise, practical, and science-oriented guidelines that have direct applicability to routine practice within ambulatory and hospital-based settings. Patient management is the book's common theme, offering insights and a comprehensive description of medical practice as we will increasingly come to understand it during this new millennium.

We have highlighted key management issues in the text by placing them in tinted boxes. In the references, a diamond (♦) denotes a key primary article, an open circle (○) denotes a key review article.

Richard C Becker MD
Joseph S Alpert MD

PART 1

Cardiovascular disease prevention

International aspects of coronary heart disease: epidemiology

YUNSHENG MA, JAMES R HEBERT, CARA B EBBELING AND IRA S OCKENE

While coronary heart disease (CHD) deaths have declined in most developed countries since the mid-1960s, CHD still remains the leading cause of death in most developed countries, such as the USA. CHD mortality is now increasing in developing countries as their populations age and adopt unhealthy lifestyles. Extensive epidemiological and clinical studies have identified the major risk factors associated with the occurrence of CHD. The major risk factors are cigarette/tobacco smoke, high blood cholesterol levels, high blood pressure, physical inactivity, and a high saturated-fat diet. Designing, planning, and implementing effective behavioral interventions and creating policies that motivate healthy behavior change remain a challenge.

INTRODUCTION

At the beginning of the twentieth century, the death rate from coronary heart disease (CHD) in the USA began to increase dramatically, reaching epidemic proportions in the mid-1960s.[1] Since 1965, age-adjusted CHD mortality has leveled off and then turned downward, declining by approximately 2–3 per cent annually (Fig. 1.1).[1] Despite this reduction, CHD remains the leading cause of death among adults in the USA and other developed countries, accounting for 30 per cent of deaths in men and 25 per cent in women.[2] Worldwide, CHD was responsible for more than 7 million deaths in 1996.[3] It is estimated that CHD will be the leading cause of death and disability in the entire world by the year 2020.[2] Thus, identifying subsets of individuals who are particularly susceptible to CHD and developing effective methods of intervention are crucial. The major modifiable risk factors for CHD are known, and targeting risk factors such as diet, smoking, and physical activity is relatively easy. However, designing, planning and implementing effective behav-ioral interventions, and creating policies that motivate healthy behavior change are much more difficult.[1]

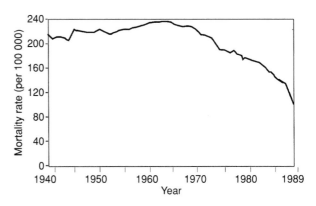

Figure 1.1 *Age-adjusted death rates for coronary heart disease in the USA, 1940–1989. (Adapted from Fetters JK, et al., Sex-specific differences in coronary artery disease risk factors, evaluation, and treatment: have they been adequately evaluated? Am Heart J 1996; **131**, 796.)*

EPIDEMIOLOGY OF CHD

International and regional variation in CHD

Since 1950, the World Health Organization (WHO) has routinely collected annual cause-of-death data from member states and countries. Currently, some 80 countries or areas are reporting cause-of-death statistics to the WHO.[4] To study the international variation and trends of CHD, the WHO initiated the Multinational Monitoring Trends and Determinants in Cardiovascular Disease (MONICA) project in 1986.[5] During 1996, the WHO published the first 5-year trend data on risk factors and incidence of CHD, made available protocols and a training manual for monitoring CHD risk factors in developing countries, and disseminated guidelines for promoting physical activity as part of a prevention strat-

egy.[6] Several other national and international CHD epidemiologic studies[7–12] also provide broad population-based comparisons, as summarized below for developed and developing countries.

DEVELOPED COUNTRIES

CHD is the leading cause of death in developed countries, and it is widely recognized as a major health concern in modern industrialized societies.[2] In 1990, a total of 10.9 million deaths occurred in the developed nations, of which 2.7 million were attributed to CHD.[13] CHD rates began increasing in North America, Europe and Australia in the early decades of the twentieth century. In many developed countries, death rates peaked in the 1960s and early 1970s, and have declined dramatically since that time, by over 50 per cent in some countries. For both men and women, the world's highest

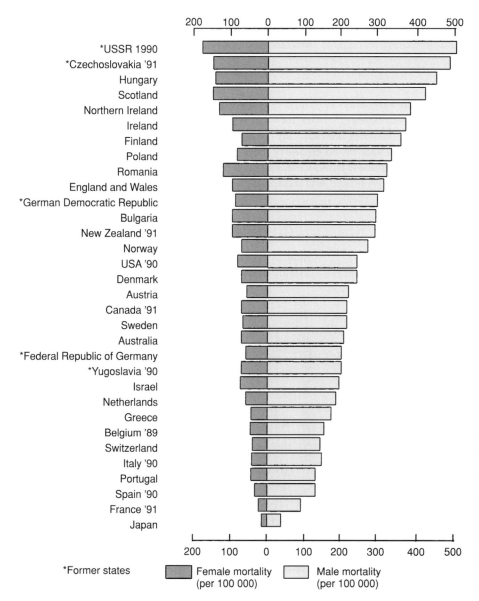

Figure 1.2 *Mortality rates for ischemic heart disease in 1992 or latest available year, age standardized to WHO European standard, age group 40–69 years. (Reprinted from Detels R, et al., Oxford textbook of public health, Vol. 3, 3rd edn. Oxford: Oxford University Press, 1997.)*

CHD mortality rates are now found in Eastern and Central Europe (Fig. 1.2), and rates are still rising in countries such as Bulgaria and Hungary.[3] In Japan, CHD mortality rates in both men and women increased from 1950 to 1970 but have decreased since 1970.[14] In the USA alone, CHD caused 487 490 deaths (i.e. 1 of every 4.7 deaths) in 1994.[15] Heart attack is the single greatest killer of men and women in the USA. Table 1.1 shows mortality rates from CHD in the Americas for a 3-year period around 1969 and a second such period around 1986. In both periods, the highest rates in the Americas were in Argentina, Canada, the USA, Trinidad and Tobago, and Uruguay. Data from North America show a declining trend for both males and females. Greater declines were evident in countries with higher initial rates.

DEVELOPING COUNTRIES

CHD mortality and morbidity are now increasing in developing countries as populations age and adopt a 'Western' lifestyle characterized by high saturated fat diets and increased rates of cigarette smoking.[3] In terms of absolute numbers of deaths in developing countries as a whole, CHD is emerging as the second leading cause.[2]

In 1990, 39.6 million deaths occurred in developing countries, 3.6 million of which were attributed to CHD. Over half of the deaths caused globally by CHD occurred in developing countries.[2] Even among countries such as Ecuador with a low rate of CHD, there have been large increases in CHD mortality over the last two decades.[1] CHD is now the predominant form of heart disease encountered in many Eastern Mediterranean countries, and hospital data indicate rising admission trends for CHD.[16]

Although the quality of vital statistics data in Africa is the poorest in the world, here too CHD appears to be emerging as an important cause of morbidity and mortality. Frequencies of CHD and related complications are relatively low in most regions, but the situation appears to be changing rapidly. For example, in the Ivory Coast, 2.2 per cent of patients with cardiovascular disorders who were admitted to medical units in 1965 had CHD, while in 1983 a frequency of 5.3 per cent was reported.[17] Likewise, autopsy studies on black South Africans in 1959 and 1976 revealed the presence of CHD in 0.9 per cent and 11.7 per cent, respectively.[18] CHD also appears to be more common in the northern African countries than in those of either Savannah or forest regions.[17]

Table 1.1 *Three-year average age-adjusted mortality rates (per 100 000) from ischemic heart disease for males and females by region of the Americas and period. (Reproduced from Nicholls, ES, Peruga A, Restrepo HE. Cardiovascular disease mortality in the Americas. World Health Stat Q 1993; **46**: 137)*

Country	Males			Females		
	1968–1970	1985–1987	%[a]	1968–1970	1985–1987	%[a]
Andean area						
Colombia	51.2	63.7	24.4	37.9	41.4	9.2
Venezuela	89.1	67.6	−24.1	56.7	42.3	−25.4
Southern Cone						
Argentina	108.3	55.2	−49.0	53.3	25.1	−52.9
Chile	68.0	54.1	−20.4	56.7	32.7	−30.0
Uruguay	103.7	66.9	−35.5	57.1	33.8	−40.8
Central America						
Costa Rica	53.4	71.2	33.3	39.3	41.7	6.1
El Salvador	14.7	37.2	153.1	13.0	24.7	90.0
Guatemala	10.1	25.2	149.5	7.1	16.5	132.4
Mexico	31.9	33.5	5.0	22.8	19.7	−13.6
Latin Caribbean						
Cuba	91.7	86.5	−5.7	67.0	63.7	-4.9
Dominican Republic	31.3	41.7	33.2	22.0	30.0	37.7
English-speaking Caribbean						
Barbados	38.7	41.0	5.9	18.2	23.7	30.2
Trinidad and Tobago	105.4	104.5	−0.9	61.8	65.0	5.2
North America						
Canada	152.3	95.0	−37.6	71.1	44.4	−37.6
United States	187.9	97.3	−48.2	92.1	50.0	−45.7

[a] Percentage change between the two 3-year periods.

Demographic characteristics

A wealth of epidemiological data provide information on a variety of demographic factors that influence CHD. Gender, age, race, and socioeconomic status are among these factors.

GENDER AND AGE

CHD is a major health concern for both men and women. As shown for the USA (Fig. 1.3), the number of Americans experiencing diagnosed heart attack annually increases with age in both genders. The annual number of heart attacks is relatively low among premenopausal women but increases sharply thereafter. Furthermore, the difference in heart attack rates between men and women becomes narrower after menopause. Narrowing of gender differences also is observed for serum cholesterol levels and blood pressure such that the CHD risk factors are higher, on average, in postmenopausal women than in men of the same age group. Two lines of evidence suggest that estrogen is an important mediator of a woman's risk of CHD.[19] First, young women with bilateral oophorectomy have an increased risk of CHD unless they are treated with estrogen.[20] Second, accumulating data from observational studies show that women who use estrogen replacement therapy after menopause have lower rates of heart disease.[21] However, potential selection bias exists in these observational studies if women who choose to take hormones are healthier and have a more favorable CHD profile than those who do not. Only a clinical trial can resolve this uncertainty. The Heart and Estrogen–Progestin Replacement Study (HERS) is the first large clinical trial evaluating secondary prevention of CHD with estrogen and progestin.[23] The results, after an average of 4.1 years follow-up, suggest that daily use of conjugated equine estrogen and medroxyprogesterone acetate in postmenopausal women with established CHD did not reduce the overall rate of CHD events.[23a] The Women's Health Initiative (WHI) is the first large primary prevention trial of estrogen with progestin.[22] Participants are not required to have CHD and are generally younger than the HERS cohort. The WHI plans to enroll 27 500 women and to report results in 2005 after 9 years of treatment. Results of the WHI and further information from HERS, as it continues CHD event surveillance, will provide more information concerning the relationship between estrogen and prevention or treatment of CHD in women.

Women in the USA are more likely to die of CHD than any other cause. Despite the apparent protective effect of endogenous estrogen production early in life, the major risk factors (i.e. cigarette/tobacco smoke, high blood cholesterol levels, high blood pressure, physical inactivity and high-fat diet) for CHD are the same for women and men. Unfortunately, teenage girls are now more likely to smoke than boys and less likely to quit, in part perhaps due to fear of weight gain. Middle-aged women tend to exercise less than middle-aged men.[3] Women taking oral contraceptives who also smoke have an increased risk of CHD.[24] Women often do not have the same attention given to prevention and treatment of CHD. Many women with CHD are diagnosed late. Studies evaluating women have shown a lower referral rate for catheterization and higher mortality rates following myocardial infarction and bypass surgery.[25,26]

RACE

Blacks and Hispanics are the two largest minority groups in the USA. In 1993, CHD death rates (per 100 000 population) were 133.0 for white males and 139.3 for black males (4.7 per cent higher as compared to whites); and 63.8 for white females and 85.7 for black females (34.3 per cent higher as compared to whites). For ages 35–74 years, the death rate from heart attack for black women is more than 38 per cent higher than that for white women.[15] The available data from the National Health Interview Survey (NHIS) (1986–1994)[27] on persons over 45 years of age showed that Hispanics had a CHD mortality rate some 20 per cent lower than that of whites. Yet, Hispanics have higher levels of several important risk factors for CHD compared to whites. These include higher relative body weights, larger central stores of adipose tissue (i.e. they are more 'apple-shaped'), lower concentrations of high-density lipoprotein cholesterol, higher triglyceride levels, higher rates of cigarette smoking, and higher rates of type II diabetes.[27] This paradox warrants further investigation.

SOCIOECONOMIC STATUS

CHD mortality shows different social patterns in different populations. In developed countries, CHD is now concentrated in the lower socioeconomic, less-educated sector of the population. Contrarily, in developing countries, CHD is more a disease of urban middle and upper

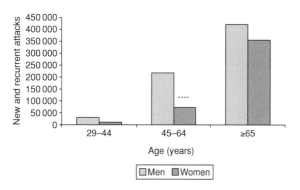

Figure 1.3 *Estimated annual number of Americans experiencing diagnosed heart attack by age and sex in the USA, 1987–1994. (Source 2000 Heart and Stroke Statistical Update, American Heart Association, National Center, Dallas, TX, 1999.)*

classes, and often is virtually unknown in the traditional country villages. Thus, most developing countries evince an urban–rural gradient wherein urban rates are like those in developed countries and rural rates are low. To a large extent, rural and urban differences simply reflect socioeconomic differences. Among the cardiovascular diseases, CHD is the leading cause of death in urban areas in many rapidly industrializing countries (e.g. China), while pulmonary heart disease is the leading cause in rural areas. There were marked differences in CHD incidence and mortality among 16 monitored regions of China, with higher rates occurring in the north than in the south.[28] A similar trend was found in India.[29] A survey in Delhi, involving the use of electrocardiographic criteria, indicated a prevalence of ischemic heart disease of 4.1 per cent in adults of both sexes in the age range 35–64 years, while the addition of history-based diagnostic criteria increased the figure to 7.6 per cent. Rural estimates based on electrocardiographic criteria yielded lower prevalence figures: 2.3 per cent in males and 1.7 per cent in females in Haryana.[30] Small towns tend to have rates that are intermediate between rural and urban.[31] Population surveys in India indicate that higher socioeconomic groups tend to have a higher prevalence of CHD.[29]

RISK FACTORS FOR CHD

Much of what we know about lifestyle and demographic risk factors for CHD comes from a variety of epidemiological studies. The Framingham (Massachusetts) Study[7] began in 1948. This study, along with other landmark prospective US epidemiological studies (Table 1.2), established the major risk factors (cigarette/tobacco smoke, high blood cholesterol levels, high blood pressure, physical inactivity and high-fat diet) for mortality and morbidity from CHD in the USA. Additional cohort studies have helped us to understand CHD determinants in greater detail. The British Civil Servants Study,[8] the Ni-Hon-San (from Nippon, Honolulu, and San Francisco) study of Japanese migrants,[9,10] the Seven Countries Study[11,12] and the MONICA project[5] have established a framework for the study of CHD from a broad population-based perspective and have provided data for international comparisons. Much of what we know regarding the roles of diet, blood lipids, physical inactivity and obesity, hypertension, cigarette smoking, alcohol, diabetes mellitus, psychosocial factors, genetic factors and family history, homocysteine, hemostatic factors and higher white blood cell count as risk factors for CHD is supported or derived from these studies.

Diet

The development of CHD represents a complex interplay of genetic and environmental factors, with diet playing a pivotal role. There is much evidence that habitual diet in populations, a culturally determined characteristic, has an important influence on the mean levels and distribution of blood cholesterol levels and, therefore, on the population risk and potential for prevention of CHD.[32]

The origin of the diet–heart hypothesis comes from multiple sources. International epidemiological studies have indicated a strong relationship between habitual

Table 1.2 *Descriptive characteristics of landmark prospective epidemiologic investigations of coronary heart disease in the USA. (Reproduced from Ockene IS, Ockene JK, eds.* Prevention of coronary heart disease. *Boston: Little, Brown and Co., 1992:6)*

Investigation	Geographic locale	Year of initiation	Sample size	Sample characteristics	Age range (years)
Framingham study[7]	Framingham, MA	1948	5127 men and women	Sample of town residents	30–62
Minnesota Business and Professional Men's Study[137]	St Paul and Minneapolis, MN	1948	281 men	Volunteers from local business	45–55
Los Angeles Heart Study[138]	Los Angeles, CA	1950	1653 men 354 women	Stratified sample of local civil service employees	21+
Albany Cardiovascular Health Center Study[139]	Albany, NY	1953	1843 men	Volunteer sample of civil service employees	<40–55+
Chicago Peoples Gas Company Study[140]	Chicago, IL	1954	3203 men	Complete sample of employees of a large public utility company	25–59
Chicago Western Electric Company Study[141]	Chicago, IL	1957	1989 men	Random sample of long-term employees of a large manufacturing corporation	40–55
Tecumseh Health Study[142]	Tecumseh, MI	1959	2328 men 2592 women	Sample of town residents	16–70+
Western Collaborative Group Study[143]	San Francisco Bay Area and Los Angeles, CA	1960	3154 men	Recruited from ten companies in California	39–59

diet, average blood cholesterol levels, and prevalence of CHD.[11] Diets of populations with a high incidence of CHD are characterized by relatively high saturated fatty acid (SFA) and cholesterol intakes and low carbohydrate intake (under 50 per cent of total caloric intake). Diets in populations having a low CHD incidence are characterized by low SFA (less than 10 per cent of calories) and high carbohydrate intakes (generally complex carbohydrates) but widely varying total fat intake (varying mainly with the proportion of dietary energy from monounsaturated and polyunsaturated fatty acids). Although cross-sectional relationships between fatty acid intakes and serum cholesterol levels tend to be weak,[33] most of the difference in mean population levels of serum total and low-density lipoprotein (LDL) cholesterol can be accounted for by differences in the fatty acid composition of habitual diets.[12] Likewise, population CHD rates can be predicted based on the average intakes of fatty acids and cholesterol.[34,35]

Comparison of a stable population with a population that emigrates to another country or a different geographical location provides a special opportunity to evaluate changes in risk factors among persons sharing similar genetic and cultural backgrounds. If this move involves a higher consumption of total and saturated fat, the population distribution of serum cholesterol shifts upward and CHD rates also rise. There are several examples of this type of international comparison. The Ni-Hon-San Study (Nippon–Honolulu–San Francisco), a study of middle-aged Japanese men who had migrated to Honolulu and San Francisco, showed saturated fat intakes of 7 per cent, 12 per cent and 14 per cent of calories in Japan, Honolulu and San Francisco, respectively. There also were concomitant differences in mean body weight of 55, 63 and 66 kg, respectively.[10] The serum cholesterol was 12 per cent and 21 per cent higher in Honolulu and San Francisco, respectively, than in Japan. The age-specific CHD mortality rates were 2–3 times greater for Japanese migrating to a setting with epidemic rates of CHD (mainland USA) compared to those

persons remaining in Japan, whereas the mortality rates were intermediate for those Japanese men who had migrated to Hawaii[9] (Fig. 1.4).

Laboratory evidence is consistent with epidemiological studies in its support of the diet–heart hypothesis. There is an extensive literature from a wide variety of animal models (rabbits, monkeys, pigs),[36,37] indicating that feeding a high-saturated fat or cholesterol-containing diet produces atherosclerotic deposits in coronary arteries.

Blood lipids

Data accumulated from observational epidemiological studies over the past several decades strongly support the contention that total serum cholesterol is a major predictive factor in the development of CHD.

There is a strong relationship between CHD incidence and mean population LDL and total cholesterol levels.[38] For example, in the Seven Countries Study, there was a correlation coefficient of 0.81 between mean serum cholesterol and CHD incidence.[12] Over the past 30 years, the mean total cholesterol level in the US population has fallen some 25 mg/dl (about 10–15 per cent of the total), a phenomenon that likely has made an important contribution to decreasing the CHD mortality rate.[39] Indeed, the Lipid Research Clinic Study estimated that a reduction on the order of 2 per cent in CHD incidence may be expected for each 1 per cent reduction in total cholesterol.[40]

As indicated in Fig. 1.5, the serum cholesterol distribution is positioned at a higher level in a country such as East Finland, where CHD is common, as compared to Japan where the incidence of CHD is low. The upward cholesterol distribution in East Finland is thought to be the reason for mass atherosclerosis and high overall incidence of CHD. A 15-year follow-up study in Finland[41] indicated a 37 per cent decline in the incidence of CHD

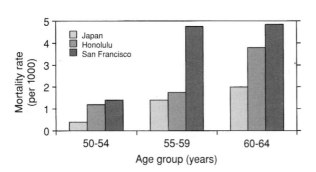

Figure 1.4 *Mortality rates from coronary heart disease in the Ni-Hon-San study. (Reprinted from Ockene IS, Ockene JK, eds. Prevention of coronary heart disease. Boston: Little, Brown and Co., 1992: 9.)*

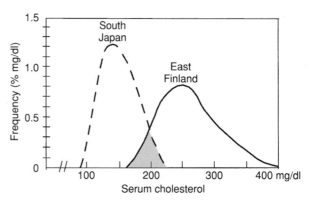

Figure 1.5 *Cultural differences in serum cholesterol level. (Reprinted from* Prevention of coronary heart disease, WHO Technical Report Series 678. Geneva: World Health Organization, 1982: 10.)*

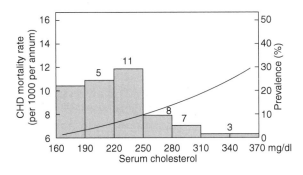

Figure 1.6 *Prevalence distribution (histogram) of serum cholesterol concentrations related to coronary heart disease mortality (line) in men aged 55–64 years. The number above each column represents an estimate of attributable deaths per 1000 population per 10-year period.* (Reprinted from Prevention of coronary heart disease, *WHO Technical Report Series 678. Geneva: World Health Organization, 1982: 11.)*

between 1972 and 1987. During the same period, the mean total cholesterol level fell by 11.8 per cent, and there also were increased intakes of antioxidants from fruits and vegetables. Reduction of serum total cholesterol probably is still the most important single target in preventing CHD in Finland, as more than 80 per cent of the population has a higher than desirable cholesterol level.

Figure 1.6 demonstrates the relationships between individual and population-level risk and serum cholesterol. Although the risk of CHD increases with serum cholesterol concentration, the vastly larger proportion of the population with moderately high cholesterol levels (as opposed to very high levels) means that the majority of CHD occurs at moderate serum cholesterol concentrations. Therefore, most CHD occurs at levels many physicians consider near-normal.

Findings from the Multiple Risk Factor Intervention Trial (MRFIT) provide additional support for the associ-

ation between serum cholesterol and CHD mortality (Fig. 1.7), in which a continuous and graded relationship between the level of serum cholesterol at the time of initial screening and CHD mortality over a 6-year follow-up period was observed. These results also suggest that a 'safe' level of cholesterol below which the risk of CHD is negligible is much lower than was previously thought. Therefore, the National Cholesterol Education Program (NCEP) has recommended universal screening of adults in the USA for hypercholesterolemia.[42]

Data from countries widely varying on diet indicate that serum cholesterol levels can be maintained at low levels from childhood. Total serum cholesterol levels at birth have similar means and ranges across many cultures.[43] However, average levels and distributions of total serum cholesterol differ widely for populations of schoolage children and these levels tend to parallel the differences found in distributions of corresponding adult populations. That is, means and distributions are found to be elevated in youth when they are elevated in adults from the same population.[43] Taken together, these observations imply that early prevention of CHD is very important and that pediatric initiation of primary CHD prevention should be encouraged.

Physical inactivity and obesity

Reviews and a comprehensive meta-analysis indicate that physical activity is inversely related to the incidence of CHD.[44,45] In fact, physical activity confounded early efforts to link diet to CHD because individuals who engage in more physical activity often tend to consume more food.[46,47] Morris[48] suggested that an inverse association between caloric intake and CHD represented the protective effect of physical activity. Powell *et al.*[44] inferred from their review of 43 studies that the relationship was causal and that the relative risk associated with physical inactivity is similar in magnitude to that associated with hypertension, hypercholesterolemia and

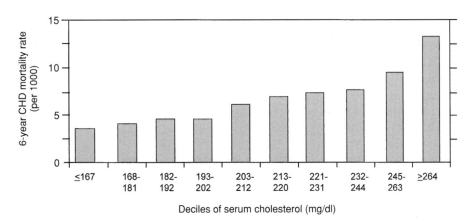

Figure 1.7 *Association between serum cholesterol and CHD mortality from MRFIT.* (Reprinted from Ockene IS, Ockene JK, eds. Prevention of coronary heart disease. *Boston: Little, Brown and Co., 1992: 21.)*

smoking. These authors also noted that the population attributable risk of a sedentary lifestyle is likely to be very high in countries such as the USA where 60–80 per cent of adults are sedentary or only irregularly active.[49] In a meta-analysis conducted by Berlin and Colditz[45] the estimated relative risk of death from CHD was 1.8 (comparing risks for the lowest versus highest levels of physical activity).

The reasons for the inverse association between physical activity and CHD may include effects on raising high-density lipoprotein (HDL)-cholesterol, reducing body weight, lowering blood pressure and improving glucose tolerance. In addition to altering these risk factors, physical activity has an overall beneficial effect on the cardiovascular system. However, heavy physical exertion has been associated with ischemic events and can occasionally result in fatal myocardial infarction, especially among people who are unaccustomed to physical activity.[50]

Obesity is a consequence of excess energy intake relative to energy expenditure, resulting in deposition of adipose tissue. Obesity must be considered a problem in terms of not only energy regulation *per se* but also metabolic sequelae. An increased prevalence of obesity and redistribution of fat from the extremities to the trunk occurs with age in many populations and with changes from rural to urban lifestyles, especially among men.[51–53] General and especially abdominal (central or truncal) obesity has been associated with an increased risk of CHD and death from all causes in both sexes across several populations.[54–57] Indicators of body fat distribution also have been related to an atherogenic lipid profile in both men and women.[58,59] Some studies have reported interpopulation differences in the association between fat distribution and blood lipids.[60–62] For example, Haffner *et al.*[62] observed that HDL-cholesterol and triglyceride levels among Mexican Americans were different from those of their Anglo counterparts, and suggested that such differences were due, in part, to differences in body fat distribution.

Physical activity is the other half of the energy balance equation that governs body weight. There appears to be consensus that physical activity is the most important determinant of weight maintenance and body weight set points.[47,63] However, as with diet, it is an aspect of lifestyle that is very difficult to change.[64] Among the more affluent portions of the industrialized nations, there has been a trend towards more intentional leisure-time activity, while simultaneously these same groups of people have progressively adopted a more healthful diet. There has been a reduction in CHD rates and levels of obesity in these groups. Exercise may elicit an increase in HDL-cholesterol and thereby exert a beneficial effect independent of its role in regulating body weight.[65] However, increases in HDL-cholesterol in response to exercise *per se* are modest compared to those associated with exercise accompanied by weight loss.[65,66]

Hypertension

Hypertension is an important risk factor for CHD. In industrialized countries, the prevalence of hypertension is as high as 25 per cent among adults.[67] The international collaborative INTERSALT Study used uniform procedures in evaluating 52 population samples from 32 countries of Africa, Asia, Europe, North America and South America.[68,69] The study found a significant relationship between median 24-hour sodium excretion (an indicator of dietary sodium intake) and the slope of the age-related systolic blood pressure increase. This relationship held over the 30-year range from 25 to 55 years of age and was similar for most developed countries. The mean systolic blood pressure increases from approximately 110–120 mm Hg at age 20 to 150–160 mm Hg at age 55. Interestingly, studies of a number of populations living a relatively traditional lifestyle have shown that an age-related increase does not necessarily have to take place. These populations include groups living at high altitude in the Andean Region and low-altitude Indian tribes of Brazil[70,71] and Costa Rica.[72] Low-blood-pressure communities, once common in rural Africa, are characterized by the absence of hypertensive subjects and a lack of increase in blood pressure with age. Such communities share a number of similarities including high carbohydrate diets, low salt consumption, lean body makeup and high levels of physical activity.[73]

A controlled, longitudinal, observational study by Poulter and colleagues[74] demonstrates the magnitude, timing, and possible causes of changes in blood pressure among Kenyan Luo migrants who moved to Nairobi, the largest urban center of Kenya, from low-blood-pressure rural communities. The authors found a statistically significant increase in systolic blood pressure, and a mean systolic and diastolic blood pressure distribution, which increased over time among those individuals living in the urbanized area as compared to those who remained in the rural zone. These changes became evident as soon as one month after migration. Progressive increases in sodium intake, body weight and stress might be important predictors of the shift in the blood pressure distribution during the urbanization process, and these factors may play a role in the further development of hypertension. A recent clinical trial offers additional support for the results of migration studies, suggesting that lifestyle (e.g. diet) is important in prevention of hypertension (Fig. 1.8).[75] In brief, it showed that a low-fat diet rich in fruits, vegetables and low-fat dairy foods elicited decreases of 5.5 and 3.0 mm Hg in systolic and diastolic blood pressure, respectively, as compared to the control diet.

Cigarette smoking

Cigarette smoking exerts many pathologic effects on the heart, as summarized in Table 1.3. Ecological analyses

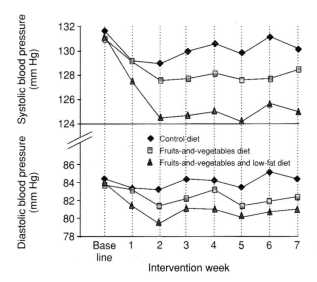

Figure 1.8 *Mean systolic and diastolic blood pressures at baseline and during each intervention week according to diet group for 379 subjects with complete sets of weekly blood pressure measurements. (Reprinted from Appel LJ, et al., A clinical trial of the effects of dietary patterns of blood pressure.* N Engl J Med *1997;* **336**: 1122.)

have shown a clear relationship between cigarette and tobacco consumption and CHD mortality. For individuals living within societies having a high CHD incidence, smoking is found consistently to be a strong and independent risk factor for myocardial infarction and sudden death.[76] The relationship between smoking and risk of CHD is continuous, being lowest in persons who never smoked, and is related to duration of the habit.[77] The correlation coefficients between mean per capita tobacco consumption for the late 1950s and the early 1960s, and CHD mortality rates in 1971 and 1973 for men and women in 19 countries were in the range of 0.44–0.50.[78] Most of the excess CHD cases attributable to smoking come from light and moderate smokers, because the

prevalence of heavy smokers is relatively low. Thirty per cent of all CHD deaths in the USA are thought to be attributable to cigarette smoking.[79] Experimentally, ischemic pain, angiographic coronary spasm and electrocardiographic abnormalities have been demonstrated during smoking in patients with compromised coronary circulation.[76] A synthesis of the available data suggests that smoking is a potent accelerator of CHD and an initiator of clinical events. In the USA, the decline in CHD mortality rates correlates with the decreasing prevalence of cigarette smoking in men. However, in women, the relationship is more difficult to demonstrate.[80] While the smoking rate in men began a steady decline in the 1950s and 1960s, it began to rise in women and did not show a decline until the late 1970s. Tragically, the prevalence of smoking among women began to rise again around 1990.[81] In a large-scale study of female nurses, approximately half of the coronary events were attributable to smoking, suggesting that smoking appears to be a particularly important risk factor in women.[82]

Interactions with other risk factors also are important, as indicated by the weak association of smoking with CHD risk in low-risk societies. The observed incidence of CHD in populations with a low prevalence of hyperlipidemia is much smaller than the risk predicted by multiple regression equations derived from the USA or northern European data.[73] Thus, in Japan, despite high levels of smoking in men, the association of smoking and CHD is relatively weak.[12] It suggests that smoking is particularly harmful in combination with other risk factors such as hyperlipidemia.

With regard to environmental tobacco exposure, the results of numerous studies[83–92] are remarkably consistent. All the studies of men yield relative risks of death from heart disease exceeding 1.0 when a non-smoking man is married to a women who smokes, with an overall risk of 1.3. All but one[84] of the studies of non-smoking women who live with a smoker yielded relative risks exceeding 1.0, with an overall average relative risk of 1.3.

Table 1.3 *Pathologic effects of smoking on the heart. (Reproduced from Tresch DD, Aronow WS.* Smoking and coronary artery disease. Clinics Geriatr Med *1996;* **12**: 24)

Component	Effects
Plasma lipids and lipoproteins	Decreased HDL; increased LDL and triglycerides
Blood cells	Increased erythrocytes and leukocytes; displacement of O_2 from hemoglobin
Platelets	Increased adhesiveness
Fibrinogen	Increased levels
Vessel endothelium damage	Increased atherogenesis
Sympathoadrenal activation	Increased myocardial O_2 demands by increased cardiac output, heart rate, and blood pressure; increased vasoconstriction.

HDL = high-density lipoprotein; LDL = low-density lipoprotein.

Alcohol

Existing data suggest that moderate alcohol consumption reduces the rate of non-fatal myocardial infarction and mortality from CHD.[93] A report from the Yugoslavia Cardiovascular Disease Study found a statistically significant inverse relationship between alcohol consumption and CHD incidence that persisted even after controlling for blood pressure, serum cholesterol levels and cigarette smoking.[94] A prospective study of 87 500 women in the USA suggested that, among middle-aged women, moderate alcohol consumption decreases the risk of CHD.[95] Similar results were obtained for both sexes in a New Zealand study.[96] The mechanism by which moderate alcohol intake 'protects' against CHD remains unclear. It has been suggested that this effect is mediated by increasing HDL cholesterol levels. On the other hand, once hepatic damage occurs in alcoholics, plasma HDL levels actually may be lower than normal. High population rates of alcohol consumption, specifically of wine, may help to explain the unusually low rates of CHD in France.[97] However, high rates of cirrhosis also are seen in France. The apparent beneficial effect of moderate alcohol intake on CHD needs further verification and recommendations for use must be balanced by knowledge of the other well-known deleterious effects of alcohol.

Diabetes mellitus

The association of clinical diabetes mellitus with CHD and atherosclerosis is documented in clinical, pathologic and epidemiological studies.[98] CHD is the most common underlying cause of death in diabetics in the USA, accounting for more than one-third of all deaths in diabetic adults 40 years of age and older. In longitudinal studies, clinical diabetes mellitus is associated with excess CHD risk. Many such cohort studies confirm the excess of fatal myocardial infarction in women with diabetes as compared to women without diabetes. The relative risk of death from CHD in type II diabetic patients compared with age-matched non-diabetic patients ranges from 1.5 to 2.5 times in men and 1.7 to more than 4.0 times in women. Diabetes essentially negates the normal premenopausal female advantage.[99] Finally, in most autopsy studies, CHD and the frequency and severity of myocardial infarction are greater in diabetics than in controls.[98] Diabetes amplifies the underlying risk of CHD in all populations, especially in racial groups such as Japanese and Native Americans for whom rates of CHD are low in non-diabetics. People with type 2 diabetes also develop CHD at a younger age and are more likely to develop congestive heart failure. Diabetic patients also have poorer outcomes after a myocardial infarction. Overall, diabetes contributes to a significant excess of CHD in all populations studied.

Psychosocial factors

Several years ago, the Type A behavior pattern (i.e. a complex mixture of traits including competitiveness, hostility and impatience) was associated with CHD morbidity and mortality.[100] However, most studies performed after 1979 have found no association, or demonstrated such an association for only one Type A behavior subscale.[101–103] Hostility (i.e. the tendency to employ antagonistic behavior, cynical cognition and angry feelings) has become the focus of attention in the research on the psychological risk factors of CHD.[104] Hostility has been shown to be related to CHD in both cross-sectional and prospective studies.[101–105] Several researchers have found that hostility predicts CHD, after controlling for age, smoking, cholesterol level and blood pressure.[106–108] A study by Gidron et al.[105] showed that certain components of hostility (e.g. aggressive-responding, cynicism and hostile affect) are better predictors of CHD than the full hostility score, but further study is needed to verify this observation. Social support is another psychosocial factor that deserves research attention. Several prospective population-based studies suggest increased social support as a factor associated with reduced risk of CHD,[109] indicating that social support is capable of moderating potentially harmful negative emotions and the cardiovascular response to psychological challenge. Several studies in Europe[110] and Japan[111] also suggest a link between psychosocial factors and CHD. However, the limitations of studies of psychosocial factors on the international level are great, as standardized methods to evaluate and classify behavior patterns and psychological states from an international perspective are largely lacking.

Genetic factors and family history of CHD

Migrants and their children tend to acquire rates of chronic diseases, including CHD, which are characteristic of their host countries,[9] suggesting that genetic factors are not the main determinant of rate differences among populations. Genetic factors are, however, important in relation to individual susceptibility, as has been confirmed by twin studies.[112,113] Both women and men are more likely to develop heart disease if their close blood relatives have had it. Entire populations may have a genetic susceptibility to the effects of particular risk factors.[114–117] For example, many people from the Indian subcontinent appear to have a phenotype that is particularly responsive to producing cholesterol from dietary precursors (i.e. saturated fatty acids) and tend to have low HDL and high triglyceride levels, placing them at greater risk as compared to other populations.[116,117] Genetic effects are especially evident in younger patients and in women. However, they may not explain all familial tendencies, given that social and behavioral risk factors also aggregate in families.

Homocysteine

Homocysteine, a product of methionine metabolism, is currently considered a risk factor for CHD.[118,119] Although the mechanism whereby homocysteine is associated with CHD is still not known, studies employing animal models suggest that high levels of homocysteine produce atherosclerosis.[120-122] In the Physicians' Health Study, subjects with homocysteine levels in the upper fifth percentile had myocardial infarction rates three times that of the rest of the cohort, suggesting that there may be a threshold level below which homocysteine is not a CHD risk factor.[118] However, data reported by Arnesen et al.[119] imply that serum homocysteine level is linearly related to risk for CHD, with no special threshold level defined risk for CHD. In the latter study, the association between serum homocysteine and CHD risk was not materially altered after adjustment for possible confounders (i.e. serum total cholesterol, HDL cholesterol, triglycerides, systolic blood pressure, the number of cigarettes smoked per day, and history of diabetes and angina pectoris), suggesting that serum homocysteine is an independent risk for CHD. Furthermore, a prospective study following patients with CHD for 4.6 years suggested that serum total homocysteine levels are a strong predictor of CHD mortality.[123]

Other risk factors: hemostatic factors and white blood cell count

The components of the coagulation cascade continue to be an important area of research. These include fibrin, which forms when cell walls are damaged and which contributes to fibrin platelet masses, and platelet aggregation.[124] Of the several hemostatic variables measured with respect to subsequent CHD risk, those that have received the most attention include fibrinogen, Factor VII and plasminogen activator inhibitor (PAI-1). Several investigators have concluded that an elevated fibrinogen level is likely to be causally associated with CHD but that circulating fibrinogen may be closely linked to smoking.[124] Factor VII levels have been shown to be a risk factor of CHD and to be lowered by reducing the consumption of dietary fat.[125] PAI-1 is a circulating inhibitor that increases the coagulability of the blood and is a risk factor for CHD.[126] Anticoagulant trials appear to demonstrate reduced short-term mortality in the hospital phase of acute myocardial infarction; however, long-term results are inconclusive. Total white blood cell (WBC) count was shown to be strongly and significantly related to CHD risk, independent of smoking status, in the Multiple Risk Factor Intervention Trial (MRFIT).[127]

Multifactorial nature of CHD

Risk factors interact with one another. There is a multiplicative contribution for each of the risk factors including cigarette smoking, hypertension and total serum cholesterol.[128] The risk ratio between the highest and lowest categories for combined risk within a population is of the order of 8–10-fold, in contrast to the risk ratios for single risk factors, which are of the order of 2–4-fold. Results from MRFIT[129,130] demonstrated that a multiple risk factor approach conferred a CHD mortality benefit after 10.5 years of follow-up. These findings provide support for early intervention on cholesterol, smoking and blood pressure for the primary prevention of CHD.

HEALTH CARE POLICY EFFORTS AND CULTURAL INFLUENCES ON THE PREVENTION OF CHD

Policy development

Traditionally, the nearly exclusive concern of physicians has been their individual patients with the major focus on individual risk behaviors related to lifestyle. However, physicians are playing an increasingly important role in both primary and secondary prevention of CHD. To some extent, this has involved the planning and development of health care policy. As for any disease, health care policy with respect to CHD should be based on: a clear understanding of the pathophysiology and epidemiology of the disease; the prevalence of important risk factors; evidence for the efficacy, effectiveness and efficiency of available interventions; and the cost and availability of resources to mount appropriate public health initiatives.

In the world at large, a crucial step in establishing policy must focus on defining the incidence and prevalence of CHD. This requires monitoring and data collection procedures that are beyond the capability of many developing countries, most of which currently have low rates of CHD. However, CHD incidence and prevalence are low because of a combination of factors, the most important of which are competing causes of morbidity and mortality (i.e. with infectious diseases predominating, many people simply do not live long enough to develop CHD) and the traditional absence of major risk factors, especially overnutrition, sedentariness and obesity. However, CHD incidence is rapidly increasing throughout the world and, as noted earlier in this chapter, will soon replace many of the traditional causes of death and disability in the developing world as the primary cause of serious illness.[2] Therefore, the prevention of CHD will need to be given an increasing priority throughout the world as these risk factor and disease patterns change.

CHD is amenable to primary prevention. The major determinants of CHD have been identified as cigarette/tobacco smoke, high blood cholesterol levels, high blood pressure, physical inactivity and a high saturated-fat diet. Therefore, anticipating trends in these risk factors and changes in overall life expectancy is necessary for formulating a cogent national policy for prevention. Community prevention programs have demonstrated the feasibility of risk factor reduction by the adoption of a healthier lifestyle at the community level.[131] In countries such as India and China, this will need to focus primarily on educating people to maintain low saturated-fat, high-fiber diets, despite media-promoted popular trends towards higher saturated fat and lower fiber Westernized alternatives.

In the USA, current policy is well articulated in the report of the National Institutes of Health (NIH) expert panel on population strategies for blood cholesterol reduction[132] and in the revised guidelines of the NCEP.[42] Recommendations are made for universal screening of adults for hypercholesterolemia and for a shift in the national diet to foods lower in saturated fat and cholesterol, with an overall goal of a population mean per cent of calories obtained from fat less than 30 per cent and from saturated fat less than 10 per cent. Public campaigns for smoking cessation and for increasing physical activity also are recommended.[132] The revised guidelines emphasize the role of the clinical approach in primary prevention of CHD. Dietary therapy remains the first line of treatment for high blood cholesterol, and drug therapy is reserved for patients who are considered to be at high risk for CHD. The revised guidelines contain the new features listed below.

1 Increased emphasis on CHD risk status as a guide to type and intensity of cholesterol-lowering therapy, including the following:
   • identification of the patient with existing CHD or other atherosclerotic diseases as being at the highest risk and establishment of lower target levels for LDL cholesterol in these patients;
   • addition of age to the list of major CHD risk factors, defined as 45 years or older in men and 55 years or older in women;
   • recommendation for delaying the use of drug therapy in most young adult men and premenopausal women with high LDL cholesterol levels who are otherwise at low risk for CHD in the near future; and
   • enhanced recognition that high-risk postmenopausal women and elderly patients, who are otherwise in good health, are candidates for cholesterol-lowering therapy.
2 More attention to low level of circulating HDL as a CHD risk factor, including the following:
   • addition of HDL cholesterol to initial cholesterol testing; and

   • consideration of HDL cholesterol levels in the choice of drug therapy.
3 Increased emphasis on physical activity and weight loss as components of therapy for hypercholesterolemia.

Secondary prevention and early treatment will need to be provided for those who have had a clinical coronary event or have developed symptoms of CHD. Secondary prevention also includes the pharmacological treatment of patients with hypertension, diabetes, hyperlipidemia and cigarette smoking.

Cardiac rehabilitation, which represents a tertiary prevention of CHD, is an essential and growing component of cardiac care. Cardiac rehabilitation is undergoing a rapid transition from a largely exercise-based orientation to more comprehensive programs that treat the entire gamut of risk factors, including components for lipid management, such as dietary intervention, smoking cessation and stress reduction. Much of the appropriate secondary prevention efforts can be best delivered through such integrated programs.

Policy implementation and cultural influences

The major risk factors for CHD (i.e. cigarette/tobacco smoke, high blood cholesterol levels, high blood pressure, physical inactivity and high saturated-fat diet) are environmental and therefore under a large degree of cultural influence. Policies to support health care are required in many sectors (e.g. economic, housing, welfare and transportation). Ideally, governments should take a leading role in formulating national strategies for the active promotion of cardiac health and the prevention and control of CHD. However, in reality, governments often are burdened by other, apparently more pressing, problems. Political expedience often runs counter to dealing with the primary prevention of chronic conditions, especially those that have not yet evinced high levels of incidence or prevalence. Although it might make sound economic sense to intervene prior to the onset of debilitating and expensive clinical disease, this normally does not occur. Effective policy will need to set into place an interlocking network of operational units. With regard to smoking, for instance, it should include taxes on tobacco, control of advertising and sales, health education in schools and workplaces, provision of non-smoking areas in public places and encouragement of public pressure against smoking. The expansion of healthy eating habits in the population may include legislation governing the content of prepared foods, subsidies for healthy products and special access to healthy foods among the most vulnerable groups. Basic training of health professionals to provide a unified voice for the health promotion effort is an important aspect of public policy.

In the USA, the NCEP was initiated as a means to prevent CHD by reducing the prevalence of hypercholesterolemia. CHD mortality has been decreased as a consequence of favorable changes in exposure to the relevant risk factors.[39] However, CHD mortality and morbidity are increasing in developing countries.[3] There are no consistent guidelines for the management of hyperlipidemia in developing countries such as those espoused by the NCEP in the USA. In part, this reflects the lag in CHD rates. However, increases in the prevalence of CHD risk factors in developing countries are a growing concern. For example, in China the traditional diet consists mainly of rice and vegetables, which are protective against CHD because they are low in saturated fat and high in fiber and complex carbohydrates. At present, with industrialization and Westernization, eating habits are changing, resulting in increases in saturated fatty acid intakes.[46] In the urban areas of China, where the pace of change is faster than in the rural areas, rates of CHD are already increasing.[28] At the same time, prevalence of smoking in China is as high as 59.3 per cent in males.[133] Estimates from 1988 showed that China is responsible for consuming 30 per cent of all cigarettes worldwide (i.e. 1.5 trillion cigarettes).[134] It has been predicted that in China alone 50 million individuals currently under 20 years of age will ultimately die of tobacco-related diseases.[135] As stated above, with increases in dietary saturated fat intake and the subsequent increases in total and LDL cholesterol, cigarette smoking will have a much greater impact on CHD rates. Anticipating these changes, governments, policy advocates, and health workers might be well advised to accord high priority to tobacco control. Unlike the West, where smoking is now associated with low socioeconomic status, smoking is more widely distributed in many developing countries, especially among males of higher socioeconomic status. Because of effect modification by dietary fat, smoking's deleterious effects on CHD may be more pronounced among the affluent. This will provide interesting challenges and opportunities to health policy planners.

RISK FACTOR SCREENING

Although beyond the scope of this chapter, it is important to note relevant factors pertaining to population-based screening. Typically, screening focuses on the early detection of disease. For CHD, the major form of screening has taken the form of detecting high serum cholesterol (in particular, LDL) levels in asymptomatic individuals.

In a country such as the USA, which has a high CHD prevalence and where acute cases can be treated aggressively (and therefore very expensively), such screening may be cost effective in adults.[136] NCEP has recommended universal cholesterol screening in the US adult population. The decision to screen in developing countries is not so clear. Sensitivity may be very low if the constellation of risk factors do not predispose large portions of the population to develop CHD. With low prevalence rates, costs of screening are high relative to the cost of other health-related measures that may render larger or more immediate benefits.

FUTURE DIRECTIONS

Health providers should play a significant role in both primary and secondary prevention of CHD. Developing countries should learn from developed countries about secondary prevention of CHD, while developed countries need to learn from developing countries about the primary intervention of CHD (e.g. maintaining low saturated-fat diets and increasing physical activity). Further research is warranted to implement and evaluate the effects of intervention programs focused on the specified risk factors. Epidemiologic and clinical research also should identify those persons likely to respond to various intervention strategies and in whom additional and possibly tailored intervention approaches can be delivered.

SUMMARY

- CHD remains a leading cause of mortality and morbidity in the USA and other developed countries.
- CHD mortality and morbidity are increasing in developing countries as populations age and adopt a 'Western' lifestyle.
- The major risk factors include cigarette/tobacco smoke, high blood cholesterol levels, high blood pressure, physical inactivity, and a high saturated-fat diet.
- Designing, planning, and implementing effective behavioral interventions and creating policies that motivate healthy behavior change remain a challenge.

ACKNOWLEDGMENTS

We thank Dr Jane Teas and Mr Thomas G. Hurley for comments on earlier drafts of this chapter.

REFERENCES

1. Ockene IS, Ockene JK, eds. *Prevention of coronary heart disease*. Boston, MA: Little, Brown and Company, 1992.
2. Murray CJL, Lopez AD. *The global burden of disease*. Boston: Harvard School of Public Health, 1996.

3. World Health Organization. *The world health report 1997*. Geneva: World Health Organization, 1997.

4. Ruzicka LT, Lopez AD. The use of cause-of-death statistics for health situation assessment: national and international experiences. *World Health Stat Q* 1990; **43**: 249–59.

5. WHO/MONICA Project Principal Investigators (prepared by Tunstall-Pedoe H). The World Health Organization MONICA Project (monitoring trends and determinants in cardiovascular disease): a major international collaboration. *J Clin Epidemiol* 1988; **41**: 105–14.

6. World Health Statistical Information System. *Division of health situation and trend assessment*. Geneva: World Health Organization, 1997.

7. Dawber T, Meadors G, Moore F. Epidemiological approaches to heart disease: the Framingham Study. *Am J Public Health* 1951; **41**: 279–86.

8. Reid D, Hamilton P, McCartney P, *et al*. Smoking and other risk factors for coronary heart disease in British civil servants. *Lancet* 1976; **2**: 979–83.

9. Marmot MG, Syme SL, Kagan A, *et al*. Epidemiolgic studies of CHD and stroke in Japanese men living in Japan, Hawaii, and California. Prevalence of coronary and hypertensive heart disease and associated risk factors. *Am J Epidemiol* 1975; **102**: 514.

10. Kato H, Tillotson J, Nichaman MZ, *et al*. Epidemiologic studies of coronary heart disease and stroke in Japanese men living in Japan, Hawaii, and California. Serum lipids and diet. *Am J Epidemiol* 1973; **97**: 372–85.

11. Keys A. Coronary heart disease in seven countries. *Circulation* 1970; **41**: 1–211.

12. Keys A. *Seven countries: a multivariate analysis of death and coronary heart disease*. Cambridge, MA: Harvard University Press, 1980.

13. *World health statistics annual 1990*. Geneva: World Health Organization, 1991.

14. Ueshima H, Tatara K, Asakura A. Declining mortality from ischemic heart disease and changes in coronary risk factors in Japan, 1956–1980. *Am J Epidemiol* 1987; **125**: 62–72.

15. *1997 Heart and Stroke Statistical Update*. Dallas, TX: American Heart Association, 1997.

16. Alwan AAS. Cardiovascular diseases in the Eastern Mediterranean Region. *World Health Stat Q* 1993; **46**: 97–100.

17. Muna WFT. Cardiovascular disease in Africa. *World Health Stat Q* 1993; **46**: 125–33.

18. World Health Statistics Quarterly. *Cardiovascular disease mortality in the developing countries*. Geneva: World Health Organization, 1993.

19. Gorodeski GI. Impact of the menopause on the epidemiology and risk factors of coronary artery heart disease in women. *Exp Gerontol* 1994; **29**: 357–75.

20. Stampfer MJ, Colditz GA, Willett WC. Menopause and heart diease: a review. *Ann N Y Acad Sci* 1990; **592**: 193–203.

21. Grodstein F, Stampfer M. The epidemiology of cornary heart disease and estrogen replacement in postmenopausal women. *Prog Cardiovasc Dis* 1995; **38**: 199–210.

22. Finnegan LP. The NIH Women's Heath Initiative: its evolution and expected contributions to women's health. *Am J Prevent Med* 1996; **12**: 292–3.

23. Schrott HG, Bittner V, Vittinghoff E, *et al*. Adherence to national cholesterol education program treatment goals in postmenopausal women with heart disease. The Heart and Estrogen/Progestin Replacement Study (HERS). *JAMA* 1997; **277**: 1281–6.

23a. Hulley S, Grady D, Bush T, *et al*. Randomized trial of estrogen plus progestin for secondary prevention of coronary heart disease in postmenopausal women. *JAMA* 1998; **280**: 605–13.

24. *Coronary heart disease: are women special?* United Kingdom National Forum for Coronary Disease Prevention, 1994.

25. Bickell NA, Pieper KS, Lee KL. Referral patterns for coronary artery disease treatment: gender bias or good clinical judgement? *Ann Intern Med* 1992; **116**: 791–7.

26. Khan SS, Nessim S, Gray R. Increased mortality of women in coronary artery bypass surgery: evidence for referral bias. *Ann Intern Med* 1990; **112**: 561–7.

27. Liao Y, Cooper RS, Cao G, *et al*. Mortality from coronary heart disease and cardiovascular disease among adult US Hispanics: findings from the National Health Interview Survey (1986 to 1994). *J Am Coll Cardiol* 1997; **30**: 1200–5.

28. *World Development Report*. New York, Oxford: World Bank, 1984.

29. Reddy KS. Cardiovascular diseases in India. *World Health Stat Q* 1993; **46**: 101–7.

30. Sapru RP. Cardiovascular and non-tuberculous chest diseases. An estimate of the size of the problem in India. *Ann Natl Acad Med Sci (India)* 1983; **19**: 179–93.

31. Dewan BD. Epidemiological study of coronary heart disease in rural community in Haryana. *Ind Heart J* 1974; **26**: 68–78.

32. Singh RB, Rastogi SS, Niaz MA, *et al*. Effect of fat-modified and fruit- and vegetable-enriched diets on blood lipids in the Indian Diet Heart Study. *Am J Cardiol* 1992; **70**: 869–74.

33. Jacobs DJ, Anderson J, Blackburn H. Diet and serum cholesterol: do zero correlations negate the relationship? *Am J Epidemiol* 1979; **110**: 77–87.

34. Shekelle RB, Shryock AM, Paul O, *et al*. Diet, serum cholesterol, and death from coronary heart disease. *N Engl J Med* 1981; **304**: 65–70.

35. Kushi LH, Lew RA, Stare FJ, *et al*. Diet and 20-year mortality from coronary heart disease – The Ireland–Boston Diet–Heart Study. *N Engl J Med* 1985; **312**: 811–18.

36. Williams JK, Anthony MS, Clarkson TB. Coronary heart disease in rhesus moneys with diet-induced coronary artery atherosclerosis. *Arch Pathol Lab Med* 1991; **115**: 784–90.

37. Reddick RL, Read MS, Brinkhous KM, *et al*. Coronary artherosclerosis in the pig. Induced plaque and platelet response. *Artherosclerosis* 1990; **10**: 541–50.

38. Report of a conference on the health effects of lipoproteins: Optimal blood lipid levels of populations. *Prevent Med* 1979; **8**: 609–759.

39. Goldman L, Cook EF. The decline in ischemic heart disease mortality rates. *Ann Intern Med* 1984; **101**: 825–36.

40. The Lipid Research Clinics Program. The Lipid Research Clinics Coronary Primary Prevention Trial Results. I. Reduction in incidence of coronary heart disease. *JAMA* 1984; **251**: 351–64.

41. Vartiainen E, Korhonen HJ, Pietinen P, *et al*. Fifteen-year trends in coronary risk factors in Finland, with special reference to North Karelia. *Int J Epidemiol* 1991; **20**: 651–62.

42. Expert Panel on Detection Evaluation and Treatment of High Blood Cholesterol in Adults. Summary of the second report of the National Cholesterol Education Program (NCEP) Expert Panel on Detection, Evaluation, and Treatment of High Blood Cholesterol in Adults (Adult Treatment Panel II). *JAMA* 1993; **269**: 3015–23.

43. Report of a conference on blood lipids in children: Optimal levels for early prevention of coronary heart disease. *Prevent Med* 1983; **12**: 725–905.

44. Powell KE, Thompson PD, Caspersen CH, *et al*. Physical activity and the incidence of coronary heart disease. *Ann Rev Public Health* 1987; **8**: 251–87.

45. Berlin JA, Colditz GA. A meta-analysis of physical activity in the prevention of coronary heart disease. *Am J Epidemiol* 1990; **132**: 612–28.

46. Campbell TC, Chen JS. Diet and chronic degenerative diseases: perspectives from China. *Am J Clin Nutr* 1994; **59**: S1153–61.

47. Romieu I, Willett WC, Stampfer MJ, *et al*. Energy intake and other determinants of relative weight. *Am J Clin Nutr* 1988; **47**: 406–12.

48. Morris JN, Marr JW, Clayton DG. Diet and heart: a postscript. *Br Med J* 1977; **2**: 1307–14.

49. Stephens T, Jacobs DR Jr, White CC. A descriptive epidemiology of leisure-time physical activity. *Public Health Rep* 1985; **100**: 147–58.

50. Steenland K. Epidemiology of occupation and coronary heart disease: research agenda. *Am J Ind Med* 1996; **30**: 495–9.

51. Okeke EC, Nanyelugo DO, Ngwu E. The prevalence of obesity in adults by age, sex, and occupation in Anambra State, Nigeria. *Growth* 1983; **47**: 263–71.

52. Mueller WH. The changes with age of anatomical redistribution of fat. *Soc Sci Med* 1982; **16**: 191–6.

53. Ramirez ME, Mueller WH. The development of obesity and anatomical fat patterning in Tokealau children. *Human Biol* 1980; **52**: 675.

54. Donahue RP, Abbott RD, Bloom E, *et al*. Central obesity and coronary heart disease in men. *Lancet* 1987; **1**: 821–4.

55. Larsson B, Svrdsudd K, Welin L, *et al*. Abdominal adipose tissue distribution, obesity, and risk of cardiovascular disease and death: 13 year follow-up of participants in the study of men born in 1913. *Br Med J* 1984; **288**: 1401–4.

56. Higgins M, Kannel W, Garrison R, *et al*. Hazards of obesity – the Framingham experience. *Acta Med Scand* 1988; **723**: 23–6.

57. Lapidus L, Bengstoon C, Larsson B. Distribution of adipose tissue and risk of cardiovasular disease and death: a 12-year follow up of participants in the population study of women in Gothemburg, Sweden. *Br Med J* 1984; **289**: 1257–61.

58. Garn SM, Sullivan TV, Hawthorne WM. Fatness dependence of skinfold ratios and its implications to fat patterning. *Ecol Food Nutr* 1987; **21**: 151–8.

59. Despres JP, Allard C, Tremblay A, *et al*. Evidence for regional components of body fatness in the association with serum lipids in men and women. *Metabolism* 1985; **34**: 967–73.

60. Durnin J, Womersley J. Body fat assessed from total body density and its estimation from skinfold thickness: measurements on 481 men and women aged from 16 to 72 years. *Br J Nutr* 1974; **32**: 77–92.

61. Seidell JC, Giocolini M, Charzewska J, *et al*. Indicators of fat distribution, serum lipids, and blood pressure in European women born in 1948. The European Fat Distribution Study. *Am J Epidemiol* 1989; **130**: 53–65.

62. Haffner SM, Stern MP, Hazuda HP, *et al*. Role of obesity and fat distribution in non-insulin dependent diabetes mellitus on Mexican American and non-Hispanic whites. *Diabetes Care* 1986; **9**: 153–61.

63. Flatt JP. Dietary fat, carbohydrate balance, and weight maintenance: effects of exercise. *Am J Clin Nutr* 1987; **45**: 296–306.

64. Williamson D, Madans J, Anda R, *et al*. Recreational physical activity and ten-year weight change in a US national cohort. *Int J Obesity Related Metabol Disord* 1993; **17**: 279–86.

65. Thompson PD, Yurgalevitch SM, Flynn MM, *et al*. Effect of prolonged exercise training without weight loss on high-density lipoprotein metabolism in overweight men. *Metabolism* 1997; **46**: 217–23.

66. Gartside PS, Khoury P, Blueck CJ. Determinants of high-density lipoprotein cholesterol in blacks and whites: the Second National Health Examination Survey. *Am Heart J* 1984; **108**: 641.

67. Marmot MG. Geography of blood pressure and hypertension. *Br Med Bull* 1984; **40**: 380–6.

68. INTERSALT Cooperative Research Group. INTERSALT Study: An international cooperative study on the relation of blood pressure to electrolyte excretion in populations. I. Design and methods. *J Hypertension* 1986; **4**: 781–7.

69. INTERSALT Cooperative Research Group. INTERSALT: An international study of electrolyte excretion and blood pressure: results for 24 hour urinary sodium and potassium excretion. *Br Med J* 1988; **297**: 319–28.

70. De Costa E, Rose GA, Klein CH, *et al.* Salt and blood pressure in Rio Grande do Sul, Brazil. *Bull Pan Am Health Organ* 1990; **24**: 159–76.

71. INTERSALT Cooperative Research Group. Appendix tables. Center-specific results by age and sex. *J Hypertension* 1989; **3**: 331–407.

72. Ruiz L, Dunbar JB, Horan MJ. Hypertension in Latin America. Special Report. Interamerican Society Proceedings. *Hypertension* 1988; Suppl. I:2.

73. Watkins LO. Coronary heart disease and coronary disease risk factors in black populations in underdeveloped countries: the case of primordial prevention. *Am Heart J* 1984; **62**: 850–62.

74. Poulter NR, Khaw KT, Hopwood BEC, *et al.* The Kenyan Luo migration study: observations on the initiation of a rise in blood pressure. *Br Med J* 1990; **300**: 967–72.

75. Appel LJ, Moore TJK, Obarzanek E, *et al.* A clinical trial of the effects of dietary patterns of blood pressure. *N Engl J Med* 1997; **336**: 1117–24.

76. Report of the Surgeon General. *The health consequences of smoking: cardiovascular disease.* Rockville, MD: US Department of Health and Human Services, Public Health Service, Office on Smoking and Health, 1983.

77. Whihelmsen L. Coronary heart disease: epidemiology of smoking and intervention studies of smoking. *Am Heart J* 1988; **115**: 242–9.

78. Stamler J. Opportunities and pitfalls in international comparisons related to patterns, trends and determinants of coronary heart disease mortality. *Int J Epidemiol* 1989; **18**: S58–66.

79. US Department of Health, Education, and Welfare: Smoking and Health. *A report of the Surgeon General.* Washington, DC: US Government Printing Office, 1979 [DHEW publication no. (PHS) 79–50066.].

80. Higgins M, Thom T. Trends in CHD in the United States. *Int J Epidemiol* 1989; **18**: S3–18.

81. Centers for Disease Control and Prevention. Cigarette smoking among adults – United States, 1995. *MMWR* 1997; **46**: 1217–20.

82. Willett WC, Green A, Stampfer MJ, *et al.* Relative and absolute excess risks of coronary heart disease among women who smoke cigarettes. *N Engl J Med* 1987; **317**: 1303–9.

83. Gillis C, Hole D, Hawthorne V, *et al.* The effect of environmental tobacco smoke in two urban communities in the west of Scotland. *Eur J Respir Dis* 1984; **65**: 121–6.

84. Lee P, Chamberlain J, Alderson M. Relationship of passive smoking on risk of lung cancer and other smoking-associated diseases. *Br J Cancer* 1986; **54**: 97–105.

85. Svendsen K, Kuller L, Martin M, *et al.* Effects of passive smoking in the Multiple Risk Factor Intervention Trial. *Am J Epidemiol* 1987; **126**: 783–95.

86. Helsing K, Snadler D, Comstock G, *et al.* Heart disease mortality in nonsmokers living with smokers. *Am J Epidemiol* 1988; **127**: 915–22.

87. Hirayama T. Lung cancer in Japan: effects of nutrition and passive smoking. In: Mizell M, Correa P, eds. *Lung cancer: causes and prevention.* New York: Verlag Chemie International, 1984: 175–95.

88. Garland C, Barrett-Connor E, Suarez L, *et al.* Effects of passive smoking on ischemic heart disease mortality of nonsmokers. *Am J Epidemiol* 1985; **121**: 645–50.

89. He Y. Women's passive smoking and coronary heart disease. *Chung Hua Yu Fang I Hsueh Tsa Chih* 1989; **23**: 19–22.

90. Humble C, Croft J, Gerber A, *et al.* Passive smoking and twenty year cardiovascular disease mortality among nonsmoking wives in Evans County, Georgia. *Am J Public Health* 1990; **80**: 599–601.

91. Butler T. The relationship of passive smoking to various health outcomes among Seventh-Day Adventists in California (abstract). *Seventh World Conference on Tobacco and Health*, 1990: 316.

92. Hole D, Gillis C, Chopra C, *et al.* Passive smoking and cardiorespiratory health in a general population in the west of Scotland. *Br Med J* 1989; **299**: 423–7.

93. Gartside PS, Khour P, Glueck CJ. Determinants of high-density lipoprotein cholesterol in blacks and whites: the Second National Health Nutrition Examination Survey. *Am Heart J* 1984; **108**: 641.

94. Kozarevic D, Demirovic J, Gordon T, *et al.* Drinking habits and coronary heart disease: The Yugoslavia cardiovascular disease study. *Am J Epidemiol* 1982; **116**: 748–58.

95. Stampfer MJ, Colditz GA, Willett WC, *et al.* A prospective study of moderate alcohol consumption and the risk of cornary disease and stroke in women. *N Engl J Med* 1988; **319**: 267–73.

96. Scragg R, Stewart A, Jackson R, *et al.* Alcohol and exercise in myocardial infarction and sudden coronary death in men and women. *Am J Epidemiol* 1987; **126**: 77–85.

97. Renaud S, Lorgeril MD. Wine, alcohol, platelets, and the French paradox for coronary heart disease. *Lancet* 1992; **339**: 1523–6.

98. West KM. *Epidemiology of diabetes and its vascular lesions.* New York: Elsevier, 1987: 375–420.

99. Barrett-Connors E, Cohn B, Wingard D, *et al.* Why is diabetes mellitus a stronger risk factor for fatal ischemic heart disease in women than in men? *JAMA* 1991; **265**: 627–31.

100. Eaker ED, Castelli WP. Type A behavior and mortality from coronary disease in the Framingham Study. *N Engl J Med* 1988; **319**: 1480–1.

101. Lahad A, Heckbert SR, Koepsell TD, *et al.* Hostility, aggression and the risk of nonfatal myocardial infarction in postmenopausal women. *J Psychosom Res* 1997; **43**: 183–95.

102. Kawachi I, Sparrow D, Spiro A III, *et al.* A prospective study of anger and coronary heart disease: the Normative Aging Study. *Circulation* 1996; **94**: 2090–5.

103. Maruta T, Hamburgen ME, Jennings CA, *et al.* Keeping hostility in perspective: coronary heart disease and the

hostility scale on the Minnesota Multiphasic Personality Inventory. *Mayo Clin Proc* 1993; **68**: 109–14.

104. Smith TW. Hostility and health: current status of psychosomatic hypothesis. *Health Psychol* 1992; **11**: 139–50.

105. Gidron Y, Davidson K. Development and preliminary testing of a brief intervention for modifying CHD-predictive hostility components. *J Behav Med* 1996; **19**: 203–20.

106. Dembroski TM, MacDougall JM, Costa PT, *et al.* Components of hostility as predictors of sudden death and myocardial infarction in the Multiple Risk Factor Intervention Trial. *Psychosom Med* 1989; **51**: 514–22.

107. Hecker MHL, Chesney MA, Black GW, *et al.* Coronary–prone behaviors in the Western Collaborative Group Study. *Psychosom Med* 1988; **50**: 153–64.

108. Shekelle R, Gale M, Ostfeld A, *et al.* Hostility, risk of coronary heart disease, and mortality. *Psychosom Med* 1983; **45**: 109–14.

109. Kaplan GA, Salonen JT, Cohen RD, *et al.* Social connections and mortality from all causes and from cardiovascular disease: prospective evidence from Eastern Finland. *Am J Epidemiol* 1988; **128**: 370–80.

110. Wrsesniewski K, Forgays DG, Bonaiuto P. Measurement of the Type A behavior pattern in adolescents and young adults: cross-cultural development of AATAB. *J Behav Med* 1990; **13**: 111–35.

111. Maeda S, Ito T. Type-A behavioral pattern as a risk factor of coronary heart diseases. *Jap Circulation J* (English edn) 1990; **54**: 457–63.

112. Feinleib M, Garrison RJ, Fabsitz R. The NHLBI twin study of cardiovascular disease risk factors: methodology and summary of results. *Am J Epidemiol* 1977; **106**: 284–95.

113. Goldbourt U, Neufeld HN. Genetic aspects of arteriosclerosis. *Arteriosclerosis* 1986; **6**: 357–77.

114. Connor WM, Cerqueira MT, Connor RW, *et al.* The plasma lipids, lipoproteins, and diet of the Tarahumara Indians of Mexico. *Am J Clin Nutr* 1978; **31**: 1131–42.

115. McMurry MP, Cerqueira MT, Connor SL, *et al.* Changes in lipid and lipoprotein levels and body weight in Tarahumara Indians after consumption of an affluent diet. *N Engl J Med* 1991; **325**: 1704–8.

116. Vardan S, Mookherjee S, Vardan S, *et al.* Special features of coronary heart disease in people of the Indian sub-continent. *Ind Heart J* 1995; **47**: 399–407.

117. Dhawan J. Coronary heart disease risks in Asian Indians. *Curr Opin Lipidol* 1996; **7**: 196–8.

118. Stamfer MJ, Malinow MR, Willett WC. A prospective study of plasma homocysteine and risk of myocardial infarction in US physicians. *JAMA* 1992; **268**: 877–81.

119. Arnesen E, Refsum H, Bonaa KH, *et al.* Serum total homocysteine and coronary heart disease. *Int J Epidemiol* 1995; **24**: 704–9.

120. McCully KS, Ragsdale BD. Production of arteriosclerosis by homocysteinemia. *Am J Pathol* 1970; **61**: 1–8.

121. Harker LA, Slichter SJ, Scott CR, *et al.* Homocystinemia,

vascular injury and arterial thrombosis. *N Engl J Med* 1974; **291**: 537–43.

122. Harker LA, Ross R, Slichter SJ, *et al.* Homocysteine-induced arteriosclerosis. The role of endothelial cell injury and platelet response in its genesis. *J Clin Invest* 1976; **58**: 531–41.

123. Nygard O, Nordrehaug JE, Refsum H, *et al.* Plasma homocysteine levels and mortality in patients with coronary artery disease. *N Engl J Med* 1997; **337**: 230–6.

124. Meade TW, Brozovich M, Chakrabartti RR, *et al.* Hemostatic function and ischemic heart disease: principal results of the Northwich Park Heart Study. *Lancet* 1986; **2**: 533–7.

125. Miller GJ, Martin JC, Mitropoulos KA. Plasma factor VII is activated by postprandial triglyceridaemia irrespective of dietary fat composition. *Atherosclerosis* 1991; **86**: 163–71.

126. Paramo JA, Colucci M, Collen D, *et al.* Plasminogen activator inhibitor in the blood of patients with coronary artery disease. *Br Med J* 1985; **291**: 573.

127. Grimm RH Jr, Neaton JD, Ludwig W. Prognostic importance of the white blood cell count for coronary, cancer and all cause mortality. *JAMA* 1985; **265**: 1932–7.

128. The Pooling Project Research Group. Relationship of blood pressure, serum cholesterol, smoking habits, relative weight and ECG abnormalities to incidence of major coronary events: final report of the Pooling Project. *J Chron Dis* 1978; **31**: 201–306.

129. Multiple Risk Factor Intervention Trial Research Group. Multiple risk factor intervention trial: risk factor changes and mortality results. *JAMA* 1982; **248**: 1465–77.

130. Multiple Risk Factor Intervention Trial Research Group. Mortality rates after 10.5 years for participants in the Multiple Risk Factor Intervention Trial. *JAMA* 1990; **263**: 1795–801.

131. Froment JW. The community-based model of life-style intervention trials. *Am J Epidemiol* 1979; **108**: 103.

132. US Department of Health and Human Services. *Report of the Expert Panel on Detection, Evaluation and Treatment of High Blood Cholesterol in Adults.* Washington DC: USDHHS, 1987.

133. Ministry of Public Health. *Smoking prevalence rate in China.* PR China: 1994.

134. Tobacco. Cigarette sales are on the up. *Tobacco* 1989; Sept.

135. Peto R. Future mortality from tobacco in China. *Shangai Symposium on Smoking and Health*, Shangai, China, 1987: 14–17.

136. Garber AM, Browner WS, Hulley S. Clinical guideline, part 2: Cholesterol screening in asymptomatic adults, revisited. *Ann Intern Med* 1996; **124**: 518–31.

137. Keys A, Taylor HL, Blackburn H. Coronary heart disease among Minnesota business and professional men followed 15 years. *Circulation* 1963; **28**: 381–95.

138. Chapman JM, Goerke LS, Dixon W. The clinical status of a population group in Los Angeles under observation for two to three years. *Am J Public Health* 1957; **47**: 33–42.

139. Doyle J, Heslin A, Hilleboe H. A prospective study of degenerative cardiovascular disease in Albany: report of three years' experience. I. Ischemic heart disease. *Am J Public Health* 1957; **47**: 25–32.

140. Stamler J, Lindberg H, Berkson D. Prevalence and incidence of coronary heart disease in strata of the labor force of a Chicago industrial corporation. *J Chronic Dis* 1960; **11**: 405–20.

141. Paul O, Lepper MH, Phelan WH. A longitudinal study of heart disease. *Circulation* 1963; **28**: 20–31.

142. Epstein FH, Ostrander LD Jr, Johnson BC. Epidemiological studies of cardiovascular disease in a total community–Tecumseh, Michigan. *Ann Intern Med* 1965; **62**: 1170–87.

143. Rosenman R, Friedman M, Straus R. A predictive study of coronary heart disease: the Western Collaborative Group Study. *JAMA* 1964; **189**: 15–22.

Primary prevention of cardiovascular disease: helping patients change lifestyle behaviors*

JUDITH K OCKENE AND IRA S OCKENE

This chapter provides information about the 'how' of intervention. Physicians and other health care clinicians want to help their patients make lifestyle changes to decrease risk for cardiovascular disease (CVD), but most lack the counseling skills needed for such intervention. This chapter emphasizes a patient-centered counseling approach which is effective and takes no more time than less effective methods of physician–patient interaction. The chapter also presents the theoretical background needed for an understanding of physician–patient interactions. Physicians need to be able to participate in an integrated approach that takes advantage of the different skills available on the health care team.

IMPORTANCE OF LIFESTYLE INTERVENTION BY THE PHYSICIAN AND OTHER CLINICIANS

Changing such lifestyle behaviors as smoking, high-fat eating patterns, little physical activity, and ineffective methods for dealing with stress can significantly decrease the risk of CVD. Likewise, improved adherence to therapeutic regimens for the treatment of hypertension, diabetes, and hyperlipidemia can prevent the development and/or progression of CVD[1] (see Table 2.1). However, changing a behavior that is detrimental to health requires knowledge, skills, and active involvement by busy clinicians and the at-risk individual in the planning and learning process.[2,3]

Physicians and other clinicians (e.g. psychologists, health educators, nurses, nutritionists, health counselors) who focus on lifestyle changes with their patients have demonstrated that they can significantly affect a patient's efforts to alter behaviors such as smoking,[4,5] diet,[6] and adherence to medical regimens.[7–9] Members of the health

Table 2.1 *Suggested target behaviors for risk behavior modification*

Dietary behaviors related to CVD
   High sodium intake (high blood pressure)
   High saturated fat intake (atherosclerosis, obesity, diabetes)
   Low fiber intake (diabetes mellitus, cardiovascular disease)
Physical inactivity
Poor medication adherence, e.g. for high blood pressure, diabetes
High stress levels and type A personality
Poor-quality relationships/supports

care team are uniquely and powerfully situated in their routine office practice to educate patients and to help them develop the skills required to make behavioral changes, playing a pivotal role in the prevention of CVD. There are clinical practice guidelines, such as those for smoking cessation (treating tobacco use and depen-

---

*This chapter is an adaptation of a chapter, 'Helping patients to reduce their risk for coronary heart disease: an overview', which appears in Ockene IS, Ockene JK, eds, *Prevention of coronary heart disease*, Little, Brown and Company, 1993.

dence),[5] and for cholesterol management, (the National Cholesterol Education Program (NCEP) clinical practice guidelines),[10] which provide strong evidence for the important role of the physician and other clinicians in lifestyle intervention. However, guidelines and education for clinicians are not enough. They need skills to help patients make changes and systems to cue them to intervene, provide them with materials for patients, and track the patients and their progress in making changes. Doctors have always been expected to teach their patients about their illnesses (the word *doctor* derives from the Latin *docere,* meaning 'to teach').[11-12] It is only a logical extension of this role that doctors should educate patients about behaviors that might cause illness in the future.

In addition to the fact that they are effective, there are several other reasons why physicians and other members of the health care team can and should play a major role in the management of patients who need to make behavioral changes. First, physicians are perceived by the general public as the most reliable and credible source of health information and advice.[13-15] Second, physicians and the health care system have contact with at least 80 per cent of the adults in the USA each year,[16] and are thus an immediately available and potent source of information regarding the prevention of CVD for over 120 million individuals. Data from the National Health Interview Survey (NHIS) also indicate that Americans visit a physician an average of 5.3 times per year.[16] Third, people think more seriously about their health and the impact of their lifestyle on it when they are in a physician's office or a hospital than at any other time. Fourth, physicians can provide a continuity of care, which allows them to reinforce messages to their patients.

Finally, patients generally do not want to go to a special program for help in altering unhealthy behaviors. More than 90 per cent of smokers who have quit smoking have done so on their own, without formal smoking intervention programs;[17] most current smokers would prefer to stop without such a program. Physicians and other clinicians in the health care setting are not perceived as special programs. They are part of the natural environment of individuals who may require help for reduction of risk for CVD.[18]

Given their effectiveness, the high credibility level of physicians and other clinicians as a source of needed health information, their high contact rate with the population at a time when people are particularly aware of their health and lifestyle behaviors, and the continuity of care that they provide, clinicians can have a significant impact on the prevention of CVD.

Overcoming barriers to physician interventions

Although physicians are generally aware of the benefits of implementing preventive interventions with their patients, national surveys of both patients and physicians indicate that a large percentage of physicians often do not intervene with lifestyle behaviors.[19] Physicians report several barriers to providing such intervention, including a belief that they are not effective in their health behavior interventions, poor intervention skills, a belief that patients do not want intervention when they are being seen for other problems, and little time to fit such intervention into their practices. Other factors more broadly associated with the practice of medicine also inhibit preventive interventions, such as non-reimbursement for these services. Also, physicians' practices generally are not set up to cue them to intervene and to facilitate integration of prevention activities with other more traditional medical needs. Finally, even though behavioral intervention for lifestyle change is of exceptional importance, there is not the same immediate gratification as with other interventions such as resuscitating a patient who has arrested.

> These barriers to implementing physician-delivered interventions for management of lifestyle change can be overcome. Physicians can achieve the skill level necessary for effective interventions with very little training. These interventions can be relatively brief (3–4 minutes) if they are focused and utilize the backup services of office staff, consultants, special programs, and supportive aids such as self-help materials. They also can be easily integrated into the out-patient encounter if effective office systems are set up to facilitate integration with other services.

Surveys have demonstrated that patients welcome their physicians' input for health behavior change; in fact, even those patients who do not alter their behaviors are more satisfied with[20] and more likely to refer other patients to those physicians who do intervene than to those who do not.[21]

Many patients and physicians are understandably concerned about the lack of reimbursement for prevention-oriented visits. However, there are legitimate billable diagnoses that physicians can use to receive reimbursement. In most cases, for example, physicians can receive reimbursement from third-party payers for patients with smoking-related problems (e.g. bronchitis). Reimbursement policies vary from state to state and among different insurers and types of policies.

Finally, physicians must have realistic expectations about the possibilities of health behavior change and adopt a new (or at least modified) mind set when dealing with lifestyle behavioral change. Change is a process which is slow and sometimes it seems as though little is accomplished. For example, smokers often quit three or four times over a period of about 5 years before they are successful in the long term.[22] From a population perspective, there have been remarkable changes in both smoking[23] and diet[24,25] in the USA over the last 20 years, and the health professions have played an important role. Throughout this chapter information is presented to address barriers to intervention and to help physicians and other clinicians to acquire the knowledge and skills needed to intervene effectively.

Physicians as part of an integrated approach to intervention

Although physicians and other clinicians in the health care system have a major role in the prevention of CVD, their intervention efforts do not exist in a vacuum. Rather, they occur in combination with health promotion education efforts implemented through the media, worksites, schools, and voluntary organizations and via legislation covering areas such as smoking in public places and food labeling. The health care system as a whole and clinicians who work in it are an integral and important part of these combined efforts.[26]

The first section of this chapter is an overview of the determinants of human behavior and behavior change, and the principles and procedures of behavior modification that physicians can use to help patients make changes in lifestyle behaviors to enhance their health and help prevent CVD. Although physicians are not expected to become experts in psychological and behavioral theories, a general understanding of the development of behavior and the factors that affect its alteration can enhance a physician's ability to help patients alter harmful behaviors. The second section addresses the practical aspects of physician-delivered interventions and the skills needed in the practice of clinical prevention. It presents strategies ranging from those that are relatively simple and can be used by clinicians who have minimal availability of time and staff to do preventive interventions to those that are more involved and require more of the clinician's time as well as that of other staff to coordinate activities and referrals. The last section addresses the special issues clinicians need to be aware of when implementing preventive interventions with special populations.

DETERMINANTS OF BEHAVIOR AND BEHAVIOR CHANGE

There are four theories which help explain the determinants of health behavior development and change and provide a foundation on which to develop effective strategies for interventions. The first, Consumer Information Processing Theory, explains the effects of knowledge on health behavior and on the factors that influence its processing. The other three theoretical models – Social Learning Theory, the Health Belief Model, and the Stages of Change Theory – present the cognitive, attitudinal, and behavioral determinants of health behav-

ior. The four theories taken together help us to understand how to promote changes in health behavior.

In this book we are interested in strategies for increasing CVD preventive behaviors and decreasing CVD-promoting behaviors. These behaviors include actions or activities that contribute to the maintenance of current good cardiovascular health and a reduction in the likelihood of developing CVD, or to the favorable alteration of the rate of progression of already-present CVD. Examples of CVD-preventive behaviors are the cessation of cigarette smoking, the alteration of eating patterns that contribute to increased weight or hyperlipidemia, and the reduction of certain types of stress responses. CVD-preventive behaviors also would include the initiation or increase in the frequency of healthy activities as part of the patient's daily routine. These activities might include an increase in physical activity or initiation of a meditation routine or adherence to a medication-taking regimen. Such behaviors make it clear that it is the patient who has responsibility for performing the action, which often requires special skills.

Consumer Information Processing (CIP) Theory[27] states that information is necessary for rational decision making and has an important influence on human behavior. However, although information is necessary, it is not sufficient to guide health actions and promote health-enhancing behaviors.[28] Thus, 87 per cent of current smokers report that they understand that smoking is harmful to their health,[29] but they continue to smoke. Most smokers also express a great desire to stop smoking but find it difficult to do so. Similarly, surveys indicate that three-quarters of US adults believe that cholesterol reduction would have an effect on CVD,[30] yet many continue to eat high-fat diets. Several minimum conditions are necessary for individuals to make use of information: it must be available; it must be wanted or believed to be useful by the consumer; and it must be able to be processed by the consumer.[28]

> Thus, the clinician must make information available and present it in such a way that it is at the level of the patient's comprehension, and the patient must be ready to hear the information and act on it.

Once individuals have the necessary information, they often lack the motivation, skills, environmental support, or resources needed to use it and to establish a new behavior as a habit, or to eliminate undesirable behaviors. These mediating factors are explained more fully by social learning theory and the health belief model, described next.

Social Learning Theory (SLT) (also referred to as social cognitive theory) is one of the best theoretical models for understanding lifestyle behaviors and methods to promote behavioral change. SLT assumes that most behaviors are learned and can therefore be unlearned or altered; that a person is able to self-manage behavior; that active participation is needed in the learning and the application of behavior-changing skills; and that behavior is dynamic and is constantly interacting with and being influenced by multiple determinants (reciprocal determinism),[31-33] with no single factor being sufficient to influence the behavior totally (see Table 2.2). The multiple and reciprocal interacting determinants of behavior include four groups of factors: personal characteristics of the individual; environmental influences; other associated behaviors; and physiologic and/or pharmacologic factors that affect addictive and/or habitual behaviors.

SLT incorporates easily applied behavior modification strategies that address the cognitive, interpersonal, and environmental influences on behavior.[33] (The specific strategies are discussed in the next section.) The clinician using these strategies can help the patient identify the triggers and reinforcements of behaviors, understand how and when they operate, and learn how to control these triggers and find reinforcements for CVD-preventive behaviors.

Three concepts in SLT are of particular importance for physicians and other health care clinicians seeking easily used interventions to educate patients and help them develop the skills and attitudes necessary to develop health-promoting behaviors. These concepts are self-efficacy, behavioral self-management, and shaping. Self-efficacy, the degree to which a person is confident of his ability to change successfully a specific behavior (e.g. to stop smoking), affects performance of that behavior independent of actual skill or knowledge. Self-efficacy is affected by past experiences of success and is alterable through behavioral strategies[3, 34] such as reaching small goals, monitoring, and self-reward.

Behavioral self-management (BSM) requires that an individual be aware that behavior is not an arbitrary occurrence but occurs as a result of identifiable factors (antecedents) that trigger, or cue, it and the consequences that reinforce it. The triggers can become linked, or conditioned, to the behavior, depending on the consequences that follow it. The consequences are either positive (pleasurable) and reinforce the occurrence of the behavior or negative (aversive), and decrease the likelihood of its occurrence. If a stressful situation triggers smoking and the smoker then feels more relaxed, the result reinforces the continued use of cigarettes. Alternatively, a stressful situation may trigger the consumption of a cup of coffee and palpitations immediately follow. In this case, the individual may decrease coffee use as a result of the aversive consequence.

Behavioral self-monitoring or the use of a special log to record occurrences of a behavior, its triggers, and consequences can help an individual become aware of his behaviors. He can then decide whether to avoid the trigger, alter it, or substitute a CVD-preventive behavior when the trigger occurs.

Alternatively, he can alter the consequences or reinforcements of the undesirable behavior to the extent that an alternative behavior is elicited and supported instead.

Shaping involves initially setting realistic, often small, attainable goals for change, so that reinforcement can be achieved quickly, in preparation for moving toward the final desired behavior.[32, 33] This gradual shaping helps facilitate the development of self-efficacy and subsequent motivation for the patient to continue to work on change. As specific steps toward the desired behavior are performed, the criterion for success and reinforcement is increased. For example, an individual who has the ultimate goal of smoking cessation may begin by cutting her number of cigarettes by 25 per cent each week for 1 or 2 weeks before quitting completely.

The Health Belief Model (HBM) focuses on cognitive and attitudinal variables[35-37] as a way of understanding a patient's motivation and the likelihood of his adhering to a particular medical regimen or implementing a health behavior change. The HBM proposes that several factors affect the likelihood that a patient will implement preventive action. Individuals are more likely to take action if they believe they are personally vulnerable or susceptible to a given condition, such as CVD; if there will be potentially serious consequences if they do not

Table 2.2 *Multiple and interacting determinants that affect health behavior*

Personal characteristics/cognitions
Demographics
Personality
Education/information
  Availability
  Believed to be useful
  Wanted by consumer
  Can be processed by consumer
Cognition (thoughts, beliefs, fears)
Belief in personal vulnerability and perceived risks of the
    behavior
  Belief in capability of changing the behavior
  Belief that behavior change will decrease risk
  Belief that benefits from change outweigh costs
Skills
  Self-management skills
  Stress reduction skills
Stage of change (readiness)

Enviroment
Social
Cultural
Economic
Political

Other behaviors, e.g. use of alcohol or coffee in a person
    trying to stop smoking

Physiologic factors, e.g. nicotine addiction

take action; if they are capable of taking action that will decrease their risk; and if the potential costs (barriers) of their taking action will be outweighed by the benefits.[37] The concepts of susceptibility and perceived risks help to explain why individuals who have already had a myocardial infarction are more likely to stop smoking or change their eating behavior than are individuals who do not yet have evidence of illness.[22] Providing information to the patient about the atherosclerotic process and its personal relevance to him or her, prior to the manifestation of signs and symptoms of disease, is important in helping the patient develop a realistic perception of personal risks and vulnerabilities.

The Stages of Change Model helps clinicians develop more realistic expectations of what can be achieved in one encounter with a patient. Behavior change is not a one-time event but a process that occurs in stages, often over an extended period of time.[38,39] Smoking cessation, for example, often takes 5–10 years and 3–4 attempts before long-term success is achieved.[38, 39] The stages of behavior change include precontemplation (not yet considering change), contemplation (thinking about and making plans to change a behavior), action (alteration of the behavior), and maintenance of the altered behavior (usually defined as having maintained the altered behavior for at least 6 months) or relapse (see Table 2.3). The stages are cyclical rather than linear, so if an individual relapses to the old behavior, he will generally cycle back to either precontemplation or contemplation.

The Stages of Change Model has two important implications for interventions by health care clinicians. First, because change is a process of several stages before eventful action takes place, clinicians, by their persistent efforts over repeated contacts, can be important resources to individuals who are at different points in the change process. Their assistance can help move the precontemplator to contemplation and the contemplator to action. Second, clinicians aware of this process do not need to become discouraged or alienate the often defensive precontemplator or embarrassed relapser. A single counseling interaction is not likely to move a precontemplator to action, but it may move him or her to the next stage, contemplation. The patient who quit smoking for 3 months and then resumed is not a failure; he or she is someone learning about what he or she needs to succeed and finding the path a bit difficult. Every patient can be reached at some level through education and persistent efforts at management. Individuals not ready or willing to change can still benefit from a brief intervention during their medical encounters to move them closer to the final goal.

> Interventions need to be targeted to the stage of the patient, his or her level of education and skills, and the social, financial, and cultural context.

The four theoretical models discussed here indicate that provision of usable information is necessary but not sufficient for behavioral change to occur (see Table 2.2). Whether an individual modifies a particular health behavior depends on several sets of factors: environmental, personal/cognitive, behavioral, and, in some cases,

Table 2.3 *Stages of behavior change and strategies to help the patient move to the next stage*

Stage	Strategies
Precontemplation Patient not yet considering change	Provide more information Help patient develop belief in ability to change (self-efficacy) Personalize assessment/feedback
Contemplation Patient thinking about and making plans to change behavior	Help patient develop skills for behavior change Provide support Help patient develop plan for behavior change Provide self-help materials
Action Patient changing behavior	Provide support Help patient prepare for possible problems
Maintenance Patient maintaining behavioral change	Help patient prepare for possible problems
Relapse Patient returning to old behavior	Help patient understand reasons for relapse Provide information about process of change Help patient make plans for next attempt Facilitate patient's belief in ability to change again Provide unconditional support

physiologic. These factors interact and determine whether an individual is ready to consider using the information available to make a change. No one factor is sufficient by itself to affect behavior. Such cognitive factors as belief in personal susceptibility, capability to make the needed change, and comprehension of the risk of disease strongly affect behavior.

Our understanding of the multiple and interacting factors that affect behavior determine the strategy clinicians can use to help patients develop CVD-preventive behaviors. These strategies, which are discussed in the next section, include methods designed to promote patients' self-efficacy, or confidence in their ability to manage their own behavior, self-management skills, and understanding of personal risk.

RECOMMENDATIONS FOR THE PRACTICE OF CLINICAL PREVENTION

The clinician's role in helping patients manage lifestyle change for the prevention of CVD involves a sequence of activities: diagnosis/assessment, treatment/intervention, plan for change, and monitoring/follow-up (Table 2.4). This sequence is similar to the clinician's actions when faced with a patient with more conventionally defined medical problems such as hypertension or chest pain. Not all risk factors can receive the same attention, given time availability, known effective interventions, patients' openness to action, and the physician's personal interests. *Physicians and other clinicians need to decide what they are willing and capable of doing and set themselves up to succeed at that level.* They also need to develop an office system that will be conducive to implementing preventive interventions.

Diagnosis/assessment involves the evaluation of CVD-risk factors, medical and family history, and relevant psychosocial, physiologic, behavioral, and demographic variables. Treatment/intervention involves, at a minimum, the physician advising the patient of the need to increase CVD-preventing behaviors and to alter CVD-promoting behaviors.

When appropriate and desired by the physician, treatment/intervention also involves an interactive counseling process where both the patient and the physician ask questions, provide information, and discuss the use of possible behavioral and pharmacological interventions. The eventual outcome of counseling is the collaborative development to negotiate a plan for change. Whether or not the physician decides to provide brief counseling, someone else in the office should be able to provide more comprehensive assistance, or the patient could be referred outside the office for assistance with behavioral change. In any case, the physician's role is crucial and one that requires coordination and a level of energy that indicates to the patient that risk reduction is of primary importance for his health. Follow-up/monitoring involves further assessment to determine whether goals have been met and whether the treatment plan developed has been implemented by the patient and is adequate to reach the goals set. Further development of goals and refinement of the treatment plan can then occur, again with the provision of continued follow-up.

Diagnosis/assessment, treatment/intervention, and monitoring/follow-up are often cyclical and ongoing. Even when lifestyle change occurs, periodic monitoring is necessary.

The physician can carry out each phase in the practice of clinical prevention. It is unlikely, however, that he or

Table 2.4 *Clinical steps in the prevention of cardiovascular disease*

Step	Physician's role

Step 1
Diagnosis/assessment
	Assess health and risks using:
	  Medical interview
	  Questionnaires
	  Laboratory tests

Step 2 Treatment/intervention	Advise need for behavioral change Provide information/personalize risk Help patient to establish motivation, understand personal strengths, and deal with barriers
Step 3 Plan for change	Negotiate goals with patient and plan strategies to achieve them
Step 4 Follow-up/maintenance	Schedule follow-up visits Provide support

she will want or have the time and/or skills to be intensively involved in the treatment of each patient. To limit the physician's involvement, other clinicians (e.g. health educators, nutritionists, nurses, psychologists) can intervene at each step, or professionals outside the office can be used for referrals. Because the cycle can become rather complex, it is important for the physician to set up an adequate office reminder and follow-up system and communication links to ensure efficiency of patient management.

There are four basic models for physician involvement, which can be used in various combinations: (1) brief physician advice; (2) brief physician counseling; (3) brief counseling with referral for comprehensive individual counseling; and (4) brief counseling with referral for group education (either one session or multiple sessions).[40] The following comprehensive overview of what the physician can do in the behavior modification process can be adapted to each physician's own needs, time, interests, and circumstances.

Step 1: Diagnosis/assessment

> The first step in the physician's role in the prevention of CVD is an assessment of the patient's health and risk status, his or her perception of the problem(s), and his or her knowledge regarding the relationship of lifestyle to CVD.

This first step of diagnosis/assessment in clinical prevention parallels the first step in diagnostic and therapeutic medicine (see Table 2.4).[41] Such an assessment uses the medical interview, questionnaires, the physical examination, and laboratory tests. Self-administered questionnaires have the advantage of increasing efficiency and standardization, are widely available, and have a high level of patient acceptability. Questionnaires also can facilitate communication. Although most of the information needed for determining a risk profile can be obtained without laboratory tests, data regarding factors such as total blood cholesterol and lipid profiles require blood tests.

A substantial number of patients are likely to have multiple high-risk lifestyle behaviors, which will be identified during the risk assessment. For patients with multiple risk behaviors, the patient and the physician need to decide which behavior to address first. (The possible options are discussed in the final section of this chapter.)

> The assessment process is one of mutual education for the patient and the physician. It provides the physician with information regarding the patient's CVD risk and an understanding of whom the patient is, his needs, knowledge, motivations, resources, barriers to change, and concerns.

Education of the patient begins during this initial assessment, as the physician and the patient engage in an interactive process.

During this interactive exchange between physician and patient, in which the patient provides much of the information, the physician provides feedback, at times paraphrasing what the patient has said, and provides additional information as required. These interviewing behaviors, which are appropriate and valuable for all physician–patient encounters, inform the patient that the physician is listening, understands his or her needs and concerns, and cares about him or her. They also allow the physician to help the patient use all the available information eventually to develop goals and a plan for altering the CVD promoting behaviors and for maintaining these changes. This process requires little extra time in the long-term care of the patient; if the physician carefully facilitates the discussion, greater understanding results and less time is needed later to clear up misconceptions and conflicts.

Step 2: Treatment/intervention

Treatment/intervention by the physician has been demonstrated to be effective for helping patients to stop smoking,[5,21] to lower cholesterol[10] and help patients with other lifestyle changes.[42] With a highly motivated patient who has personal resources and a positive history of change, such treatment by the physician usually requires very little time. However, additional time for education is needed for even the most motivated patient if he or she has few resources, little support, substantial problems in daily living, low confidence in his or her ability to alter behavior, and multiple risk behaviors. The physician needs to decide how much time intervention will take, how much time he or she is willing to devote, and whether a referral to a specialist is appropriate. At the very least, the physician must emphasize the patient's risk and the importance of the need for change. Even when making a referral, the physician needs to take at least a few minutes to make sure the patient understands the reason for the referral and that the physician plans to continue to follow the progress made and will be available if problems occur.

Whether the physician himself works with the patient or refers the patient to an outside resource, he or she needs to convey several consistent brief messages that have a strong scientific basis:

- Behavior change is a process, not a one-time event. It often proceeds through several gradual changes from first becoming aware of the need to change to finally making the complete change.
- Behavior change often takes several attempts before long-term maintenance of the change occurs.
- A return to an old behavior is not a failure. It can be used as a learning experience to help you prepare for the next time you make the change.

- Many methods can help you change a behavior. The best method to use is the one you choose for yourself, based on your own experiences.

> The major intervention strategy used in treatment to help patients make lifestyle changes is education, which is more than just the delivery of information or the transfer of facts.[11]

The National Task Force on Training Family Physicians in Patient Education[43] defined patient education as a process of influencing patient behavior to produce the changes in knowledge, attitudes, and skills needed to maintain or improve health. This process includes providing information, and interpreting and integrating it in such a way as to bring about attitudinal or behavioral changes to benefit patient health.

Attention to factors such as the social, political, and cultural environment, cognitions (thoughts), and skills, each of which mediate the relationship between knowledge and action, is needed if maximal change is to occur. This attention requires the use of a wide variety of strategies in patient education, including providing information, patient-centered counseling, discussion, and behavior modification. Although this may sound somewhat foreboding, the strategies are easily learned and can fit into the framework of the typical office encounter. While they are unlikely to use all approaches in their encounters with patients, it is important that physicians be aware of which approaches have been demonstrated to be efficacious in behavioral interventions. It is also important to accept that for some patients, problems in their social environment and difficulties in their daily lives may preclude their ability and desire to make CVD-preventing changes. Of course, final responsibility for change lies with the patient, who may have priorities at the time of the encounter other than changing lifestyle behaviors.

PROVIDING INFORMATION

> If the physician does nothing else, a necessary step in treatment/intervention is to use the information gathered during assessment and advise the high-risk patient of the value of reducing his or her CVD risk by modifying certain behaviors.

An understanding of the patient can be used to personalize the approach and make it particularly relevant to the patient and his or her situation. Thus, the most important information needed for advising a patient to change lifestyle behaviors comes from the patient.

The physician can provide information verbally or through written self-help materials. Alternatively the patient can be referred to other health professionals for additional information or more intensive intervention.

Depending on the preference and the needs of the patient, the physician, and the health care setting, the physician can use a combination of these approaches to provide information. A wide variety of informational and self-help materials regarding changes in various health behaviors is available for distribution to patients free of charge or for a nominal cost. These materials are published by several agencies, including the American Heart Association (AHA), the American Cancer Society (ACS), the National Heart Lung and Blood Institute (NHLBI), the American Lung Association (ALA), and the National Cancer Institute (NCI). The materials used should correspond to the social, cultural, and educational level of the patient. The AHA, ACS and ALA have state and regional offices, which can provide assistance and information.

PATIENT-CENTERED COUNSELING

The physician who desires to go beyond a 2-minute personal advice session and the provision of information can engage in brief patient-centered behavioral counseling. If the physician does engage in such counseling, advice giving and the provision of information can be integrated into the counseling approach and do not need to precede it. Patient-centered counseling can take anywhere from 2 to 3 additional minutes, if it is focused on a particular concern and ancillary materials or resources are used, to 10–15 minutes for the physician who wishes to or is able to spend more time with the patient. The most important aspect of patient-centered counseling, no matter how much time is spent, is that it emphasizes the importance of the patient's input in developing an effective plan for change and strategies for altering behaviors.

It is difficult to separate the assessment from the counseling intervention process, which largely entails further exploration of the patient's resources, motivations, strengths, problem areas, and behavioral patterns in relation to the targeted behavior. However, the goal shifts from simple assessment to a facilitative role for the physician. Through discussion and exploration of the way in which the patient can make the needed changes, the physician can help the patient gain greater self-awareness and can act as a catalyst for change. Table 2.5 summarizes the topics that should be covered in patient-centered counseling.

The counseling process provides a systematic approach for working with a patient in which the physician asks a series of questions that focus on the development of positive self-efficacy in the patient (i.e. a belief in one's ability to implement the behavioral change) and on the development of a plan for change. Every individual has strengths, resources, and past experiences that can be used to help make the needed health-related changes. If necessary, further information can be provided regarding effective behavioral strategies to be used to promote

Table 2.5 *Physician-delivered counseling steps and sample questions*

Step	Sample questions
1. Advise change Personalize risks of CVD and benefits of altering behaviors.	
2. Assess motivation	How do you feel about your diet? About the stresses in your life? How do you feel about changing this? What reasons or motivations would you have for changing this? Are you thinking about altering your diet in the next 6 months?

3. Assess past experiences with behavioral change	Did you ever (stop smoking) before?
	   If yes: When and why did you stop? How did you stop? What problems did you have? What helped? When and why did you start again?
	   If no: Have you made any other positive changes in your lifestyle (diet, physical activity)? How? Any problems? What helped you?

4. Discuss problems/barriers	In what situations do you most want to eat sweets? What possible problems are you concerned about if you stop?
5. Discuss resources	What might you do to help deal with possible problems? What might you do instead of overeating in situations when you usually overeat or eat unnecessarily?
6. Develop plan for change	Now that we have discussed your physical activity, what plans would you like to make to increase it?

If patient decides to change behavior:
   Negotiate behavioral goals
   Set timeline
   Review strategies for change
   Provide self-help materials (discuss these at next regularly scheduled visit)
   Refer patient to outside resource if indicated
If patient decides not to change or is unsure:
   Discuss other related goals (e.g. relaxation approaches, physical activity program) instead of endpoint goal (e.g. diet change).
   Provide self-help materials (discuss these at next regularly scheduled visit)	

7. Schedule follow-up contact
   Monitor progress to determine if goals have been met
   Determine future goals and revise plan
	What part of your plan was helpful?
	What part did you have problems with?

the target behavior. The effect of these strategies can be monitored in follow-up, and the treatment plan can be adjusted as needed.

The physician–patient interaction is different in the counseling for behavior change encounter from that which typically occurs in traditional medical treatment. In the latter situation the patient's role is often one of cooperation and dependence; in the counseling relationship the patient is actively involved in diagnosis and treatment, and the relationship is collaborative.

Despite the active involvement of the patient, the physician must still assume clinical responsibility. He sets the tone for the encounter – mutual exchange of information where both the physician's and the patient's participation is optimal.[44] The physician also needs to remain ultimately in control of the process to facilitate progression along a sequence of interchangeable steps designed to help the patient make the needed changes.

The success of counseling depends on the collaboration between patient and physician and on the physician's ability to facilitate the process and help keep the patient on target.

Topics in patient-centered counseling

The topics to be addressed in patient-centered counseling are suggested in a particular sequence. However, the sequence and the emphasis can be changed to fit the style of the physician and those needs and behaviors unique to the patient. For example, intervention in smoking often emphasizes exploring past changes, while counseling for alteration in eating patterns might be more effective if present patterns are emphasized. As the physician becomes more comfortable with the counseling approach, he or she should adapt it to his or her own needs, time constraints, and style.

The first topic that might be addressed is the patients' desire and motivation to change their behavior. It is important to determine the patients' reasons for wanting to change, which may be different from the physicians' reasons for wanting the patients to make a change. For example, patients may be more concerned about the impact of their eating behavior on their weight than on the risk of disease. Without a clear motivation for making the needed changes, it is unlikely that change will take place. For some patients, however, lack of motivation may be related to a lack of confidence in their ability to make the needed change. Therefore, even for patients who do not express strong motivation for change, it may be useful to go to the second topic, exploration of past experiences with change, to help them focus on past successes, no matter how small.

Most individuals who have made lifestyle changes in the past have returned to their old behaviors. For example, 80 per cent of all smokers have stopped in the past.[22] The past behavior modification should be positively reinforced, no matter how brief the period of change. The physician can help patients focus on the resources they used and the positive feelings that came from being a non-smoker. This can help patients become aware of their ability to stop smoking and help motivate them to try again. After addressing past experiences with patients who were not initially motivated to make a change, the physician can return to assessing motivation and determine whether the patients are now motivated to make a smaller change. Small successes help to shape positive self-efficacy.

Exploration of past experiences with change also can reveal problems that need to be prepared for and dealt with and the resources available to handle problems. What led to the stopping of a physical activity program? What was most difficult about starting one? How did the patients try to overcome lack of motivation when they were exercising regularly? What worked? What didn't?

The third and fourth topics, problems experienced and resources utilized, should be used to provide information about resources for the current effort. Ask the patients what most concerns them about making the change at the present time. Once again, it is important for the physician to focus initially on the patients' perspective and then add his or her own perspective, as needed. Reticent patients can be asked open-ended questions about behaviors that they might substitute for an

---

My reasons for (losing weight, increasing physical activity, stopping smoking) are:

1.

2.

3.

4.

Steps I will take to help me (lose weight, increase physical activity, stop smoking) are:

1.

2.

3.

4.

I am responsible for this decision and understand that my own commitment to

_____ is of primary importance.

I will return in _____ weeks or I will be telephoned in _____ weeks to see/to speak

to Dr. _____ on _____ at _____.
                                        (DATE)   (TIME)

_____   _____
(MY SIGNATURE)   (TODAY'S DATE)

Figure 2.1 *Sample plan for change. (Source: PDSIP Training Manual © 1990.)*

_____
(PHYSICIAN'S SIGNATURE)

unwanted behavior: 'What do you do to relax besides eating sweets?' If the patient cannot think of anything, a more focused question such as: 'Have you ever used physical activity to help you relax?' or 'Have you ever used deep breathing as a relaxation approach?', is useful.

> The counseling approach should lead to a plan for change. No encounter should end without a plan, no matter how small the goal.

The plan may focus on immediate goals: not shopping when hungry, walking 10 minutes each morning, or simply learning a relaxation technique. Optimally this plan should be written and signed (see Fig. 2.1), indicating commitment from both the physician and the patient. Finally, end with an arrangement for follow-up.

Behavior modification strategies

During the treatment/intervention phase the patient may need assistance in developing new skills. Several behavior modification strategies can be used to help the patient develop the skills and new behaviors needed for alteration of CVD-promoting behaviors. Changes that depend only on the provision of information or personal support alone often do not result in long-lasting behaviors.[45] The patient may need assistance in developing new behaviors. As noted previously, behavior modification strategies are based on social learning theory concepts[31–33] of self-efficacy, shaping, and behavioral self-management. Health care clinicians can use the following five key strategies as treatment options with the patient who needs to make lifestyle changes. Not all strategies are appropriate for each patient or problem. Deciding on the appropriate strategy for a given patient comes from knowledge of the patient and an understanding of the problem.

Behavioral self-monitoring

The individual uses a special log (behavioral record) to record each occurrence of the behavior that has been targeted for change (e.g. smoking), the triggers (antecedents) that cue the urge to perform the behavior, and the rewards or incentives (consequences) that follow it (Fig. 2.2).

Name: _____ Date: _____

Record each time you snack between meals (physical activity) (smoke)

	Time	Place	Activity	With Whom	Need* Rating
1.					
2.					
3.					
4.					
5.					
6.					
7.					
8.					
9.					
10.					
11.					
12.					
13.					
14.					
15.					
16.					
17.					
18.					
19.					
20.					

* Estimate how much you need the snack (cigarette) on a scale of 1 to 5. 1 = very important (cannot do without), 5 = least important (can do without).

Figure 2.2 *Behavioral record.*

Self-monitoring by the patient provides both the patient and the physician with additional information and insight about the behavior targeted for change and allows the individual to engage in behavioral self-management.

The individual can then choose to avoid or alter the trigger in some way or substitute a CVD-preventive behavior when the trigger occurs (e.g. do slow deep breathing instead of eating) and/or develop rewards or incentives for substituting CVD-preventive behaviors.

Stimulus control

The information from the self-monitoring records can be used to identify situations or thoughts that have been conditioned to the unwanted behavior and now trigger it. The patient can then decide how to avoid that trigger, as a way to change the behavior. For example, an individual who eats sweets when they are available in the home may decide not to buy any for a week and request that other household members help by not bringing any into the home.

Incentives

Rewards, or incentives, are developed for meeting predefined behavioral goals.

Investigators have demonstrated that self-reward strategies, when used as consequences of the performance of a specific behavior, reinforce its occurrence and maintenance better than do self-punishment strategies.[46]

Rewards should be provided close to the time that the goal is met. If a patient's goal is to walk 10 minutes each day for the next 3 days, a reward might be to purchase a magazine which he or she likes but usually does not allow him/herself to buy after he or she has completed the 3 days. Incentives must be developed by the patient, be pleasurable, and be used often and repeatedly to reinforce and shape the desired behavior.

One of the difficulties of discontinuing a CVD-promoting behavior or initiating a CVD-preventive behavior is that most of the positive consequences of the healthy behavior are often experienced only in the future (e.g. good health or feeling better), whereas the immediate consequences are often negative (e.g. feeling anxious). Conversely, the positive consequences of an unhealthy behavior (e.g. drinking alcohol) are often immediate (e.g. being able to forget stressful events), and the negative consequences are experienced only in the long term (e.g. dying prematurely). This pattern often makes it difficult for patients to reach their desired behavioral goals because they lack the necessary reinforcements for behavior change.[47] It is important for the physician briefly to explore with the patient immediate positive and meaningful consequences of the CVD-

preventive behavior. For example, a parent of a young child may see being a good role model as a positive short-term consequence of smoking cessation.

Substituting CVD-preventive behaviors

The vast majority of individuals offer the need to increase relaxation or reduce stress or boredom as a primary reason for smoking or overeating. Even individuals who can readily identify other ways of relaxing, such as physical activity, reading, or socializing, may not think they are capable of doing without cigarettes or food to handle the moment-to-moment stresses from which smoking or eating provide quick relief.

Deep breathing, simple meditation, physical activity, and physical exercise are relaxation techniques that can be used as substitutes and serve as effective functional equivalents for smoking or food in that they provide brief breaks from ongoing concerns, can be used under many circumstances, and seem to be physiologically effective.

Training in stress-reduction techniques can be done relatively quickly, particularly if aided by the use of an audiotape.

Contracts

After a review of goals and the means by which to reach these, putting the details into a written behavioral plan for change may help the individual to keep them in mind, particularly if no further treatment contact is possible. Such a plan or contract underlines the seriousness of the endeavor and provides the patient with something to refer to after the encounter. The plan should indicate the steps for change, the timetable proposed, the reasons for changing the behaviors, and a plan for follow-up (see Fig. 2.1).

Step 3: Negotiate a plan for change

Patient-centered counseling facilitates the development of a collaborative plan for change. Since most of the changes involved in risk reduction and prevention require the patient's voluntary cooperation and assumption of responsibility, successful outcomes require the patient to take a more active role in decision making and planning for change than usually occurs in a physician–patient interaction, with the physician acting as educator and counselor.[48–49] Individuals are more likely to initiate and maintain changes in their behavior if they have participated actively in developing the goals and plans for change.[2,50]

Some patients may be ready to change, and the patient and the physician may decide that the time is right for the patient to put effort into changing a particular behavior. In other cases they may decide that the time is not appropriate. Patients may have pressing social or financial problems that make it difficult for them to attend to lifestyle alteration. They may want to wait until they are able to bring these problems under control. Alternatively, they may decide that attending to the health behavior problems will provide them with a better sense of self, since they may be able to do something positive for their health while they may not be able to do anything about their other problems. For patients who decide that the time is not right for change, the physician may want to set up a subsequent appointment 2–3 months later to discuss the problem again. It is important not to let the issue drop or be deferred for too long.

REFERRING PATIENTS FOR ASSISTANCE

> The physician's assessment of the patient during the diagnosis/assessment and the treatment/intervention phases may lead him to conclude that specialized attention or more advanced, time-consuming efforts are needed to help the patient make the necessary behavioral changes or deal with other life problems.

Such patients may be very dependent on food or cigarettes for relief of negative feelings; or they may be slower in learning and require the services of a specialist. For example, a very obese individual may require a highly structured long-term program to lose weight and maintain the loss, which would be beyond the resources of most physicians' offices. The physician can still fill a very important role, however, by providing continued support and continuity of follow-up. Some problems requiring referral can be identified easily during the initial session, while others may take more than one visit to recognize.

When making a referral, the physician needs to indicate to the patient the reason for the referral, and should emphasize his or her continued involvement in the patient's care. Patients are often hesitant to obtain specialized help because they are concerned that this need indicates that they are 'sick' or too incompetent to handle their own problems. Discussion of these concerns is necessary if a successful referral is to be made. Specialists in prevention, such as health psychologists involved in intervention with medical patients, are often affiliated with medical clinics. Many patients would prefer to see a specialist such as a psychologist in a medical setting rather than a mental health setting. The physician needs to write out a referral to the specialist or agency indicating the specific problems, the information that has been gathered, and the reason for the referral. He or she also needs to develop a mechanism in his or her office system to ensure that he or she is kept aware of what occurs as a result of the referral.

It is important for physicians to have psychologists, nutritionists, nurses, and other health care clinicians and special intervention programs identified for appropriate referral. In general such programs and specialists are available in medical centers and medical schools, often in specialized departments of behavioral medicine or nutrition. Psychologists specializing in behavioral medicine also can be found in universities or colleges with psychology departments that have a concentration in health psychology. Names of individuals who specialize in interventions for risk factor-related changes can be obtained through local voluntary organizations. Most communities also have special group programs that help patients make health-related changes and local offices of the AHA, ACS, and ALA often have group programs available for lifestyle modification. In addition, many local hospitals, health departments, and community health centers sponsor programs for smoking cessation, dietary change, physical activity, and stress reduction.

A member of the physician's staff can develop a listing of programs or specialists in particular in the geographic area to provide to patients. While the effort is initially time consuming, the long-term payoff is substantial. Only those programs consistent with the physician's message should be included on this list. If the patient is referred to a program, it is necessary for the physician to know if the patient kept the appointment, what recommendations were made, and the outcomes.

Step 4: Follow-up/monitoring

> Follow-up by the physician or a staff member should occur within a few weeks of the initial visit, ideally in person, but follow-up by telephone is acceptable.

The time frame for follow-up is determined by the behavioral goals. If achievements are to be reinforced and problems identified, follow-up must be done while motivation to change is still high. Successful behavior change is not easy, and if follow-up does not occur for several months, it is likely that the process will need to be started over. Sending a letter that reiterates the goals and the plan immediately after the visit can be a useful procedure (Fig. 2.3 shows a sample letter.) This letter serves as a reminder to the patient and reinforces how important the physician thinks the behavior change is. Follow-up permits the physician and the patient to determine whether the plan for change is helpful and whether there are problems in meeting the negotiated goals. As part of this encounter, problem solving can occur and negotiation can again take place for new or revised goals and plans. The patient with multiple lifestyle health-related problems will need considerable follow-up to work through all the problem areas.

A major problem in behavioral change is that relapse or a return to old behaviors often occurs. For example, 70 per cent of all smokers who stop smoking return to smoking within 6 months.[39] Implementation of new behaviors is generally easier than their long-term maintenance. For most patients it is not realistic to expect that

Note: This letter is addressed to patients with high cholesterol. Follow-up letters can be used for any behaviors.

Dear _____:

At your recent visit we discussed the importance of finding a method to decrease your intake of foods high in cholesterol and saturated fat. Any method you choose can be helpful to you as long as you make a firm decision to alter your eating pattern. At the visit you indicated that you would:

1. (note steps agreed upon)_____

2. _____

3. _____

When you lower your cholesterol, important health benefits can be achieved. Your risk of developing cardiovascular disease will be decreased. If you would like further assistance, please call _____ at our office. As your physician, I encourage all efforts that you may want to make to lower your cholesterol. I wish you success.

Sincerely,

_____
(Physician's Name)

Figure 2.3 *Sample follow-up letter for preventive interventions.*

brief one-session interventions will produce successful long-term outcomes. Hypertension control is a more traditional medical example of the need for continued intervention of some type. It would be unusual for a physician to treat a patient's hypertension and then not follow-up to evaluate the treatment plan and its effects. Continued follow-up and reinforcement of some kind are likewise important for behavioral risk factors. The behavioral and counseling strategies used in the intervention phase also can be used in maintenance or relapse prevention. A relapse prevention strategy as a specific treatment component was developed by Marlatt, Gordon, and McClellan[51] to deal with preventing relapse in alcohol abuse and has been extended to other behaviors.

Relapse prevention is an approach that is consistent with social learning theory concepts and encourages patients to strengthen coping, self-management, and problem-solving skills. Five key elements, which are summarized below, can provide preparation for maintaining new behaviors. The physician can review these elements with the patient; they are also often addressed in self-help materials.

IDENTIFYING TRIGGERS OF HIGH-RISK SITUATIONS

Situations formerly associated with the behavior can trigger urges to return to the behavior, even though initial change has occurred. Thus, identification of high-risk situations can help patients predict problems and prepare for them. The following types of situations are ones in which individuals are most likely to slip:

- situations involving negative emotional states such as anger, frustration, or stress;
- situations involving positive emotional states – being relaxed and in a good mood and often involving the consumption of alcohol;
- situations in which the individual sees others engaging in the old behavior, such as smoking cigarettes.

Patients should be reassured that cravings or urges to re-engage in the old behavior are normal and are to be expected rather than an indication of poor motivation or lack of will power. Patients who deny any significant difficulties may find themselves much more vulnerable to urges to return to their earlier behaviors.

COPING REHEARSAL

The outcome of exposure to high-risk situations is determined by whether the individual produces a healthy coping response that does not involve the old behavior. Use of imagery or hypnotherapy techniques may be valuable if the patient cannot easily visualize handling the high-risk situations. Once the individual has identified high-risk situations, he or she can develop and mentally rehearse specific strategies that can prevent a slip that might lead to a full relapse.

IDENTIFYING AND COMBATING RESUMPTIVE THINKING

Patients may have habitual rationalizations to justify behavioral lapses or resumption of old behaviors. Identification of these rationalizations ahead of time can help guard against relapse by increasing awareness and by returning a sense of control to the patient. The following rationalizations are examples of resumptive thinking:

- Nostalgia – 'I remember how nice it was when I didn't feel like I had to take a walk and could just sit and relax before dinner.'
- Testing oneself – 'I bet I could eat just one cookie with my coffee.'
- Crisis – 'I know I'll deal with this better if I take a drink.'

Combating resumptive thinking may require rehearsal of counter thoughts:

- Challenging – 'Taking just one cookie may be an excuse for returning to overeating. I do not need to test myself.'
- Visualization of benefits – 'I want to be able to play tennis without collapsing.'
- Distractions – 'I think I'll go call a friend instead.'

AVOIDING THE ABSTINENCE VIOLATION EFFECT

The abstinence violation effect (AVE) is a common emotional response to a slip or a lapse in the face of personal commitment to change. Accompanying thoughts such as 'I blew it' appear to predict a decision to give up the commitment entirely and to resume the avoided behavior. Discussion with a patient of this predictable response appears to decrease the problem. Consequently patients should be acquainted with the following points:

- anticipating the AVE will help to reduce its impact;
- a slip is not the same as a relapse;
- a slip can be a learning experience;
- slips often lead to relapse if not dealt with quickly.

ENCOURAGING SUPPORT

Other relapse prevention strategies include encouraging the patient to enlist the support of family, friends and co-workers.

> The stronger the patient's support system, the more likely it is that he or she will maintain the new behavior.

The patient's spouse may benefit from encouragement to provide positive rather than nagging support. It is important that neither the physician nor the patient become discouraged or angry if relapse occurs. A characteristic of successful long-term maintenance is that

there is a history of having made changes in the past.[39] Each attempt can be viewed as a small gain on the way to final success.

Summary of the practice of clinical prevention

As noted in the introduction to this section, the physician may be able to and desirous of implementing each of the phases of the practice of clinical prevention. Alternatively, part of each phase can be carried out by referrals to consultants, programs or agencies, or other office personnel can assist. Considering the various possible combinations of clinicians who may assist in assessment and intervention, it is necessary that an adequate communication and office monitoring system be set up to assure that there are no gaps in the process and that all required communications occur.

> For the patients who have only one lifestyle behavior to change, good skills, strong motivation to make changes, and strong support systems, much of the preventive sequence can be accomplished in 3–10 minutes, depending on the level of physician involvement and use of ancillary materials, during two or three visits.

The first visit would include diagnosis/assessment and possible treatment/intervention. If laboratory tests are used, then treatment/intervention and development of a plan for change will need to be defined to take place during visit two. However, there are likely to be enough data available during visit one for an initial plan to be negotiated and strategies for change identified. Visits two and three and possibly a fourth visit are needed to address follow-up and assessment, and possible revision of the negotiated plan for change. Patients with multiple lifestyle behaviors to change or more difficult patients will require more time and/or greater reliance on other intervention specialists.

Physicians with little practice can quickly learn the skills needed for patient management and education for clinical prevention. Studies have demonstrated that the development of such skills can occur within 1–2 hours and can lead to more effective patient intervention.[4]

CLINICAL PREVENTION FOR SPECIAL POPULATIONS

Difficult-to-reach patients

Patients of lower socioeconomic status who may also be unemployed or homeless are generally difficult to reach for CVD-preventive interventions and often face multiple obstacles to making needed changes. Patients with psychiatric disorders and drug and alcohol abusers also prove difficult for intervention and require special attention. Individuals in each of these groups have difficulty seeing beyond the needs of the day and have little energy to make changes that would lead to health benefits in the more distant future. Minimal resources and poor skills also may make it difficult for these individuals to obtain the help they need. Poor comprehension may make it difficult for them to apply health-related information to themselves, and disrupted social and family environments make it hard for them to adhere to programs and plans that require focused attention. These substantial obstacles require attention and an approach that is sensitive to the patient's needs.

> Preventive efforts aimed at homeless individuals are especially important since they have a high prevalence of CVD-promoting behaviors, such as smoking.

Results of a study by Dr Lori Fantry, an internist who provided medical services in the shelters in Worcester, Massachusetts, demonstrated that there is a subgroup of homeless individuals with a high desire to stop smoking and a high confidence level in their ability to do so.[52] Health-related intervention efforts for the homeless population should be specifically targeted toward their needs and can be successful if provided at sites such as shelters, city hospital clinics, and soup kitchens, which are easily accessible to them.[52]

> The physician in encounters with difficult-to-reach patients can become aware of their special problems and belief systems and help to direct them to appropriate agencies for assistance if indicated.

It is important for the physician not to be pulled into a sense of hopelessness and helplessness. He can help the patient see that options are available, including obtaining the help needed for dealing with problems in daily living. The physician also must not make the assumption that a patient with difficult problems would not be interested in making health-related changes. Some patients in difficult life situations actually view health behavior change as something positive that they can do for themselves, no matter how small. For those patients with chronic life problems who make small changes, there is an increase in their self-efficacy and belief in their ability to effect change. Such an increase in self-efficacy can help patients make other changes in their lives as well.

Patients with chronic psychiatric problems and drug or alcohol abusers present special problems. Research examining treatment options for health behaviors in these populations has not been done in spite of the substantial evidence of an unusually high incidence of poor health behaviors. Treatment of health behaviors in these complicated patients usually requires much individualized attention and longer follow-up.

Minority patients

Patients from minority groups are often at greater risk for obesity, non-insulin-dependent diabetes, and hypertension than those from white populations. However, patients from minority groups are often also more difficult to reach because of the physician's lack of awareness, of their health beliefs and cultural values, and because these individuals often have fewer financial and educational resources. Clinicians should familiarize themselves with the health-belief systems of the minority populations they serve so they can provide these patients with adequate information.

Elderly patients

Lifestyle modification in the elderly patient has been demonstrated to be beneficial.[53-56] However, elderly patients often present with special needs that may interfere with CVD-preventive interventions. Some elderly individuals have poor social support systems, difficulty engaging in physical activity, the need to adhere to regimens for other medical problems, depression, and other chronic problems. These possible obstacles require attention and a sensitive approach. The physician can direct the patient to the appropriate services for assistance. It is important not to assume that the elderly patient, especially the vigorous healthy individual, is not interested in lifestyle modification. The elderly patient experiencing other chronic problems is also a possible candidate for lifestyle modification, and this possibility needs to be assessed.

Patients with multiple risk behaviors

Patients with multiple risk behaviors require special consideration for intervention decisions. The presence of multiple risk behaviors may pose obstacles to change or, alternatively, may increase the individual's motivation and subsequent improvement in each of the behaviors. Several studies have found that individuals who quit smoking are also more likely to lower their cholesterol and blood pressure and practice other health-promoting behaviors than those individuals who continue to smoke.[57-59] Of course the former may be more health conscious at the outset. However, changes in some behaviors, for example, increased physical activity or use of meditation, can help individuals implement changes in other behaviors such as smoking cessation and reduced food intake.

> For the patient with multiple problems the patient and the physician need to decide which behavior to address first, following one of three approaches:

- start with alteration of one risk behavior; once that is under control, focus on another risk behavior;
- work equally on all risk behaviors at the same time;
- focus attention on one risk behavior and at the same time make small changes in another one.

With the first approach an optimal way to proceed is to work first with the behavior the patient believes he or she is most capable of changing and most interested in changing. However, if the physician thinks a particular behavior has a significantly greater effect on the patient's health, for example, smoking 40 cigarettes a day compared to being 10 pounds overweight, then the physician needs to indicate this to the patient and negotiate regarding the first risk behavior to be addressed. It has been our experience that many patients who smoke and are also overweight most commonly choose weight control as their initial target, because they perceive it to be easier; in reality long-term success rates are much greater for smoking cessation.[39] The second approach requires a highly motivated patient with good resources and a supportive environment. The third approach is useful for the patient who may need to stop smoking and at the same time alter his or her eating patterns because of a concern for possible weight gain. The patient may decide that along with stopping smoking he or she will monitor his or her sweet intake and start a physical activity program, but not focus on weight loss.

Whatever approach is chosen, the physician and the patient must weigh the costs against the benefits. The physician's role is to express what he or she sees as optimal and help direct the patient to set realistic goals. The physician must also be sensitive to the fact that, for some patients, the cost of change may outweigh any benefits.

Costs of lifestyle change

For some patients behavioral change can lead to deleterious consequences as well as benefits. Altering lifelong habits can, for a small number of patients, cause anxiety, irritability, and, in the case of smoking cessation, weight gain (which is generally moderate[39]), especially for the patient with poor resources and other problems in daily living. Important social networks can be disrupted by the cessation of smoking or alcohol abuse or by the implied criticism of others seen in such actions as the initiation of a vigorous diet alteration and physical activity program.

For some individuals detrimental effects may outweigh the benefits of change, at least in the short term, and make such change difficult. The physician can take the following steps to minimize such difficulty:

- identify clearly the target goals that are likely to decrease risk;
- analyze both the benefits and the expected costs of a particular lifestyle change;
- identify a range of alternative approaches that might reduce the cost of achieving particular goals;
- negotiate with the parties involved to reach consensus on the importance of a change and the best approach(es) to achieve maximum benefit based on the energy and the resources available;
- identify the conditions under which intervention to achieve a particular goal is not warranted because of an anticipated high cost/benefit ratio or because it produces irreconcilable social dilemmas;
- monitor progress periodically to reassess the balance of costs and benefits in light of changing circumstances and the response to the intervention.

As we encourage patients to make lifestyle changes beneficial to their health, it is equally important to avoid creating a nation of people who are hypochondriacs and overly health-conscious. Barsky points out that, although life expectancy has increased remarkably (a 6.5-year increase from 1950 to the mid-1980s), the proportion of people living in the USA who are satisfied with their health has fallen from 61 per cent in the 1970s to 55 per cent in the mid-80s.[60] People now report more frequent and longer-lasting episodes of serious disability than they did 60 years ago, and there has been a continuous decline in the proportion of people who report no symptoms. Dr Barsky concludes, 'There appears to have been a progressive decline in our threshold and tolerance for mild disorders and symptoms.'

This is not a simple problem. An almost inevitable consequence of continuously reminding people to think about their health, to eat better, to avoid various noxious behaviors, and to run to the emergency room for thrombolytic therapy at the first hint of chest pain is a nation of people preoccupied with the state of their bodies. As we encourage people to make beneficial changes, we also must avoid using scare tactics, and we should emphasize a patient's current state of health rather than the dire potential for disease. It is at times a difficult balance to achieve, but an important one.

OVERVIEW

This chapter began by noting that, while physicians are aware of the benefits of preventive interventions, they often do not provide such interventions. The reasons for such failures include:

- low perceived efficacy;
- lack of skills;
- concern that patients do not welcome such interactions;
- lack of time;
- lack of reimbursement;
- lack of practice organization to facilitate such interventions;
- little self-gratification from such efforts.

Throughout this chapter, information has been presented that indicates that physicians can be effective by using brief interventions that are direct and supportive of the patients' efforts. This approach accepts that patients do welcome physician interventions, that they usually want to make the needed changes, and that they often have the resources to do so. The physician's role as counselor and educator is to help the patient become aware of the need for change and of his or her own personal resources, and to help him or her find ways to make the needed changes. The physician must also learn to enlist the services of other office staff, consultants, and outside programs. He or she must be aware of the available services and able to make an effective referral. To close the intervention loop and ensure that prevention is addressed, an office system must be set up that facilitates support, integration with other services, and follow-up. While reimbursement for these services is not likely to change in the near future, there are legitimate billing practices that allow for reimbursement of risk behavior intervention. Physicians need to become aware of how to maximize such reimbursement.

Regarding gratification for the physician's prevention efforts, the physician must have realistic expectations of what can be accomplished. Behavioral change is often a slow process as people move through stages of change. It is important to be aware that significant risk behavior changes have occurred in this country and that the physician is an important part of the national effort.

The ability to think in terms of large numbers of patients as well as the individual patient, a public health perspective often foreign to usual physician practice, is very helpful. A 5 per cent decrease in the blood cholesterol level is small and often ungratifying when seen from the perspective of the individual physician–patient relationship. However, a 5 per cent decrease in cholesterol yields a 10 per cent decrease in risk,[25] and a 10 per cent decrease in risk in a disease that causes 500 000 deaths a year is an annual savings of 50 000 lives: gratifying indeed when seen from such a population perspective. Similarly if increased physician efforts double or triple smoking cessation rates (i.e. from 5 per cent to 15 per cent), a magnitude of impact found in several physician-delivered intervention studies, such an effect is of tremendous clinical and public health importance. The physician, however, may be more aware of the 85 per cent of his or her smoking patients who continue to smoke.

It is also necessary to accept that once a patient becomes ill, all medicine usually has to offer is palliation. We cure very few adult diseases, and the knowledgeable physician understands that the cost of such therapy is extraordinary. Patients who remain healthy because the physician successfully helped them to stop smoking may never appreciate that because of the counseling, they are well and active instead of having prematurely suffered a myocardial infarction. However, for the prevention-oriented physician who understands the positive consequences of risk behavior modification, the rewards can be great.

SUMMARY

- Members of the health care team are uniquely situated in their routine office practice to educate patients and help them develop the skills needed to make behavioral changes, playing a pivotal role in the prevention of cardiovascular disease (CVD).
- Health care providers need guidelines/education regarding CVD prevention and office systems which remind them to intervene, provide them with the necessary materials, integrate their interventions with other services, and facilitate patient follow-up.
- Interventions by multiple providers significantly enhance health behavior change outcomes. Therefore use of intervention teams can be very effective.
- The physician's role as counselor and educator is to help the patient become aware of the need for change, and to help him or her find ways to succeed.
- Phases of clinical CVD prevention are similar to the following phases of any medical encounter: (1) diagnosis/assessment; (2) treatment/intervention; (3) negotiation of a plan for change; and (4) follow-up/monitoring.
- Patient-centered counseling, in which the patient is an active part of the encounter, is the best way to educate patients about CVD-related behaviors and the strategies for changing them.
- Behavior change is a process, not a one-time event, and proceeds through several phases. It often takes several attempts before long-term change occurs.
- Many methods can help patients to change behaviors. The best method is the one that the patient and the provider agree upon based on the patient's experiences, skills and resources.

REFERENCES

1. Stamler J. Coronary heart disease: Doing the 'right things' (editorial). *N Engl J Med* 1985; **12**: 1053–5.

2. Haggerty RJ. Changing lifestyles to improve health. *Prevent Med* 1977; **6**: 276–89.

3. Bandura A. Self-efficacy: toward a unifying theory of behavioral change. *Psychol Rev* 1977; **84**: 191–215.

♦4. Ockene JK, Quirk M, Goldberg RJ, *et al*. A residents' training program for the development of smoking intervention skills. *Arch Intern Med.* 1988; **148**: 1039–45.

5. Fiore MC, Bailey WC, Cohen SJ, *et al. Smoking cessation: clinical practice guideline* no. 18. Rockville, MD: US Department of Public Health and Human Services, Public Health Service, Agency for Health Care Policy and Research, 1996. AHCPR #96-0692.

6. Mojonnier ML, Hall Y, Berkson DM, *et al*. Experience in changing food habits of hyperlipidemic men and women. *J Am Diet Assoc.* 1988; **77**: 140–8.

7. Dunbar J. Assessment of medication compliance: a review. In: Haynes RB, Mattson ME, Engebretson TO, eds. *Patient compliance to prescribed antihypertensive medication regimen*. Bethesda, MD: USDHHS, 1980. (Publ. no. (NIH) 81-2102).

8. Greenfield S, Kaplan SH, Ware JE, Yano EM, Frank HJL. Patients' participation in medical care; effects on blood sugar control and quality of life in diabetes. *J Gen Intern Med* 1988; **3**: 448–57.

9. Schulman BA. Active patient orientation and outcomes in hypertensive treatment: application of a socio-organizational perspective. *Med Care* 1979; **17**(3): 267–80.

♦10. Ockene IS, Hebert JR, Ockene JK, Sapeira GM, Stanek E, Nicholosi R, Merriam PA, Hurley TG. Effect of physician-delivered nutrition counseling training and a structured office-support program on saturated fat intake, weight, and serum lipid measurements in a hyperlipidemic population: the Worcester-Area Trial for Counseling in Hyperlipidemia (WATCH). *Arch Intern Med* 1999; **159**: 725–31.

○11. Canfield RE. Role preparation: The physician as a teacher of patients. *Med Educ Care* 1973; **48**: 79–87.

12. Brunton SA. Physicians as patient teachers. *West J Med* 1984; **151**: 855–60.

13. US Department of Health Education and Welfare. *Healthy people. The Surgeon General's report on health promotion and disease prevention*. Washington, DC: Public Health Service, 1979. DHEW(PHS) Publ. 79-55071A.

14. Glynn TJ, Manley MW, Cullen JW, Mayer WJ. Cancer prevention through physician intervention. *Semin Oncol* 1990; **17**: 391–401.

15. Ford AS, Ford WS. Health education and the primary care physician: the practitioner's perspective. *Soc Sci Med* 1983; **17**: 1505–12.

16. National Center for Health Statistics. *Health, United States, 1987*. Hyattsville, MD: USDHHS, PHS, 1988. USDHHS publ. no. (PHS) 88-1232.

○17. Fiore MC, Novotny TE, Pierce JP, *et al*. Methods used to quit smoking in the United States: do cessation programs help? *JAMA* 1990; **263**: 2760–5.

18. Ockene JK. Towards a smoke-free society. *Am J Public Health* 1984; **74**: 1198–200.

19. Ockene JK. Physician-delivered interventions for smoking cessation: strategies for increasing effectiveness. *Prevent Med* 1987; **16**: 723–37.

20. Bertakis KD. The communicating of information from physician to patient: a method for increasing patient retention and satisfaction. *J Family Pract* 1977; **5**: 217–22.

21. Ockene JK, Kristeller J, Goldberg R, *et al*. Increasing the efficacy of physician-delivered smoking intervention: a randomized clinical trial. *J Gen Intern Med* 1991; **6**: 1–8.

22. US Department of Health and Human Services. *Reducing the health consequences of smoking: 25 years of progress. A report of the Surgeon General*. Rockville, MD: PHS, Centers for Disease Control, Center for Chronic Disease Prevention and Health Promotion, Office of Smoking and Health, 1989. USDHHS publ. no. (CDC) 89-8411.

23. Centers for Disease Control and Prevention. Cigarette smoking among adults – United States, 1995. *MMWR* 1997; **46**: 1217–20.

24. National Center for Health Statistics, National Heart Lung and Blood Collaborative Lipid Group. Trends in serum cholesterol levels among US adults aged 20 to 74 years: data from the national Health and Nutrition Examination Surveys, 1960 to 1980. *JAMA* 1987; **257**: 937–42.

25. The Lipid Research Clinics Program. The lipid research clinics coronary primary prevention trial results: I. Reduction in incidence of coronary heart disease. *JAMA* 1984; **251**: 351–64.

26. Ockene JK. Smoking intervention: the expanding role of the physician. *Am J Public Health.* 1987; **77**(7): 782–3.

27. Bettman JR. *An information processing theory of consumer choice*. Reading, MA: Addison-Wesley, 1979.

28. Rudd J, Glanz K. How individuals use information for health action and consumer information processing. In: Glanz K, Lewis FM, Rimer BK, eds *Health behavior and health education: theory, research and practice*. San Francisco: Jossey-Bass, 1990.

29. American Lung Association. *Survey of attitudes toward smoking*. Princeton, NJ: Gallup Organization, 1985.

30. Schucker B, Bailey K, Heimbach JT, *et al*. Change in public perspective on cholesterol and heart disease: results from two national surveys. *JAMA* 1987; **258**: 3527–31.

31. Mischel W. Toward a cognitive social learning

reconceptualization of personality. *Psychol Rev* 1973; **80**: 252–83.

32. Bandura A. *Social learning theory*. Englewood Cliffs, NJ: Prentice-Hall, 1977.

33. Bandura A. *Social foundation of thought and action: a social cognitive theory*. Englewood Cliffs, NJ: Prentice-Hall, 1986.

34. Bandura A, Schunk DH. Cultivating competence, self-efficacy and interests through proximal self-motivation. *J Pers Soc Psychol* 1981; **41**: 586–98.

35. Rosenstock IM. What research in motivation suggests for public health. *Am J Public Health.* 1960; **50**: 295–301.

○36. Becker MH. The health belief model and personal health behavior. *Health Educ Monographs.* 1974; **2**: 324–473.

37. Rosenstock IM. The health belief model: explaining health behavior through expectancies. In: Glanz K, Lewis FM, Rimer BK, eds *Health behavior and health education: theory, research, and practice*. San Francisco: Jossey-Bass, 1990.

38. Prochaska J, DiClemente C. Stages and processes of self-change of smoking: toward an integrative model of change. *J Consult Clin Psych* 1983; **51**: 390–5.

39. US Department of Health and Human Services. *The health benefits of smoking cessation: A report of the Surgeon General*. Washington, DC: US Government Printing Office, 1990, (CDC)90-8416.

40. Glanz K. Nutrition education for risk factor reduction and patient education: a review. *Prev Med* 1985; **14**: 721–52.

41. Stokes J, Noren J, Shindell S. Definition of terms and concepts applicable to clinical preventive medicine. *J Commun Health* 1982; **8**: 33–40.

42. Ockene JK, McBride P, Sallis J, Bonollo DP, Ockene IS. Synthesis of lessons learned from cardiopulmonary preventive interventions in healthcare practice settings. *Ann Epidemiol* 1997; **S7**: S32–S45.

43. Fass MF, Vahldieck LM, Meyer DL. *Teaching patient education skills: a curriculum for residents*. Kansas City, MO: Society of Teachers of Family Medicine, 1983.

44. Lazare A, Eisenthal S, Frank A. A negotiated approach to the clinical encounter. II. Conflict and negotiation. In: Lazare A, ed. *Outpatient psychiatry: diagnosis and treatment*. Baltimore: Williams & Wilkins, 1979.

45. Stunkard AJ. Behavioral medicine and beyond: the example of obesity. In: Pomerleau OF, Brady JP, eds *Behavioral medicine: theory and practice*. Baltimore: Williams & Wilkins, 1979.

46. Mahoney MJ, Moura NCM, Wade TC. Related efficacy of self-reward, self-punishment, and self-monitoring techniques for weight loss. *J Consult Clin Psychol* 1973; **40**: 404–7.

47. Russell ML. *Behavioral counseling in medicine*. New York: Oxford University Press, 1984.

48. Demak MM, Becker MH. Current perspectives on the changing patient-provider relationship: charting the future of health care. *Patient Educ Couns* 1987; **9**: 5–24.

49. Carter WB, Belcher DW, Inui TS. Implementing preventive care in clinical practice: Problems for managers, clinicians, and patients. *Med Care Rev* 1981; **38**: 195.

50. Green LW. Modifying and developing health behavior. *Annu Rev Public Health* 1984; **5**: 215–36.

51. Marlatt A, Gordon J, McClellan W. Current perspectives: Patient education in medical practice. *Patient Educ Couns* 1986; **8**: 151–63.

52. Fantry LS. Unpublished report, 1990.

53. Castelli WP, Wilson PWF, Levy D, *et al*. Cardiovascular risk factors in the elderly. *Am J Cardiol* 1989; **63**: 12H–19H.

54. Gordon DJ, Rifkind BM. Treating high blood cholesterol in the older patient. *Am J Cardiol* 1989; **63**: 48H–52H.

55. Hermanson B, Omenn GS, Kronmal RA, *et al*. Beneficial six year outcome of smoking cessation in older men and women with coronary artery disease: results from the CASS registry. *N Engl J Med* 1988; **319**: 1365–9.

♦56. Kafonek SD, Kwiterovich PO. Treatment of hypercholesterolemia in the elderly. *Ann Intern Med* 1990; **112**: 723–5.

57. Orleans CT, Shipley RA, Wilbur C, *et al*. Wide-ranging improvements in employee health lifestyle and well-being accompanying smoking cessation in the Live for Life program. *Annual Meeting of the Society of Behavioral Medicine*, Baltimore, MD, 1983.

58. Schoenenberger JC. Smoking change in relation to changes in blood pressure, weight, and cholesterol. *Prevent Med* 1982; **11**: 441–53.

59. Tuomilehto J, Nissinen A, Puska P, *et al*. Long-term effects of smoking cessation on body-weight, blood pressure and serum cholesterol in the middle-aged population with high blood pressure. *Addict Behav* 1986; **11**: 1–9.

60. Barsky AJ. The paradox of health. *N Engl J Med.* 1988; **318**: 414–8.

National efforts to reduce coronary disease-related mortality

COSTAS T LAMBREW

Cardiovascular disease continues to be the major cause of death in the USA. Guidelines/benchmarks are available against which the process can be evaluated. Benchmarks, data, and a feedback mechanism are necessary to effect change as part of a continuous quality improvement process. Improvements in the care of patients with cardiovascular disease can be effected, while protecting confidentiality. Changes in process should lead to changes in outcomes. No change can occur unless data are collected, reviewed regularly and compared with benchmarks and/or aggregated comparison practice of other physicians or hospitals.

INTRODUCTION

Mortality from cardiovascular disease has declined substantially over the last 25 years. Between 1983 and 1993, there was a decrease in deaths by 23.1 per cent. However, given the rise in total US population and the aging of America, its people survive longer only to die of cardiovascular disease. Therefore, the actual number of deaths during this period declined only by 3.8 per cent.[1] Furthermore, management of symptoms in patients with established cardiovascular disease and reduction of recurring morbid events has occurred because of earlier, more accurate identification of abnormalities in anatomy and physiology, and treatment with a remarkable armamentarium of medications and mechanical interventions which have become available through investigative efforts in the last 30 years.

However, cardiovascular disease continues to be the major cause of death and disability in this country, significantly exceeding mortality from cancer of all types in both men and women. Efficacy of drugs and interventions as demonstrated in clinical trials does not necessarily translate into effectiveness in reducing mortality

and morbidity in clinical practice. Drugs and mechanical interventions must be used for appropriate indication in order to be effective. Clinical effectiveness of these remarkable therapeutic interventions cannot be assured unless data are available on our use that would identify voids in use, inappropriate use and the relationship of use to outcomes. Therefore, it is imperative that a continuing quality improvement effort consisting of three major components be available to each practitioner, in every institution, if patients are to derive maximal effectiveness from the remarkable progress we have made in identification and treatment of these patients. First, there must be evidence-based benchmarks or guidelines against which we compare practice and deviations from practice. Second, there must be data that track practice, including process and outcomes, objectively. Finally, there must be a feedback of these data to practitioners and comparisons to benchmarks, the practice of others, and trends in practice over time, which would lead to changes in practice, which, in turn, should be expected to affect outcomes.

The goal of this chapter will be to identify evidence-based benchmarks, to give examples of how data are collected and used to improve practice, and to discuss appropriate feedback mechanisms that are not a threat to professional integrity, which cause physicians and nurses to modify practice on behalf of the patient.

GUIDELINES

It is fortunate that there are excellent clinical guidelines that have been developed given the large number of well-conducted clinical cardiology trials which have investigated efficacy of various drugs and interventions. Guidelines provide a frame of reference for the practitioner for appropriate treatment. They are not rigid, and in all instances must be used with the appropriate clinical judgment that is brought to bear on the care of the patient by the physician. They must be based on evidence. Furthermore, the validity of the studies that have found a drug or intervention to be effective must be evaluated by expert panels that develop these recommendations. In some instances, where evidence is lacking, recommendations may be made on the basis of a consensus of experts in the field. There should also be levels of recommendation based on efficacy indicating definite effectiveness, possible effectiveness as well as possible harmful effects when used under defined clinical conditions.

The National Heart, Lung and Blood Institute has been involved in the development of guidelines for the treatment of cardiovascular disease since 1972 when the National High Blood Pressure Education Program was developed. Since their initial publication, the guidelines have undergone revisions with a fifth consensus document on definition of hypertension, thresholds for treatment and recommendations regarding treatment published in 1993.[2] Despite its high prevalence and acknowledged relationship to morbidity and mortality, only about one-half of identified hypertensives are actively treated. Lack of intervention may, in part, be attributed to the fact that many identified hypertensives remain asymptomatic for a substantial period of time and are therefore reluctant to modify their lifestyle or take medications. Nevertheless, these guidelines give a stepwise approach to appropriate use of very effective medications which have become available for the treatment of hypertension over the course of the past 20 years, and should be used as a benchmark for appropriate treatment.

There is now compelling evidence that treatment of dyslipidemia in patients with known cardiovascular disease will reduce subsequent mortality and recurring morbid events, including the need for revascularization. There is also compelling evidence that in patients at risk who have not developed symptomatic coronary disease, aggressive management of hyperlipidemia will reduce subsequent mortality as well as morbidity. Unfortunately, the majority of patients leaving hospital following acute myocardial infarction, coronary bypass surgery, or percutaneous transluminal coronary angioplasty for symptomatic coronary disease do not receive lipid-lowering therapy following discharge. The National Cholesterol Education Program defines indications and thresholds for treatment and makes recommendations for appropriate use of the remarkably effective drugs that have become available for the treatment of dyslipidemias.[3]

The National Heart Attack Alert Program (NHAAP) is the latest in this line of National Heart, Lung and Blood Institute programs to address issues and present recommendations for the treatment of patients with cardiovascular disease. It specifically focuses on the patient with acute myocardial infarction (AMI) and is based on the recommendations of experts in cardiology, epidemiology, emergency medical services, emergency medicine and patient education. These experts convened in 1991 to consider barriers to early identification and treatment of such patients, given the compelling evidence that myocardial salvage and related reduction in mortality from acute myocardial infarction is a time-dependent function of early reperfusion. The ultimate goal is that patients with symptoms of AMI will receive appropriate therapy within 1 hour after symptom onset. This is not felt to be imminently possible, given patient-mediated delay, which requires appropriate education of both the community at large in the recognition and early action relating to symptoms of AMI, and patients with known cardiovascular disease at high risk of AMI.

The first recommendations of the NHAAP related to inordinate delays between patient arrival and treatment in the emergency department. The Sixty (60) Minutes to Treatment Working Group identified processes of care in the emergency department which inappropriately delayed identification and initiation of reperfusion therapy in such patients. It proposed that changes in process could only occur if time between emergency department arrival (door) and initiation of treatment with a thrombolytic drug in appropriate patients (drug) be tracked on each patient as the basis for reducing time to treatment. It also identified two other critical intervening time points, data (time of recording of the electrocardiogram (ECG) with ST segment elevation as the trigger for consideration of reperfusion) and decision (time when the decision is made to initiate reperfusion therapy as indicated by order entry) as important time points to also be tracked.

It recommended a 30-minute door–drug time as a goal in the identification and treatment of patients with clear-cut symptoms of AMI with ST segment elevation on the ECG and no contraindications.[4]

Other recommendations from the NHAAP address the physician's role in minimizing prehospital delay in patients at high risk for AMI, specifically those 11 million patients with known cardiovascular disease whose risk of AMI is 5–7 times that of the population at large.[5] A study to develop a community intervention that would promote early recognition by patients of symptoms consistent with acute cardiac ischemia and early action by them to call 911 is currently being evaluated in five paired communities throughout the country. An evidence-based evaluation of technologies for identifying acute cardiac ischemia in the emergency department has been completed which raises significant questions as to current process and to sensitivity and specificity of the usual studies for identifying patients with cardiac ischemia when applied to a relatively low-risk group of patients presenting to emergency departments with chest pain.[6] Working groups representing the coordinating committee of 38 organizations have also published recommendations for staffing and equipping emergency medical services systems, emergency medical dispatching, and 911 implementation.

Finally, the American College of Cardiology (ACC) and the American Heart Association (AHA) have engaged in the preparation of guidelines in cardiovascular disease since 1980. Under the direction of the ACC/AHA Task Force on Practice Guidelines, Guidelines for the Early Management of Patients with Acute Myocardial Infarction were introduced in 1990 and because of rapid changes in knowledge and clinical experience in the course of the past 5 years, they were revised again beginning with the task force that convened in 1994 and published its recommendations in November of 1996[7] with revisions most recently in 1999. These evidence-based guidelines consider the strength of the evidence that is the basis for the recommendations, ranging from the strongest evidence (data derived from multiple randomized clinical trials involving large numbers of individuals) to the least strong evidence (consensus opinion of experts as a primary source of a recommendation, given lack of compelling data). There are three levels of recommendation, which are listed below.

- Class 1: Conditions for which there is evidence and/or general agreement that a given procedure or treatment is beneficial, useful and effective.
- Class 2: Conditions for which there is conflicting evidence and/or divergence of opinion about usefulness/efficacy of a procedure or treatment, with two subclasses – Class 2A, when evidence is in favor of usefulness or efficacy, and Class 2B, when usefulness, efficacy is less well established by evidence or opinion.
- Class 3: Conditions for which there is evidence and/or general agreement that a procedure/treatment is not useful, effective and, in some cases, may be harmful.

These recommendations cover prehospital care, initial recognition and management in the emergency department, and hospital management. They also include a detailed analysis of the rationale and approach for phar-macotherapy and, finally, recommendations in preparation for discharge from the hospital and for long-term management. It is imperative that every practitioner be familiar with these recommendations since they do constitute benchmarks that must be utilized in determining effectiveness of care for patients with acute myocardial infarction.

PROGRAMS TO MODIFY AND IMPROVE PRACTICE AND OUTCOMES

While guidelines are the basis for improving practice in the care of patients with cardiovascular disease, no individual physician and institution can evaluate the effectiveness with which these guidelines are appropriately applied, unless data are gathered systematically on all patients that would track the appropriateness and frequency with which interventions are used, and compare these data against the benchmarks from the guidelines. There will be deviations from these guidelines that become obvious when considering patient data, and these should be investigated and justified. These deviations may result in significant changes in practice that would result in improved efficiency and outcome. Generally, change cannot be appreciated and may not be significant unless enough time, perhaps 3–6 months, elapses between comparison points. Quarterly analysis of data that would allow practices and outcomes to be tracked from quarter to quarter are meaningful. Comparisons may be made to prior quarters and, in some databases, comparisons can be made to other hospitals in the region and/or to a national sample. To be credible, compliance with guidelines should result in change as reflected in improved efficiency and better patient outcomes.

There are a number of models that have been developed that have utilized databases to track practice and to feed those data back to the physician and to hospitals for the purpose of modifying practice on behalf of the patient. The feedback loop is imperative if change is to be effected, but must be non-threatening and confidential as it relates to the practice of individual physicians and institutions when compared with the experience of an aggregate, non-identified peer group or other non-identified hospitals.

The Maine Medical Assessment Foundation Program is one such model. Lest there be an illusion that practice profiling activity and organized quality improvement programs are new, this program began in 1975 when Dr John Wennberg of Dartmouth Medical School, in conjunction with Dr Daniel Hanley of the Maine Medical Association, began to work in the State of Maine, utilizing Maine total hospital discharge data to construct 31 Maine hospital service areas and to analyze variation and population-based hospital use rates, and variations in the application of medical and surgical procedures between these areas.[8] It has been found that the frequency with which these procedures are performed varies significantly in certain localities, and high utilization of procedures bears no relationship to differences in incidence of disease. The intervention consists of presenting these data to the physicians in the high utilization area. Individual physicians are not identified by name and those data are compared to aggregate data for physicians practicing in other hospital service areas throughout the state. Over the years, there has been a consistent response to the intervention, specifically, a significant decrease in the frequency with which these procedures are performed in the targeted area, and the flattening of the utilization rate compared to other service areas in the State. In the case of cardiovascular disease, there was one service area in which the chances of having a cardiac catheterization and subsequent revascularization was about three times greater per thousand population than in two other urban hospital service areas. Following the intervention and presentation of the data to the cardiologists in that hospital service area and sharing of data that showed no differences in discharge rates for AMI and congestive heart failure from other hospital service areas, there was a 33 per cent decrease in the frequency of diagnostic left heart catheterization and coronary angiography within 6 months of the presentation of data.[9] The very feedback of data to involved physicians caused them to appraise their practice critically when comparing their procedure utilization rate with those of their peers dealing with the same population of patients with coronary heart disease.

The Northern New England Cardiovascular Study Group (NNECDSG) was established in 1987 by the surgeons from the three institutions in Maine, New Hampshire, and Vermont performing cardiac surgery for the purpose of developing a registry of all coronary artery bypass graft and valve surgical procedures performed in the Northern New England area. Since that time, it has been expanded by two other centers that have developed cardiac surgical programs. It therefore has collected data through this registry on all patients in these three states who undergo these procedures and all data have been validated and analyzed. Through 1 July, 1993, data were available on 15 085 consecutive coronary artery bypass graft surgeries done by all 23 of the surgeons performing these procedures in these states. When mortality was adjusted for patient variables, significant mortality differences within and between hospitals remained, which were not explained by these patient variables and were therefore probably related to individual surgeon's procedure and differences in process between hospitals. Between 1990 and 1991, data were fed back so that individual surgeons could compare themselves to the aggregate experience of all other surgeons within the institution and the aggregate experience of surgeons within each of the other four institutions. Site visits of an observer group composed of a cardiac sur-

geon, an anesthesiologist, a perfusionist, and an operating room nurse, visited each institution to observe the process and make comments on the differences in the process from the other institutions. Principles and practices related to continuing quality improvement were also shared with the surgeons in each hospital and at the group meetings, which take place on a quarterly basis. Following the intervention and the above process, 24 per cent fewer deaths were observed compared to predicted mortality. Variance between and within institutions decreased significantly and flattened. Therefore, once again, sharing of these differences, as reflected by credible data, with the practicing surgeons caused them to examine their process and their outcomes critically compared to those of their peers and to make changes that resulted in improved patient outcomes.[10]

Both of the above efforts have been voluntary. They have not been supported by government grants. Physicians have been responsible for development of the programs, including development of the database, analysis of the data, review of these analyses and the feedback process. In every instance, confidentiality of individual physician performance has been maintained and the sharing of data has been a true peer-review process. Administrations have not been aware of individual physician performance and only chiefs of departments are aware of the identity of individual physicians. Physicians cooperated in providing accurate data since they knew that their performance would remain confidential and would not be shared with either administrative or outside sources. Since this becomes a peer-review, quality-improvement process, the confidentiality of review of these data becomes protected from discovery. This process has been emulated by many hospitals on a smaller scale but in all instances there is a benefit to having available aggregate experience from national databases for the purpose of comparing individual and institutional outcomes to an external benchmark.

There are several national models that have gathered data on patients with AMI for the purpose of providing feedback to institutions and participating physicians on the process of care as well as on outcomes. The first and largest of these is the National Registry of Myocardial Infarction (NRMI). The NRMI is a voluntary, prospective, Phase 4 observational study, or registry of myocardial infarction. The purpose of this study is to collect, analyze, and disseminate data through the establishment of a large national database. The database is designed to monitor hospital experience with processes of care for AMI, as well as outcomes, and to provide individual hospitals with a summary of their data on a quarterly basis to assist them in their assessment of care for these patients and offer them the opportunity to compare their experience with those of like hospitals, hospitals in the same region or state, and a national sample. It was established in 1990.[11] NRMI-1 enrolled 354 435 patients from 1246 participating hospitals throughout the USA through 30 September 1994. NRMI-2, which utilized an expanded two-page case report form designed to collect additional data on risk factors, resource utilization and safety began in June of 1994 and through December 1996, had enrolled 401 427 patients from 1515 participating hospitals.

Each hospital receives a quarterly report detailing demographic characteristics of the patient population, process of care, including door to drug time, drugs used, the percentage of patients receiving these drugs, the patients undergoing various diagnostic procedures during the course of hospitalization, as well as complications and outcomes as reflected in mortality and need for revascularization procedures. Each institution is able to compare itself with aggregate data from hospitals in the same state or region as well as to the national sample, for each parameter of analysis. It is also possible, on a national level, through analyses initiated by investigators and a National Scientific Advisory Board, to track national practice patterns, adherence to guidelines and outcomes. These analyses and data are presented at National Investigator's Meetings to physician investigators and database coordinators, at national scientific meetings and published in peer-reviewed journals. These analyses further close the feedback loop in terms of providing data to participants on their performance compared to a regional or national sample, and to national organizations such as the NHAAP and the ACC and AHA on implementation of their recommendations and guidelines.

The NRMI is supported financially by Genentech, Inc., but all data that are submitted by hospital coordinators are entered and analyzed independently by Clintrials Research of Lexington, Kentucky. The integrity of the database and the conclusions from analyses derived from these data are maintained by a nationally respected Scientific Advisory Council. The feedback of data to participating hospitals has resulted in significant changes in the care of patients with AMI as demonstrated by trends of data tracked on a quarterly basis from the national sample over a period of several years. Significant problems in the process of care which have delayed early identification and treatment of patients with AMI have been identified and then tracked to document and demonstrate effective change as a result of the feedback of data. Door to drug time has decreased from 60 median minutes in 1990 to 38 minutes in 1997.

The Cooperative Cardiovascular Project (CCP) is sponsored by the Health Care Finance Administration (HCFA) and is a quality improvement project that involves more than 220 000 Medicare patients with AMI. It involves 100 per cent audit of such Medicare patients with AMI to determine patterns of use of recommended therapies and interventions as developed by expert panels as well as by the ACC/AHA Guidelines Panel. A pilot study in 16 000 such patients conducted in four states was reported in 1995, and determined the extent to which various therapies were underused and thereby led to the national project.[12] Peer-review organizations throughout the USA are reporting the results of these audits to each hospital as a continuous quality improvement project which replaces previously utilized case review, which concentrated on identification of deficiencies in patient care and was looked upon as punitive action as opposed to constructive positive recommendation. The current process emphasizes a profile of practice on the basis of solid data and reporting back of these data to participating hospitals for the purpose of allowing them to study their practice against nationally accepted indicators of quality of care and outcomes in the Medicare population. Each peer-review organization expects a response from the hospitals who are sent the report. Results from this analysis and those of the NRMI reveal surprising deficiencies in practice relating to patients with AMI but, over time, because of the feedback mechanism of providing data to participating physicians and hospitals, improvement in practice and a resultant improvement in patient outcomes have occurred. The remarkable variability in practice between regions of the country, such as the use of primary percutaneous transluminal coronary angioplasty (PTCA) or reperfusion therapy, and the use of diagnostic cardiac catheterization and coronary angiography prior to hospital discharge, from the analyses is striking. Data from the NRMI support the findings from the clinical trials that mortality reduction is related to early reperfusion and that delays in initiation of thrombolytic therapy or of angioplasty result in substantial statistically significant increases in mortality. The NRMI also has found that in the real world, primary PTCA for AMI is not being implemented within 60 minutes, which was the Primary Angioplasty in Myocardial Infarction Trial (PAMI) standard, and that in the majority of patients, balloon dilatation is delayed more than 2 hours after hospital arrival, with a concomitant increase in mortality.[13] Thus, these registries critically examine the implementation of findings from clinical trials and indeed document deficiencies in care which when fed back to participating physicians and hospitals can be the basis for implementation of changes in process that result in improved care and outcomes over time.

SUMMARY

- National evidence-based guidelines are available to inform the care of patients with cardiovascular disease.
- The availability of guidelines cannot improve care unless performance measures based on the guidelines are used to collect data on guidelines compliance and the impact on patient outcomes.
- Data that profile practice can be used in a practice, clinic or hospital to effect longitudinal improvement in compliance with guidelines, and to benchmark practice against other hospitals and practices.
- Critical to the process of quality improvement is the feedback of these data to health practitioners and hospitals in a confidential, constructive, peer-review process that will encourage physicians to modify practice without embarrassment or threat of sanctions.
- The process as applied in the models cited in this chapter has resulted in improved care for patients with cardiovascular disease with concomitant improvement in patient outcomes.
- The process of quality improvement must be applied to the care of all of our patients in the future.

REFERENCES

1. American Heart Association. *Heart and stroke facts: 1996 statistical supplement*. Dallas: American Heart Association, 1996: 1–23.
2. Joint National Committee on Detection, Evaluation, and Treatment of High Blood Pressure. The Fifth Report of the Joint National Committee on Detection, Evaluation and Treatment of High Blood Pressure (JNC V). *Arch Intern Med* 1993; **153**: 154.
3. National Cholesterol Education Program. Second Report of the Expert Panel on Detection, Evaluation and Treatment of High Blood Cholesterol in Adults (Adult Treatment Panel Two). *Circulation* 1994; **89**: 1329.
4. National Heart Attack Alert Coordinating Committee, 60 Minutes to Treatment Working Group. Emergency department: rapid identification and treatment of patients with acute myocardial infarction. *Ann Emergency Med* 1994; **23**: 311–29.
♦ 5. Dracup K, Alonzo A, Atkins JM, *et al*. Working Group on Educational Strategies to Prevent Prehospital Delay in Patients at High Risk for Acute Myocardial Infarction. The physician's role in minimizing prehospital delay in patients at high risk for acute myocardial infarction: recommendations from the National Heart Attack Alert Program. *Ann Intern Med* 1997; **126**: 645–51.
♦ 6. Selker HP, Zalenski RJ, Antman EM, *et al*. An evaluation of technologies for identifying acute cardiac ischemia in the emergency department: A report from a National Heart Attack Alert Program Working Group. *Ann Emerg Med* 1997; **29**: 13–87.
7. Ryan TJ, Anderson JL, Antman EM, *et al*. ACC/AHA Guidelines for the Management of Patients with Acute Myocardial Infarction: A Report of the American College of Cardiology/American Heart Association Task Force on Practice Guidelines (Committee on Management of Acute Myocardial Infarction). *J Am Coll Cardiol* 1996; **28**: 1328–428.
8. Wennberg JE, Gittelsohn AM. Health care delivery in Maine I: patterns of use of common surgical procedures. *J Maine Med Assoc* 1975; **66**: 123–30.
9. Keilson L, Soule R, Lambrew C, Kellett M. The influence of peer groups upon angioplasty and bypass surgery in Maine. *Circulation* 1994; **904**: 1–92.
10. O'Connor GT, Plume SK, Olmstead EM, *et al*. for the Northern New England Cardiovascular Study Group. A regional intervention to improve the hospital mortality associated with coronary artery bypass graft surgery. *JAMA* 1996; **275**: 841–6.
♦ 11. Rogers WJ, Bowlby LJ, Chandra NC, French WJ, Gore JM, Lambrew CT for the National Registry of Myocardial Infarction (NRMI) Investigators. Treatment of myocardial infarction in the United States (1990–1993). *Circulation* 1994; **90**: 2103–14.
12. Ellerbeck EF, Jencks SF, Radford MJ, *et al*. Quality of care for Medicare patients with acute myocardial infarction: a four-state pilot study from the Cooperative Cardiovascular Project. *JAMA* 1995; **273**: 1509–14.
13. Cannon CP, Lambrew CT, Tiefenbrunn AJ, *et al*. for the NRMI-2 Investigators. Influence of door–balloon time on mortality in primary angioplasty. Results in 3,648 patients in the Second National Registry of Myocardial Infarction (NRMI-2). *J Am Coll Cardiol* 1996; **27** (Suppl A): 389A.

4

The women's health initiative: focus on risk factors and diagnostic approach to suspected coronary artery disease

KAREN B JAMES

The impact of coronary artery disease in women has gained increasing attention over the years. The realization that coronary atherosclerosis is a significant health problem in females has led to a proliferation of gender-specific research. This substantial body of data now allows us to evaluate each of the risk factors for coronary heart disease in women, and to make specific preventative and therapeutic recommendations.

INTRODUCTION AND OVERVIEW

There are inherent gender differences in the pattern of coronary artery disease between men and women. Coronary heart disease is more age-dependent in women, exhibiting a 40-fold rise in 75–84-year-olds.[1]

Lipids are affected by hormones in women. Estrogen raises high-density lipoprotein (HDL) cholesterol, which is cardioprotective. At menopause, low-density lipoprotein (LDL) cholesterol rises significantly.[2] Lipid-lowering therapy is beneficial in women when indicated.[3] Also, in the past three decades, the number of female smokers 60 years and older has risen markedly. Tobacco use exerts it cardiotoxic effects acutely via thromboembolic effects.[4,5]

The higher prevalence of diabetes in women helps explain in part the higher mortality rates following myocardial infarction and revascularization procedures.[6,7] Similarly, females have a higher prevalence of obesity than males.[8] Increasing weight parallels increased risk of coronary events.[9] Exercise, on the other hand, is associated with a lower cardiovascular risk, with attendant decreases in blood pressure, obesity, and lipid levels.[10–12]

Postmenopausal hormone replacement therapy remains in the limelight owing to the well-demonstrated beneficial cardiovascular effects of estrogen. Major effects of estrogen include raising of HDL levels as well as probable direct beneficial effects on the coronary arterial wall.[13] An area of concern with long-term estrogen use, however, is the increased incidence of breast cancer after 10 years of use.[14]

Exercise electrocardiography in women is often associated with false-positive studies. Useful non-invasive diagnostic tests in females include exercise and pharmacologic radionuclide testing. Stress echocardiography is also quite accurate and cost effective in women.[15] Coronary angiography and revascularization should be pursued aggressively in women when indicated by significant evidence of ischemic burden, if the benefits of invasive therapy outweigh medical treatment.

Coronary artery disease is the leading cause of death

in American women, accounting for over 250 000 deaths yearly.[16] In previous years, most of the data on atherosclerotic heart disease was derived from studies consisting predominantly of men. More recently, large randomized trials have been under way specifically to address questions regarding women's health and coronary artery disease, including the Heart and Estrogen/Progestin Replacement Study (HERS) and the Women's Health Initiative (WHI).

This chapter addresses gender differences in coronary heart disease and reviews the impact of risk factors, including hormonal status, on women. The diagnostic evaluation for coronary heart disease in women is discussed as well.

GENDER DIFFERENCES IN CORONARY ARTERY DISEASE AND HISTORICAL LANDMARKS

The Framingham studies were among the earliest to point out striking differences between men and women in a 26-year follow-up. The mean age at which women present with initial symptoms of coronary artery disease is 10 years greater than that at which men present with the same symptoms.[17] The mean age of women's first myocardial infarction is 20 years greater than that for men.[17] Given that the average life expectancy of women is 6 years greater than that for men, more women live to old age, when coronary artery disease is more prevalent. Coronary heart disease is significantly more age-dependent in women, with a 40-fold increase in coronary morbidity in the age range of 75–84 years, as compared with 35–44-year-olds.[1]

The incidence of hypertension is lower in women than men under 45; this reverses at age 45.[17] Diabetes mellitus is more prevalent in women, and imparts a two-fold greater risk of coronary heart disease in women.[17] At the age of menopause, high-density lipoprotein (HDL) cholesterol does not significantly change, but low-density lipoprotein (LDL) and total cholesterol rise. Indeed hormonal changes in the lifetime of a woman, related to oral contraceptives, pregnancy, hysterectomy, or menopause, help to explain some of the gender-related differences in heart disease, as will be discussed later.

Angina

The Framingham data showed that women developed angina twice as often as myocardial infarction, leading to the early impression that angina in women was benign.[17] However, later angiographic data from the Cleveland Clinic revealed that only 50 per cent of premenopausal women with angina had angiographically significant coronary artery disease.[18] Similarly, the Coronary Artery Surgery Study (CASS) data showed that 50 per cent of

women with 'angina' had minimal or no coronary artery disease, as compared with 17 per cent of men with angina having normal angiograms.[19] In contrast, other cardiac causes of chest pain, such as coronary spasm and microvascular angina (Syndrome X), are more common in women.

Acute coronary syndromes

The clinical trial TIMI IIIB examined gender differences in unstable angina and non-Q myocardial infarction in 497 men and 976 men.[20] In both acute syndromes, women were older than men with more co-morbidities. Outcomes were related to the severity of coronary artery disease rather than to gender. Women had more unstable angina than men, possibly related in part to trial eligibility.

Silent ischemia

Silent myocardial ischemia in men and women was assessed as part of CASS, utilizing exercise stress testing.[21] The patients were divided into three groups, based on their stress test results: those with silent ischemia, symptomatic ischemia, or no ischemia. In both genders with silent ischemia, the 12-year survival rate was related to the severity of coronary artery disease. Survival at 12 years was enhanced by coronary bypass surgery in men with silent ischemia and three-vessel disease but not in women (61 per cent vs 45 per cent, respectively), compared with medical therapy.[21]

Myocardial infarction

The Framingham data reported increased mortality for myocardial infarction as the initial cardiac presentation in women over men (39 per cent vs 31 per cent, respectively).[22] Similarly, the occurrence of death with the presenting myocardial infarction was more frequent in women than men (68 per cent vs 49 per cent).[22] The 1-year mortality following myocardial infarction was higher in women at 45 per cent than men (10 per cent) in the Framingham data, as were reinfarction rates (40 per cent women vs 13 per cent men).[23] The older age at presentation in women may partially explain the discrepancies.

The MILIS (Multicenter Investigation of Limitation of Infarct Size) Study reported that non-Q myocardial infarctions occur more frequently in women.[24] The study also reported that women have higher left ventricular ejection fractions after myocardial infarctions, which should lead to a better prognosis. However, this was not found to be true; women in fact had a higher hospital mortality at 13 per cent as compared with men (7 per cent), indicating that other factors besides ventricular function adversely affect outcome in women. Similarly, although the benefit of thrombolysis was shown for both genders, mortality rates for women were still double those for men at 1 year (29.8 per cent *vs* 15.2 per cent, respectively).[25] Fortunately, other post-infarction therapies have shown equal gender benefits. These include beta blockade as well as aspirin use (International Study of Infarct Survival (ISIS) Study).[26,27]

Ventricular arrhythmias

The Framingham data showed a lower frequency of sudden death in all coronary deaths in women (39 per cent) as contrasted with men (50 per cent).[17] With regard to ventricular arrhythmias, the Multicenter Postinfarction Research Trials found that frequent premature contractions and runs of ventricular tachycardia portended unfavorable prognosis for men but not women.[28] In survivors of cardiac arrest due to coronary artery disease, ventricular tachycardia and fibrillation have been found to be less frequently inducible in women than men during programmed electrophysiologic testing as well.[29]

Left ventricular dysfunction

Left ventricular function in women is generally better than men at any age due to the older age in women at which coronary heart disease occurs. Surprisingly, however, left ventricular function is not the powerful predictor of outcome of revascularization in women as it is in men.[30] For example, following coronary angioplasty, preserved ventricular function is a powerful predictor of outcome for men but not women.[31] Similarly, the CASS data indicated that women have a greater perioperative mortality than men (4.5 per cent *vs* 1.9 per cent, respectively), despite preserved ejection fraction in women.[30]

Coronary artery bypass surgery

The CASS studies also have shown that women have a higher 15-year mortality following bypass surgery (52 per cent) than men (48 per cent), $P = 0.004$.[32] However, analysis by Rahimtoola indicated that patient-related factors rather than gender are the actual predictors of survival 15–18 years postoperatively.[33] The specific patient-related factors were older age, previous bypass surgery, previous myocardial infarction, and diabetes mellitus. He concluded that coronary artery bypass surgery should therefore not be denied or delayed in women with the appropriate indications.

Psychosocial differences

Following myocardial infarction, women have a higher incidence of depression, anxiety, guilt, and sexual dysfunction than men, with a lower return to work rate, as well.[34] Fewer women also attend cardiac rehabilitation after infarction, and have higher attrition rates.[35] In the general US population, the support system appears weaker for older women, in that three out of four men aged 65 or older are married, whereas three out of five women in the same age group are without spouses.[34] Poverty rates for elderly women are roughly 19 per cent, among the highest in any US age group.

Gender differences with regard to medical care access

The earlier data from Framingham, Cleveland Clinic, and CASS had shown lower incidence of myocardial infarction in women with chest pain as well as a much lower incidence of atherosclerosis by coronary angiography.[17,18] These earlier findings may have contributed to the many reasons why angina in women was viewed as a relatively benign process.

Tobin reported that, in the presence of an abnormal exercise radionuclide study, physicians referred men for coronary angiography ten times more than women.[36] Similarly, by review of hospital discharge records in Massachusetts and Maryland, it was found that 15–28 per cent more men than women were referred for coronary angiography; and that 27–45 per cent of men had better outcomes following bypass surgery than females.[37] It remains unclear whether less aggressive evaluation, older age, smaller coronary arteries, emergent presentations, or a combination of factors, explains the excess mortality in women following bypass surgery.

The Survival and Ventricular Enlargement (SAVE) Study reported that 27 per cent of men *vs* 15 per cent of women had undergone coronary angiography in the past before myocardial infarction.[38] Similarly, 12 per cent of men with infarction had previously undergone bypass surgery as contrasted with 6 per cent of the women.

Fortunately, by the 1980s, the performance of coronary angiography in women had doubled, while bypass surgeries in women tripled. Of note, some of the earlier age-based restrictions of care (such as in thrombolysis) precluded older women.

RISK FACTORS FOR CORONARY ARTERY DISEASE IN WOMEN

Lipids

Lipoproteins are large macromolecules containing a core of lipid, triglyceride, and esterified cholesterol, surrounded by a protein shell. They transport lipids in the bloodstream. Chylomicrons and very-low-density lipoprotein (VLDL) carry the majority of triglycerides. The low-density lipoprotein and high-density proteins are of major interest in coronary heart disease; these transport more cholesterol and protein and much less triglyceride. Oxidized or altered LDL *in vitro* has been shown to convert scavenger cells to foam cells and is associated with increased atherosclerotic risk. HDL, in contrast, clears cholesterol from foam cells and is associated with lower risk of coronary heart disease.[39]

Lipoproteins differ between men and women at any given age, largely due to hormonal effects. Estrogen raises HDL and triglycerides, while lowering LDL; androgens have the opposite effect.[40] It is not surprising, then, that women have a higher HDL than men throughout the life cycle.

At puberty, HDL levels drop in males as androgen levels rise (Table 4.1).[41] During pregnancy, both HDL and LDL rise. This is likely owing to the rise in both estrogen and progesterone. At the menopause, HDL falls slightly. On the other hand, LDL levels rise in females around the age of 55. Thereafter, women have higher LDL levels than their male counterparts.

In women, as in men, cardiac risk rises with higher LDL and declines with increases in HDL. However, HDL is a more potent predictor of risk in women than men.[42] On the other hand, LDL is not as strong a predictor in females. It is possible that estrogen interferes with LDL uptake in the arterial wall, based on primate data.[43] In postmenopausal women, triglycerides are an independent predictor of cardiac risk, although they are not in men and younger women.[44]

Lipoprotein A (Lp(a)) is a lipoprotein that has received attention in recent years. It is known to be a risk factor for coronary artery disease in men. More recently, a Swedish study assessed Lp(a) in 292 females followed for subsequent angina or myocardial infarction.[45] After controlling for other risk factors, Lp(a) was found to be a determinant for coronary artery disease in both pre-menopausal and postmenopausal women. The odds ratios were 5.1 and 2.4 for angina and myocardial infarction, respectively.

In terms of treatment of hyperlipidemia, many of the prior trials on cholesterol lowering excluded women. However, a meta-analysis was performed of three European trials (Newcastle, Edinburgh, and Finnish Mental Hospital) that included women.[46] This analysis indicated that there is equivalent cholesterol lowering in both genders, associated with equivalent reductions in cardiac death rates.

The SCRIP (Stanford Coronary Risk Intervention Project) studied the effects of intensive risk factor medication in both genders, with angiographic follow-up at 4 years.[3] Risk-factor modification consisted of low-fat diet, exercise, weight reduction, smoking cessation, and lipid-lowering medication. The study found that there was a 47 per cent decrease in the rate of narrowing of diseased coronary arteries in the treated group, favorably affecting both genders.

In the CCAIT (Canadian Coronary Atherosclerosis Intervention Trial) study, lovastatin *vs* placebo was evaluated in women.[47] When studied 2 years later, angiographic progression was 59 per cent *vs* 28 per cent in untreated *vs* treated women ($P = 0.031$). New atherosclerotic lesions were found in 4 per cent of the treated females *vs* 45 per cent of the untreated ($P < 0.001$).

Tobacco use

Smoking is an independent risk factor for coronary artery disease in women. Since 1965, the number of woman 60 years and older who began smoking as teenagers has increased tenfold.[48] More women inhale than was the practice prior to 1965. Tobacco use is associated with educational level in women: in those with <12 years of education, 37 per cent smoke. In females with ≥16 years of education, 26 per cent use tobacco.[49]

Half of all cases of coronary heart disease in women aged 30–55 is attributable to tobacco use.[50] In the Nurses' Health Study, 30–55-year-old women smokers had a three-fold increased risk of myocardial infarction as compared with non-smokers.[50] The Framingham studies indicate a relative risk for smokers aged 50–59 of 1.9 in women and 1.8 in men.[51]

Studies on smoking in general reveal that the risk of coronary artery disease in females increases with the number of cigarettes smoked. Indeed, risk of coronary heart disease is twofold higher in females who smoke as little as 1–4 cigarettes daily.[50]

Low-yield cigarettes, touted as containing less nicotine and carbon monoxide, were popular among women in the past. However, subsequent data have shown that there is no decrease in risk of non-fatal first myocardial infarction in women who smoke low-yield as compared with regular cigarettes.[52]

Table 4.1 *Effects of hormonal events on lipids*

Lipid		Puberty (female)	Puberty (male)	Pregnancy	Menopause
Total cholesterol	→		↑	↑	↑
LDL cholesterol	→		↑	↑	↑
HDL cholesterol	→		↓	↑	↓

→ = no effect; ↓ = decreased; ↑ = increased.

Smoking causes acute arterial injury.[53] The components of cigarette smoke cause increased platelet aggregability and fibrinogen, which predispose to thrombosis and endothelial dysfunction.[4] Plasminogen is lower in smokers.[54] Smoking in females leads to increased levels of dehydroepiandrosterone (DHEA) and androstenedione with a menopause that occurs 1–2 years earlier than in non-smokers.[55]

Oral contraceptive use in conjunction with smoking has been shown to be associated with a significant increase in cardiac events.[56] The relative risk of myocardial infarction in female smokers on oral contraceptives is increased 20–30-fold. The mechanism appears to be thromboembolic as both tobacco and oral contraceptives lead to clotting via both platelet and coagulation mechanisms.[57,58]

SMOKING CESSATION

Women smokers have lower 'quit' rates than men.[59] Women stop smoking at 0.33 percentage points per year, as compared with 0.84 percentage points per year for men. It is theorized that weight gain may account for some of the cessation failures. Almost 80 per cent of successful smoking quitters gain weight – particularly women.[60] The average weight gain is 4–6 pounds, although 3.5 per cent of quitters gain over 20 pounds! There are therefore social implications in younger female smokers, in particular, to continue tobacco use in order to remain thin.

Smoking cessation can be approached with behavioral and/or pharmacologic methods. Up to 95–99 per cent of quitters of both genders do so 'on their own', underscoring the importance of strong self-motivation to stop.[61] Strong social support from significant others is especially important for women smokers. Nicotine replacement therapy is often used to diminish withdrawal symptoms. It reduces irritability, anxiety, and partially ameliorates the weight gain. Both chewing gum and transdermal preparations are available. With either approach, a gradual weaning program is used. Non-nicotine preparations such as bupropion hydrochloride are also utilized to aid tobacco cessation.

Of note is the fact that only 4 per cent of smokers remain free of relapse.[61] Few people succeed on the first try; usually 3–4 attempts are required. The media has certainly played a powerful role in promoting tobacco use. In certain groups of women, smoking represents a symbol of women's rights and equality in the workplace.

Diabetes mellitus

Both males and females with diabetes have more adverse risk factors for coronary artery disease than non-diabetics. Framingham data revealed that diabetic females were more obese and hypertensive, and had lower HDL levels than non-diabetic women.[62] The relative risk of cardiac events for diabetic women aged 45–74 was 2.0 as contrasted with non-diabetic females.[63] The Nurses' Health Study yielded similar findings in that a 3–7-fold increase in cardiovascular events was seen in diabetic women.[64]

Patients with long-standing diabetes exhibit atherosclerosis of both the large epicardial coronary arteries as well as microangiopathic changes. Compared to non-diabetics, the coronary atherosclerosis is more diffuse. The tendency for thrombosis is greater in diabetics.[65] The platelets are hyperaggregable. Fibrinolysis is impaired as evidenced by levels of tissue plasminogen activator and plasminogen activator inhibitor.[66] Fibrinogen is elevated and appears to correlate with blood glucose levels.[67]

The higher prevalence of diabetes in females helps to explain the difference in postinfarction mortality in women as compared with men. For in-hospital and 1-year mortality following myocardial infarction, diabetes was found to be a significant predictor of outcome for women (RR = 1.7, 95 per cent confidence interval (CI) 1.10–2.53) as compared with men (RR = 0.96, 95 per cent CI 0.69–1.34).[68]

In the MILIS study, in-hospital mortality for females exceeded males by 6 per cent.[69] The independent predictors of outcome for women were age, hypertension, diabetes, and heart failure. The SAVE study showed that for patients hospitalized after acute infarction, 31 per cent of the women were diabetic as compared with only 19.9 per cent of the men.[70]

In women who survive myocardial infarction and are candidates for revascularization, diabetes adds to the risks.[6,7] Compared to males undergoing angioplasty or coronary bypass surgery, women are far more prone to suffer from diabetes and its associated vascular complications.

Owing to the increased risk of coronary artery disease and silent ischemia, diabetic women should be counseled regarding risk reduction strategies, and should undergo periodic non-invasive screening for ischemia.

Currently, the data remain insufficient as to whether strict control of hyperglycemia can retard the progression of atherosclerosis in diabetics.

Obesity

Obesity has been defined as an excess of body fat with increase in fat cell size.[71] Normal body fat content is 15–20 per cent of body weight for men and 20–25 per cent for women.[72] For women, obesity is defined as ≥ 27.3 kg/m^2 in body mass index.[73] Distribution of body fat influences cardiac health. Fat in the waist, abdomen, and upper torso is more metabolically active. A waist-to-hip ratio > 0.80 in women or 0.95 in men is associated with increased cardiovascular risk.[74]

Overall, women have a higher prevalence of obesity than men – 23.8 per cent of American women are overweight.[8] American black women have twice the prevalence of obesity as caucasians. Low socioeconomic status and educational level are also associated with obesity.[75] Genetic factors, environmental dietary factors, and physical inactivity all also affect obesity.

Relatively few prospective studies have investigated the association between obesity and coronary heart disease in women. The American Cancer Society study revealed an association between weight and coronary heart disease mortality. Grossly obese women (> 140 per cent above the average) had a twofold increase in cardiac mortality.[76] In the Framingham data, weight was directly related to risk of cardiovascular disease in both genders.[77] The Nurses' Health Study showed a linear increase in risk in both fatal and non-fatal coronary events with increasing weight.[9]

From a hemodynamic standpoint, obesity is associated with elevated preload, increased cardiac output, and expanded plasma volume, as well as higher stroke volume and left ventricular filling pressure.[78] Eccentric left ventricular hypertrophy occurs.[79] Weight reduction improves hemodynamics and can even reverse the hypertrophy.[79]

Obesity unfavorably affects risk-to-benefit ratio in both genders for revascularization procedures.[80] Given women's known higher risks for both coronary angioplasty and bypass surgery, it is likely that concomitant obesity only worsens the risk.

In terms of treatment, thorough elevation for any treatable factors in obesity is essential. Dietary restriction remains the first line of therapy, although recidivism is common. Weight loss does lead to improvement in glucose tolerance, lipids, and blood pressure.

The Nurses' Health Study recently reported its long-term follow-up on obesity.[81] The study found that higher levels of body weight still within 'normal' range, as well as modest gains after the age of 18, appear to increase the risk of cardiovascular disease in middle-aged women. These data provide evidence that current US weight guidelines may be falsely reassuring.

Exercise

In the past, only 5 of 43 studies examining the relationship between activity and coronary heart disease reported data on women.[82] Of these, three reported a relative increase in risk of low activity levels for angina, myocardial infarction, and cardiac death. Two other studies (Framingham and Goteburg) failed to show a significant association between exercise levels and coronary deaths in women.

Blair et al. studied 3120 women, evaluating mortality as predicted by maximal treadmill performance.[83] The least-fit women had a 4.7 relative risk for all-cause mortality compared to the most physically fit. The study suggested that moderate physical fitness can provide a substantial decrease in the risk of death in women.

Physical exercise can have beneficial effects on various risk factors for coronary artery disease. In one large study, low-fitness middle-aged women who were normotensive had a 1.52 relative risk of developing hypertension over 4 years, as compared with highly physically fit women.[84] Similarly, Urata et al. reported decreases of 15 and 10 mm Hg (in systolic and diastolic pressures, respectively) following 10–20 weeks of moderate exercise by hypertensive men and women.[85]

Shangold has suggested that inactivity is the most common cause of obesity in women.[86] Women who are normal weight or < 20 per cent overweight can often exercise sufficiently to control their weight. Aerobic exercise increases lean body mass and decreases body fat.[87] Walking promotes loss of abdominal fat in particular. In addition, regular physical exercise is related to glucose tolerance, insulin sensitivity, and prevalence of diabetes in both genders.

With regard to lipids, regular exercise exerts its primary effect on HDL cholesterol and triglycerides. Physical fitness, based on treadmill exercise time, has been shown to be significantly related to HDL levels in women aged 18–65.[88] The association was independent of age and weight.

In order to raise HDL, exercise intensity needs to be fairly high. Notelovitz reported that 3–4 months of fairly strenuous exercise (running 10–15 miles/week or walking 30 miles/week) is necessary to increase HDL levels.[89] Kokkinos et al. similarly reported that moderate fitness (equivalent to 10 metabolic equivalents) is required to improve the cardiac risk profile in women.[90]

Clinical trials have shown that exercise rehabilitation reduces cardiovascular mortality by 23–25 per cent.[91] However, women specifically were not focused upon in most trials. Therefore, the definite impact of cardiac rehabilitation on females in terms of mortality remains unclear.

In terms of emotional well-being, Lavie and Milani found that cardiac rehabilitation led to significant improvement in many behavioral traits and measures of quality of life.[92] However, depression and hostility were not significantly reduced. Nonetheless, their data reaffirm that women should routinely be referred to cardiac rehabilitation programs.

Hormones

Certainly the area of most intense attention in women's health and coronary heart disease in recent years has been on the risks and benefits of postmenopausal hormone replacement therapy. The menopausal transition is a period of hormonal changes, as follicle stimulating hormone (FSH) starts to rise. FSH levels above 40 mlU/mL signify a menopausal state. The mean age of menopause is 51.4 years, although the perimenopausal period can span 5 or more years.[93] Clinically, the perimenopausal period is accompanied by changes in menstrual pattern, increased rate of bone loss, and vasomotor instability. The most significant hormonal changes are marked reductions in E_2 (estradiol) and E_1 (estrogen).[94] E_2 is reduced more than E_1, because it is dependent on ovarian secretion. E_1, on the other hand, is produced primarily by peripheral aromatization from androgens.

It is well accepted that estrogen deprivation increases cardiovascular risk in women. Framingham data have shown that the risk of cardiovascular disease is three times lower in women than men prior to menopause. It is nearly equal in both genders in the 75–79 age range, in contrast. Premature menopause before the age of 35 has been shown to be associated with a 2–3-fold increase in the risk of myocardial infarction.[95] Similarly, oophorectomy prior to age 35 increases myocardial infarction risk sevenfold.[96] What explains this increased risk?

When potential reasons for the gender differences in coronary heart disease as a function of age are scrutinized, the most relevant finding is that total cholesterol rises at an accelerated rate following menopause.[97] The increase of total cholesterol is due primarily to increases in the LDL. In the Framingham study, HDL did not decrease after menopause, although total, LDL, and VLDL cholesterol did rise.[95] Other studies, however, have suggested some HDL decreases after menopause.[98]

In terms of 'physiologic' hormone replacement therapy, doses of estrogen are utilized that should theoretically not expose a woman to any more steroid than would occur endogenously during a normal menstrual cycle. Natural estrogens either cause no change in blood pressure or lower it in most users.[99] There also do not appear to be any deleterious effects of natural estrogen replacement on carbohydrate metabolism.[100] In fact, postmenopausal estrogen users have been reported to have a reduced frequency of diabetes, as estrogen may be beneficial in improving insulin action.[100] Lastly, as contrasted with older generations of oral contraceptives, there is no increased thromboembolic risk with estrogen replacement in most women with normal coagulation systems.[101]

From a lipid standpoint, postmenopausal estrogens are cardioprotective. Their principal action is to raise HDL cholesterol;[102] lowering of LDL is more variable. Other beneficial lipid effects include a lower VLDL/triglyceride ratio, increased clearance of intermediate-density lipoprotein (IDL) and LDL via an upregulated LDL receptor, diminished penetration and degradation of LDL in the arterial wall, and inhibition of

LDL oxidation by estrogen.[103] The only potential concern with oral estrogen use is hypertriglyceridemia. Because the lipoprotein changes are felt to be dose dependent, it has been suggested that by keeping estrogen doses low, triglyceride levels will be kept to a low percentage.

A growing body of data supports the notion that estrogen's beneficial effects are mediated directly on the arterial wall.[13] When studied in macaque monkeys, in animals challenged with acetylcholine, the coronary arteries of non-treated monkeys constricted characteristic of endothelial damage due to atherosclerosis, whereas monkeys with estrogen replacement did not. These data suggest that estrogen may affect production of endothelial-derived relaxing factor and other similar substances. Estrogen may also favorably alter prostacyclin–thromboxane balance.[104] Other coagulation effects of estrogen include lower plasminogen activator inhibitor levels in women with higher estrogen levels, as noted in recent analysis of Framingham data.[105]

CARDIOPROTECTIVE EFFECTS OF ESTROGENS

Numerous studies on postmenopausal estrogen use have shown that there is a significant reduction in risk of cardiovascular disease when fatal or non-fatal myocardial infarction are the end points.[106,107] The calculated relative risk by meta-analyses was 0.56 (0.5–0.61). This translates into 5250 lives saved for every 100 000 estrogen users aged 50–75, or 333 lives annually. Among women with greater than 70 per cent coronary occlusion, the 10-year survival is significantly greater (97 per cent) in estrogen users than non-users (65 per cent).[108]

Recently, Sullivan et al. studied postmenopausal hormone replacement in 1098 women who had undergone coronary bypass surgery.[109] Ten-year survival was 81.4 per cent in users and 65.1 per cent in non-users (P = 0.0001). The women who did not use estrogen were older, had more diseased vessels, lower ejection fractions, and more prior myocardial infarctions.

Gorsky et al. calculated risks in a hypothetical cohort of 10 000 women aged 50 using estrogens, using data from longitudinal studies.[110] They extrapolated that estrogen use for 25 years would decrease fatal coronary events by 48 per cent, decrease deaths from hip fracture by 49 per cent, increase deaths from breast cancer by 21 per cent, and increase deaths by endometrial cancer by 207 per cent.

More recently, the Nurses' Health Study found the current hormone users had a lower risk of death (RR 0.63) than women who had never used hormones.[14] However, the apparent benefit decreased with long-term use after 10 or more years, owing to the increase in mortality from breast cancer in long-term users. The breast cancer risk increased by 43 per cent after 10 years of hormone use.

Although the cardioprotective effects of estrogens are unquestionable, the concern regarding breast cancer risk is growing. Two large-scale studies on these issues are in progress, the Heart and Estrogen/Progestin Replacement Study,[111] and the Women's Health Initiative. These studies should yield further answers as they complete in the years 2000 and 2005, respectively. Preliminary data from the HERS Trial are suggesting an increased risk of breast cancer in postmenopausal women treated with a prolonged course of the estrogen plus medroxyprogesterone acetate combination.

DIAGNOSTIC APPROACH TO CORONARY DISEASE IN WOMEN

As discussed earlier, premenopausal women have a lower incidence of angiographic coronary disease for symptoms of chest pain, with a greater prevalence of noncoronary causes of chest pains. The utility of the various diagnostic tests for coronary heart in women is reviewed.

Exercise testing

The exercise electrocardiogram (ECG) has lower sensitivity in women than men for multiple reasons, including a higher prevalence of resting ECG changes; a lesser likelihood of exercise to adequate intensity; and the presence of associated conditions that alter repolarization, such as mitral valve prolapse. Gender differences also obtain in exercise testing a prognostic value. When the predictive value of exercise testing was analyzed in men and women in the CASS study, it was determined that only in men did exercise testing identify the high-risk subset whose survival was enhanced by coronary artery bypass surgery.[112]

Hung et al. reported a 93 per cent occurrence of abnormal exercise ECG in women with multivessel coronary artery disease as compared with 43 per cent of women with single-vessel disease.[113] Thus, the test is useful in detecting severe multivessel disease in females who exercise adequately. Because of the low prevalence of coronary artery disease, a negative test in women who exercise to adequate intensity has a high specificity for the absence of significant coronary artery disease. Thus, normal results are useful, but abnormal results may be falsely positive.

Exercise radionuclide testing

When the resting ECG is abnormal in women, exercise radionuclide perfusion testing will be helpful. In a study of 60 females using angiographic correlation, Friedman reported a sensitivity of 75 per cent and a specificity of 97 per cent for stress thallium scintigraphy, as compared with 32 per cent and 41 per cent for exercise electrocardiography, respectively.[114] The lesser sensitivity of thallium scintigraphy in women reflects the decreased prevalence of multivessel disease. Also, breast tissue creates artifact which can to some extent be corrected. It is hopeful that newer high-energy perfusion agents, such as technetium-99m sestamibi, may produce less soft-tissue attenuation.[115] In terms of other exercise radionuclide modalities, stress ventriculography has been evaluated in the past and had been shown to have poor sensitivity and specificity in women.[116]

Pharmacologic radionuclide perfusion testing

Pharmacologic nuclear studies, using dipyridamole or adenosine, are other modalities for assessing for ischemia in women. Amanullah et al. recently evaluated the diagnostic efficacy of adenosine ^{99m}Tc sestamibi single-photon emission computed tomography (SPECT) in females.[117] Among catheterized women, the sensitivity, specificity, and predictive accuracy for detecting coronary artery stenosis $\geq$ 50 per cent were 93, 78, and 88 per cent, respectively. They further found that adenosine ^{99m}Tc sestamibi was effective in detecting coronary artery disease in women irrespective of presenting symptoms or pretest likelihood.

Stress echocardiography

Stress echocardiography can be performed with either exercise or a pharmacologic agent such as dobutamine, in conjunction with echocardiographic imaging to assess for new regional wall motion abnormalities indicative of ischemia. In one small series of women with a high prevalence of coronary disease, exercise echocardiography showed a sensitivity and specificity of 86 per cent.[118] More recently, Marwick et al. compared exercise echocardiography and electrocardiology and found that exercise echocardiography is more specific for diagnosing coronary artery disease in women and is a cost-effective approach because of the avoidance of inappropriate angiography.[15]

Recommendations: non-invasive testing

Exercise electrocardiography appears to be cost effective in the diagnostic evaluation of females with typical angina and a normal resting ECG (Fig. 4.1).[119] However, if a woman has probable or atypical angina and/or an abnormal resting ECG, nuclear studies or stress echocardiography are indicated. Either are roughly equivalent in accuracy.[115] In contrast, the low pretest likelihood of coronary artery disease in women with non-specific chest pain syndromes precludes any added usefulness of non-invasive testing. In those women with abnormal non-invasive results indicating significant ischemia, coronary angiography should be pursued.

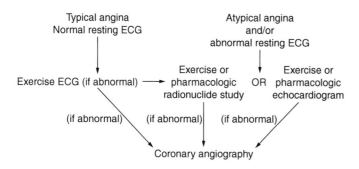

Figure 4.1 *Evaluation of suspected coronary artery disease in women.*

TREATMENT OPTIONS AND OVERVIEW

As previously discussed in this chapter, risk factor modification plays an important role in the prevention of heart disease in women. Specific areas include lipid control with diet and medication if needed; smoking cessation; conscientious control of weight and diabetes; and regular aerobic exercise.

The final recommendations regarding postmenopausal hormone use in relation to cardiac benefit versus breast cancer risk should be available in several more years, pending completion of several, large, prospective trials. Until then, the decision regarding hormone replacement therapy should remain an individualized one between patient and physician, based on a woman's relative risk profiles for coronary heart disease and breast cancer.

With regard to aspirin, data from Israel on 2418 women with coronary artery disease showed benefit with aspirin use.[120] Those who particularly benefited were older women, diabetics, symptomatic women, or those who had had a previous myocardial infarction. The study showed reduced mortality among women aspirin users with coronary heart disease. The role of aspirin in healthy women, however, remains under study and should be answered soon by the Women's Health Study.[121]

Antioxidant vitamins have been studied in heart disease, owing to basic research, which has shown that they either inhibit oxidation of LDL cholesterol or its uptake into coronary artery endothelium.[121] The Iowa Women's Health Study evaluated 34 486 postmenopausal women and found that the intake of vitamin E from food is inversely associated with coronary heart disease death.[122] They noted that women can lower their risk without using vitamin supplements; dietary measures alone sufficed.

Lastly, a word about alcohol: low to moderate daily alcohol consumption provides protection against coronary artery disease in both genders.[121] In the Nurses' Health Study, women who consumed one glass of wine daily had a 40 per cent reduction in coronary heart disease risk. The possible mechanisms for alcohol giving cardiac protection include increased HDL levels, increased ratio of prostacyclin to thromboxane, increased tissue plasminogen activator levels, and reduced platelet aggregation.[121] However, some data suggest alcohol use may increase the risk of breast cancer.[123] Therefore, recommending that women consume moderate amounts of alcohol to prevent heart disease is currently unwarranted.

FUTURE DIRECTIONS

Our knowledge of heart disease in women has undergone much evolution since the earlier misconceptions that originated prior to angiographic literature. Many of the previous biases in access of women to evaluation of suspected coronary heart disease have been abolished as the body of gender-specific data continues to grow. The unique protective effect of estrogen on heart disease has been intensely investigated. An exciting area of future focus will be the ultimate findings of risks and benefits of postmenopausal hormone replacement, especially with regard to the breast cancer dilemma. The years 2000 and 2005 will hopefully yield answers to these very pivotal questions as the HERS and the WHI studies conclude.

SUMMARY

- Several large-scale studies indicate that lipid-lowering medications slow the progression of atherosclerosis in women.
- Up to 95–99 per cent of women who stop smoking do so on their own, underscoring the importance of self-motivation.
- Owing to increased risk of coronary heart disease in diabetic women, they should undergo risk-factor modification and periodic non-invasive screening for ischemia.

- Higher levels of body weight still within the 'normal' range, as well as weight gain after age 18, increase cardiovascular risk in middle-aged women.
- Moderate physical fitness can provide a substantial reduction in risk of cardiovascular death in women.
- Postmenopausal hormone replacement is beneficial from a cardiac standpoint; this must be weighed against the increased risk of breast cancer following prolonged use of estrogen/progesterone combinations.

REFERENCES

1. Johansson S, Vedin A, Wilhelmsson C. Myocardial infarction in women. *Epidemiol Rev* 1983; **5**: 67.
○2. Matthews KA, Meilahn E, Kuller LH. Menopause and risk factors for coronary artery disease. *N Engl J Med* 1989; **321**: 641–6.
3. Haskell WL, Alderman EL, Fair JM, *et al.* Effects of multiple risk factor reduction on coronary atherosclerosis and clinical cardiac events in men and women with coronary artery disease. *Circulation* 1994; **89**: 975–90.
○4. Hawkins RI. Smoking, platelets and thrombosis. *Nature* 1972; **236**: 450–2.
5. Meade TW, Imeson J, Stirling Y. Effects of changes in smoking and other characteristics on clotting factors and the risk of ischemic heart disease. *Lancet* 1987; **2**: 986–8.
6. Holmes DR, Holubkov R, Vliestra RE. Comparison of complications during percutaneous transluminal coronary angioplasty from 1977 to 1981 and from 1985 to 1986: The National Heart, Lung, and Blood Institute PTCA registry. *J Am Coll Cardiol* 1988; **12**: 1149–55.
7. Eaker ED, Kronmal B, Kennedy JW, Davis K. Comparison of the long-term, post-surgical survival of women and men in the Coronary Artery Surgery Study (CASS). *Am Heart J* 1989; **117**: 71–81.
8. Cooppan R, Flood TM. Obesity and diabetes. In: Marble A, Krall LP, Bradley RF, Christlieb AR, Soeldner JS, eds *Joslin's diabetes mellitus*. Philadelphia: Lea and Febiger, 1985: 373–9.
9. Manson JE, Colditz GA, Stampfer MJ. A prospective study of obesity and risk of coronary heart disease in women. *N Engl J Med* 1990; **32**: 882–9.
10. Saar E, Chayot R, Meyerstein N. Physical activity and blood pressure in normotensive young women. *Eur J Appl Physiol* 1986; **55**: 64–7.
11. Marti B, Salonen JT, Tuomilehto J. 10-year trends in physical activity in the eastern Finnish adult population. Relationship to socioeconomic and life-style characteristics. *Acta Med Scand* 1988; **224**: 195–203.
12. Moore CE, Hartung GH, Mitchell RE. The relationship of exercise and diet on high-density lipo-protein cholesterol levels in women. *Metabolism* 1983; **32**: 189–96.
13. Williams JR, Adams MR, Herrington DM. The effects of short-term estrogen treatment on vascular responses of coronary arteries. *Circulation* 1991; **84**(suppl II): II–272.
14. Grodstein F, Stampfer MJ, Colditz GA, *et al.* Postmenopausal hormone therapy and mortality. *N Engl J Med* 1997; **336**: 1769–75.
15. Marwick TH, Anderson T, Williams J, Haluska B, Melin JA, Pashkow F, Thomas JD. Exercise echocardiography is an accurate and cost-efficient technique for detection of coronary artery disease in women. *J Am Coll Cardiol* 1995; **26**: 335–41.
16. Wenger NK. Coronary disease in women. *Annu Rev Med* 1985; **36**: 285–94.
♦17. Lerner DJ, Kannel WB. Patterns of coronary heart disease morbidity and mortality in the sexes: a 26-year follow-up of the Framingham population. *Am Heart J* 1986; **111**: 383–90.
♦18. Proudfit WL, Welch CC, Siqueira C. Prognosis of 1000 young women studied by coronary angiography. *Circulation* 1981; **64**: 1185–90.
19. The Principal Investigators of CASS and their associates. The National Heart, Lung, and Blood Institute Coronary Artery Surgery Study (CASS). *Circulation* 1981; **63**(suppl I): I–1.
♦20. Hochman JS, McCabe CH, Stone PH, *et al.* Outcome and profile of women and men presenting with acute coronary syndromes: a report from TIMI III B. *J Am Coll Cardiol* 1997; **30**: 141–8.
21. Weiner DA, Ryan TJ, Parsons L, Fisher LD, Chaitman BR, Sheffield LT, Tristani FE. Significance of silent myocardial ischemia during exercise testing in women: report from the Coronary Artery Surgery Study. *Am Heart J* 1995; **129**: 465–70.
22. Kannel WB, Abbott RD. Incidence and prognosis of myocardial infarction in women: the Framingham study. In: Eaker ED, Packard B, Wenger NK, *et al.* eds *Coronary heart disease in women*. New York: Haymarket Doyma, 1987: 208.
23. Kannel WB, Sorlie P, McNamara PM. Prognosis after initial myocardial infarction: the Framingham study. *Am J Cardiol* 1979; **44**: 53–9.
24. Tofler GH, Stone PH, Muller JE. Effects of gender and race on prognosis after myocardial infarction: adverse prognosis for women, particularly black women. *J Am Coll Cardiol* 1987; **9**: 473–82.
25. Gruppo Italiano per lo Studio della Strepochinasi nell'Infarto Miocardico (GISSI). Long-term effects of intravenous thrombolysis in acute myocardial infarction: final report of the GISSI study. *Lancet* 1987; **2**: 871–4.

26. Pedersen TR. Six-year follow-up of the Norwegian Multicenter Study on timolol after acute myocardial infarction. *N Engl J Med* 1985; **313**: 1055–8.

27. ISIS-2 (Second International Study of Infarct Survival) Collaborative Group. Randomized trial of intravenous streptokinase, oral aspirin, both, or neither among 17,187 cases of suspected acute myocardial infarction: 1515–2. *Lancet* 1988; **2**: 349–60.

28. Moss AJ, Carleen E, and the Multicenter Postinfarction Research Group. Gender differences in the morality risk associated with ventricular arrhythmias after myocardial infarction. In: Eaker ED, Packard B, Wenger NK, *et al.* eds *Coronary heart disease in women*. New York: Haymarket Doyma, 1987: 204.

29. Vaitkus PT, Kindwall KE, Miller JM. Influence of gender on inducibility of ventricular arrhythmias in survivors of cardiac arrest with coronary artery disease. *Am J Cardiol* 1991; **67**: 537–9.

30. Kennedy JW, Kaiser GC, Fisher LD. Clinical and angiographic predictors of operative mortality from the collaborative study in coronary artery surgery (CASS). *Circulation* 1981; **63**: 793–802.

31. Cowley MJ, Mullin SM, Kelsey SF. Sex differences in early and long-term results of coronary angioplasty in the NHLBI PTCA Registry. *Circulation* 1985; **71**: 90–7.

32. Davis KB, Chaitman B, Ryan T, Bittner V, Kennedy W. Comparison of 15-year survival for men and women after initial medical or surgical treatment for coronary artery disease: a CASS registry study. *J Am Coll Cardiol* 1995; **25**: 1000–9.

33. Rahimtoola SH, Bennett AJ, Grunkemeier GL, Block P, Starr A. Survival at 15 to 18 years after coronary bypass surgery for angina in women. *Circulation* 1993; **88**: 71–8.

34. Fisher LD, Kennedy JW, Davis KB. Association of sex, physical size, and operative mortality after coronary artery bypass in Coronary Artery Surgery Study (CASS). *J Thorac Cardiovasc Surg* 1982; **84**: 334–41.

35. Oldridge NB, LaSalle D, Jones NL. Exercise rehabilitation of female patients with coronary artery disease. *Am Heart J* 1980; **100**: 755–7.

36. Tobin JN, Wassertheil-Smoller S, Wexler JP. Sex bias in considering coronary bypass surgery. *Ann Intern Med* 1987; **107**: 19–25.

37. Ayanian JZ, Epstein AM. Differences in the use of procedures between women and men hospitalized for coronary heart disease. *N Engl J Med* 1991; **325**: 221–5.

38. Steingart RM, Packer M, Hamm P. Sex differences in the management of coronary artery disease. *N Engl J Med* 1991; **325**: 226–30.

○39. Mahley RW, Innerarity TL, Rall SC, Jr. Plasma lipoproteins: apolipoprotein structure and function. *J Lipid Res* 1984; **25**: 1277–94.

40. Seed M. Sex hormones, lipoproteins, and cardiovascular risk. *Atherosclerosis* 1991; **90**: 1–7.

41. Rifkind BM, Segal P. Lipid Resource Clinics reference values for hyperlipidemia and hypolipidemia. *JAMA* 1983; **250**: 1869–72.

42. Gordon DJ, Probstfield JL, Garrison RF. High-density lipoprotein cholesterol and cardiovascular disease: four prospective studies. *Circulation* 1989; **79**: 8–15.

43. Eaker ED, Castelli WP. Coronary heart disease and its risk factors among women in the Framingham study. In: Eaker ED, Packard B, Wenger N, *et al.* eds *Coronary heart disease in women*. New York: Haymarket Doyma, 1987: 122–30.

44. Castelli WP. The triglyceride issue: a view from Framingham. *Am Heart J* 1986; **112**: 432–37.

45. Orth-Gomér K, Mittleman MA, Schenck-Gustafsson K, *et al.* Lipoprotein (a) as a determinant of coronary heart disease in young women. *Circulation* 1997; **95**: 329–34.

46. Rossouw JF. International trials (abstract). *Cholesterol and heart disease in older persons and in women*, June 18–19, 1990. Besthesda, MD: National Heart, Lung, and Blood Institute, National Institutes of Health.

47. Waters D, Higginson L, Gladstone P, Boccuzzi SJ, Cook T, Lespérance J. Effects of choleterol lowering on the progression of coronary atherosclerosis in women. *Circulation* 1995; **92**: 2404–10.

48. US Department of Health and Human Services. *Reducing the health consequences of smoking for women: a report of the Surgeon General*. DHHS Publication no. (CBC) 89–8411. Washington, DC: US Government Printing Office, 1989.

49. National Center for Health Statistics. *Health, United States, 1990*. Hyattsville, MD: Public Health Service, 1991.

50. Willett WC, Green A, Stampfer MJ. Relative and absolute excess risks of coronary heart disease among women who smoke cigarettes. *N Engl J Med* 1987; **317**: 1303–9.

51. Eaker E, Packard B, Thoma TJ. Epidemiology and risk factors for coronary heart disease in women. In: Douglas PS, ed. *Heart disease in women*. Cardiovascular Clinics. Philadelphia, F.A. Davis, 1989: 120–45.

52. Colditz GA, Bonita R, Stampfer MJ. Cigarette smoking and risk of stroke in middle-aged women. *N Engl J Med* 1988; **318**: 937–41.

53. Sarma JSM, Tillmanns H, Ikeda S. The effect of carbon monoxide on lipid metabolism of human coronary arteries. *Atherosclerosis* 1975; **22**: 193–8.

54. Dolevall A, Khutti J, Teger-Nilsson A. Platelet reactivity, fibrinogen and smoking. *Eur J Haematol* 1987; **38**: 55–9.

55. McKinlay SM, Bifano NL, McKinlay JB. Smoking and age at menopause in women. *Ann Intern Med* 1985; **103**: 350–6.

56. Stampfer MJ, Willett WC, Colditz GA. Past use of oral contraceptives and cardiovascular disease: a meta-analysis in the context of Nurses' Health Study. *Am J Obstet Gynecol* 1990; **163**: 285–91.

57. Stadel BV. Oral contraceptives and cardiovascular disease. *N Engl J Med* 1981; **305**: 672–7.

58. Mileikowsky GN, Nadler JL, Huey F. Evidence that smoking alters prostacyclin formation and platelet aggregation in women who use oral contraceptives. *Am J Obstet Gynecol* 1988; **1598**: 1547–52.

59. Massey JT, Moore TF, Parson VL. *Design and estimation for the National Health Interview Survey 1985–1994.* Series II, No. 110. Hyattsville, MD, August, 1989.

60. Klesges RC, Eck LH, Clark E. The effects of smoking cessation and gender on dietary intake, physical activity, and weight gain. *Int J Eating Disorders* 1990; **9**: 435–46.

61. US Department of Health and Human Services. *The health benefits of smoking cessation. A report of the Surgeon General.* US DHHS Publication (CDC), 90–8416. Atlanta, GA: Centers for Disease Control, 1990.

62. Gordon T, Castelli WP, Hjortland MC. Diabetes, blood lipids, and the role of obesity in CHD risk for women. The Framingham study. *Ann Intern Med* 1977; **87**: 393–7.

63. Kannel WB, D'Agostino RB, Wilson PWF. Diabetes, fibrinogen, and risk of cardiovascular disease: the Framingham experience. *Am Heart J* 1990; **120**: 672–6.

64. Manson JE, Colditz GA, Stampfer MJ. A prospective study on maturity-onset diabetes mellitus and risk of coronary heart disease and stroke in women. *Arch Intern Med* 1991; **151**: 1141–7.

♦65. Ridker PM, Hennekens CH. Hemostatic risk factors for coronary heart disease. *Circulation* 1991; **83**: 1098–100.

66. Juhan-Vague I, Vague PH, Alessi MC. Relationships between plasma insulin, triglyceride, body mass index, and plasminogen activator inhibitor. *Diabet Metab* 1987; **13**: 331–6.

67. Kannel WB, Wolf PA, Castelli WP. Fibrinogen and risk of cardiovascular disease: the Framingham study. *JAMA* 1987; **258**: 1183–6.

68. Greenland P, Reicher-Reiss H, Goldbourt U, Behar S, Israeli SPRINT Investigators. In-hospital and 1-year mortality in 1524 women after myocardial infarction: comparison with 4315 men. *Circulation* 1991; **83**: 484–91.

69. Tofler GH, Stone PH, Muller JE. Effects of gender and race on prognosis after myocardial infarction: adverse prognosis for women, particularly black women. *J Am Coll Cardiol* 1987; **9**: 473–82.

70. Steingart RM, Packer M, Hamm P. Sex differences in the management of coronary artery disease. *N Engl J Med* 1991; **325**: 226–30.

71. Durnin JVGA, Wormesly J. Body fat assessed from total body density and its estimation from skinfold thickness: measurements of 481 men and women aged 17 to 72 years. *Br J Nutr* 1974; **32**: 77–82.

○72. Keys A. Overweight, obesity, coronary heart disease and mortality. *Nutr Rev* 1980; **38**: 297–307.

73. National Institutes of Health Concensus Development Panel on the Health Implications of Obesity. Health implications of obesity: National Institute of Health concensus development conference statement. *Ann Intern Med* 1985; **103**: 1073–7.

74. Kissebah AH, Vydelingum N, Murray R. Relation of body-fat distribution to metabolic consequences of obesity. *J Clin Endocrinol Metab* 1982; **54**: 254–60.

75. Stunkard AJ. Obesity and the social environment: current status, future projects. In: Bray G ed. *Obesity in America.* US DHEW Publication NIH 79–359. Washington, DC: US Government Printing Office, 1979: 206.

76. Lew EA, Gaefinkel L. Variations in mortality by weight among 750,000 men and women. *J Chron Dis* 1979; **32**: 563–76.

77. Hubert HB, Fernlieb M, McNamara PM. Obesity is an independent risk factor for cardiovascular disease: a 26-year follow-up of participants in the Framingham Heart Study. *Circulation* 1983; **249**: 2199–203.

78. DeDevitis O, Fazio S, Petitto M, Maddalena G, Contaldo F, Mancini M. Obesity and cardiac function. *Circulation* 1981; **64**: 477–82.

♦79. MacMahon SW, Wilcken DEL, Macdonald GJ. The effect of weight reduction on left ventricular mass: a randomized controlled trial in young, overweight hypertensive patients. *N Engl J Med* 1986; **314**: 334–9.

80. O'Connor GT, Olmstead EM, Coffin LH, *et al.* for the Northern New England Cardiovascular Disease Study Group. Gender and in-hospital mortality associated with coronary artery bypass grafting. *Circulation* 1991; **83**: 723A.

81. Willett WC, Manson JE, Stampfer MJ, Colditz GA, Rosner B, Speizer FE, Hennekens CH. Weight, weight change, and coronary heart disease in women. *JAMA* 1995; **273**: 461–5.

82. Powell KE, Thompson PD, Caspersen CJ. Physical activity and the incidence of coronary heart disease. *Ann Rev Public Health* 1987; **8**: 253–87.

♦83. Blair SN, Kohl HW, Paffenbarger RS. Physical fitness and all-cause mortality. A prospective study of healthy men and women. *JAMA* 1989; **262**: 2395–401.

84. Blair SN, Goodyear NN, Gibbons LW. Physical fitness and incidence of hypertension in healthy normotensive men and women. *JAMA* 1984; **252**: 487–90.

85. Urata H, Tanabe Y, Kiyonaga A. Antihypertensive and volume-depleting effects of mild exercise on essential hypertension. *Hypertension* 1987; **9**: 245–52.

86. Shangold MM. Exercise in the menopausal woman. *Obstet Gynecol* 1990; **75**: 53S–58S.

87. Brownell KD, Rubin CJ, Smoller JW. Exercise and regulation of body weight. In: Shangold M, Mirkin G, eds *Women and exercise.* Philadephia: F.A. Davis, 1988: 40–54.

88. Gibbons LW, Blair SN, Cooper KH. Association between coronary heart disease risk factors and physical fitness

in healthy adult women. *Circulation* 1983; **67**: 977–83.

89. Notelovitz M. Exercise and health maintenance in menopausal women. *Ann N Y Acad Sci* 1990; **592**: 204–20.

90. Kokkinos PF, Holland JC, Pittaras AE, Narayan P, Dotson CO, Papademetriou V. Cardiorespiratory fitness and coronary heart disease risk factor association in women. *J Am Coll Cardiol* 1995; **26**: 358–64.

91. May GS, Eberlein KA, Furberg CD. Secondary prevention after myocardial infarction: a review of long term trials. *Prog Cardiovasc Dis* 1982; **24**: 331–52.

92. Lavie CJ, Milani RV. Effects of cardiac rehabilitation and exercise training on exercise capacity, coronary risk factors, behavorial characteristics, and quality of life in women. *Am J Cardiol* 1995; **75**: 340–3.

93. Sherman BM, West JH, Korenman SG. The menopausal transition: analysis of LH, FSH, estradiol and progesterone concentrations during menstrual cycles of older women. *J Clin Endocrinol Metab* 1976; **42**: 629–36.

94. Grodin JM, Siiteri PK, MacDonald PC. Source of estrogen production in postmenopausal women. *J Clin Endocrinol Metab* 1973; **36**: 207–14.

95. Kannel WB, Hjortland MC, McNamara PM. Menopause and the risk of cardiovascular disease: the Framingham study. *Ann Intern Med* 1976; **85**: 447–52.

96. Rosenberg L, Hennekens CH, Rosner B. Early menopause and the risk of myocardial infarction. *Am J Obstet Gynecol* 1981; **139**: 47–51.

97. Kannel WB, Gordon T. Cardiovascular effects of the menopause. In: Mishell DR Jr, ed. *Menopause: physiology and pharmacology*. Chicago: Year Book, 1987: 91.

98. Matthews KA, Meilahn E, Kuller LH. Menopause and risk factors for coronary heart disease. *N Engl J Med* 1989; **321**: 641–6.

99. Mashchak CA, Lobo RA. Estrogen replacement therapy and hypertension. *J Reproduct Med* 1985; **30** (suppl 10): 805–10.

100. Ballejo G, Saleem TH, Khan-Dawood FS. The effects of sex steroids on insulin binding by target tissues in the rat. *Contraception* 1983; **28**: 413–22.

101. Notelovitz M, Ware M. Coagulation risks with postmenopausal oestrogen therapy. In: Studd J, ed. *Progress in obstetrics and gynecology*, Vol. 2. Edinburgh: Churchill Livingstone, 1982.

102. Lobo RA. Effects of hormonal replacement on lipids and lipoproteins in postmenopausal women. *J Clin Endocrinol Metab* 1991; **73**: 925–30.

103. Knopp RH, Zhu X, Bonet B. Effects of estrogens on lipoprotein metabolism and cardiovascular disease in women. *Atherosclerosis* 1994; **110**(suppl.): S83–91.

104. Steinleitner A, Stanczyk FZ, Levin JH. Decreased in vitro production of 6-keto-prostaglandin F_1 alpha by uterine arteries from postmenopausal women. *Am J Obstet Gynecol* 1989; **161**: 1677–81.

105. Gebara OCE, Mittleman MA, Sutherland P, *et al.* Association between increased estrogen status and increased fibrinolytic potential in the Framingham offspring study. *Circulation* 1995; **91**: 1952–8.

106. Bush TL. Noncontraceptive estrogen use and risk of cardiovascular disease: an overview on critique of the literature. In: Korenman SG, ed. *The menopause, biological and clinical consequences of ovarian failure: evolution and management*. Norwell, MA: Serono Symposium, 1990: 211.

107. Stampfer MJ, Willett WC, Colditz GA. Past use of oral contraceptives and cardiovascular disease: a meta-analysis in the context of the Nurses' Health Study. *Am J Obstet Gynecol* 1990; **163**: 285–91.

108. Sullivan JM, Vander Zwaag R, Hughes JP. Estrogen replacement and coronary artery disease. *Arch Intern Med* 1990; **150**: 2557–62.

109. Sullivan JM, El-Zeky F, Zwaag RV, Ramanathan KB. Effect on survival of estrogen replacement therapy after coronary artery bypass grafting. *Am J Cardiol* 1997; **79**: 847–50.

110. Gorsky RD, Koplan JP, Peterson HB, Thacker SB. Relative risks and benefits of long-term estrogen replacement therapy: a decision analysis. *Obstet Gynecol* 1994; **83**: 161–6.

111. Grady D, Wenger NK, Herrington D, *et al.* The Heart and Estrogen/progestin Replacement Study. *Ann Intern Med* 2000; **132**: 689–96.

112. Weiner DA, Ryan TJ, Parsons L, Fisher LD, Chaitman BR, Sheffield LT, Tristani FE. Long-term prognostic value of exercise testing in men and women from the coronary artery surgery (CASS) registry. *Am J Cardiol* 1995; **75**: 865–70.

113. Hung J, Chaitman BR, Lam J. Noninvasive diagnostic test choices for the evaluation of coronary disease in women: a multivariate comparison of cardiac fluorscopy, exercise electrocardiography, and exercise thallium myocardial perfusion scintigraphy. *J Am Coll Cardiol* 1984; **4**: 8–16.

114. Friedman TD, Greene AC, Iskandrian AS. Exercise thallium-201 myocardial scintigraphy in women: correlation with coronary arteriography. *Am J Cardiol* 1982; **49**: 1632–7.

115. Douglas PS, Ginsburg GS. The evaluation of chest pain in women. *N Engl J Med* 1996; **334**: 1311–15.

116. Greenberg PS, Berge RD, Johnson KD. The value and limitation of radionuclide angiography with stress in women. *Clin Cardiol* 1983; **6**: 312–17.

117. Amanullah AM, Kiat H, Friedman JD, Berman DS. Adenosine technetium-99m sestamibi myocardial perfusion SPECT in women: diagnostic efficacy in detection of coronary artery disease. *J Am Coll Cardiol* 1996; **27**: 803–9.

118. Sawada SG, Ryan T, Fineberg NS. Exercise echocardiographic detection of coronary artery disease in women. *J Am Coll Cardiol* 1989; **14**: 1440–7.

119. Chaitman BR, Bourassa MG, Lam J. Noninvasive
diagnosis of coronary heart disease in women. In:
Eaker ED, Packard B, Wenger NK, *et al*. eds *Coronary
heart disease in women*. New York: Haymarket Doyma,
1987: 222.

120. Harpaz D, Benderly M, Goldbourt U, Kishon Y, Behar S.
Effect of aspirin on mortality in women with
symptomatic or silent myocardial ischemia. *Am J
Cardiol* 1996; **78**: 1215–19.

♦121. Rich-Edwards JW, Manson JE, Hennekins CH, Buring JE.
The primary prevention of coronary heart disease in
women. *N Engl J Med* 1995; **332**: 1758–66.

122. Kushi LH, Folsom AR, Prineas RJ, Mink PJ, Wu Y,
Bostick RM. Dietary antioxidant vitamins and death
from coronary heart disease in postmenopausal
women. *N Engl J Med* 1996; **334**: 1156–62.

123. Longnecker MP. Alcoholic beverage consumption in
relation to risk of breast cancer: meta-analysis and
review. *Cancer Causes Control* 1994; **5**: 73–82.

PART 2

Urgent and emergency management of cardiovascular disorders

5

Emergency department approach to acute myocardial infarction

GARY B GREEN AND EDWARD BESSMAN

Due to the time-dependent nature of acute myocardial infarction (AMI) therapy, the pre-hospital and emergency department (ED) environments are critical components of the Emergency Cardiac Care (ECC) system. The aims of the ECC system are to ensure immediate evaluation of all patients with symptoms of possible ischemia, optimize utilization of early revascularization therapies, and reduce to zero the number of patients leaving the ED with unrecognized AMI. Early and complete recognition of AMI is accomplished by maintaining a high level of vigilance and through implementation of evidence-based evaluation protocols which incorporate history, ECG and laboratory data for diagnosis and risk stratification. The primary goal of therapy in AMI is rapid reperfusion of the infarct-related artery. When appropriate criteria are met, early angiographic intervention (goal <60 minutes) or fibrinolytic therapy (goal <30 minutes) dramatically improve survival. Aspirin, beta-blockers and other adjuvent therapies may also lower mortality and should be considered.

INTRODUCTION

In recent years, the care of patients presenting to the emergency department (ED) with symptoms of acute myocardial ischemia has been virtually revolutionized. Although the dramatic changes that have occurred were perhaps initiated by the advent of fibrinolytic therapy, they have by no means been limited to this treatment. Significant advances have also taken place in many other areas relevant to emergency cardiac care (ECC).* Development of improved diagnostic technologies such as rapid assays for serum markers of myocardial injury, more sophisticated monitoring devices and cardiac imaging techniques now allow rapid, accurate diagnosis as well as early risk assessment in the ED. Additionally,

the spectrum of therapies available for treatment of patients with acute myocardial ischemia continues to expand rapidly. Further, since the efficacy of these therapies is frequently time dependent, increasingly complex management decisions must be made soon after presentation while the patient is still in the ED. In combination, these events have prompted fundamental changes in the scope, depth and even the goals of ECC.

In this chapter, we will provide a broad overview of modern ECC systems that are likely to benefit both clinicians and system planners. We begin with a topic of fundamental importance to both groups, a discussion of the unique environment in which emergency cardiac care is delivered and the implications of this environment toward ECC system structure and function. The major components of an ECC system are then described,

---

* The term 'emergency cardiac care' encompasses a spectrum of practice including but not limited to the evaluation and treatment of patients with acute myocardial ischemia in the ED. However, for the purpose of this discussion, it is used in this chapter to refer specifically to the care of those presenting to the ED with symptoms suggesting possible ischemia.

including the establishment of patient-oriented goals, care plans, indicators, and resource needs. Subsequently, a comprehensive description of relevant clinical considerations is given by following the course of patient care from the prehospital setting, through initial ED evaluation, data gathering and decision making, and including a detailed review of up-to-date recommendations concerning therapy for patients with confirmed or suspected acute myocardial infarction (MI).

EMERGENCY CARDIAC CARE SYSTEM MANAGEMENT

Unique environment of ECC

The implementation of any effective clinical practice is dependent on more than technical expertise concerning therapeutic interventions. Attention to system requirements must also be maintained in order to optimize patient care in all practice settings. It is clear that specific material needs must be met, such as appropriate facilities and equipment and adequately trained personnel. However, other system requirements, such as goal setting, establishment of care plans and system evaluation may have an equal impact on patient outcomes. This is especially true for ECC, owing to both the unique nature of the ED environment and considerations inherent to the care of patients with possible ischemia. For example, the utility of written protocols governing rapid triage, evaluation and disposition of chest pain patients is mandated both by the need for early identification of eligibility for time-dependent therapies and by the ever-present time constraints of multiple patient management in a busy ED. Some of the system characteristics unique to the delivery of ECC are therefore listed and summarized here, followed by a discussion of the various requirements of an effective ECC system.

EVALUATION OF UNDIFFERENTIATED PATIENTS

Unlike most other clinical settings, ED patients generally present soon after onset of their symptoms and without previous evaluation. In most patients, symptoms represent stable or slowly progressive processes. However, in some, initially similar presentations are due to rapidly progressive, immediately life-threatening pathology which requires immediate action. Therefore, emergency physicians must consider and actively exclude life-threatening conditions in all patients even when these diagnoses are statistically improbable.

ATYPICAL PRESENTATIONS

Most patients presenting to EDs with chest pain do not have acute myocardial ischemia. However, patients with ischemic syndromes often present atypically, with symptoms identical to those of patients with more benign processes. Additionally, symptoms of many non-cardiac diseases, such as gastroesophageal reflux and musculoskeletal pain syndromes often mimic ischemic symptoms. Owing to these facts, an accurate diagnosis cannot be reliably determined based on the information available during a brief ED stay. Therefore, the emergency physician must constantly weigh the risks of inadvertently discharging a patient with an atypical presentation of acute myocardial ischemia against the possibility of a costly in-patient evaluation of a patient without a true cardiac emergency.

CONCERN ABOUT PATIENT FLOW

Unlike other areas of the hospital, the entry of patients into the ED is difficult to control. New patients arrive at all times and must be evaluated with minimal delay. Therefore, in order to deliver quality care, patient flow through the department must be actively managed. As a result, the emergency physician often treats several patients simultaneously and must adjust the time attending to each patient not only according to acuity and complexity, but also according to the volume and acuity of other patients in the ED.

TIME-DEPENDENT NATURE OF TREATMENT

Fibrinolytic trials have clearly demonstrated that the magnitude of the mortality benefit gained by coronary artery reperfusion is time dependent. Percutaneous coronary intervention (PCI) and newer anti-ischemic therapies, such as antiplatelet and antithrombin agents, are also likely to be more beneficial when initiated soon after presentation.[1,2] Therefore, specific system components, such as continuous time-to-treatment monitoring, which can effectively identify and reduce treatment delays, are critical components of a successful ECC system.

MULTIDISCIPLINARY TEAM APPROACH

The care of patients with symptoms of acute myocardial ischemia is multidisciplinary and decentralized. Over the course of hours (or even minutes), the site of care delivery may change from the patient's home to an ambulance, from ambulance to the ED, and from the ED to an in-patient bed (or perhaps the catheterization laboratory). Similarly, the provider accepting responsibility for the patient is also likely to transition several times within the initial hours after symptom onset. Owing to this fact, extra care must be taken to avoid conflict and to prevent fragmentation of care. Incorporation of all involved personnel into a multidisciplinary team will ensure maintenance of a high level of care. The team should consist of emergency physicians and cardiologists as well as representatives of prehospital care providers, nursing, pharmacy, laboratory medicine, radiology, and administrators. The purpose of the team is to establish a working relationship which will allow the translation of common care goals into specific policies and procedures, to ensure availability of adequate resources and to provide a mechanism for ongoing system evaluation and improvement.

ECC system requirements

TREATMENT GOALS

Owing to the diversity and complexity of care in the ED environment and the multidisciplinary nature of emergency medicine, it is not surprising that competing agendas sometimes coexist. For example, valid concerns about patient flow through the department, limitations on physician and nurse staffing and cost containment may all require attention. It is therefore of utmost importance that the over-riding goal of all members of the care team and of all patient care activities be clearly articulated and remain a focus at all times. A relevant set of outcome-centered goals should be written, promoted and actively pursued. These goals must be consistent with current standards of care, generate broad-based support, yet be specific enough to allow development of detailed patient care protocols.

The most obvious and most frequently articulated goal concerning the care of patients with suspected MI is reducing the time from patient arrival to fibrinolytic administration (door-to-needle time). Reduction and maintenance of an appropriately brief door-to-needle time must be a primary goal of every ED's cardiac care program and requires a concerted effort from all members of the care team. However, it must be emphasized that patients with chest pain are a diverse group and 10 per cent or less may actually be experiencing an acute MI and only 5 per cent may meet established criteria for fibrinolytic therapy.[3] Therefore, goals must also be expressed and policies directed towards optimizing the outcomes of all patient subgroups. In addition, a complementary set of key indicators should be established and monitored on an ongoing basis in order to determine policy compliance. These data should be periodically reviewed and utilized to drive system adjustments and targeted interventions in a continuous process of quality improvement. Examples of appropriate patient-centered goals and outcome measures for an emergency cardiac care program are listed in Table 5.1. Specific examples are briefly discussed below.

Immediate evaluation of chest pain patients

In a busy ED, physicians, nurses and other staff must divide their attention between a large number of patients. It is essential that the time-dependent nature of optimal treatment be widely recognized. Triage protocols should establish all patients with chest pain or other symptoms of possible ischemia as a high priority and mandate immediate physician evaluation and avoidance of possible delays due to registration, insurance authorization or other administrative matters. Upon arrival, standing orders should stress basic evaluation and treatment measures, such as vital signs, cardiac monitoring, placement of an intravenous line and oxygen administration. Other documented causes of treatment delay include the need for a specific physician request to obtain the initial 12-lead electrocardiogram (ECG) and delays in physician interpretation.[4] The American Heart Association/American College of Cardiology guidelines recommend completion of the initial ECG and a targeted clinical examination by the ED physician within 10 minutes of patient arrival.[1]

Optimize utilization of early reperfusion therapies

Maximizing the appropriate utilization of fibrinolytics and PCI should be the goal of every ECC system. Adequate resources must be allocated to allow identifica-

Table 5.1 *Examples of patient-centered goals of an emergency cardiac care program*

Aim	Outcome measure	Goal
Immediate patient evaluation	ECG interpretation and targeted examination	10 minutes from arrival
Optimal utilization of revascularization therapies	Patients meeting revascularization criteria (by audit) Thrombolytics and primary PCI utilization	100 per cent utilization in eligible patients
Reduction of treatment delay	Time to treatment: thrombolytics Time to catherization: PCI	30 minutes 60 minutes
Zero tolerance for 'missed' MI	Number of undiagnosed MIs (identified by routine follow-up phone calls, medical record audit)	0 missed MIs per year
Reduction in cost of excluding MI in low-risk patients	Percentage of CCU 'rule-out MI' patients with MI	10 per cent reduction without increase in adverse events

ECG = electrocardiogram; PCI = percutaneous coronary intervention; MI = myocardial infarction; CCU = coronary care unit.

tion and removal of any obstacles to successful candidate identification and treatment initiation. Specific interventions may be required to ensure widespread agreement and understanding of treatment protocols among all staff. Goals regarding revascularization of MI patients should focus on maximizing utilization (treatment of 100 per cent of ideal candidates) as well as on minimizing treatment delay. Guidelines from the National Heart, Lung and Blood Institute recommend a goal of 30 minutes from patient arrival in the ED for initiation of fibrinolytics ('door-to-needle time') and a goal of 60 minutes for time from patient arrival to initiation of cardiac catheterization ('door-to-catheterization time') in those institutions utilizing primary PCI.[1] Many causes of fibrinolytic treatment delay have been recognized (Table 5.2). The use of a time-to-treatment flow sheet (Fig. 5.1) for all reperfusion candidates serves as a continuous reminder of the importance of avoiding treatment delays as well as a surveillance tool to allow monitoring of protocol compliance and identification of problem areas.

Table 5.2 *Factors leading to fibrinolytic treatment delay*

Delay in seeking care
Ignorance of symptom significance
Denial
Previous MI or angina symptoms
Alone at time of symptoms
Attempts at contacting private physician or HMO

Delay in triage arrival
Transport delays
Parking
Prolonged prehospital evaluation
Registration

Delay in decision making
Decision to obtain ECG
Interpretation of ECG
Diagnostic and therapeutic interventions
Political (cardiology consultation)

Delay in treatment initiation
Physician–nurse communication
Obtain drug from pharmacy
Preparation of agent

MI = myocardial infarction; HMO = health maintenance organization; ECG = electrocardiogram.

Zero tolerance for 'missed' MI

It is estimated that 2–10 per cent of MI patients are inappropriately discharged from the ED.[5-8] Although in some of these cases diagnostic findings are neglected, many of these patients present with atypical symptoms and non-diagnostic ECGs.[9] These 'missed MI' patients suffer a higher mortality compared to those admitted to the coronary care unit (CCU)[9,10] and this patient group accounts for 20 per cent of malpractice awards against

Clock time

__:__ **Time 0:** Symptom onset

__:__ **Time 1:** 'Door' (arrival at triage)

__:__ **Time 2:** Initial ECG obtained

__:__ **Time 3:** 'Decision' (fibrinolytic ordered)

__:__ **Time 4:** 'Drug' (fibrinolytic infusion started)

Time 2 – time 1 = ____ minutes (goal = 10 minutes)

Time 3 – time 2 = ____ minutes

Time 4 – time 3 = ____ minutes

'Door-to-drug' time = Time 4 – time 1 = ____ minutes (goal = 30 minutes)

Symptom onset to drug time = Time 4 – time 0 = ____ minutes

Figure 5.1 *Time to treatment flow sheet for fibrinolytics in acute myocardial infarction.*

emergency physicians.[11] System planners and clinicians must take a prospective, proactive approach to this problem and should adopt strategies to monitor and reduce the number of 'missed' MIs. Several approaches have been suggested that include routine 'screening' of chest pain patients deemed safe for discharge using a single sample rapid CK-MB test[5] and/or routine referral for follow-up in a 'chest pain clinic' within 24 hours after discharge.[12] The use of an ED cardiac evaluation unit to observe and exclude MI in low-risk patients is becoming increasingly common and also may reduce the number of missed MIs. However, these units are generally utilized for patients whose risk of MI, although low, has been recognized by the clinician and who would have otherwise been admitted. The use of observation units to prevent 'missed' MIs may require a level of resource utilization that is not cost effective.[13]

CARE PLANS

The value of a written plan which establishes guidelines for the delivery of care to patients with a specific diagnosis or complaint has been increasingly advocated. These plans, which may be referred to by various names (clinical protocols, care maps, critical pathways) and are structured in differing formats (algorithm, chart, or written document), have recently been developed and applied at departmental, institutional, and national levels. Utilization of a protocol-based approach to guide the care of ED patients with suspected ischemia or MI offers several advantages. Most importantly, they promote the use of a standardized, systematic approach to a complex clinical problem. The protocols are generally written by clinicians with expertise in the field according to recent literature and therefore represent the state of the art. They are commonly developed using a multidisciplinary approach, thus ensuring that all available knowledge and resources will be utilized in the patient's best interest. Care plans may address a particular aspect of patient care or may be longitudinal and comprehensive in nature. In whatever form they take, care plans should also include identification of key indicators to allow monitoring of patient outcomes, resource utilization, and protocol compliance.

FACILITIES AND PERSONNEL

Facilities must allow convenient delivery of the required spectrum of diagnostic and therapeutic modalities, accessibility for a high intensity of provider–patient interactions and resuscitation capabilities. In high-volume EDs, designation of a specific area as a chest pain unit with distinct monitors, equipment and staff may facilitate care, while in lower volume centers, an appropriately stocked mobile 'cardiac cart' may be adequate. Continuous cardiac monitoring, immediate radiography including portable chest radiography and 'stat' measurement of myocardial markers should be available. Recommendations for the design of ED chest pain units are available from the American College of Emergency Physicians and the American Institute of Architects.[14,15]

Adequate staffing must be present at all times in order to allow for the immediate evaluation of patients with chest pain upon presentation. All ED staff, including registration clerks and other clerical workers must be trained in the importance of avoiding delay in the evaluation of these patients. Additionally, nursing personnel should receive specific training in Advanced Cardiac Life Support and arrhythmia recognition. Educating nurses in 12-lead ECG interpretation may also facilitate early recognition of patients with MI and other acute ischemic syndromes.

CLINICAL CONSIDERATIONS

PREHOSPITAL CARE

Approximately half of all patients with MI are transported to the hospital by ambulance. For these patients, prehospital evaluation and transport can contribute significantly to delays in reperfusion therapy. Conversely, specific prehospital interventions also have the potential to significantly reduce treatment delays.[16,17] Owing to its pivotal role, considerable attention has been devoted to prehospital care of patients with MI. It is imperative that every ED-based ECC program includes a program of coordination with prehospital care officials for protocol development and provider education. Additionally, efforts must be directed at maintaining a collaborative atmosphere and free communication between prehospital and in-hospital providers to facilitate constructive feedback.

Multiple studies have established the feasibility and positive impact of obtaining a 12-lead ECG in the prehospital setting.[16–18] Acquisition of an ECG increases the time spent in the field by approximately 4 minutes and can be transmitted to the ED in 70 per cent of eligible patients.[19] The goal of obtaining the ECG in the prehospital setting is to allow the emergency department to identify potential fibrinolytic candidates prior to patient arrival and thereby decrease the time to treatment. Investigations of prehospital 12-lead ECGs have demonstrated significant reductions in hospital-based time-to-treatment, ranging from 20 to 40 minutes saved.[16,17] Although a mortality reduction has not yet been demonstrated and the applicability of these studies to all populations and practice settings has been challenged, the National Heart, Lung and Blood Institute's National Heart Attack Alert Program Working Group supports this intervention.[20]

> Prehospital ECG eligibility criteria include cooperative adult patients with a complaint of chest pain or other heart attack symptoms with systolic blood pressure greater than 90 mm Hg, and without malignant arrhythmias.[21]

The prehospital administration of fibrinolytic therapy has also been studied in numerous trials. Although several investigations outside of the USA support prehospital thrombolytic administration,[22,23] US data show a reduction in treatment delay without a survival benefit.[24] Based on existing data, the National Heart Attack Alert Program Working Group suggests that prehospital fibrinolytic administration may be of benefit in regions where the resultant reduction in treatment delay would be 1 hour or more. In other regions, an additional clinical benefit may be obtained without fibrinolytic administration utilizing prehospital ECG acquisition in conjunction with completion of an eligibility checklist (Fig. 5.2) in order to identify ideal candidates prior to ED arrival.[20]

REGISTRATION AND TRIAGE

Efforts are required to minimize delay between the patients arrival at the entrance to the ED and their clinical evaluation. Patients with MI symptoms should be directly referred to triage personnel prior to obtaining registration or insurance information. The challenge of correctly identifying and prioritizing patients with MI in a busy ED should not be underestimated. Of patients presenting with chest pain, only 5 per cent may be ideal candidates for fibrinolytic therapy.[3] Owing to this low yield and the constant presence of competing high-priority patients, continuous reinforcement and monitoring are necessary to maintain the level of vigilance required to avoid treatment delay among those needing

Yes		No
☐	Currently having chest pain	☐
☐	Time since pain onset	
☐	Pain onset <12 hours	☐
☐	Pain >20 minutes, <6 hours	☐
☐	Alert and oriented	☐
☐	Cooperative for ECG	☐
☐	Age >30 _____	☐
	Gender (M/F) _____	
	BP right arm _____	
	BP left arm _____	
☐	Systolic BP >60, <180	☐
☐	Difference in systolic	
	BP <20 between R & L arm	☐
☐	Dystolic BP <110	☐

_____	Stroke, seizures, brain surgery, head trauma	_____
_____	Central lines < 2 weeks	
	Trauma < 2 weeks; or PCI < 1 month	_____
_____	Previous fibrinolytic Rx	_____
_____	Takes warfarin, coumadin	_____
_____	Known bleeding problems	_____
_____	GI bleed in last 2 months	_____
_____	Surgery in last 2 months	_____
_____	Jaundice, hepatitis, kidney failure	_____
_____	Colitis, Crohn's enteritis	_____

Times

Pain onset	___:___
Arrived at scene	___:___
ECG performed	___:___
ED arrival	___:___

Modified from MITI Study.

Figure 5.2 *Prehospital chest pain checklist. ECG = electrocardiogram; BP = blood pressure; PCI = percutaneous coronary intervention; Rx = treatment.*

immediate reperfusion. Once recognized at triage, patients with myocardial ischemia should receive only vital signs and a brief targeted history and examination before transfer to a monitored bed and entry into the ECC protocol. Reperfusion candidates brought to the ED by ambulance may benefit from direct transport to a monitored ED bed without stopping for registration or triage.[4] The ED physician should be notified immediately upon patient arrival.

Initial physician assessment

HISTORY

A comprehensive history is a key element in evaluating patients with chest pain. Information obtained will provide more diagnostic and prognostic data than will the physical examination, the ECG, and laboratory tests. Identification and integration of specific characteristics related to the patient's presenting symptoms enables the clinician to formulate a semiquantitative probability estimate of acute myocardial ischemia (Table 5.3). In addition, information from the history, especially when supplemented by ECG and laboratory data, permits early and accurate stratification of patients on the basis of the subsequent short-term risk of adverse events. The combination of diagnostic and prognostic information obtained from an optimal history will allow the clinician to make accurate and rapid treatment and disposition decisions.

Although an integral component of early assessment, relying on the patient's description of symptoms for decision making also has limitations. The frequency of atypical presentations and the overlapping spectrum of symptoms caused by thoracic pathologies make it possible for patients with differing diseases to present with similar symptoms. Conversely, patients with identical pathologies may experience completely different symp-

Table 5.3 *Characteristics of ischemic and non-ischemic chest pain syndromes*

Characteristic	Less suggestive of ischemia	More suggestive of ischemia
Quality	Sharp (somatic)	Vague (visceral)
Location	Lateral ribs Costochondral junction	Substernal
Pattern	Sudden onset	Gradual onset
Duration	Very brief (seconds) or prolonged (>12 hours)	Minutes to hours
Exacerbated by	Body movement Breathing (respirophasic) or palpation	Exertion[a]
Radiation	Absent; to legs or abdomen	Jaw, arm, shoulder
Associated symptoms	Absent	Dyspnea, nausea/vomiting, diaphoresis, lightheadedness

[a]Symptoms of myocardial infarction can begin at rest or following exertion.

Table 5.4 *Life-threatening causes of chest pain and their typical clinical characteristics*[a]

Diagnosis	Quality of pain	Radiation	Associated symptoms
Acute myocardial infarction	Vague, pressure-like	Arm, neck, jaw	Diaphoresis, dyspnea, lightheadedness, nausea/vomiting
Pulmonary embolism	Sudden, sharp, pleuritic	—	Dyspnea, syncope
Aortic dissection	Tearing	Back	Neurologic symptoms
Acute pericarditis	Sharp, positional	Left trapezious ridge	Dyspnea
Pneumothorax	Sudden, sharp, pleuritic	—	Dyspnea

[a] Many patients present with atypical presentations.

toms. Utilization of a structured, systematic approach to history taking will ensure collection of useful information.

The clinician should have priorities in interviewing a patient with chest pain. The initial moments of the physician–patient interaction must progress rapidly to determine if he or she is dealing with a life-theatening event and the need for an immediate intervention, such as airway management or other resuscitative measures. If no urgent life-saving intervention is required, a more complete history should then be elicited. If the presentation is consistent with an acute ischemia syndrome, further details should be elicited to differentiate between acute MI, unstable angina, and stable angina pectoris. Additionally, in all patients with suspected MI, specific questions should be directed at identification of indications and contraindications for fibrinolytic therapy and further risk assessment.

DIFFERENTIAL DIAGNOSIS

When evaluating a patient with chest pain it is important to consider the possibility of acute myocardial ischemia. However, during the initial assessment it is equally important not to overlook other life-threatening causes of chest pain (Table 5.4). Aortic dissection and pulmonary embolism result in high mortality when not recognized and treated early in their course.

After all potentially life-threatening causes of chest pain have been excluded, more benign conditions should be considered. The differential diagnosis of chest pain is broad and includes pathology of many different organ systems (Table 5.5).

PHYSICAL EXAMINATION

The physical examination is a vital component in evaluating patients with chest pain. In the setting of acute MI many patients will be tachycardic due to increased sympathetic tone, however bradycardia may occur among patients with inferior ischemia or in those already taking beta-blockers. In patients with myocardial ischemia, car-

Table 5.5 *Differential diagnosis of chest pain*

1. Cardiac
Myocarditis
Ischemic syndromes
    Acute myocardial infarction
    Stable angina
    Unstable angina
    Variant angina (coronary vasospasm)
Pericarditis
Valvular disease
    Aortic stenosis
    Mitral valve prolapse
    Hypertrophic obstruction cardiomyopathy

2. Gastrointestinal
Biliary colic
Esophageal spasm
Esophagitis/gastritis
Gastric/duodenal ulcer
Gastroesophageal reflux disease (GERD)
Mallory–Weiss tear

3. Musculoskeletal
Cervical radiculopathy
Costochondritis
Muscle strain/spasm

4. Neurologic
Herpes Zoster

5. Pulmonary
Bronchitis
Bronchospasm
Empyema
Pleural effusion
Pleuritis
Pneumonia
Pneumothorax
Pulmonary edema
Pulmonary embolism
Pulmonary hypertension

6. Vascular
Aortic dissection
Pulmonary embolism
Pulmonary hypertension

diac auscultation may reveal a diminished S_1, a paradoxically split S_2, and/or S_3 or S_4 gallops due to changes in ventricular function and compliance. The physical examination may also uncover non-ischemic causes of chest pain (e.g. pericarditis) or non-cardiac conditions (e.g. aortic dissection). The clinician must also carefully seek evidence of emerging complications of myocardial infarction. For example, the presence of worsening pulmonary congestion and jugular venous distention soon after symptom onset suggests pump failure and is an important prognostic marker while a new murmer may indicate papillary muscle dysfunction or ventricular septal rupture.

ELECTROCARDIOGRAPHY

The ECG remains the single most important diagnostic test in the evaluation of patients with chest pain. The role of the ECG is multifaceted. Of principal importance is the ability to aid in making the diagnosis of MI and acute ischemia (Fig. 5.3) as well as determining the region of myocardium affected (Table 5.6). In addition to yielding diagnostic information, the ECG may pro-

Table 5.6 *Electrocardiogram (ECG) localization of regional ischemia*

ECG leads affected	Myocardial region
II, III, aVF	Inferior
V_1–V_3	Anteroseptal
I, aVL, V_4–V_6	Lateral
V_1–V_6	Anterolateral
V_1–V_2 (tall R wave, ST depression)	Posterior
V_3R–V_4R	Right ventricle

vide equally important prognostic data. Further, the ECG may be useful in identifying certain non-ischemic causes of chest pain, such as arrhythmias, acute pericarditis or pulmonary embolism.

It is suggested that all patients with 'ischemic type' pain have a 12-lead ECG performed within 10 minutes of arrival in the emergency department[1] under standing orders, and that the ECG be handed directly to the treating physician for immediate interpretation.[4]

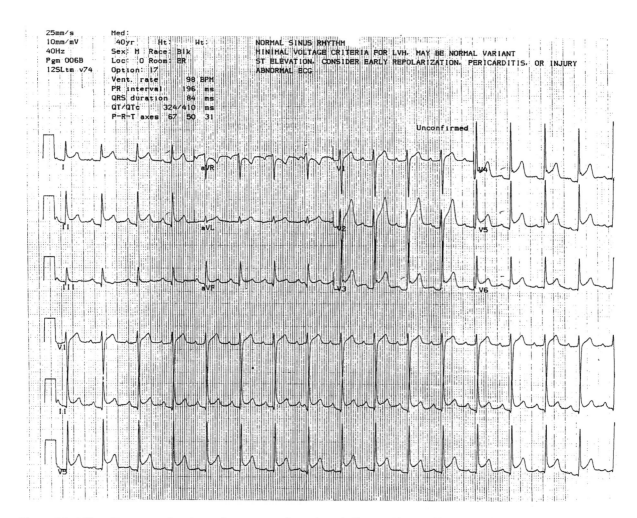

Figure 5.3 *Diffuse ST segment elevation and PR segment depression. Findings consistent with acute pericarditis.*

Although the ECG is a critical guide to therapy when abnormal, a normal or non-specific ECG, in and of itself, does not exclude myocardial ischemia or infarction. Among patients presenting to the ED with acute myocardial infarction, only 50 per cent will have diagnostic changes on the initial ECG.[25] Serial ECGs, even over several hours during the patient's ED stay, will increase the sensitivity of the ECG for the detection of MI,[26] as will including right-sided, posterior,[27] or 22-lead electrocardiography.[28] The use of continuous 12-lead ST-segment monitoring in the ED may also aid in the detection of patients with transient and and/or silent ischemia.[29]

Risk stratification based on the initial ECG has also been suggested as a method to improve ED decision making. Although the initial ECG can not exclude the diagnosis of MI, stable ED patients whose initial ECG is without ischemic changes are at low risk of subsequent life-threatening complications and therefore can usually be managed in a non-intensive care setting.[30,31]

SERUM MARKERS OF MYOCARDIAL INJURY

Cardiac enzymes and markers of myocardial injury are valuable tools for assessing patients with chest pain. Early discussions of CK-MB use in the ED focused on legitimate, but perhaps exaggerated, concerns about the dangers of misinterpretation of a single negative enzyme measurement in the ED. In the past, owing to the fear of patients with MI being inappropriately discharged after a single negative CK-MB, experienced clinicians had warned against the use of CK-MB testing in the ED.[32,33] These recommendations were challenged in 1987 when investigations demonstrated that serial CK-MB measurement in the ED was able to identify patients with MI that would otherwise have been missed.[8,9] During the

same time period, advances in laboratory techniques enabled the development of more rapid and accurate CK-MB testing methods, which allowed reporting of results within the time frame required for decision making in the ED.[5] Current practice supports myocardial marker measurement during the initial ED evaluation for three distinct purposes (Table 5.7); (1) to confirm suspected MI in patients with non-diagnostic ECGs within the first hours after presentation;[33–38] (2) to identify patients with otherwise unrecognized MI from among those with atypical presentations;[5,8,39] and (3) to risk stratify patients early in their ED course.[40–43]

Early diagnosis of MI

A single CK-MB measurement upon ED presentation has a sensitivity for MI of less than 60 per cent and therefore has limited diagnostic utility.[32,33] However, by utilizing rapid serial CK-MB sampling sensitivities for MI of 80–96 per cent among ED patients within 3 hours of presentation can be achieved.[34–36] Owing to its earlier release into serum after coronary occlusion, the heme-containing protein, myoglobin, may be even better suited for this purpose. Studies of early serial sampling of myoglobin for the detection of MI have demonstrated an initial, single sample sensitivity of 62 per cent, increasing to a sensitivity of 100 per cent at 2 hours after presentation.[37,38]

Identification of 'missed MI'

Although low diagnostic sensitivity does not allow the exclusion of MI based on a single cardiac enzyme, early CK-MB testing can be used to identify some patients with clinically unsuspected MI. Nationwide, 2–7 per cent of patients presenting to the ED with MI are inadvertently discharged to home.[5,6,8] Many of these patients have atypical symptoms and non-specific ECGs. Routine use of early CK-MB measurement has been shown to

Table 5.7 *Emergency department utilization of cardiac markers to determine myocardial injury*

Purpose	Marker	Timing of samples (hours from presentation)	n	Reference
Initial ED evaluation				
Early MI diagnosis	CK-MB	0, 3	183	34
	CK-MB	0, 1, 2, 3	313	35
	CK-MB	0, 1–2, 3	616	36
	Myoglobin	0, 3	59	37
	Myoglobin	0, 1, 2	198	38
Identification of 'missed' MI	CK-MB	Single sample	271	5
	CK-MB	0, 3	1042	39
Early risk stratification	CK-MB	0, 2	449	40
	CK-MB	0, 2	5120	41
	Troponin T	Single sample	113	42
	Troponin T	Single sample	292	43

MI = myocardial infarction; CK-MB = creatine kinase myocardial band.

identify some patients with MI that would otherwise not be suspected.[5,8] These observations suggest that patients with symptoms suggestive of myocardial ischemia who are to be sent home or admitted to non-monitored beds should undergo prerelease 'screening' for MI using a myocardial marker.

Risk stratification

As the number of available treatment options for individuals suffering acute ischemic events continues to grow, clinicians must be able to determine the overall risk–benefit relationship for individual patient subsets. Among 5120 patients enrolled from 53 EDs in the National Cooperative CK-MB Project, the relative risk of subsequent complications was 16.1 among those with a positive CK-MB compared to those with a negative test (regardless of final diagnosis).[41] Early single sample ED measurement of cardiac troponin T[43] and troponin I[44] have also demonstrated the ability to predict subsequent adverse events during the 14-day period following ED arrival.

COMPUTERIZED DECISION AIDS

In an effort to enable more accurate disposition decisions and thereby reduce mounting health care costs,[45,46] several investigators have developed computerized decision aids or computer-based triage protocols for ED

patients with chest pain.[47–51] Although the more recent proliferation of ED-based chest pain centers now provides a more cost effective alternative to admission for many patients, these units do not preclude the potential usefulness of an instrument capable of accurately estimating the probability of acute ischemia being present at the time of presentation.

One well-known computer-derived decision aid developed by Goldman *et al.* applied recursive partitioning to clinical and ECG data in order to derive and prospectively validate an algorithm that could stratify ED patients into groups with variable likelihood of acute MI (Fig. 5.4).[47] When tested hypothetically, the protocol improved the specificity of CCU triage decisions without affecting sensitivity. However, a prospective study evaluating the impact of utilizing this algorithm in the ED did not result in a significant decrease in CCU admission rates.[48]

Pozen *et al.* utilized a multivariate analysis to develop a predictive instrument for the detection of acute ischemic heart disease. In a multicenter trial, the instrument was able to reduce the number of CCU admissions (among patients without acute ischemia) by 30 per cent without any change in sensitivity.[49] This work has subsequently been expanded by Selker *et al.*, who developed a 'time-insensitive' predictive instrument designed to aid in prospective decision making as well as retrospective

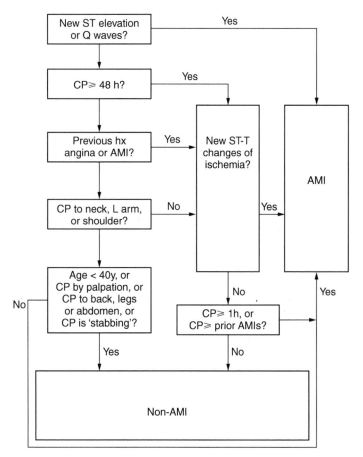

Figure 5.4 *An abridged version of the Goldman algorithm for triaging emergency department patients with chest pain.*[47] *CP = chest pain; L = left; y = years; AMI = acute myocardial infarction.*

analysis.[50] A small prospective trial has been reported that utilized an ECG recording device to automatically deliver the instrument's output to the emergency physician.[52,53] In this study, use of the device by novice physicians resulted in a 19 per cent (0.7 hour) decrease in the time from presentation to disposition, but no change in decision appropriateness or mortality. More recently, the results of a large multicenter prospective trial utilizing the instrument has been reported to reduce CCU admissions by 26 per cent and increase ED discharges to home by 48 per cent across all hospitals studied.[54] Baxt *et al.* has reported the development of an instrument to predict MI among ED patients with anterior chest pain based on an artificial neural network. When applied hypothetically, this model predicted MI with greater sensitivity and specificity than physician judgement alone or other predictive instruments.[51] When prospectively validated, model performance remained superior to the treating physician's assessment.[55]

THERAPY

Treatment of acute myocardial infarction (AMI) in the emergency department is aimed at limiting infarct size and preventing or managing complications. AMI represents the end point of a spectrum of acute coronary syndromes precipitated by myocardial ischemia. The mildest form is angina pectoris; progressively more serious entities include unstable angina, non-ST segment elevation MI and ST-segment elevation AMI.[56]

A patient who presents to an ED with chest pain can be placed conceptually into one of four categories: (I) probably non-cardiac; (II) possibly cardiac; (III) unstable angina/non-ST segment elevation AMI; and (IV) AMI. Initial triage decisions are based on the history, physical examination and the 12-lead ECG (Fig. 5.5).[1] The goal is to rapidly identify category IV (AMI) patients and administer reperfusion therapy to ideal candidates.[57] Category III patients are admitted to the hospital for

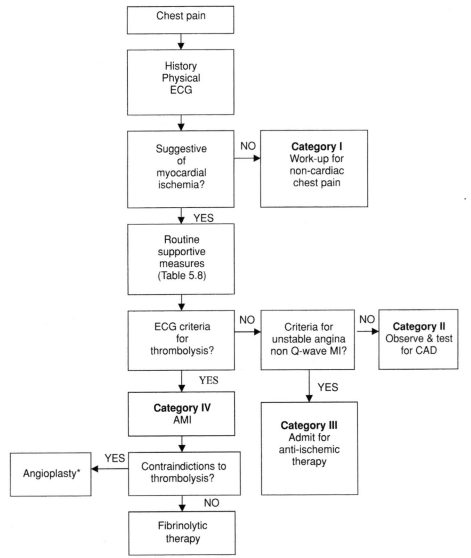

Figure 5.5 *Emergency department chest pain management algorithm. *In experienced hands, angiographic intervention may be more effective than thrombolytic therapy.*

optimal anti-ischemic therapy, while category II patients are observed and undergo appropriate testing to confirm or exclude a cardiac cause for their symptoms. Category I patients are treated according to their specific needs.

Initial therapy

Several routine measures should be undertaken in patients with suspected myocardial ischemia (Table 5.8).

Table 5.8 *Routine measures for all patients with chest pain*

Intravenous access
Supplemental oxygen
Continuous electrocardiographic (ECG) monitoring
Nitroglycerine
Analgesia (morphine)
Aspirin

INTRAVENOUS ACCESS

All patients should have at least one intravenous (iv) line or saline lock. Other measures should *not* be delayed while attempting iv access.

OXYGEN

All patients should receive supplemental oxygen for the first 2 or 3 hours. However, there is no evidence that oxygen is beneficial beyond this time in uncomplicated patients.

ELECTROCARDIOGRAPHIC MONITORING

Continuous ECG monitoring is recommended to allow early recognition of cardiac rhythm abnormalities. The most common cause of death during the first 2 hours of AMI is ventricular arrhythmias, specifically ventricular fibrillation (VF).[58] Immediate treatment is potentially life-saving.

NITROGLYCERINE

Nitroglycerine (TNG) is a veno- and arteriolar vasodilator and, as a result, reduces both preload and afterload. It is also a coronary arterial dilator. This combination of effects causes TNG to lower myocardial oxygen demand while simultaneously improving oxygen supply. Although its impact on survival is limited, particularly in the reperfusion era, NTG is used commonly as initial therapy for ischemic chest pain.[59] TNG may be given as sublingual tablets or iv infusion. The most serious side effect of TNG is hypotension and reflex tachycardia, both of which can worsen myocardial ischemia.

ANALGESIA

The pain and anxiety associated with AMI causes a release of epinephrine (and other catecholamines),

increasing myocardial oxygen consumption and irritability. TNG alone may not provide complete pain relief, and does not treat anxiety. For these reasons, morphine sulfate is recommended in increments of 2–4 mg iv. When titrated to effect, morphine is generally safe. Potential adverse effects include respiratory depression and hypotension. The former can be treated by giving naloxone, a specific morphine antagonist, and the latter by giving iv fluids.

ASPIRIN

Aspirin inhibits the ability of platelets to aggregate and has been shown to reduce mortality. Thus, its routine use is recommended.[60] Side effects such as gastrointestinal upset are not uncommon, but can readily be managed. Serious allergic reactions (angioedema, anaphylaxis, bronchospasm) are rare but when present preclude the use of aspirin. In this instance clopidogrel is recommended.

REPERFUSION THERAPY

In most cases of AMI, the precipitating event is occlusion of a coronary artery by thrombus.[61] Current treatment strategies are designed to address the component parts of coronary arterial thrombi – platelets, coagulation proteins, and fibrin. Aspirin, as noted above, inhibits platelet aggregation; anticoagulants prevent clot formation and extension; fibrinolytics promote clot lysis; and PCI or bypass surgery can be used to mechanically restore blood flow to the myocardium (Table 5.9).

Table 5.9 *Myocardial reperfusion strategies*

Aspirin
Inhibits platelet aggregation

Anticoagulants/antithrombotics
Inhibit thrombus formation and extension

Fibrinolytics
Dissolve thrombus

Angioplasty/coronary artery bypass surgery
Mechanical restoration of myocardial blood flow

ANTICOAGULANTS/ANTITHROMBOTICS

In spite of its theoretical value, there is modest evidence supporting the benefit of heparin in AMI. Its use is recommended in selected circumstances:[1] (1) patients undergoing PCI or surgical bypass; (2) patients not eligible for fibrinolytic therapy; and (3) patients at risk for systemic emboli.

The major complication of heparin therapy is bleeding. The risk of bleeding can be minimized by dosing heparin based on weight and by following the activated partial thromboplastin time (aPTT). Recent studies have focused on the potential benefit of alternative anticoagulants and platelet antagonists, including low-molecular weight heparin,[62] hirudin[63] and abciximab.[64] The LMWH compounds and GPIIb/IIIa antagonist appears particularly promising.

Warfarin and other coumarin derivatives interfere with the synthesis of vitamin K-dependent clotting factors. Warfarin is given orally, thus providing a mechanism for long-term anticoagulation and should be considered in the following clinical settings:[1] (1) for secondary prevention of MI in patients unable to take daily aspirin; (2) for post-MI patients with atrial fibrillation; and (3) for patients with left ventricular thrombus or extensive wall motion abnormalities. Bleeding is the major risk of warfarin therapy, which can be prevented by careful attention to coagulation measurements (e.g. prothrombin time).

FIBRINOLYTIC THERAPY

There are five fibrinolytic agents approved by the FDA for intravenous administration in AMI:[65] streptokinase (SK); anisoylated plasminogen streptokinase activator complex (APSAC or anistreplase); recombinant tissue-type plasminogen activator (alteplase or r-TPA); reteplase (r-PA); and tNK-tPA. There are significant differences between these agents with respect to circulating half-life, systemic fibrinogen depletion (clot specificity), antigenicity, rate of coronary recanalization and reocclusion, risk of intracerebral hemorrhage (ICH), dose, technique of administration, and cost (Table 5.10).

There have been large scale, multicenter, international, randomized trials comparing fibrinolytic strategies; however, the dominant theme in the ED is reducing time-to-treatment, preferably to 30 minutes or less.[66]

Eligibility criteria for fibrinolytic therapy relate primarily to stratifying patients to maximize potential benefit and minimize complications. The greatest risk of fibrinolytic therapy is bleeding.[67] Intracranial hemorrhage is the most serious complication and up to two-thirds of patients will die.[68] The risk of ICH is increased with hypertension, either by history or on presentation. Thus, fibrinolytics are relatively contraindicated in hypertensive patients with low-risk AMI (inferior ST elevation, or ST depression only). Table 5.11 summarizes the contraindications and cautions for fibrinolytic therapy in AMI.[69,70]

The following guidelines for fibrinolytic therapy are the recommendations of the ACC/AHA.[1]

- Fibrinolytic therapy generally beneficial:
  - ST-segment elevation > 0.1 mV in two or more contiguous leads, 12 hours or less from onset of symptoms and age less than 75 years old.
  - LBBB obscuring ST-segment analysis in the face of a history suggestive of AMI.
- Fibrinolytic therapy probably beneficial:
  - ST-segment elevation and age 75 years or greater.
- Fibrinolytic therapy possibly beneficial:
  - ST-segment elevation and time-to-therapy greater than 12–24 hours.
  - Presenting blood pressure > 180 mm Hg systolic or 110 diastolic in the face of high-risk AMI.
- Fibrinolytic therapy not beneficial, possibly harmful:
  - ST-segment elevation and time-to-therapy > 24 hours, ischemic pain resolved.
  - ST-segment depression only.

PERCUTANEOUS CORONARY INTERVENTION

For AMI, PCI can either be *primary* (instead or in place of thrombolysis) or *salvage* (when PCI has failed).[71]

Theoretical advantages of PCI compared to thrombolysis include direct reopening of the infarct-related vessel,

Table 5.10 *Comparison of fibrinolytic agents*

Agent	Dosing	Cost	Clot specific	Allergic reactions (%)	Reperfusion rate (%)	ICH[a] rate (%)	Lives saved per 100 treated
SK	1.5 million units over 30–60 minutes	$ 280.00	No	4	40	0.3	2.5
APSAC	30 mg over 5 minutes	$1700.00	No	4	60	0.6	2.5
r-TPA	15 mg bolus, then 50 mg over 30 minutes, then 35 mg over 60 minutes	$2200.00	Yes	No	79	0.6	3.5
r-PA	2 boluses of 10 units 30 minutes apart	$2100.00	Yes	No	83	0.6	—
tNK-tPA	0.5 mg/kg (max 50 mg for patients > 90 kg)	$2200.00	Yes	No	79	0.8	—

[a] Intracranial hemorrage.

SK = streptokinase; APSAC = anisoylated plasminogen streptokinase activator complex; r-TPA = alteplase; r-PA = reteplase; tNK-tPA = tenecteplase.

Table 5.11 *Contraindications and cautions for fibrinolytic use in myocardial infarction*

Contraindications

Previous hemorrhagic stroke at any time; other strokes or cerebrovascular events within 1 year

Known intracranial neoplasm, aneurysm or AV malformation

Active internal bleeding (does not include menses)

Pregnancy

Cautions/relative contraindications

Severe uncontrolled hypertension on presentation (blood pressure > 180/110 mm Hg); especially in low-risk acute myocardial infarction

Current use of anticoagulants in therapeutic (INR > 2–3); known bleeding diathesis

Recent trauma (within 2–4 weeks), including head trauma or traumatic or prolonged (>10 minutes) CPR or major surgery (<3 weeks)

Non-compressible vascular puncture or organ biopsy (within 4 weeks)

Recent (within 2–4 weeks) internal bleeding

For streptokinase/anistreplase: prior exposure (especially within 5 days–2 years) or prior allergic reaction to streptokinase

Active peptic ulcer

History of chronic poorly controlled hypertension

AV = arteriovenous; INR = international normalized ratio; CPR = cardiopulmonary resuscitation.

---

avoidance of systemic fibrin depletion, and delineation of coronary anatomy. Disadvantages are cost, need for specially trained personnel and facilities, and potentially longer time-to-patency. A number of studies have been done to compare PCI to thrombolysis for primary therapy of AMI, but to date they have been small. A recent meta-analysis pooled 2023 patients from nine trials in order to have greater statistical power. In this study, there was a borderline statistical benefit of PCI over thrombolysis when the end point was mortality. When both death and rate of AMI were considered, PCI had a clear advantage over thrombolysis (relative risk = 0.2, $P = 0.001$).[72] However, considering that in excess of 100 000 patients have been enrolled in the various thrombolytic trials, the data for PCI are quite limited, and the need for further study is apparent.

Complications of PCI include bleeding at the site of needle puncture, AMI precipitated by balloon inflation, failure to relieve obstruction, reocclusion, and rupture of the coronary artery. The latter event can be catastrophic and requires urgent open heart surgery to repair. For that reason, current guidelines recommend that PCI be performed by experienced personnel, in facilities where emergent access to cardiac surgery is available.[73] However, studies are under way to evaluate the safety and efficacy of PCI in hospitals without cardiac surgery, and broader guidelines may be forthcoming as a result. The role for PCI in AMI will continue to evolve as experience accumulates and newer techniques and strategies are introduced.

CORONARY ARTERY BYPASS GRAFT (CABG) SURGERY

The first coronary bypass surgery was performed in 1964, and within a few years the surgical technique had been refined and standardized. Prior to the advent of fib-rinolytic therapy and PCI, CABG was the only revascularization technique available for AMI. Currently, however, emergency CABG is restricted primarily to circumstances where thrombolysis and/or PCI have failed or are not appropriate.[74]

Anti-ischemic therapy and mortality reduction

There are a number of pharmacologic adjuncts that are used in the treatment of patients with myocardial ischemia and infarction.

β-ADRENORECEPTOR BLOCKING AGENTS

β-Blockers have several potentially beneficial effects on the heart that include a decrease in the force and rate of contraction, and slowing the rate of myocardial depolarization. These actions serve to decrease myocardial oxygen demand. In addition, the decrease in heart rate prolongs diastole and can increase myocardial oxygen delivery, particularly to the penumbra of ischemic tissue surrounding an area of infarction. As a result, β-blockers reduce infarct size and the incidence of complications in patients not given fibrinolytics[75] and reduce the rate of reinfarction in patients who are treated with fibrinolytics.[76] However, these beneficial effects have only been seen in patients given β-blockers early in the course of their infarction (less than 12 hours). Complications from β-adrenoreceptor blocking agents include hypotension, congestive heat failure, and heart block. β-Blockers can also cause bronchoconstriction. The contraindications/cautions to the use of β-blockers in AMI are presented in Table 5.12.

The β-adrenoreceptor blocking agents that have been studied in AMI are atenolol and metoprolol. Atenolol is

Table 5.12 *Contraindications/cautions to β-adrenoreceptor blocking agents in acute myocardial infarction*

Heart rate less than 60 beats/minute
Systolic blood pressure less than 100 mm Hg
Moderate or severe left ventricular failure (Killip class II or greater)
Signs of peripheral hypoperfusion
First-degree atrioventricular block with PR interval >0.25
Second- or third-degree atrioventricular block
Severe chronic obstructive pulmonary disease
Wheezing or a history of asthma
Severe peripheral vascular disease
Insulin-dependent diabetes mellitus

given in two doses of 5 mg intravenously, 10 minutes apart, followed in 15 minutes by an oral dose of 50 mg. Metoprolol is given intravenously as three doses of 5 mg each at 5–10 minute intervals, followed in 15 minutes by an oral dose of 25–50 mg given every 6 to 12 hours depending on heart rate and blood pressure response.

ANGIOTENSIN-CONVERTING ENZYME (ACE) INHIBITORS

ACE inhibitors have been used for years to control elevated blood pressure. More recently, they have been studied for their cardioprotective effects in AMI. ACE inhibitors have been shown to reduce the incidence of CHF and reinfarction and to reduce mortality when given on a long-term basis following AMI.[77] The GISSI-3 study assessed the effects of oral lisinopril in over 19 000 patients,[78] and ISIS-4 studied captopril in over 58 000 patients.[59] A meta-analysis of these two large trials combined with a number of smaller trials, with a total of over 100 000 patients, reported an absolute reduction of 4.6 deaths per 1000 patients treated with ACE inhibitors.[79] A subgroup analysis suggested that the benefits were greatest in patients at highest risk of death (e.g. anterior MI, CHF, previous infarction), but that all patients may benefit from early use of ACE inhibitors.

Ace inhibitors can precipitate hypotension and renal failure. Use should also be avoided when the systolic blood pressure is less than 100 mm Hg or when bilateral renal artery stenosis is present. Furthermore, all agents should be administered orally, since the only trial of an intravenous ACE inhibitor (enalapril) had to be terminated prematurely due to excess morbidity.[80]

There are a variety of ACE inhibitors available for clinical use. Lisinopril (GISSI-3) is given as a 5 mg oral dose (2.5 mg for blood pressure <120 mm Hg) initially and at 24 hours, then 10 mg daily. Captopril therapy (ISIS-4) is initiated with a 6.25 mg oral dose, followed by 12.5 mg after 2 hours, then 25 mg at 12 hours and continued at 50 mg twice a day.

MAGNESIUM

There is considerable experimental evidence that magnesium may be beneficial in cardiovascular disease.[81] Nevertheless, the role of magnesium for cardioprotection in AMI remains controversial. Several small studies, when considered independently and after a meta-analysis, suggested a decrease in both short- and long-term mortality.[82] However, the ISIS-4 trial, which at 58 050 subjects was 20 times the size of the largest of the smaller trials (LIMIT-2), did not reveal benefit.[59] Nevertheless, further analysis suggests that magnesium may be beneficial if given early,[83] especially to the sickest patients[84] and to those who do not qualify for thrombolysis.[85] Additional investigation will be necessary to clarify the issue.

CALCIUM CHANNEL BLOCKERS

There are three commonly used calcium channel blocking agents: nifedipine, verapamil and diltiazem. All are available for oral use in both immediate and sustained-release preparations. The latter two can be given intravenously as well. The calcium channel blockers are used to treat hypertension and angina and there was hope that these drugs would reduce mortality in the setting of AMI. However, after a number of studies, there is no evidence that these agents reduce mortality in AMI or decrease the rate of reinfarction.[86] Furthermore, several studies have suggested increased mortality when these agents are used, particularly immediate release nifedipine, and especially when left ventricule (LV) dysfunction is present.[87,88]

The consensus of the American College of Cardiology/American Heart Association is that calcium channel blockers are overused in the setting of AMI and that β-blockers represent a better choice.[1] Calcium antagonists may be considered for intravenous use for relief of ongoing ischemia or control of rapid atrial fibrillation when β-blockers are ineffective or contraindicated.

Treatment of complications

The major complications associated with MI are arrhythmias and low-output syndromes or 'pump failure'.[89]

Arrhythmias

Ventricular tachycardia (VT)/Ventricular fibrillation (VF)

VF is the most common cause of death early in the course of AMI.[58] In response to ischemia, the myocardium becomes electrically irritable. This is worsened by the release of endogenous catecholamines associated with the pain and anxiety of an MI and further exacerbated by a number of metabolic derangements, including acidosis, hypomagnesemia and hypokalemia. VF is usually, but not always, preceded by VT. The mechanism of VT/VF is thought to be micro-re-entry where an irritable focus of myocardium depolarizes repeatedly in a short circuit effect.[90] VF is a 'non-perfusing rhythm', whereas pulse and blood pressure may or may not be maintained during VT.

Treatment is directed toward abolishing the re-entrant electrical activity, and then aggressively searching for and correcting any aggravating factors. Unstable patients should be treated with an electrical countershock. Stable patients should be treated with the appropriate medication per ACLS guidelines.

Atrial fibrillation (AF)/Supraventricular tachycardia (SVT)

In the setting of suspected AMI, AF, atrial flutter and SVT can be addressed together, since their hemodynamic effects and initial treatments are similar. AF is by far the most common of the three, occurring in about 15 per cent of all AMI patients.[91] The basic problem produced by these rhythms is a rapid ventricular rate, which increases myocardial oxygen demand and therefore worsens ischemia. Too rapid a rate will also interfere with cardiac filling and thus decrease cardiac output, as does the loss of a coordinated atrial contraction.

Treatment is directed toward controlling ventricular rate, and in an unstable patient the treatment of choice is electrical cardioversion. The rationale for cardioversion is straightforward: a patient with worsening ischemia or hypotension requires immediate termination of the arrhythmia. Digoxin is used to slow conduction through the atrioventricular (AV) node, but its effects may not be seen for several hours. β-Blockers and calcium channel blockers with AV node suppressing activity can be used to control ventricular response. Caution is encouraged in patients with heart failure and hypotension. The treatment of choice for SVT in non-AMI patients is adenosine, which briefly interrupts impulse propagation through the AV node and terminates re-entrant arrhythmias. There is limited data regarding its use in the setting of AMI.[56]

Bradyarrhythmias

A slow heart rate, or bradyarrhythmia, can be caused by several abnormalities ranging from sinus node dysfunction to complete AV block. Sinus bradycardia is common in AMI, especially those involving the inferior wall. The primary mechanism is increased parasympathetic (vagal) tone, which suppresses automaticity of the SA node and slows conduction through the AV node. If the rate is slow enough, the patient may experience hypotensive or worsening ischemia. Sinus bradycardia generally responds promptly to treatment and is not an independent marker for increased mortality.[56]

Heart block is divided into first, second, and third degree, with a few subtypes and other conduction abnormalities. There is increased mortality in patients with heart block, because of its association with more extensive myocardial damage. Treatment does not have an impact on long-term survival.[92] Treatment protocols for bradyarrhythmias can be summarized as follows.[89]

- Atropine counteracts the effects of increased vagal tone and is a first line therapy for most bradyarrhythmias.
- Transcutaneous pacing – as a temporizing measure, a slow rhythm may respond to external pacing. This modality is particularly suited for high risk patients at risk for bradyarrhythmias.
- Temporary transvenous pacing – a more dependable pacing method where the pacemaker electrode is introduced percutaneously into a central vein and advanced into the right ventricle. The pacemaker generator itself remains external.
- Permanent implanted pacemaker – reserved for patients who have symptomatic or high-grade conduction abnormalities that persist beyond the acute infarction phase.

Pump failure

Pump failure can be viewed conceptually as forward failure and/or backward failure. In forward failure, the heart is unable to deliver an adequate volume of blood for vital organ perfusion. Clinical findings include low blood pressure, weak pulse, cool and clammy skin, decreased urine output, anxiety and confusion. With backward failure, the heart is unable to accommodate the volume of blood being returned to it, causing passive congestion in the lungs and peripheral venous system. Either or both ventricles can fail, but most commonly it is the left ventricle. LV failure in the setting of AMI can be the result of infarction of a substantial portion of myocardium, widespread ischemia, or rupture of a portion of the heart weakened by infarction.

The most common cause of RV failure is LV failure, with a resultant increase in pulmonary pressures and thus increased RV afterload. However, in AMI, RV infarction can precipitate RV failure. Failure of the RV to deliver an adequate volume of blood to the LV results in systemic hypotension, which is often profound. RV infarction is generally a complication of inferior wall MI and is associated with a substantially greater mortality than IMI without RV infarction (31 per cent vs 6 per cent).[93]

When heart failure is precipitated by myocardial ischemia or infarction, anti-ischemic and reperfusion strategies are indicated. Other specific therapies may be beneficial and are discussed below.

Diuretics

Furosemide and bumetanide are potent agents that can be given intravenously to promote disuresis. Complications include hypokalemia, hypomagnesemia, and hypotension.

Inotropes/vasopressors

Inotropic agents, including dobutamine, dopamine, amrinone and milrinone may be required in patients with pump failure (forward or backward). Vasopressors like norepinephrine, vasopressin and high-dose dopamine are indicated for the treatment of refractory pump failure and septic shock.[1,56,89]

Left ventricular assist devices

Intra-aortic counterpulsation should be considered for patients with cardiogenic shock as a bridge to revascularization or surgical treatment of mechanical defects (e.g. mitral insufficiency, ventricular septal defect).[94] Left ventricular or bi-ventricular assist devices are a consideration in transplant candidates or as destination therapy.

Urgent surgical repair

Urgent surgical repair of an infarct-related mechanical defect may be life saving. Clinical scenarios include rupture of a papillary muscle leading to severe mitral regurgitation, ventricular septal defect, and ventricle free wall rupture. Surgical mortality varies with the nature of the defect, condition of the heart, and existing comorbid factors.

SYSTEM MANAGEMENT

Owing to the unique environments of the prehospital and emergency department settings as well as the time-dependent nature of the evaluation of patients with possible AMI, attention to the specific characteristics of an emergency cardiac care system are critical to optimize patient outcomes. The most important component of this system is utilization of a multidisciplinary approach, with appropriate care planning and coordination between prehospital, emergency department and in-patient providers. Whenever possible, clinical practice should be based on written outcome-centered goals. Key indicators linked to these goals should be continuously monitored.

The most fundamental goals of the emergency cardiac care system are to ensure the immediate evaluation of all patients with symptoms of possible acute myocardial ischemia, to optimize the utilization of early revascularization therapies, and to reduce to zero the number of patients leaving the emergency department with unrecognized AMI.

CLINICAL CONSIDERATIONS

Patient history and the initial ECG provide the most critical data for ED decision making. All patients presenting to an ED with 'ischemic type' chest pain should have a 12-lead ECG performed within 10 minutes of arrival (under standing orders) and the ECG should be handed directly to the treating physician for immediate interpretation. Acquisition of a 12-lead ECG in the prehospital setting can further reduce the time to diagnosis and reperfusion therapy.

The patient's history provides the most useful data for both diagnosis and prognosis. However, owing to the wide variation in presentations among patients with myocardial ischemia, the history alone does not provide adequate information to exclude the possibility of infarction.

During the initial evaluation of patients with chest pain, it is imperative that the clinician maintains a high index of suspicion for other life-threatening conditions that may mimic myocardial ischemia. Pulmonary embolism, aortic dissection, pneumothorax and pericardial tamponade should be considered and excluded.

Utilization of laboratory measurements of myocardial injury provides data supplemental to the history and physical examination and enables more accurate and rapid treatment and disposition decisions. The use of myocardial markers has been shown (1) to facilitate the early diagnosis of AMI in patients with non-diagnostic ECGs, to identify patients with AMI who would otherwise go unrecognized; and (2) to provide prognostic information.

Therapy

Patients with ischemic chest pain should receive intravenous access, oxygen and ECG monitoring. Aspirin, nitroglycerin and morphine are generally of benefit and should be considered in the absence of contraindications.

The primary goal of therapy in AMI is rapid reperfusion of the infarct-related artery. This may be done using a fibrinolytic agent (goal: door-to-drug time < 30 minutes) or by direct PCI (goal: door-to-catheterization time < 60 minutes). In the absence of strong contraindications, fibrinolytic therapy is generally beneficial in patients whose ECG shows ST-segment elevation > 0.1 mV in two or more contiguous leads, 12 hours or less from onset of symptoms and age less than 75 years old, or in those with new or presumed new left bundle branch block obscuring ST-segment analysis in the face of a history suggestive of AMI. Fibrinolytic therapy is also probably beneficial in patients greater than 75 years old with ST-segment elevation.

Several adjuvant therapies may offer significant benefits in lowering mortality and morbidity among patients with AMI and should be considered for use in the ED. Among these agents are antithrombin and antiplatelet drugs, β-blockers, and ACE-inhibitors.

SUMMARY

- The unique characteristics of emergency cardiac care systems must be understood to optimize the care of patients presenting with possible myocardial ischemia.
- The structure and function of emergency cardiac care systems should be driven by a set of well-defined, measurable, patient-centered goals.
- Management protocols for patients with possible acute myocardial ischemia or infarction should be developed using a multidisciplinary approach.
- Acute myocardial ischemia is only one of several potentially life-threatening causes of chest pain. Other diagnoses must be routinely and systematically excluded.
- The history is the single most important tool in evaluating the patient with possible myocardial ischemia, but as atypical presentations are frequent, this must be considered in conjunction with all available data.
- The electrocardiogram and serum markers of myocardial injury are valuable aids for diagnosis and decision making in the emergency department.
- All patients suspected of having acute myocardial ischemia must have certain routine, life-saving measures instituted upon arrival including intravenous access, oxygen and electrocardiographic monitoring.
- Early re-establishment of adequate coronary blood flow is the primary goal of therapy for all patients with acute myocardial infarction.
- A thorough knowledge of current indications and therapeutic affects of available thrombolytic, antithrombin, and antiplatelet agents as well as invasive revascularization techniques is essential.
- Drugs, such as β-adrenergic blocking agents and angiotensin-converting enzyme inhibitors, may also be of benefit.

REFERENCES

1. Ryan TJ, Anderson JL, Antman EM, *et al*. ACC/AHA guidelines for the management of patients with acute myocardial infarction: a report of the American College of Cardiology/American Heart Association Task Force on Practice Guidelines (Committee on Management of Acute Myocardial Infarction). *J Am Coll Cardiol* 1996; **28**: 1328–419.

2. Braunwald E, Mark DB, Jones RH, *et al*. *AHCPR clinical practice guideline #10: Unstable angina; diagnosis and management*. AHCPR Publication #94–0602. US Department of Health and Human Services. May, 1994 (amended).

3. Ornato JP: Problems faced by the urban emergency department in providing rapid triage and intervention for the patient with suspected acute myocardial infarction. *Heart Lung* 1991; **20**: 584.

4. National Heart Attack Alert Program Coordinating Committee, 60 minutes to treatment working group. Emergency department: rapid identification and treatment of patients with acute myocardial infarction. *Ann Emerg Med* 1994; **23**: 311–29.

○5. Green GB, Hansen KN, Chan DW, *et al*. The potential utility of a rapid CK-MB assay in evaluating emergency department patients with possible myocardial infarction. *Ann Emerg Med* 1991; **20**: 954–60.

6. Tierney WM, Fitzgerald J, McHenry R, *et al*. Physicians' estimates of the probability of myocardial infarction in emergency room patients with chest pain. *Med Decision Making* 1986; **6**: 12–17.

7. Eisenberg JM, Horowitz LN, Busch R, *et al*. Diagnosis of acute MI in the emergency room. *J Community Health* 1979; **4**: 190–8.

8. Hedges JR, Rouan GW, Toltzis R, *et al*. Use of cardiac enzymes identifies patients with acute MI otherwise unrecognized in the emergency department. *Ann Emerg Med* 1989; **18**: 1029–34.

○9. Lee TH, Rouan G, Weisberg M, *et al*. Patients with acute myocardial infarction sent home from the emergency room: clinical characteristics and natural history. *Am J Cardiol* 1987; **60**: 219–24.

10. Baxt WG. Use of an artificial neural network for the diagnosis of myocardial infarction. *Ann Intern Med* 1991; **115**: 843–8.

11. Rusnack RA, Stair TO, Hansen D, *et al*. Litigation against the emergency physician: common features in cases of missed myocardial infarction. *Ann Emerg Med* 1989; **18**: 1029–34.

12. Rouan GW, Hedges JR, Toltzis R, Goldstein-Wayne B, Brand D, Goldman L. A chest clinic to improve the follow-up of patients released from an urban university teaching hospital emergency department. *Ann Emerg Med* 1987; **16**: 1145–50.

13. Gibler WB, Runyon JP, Ley RC, *et al*. A rapid diagnostic and treatment center for patients with chest pain in the emergency department. *Ann Emerg Med* 1995; **25**: 1–8.

14. Donavan MR, Keeler ML. The chest pain ED. In: Riggs L Jr, ed. *Emergency department design*. Dallas, TX: American College of Emergency Physicians, 1993: 277–83.

15. American Institute of Architects Committee on Architecture for Health. *1992–1993 guidelines for construction and equipment of hospitals and medical facilities*. Washington, DC: American Institute of Architects Press, 1993.

16. Kereiakes DJ, Gibler WB, Martin LH, *et al*. Relative importance of emergency medical system transport and the prehospital electrocardiogram on reducing hospital time delay to therapy for acute myocardial infarction. *Am Heart J* 1992; **23**: 835–40.

17. Karagounis L, Ipsen SK, Jessop MR, *et al*. Impact of field-transmitted electrocardiography on time to in-hospital therapy in acute myocardial infarction. *Am J Cardiol* 1990; **66**: 786–91.

18. Grim P, Feldman T, Martin M, *et al*. Cellular telephone transmission of 12-lead electrocardiograms for ambulance to hospital. *Am J Cardiol* 1987; **60**: 715–20.

19. Aufderheide TP, Hendley GE, Woo J, *et al*. A prospective evaluation of prehospital 12-lead ECG application in chest pain patients. *J Electrocardiol* 1992; **24S**: 8–13.

♦20. Selker HP, Zalenski RJ, Antman EM, *et al*. An evaluation of technologies for identifying acute cardiac ischemia in the emergency department: a report from a national heart attack alert program working group. *Ann Emerg Med* 1997; **29**: 13–87 (20–24).

21. Aufderheide TP, Keelan MH, Hendley GE, *et al*. Milwaukee prehospital chest pain project: feasibility and accuracy of prehospital thrombolytic candidate selection. *Am J Cardiol* 1992; **69**: 991–6.

22. Rawles J, on behalf of the GREAT Group. Halving of mortality at 1 year by domiciliary thrombolysis in the Grampian region early anistreplase trial. *J Am Coll Cardiol* 1994; **23**: 1–5.

23. The European Myocardial Infarction Project Group: Prehospital thrombolytic therapy in patients with suspected acute myocardial infarction. *N Engl J Med* 1993; **329**: 383–9.

24. Weaver WD, Cerqueira M, Hallstrom AP, *et al*; Prehospital initiated vs hospital initiated thrombolytic therapy. The myocardial infarction and intervention trial. *JAMA* 1993; **270**: 1211–16.

25. McGuiness JB, Begg TB, Semple T. First electro-cardiogram in recent myocardial infarction. *Br Med J* 1976; **2**: 449–51.

26. Silber SH, Leo PJ, Katapadi M. Serial electro-cardiograms for chest pain patients with initial nondiagnostic electrocardiograms: implications for thrombolytic therapy. *Acad Emerg Med* 1996; **3**: 147–52.

27. Zalenski RJ, Rydman RJ, Sloan EP, *et al*. Value of posterior and right ventricular leads in comparison to the standard 12-lead ECG in evaluation of ST-segment elevation in suspected acute myocardial infarction. *Am J Cardiol* 1997; **79**: 1579–85.

28. Justis DL, Hession WT. Accuracy of 22-lead ECG analysis for diagnosis of acute myocardial infarction and coronary artery disease in the emergency department: a comparison with 12-lead ECG. *Ann Emerg Med* 1992; **21**: 1–9.

29. Fu GY, Joseph AJ, Antalis G. Application of continuous ST-segment monitoring in the detection of silent myocardial ischemia. *Ann Emerg Med* 1994; **23**: 1113–15.

30. Brush JE, Brand DA, Acampora D, Chalmer B, Wackers F. Use of the initial electrocardiogram to predict in-hospital complications of acute myocardial infarction. *N Engl J Med* 1985; **312**: 1137–41.

31. Zalenski RJ, Rydman RJ, Sloan EP, Caceres L, Murphy DG, Cooke D. The emergency department ECG and hospital complications in myocardial infarction patients. *Acad Emerg Med* 1996; **3**: 318–25.

32. Lee TH, Cook EF, Weisberg M. Acute chest pain in the emergency room: identification and examination of low risk patients. *Arch Intern Med* 1985; **145**: 65–9.

33. Eisenberg JM, Horowitz LN, Busch R, Arvan D, Rawnsley H. Diagnosis of acute myocardial infarction in the emergency room: a prospective assessment of clinical decision making and the usefulness of immediate cardiac enzyme determination. *J Community Health* 1979; **4**: 190–8.

♦34. Gibler WB, Lewis LM, Erb RE, *et al*. Early detection of acute myocardial infarction in patients presenting with chest pain and nondiagnostic ECGs: serial CK-MB sampling in the emergency department. *Ann Emerg Med* 1990; **19**: 1359–66.

35. Marin MM, Teichman SL. Use of rapid serial sampling of creatine kinase MB for very early detection of myocardial infarction in patients with acute chest pain. *Am Heart J* 1992; **123**: 354–61.

36. Gibler WB, Young GP, Hedges JR, *et al*. The Emergency Medicine Cardiac Research Group: acute myocardial infarction in chest pain patients with nondiagnostic ECGs: serial CK-MB sampling in the emergency department. *Ann Emerg Med* 1992; **21**: 504–12.

37. Gibler WB, Gibler CD, Weinshenker E, *et al*. Myoglobin as an early indicator of acute myocardial infarction. *Ann Emerg Med* 1987; **16**: 851–6.

38. Tucker JF, Collins RA, Anderson RA, *et al*. Accuracy of serial serum CK, CK-MB, and myoglobin levels in the emergency department evaluation of acute myocardial infarction. In: *Myoglobin: an aid in the early detection of myocardial infarction*. Baxter Diagnostic Inc., 1994: 12.

39. Hedges JR, Gibler WB, Young GP, *et al*. Multicenter study of creatine kinase MB use: effect on chest pain clinical decision making. *Acad Emerg Med*; **3**: 7–15.

40. Hedges JR, Young GP, Henkel GF, *et al*. Early CK-MB elevations predict ischemic events in stable chest pain patients. *Acad Emerg Med* 1994; **1**: 9–16.

41. Hoekstra JW, Hedges JR, Gibler WB, *et al*. Emergency department CK-MB: a predictor of ischemic complications. *Acad Emerg Med* 1994; **1**: 17–28.

◆42. Hamm CW, Ravkilde J, Gerhardt W, *et al.* The prognostic value of serum troponin T in unstable angina. *N Engl J Med* 1992; **327**: 146–50.

43. Green GB, Beaudreau R, Chan DW, McGreivy TS, Baskerville M, Kelen GD. Troponin T for risk stratification of ED patients with possible myocardial ischemia. *Ann Emerg Med* 1998; **31**: 19–29.

44. Green GB, Li DJ, Bessman ES, Cox JL, Kelen GD, Chan DW. The prognostic significance of troponin I and troponin T. *Acad Emerg Med* 1998; **5**: 758–67.

45. Schor S, Behar S, Modan B, *et al.* Disposition of presumed coronary patients from an emergency room: a follow-up study. *JAMA* 1976; **236**: 941–3.

46. Selker HP, Griffith JL, Dorey FJ, *et al.* How do physicians adapt when the coronary care unit is full? *JAMA* 1987; **257**: 1181–5.

47. Goldman L, Cook EF, Brand DA, *et al.* A computer protocol to predict myocardial infarction in emergency department patients with chest pain. *N Engl J Med* 1988; **318**: 797–803.

48. Lee TH, Pearson SD, Johnson PA, *et al.* Failure of information as an intervention to modify clinical management in a time-series trial in patients with acute chest pain. *Ann Intern Med* 1995; **122**: 434–7.

49. Pozen MW, D'Agostino RB, Selker HP, *et al.* A predictive instrument to improve coronary care unit admission practices in acute ischemic heart disease: a prospective multicenter clinical trial. *N Engl J Med* 1984; **310**: 1273–8.

◆50. Selker HP, Griffith JL, D'Agostino RB. A tool for judging coronary care unit admission appropriateness, valid for both real-time and retrospective use: a time-insensitive predictive instrument (TIPI) for acute cardiac ischemia. *Med Care* 1991; **29**: 610–27.

51. Baxt WG. Use of an artificial neural network for the diagnosis of myocardial infarction. *Ann Intern Med* 1991; **115**: 843–8.

52. Sarasin FP, Reymond JM, Griffith JL, *et al.* Impact of the acute cardiac ischemia time-insensitive predictive instrument (ACI-TIPI) on the speed of triage decision making for emergency department patients presenting with chest pain. *J Gen Intern Med* 1994; **9**: 187–94.

53. Selker HP, D'Agostino RB, Laks MM. A predictive instrument for acute ischemic heart disease to improve coronary care unit admission practices: a potential on-line tool in a computerized electrocardiograph. *J Electrocardiog* 1988; **21**: S11–17.

54. Griffith JL, Beshanshy JR, Selker HP, for the TIPI working group. A multi-center prospective test of electrocardiograph generated ACI-TIPI predictions for acute cardiac ischemia. *J Invest Med* 1995; **43**: 215A (abstract).

55. Baxt WG. Prospective validation of an artificial neural network for identifying the presence of acute myocardial infarction. *Acad Emerg Med* 1994; **1**: A5 (abstract).

56. Antman EM, Braunwald ED. Acute myocardial infarction. In: Braunwald ED, ed. *Heart disease: A textbook of cardiovascular medicine*, 5th edn. Philadelphia: WB Saunders, 1997: 1185.

57. Hermens WT, Willems GM, Nijssen KM, Simoons ML. Effect of thrombolytic treatment delay on myocardial infarct size. *Lancet* 1992; **340**: 1297(letter).

58. Gunby P. Cardiovascular disease remains nation's leading cause of death. *JAMA* 1992; **267**: 335.

◆59. ISIS-4: a randomized factorial trial assessing early oral captopril, oral mononitrate, and intravenous magnesium sulphate in 58,050 patients with suspected acute myocardial infarction. *Lancet* 1995; **345**: 669–85.

◆60. ISIS-2 (Second International Study of Infarct Survival) Collaborative Group. Randomized trial of intravenous streptokinase, oral aspirin, both, or neither among 17,187 cases of suspected acute myocardial infarction: ISIS-2. *Lancet* 1988; **2**: 349–60.

61. Mizuno K, Satomura K, Miyamoto A, *et al.* Angioscopic evaluation of coronary-artery thrombi in acute coronary syndromes. *N Engl J Med* 1992; **326**: 287–91.

62. Garfunkel EP, Manos EJ, Mejail RI, *et al.* Low molecular weight heparin versus regular heparin or aspinin in the treatment of unstable angina and silent ischemia. *J Am Coll Cardiol* 1995; **26**: 313–18.

63. Antman EM. Hirudin in acute myocardial infarction: thrombolysis and thrombin inhibition in myocardial infarction (TIMI) 9B trial. *Circulation* 1996; **94**: 911–21.

◆64. Tcheng JE. Glycoprotein IIb/IIIa receptor inhibitors: putting the EPIC, IMPACT II, RESTORE, and EPILOG trials into perspective. *Am J Cardiol* 1996; **78**: 35–40.

65. Sherry S. *Fibrinolysis, thrombosis, and hemostasis: concepts, perspectives, and clinical applications.* Philadelphia: Lea & Febiger; 1992: 119–60.

66. Fendrick AM, Ridker PM, Bloom BS. Improved health benefits in increased use of thrombolytic therapy. *Arch Intern Med* 1994; **154**: 1605–9.

67. Sane DC, Califf RM, Topol EJ, *et al.* Bleeding during thrombolytic therapy for acute myocardial infarction: mechanisms and management. *Ann Intern Med* 1989; **111**: 1010–22.

68. Fibrinolytic Therapy Trialists' Collaborative Group (FTT). Indications for fibrinolytic therapy in suspected acute myocardial infarction: collaborative overview of early mortality and major morbidity results from all randomized trails of more than 1000 patients. *Lancet* 1994; **343**: 311–22.

69. Anderson JL, Karagounis LA. Does intravenous heparin or time-to-treatment/reperfusion explain differences between GUSTO and ISIS-3 results? *Am J Cardiol* 1994; **74**: 1057–60.

70. Cannon CP, McCabe CH, Diver DJ, *et al.* Comparison of front-loaded recombinant tissue-type plasminogen activator, anistreplase and combination thrombolytic therapy for acute myocardial infarction: results of the

thrombolysis in MI (TIMI) 4 trial. *J Am Coll Cardiol* 1994; **24**: 1602–10.

71. Lincoff AM, Topol EJ. Interventional catheterization techniques. In: Braunwald ED, ed. Heart disease: a textbook of cardiovascular medicine, 5th edn. Philadelphia: WB Saunders, 1997: 1366–9.

72. Simes JR, Weaver DW, Ellis SG, *et al*. Overview of the randomized trials of primary PTCA and thrombolysis in acute myocardial infarction. *Circulation* 1996; **94**(suppl): I-331 (abstract).

73. Ryan TJ, Bauman WB, Kennedy JW, *et al*. ACC/AHA guidelines for percutaneous transluminal coronary angioplasty; a report of the ACC/AHA task force on the assessment of diagnostic and therapeutic cardiovascular procedures (subcommittee on percutaneous transluminal coronary angioplasty). *J Am Coll Cardiol* 1993; **22**: 2033–54.

74. Kirklin JK, Akins CW, Blackstone EH, *et al*. Guidelines and indications for coronary artery bypass graft surgery; a report of the ACC/AHA task force on assessment of diagnostic and therapeutic cardiovascular procedures (subcommittee on coronary artery bypass graft surgery). *J Am Coll Cardiol* 1991; **17**: 543–89.

75. Yusef S, Peto R, Lewis J, Collins R, Sleight P. Beta blockade during and after myocardial infarction: an overview of the randomized trials. *Prog Cardiovasc Dis* 1985; **27**: 335–71.

76. The TIMI Study Group. Comparison of invasive and conservative strategies after treatment with intravenous tissue plasminogen activator in acute myocardial infarction: results of the Thrombolysis in Myocardial Infarction (TIMI) phase II trial. *N Engl J Med* 1989; **320**: 618–27.

♦77. Pfeffer MA, Braunwald E, Moye LA, *et al*. Effect of captopril on mortality and morbidity in patients with left ventricular dysfunction after myocardial infarction: results of the survival and ventricular enlargement trial (SAVE). *N Engl J Med* 1992; **327**: 669–77.

78. GISSI-3 Study Group. Effects of lisinopril and transdermal glyceryl trinitrate singly and together on 6-week mortality and ventricular function after acute myocardial infarction. *Lancet* 1994; **343**: 1115–22.

79. Latini R, Maggioni AP, Flather M, Sleight P, Tognoni G. ACE-inhibitor use in patients with myocardial infarction: summary of evidence from clinical trials. *Circulation* 1995; **92**: 3132–7.

80. Sigurdsson A, Swedberg K. Left ventricular remodelling, neurohormonal activation and early treatment with enalapril (CONSENSUS II) following

myocardial infarction. *Eur Heart J* 1994; **15**(suppl 1B): 14–19.

81. Arsenian MA. Magnesium and cardiovascular disease. *Prog Cardiovasc Dis* 1993; **35**: 271–310.

○82. Antman EM, Lau J, Kupelnick B, Mosteller F, Chalmers TC. A comparison of results of meta-analyses of randomized control trials and recommendations of clinical experts: treatments for myocardial infarction. *JAMA* 1992; **268**: 240–8.

83. Antman EM. Magnesium in acute MI: timing is critical. *Circulation* 1995; **92**: 2367–72.

84. Antman EM. Randomized trials of magnesium in acute myocardial infarction: big numbers do not tell the whole story. *Am J Cardiol* 1995; **75**: 391–3.

85. Schechter M, Hod H, Chouraqui P, Kaplinsky E, Rabinowitz B. Magnesium therapy in acute myocardial infarction when patients are not candidates for thrombolytic therapy. *Am J Cardiol* 1995; **75**: 321–3.

86. Held P, Yusuf S, Furberg CD. Calcium channel blockers in acute myocardial infarction and unstable angina: an overview. *Br Med J* 1989; **229**: 1187–92.

87. Opie LH, Messerli FH. Nifedipine and mortality: grave defects in the dossier. *Circulation* 1995; **92**: 1068–73.

88. Held PH, Yusuf S. Effects of beta-blockers and calcium blockers in acute myocardial infarction. *Eur Heart J* 1993; **14**(suppl F): 18–25.

89. Cummins RO, ed. *Textbook of advanced cardiac life support*. American Heart Association, 1994.

90. Campbell RWF. Arrhythmias. In: Julain DG, Braunwald E, eds *Management of acute myocardial infarction*. London: WB Saunders, 1994: 223–40.

91. Madias JE, Patel DC, Singh D. Atrial fibrillation in acute myocardial infarction. A prospective study based on data from a consecutive series of patients admitted to the coronary care unit. *Clin Cardiol* 1996; **19**: 180.

92. Berger PB, Ruocco NA Jr, Ryan TJ, Frederick MM, Jacobs AK, Faxon DP. Incidence and prognostic implications of heart block complicating inferior myocardial infarction treated with thrombolytic therapy; results from TIMI-II. *J Am Coll Cardiol* 1992; **21**: 533–40.

♦93. Zehender M, Kasper W, Dauder E, *et al*. Right ventricular infarction as an independent predictor of prognosis after acute inferior myocardial infarction. *N Engl J Med* 1993; **328**: 981–8.

94. Bengtson JR, Kaplan AJ, Pieper KS, *et al*. Prognosis in cardiogenic shock after myocardial infarction in the interventional era. *J Am Coll Cardiol* 1992; **20**: 1482–9.

6

Observation units, clinical decision units, and chest pain centers

WILLIAM R LEWIS AND EZRA A AMSTERDAM

Studies during the last several decades have demonstrated that low-risk patients presenting with chest pain can be recognized by clinical criteria, including the history, physical examination and initial electrocardiogram (ECG).[1-3] Management of these patients differs fundamentally from that of high-risk patients who require urgent initiation of time-dependent coronary reperfusion therapy and other anti-ischemic modalities. To fulfill the dichotomous therapeutic requirements of both high- and low-risk patients presenting with chest pain, innovative strategies have been developed that include management guidelines, clinical algorithms, predictive instruments, chest pain observation units and new diagnostic technologies. The objectives of these methods are: 1) triage of high-risk patients into fast track therapy and 2) recognition of low-risk patients for assignment to more deliberate evaluation and treatment. Avoidance of unnecessary admissions is a major goal in the latter group. This chapter presents the current status of evolving methods to achieve these clinical objectives, with the focus on identification and management of low-risk patients.

INTRODUCTION

Safe, cost-effective management of patients presenting to the emergency department (ED) because of chest pain compatible with myocardial ischemia continues to present a major clinical challenge.[1-3b] Current standards mandate rapid institution of proven therapy for reduction of mortality and morbidity of patients with acute coronary syndromes.[4,5] However, in most patients presenting to the ED with chest pain, this symptom is related to disorders without fatal potential, such as musculoskeletal, gastroesophageal or anxiety syndromes,[1,2] in which an erroneous impression of myocardial ischemia can prompt unwarranted hospital admission, resulting in unnecessary tests and major costs. The balance of these opposing factors has traditionally favored a low threshold for admission for chest pain of possible cardiac origin because of primary concern for patient welfare, as well as litigation potential for failure to detect a coronary event. This approach is consistent with the directive of early innovators of the coronary care unit (CCU) that 'Patients should be admitted to the CCU solely on suspicion of having an acute myocardial infarction'.[6]

A low threshold for admission of these patients has also been supported by reports of a 2–10 per cent rate of missed myocardial infarction (MI) in patients discharged from the ED.[7,7a]

Underscoring this problem are data that failure to diagnose MI is the leading cause of malpractice awards against emergency medicine physicians, accounting for 21 per cent of total litigation costs to this group.[8] However, application of a low threshold for admission has resulted in annual hospitalization of two million patients in whom a coronary event is diagnosed in less than 20 per cent[9] at a cost of more than $10 billion.[10] The term 'rule-out MI', or 'ROMI', has traditionally been applied to patients admitted for findings suggestive, but not diagnostic, of acute MI and these patients comprise the great majority of those admitted for evaluation of chest pain.[9]

> Studies during the last several decades have demonstrated that low-risk patients presenting with chest pain can be recognized by clinical criteria, including the history, physical examination and initial electrocardiogram (ECG).[1–3b] Management of these patients differs fundamentally from that of high-risk patients who require urgent initiation of time-dependent coronary reperfusion therapy and other anti-ischemic modalities.

To fulfill the dichotomous therapeutic requirements of both high- and low-risk patients presenting with chest pain, innovative strategies have been developed that include management guidelines, clinical algorithms, predictive instruments, chest pain observation units, and new diagnostic technologies.

> The objectives of these methods are: (1) triage of high-risk patients into fast track therapy; and (2) recognition of low-risk patients for assignment to more deliberate evaluation and treatment.

Avoidance of unnecessary admissions is a major goal in the latter group. This chapter presents the current status of evolving methods to achieve these clinical objectives, with the focus on identification and management of low-risk patients.

BASIC APPROACH TO THE PATIENT WITH ACUTE CHEST PAIN

Figure 6.1 depicts the diagnostic spectrum of patients presenting to the emergency department with non-traumatic chest pain compatible with myocardial ischemia. Although the final diagnosis requires complete evaluation, management begins with the initial clinical assessment, in which the key factors are the history, physical examination and ECG. Blood is also obtained for measurement of cardiac serum markers (Table 6.1, Fig. 6.2).

As indicated in Fig. 6.1, the ECG is the critical determinant in the early differentiation of patients presenting with chest pain. ST-segment elevation reflects evolving Q-wave MI, which identifies potential candidates for coronary reperfusion therapy. These patients should be rapidly triaged into a fast-track protocol to facilitate reperfusion and other therapy if clinically appropriate. Patients with *non-Q MI* and *unstable angina* may have ECG changes consistent with ischemia, non-specific ECG abnormalities or normal findings (non-ST elevation). Differentiation between non-Q MI and unstable angina, syndromes on the pathophysiologic continuum of myocardial ischemia,[11] is based on elevation of serum markers of cardiac injury (Table 6.1, Fig. 6.2) in the former. This distinction can only be made retrospectively

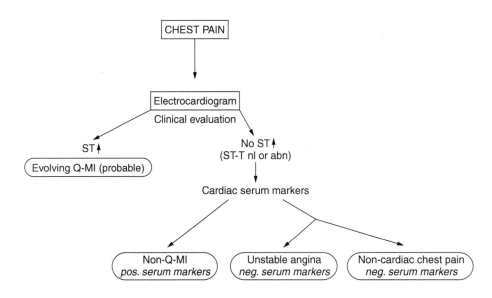

Figure 6.1 *Initial classification of patients presenting with chest pain. MI = myocardial infarction; nl = normal; abn = abnormal; pos. = positive; neg. = negative.*

Table 6.1 *Serum markers of acute myocardial infarction. (Adapted with permission from Ryan TJ, Anderson JL, Antman EM, et al. ACC/AHA guidelines for the management of patients with acute myocardial infarction. A report of the American College of Cardiology/American Heart Association Task Force on Practice Guidelines (Committee on Management of Acute Myocardial Infarction).* J Am Coll Cardiol *1996;* **28**: *1328–1428. © 1996 by the American College of Cardiology and American Heart Association, Inc.)*

| | | Cardiac traponins | | | | |
	Myoglobin	cTnI		cTnT	CK-MB	MB isoforms
Molecular weight (kDa)	17	23		33	86	86
First detectable (hours)	1–2		2–4		3–4	2–4
100% sensitivity (hours)	4–8		8–12		8–12	6–10
Peak (hours)	4–8		10–24		10–24	6–12
Duration (days)	(0.5–1.0)	5–10		5–14	2–4	0.5–1.0

cTnI = cardiac specific troponin I; cTnT = cardiac specific troponin T; CK-MB = myocardial band of creatine kinase.

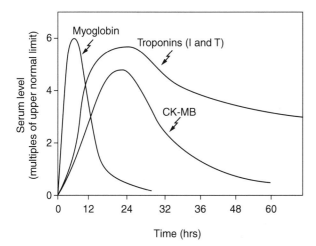

Figure 6.2 *Patterns of evolution of serum markers after onset of myocardial necrosis. (Reproduced with permission from Amsterdam EA, Lewis WR, Yadlapalli S. Evaluation of low risk patients with chest pain in the emergency department.* Cardiol Rev *1999;* **7**: *17–26.)*

because of the lag in elevation of serum markers after infarction. In addition, this differentiation has become blurred in that 20 per cent or more of patients with the diagnosis of unstable angina and negative creatine kinase myocardial band (MB) levels have elevated troponin values.[12]

> The presence of ECG evidence of ischemia defines high clinical risk among these patients and is an indication for anti-ischemic therapy and admission to either the cardiac care unit or telemetry unit, depending on the patient's clinical status (symptoms, blood pressure, cardiac rhythm, evidence of cardiac failure), prior evidence of coronary artery disease (CAD), or coronary risk profile in the absence of documented CAD.

Absence of ECG alterations and normal serum markers may occur in low-risk patients with unstable angina and is common in patients with *non-cardiac chest pain*. Stable angina must also be considered in this group. Depending on the clinical status of these patients at the time of presentation, they may undergo observation in a short-stay unit or be discharged directly from the ED.

> Further evaluation by non-invasive testing is usually performed either before discharge or shortly thereafter.

Finally, many patients in the low-risk group will have non-cardiac chest pain and the main etiologies of this problem must be considered in them.[2,3a]

> Regardless of the ultimate diagnosis (non-Q MI, low-risk unstable angina, stable angina or non-cardiac chest pain), patients identified as low risk on presentation by the foregoing clinical criteria (prior to serum marker data) do not require direct admission for intensive cardiac care and can be observed in a telemetry unit or short-stay unit while further evaluation by ECG monitoring and measurement of serum markers is performed for a 6–12-hour period, depending on institutional practice and the specific factors in the individual patient.

If serum markers are positive, the diagnosis becomes non-Q MI and the patient is admitted to the in-patient service. A negative evaluation allows early discharge with further assessment for myocardial ischemia by functional testing either before or shortly after discharge. Shorter observation periods are usually associated with predischarge functional testing to provide a further margin of safety. In our ED, we perform immediate exercise testing (IET) in patients identified as low risk with or without measurement of serum markers, depending on the indications in the individual patient. Because

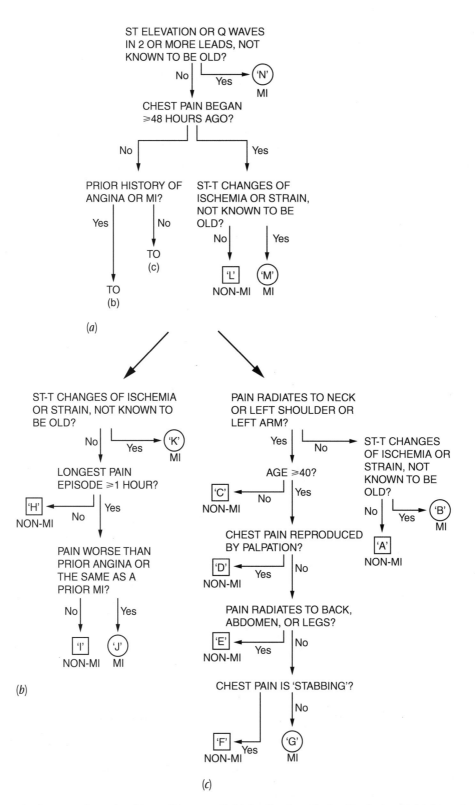

Figure 6.3 *Elements of a computer protocol to predict myocardial infarction in patients with chest pain. (a) Computer protocol for the evaluation of patients with acute chest pain in the emergency department. (b) Questions to be asked of patients with a history of angina or myocardial infarction who do not have new ST-segment elevation or Q waves and whose pain began less than 48 hours previously. MI = myocardial infarction. (c) Questions to be asked of patients with no history of angina or myocardial infarction and no new ST-segment elevation or Q waves on the electrocardiogram whose pain began less than 48 hours previously. (Reproduced with permission from Goldman L, Cook EF, Brand DA, et al. A computer protocol to predict myocardial infarction in emergency department patients with chest pain. N Engl J Med 1988; **318**: 797–803. Copyright © 1988 Massachusetts Medical Society. All rights reserved.)*

patients identified as low risk comprise the majority of those presenting with chest pain,[2,3,9,13] each of these strategies has the potential to afford enhanced cost-effective management by avoiding unnecessary admissions and improving utilization of resources while maintaining proper patient care.

CLINICAL IDENTIFICATION OF LOW RISK

Evidence that low-risk patients can be recognized by clinical factors at the time of presentation in the ED has accumulated over the last several decades. In patients admitted for ROMI, those with a probability of less than 5 per cent for acute MI were identified by the type of chest pain, cardiac history and initial ECG.[13] Extension of this approach to over 10 000 such patients showed that the initial clinical assessment could distinguish those with less than 1 per cent probability of major complications.[14] The ECG alone provides important prognostic data. Thus, Schroeder and colleagues reported that, in patients admitted with chest pain in whom MI was ruled out, ECG evidence of ischemia was associated with a 1-year mortality similar to that of MI patients.[15] Moreover, Gazes et al. reported that a normal ECG in patients admitted for 'preinfarction angina' was associated with benign early and late outcomes, while ECG evidence of ischemia correlated with markedly increased cardiac morbidity and mortality.[16] The utility of the initial ECG in patients admitted for ROMI was confirmed by Brush et al., who found that a normal or near-normal ECG on admission was associated with a 0.6 per cent occurrence of serious complications during hospitalization compared with a 14 per cent incidence in patients with abnormal ECGs.[17] An important concept to emerge from these studies is that, while the etiology of chest pain is frequently elusive, the ability to determine the patient's risk for cardiac morbidity and mortality can promote appropriate management.

Predictive instruments

The prognostic utility of clinical predictors in patients with chest pain has been further refined by computer analysis. The Goldman Chest Pain Protocol is a computer-derived decision aid developed from prospectively collected data on 1379 patients[18] and subsequently confirmed in 4770 patients[19] (Fig. 6.3). The protocol was shown to have the same sensitivity for predicting acute MI as the admitting physician's clinical judgment, but was more specific. This indicates that the protocol was superior for predicting the absence of acute MI compared to physicians' clinical impressions. Use of the protocol could therefore allow for triage of low-acuity patients, typical of the ROMI population, to intermediate care beds with a potential for approximately $85 mil-

lion annual cost savings. However, a prospective clinical trial of this instrument failed to confirm the predicted cost savings, since rates of admission during intervention and control periods were unchanged for the hospital (52 per cent and 51 per cent, respectively) and the cardiac care unit (each 10 per cent).[20]

Another computer program, the Original Acute Coronary Ischemia Predictive Instrument, yields a patient's probability (from 0 to 100 per cent) of having acute coronary ischemia (ACI). A pilot study[21] and a large validation trial were carried out.[22] The latter was multicenter and included 2801 patients. Of 59 clinical features studied, seven factors were selected for their predictive accuracy: presence or absence of chest pain or left arm pain/discomfort, chest or left arm discomfort as the primary presenting symptom, history of MI, history of nitroglycerine use for chest pain, ECG ST-segment flattening in two or more leads, ECG ST-segment elevation or depression of 1 mm or greater in two or more leads, and ECG T-wave inversion in two or more leads. The original ACI predictive instrument can be programmed into a hand-held calculator or carried as a printed table (Table 6.2).[23]

> Studies of this instrument's performance have shown increased specificity in diagnosing ACI without a change in sensitivity. Cardiac care unit admission rates were significantly lower for patients without ACI by further evaluation during experimental periods compared to control periods (17 per cent *vs* 24 per cent, respectively).

In addition, the rate of direct discharges from the ED increased from 44 to 51 per cent with use of the predictive instrument. For patients with less than a 50 per cent likelihood of having ACI, there was a 22 per cent reduction in the rate of false-positive diagnoses during experimental periods, whereas there was no change for patients having a greater than 50 per cent likelihood of having ACI. The original ACI predictive instrument has since been modified for time insensitivity so that it can be used for retrospective analysis of patients and can be included in computer-generated ECG readings. When the instrument was included in the computer-generated ECG reading of 10 689 patient in 10 hospitals, there was a significant reduction in overutilization of resources.[24,25] For patients without cardiac ischemia evaluated by unsupervised residents, use of ACI-TIPI was associated with a 32 per cent reduction in CCU admissions; a 20 per cent reduction in telemetry unit admissions; and a 25 per cent increase in discharges to home. Among patients with stable angina, in hospitals with high-capacity telemetry units, use of ACI-TIPI was associated with a reduction in telemetry unit admissions from 68 per cent to 59 per cent, and an increase in emergency department discharges to home from 10 per cent to 21 per cent. Among patients with acute myocardial infarc-

Table 6.2 *The predictive instrument's probabilities (%) of acute ischemic heart disease for emergency department patients. (Reproduced with permission from McCarthy BD, Wong JB, Selker HP. Detecting acute cardiac ischemia in the emergency department; a review of the literature. J Gen Int Med 1990; 5: 365–73.)*

	Electrocardiogram (ECG) abnormality					
	STØ TØ (%)	ST↔ TØ (%)	STØ T↑↓ (%)	ST↑↓ TØ (%)	ST↔ T↑↓ (%)	ST↑↓ T↑↓ (%)
A Chief complaint of chest pain or pressure, or left arm pain						
No heart attack *and* no NTG use	19	35	42	54	62	78
Either heart attack *or* NTG use (not both)	27	46	53	64	73	85
Both heart attack *and* NTG use	37	58	65	75	80	90
B Complaint of chest pain or pressure, or left arm pain, but not chief complaint						
No heart attack *and* no NTG use	10	21	26	36	45	64
Either heart attack *or* NTG use (*not both*)	16	29	36	48	56	74
Both heart attack *and* NTG use	22	40	47	59	67	82
C No complaint of chest pain or pressure, or left arm pain						
No heart attack *and* no NTG use	4	9	12	17	23	39
Either heart attack *or* NTG use (*not both*)	6	14	17	25	32	51
Both heart attack *and* NTG use	10	20	25	35	43	62

A, B, and C group patients by whether chest pain and/or left arm pain is present and whether this is the chief complaint. 'Heart attack' indicates a history of heart attack, and 'NTG' indicates a history of nitroglycerin use, ST↔ refers to ST-segment 'straightening, flattening, or barring'; ST↑↓ refers to ST-segment elevation or depression of at least 1 mm; ST Ø refers to the absence of any of these findings; T↑↓ refers to 'hyperacute' (at least 50 per cent of the R-wave amptitude) T-waves or inverted T-waves depressed at least 1 mm; T Ø refers to the absence of either of these findings. Notice that ECG changes must be present in at least two leads, excluding aV$_R$.

tion or unstable angina, use of ACI-TIPI did not change appropriate admission (96 per cent) to the CCU or telemetry units.

Thus the ACI predictive instrument, similar to the Goldman Chest Pain Protocol, is most helpful for accurately triaging patients with a lower risk of having ACI to appropriately lower levels of care.

CLINICAL PRACTICE GUIDELINES, CRITICAL CARE PATHWAYS, ALGORITHMS, AND PROTOCOLS

Guidelines are a recent development in medical practice and their growth has been particularly rapid in cardiology in relation to the profusion of diagnostic methods and therapeutic modalities in this field.[3a] Guidelines are a means of achieving uniformly high standards of patient management through the most effective utilization of resources.

They are not meant to replace the physician's clinical judgment but rather to provide a frame of reference within which to consider proven or recommended therapy and to identify questionable practices.

By prospectively outlining management of specific clinical conditions, guidelines reduce the likelihood of omission of important treatments, a problem of major magnitude in the current therapy of cardiovascular disease.[26] Because of differences in resources, personnel and expertise, cardiology practice guidelines have also been developed by, and tailored to, the needs of local groups and individual institutions. The recently published guidelines of the American Heart Association/American College of Cardiology (AHA/ACC) for management of patients with acute MI[27] include the spectrum of acute coronary syndromes and are an important contribution to the management of patients considered in this chapter.

Methods closely related to guidelines include *algorithms, protocols, and critical care pathways*.[3a] These terms are frequently used interchangeably and all provide recommendations for diagnosis and treatment of acute and chronic cardiac disease. Critical pathways are similar to management algorithms but they may lack the detail of the latter.

A management plan presented as a critical pathway for triage of low-risk patients with chest pain is shown in Fig. 6.4.[28]

Protocols are typically more specific in providing a detailed, daily chronology of recommendations for management of acute cardiac conditions such as chest pain. Guidelines such as those developed by the AHA/ACC, on the other hand, present a broader perspective and classify each management option in terms of the level of the

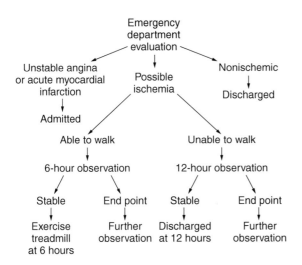

Figure 6.4 *A critical pathway for management of patients with chest pain. (Reproduced with permission from Nichol G, Walls R, Goldman L, et al. A critical pathway for management of patients with acute chest pain who are at low risk for myocardial ischemia: recommendations and potential impact. Ann Intern Med 1997; **127**: 996–1005.)*

supportive evidence: class I (supported by clinical trial data); class II (data generally supported but to a variable degree); and class III (evidence not supported).[27] Additional tools useful in the actual implementation of the broad strategy presented by guidelines include preprinted order sheets and guideline reminders

1. Admit to emergency department.
2. Diagnosis: chest pain.
3. Vital signs: on admission, then Q 15 minutes × 4, Q 30 minutes × 2, Q 1 hour (blood pressures to be taken in both arms).
4. Electrocardiogram: on admission, then Q 30 minutes × 2 and PRN chest pain.
5. Allergies.
6. Diet: NPO except sips with medications.
7. Telemetry monitoring.
8. Start 18 gauge iv with normal saline at TKO.
9. Cardiac serum markers (myoglobin, CK with MB, Troponin I or T).
10. Serum electrolytes, amylase, lipase, CBC with differential.
11. Chest x-ray: rule out aortic dissection, pneumonia, pulmonary embolism, cardiomegaly.
12. Stool guaiac.

PRN = as circumstances require; NPO = nothing per os; iv = intravenous; TKO = to keep open; CBC = complete blood count.

Figure 6.5 *Example of orders for patients admitted to the emergency department.*

attached to the patient's chart for daily review by physicians and nurses.[29]

Figures 6.5 and 6.6 are examples of preprinted order sheets for the ED and short-stay unit, respectively.

1. Admit to observation unit.
2. Diagnosis: chest pain.
3. Condition: fair.
4. Vital signs: Q 4 hours.
5. Allergies.
6. Diet: low fat, low cholesterol.
7. Activity: bed rest with bathroom privileges.
8. Maintain 18 gauge iv with normal saline at TKO.
9. Cardiac serum markers Q 3 hours × 3.
10. Electrocardiogram: Q 3 hours × 3 and PRN chest pain.
11. Aspirin 325 mg PO (chewed).
12. Nitroglycerin paste 1″ to chest wall Q 6 hours.

When cardiac serum markers are abnormal:
13. Metoprolol 5 mg iv Q 5 minutes × 3, then 50 mg PO followed by 50 mg PO Q 12 hours.
14. Admit to in-patient service.

For dynamic ST-segment changes.
15. Change nitroglycerin paste to nitroglycerin iv 30 mcg/min and titrate to 100 mcg keeping systolic blood pressure greater than 100 mm Hg.
16. Heparin intravenous bolus, 5000 units, followed by 10 units/kg per hour drip.
17. Admit to in-patient service.

TKO = to keep open; PRN = as circumstances require; PO = per os; iv = intravenous.

Figure 6.6 *Example of orders for patients admitted to short-stay unit.*

Utility of guidelines

Although the ultimate role of guidelines in patient management is still uncertain,[30] several reports have documented their utility in reducing hospital stay while maintaining the quality of patient care. One study of low-risk chest pain patients admitted to a health maintenance organization hospital demonstrated a 22 per cent reduction in overall length of stay (1.96 *vs* 2.51 days) and a 17 per cent reduction in intermediate care unit length of stay (28.2 *vs* 33.9 hours).[31] In a study of low-risk patients admitted to a CCU, guideline reminders for physicians were associated with a 25 per cent reduction in length of stay (2.63 *vs* 3.54 days) and a saving of $1397 per patient.[29] No differences were found in complication rates, health status or patient satisfaction one month after hospital discharge. In a retrospective analysis to determine the potential utility of a critical pathway (Fig. 6.4) in low-risk patients with chest pain, it was suggested that this strategy might safely reduce the number of hospital admissions (17 per cent) and days of hospitalization (11 per cent) for this population.[28]

Dissemination of practice guidelines can be achieved through multiple methods of communication, including educational conferences, memoranda, written feedback, endorsement and support of opinion leaders such as the department chairman or clinical division chief, and nursing-initiated prompting.[32,33] In our institution, guidelines for management of patients with acute cardiac conditions have been developed jointly by the director of the CCU, chief of clinical cardiology, and nurse manager of the cardiac care unit. These guidelines are presented to the cardiology faculty and nursing staff for feedback, affording the opportunity for all staff to participate in the development process and thereby increasing the likelihood of implementation. The guidelines are also available in the CCU nursing station for inclusion in patients' charts and nurses are encouraged to meet with physicians during rounds to consider patient care, using the guidelines to prompt discussion.

Application of guidelines

The process described in a previous section (Basic approach to the patient with acute chest pain) and in Fig. 6.1 represents a simple form of algorithm, in that it provides a general approach to initial consideration of patients with chest pain. A more detailed algorithm from the ACC/AHA guidelines is shown in Fig. 6.7.[27] This plan specifies diagnostic methods and treatments with the time points at which they are to be achieved for optimal care. The cornerstone of contemporary management of acute MI is rapid institution of reperfusion therapy, as indicated in the left side of the algorithm. To achieve the goals of the National Heart Attack Alert Program (interpretation of the ECG within 10 minutes of arrival in the ED and reperfusion therapy within 30 minutes of arrival in appropriate patients (Fig. 6.7),[27] each institution requires a standard action plan and specific staff assignments to coordinate activity from the time the patient with chest pain enters the ED. The further management of acute MI is described elsewhere in this text.

Because the first priority in patients presenting to the

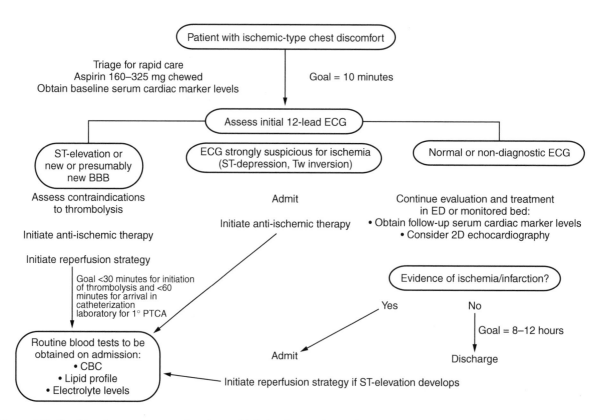

Figure 6.7 *Algorithm for management of patients with ischemic-type chest pain in the emergency department. BBB = bundle branch block; ECG = electrocardiogram; CBC = complete blood count; Tw = T wave; PTCA = percutaneous transluminal coronary angioplasty. (Reproduced with permission from Ryan TJ, Anderson JL, Antman EM, et al. ACC/AHA guidelines for the management of patients with acute myocardial infarction. A report of the American College of Cardiology/American Heart Association Task Force on Practice Guidelines [Committee on Management of Acute Myocardial Infarction]. J Am Coll Cardiol 1996; 28: 1328–428. © 1996 by the American College of Cardiology and American Heart Association, Inc.)*

ED with chest pain is rapid identification of high-risk patients, it is important to describe the actual steps in this process. They may differ among institutions but they should achieve the same ends. Adults with non-traumatic chest pain who arrive by ambulance or those who report to the registration desk of the ED should be taken directly to an ED bed, and an ECG obtained immediately by a nurse or technician dedicated to this task.

A physician should be readily available for interpretation of the ECG, which should be accomplished within 10 minutes of patient arrival. During this interval, vital signs are obtained and a screening history and physical examination are performed. If the ECG reveals ST-segment elevation fulfilling criteria for reperfusion therapy and there are no contraindications, this therapy is initiated (Fig. 6.7).

Representative admitting orders for additional, early ED management are shown in Fig. 6.5. It is mandatory that the responsible ED physician be an expert in ECG interpretation of acute MI, myocardial ischemia, and entities such as early repolarization and pericarditis that may confound ECG recognition of acute MI. Where practical, cardiology consultation should be sought if the ECG is questionable, but it is essential not to delay therapy for confirmation of ECG findings that are clear. The staff members (nurse, technician) assigned to certain of the early steps in management should be skilled, dedicated to the tasks, and immediately available. Although the ACC/AHA guidelines recommend virtually immediate administration of aspirin (Fig. 6.7), we believe it is reasonable to wait for assessment of the ECG to avoid use of this drug in patients with chest pain possibly related to etiologies such as peptic ulcer disease and aortic dissection, in which aspirin could have important adverse effects. If the ECG reveals no ST-segment elevation but is consistent with ischemia, anti-ischemic therapy, as described elsewhere in this text, is initiated and the patient is admitted to the in-patient service (Fig. 6.7). By contrast, the low-risk group, characterized by stable clinical status and an ECG that is non-diagnostic, normal or unchanged from a previously abnormal one, is observed by an initial short-stay process, including measurement of cardiac serum markers and the results of this evaluation determine final management. Orders for management of patients admitted for observation are shown in Fig. 6.6. The use of new approaches for early stratification of low-risk patients is described in detail later in this chapter.

CHEST PAIN EMERGENCY UNITS

In response to the challenge to facilitate urgent therapy in acute MI and also provide safe, cost-effective care for low-risk patients presenting with chest pain, specialized units have been developed in or near the ED.[34-37] These units are variably referred to as chest pain emergency room, chest pain evaluation unit, chest pain center, chest pain observation unit, or short-stay unit. Their purpose is to provide an integrated approach to the patient with chest pain that affords early identification of clinical risk followed by rapid triage of high-risk patients to urgent anti-ischemic therapy[3a-5] and low-risk patients to further evaluation.[34,38-41] The units vary in form but they usually involve dedicated personnel, equipment, and space. However, this approach is based less on physical structure than on a process implemented by the coordinated efforts of medical, nursing, and technical personnel. The objectives of the units are also flexible in that the focus of some is the high-risk patient,[42] while others aim primarily at decreasing unnecessary admissions of low-risk patients through the use of recently proposed strategies.[3a,34,38-41]

The units dedicated to management of low-risk patients have lower nurse–patient ratios than intensive care units, but they require continuous ECG monitoring and their personnel should be well versed in treating cardiac emergencies. Our chest pain service is staffed by internists who are skilled in assessing cardiac disease, interpreting ECGs, and performing treadmill tests. However, they also exercise a broad perspective in approaching low-risk patients with chest pain. This is essential, since the majority of these patients do not have a cardiac etiology of their symptoms.[2] It is also essential to consider other high-risk conditions in these patients, such as pulmonary embolism or aortic dissection.[2] These units are potentially economical because they provide appropriate care at reduced cost, decrease patients' length of stay, and prevent unnecessary admissions to the cardiac intensive care and telemetry units. Initial reports have demonstrated the utility of these units in identifying patients who are candidates for early discharge and they appear to be cost effective. A randomized study compared 50 low-risk patients admitted to routine hospital care with 50 similar patients managed by a short-stay unit to rule out MI.[41] Cost at 30 days for conventional care was $2253 per patient compared to $1237 in short-stay patients. Comparison of clinical outcomes was precluded by the small study cohort. Gaspoz et al.[39] demonstrated similar complication rates in 592 patients admitted to a chest pain evaluation unit and in 924 comparable patients admitted to either the cardiac care unit, a step-down unit or hospital wards. However, cost at 6 months was less than one-half to one-sixth for patients initially managed in the chest pain unit. To maintain the cost effectiveness of these units, physicians must guard against the tendency for overuse and refrain from referral of patients of such low risk that they should properly be discharged directly from the ED without assessment in a short-stay unit.

We utilize our chest pain observation unit for low-risk patients who are not candidates for immediate treadmill testing. This group includes patients who require further monitoring based on the initial clinical assessment and those who are unable to exercise or have resting ECG abnormalities unrelated to ischemia (e.g. pacemaker rhythm) that preclude interpretation of the exercise ECG.

They are managed according to the right-hand pathway in Fig. 6.7.[27] If serum markers are positive, they are admitted to the in-patient service; if the markers are negative, non-invasive cardiac stress imaging is performed within the first 24 hours to assess for myocardial ischemia. The results of this test determine subsequent management.

CARDIAC SERUM MARKERS

Cardiac serum markers are the most sensitive method for detecting myocardial damage and the degree of elevation of the marker, particularly of the troponins, is a strong predictor of clinical outcome.[12] The measurement of serum markers in patient evaluation is based on the release of these macromolecules into the blood within several hours of myocardial injury (Fig. 6.2).

Therefore, detection of increased serum concentrations of these substances, in the absence of other causes, is definitive evidence of acute MI.

The most widely employed of these markers for detecting MI has been creatine kinase (CK) and its cardiac isoenzyme, the myocardial band (MB) of CK. Until recently, the latter has been the standard biochemical indicator of MI. Other serum markers of cardiac injury include the cardiac troponins, myoglobin, and CK-MB subforms. These indicators have a high sensitivity for detecting acute MI but they have important limitations as a basis for the initial decision to admit or discharge a patient with chest pain. Their primary drawback is that, with the possible exception of the troponins, they detect MI but provide no information on ischemia. However, although the majority of low-risk patients with chest pain do not have MI,[2,3,9,13] detection of myocardial ischemia is a major concern in this group. In addition, CK-MB, which has greater sensitivity and specificity than total CK for detecting MI, does not rise significantly in most patients for 4–6 hours after MI onset and up to 12 hours may be necessary for exclusion of MI with confidence.[43] Although myoglobin is released as early as 2 hours after cardiac injury, it has an unacceptably low specificity based on its high concentration in skeletal muscle and elevation in renal insufficiency.[44] CK-MB subforms (modifications of CK-MB and CK-MM after

their release into plasma), which become positive earlier than CK-MB, are more sensitive and specific than the latter for detecting MI,[45] but they are not yet suitable for general use because of technically demanding methodology.

Both cardiac troponin I and troponin T have demonstrated superior sensitivity and specificity for detecting MI than CK-MB but their appearance times are similar to the latter marker.[7,46]

However, the troponins have attracted considerable attention because of their capacity to predict the risk of cardiac complications in patients with myocardial ischemia without infarction.[12,47,48]

These findings stem primarily from studies in high-risk patients,[47,48] whereas recent observations suggest some limitation in the predictive value of the troponins in lower risk populations.[49,50] Current experience indicates that, in the decision to admit or discharge a low-risk patient from the ED, the troponins should be utilized as part of the total patient assessment that includes the history, physical examination, and ECG. In this regard, prudence dictates that, in these cases, more than one troponin value should be obtained and that one of these should be obtained at least 6 hours after the onset of symptoms.[12,49,50] Thus, while currently available serum markers of cardiac injury are key elements in evaluating patients with chest pain, they have important limitations in identifying those who are appropriate for discharge from the ED, including delayed appearance of abnormal findings, relatively low specificity, failure to detect myocardial ischemia, and/or complex analytic methodology.

EARLY NON-INVASIVE CARDIAC TESTING

The most frequently employed of these methods for evaluation of patients presenting with chest pain are echocardiography, myocardial scintigraphy and exercise testing. These techniques are still under investigation and their applicability will be determined by their utility, cost, and adaptability to the needs and resources of each institution. The current status of each of these methods is described below.

Echocardiography

Impairment of left ventricular segmental wall motion is apparent almost immediately after the onset of myocardial ischemia, preceding symptoms and ST-segment alterations.[51] Therefore, detection of cardiac wall motion abnormalities is potentially more sensitive than the history, physical examination, and ECG for identification of myocardial ischemia. Echocardiography is highly reliable for assessing cardiac wall motion and, thus, it has been utilized for diagnosis and risk assessment in patients presenting to the ED with symptoms suggestive of myocardial ischemia. In patients with acute Q-wave MI, echocardiography is comparable to invasive left ventriculography for detecting wall motion abnormalities.[52] However, the utility of echocardiography in the low-risk population with chest pain of uncertain etiology and a non-diagnostic initial presentation is less well established. Table 6.3 depicts the results of five studies in patients presenting with chest pain and non-diagnostic ECGs in whom echocardiography was used to predict cardiac events by detection of resting wall motion abnormalities.[53–57] Although four of these reports indicated a high positive predictive value for this technique, the overall event rate in these studies was approximately 50 per cent. In these high-risk populations, the positive predictive value of a test for ischemia/infarction will be augmented compared to that in typical low-risk ROMI patients. Thus, in the study of Sabia et al. in which the cardiac event rate was 16 per cent, the positive predictive value of a resting wall motion abnormality was only 31 per cent[53] (Table 6.3). In another report with a similarly low cardiac event rate, echocardiography did not add to a 3-hour evaluation consisting of clinical assessment and cardiac serum enzymes.[58]

It is also noteworthy that, in all the aforementioned investigations, the patients with false-negative echocardiographic findings had non-Q wave MI or unstable angina, reflecting the limited sensitivity of wall motion abnormalities for identification of this population.

The latter group is typical of the minority of low-risk patients who have ischemic events.

There are several factors that limit the value of echocardiography for detecting patients in the ROMI population who are at risk for a cardiac event. The examination is highly dependent on skilled, experienced personnel for adequate data acquisition and reliable interpretation. According to the Task Force of the American College of Cardiology on training in echocardiography, a minimum of 6 months of training is required to become an independent reader.[59] Therefore, highly specialized physicians, technical personnel and equipment are required for dedicated use in the ED. Further, although ventricular wall motion abnormalities associated with ischemia may persist for prolonged periods, they may also resolve in as little as 2 hours.[60] As previously noted, patients with non-Q MI and unstable angina may have no discernible abnormalities of wall motion. In this regard, studies in animals have demonstrated that wall motion abnormalities may not be detected when infarction involves less than 20 per cent of ventricular wall thickness[61] or less than 12 per cent of left ventricular circumference.[62] Finally, echocardiography provides no information on the age of a wall motion abnormality, reducing its utility in patients with known CAD or other cardiac disease.

New echocardiographic approaches may overcome some of these limitations. Dobutamine stress echocardiography performed in the ED in 26 low-risk patients revealed wall motion abnormalities in only three, none of whom had a cardiac event.[63] Further studies are necessary to clarify the significance of positive results with this method. A second technique under investigation is analysis of variation in the scatter of acoustic signals during ischemia (ultrasonic tissue characterization).[57] This method has been as accurate as wall motion analysis for detection of cardiac events and it may thereby enhance the utility of resting echocardiography. A third strategy that may be useful for identification of myocardial ischemia is contrast echocardiography in which areas of reduced myocardial perfusion are recognized by diminished echo density.[64] This method has not yet been used for risk stratification of patients in the ED. In sum-

Table 6.3 *Predictive accuracy of echocardiography in patients presenting with acute chest pain. (Reproduced with permission from Amsterdam EA, Lewis WR, Yadlapalli S. Evaluation of low risk patients with chest pain in the emergency department: value and limitations of recent methods.* Cardiol Rev *1999;* **7***: 17–26.)*

	n		Event+	Event−	PPV (%)	NPV (%)
Sabia et al.[53]	169	RWA+	27	60	31	
		RWA−	2	80		98
Peels et al.[54]	35	RWA+	18	3	86	
		RWA−	2	12		86
Sasaki et al.[55]	46	RWA+	17	1	94	
		RWA−	6	22		79
Horowitz et al.[56]	65	RWA+	34	2	94	
		RWA−	2	27		93
Saeian et al.[57]	60	RWA+	22	3	88	
		RWA−	2	33		94

n = number of patients; RWA+ = Regional wall motion abnormality present; RWA− = no regional wall motion abnormality; Event+ = coronary event present; Event− = no coronary event; PPV = positive predictive value; NPV = negative predictive value.

mary, resting echocardiography lacks sufficient sensitivity to be of clinical utility in the low-risk ROMI patient in the ED, leading the National Heart Attack Alert Program Working Group to conclude that 'false-negative rates in the prospective studies are too high to be safe'.[65] Although the newer methods have increased sensitivity, they do not obviate the logistical problems related to personnel and equipment dedicated to the ED or the issue of cost effectiveness.

Electron beam computed tomography

Only one study of this technique for use in a chest pain unit has been performed to date,[65a] in which 105 patients without known coronary artery disease, non-diagnostic ECGs, and a negative initial cardiac enzyme underwent electron beam computed tomography (EBCT) within 24 hours of admission and prior to other cardiac work-up. The population was limited to men <55 and women <65 years of age. Fifty-eight patients subsequently underwent treadmill exercise testing, 25 underwent coronary arteriography, 19 had stress nuclear scintigraphy, and 11 had resting echocardiography. Results of the EBCT were compared to the other studies, and EBCT was considered to have 100 per cent sensitivity and 63 per cent specificity. The age of the population was limited because coronary artery calcifications increase with age and may lead to false positive studies. With a 100 per cent sensitivity in this study, EBCT appears to be promising as a screening tool for excluding the presence of coronary artery disease. Further studies are required to see if EBCT can risk stratify patients with coronary disease as accurately as other commonly used tests.

Myocardial scintigraphy

This method utilizes the radioactive tracers, thallium-201 (^{201}Tl) or sestamibi technetium-99m (sestamibi), to assess myocardial perfusion. Defects of regional myocardial perfusion result from myocardial ischemia or scar tissue following MI. The property of delayed redistribution that characterizes ^{201}Tl allows comparison of early and late perfusion images to distinguish myocardial ischemia from old MI. A fixed defect (present on both early and late imaging) is consistent with MI, whereas a reversible defect (one that normalizes on delayed imaging) reflects ischemia. Imaging with ^{201}Tl can be performed with a portable gamma camera in the ED but the relatively low-energy photons of this tracer may produce images with less resolution than those obtained with the higher energy of sestamibi. The isotope can also be injected in the ED and the patient then brought to the nuclear medicine department for imaging.

The first three studies[66–68] shown in Table 6.4 utilized rest ^{201}Tl scintigraphy in the ED for evaluation of patients with chest pain. These studies, which are listed in order of increasing cardiac events, have high negative predictive values but the positive predictive value increases as the proportion of patients with cardiac events rises. The study group of Henneman et al. is most representative of patients presenting to the ED with chest pain of diagnostic uncertainty,[66] leading to the correspondingly poor positive predictive value of 6 per cent with ^{201}Tl and 11 per cent when combined with first-pass radionuclide angiography. The negative predictive value was 95 per cent, consistent with the low incidence of disease. The retrospective report of van der Wieken and co-workers is typical of a high-risk population with Q-wave MI.[68] Resting ^{201}Tl scintigraphy within 12 hours of presentation with chest pain and a non-diagnostic ECG had favorable negative and positive predictive values (84 per cent and 91 per cent, respectively). The small study of Mace had an intermediate rate of disease and an intermediate positive predictive value.[67]

Sestamibi does not redistribute over time. Thus, after injection of this isotope, imaging can be delayed, allowing for stabilization and treatment of the patient between isotope administration and initial imaging. The last four studies in Table 6.4 utilized sestamibi and are arranged in order of increasing incidence of clinical events.[67–70] As was observed with ^{201}Tl,[66–68] the negative predictive value is consistently high but the positive predictive value is directly related to the frequency of disease. Tatum et al. prospectively evaluated over 1100 patients presenting to the ED with acute chest pain and performed myocardial scintigraphy in the 438 patients in the low-to-moderate risk subgroup, in which the cardiac event rate was 9 per cent, which is typical of a ROMI population.[69] Accordingly, the negative predictive value of sestamibi imaging was 98 per cent and the positive predictive value was 37 per cent. As the event rates in the remaining studies in Table 6.4 progressively rise from 15[70] to 42[71] and 58 per cent,[72] the positive predictive value increases from 43 to over 86 per cent with excellent negative predictive values. The cost effectiveness of myocardial scintigraphy performed with sestamibi in the ED was determined prospectively in 50 patients presenting with chest pain, non-diagnostic ECGs, and normal initial cardiac enzymes and it was concluded that this strategy yielded a saving of $785 per patient.[73]

> From these studies, it is clear that myocardial rest scintigraphy by ^{201}Tl and sestamibi have excellent negative predictive values in the early assessment of patients presenting with chest pain and non-diagnostic ECGs. Their positive predictive value, however, is highly dependent on the pretest probability of disease in the population tested.

Initial studies suggest that this strategy is cost effective. However, several factors limit the utility of early scintigraphy. In most institutions, the availability of myocardial

Table 6.4 *Predictive accuracy of myocardial scintigraphy in patients presenting with acute chest pain. (Reproduced with permission from Amsterdam EA, Lewis WR, Yadlapalli S. Evaluation of low risk patients with chest pain in the emergency department: value and limitations of recent methods.* Cardiol Rev *1999; **7**: 17–26.)*

	n		Event+	Event–	PPV (%)	NPV (%)
Henneman *et al.*[66]	47	PD+	1	17	6	
		PD–	3	26		90
Mace[67]	20	PD+	5	1	83	
		PD–	0	14		100
Van der Wieken *et al.*[68]	149	PD+	59	11	84	
		PD–	7	72		91
Tatum *et al.*[69]	438	PD+	37	63	37	
		PD–	7	331		98
Hilton *et al.*[70]	102	PD+	14	18	43	
		PD–	1	69		98
Varetto *et al.*[71]	64	PD+	27	3	90	
		PD–	0	34		100
Gregoire and Theroux[72]	45	PD+	25	4	86	
		PD–	1	15		94

n = number of patients; PD+ = perfusion defect present; PD– = no perfusion defect; Event+ = coronary event present; Event– = no coronary event; PPV = positive predictive value; NPV = negative predictive value.

scintigraphy is circumscribed and this method entails complicated logistics involving personnel and equipment that are often located some distance from the ED. These considerations preclude the use of ^{201}Tl in most centers because of the isotope's expense, short half-life and the necessity for immediate imaging after injection. Sestamibi lacks several of these limitations and may prove superior for use in the ED. Current practice in some institutions is to inject low-risk patients with sestamibi in the ED during chest pain, initiate therapy, and perform myocardial scintigraphy after further initial management. According to the Working Group of the National Heart Attack Alert Program, available data suggest that rest myocardial scintigraphy in the ED is a promising approach to evaluation of selected patients with chest pain but cannot yet be recommended for general use.[65]

Immediate exercise stress testing

In its Evaluation of Technologies for Identifying Acute Cardiac Ischemia in the Emergency Department, the National Heart Attack Alert Program Working Group appropriately indicated that 'ECG stress testing in the ED cannot be recommended in the absence of additional data demonstrating safety and effectiveness'.[65] This important admonition reflects the well-established mandate for prudence in stress testing of any patient who may have underlying cardiac disease. Although exercise testing in stable patients with CAD has been associated with a very low complication rate (mortality <0.01 per cent, morbidity <0.05 per cent),[74] patients with active chest pain present a greater potential for adverse reactions. However, based on evidence supporting the utility

of the clinical assessment in identifying a low-risk group among patients presenting to the ED with chest pain,[2,3,13,14,16,17] we have successfully performed immediate treadmill testing in selected patients to identify those requiring admission, and those who can be safely discharged from the ED and undergo further evaluation as out-patients.

Our experience in a large, heterogeneous patient population has demonstrated the safety and utility of immediate exercise testing when employed by qualified physicians in carefully selected patients.[2,3,39,40,73]

Our approach has evolved from its inception in which immediate exercise testing was performed only by cardiologists, and patients with a history of CAD were excluded.[38] Our initial report demonstrated that this strategy was practical and safe with the potential for major cost savings.[38] This experience provided the basis for extending our system to its current scope. Immediate exercise testing is now performed by internists trained in exercise testing with close consultation available by cardiologists, a history of CAD is no longer a contraindication and serial serum markers are not measured prior to testing,[40] but a single serum marker is measured in most patients. The safety of this method is predicated on judicious implementation which entails careful patient selection and rigorous adherence to guidelines for performing the exercise test. Criteria for patient selection for immediate exercise testing are listed in Table 6.5. Evaluation in the ED includes complete history, cardiac risk-factor profile, physical examination with bilateral upper extremity blood pressure measurements, and chest roentgenogram in order to exclude patients with clinical evidence of conditions such as pulmonary

Table 6.5 *Selection criteria for immediate exercise test. (Reprinted with permission from Amsterdam EA, Lewis WR, Yadlapalli S. Evaluation of low risk patients with chest pain in the emergency department: value and limitations of recent methods. Cardiol Rev 1999; 7: 17–26.)*

Chest pain suspicious for myocardial ischemia
Able to exercise
Electrocardiogram (ECG) – normal, minor ST-T changes, or no change from previous abnormal ECG
Hemodynamically stable, no arrhythmia
A single negative serum marker is required in most patients

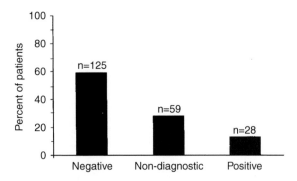

Figure 6.8 *Results of immediate treadmill testing in the emergency department (n = 212). (Reproduced with permission from Kirk JD, Turnipseed S, Lewis WR, et al. Evaluation of chest pain in low risk patients presenting to the emergency department: the role of immediate exercise testing. Ann Emerg Med 1998; 32: 1–7.)*

embolism, aortic dissection and other intrathoracic or intra-abdominal processes. The procedure and end points are shown in Table 6.6.

Table 6.6 *Immediate exercise test procedure and end points. (Reprinted with permission from Amsterdam EA, Lewis WR, Yadlapalli S. Evaluation of low risk patients with chest pain in the emergency department: value and limitations of recent methods. Cardiol Rev 1999; 7: 17–26.)*

Modified Bruce treadmill protocol[a]
Symptom-limited
Other end points – ischemia, ↓ blood pressure, arrhythmia
Positive result – ≥1.0 mm horizontal ST-segment shift
Non-diagnostic result – <85% maximum predicted heart rate with no ST shift

[a] Includes two initial 3-minute stages (1.7 mph, 0% grade and 1.7 mph 5% grade) prior to the standard Bruce protocol.

Our results in over 200 patients evaluated by this method are depicted in Fig. 6.8.[40] A majority had negative tests, approximately one-fourth had non-diagnostic tests, only 13 per cent had positive results and there were no adverse effects of the procedure. Patients with positive tests were admitted for further evaluation which revealed that slightly more than half (57 per cent of positives) were true positives. Patients with negative tests and a majority of those with non-diagnostic results who achieved a peak heart rate of ≥ 75 per cent of maximum predicted (54 per cent of patients) were discharged for further out-patient evaluation. Follow-up in these patients at 30 days revealed no mortality or ischemic events. During evaluation, three patients with occult MI underwent stress testing. Following admission, their serum CK-MB patterns indicated elevations prior to the test with no apparent alteration in enzyme evolution related to the test. The MIs were non-Q and unassociated with complications. Our experience in 100 consecutive patients with known CAD has suggested that this method is also safe and cost-effective in this group.[75]

Our results demonstrate that, in selected low-risk patients presenting with chest pain, immediate exercise testing can safely stratify this group into those that can be discharged and those requiring admission. Our total experience in over 1000 patients has been consistent with that described above in that less than 15 per cent of patients have positive tests, of which slightly more than half are true positives. This approach has been equally applicable in men and women over a wide age range.

Caution and selectivity must be exercised when utilizing immediate exercise stress testing. The patient must be able to perform an exercise test and the resting ECG must be devoid of abnormalities that preclude interpretation of exercise-induced ischemia.

> Although we have had no complications of this procedure, there is a small but real possibility of stress testing patients with acute MI.

This should be reducible to a negligible level by utilizing cardiac troponin measurements obtained over several hours[49,50] before the stress test. However, this modification would alter the strategy from immediate exercise testing to that of a short-stay observation unit,[41,76,77] which would provide an added margin of safety while introducing increased logistical factors and cost. In this regard, each institution must decide which of the evolving new approaches to assessing the low-risk patient with chest pain is most suitable to its needs and resources.[65]

CLINICAL OVERVIEW

Current standards of care mandate rapid institution of therapy for patients with acute coronary syndromes.

However, the majority of patients presenting to the ED with chest pain are at low risk for a coronary event and its complications. Appropriate management of this group is less intensive and many may not require admission. Recent studies have shown that these low-risk patients can be identified by clinical criteria on presentation, including history, physical examination, and initial ECG. Avoidance of unnecessary admission in these patients has the potential for major cost savings while maintaining effective patient care. Recent innovative approaches to the management of low-risk patients presenting with chest pain have included the application of practice guidelines and related processes, short-stay observation units, new cardiac serum markers, and early non-invasive studies (echocardiography, myocardial scintigraphy, exercise testing). Initial reports suggest that most of these methods have the potential for reducing cost and preserving quality of care.

An increasingly employed approach to the management of low-risk patients presenting with chest pain entails early identification in the emergency department and an abbreviated period of monitoring (6–12 hours), while cardiac serum markers are determined. Monitoring is performed, depending on the institution, either in the emergency department, a separate short-stay observation unit or a hospital telemetry unit. Patients in whom serum markers are positive are then admitted to the in-patient service. Stable patients with negative findings can be discharged after the short-stay protocol with further non-invasive evaluation to detect myocardial ischemia performed either before or shortly after discharge. The availability of cardiac troponins has improved the utility of serum markers for detecting MI and for identifying increased risk of cardiac complications in patients with chest pain without infarction. However, several requirements should be fulfilled for reliable use of troponins in selecting candidates for discharge after an abbreviated observation period. These include: (1) use of these markers in conjunction with the basic clinical assessment by history, physical examination, and ECG; (2) measurement of more than one troponin value during the monitoring period; and (3) determination of at least one troponin value $\geqslant 6$ hours after the onset of symptoms.

Non-invasive testing in the ED is being evaluated to assess low-risk patients with chest pain. Experience at our institution indicates that early treadmill testing of selected low-risk patients is safe and effective for stratifying this group into those who can be discharged and those who require admission. Limitations of early treadmill testing are its dependence on patients' ability to exercise, the need for a baseline ECG devoid of abnormalities that impair interpretation of exercise-induced ischemia and the possibility of testing a patient who is having a coronary event. Echocardiography has been limited by a poor positive predictive value in the low-risk population and a high false-negative rate in the sub-

group with unstable angina and non-Q infarction. Newer echocardiographic approaches are under investigation, including dobutamine echocardiography, ultrasonic myocardial tissue characterization and contrast echocardiography. Myocardial scintigraphy with sestamibi is promising in that it allows injection of the isotope in the emergency department and stabilization of the patient before imaging in the nuclear medicine department. Scintigraphy has excellent negative predictive value but its positive predictive value is dependent on the pretest probability of disease, which is typically modest in patients with chest pain who are identified as low risk by clinical criteria on presentation. In addition, scintigraphy is limited by expense, logistics, and availability.

Each of the foregoing approaches to managing low-risk patients presenting chest pain continues to evolve and undergo further investigation. It is likely that no single method will fulfill the needs of every institution in providing cost-effective, high-quality care in these patients. Selection of one or more of these approaches will be based on demonstrated utility and the individual requirements, resources, and expertise of each institution.

FUTURE DIRECTIONS

Recent innovations in the management of low-risk patients presenting with chest pain have the potential to maintain quality of care while reducing unnecessary cost. At this time, however, these approaches must be considered investigational. Although initial reports suggest that improved cost effectiveness is achievable by the short-stay process, this finding requires confirmation by further studies. A critical determinant of this goal will be avoidance of over-referral of patients in whom cardiac risk is so low that direct discharge from the ED is appropriate and the newer methods are not indicated. Practice guidelines and related tools, which are being increasingly utilized, also require demonstration of utility to support continued application. It is essential that new cardiac markers, such as the troponins, be applied prudently in assessing low-risk candidates for early discharge after an abbreviated monitoring period. Further, their utility in predicting cardiac complications in these low-risk patients requires further study. Above all, the troponins must be applied in conjunction with the total clinical evaluation. CK-MB subforms, reported to have both greater accuracy and earlier appearance kinetics in detecting myocardial necrosis than current serum markers, may contribute to the initial assessment of low-risk patients. Current studies of non-invasive cardiac testing in the ED have had variable results in terms of predictive accuracy, cost effectiveness, and applicability. Newer methods to improve the utility of both echocardiography and myocardial scintigraphy in the ED for risk stratification of patients with chest pain require further investigation before these approaches are considered for wider application. Early treadmill testing, which is a promising method, is limited to patients with basically normal electrocardiograms who can exercise. Newer, more sensitive electrocardiographic monitoring techniques for detection of ischemia, such as chaos analysis,[65] are under current investigation. Fundamental to the assessment of all new methods will be analysis not only of their accuracy, but also their cost effectiveness and potential for general application in institutions with variable resources and expertise.

SUMMARY

- Low-risk patients presenting to the emergency department with chest pain can be identified by clinical criteria (history, physical examination, electrocardiogram).
- Low-risk patients presenting with chest pain can be observed by a short stay protocol for 6–12 hours while cardiac serum markers are obtained as a basis for further management.
- Chest pain emergency or observation units are dedicated to rapid triage of high-risk patients with chest pain to urgent therapy and/or management of low-risk patients who do not require initial in-patient management.
- Cardiac troponins are the most accurate serum markers for myocardial infarction and risk of complications in patients with myocardial ischemia, but their use in selecting low-risk patients for discharge from the emergency department requires ⩾2 negative values, at least one of which should be ⩾6 hours after the onset of symptoms.
- Resting echocardiography has limited value in assessing low-risk patients with chest pain; resting myocardial scintigraphy has excellent negative predictive value but its positive predictive value is limited in the low-risk population.
- Initial studies of predischarge exercise testing after an abbreviated protocol to rule out myocardial infarction has been safe and cost effective in the management of low-risk patients with chest pain.

ACKNOWLEDGMENT

The authors gratefully acknowledge the skilled administrative assistance of Shirl Fischer.

REFERENCES

1. Rutledge JC, Amsterdam EA. Differential diagnosis and clinical approach to the patient with acute chest pain. Cardiovascular emergencies. In: Ram CVS, ed. *Cardiology clinics* 2, Philadelphia: WB Saunders, 1984: 257–68.

○2. Lewis WR, Amsterdam EA. Chest pain. In: Gershwin ME, Hamilton ME, eds *The pain management handbook: a concise guide to diagnosis and treatment*. Totowa, NJ: Humana Press, 1998: 79–115.

○3. Lewis WR, Amsterdam EA. Evaluation of the patient with 'rule out myocardial infarction'. *Arch Intern Med* 1996; **156**: 41–5.

3a. Hutter AM Jr, Amsterdam EA, Jaffe AS. 31st Bethesda Conference. Emergency Cardiac Care. Acute coronary syndromes: chest discomfort evaluation in the hospital. *J Amer Coll Cardiol* 1999; **35**(4): 853–62.

3b. Lee TH, Goldman L. Evaluation of the patient with acute chest pain. *New Engl J Med* 2000; **342**: 1187–95.

4. Fibrinolytic Therapy Trialists' (FTT) Collaborative Group. Indications for fibrinolytic therapy in suspected acute myocardial infarction: collaborative overview of early mortality and major morbidity results from all randomised trials of more than 1000 patients. *Lancet* 1994; **343**: 311–22. (Erratum appears in *Lancet* 1994; **343**: 742).

5. Braunwald E, Jones RH, Mark DB, *et al.* Diagnosing and managing unstable angina. Agency for Health Care Policy and Research. *Circulation* 1994; **90**: 613–22.

6. Lown B, Vasaux C, Hood WB Jr, *et al.* Unresolved problems in coronary care. *Am J Cardiol* 1967; **20**: 494–508.

○7. Jesse RL, Kontos MC. Evaluation of chest pain in the emergency department. *Curr Prob Cardiol* 1997; **22**: 149–236.

7a. Pope JH, Aufderheide TP, Ruthazer R, Woolard RH, Feldman JA, Beshansky JR, Griffith JL, Selker HP. Missed diagnoses of acute cardiac ischemia in the emergency department. *New Engl J Med* 2000; **342**: 1163–70.

8. Karcz A, Holbrook J, Burke MC, *et al.* Massachusetts emergency medicine closed malpractice claims: 1988–1990. *Ann Emerg Med* 1993; **22**: 553–9.

9. Karlson BW, Herlitz J, Wiklund O, *et al.* Early prediction of acute myocardial infarction from clinical history, examination and electrocardiogram in the emergency room. *Am J Cardiol* 1991; **68**: 171–5.

10. Roberts R, Kleiman NS. Earlier diagnosis and treatment of acute myocardial infarction necessitates the need for a 'new diagnostic mind-set'. *Circulation* 1994; **89**: 872–81.

11. Fuster V, Badimon L, Badimon JJ, *et al.* The pathogenesis of coronary artery disease and the acute coronary syndromes (1). *N Engl J Med* 1992; **326**: 242–50.

12. Hamm CW, Goldmann BU, Heeschen C, *et al.* Emergency room triage of patients with acute chest

pain by means of rapid testing for cardiac troponin T or troponin I. *N Engl J Med* 1997; **337**: 1648–53.

♦13. Lee TH, Cook EF, Weisberg M, *et al.* Acute chest pain in the emergency room. Identification and examination of low-risk patients. *Arch Intern Med* 1985; **145**: 65–9.

♦14. Goldman L, Cook EF, Johnson PA, *et al.* Prediction of the need for intensive care in patients who come to the emergency departments with acute chest pain. *N Engl J Med* 1996; **334**: 1498–504.

15. Schroeder JS, Lamb IH, Hu M. Do patients in whom myocardial infarction has been ruled out have a better prognosis after hospitalization than those surviving infarction? *N Engl J Med* 1980; **303**: 1–5.

16. Gazes PC, Mobley M, Faris HM, *et al.* Preinfarctional (unstable) angina – a prospective study – ten year follow-up: prognostic significance of electrocardiographic changes. *Circulation* 1973; **38**: 331–7.

♦17. Brush JE, Brand DA, Acampora D, *et al.* Use of the initial electrocardiogram to predict in-hospital complications of acute myocardial infarction. *N Engl J Med* 1985; **312**: 1137–41.

18. Goldman L, Weinberg M, Weisberg M, *et al.* A computer-derived protocol to aid in the diagnosis of emergency room patients with acute chest pain. *N Engl J Med* 1982; **307**: 588–96.

19. Goldman L, Cook EF, Brand DA, *et al.* A computer protocol to predict myocardial infarction in emergency department patients with chest pain. *N Engl J Med* 1988; **318**: 797–803.

20. Lee TH, Pearson SD, Johnson PA, *et al.* Failure of information as an intervention to modify clinical management. A time-series trial in patients with acute chest pain. *Ann Intern Med* 1995; **122**: 434–7.

21. Pozen MW, D'Agostino RB, Mitchell JB, *et al.* The usefulness of a predictive instrument to reduce inappropriate admissions to the coronary care unit. *Ann Intern Med* 1980; **92**: 238–42.

○22. Pozen MW, D'Agostino RB, Selker HP, *et al.* A predictive instrument to improve coronary-care-unit admission practices in acute ischemic heart disease. A prospective multicenter clinical trial. *N Engl J Med* 1984; **310**: 1273–8.

23. McCarthy BD, Wong JB, Selker HP. Detecting acute cardiac ischemia in the emergency department: a review of the literature. *J Gen Intern Med* 1990; **5**: 365–73.

24. Selker HP, Griffith JL, D'Agostino RB. A time-insensitive predictive instrument for acute myocardial infarction mortality: a multicenter study. *Med Care* 1991; **29**: 1196–211.

25. Selker HP, Beshansky JR, Griffith JL, *et al.* Use of the acute cardiac ischemia time-insensitive predictive instrument (ACI-TIPI) to assist with triage of patients with chest pain or other symptoms suggestive of acute cardiac ischemia. A multicenter, controlled clinical trial. *Ann Intern Med* 1998; **129**(11): 845–55.

26. Pearson TA, McBride PE, Miller NH, *et al.* 27th Bethesda Conference: Matching the intensity of risk factor management with the hazard for coronary disease events. Task Force 8. Organization of preventive cardiology service. *J Am Coll Cardiol* 1996; **27**: 1039–47.

27. Ryan TJ, Anderson JL, Antman EM, *et al.* ACC/AHA guidelines for the management of patients with acute myocardial infarction. A report of the American College of Cardiology/American Heart Association Task Force on Practice Guidelines (Committee on Management of Acute Myocardial Infarction). *J Am Coll Cardiol* 1996; **28**: 1328–428.

28. Nichol G, Walls R, Goldman L, *et al.* A critical pathway for management of patients with acute chest pain who are at low risk for myocardial ischemia: recommendations and potential impact. *Ann Intern Med* 1997; **127**: 996–1005.

29. Weingarten SR, Riedinger MS, Conner L, *et al.* Practice guidelines and reminders to reduce duration of hospital stay for patients with chest pain. An interventional trial. *Ann Intern Med* 1994; **120**: 257–63.

30. Worrall G, Chaulk P, Freake D. The effects of clinical practice guidelines on patient outcomes in primary care: a systematic review. *Can Med Assoc J* 1997; **156**: 1705–12.

31. Weingarten S, Agocs L, Tankel N, *et al.* Reducing lengths of stay for patients hospitalized with chest pain using medical practice guidelines and opinion leaders. *Am J Cardiol* 1993; **71**: 259–62.

32. Lomas J, Anderson GM, Domnick-Pierre K, *et al.* Do practice guidelines guide practice? The effect of a consensus statement on the practice of physicians. *N Engl J Med* 1989; **321**: 1306–11.

33. Lomas J, Enkin M, Anderson GM, *et al.* Opinion leaders vs audit and feedback to implement practice guidelines. Delivery after previous cesarean section. *J Am Med Assoc* 1991; **265**: 2202–7.

34. Mikhail MG, Smith FA, Gray M, *et al.* Cost-effectiveness of mandatory stress testing in chest pain center patients. *Ann Emerg Med* 1997; **29**: 88–98.

35. Zalenski RJ, Rydman RJ, McCarren M, *et al.* Feasibility of a rapid diagnostic protocol for an emergency department chest pain unit. *Ann Emerg Med* 1997; **29**: 99–108.

36. Rydman RJ, Zalenski RJ, Roberts RR, *et al.* Patient satisfaction with an emergency department chest pain observation unit. *Ann Emerg Med* 1997; **29**: 109–15.

37. Tatum JL, Jesse RL, Kontos MC, *et al.* Comprehensive strategy for the evaluation and triage of the chest pain patient. *Ann Emerg Med* 1997; **29**: 116–25.

♦38. Lewis WR, Amsterdam EA. Utility and safety of immediate exercise testing of low-risk patients admitted to the hospital for suspected acute myocardial infarction. *Am J Cardiol* 1994; **74**: 987–90.

39. Gaspoz JM, Lee TH, Weinstein MC, *et al.* Cost-

effectiveness of a new short-stay unit to 'rule out' acute myocardial infarction in low risk patients. *J Am Coll Cardiol* 1994; **24**: 1249–59.

♦40. Kirk JD, Turnipseed S, Lewis WR, *et al.* Evaluation of chest pain in low risk patients presenting to the emergency department: the role of immediate exercise testing. *Ann Emerg Med* 1998; **32**: 1–7.

41. Gomez MA, Anderson JL, Karagounis LA, *et al.* An emergency department-based protocol for rapidly ruling out myocardial ischemia reduces hospital time and expense: results of a randomized study (ROMIO). *J Am Coll Cardiol* 1996; **28**: 25–33.

42. Higgins GL III, Lambrew CT, Hunt E, *et al.* Expediting the early hospital care of the adult patient with nontraumatic chest pain: impact of a modified ED triage protocol. *Am J Emerg Med* 1993; **11**: 576–82.

43. Lee TH, Rouan GW, Weisberg MC, *et al.* Sensitivity of routine clinical criteria for diagnosing myocardial infarction within 24 hours of hospitalization. *Ann Intern Med* 1987; **106**: 181–6.

44. de Winter RJ, Koster RW, Sturk A, *et al.* Value of myoglobin, troponin T, and CK-MB mass in ruling out an acute myocardial infarction in the emergency room. *Circulation* 1995; **92**: 3401–7.

45. Puleo PR, Meyer D, Wathen C, *et al.* Use of a rapid assay of subforms of creatine kinase-MB to diagnose or rule out acute myocardial infarction. *N Engl J Med* 1994; **331**: 561–6.

46. Katus HA, Remppis A, Neumann FJ, *et al.* Diagnostic efficiency of troponin T measurements in acute myocardial infarction. *Circulation* 1991; **83**: 902–12.

47. Ohman EM, Armstrong PW, Christenson RH. Cardiac troponin T levels for risk stratification in acute myocardial ischemia. *N Engl J Med* 1996; **335**: 1333–41.

♦48. Antman EM, Tanasijevic MJ, Thompson B, *et al.* Cardiac-specific troponin I levels to predict the risk of mortality in patients with acute coronary syndromes. *N Engl J Med* 1996; **335**: 1342–9.

49. Polanczyk CA, Lee TH, Cook EF, *et al.* Cardiac Troponin I as a predictor of major cardiac events in emergency department patients with acute chest pain. *J Am Coll Cardiol* 1998; **32**: 8–14.

50. Amsterdam EA, Lewis WR. Identification of low risk patients with chest pain in the emergency department: another look at cardiac troponins. *J Am Coll Cardiol* 1998; **32**: 15–16.

51. Hauser AM, Gangadharan V, Ramos RG, *et al.* Sequence of mechanical, electrocardiographic and clinical effects of repeated coronary artery occlusion in human beings: echocardiographic observations during coronary angioplasty. *J Am Coll Cardiol* 1985; **5**: 193–7.

52. Lundgren C, Bourdillon PD, Dillon JC, *et al.* Comparison of contrast angiography and two-dimensional echocardiography for the evaluation of left ventricular regional wall motion abnormalities after acute myocardial infarction. *Am J Cardiol* 1990; **65**: 1071–7.

53. Sabia P, Afrookteh A, Touchstone DA, *et al.* Value of regional wall motion abnormality in the emergency room diagnosis of acute myocardial infarction. A prospective study using two-dimensional echocardiography. *Circulation* 1991; **84**: 185–192.

54. Peels KH, Visser CA, Kupper AJF, *et al.* Value of 2D-echocardiography for immediate detection of coronary artery disease in the emergency room. *Circulation* 1988; **78**: II–463.

55. Sasaki H, Charuzi Y, Beeder C, *et al.* Utility of echocardiography for the early assessment of patients with nondiagnostic chest pain. *Am Heart J* 1986; **112**: 494–7.

56. Horowitz RS, Morganroth J, Parrotto C, *et al.* Immediate diagnosis of acute myocardial infarction by two-dimensional echocardiography. *Circulation* 1982; **65**: 323–9.

57. Saeian D, Rhyne T, Sagar K. Ultrasonic tissue characterization for diagnosis of acute myocardial infarction in the coronary care unit. *Am J Cardiol* 1994; **74**: 1211–15.

58. Levitt MA, Promes SB, Bullock S, *et al.* Combined cardiac marker approach with adjunct two-dimensional echocardiography to diagnose acute myocardial infarction in the emergency department. *Ann Emerg Med* 1996; **27**: 1–7.

59. Stewart WJ, Douglas PS, Sagar K, *et al.* Echocardiography in emergency medicine: a policy statement by the American Society of Echocardiography and the American College of Cardiology. *J Am Soc Echocardiog* 1999; **12**: 82–4.

60. Jeroudi MO, Cheirif J, Habib G, *et al.* Prolonged wall motion abnormalities after chest pain at rest in patients with unstable angina: a possible manifestation of myocardial stunning. *Am Heart J* 1994; **127**: 1241–50.

61. Lieberman AN, Weiss JL, Jugdutt BL, *et al.* Two-dimensional echocardiography and infarct size: relationship of regional wall motion and thickening to the extent of myocardial infarction in the dog. *Circulation* 1981; **63**: 739.

62. Kaul S. Echocardiography in coronary artery disease. *Curr Prob Cardiol* 1990; **15**: 233.

63. Trippi JA, Kopp G, Lee KS, *et al.* The feasibility of dobutamine stress echocardiography in the emergency department with telemedicine interpretation. *J Am Soc Echocardiog* 1996; **9**: 113–8.

64. Sakuma T, Hayashi Y, Shimohara A, *et al.* Usefulness of myocardial contrast echocardiography for the assessment of serial changes in risk area in patients with acute myocardial infarction. *Am J Cardiol* 1996; **78**: 1273–7.

○65. Selker HP, Zalenski RJ, Antmen EM, *et al.* An evaluation of technologies for identifying acute cardiac ischemia in the emergency department: a report from a National Heart Attack Alert Program Working Group. *Ann Emerg Med* 1997; **29**: 13–87.

65a. Laudon DA, Vukov LF, Breen JF, Rumberger JA, Wollan PC, Sheedy PF. Use of electron-beam computed tomography in the evaluation of chest pain patients in the emergency department. *Ann Emerg Med* 1999; **33**: 15–21.

66. Henneman PL, Mena IG, Rothstein RJ, *et al.* Evaluation of patients with chest pain and nondiagnostic ECG using thallium-201 myocardial planar imaging and technetium-99 first-pass radionuclide angiography in the emergency department. *Ann Emerg Med* 1992; **21**: 545–50.

67. Mace SE. Thallium myocardial scanning in the emergency department of chest pain. *Am J Emerg Med* 1989; **7**: 321–8.

68. Van der Wieken LR, Kan G, Belfer AJ, *et al.* Thallium-201 scanning to decide CCU admission in patients with non-diagnostic electrocardiograms. *Int J Cardiol* 1983; **4**: 285–95.

♦69. Tatum JL, Jesse RL, Kontos MC, *et al.* Comprehensive strategy for the evaluation and triage of the chest pain patient. *Ann Emerg Med* 1997; **29**: 116–25.

70. Hilton TC, Thompson TC, Williams HJ, *et al.* Technetium-99m sestamibi myocardial perfusion imaging in the emergency room evaluation of chest pain. *J Am Coll Cardiol* 1994; **23**: 1016–22.

71. Varetto T, Cantalupi D, Altieri A, *et al.* Emergency room technetium-99m sestamibi imaging to rule out acute myocardial ischemic events in patients with nondiagnostic electrocardiograms. *J Am Coll Cardiol* 1993; **22**: 1804–8.

72. Gregoire J, Theroux P. Detection and assessment of unstable angina using myocardial perfusion imaging: comparison between technetium-99m sestamibi SPECT and 12-lead electrocardiogram. *Am J Cardiol* 1990; **66**: 42E–6E.

73. Weissman IA, Dickinson CZ, Dworkin HJ, *et al.* Cost-effectiveness of myocardial perfusion imaging with SPECT in the emergency department evaluation of patients with unexplained chest pain. *Radiology* 1996; **199**: 353–7.

74. Stuart RJ Jr, Ellestad MH. National survey of exercise stress testing facilities. *Chest* 1980; **77**: 94–7.

75. Lewis WR, Amsterdam EA, Turnipseed S, Kirk JD. Immediate exercise testing of low risk patients with known coronary artery disease presenting to the emergency department with chest pain. *J Am Coll Cardiol* 1999; **33**: 1843–7.

○76. Amsterdam EA, Lewis WR, Yadlapalli S. Evaluation of low risk patients with chest pain in the emergency department: value and limitations of recent methods. *Cardiol in Rev* 1999; **7**: 17–26.

77. Polanczyk CA, Johnson PA, Hartley LH, *et al.* Clinical correlates and prognostic significance of early negative exercise tolerance test in patients with acute chest pain seen in the hospital emergency department. *Am J Cardiol* 1998; **81**: 288–92.

7

Recognition, evaluation, and management of hypotension and cardiogenic shock

JOHN FOLEY AND RICHARD C BECKER

The maintenance of vital organ perfusion is an absolute prerequisite for normal function and biologic homeostasis. Abnormalities in myocardial performance (inotropy), atrioventricular synchrony, ventricular filling (preload), wall stress (afterload), and arteriolar tone (peripheral vascular resistance) can lead to hypotension and hypoperfusion – collectively referred to as shock. A clinician's ability to recognize preshock and overt shock states, and to institute therapy promptly are important determinants of patient outcome.

INTRODUCTION

Hypotension and shock are most often caused by a marked reduction in myocardial performance that, in essence, is inadequate for existing metabolic requirements. Prompt recognition, stabilization, diagnostic evaluation, and treatment are absolute prerequisites for patient survival.

DETERMINANTS OF A NORMAL SYSTEMIC BLOOD PRESSURE

Systemic blood pressure is determined by the volume of blood ejected into the systemic circulation (cardiac output) and by the peripheral vascular resistance. Therefore, disturbances in blood pressure are caused by either a reduced cardiac output (the hallmark of cardiogenic shock) or a reduced peripheral vascular resistance (the hallmark of septic, neurogenic and anaphylactic shock). Since the differentiation of isolated systemic hypotension and the development of overt shock is determined by the existence of tissue hypoperfusion in the latter

state, it is imperative to consider systemic (vital organ) blood flow (cardiac output and overall perfusion pressure) as the central focus of this discussion. Figure 7.1 summarizes several key concepts of flow (cardiac output) as influenced by cardiac 'pump' parameters (stroke volume and heart rate) as well as 'pressure over resistance'. This formula should serve as the starting point for understanding and managing hypotension, hypoperfusion, and shock.

Peripheral vascular resistance

Peripheral vascular resistance varies inversely with the fourth power of the arteriolar (resistance vessels) radius. Therefore, vascular resistance is determined by vascular tone, which is directly influenced by:

1 metabolic and mechanical autoregulatory mechanisms (adenosine is the primary metabolic regulator);
2 neurogenic constrictor influences operating through norepinephrine;
3 neurogenic vasodilator influences operating through acetylcholine and histamine;

$$\text{Cardiac output (C.O.)} = \text{Flow} = \frac{\text{Pressure}}{\text{Resistance}}$$

$$\text{C.O.} = \text{Flow} = \frac{\text{MAP-CVP}}{\frac{8\,\eta\,L}{\Pi\,\Gamma^4}}$$

η = viscosity
L = Length of vessels (constant)

Map = Mean Arterial Pressure
CVP = Central Venous Pressure
Γ = Radius of Resistance Vessels

$$\text{C.O.} = \text{Flow} = \text{Stroke volume} \times \text{Heart rate} = (\text{MAP-CVP}) \times \frac{\Pi}{8}\,\frac{1}{\eta}\,\frac{\Gamma^4}{L}$$

→ Preload
→ Afterload
→ Contractility

Figure 7.1 *Important concepts in understanding cardiac performance, the determinants of systemic blood pressure, and end-organ perfusion.*

Table 7.1 *Determinants of cardiac performance*

Preload (ventricular filling)
Venous return
Total blood volume
Intrathoracic pressure
Intrapericardial pressure
Atrial contribution (i.e. contraction)

Afterload (ventricular wall stress; impedance)

Contractility (intrinsic activity of myocardium)
Sympathetic nervous system
Circulating catecholamines
Local environment (anoxia, ischemia, acidemia)
Contractile mass
Inotropic stimulation

Heart rate

4 circulating and locally released vasoactive substances, including catecholamines, angiotensin II, bradykinin, and prostaglandins.

The autonomic nervous system plays a prominent role in maintaining systemic blood pressure and organ perfusion because it directly influences both cardiac output and peripheral vascular resistance.

Blood volume

An adequate intravascular volume is required to maintain systemic blood pressure. This is accomplished primarily through the renin–angiotensin–aldosterone system; other contributors include arginine vasopressin and atrial natriuretic polypeptide.

Cardiac performance

The three primary determinants of cardiac performance are preload, afterload, and contractility. As cardiac output is the product of heart rate and stroke volume, the former is considered to be a fourth determinant of cardiac performance (Table 7.1).

Preload

In the intact heart, ventricular end-diastolic wall stress or tension is analogous to the preload of isolated muscle and ultimately determines the resting length of the sarcomeres. Preload is determined largely by venous return, total blood volume and its distribution, and atrial contraction. Because ventricular filling occurs predominantly during diastole of the cardiac cycle, the rate of relaxation, dimensions of the ventricular cavities, the thickness of the ventricular walls, and the intrinsic mechanical properties of cardiac tissue are considered the main determinants of passive volume loading.

Afterload

When applied to the intact ventricle, afterload can be defined as the tension, force, or stress (force per unit of cross-sectional area) acting on the fibers in the ventricular wall after the onset of shortening. Afterload is determined largely by peripheral vascular resistance, the physical characteristics of the arterial tree, and the volume of blood contained within the circulatory system at the onset of ventricular ejection. When ventricular function is impaired or preload is reduced, afterload becomes a vital determinant of systemic blood pressure.

Inotropic state (contractility)

The force of myocardial contraction is generally influenced by altered Ca^{2+} availability to the myofilaments or through an alteration in myofilament Ca^{2+} sensitivity. Following inotropic stimulation the ventricular force–velocity relation is increased (shifted upward) as is the diastolic volume–pressure curve. Factors that modify contractility of the myocardium include sympathetic activity, circulating catecholamines, increased heart rate (force–frequency relation), exogenous inotropic agents (cardiac glycosides, sympathomimetic agents), physiological and pharmacological depressants (ischemia, anoxia, acidosis, β-adrenergic blocking agents), and loss of contractile mass (myocardial infarction, cardiomyopathy).

Heart rate

Accelerating the frequency of ventricular contraction increases stroke power (rate of performance of stroke work) at any given filling volume and pressure, a finding consistent with an improvement in myocardial contractility. Since, at a constant stroke volume, cardiac output is linearly related to heart rate, the latter is a vital means to compensate for changes in contractility.

HYPOTENSION AND SHOCK

Shock is best defined as a syndrome, i.e. a recognizable collection of symptoms, signs, and laboratory abnormalities, which results from systemic *hypoperfusion* associated with widespread cellular and organ dysfunction. Patients are usually hypotensive and the cardiac output is frequently decreased; however, in some shock states cardiac output is normal (inappropriately low) despite hypotension and/or evidence of tissue hypoperfusion.[1]

The key distinguishing feature between hypotension and shock is the presence of tissue hypoperfusion. In essence, cellular and end-organ hypoperfusion are responsible for the metabolic, inflammatory, and biochemical abnormalities that so strongly influence clinical outcome. For this reason, hypotension represents a serious, yet reversible, early warning sign that can progress to irreversible damage of vital organs.

Etiologies

A number of conditions and disease can cause hypotension and shock (Table 7.2). The pathophysiologic basis of shock can be considered as falling into one or more of the following categories: 'pre-heart' (volume-related), 'heart' (cardiac-related), or 'post-heart' (resistance-related). As previously described, the most common abnormality underlying shock is impaired myocardial performance (Tables 7.3 and 7.4). Other initiating processes leading to shock include hypovolemia, e.g. hemorrhage or severe dehydration; maldistribution of blood volume, e.g. adverse reactions to anesthetic agents or vasodilators; increased resistance to blood flow in the systemic or pulmonary circulation, e.g. myxoma, coarctation of the aorta, pulmonary embolism; decreased arteriolar tone or abnormal capillary function, e.g. anaphylaxis, adult respiratory distress syndrome (ARDS); and arteriovenous shunting of blood, e.g. sepsis, pneumonia, peritonitis.

Table 7.2 *Primary or initiating pathobiologic mechanisms in shock states*

Depressed myocardial performance
Reduced or maldistributed intravascular volume
Increased resistance to blood flow in the systemic or pulmonary circulation
Decreased arteriolar tone in the systemic resistance bed
Abnormal capillary function (increased permeability)
Arteriovenous shunting of blood

Table 7.3 *Etiologies of cardiogenic shock*

Acute myocardial infarction
Reduced left ventricular performance (systolic, diastolic)
Ventricular septal rupture (acute)
Mitral regurgitation (acute)
Ventricular free-wall rupture

Other cardiac disorders associated with impaired ventricular function
Dilated cardiomyopathy/severe myocarditis
End-stage valvular heart disease (aortic stenosis, mitral stenosis, aortic regurgitation, mitral regurgitation)
Myocardial depression in septic shock
Tachyarrhythmia or bradyarrhythmia
Following cardiopulmonary bypass

Cardiac obstruction or compression
Cardiac tamponade
Pericardial constriction
Pulmonary embolism
Pulmonary hypertension
Coarctation of the aorta
Cardiac myxoma
Hypertrophic obstructive cardiomyopathy
Tension pneumothorax

Hypovolemia related to cardiovascular pathology
Ruptured aortic aneurysm
Aortic dissection
Hemorrhagic shock

Table 7.4 *Functional approach to cardiogenic shock based on determinants of cardiac performance*

Decreased preload ('pre-heart')
Right ventricular infarction
Cardiac tamponade
Pulmonary embolism
Hypovolemia resulting from blood loss, e.g. ruptured aneurysm
Cardiac myxoma
Tension pneumothorax
Mitral stenosis
Tachyarrhythmias, advanced (A-V) conduction defects

Impaired contractility (relative or absolute) ('heart')
Acute myocardial infarction
Dilated cardiomyopathy
Mitral insufficiency
Aortic insufficiency
Ventricular septal rupture
Bradyarrhythmias

Excessive afterload ('post-heart')
Malignant hypertension
Coarctation of the aorta
Aortic stenosis
Hypertrophic obstructive cardiomyopathy

[a]Preload may also be reduced.

Persistent hypotension accompanied by cellular hypoperfusion produces an adverse metabolic environment that, in many instances, facilitates further compromise. Increased levels of circulating catecholamines lead to systemic arteriolar vasoconstriction that further impairs tissue perfusion. A variety of vasoactive substances are also released including histamine, bradykinin, serotonin, prostaglandins, endorphins, proteases, oxygen-derived free radicals, activated complement components, and tumor necrosis factor. Excessive nitric oxide production by endothelial cells and macrophages contributes to the hypotensive effect produced by tumor necrosis factor.

Compensatory mechanisms

Systemic hypotension with accompanying tissue hypoperfusion leads to activation of a number of intrinsic defense mechanisms that attempt to restore circulatory homeostasis and preserve vital organ perfusion (Table 7.5). To maximize cardiac output and tissue perfusion, stroke volume, and heart rate must increase. In the early phases of shock these compensatory mechanisms are more or less successful in preserving cardiac output, and a marginally adequate systemic blood pressure. If the shock state persists, gradual erosion in the efficacy of compensatory mechanisms develops. Finally, as the shock state worsens, compensatory mechanisms become ineffective, and irreversible shock supervenes.

Mortality from shock increases progressively in direct relationship to the severity and duration of the syndrome. The major homeostatic defense mechanism in shock is activation of the sympathetic nervous system. The signal for activation of increased adrenergic nervous activity is decreased cardiac output and systemic arterial blood pressure.[2] A decline in either systemic arterial blood pressure or blood volume activates stretch baroreceptors in the aortic arch, carotid sinus, and splanchnic arterial bed.[3,4] Volume-sensitive baroreceptors within the heart can also be activated. Increased signals from these baroreceptors to the central nervous system lead to increased sympathetic nerve efferent responses and decreased parasympathetic activity. A number of different peripheral events are produced by increased sympathetic tone:

1 arteriolar vasoconstriction with decreased perfusion to skin, skeletal muscle, kidney, and splanchnic bed;
2 increased heart rate and myocardial contractility;
3 venoconstriction with increased venous return and central blood volume;
4 increased release of adrenal hormones;[5]
5 activation of the renin-angiotensin–aldosterone axis.[6]

Activation of the renin–angiotensin–aldosterone system produces immediate arteriolar vasoconstriction and increases both circulatory blood volume and cardiac output through sodium and water retention.[7] Simultaneous release of arginine vasopressin from the posterior pituitary also occurs in the setting of hypotension and shock. Vasopressin binds to specific receptors in the splanchnic, renal, and other vascular beds, further increasing peripheral vascular resistance and intravascular volume.[8]

Another compensatory mechanism that is observed in response to decreased cardiac output is transcapillary refill. This factor involves the decrease in capillary hydrostatic pressure that results from adrenergic vasoconstriction of the precapillary sphincters. Decreased luminal capillary hydrostatic pressure favors movement of fluid and solutes from the interstitial space into the capillary, thereby increasing circulating blood volume.[9]

Contraregulatory mechanisms

A variety of systemic mechanisms that are initiated in response to shock can actually augment or amplify the effects of the shock state, ultimately contributing to the irreversible, fatal nature of the syndrome. The first of the potentially detrimental responses is loss of adrenergic-mediated peripheral vascular tone (Table 7.6).[10–17] Other microcirculatory phenomena that

Table 7.5 *Compensatory responses in shock states*

1. Preservation of coronary and cerebral perfusion at the expense of skin, skeletal muscle, kidney, and splanchnic perfusion

2. Preservation of cardiac output through increased sympathetic nervous system activity, increased heart rate, and myocardial contractility

3. Preservation of intravascular volume: vasoconstriction (venous, arteriolar), activation of the renin–angiotensin–aldosterone system

Table 7.6 *Contraregulatory mechanisms in shock states*

Factors associated with a loss of peripheral vascular tone
Acidemia
Decreased central sympathetic nervous system activity resulting from cerebral ischemia
Catecholamine depletion from vascular smooth muscle nerve endings
Antiadrenergic actions of increased endorphin concentrations
Release of nitric oxide and vasodilating prostaglandins

Factors associated with decreased cardiac performance
Acidemia
Inappropriate bradycardia
Circulating myocardial depressant factors
Decreased coronary arterial perfusion

accentuate the shock state include increased capillary permeability, obstruction of the microvasculature by platelet and white cell aggregates, decreased red blood cell deformability, and swelling of endothelial cells.[18–21]

Studies in both animal models and in humans support the concept of progressive myocardial depression during shock. The following factors contribute to a derangement in cardiac performance:

1 a decrease in coronary arterial perfusion secondary to systemic hypotension and increased coronary arterial tone mediated by circulating coronary arterial vasoconstrictors (leukotrienes);
2 presence in the blood of circulating myocardial depressant substances, e.g. tumor necrosis factor;[22–25]
3 inappropriate bradycardia from vagal stimulation – activation of inhibitory cardiac vagal afferent nerve fibers following vigorous myocardial contraction around nearly empty cardiac chambers;[26]
4 acidosis-mediated down-regulation (responsiveness of β-adrenergic receptors).

Progressive end-organ hypoperfusion augments the shock state in several ways. Increased pulmonary capillary permeability and respiratory muscle fatigue lead to hypoxemia and respiratory failure (ARDS).[27] Acute renal failure, most often from acute tubular necrosis, is a common event in patients with shock. Metabolic acidosis and hyperkalemia often accompany acute renal failure.[28,29] Splanchnic vasoconstriction with visceral ischemia can lead to erosive gastritis, pancreatitis, acalculous cholecystitis, and loss of the barrier function of the gastrointestinal tract, predisposing to bacteremias.[30]

Hepatic hypoperfusion can result in centrilobular liver necrosis (so-called shock liver) characterized by modest elevations in serum bilirubin and alkaline phosphatase and marked increases in serum transaminase values.[31] Cerebral hypoperfusion can lead to restlessness, agitation, mental obtundation, and even coma. Cerebral infarction in a 'watershed' distribution may also occur.

Patients with shock can develop disseminated intravascular coagulation (DIC); however, DIC most often occurs in the setting of septic or endotoxic shock and rarely is a feature of cardiogenic shock. A wide variety of derangements of immune function have been described in patients with shock states.[32–35]

Clinical presentation: characteristic features

The two cardinal manifestations of shock that enable the clinician to establish a diagnosis are: (1) *hypotension*, and (2) *hypoperfusion*. Hypotension is usually defined as a blood pressure less than 90 mm Hg, although patients may have evidence of hypoperfusion with systemic blood pressures above 90 mm Hg if previous basal values were *above* the usual normal range. Indeed, a relative

state of hypotension and hypoperfusion may coexist if the mean arterial pressure is ≥30 mm Hg below the baseline value.

The existence of hypoperfusion is suggested from one or more by one of the following: (1) altered mental status – restlessness, agitation, obtundation; (2) cold, clammy skin; and (3) reduced urine output (below 30 mL/h).

CARDIOGENIC SHOCK

Epidemiology

Cardiogenic shock complicates 5–15 per cent of all acute myocardial infarctions (MI). Information derived from the Worcester Heart Attack Study suggests that the incidence of cardiogenic shock as a complication of MI has remained relatively constant over the past decade, averaging 7.5 per cent of the cases. Despite recent technological advances in the diagnosis and treatment of patients with acute MI, in-hospital and long-term mortality remains very high (Figure 7.2). In-hospital case fatality rates in various series range from 70 per cent to nearly 100 per cent. For the survivors, the 5-year survival rate following discharge from the hospital is approximately 40 per cent.[36–42]

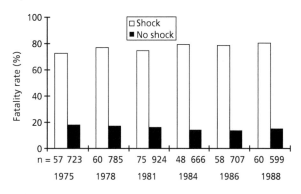

Figure 7.2 *The mortality for patients with myocardial infarction complicated by cardiogenic shock has not changed substantially over the years. The average in-hospital death rate has remained between 70 per cent and 80 per cent. (Reproduced with permission from Goldberg et al. Cardiogenic shock resulting from acute myocardial infarction: a fourteen year community-wide perspective. N Engl J Med 1991; 325: 1117–22.)*

Pathophysiologic features

Many of the conditions associated with cardiogenic shock are characterized by depressed left and/or right ventricular function. Less common are conditions that cause cardiac compression and inadequate ventricular filling or severe ventricular inflow or outflow obstruction (left atrial myxoma and coarctation of the aorta). Intravascular hypovolemia secondary to blood loss (ruptured aortic aneurysm) may lead to shock.

Acute myocardial infarction

Cardiogenic shock, a potentially life-threatening complication of MI (Table 7.7), is most often caused by either permanent (necrosis) or transient (ischemia-mediated or stunned) myocardial dysfunction (systolic, diastolic).[43,44] If untreated, progressive arterial hypoxemia and decreased cardiac output lead to metabolic acidosis and further depression of left ventricular performance. A vicious downward spiral rapidly ensues: left ventricular dysfunction leads to worsening cardiac output, hypotension and arterial hypoxemia, which in turn decreases myocardial perfusion pressure, thereby further depressing left ventricular performance.

Table 7.7 *Pathogenesis of cardiogenic shock after acute myocardial infarction*

Extensive left ventricular dysfunction
Myocardial infarction (MI) with extension or ischemic dysfunction
Massive MI (greater than 40% of left ventricle (LV))
Small MI in the presence of a prior large infarction
Small/moderate size MI with metabolic acidosis or arrhythmias

Mechanical defects
Rupture of ventricular septum
Rupture of part or all of papillary muscle
Rupture of free ventricular wall
Ischemic dysfunction of papillary muscle resulting in severe mitral regurgitation
Right ventricular infarction

Mechanical defects can also lead to cardiogenic shock. Papillary muscle rupture accounts for 5 per cent of all cardiac ruptures while ventricular septal and free wall ruptures account for 10 and 85 per cent, respectively. The posteromedial papillary muscle is 5–10 times more prone to ischemia, infarction, and/or rupture compared with the anterolateral papillary muscle, most likely because it is served by only one coronary artery. Thus, clinically important mitral regurgitation occurs more commonly in patients with inferoposterior myocardial infarction.

Rupture of the interventricular septum occurs with both anterior and inferoposterior myocardial infarction. Multivessel coronary artery disease is common, but single-vessel disease can also lead to this complication. Rupture of the septum can occur anywhere between 1 and 14 days after infarction; however, this complication usually develops 3–7 days after infarction. Thrombolytic therapy appears to accelerate rupture events to within the first 24–48 hours.[45]

Cardiogenic shock is usually considered a sequela of ST segment elevation MI; however, data derived from GUSTO IIb (Global Use of Strategies to Open Occluded Coronary Arteries)[46] show that shock, although less common in patients with non-ST segment elevation MI (odds ratio 0.58), does occur and is associated with a mortality approaching 75 per cent. In contrast to patients with ST segment elevation MI who develop shock, those without ST segment elevation are older, more frequently have diabetes mellitus, and experience recurrent myocardial ischemia or infarction prior to the event.

Right ventricular infarction

Although right ventricular infarction may complicate up to one-third of inferoposterior left ventricular infarcts, the volume of injured right ventricular myocardium is usually small to moderate.[47] An occasional patient with inferoposterior infarction develops extensive ischemia or necrosis of the right ventricle with resultant cardiogenic shock. These patients have clinical features of isolated right-sided heart failure; jugular venous distention, clear lungs, right ventricular S_3 and S_4, and hepatic congestion. Kussmaul's sign (inspiratory increase in jugular venous pressure) may be seen. Cardiac output is markedly depressed (usually less than 2.0 L/min per m²); pulmonary capillary wedge pressure is normal or slightly elevated. Right atrial pressure is significantly elevated and exceeds pulmonary capillary wedge pressure while pulmonary arterial pressure is surprisingly normal. Pulmonary arterial pulse pressure is diminished (usually less than 15–20 mm Hg). The hemodynamic findings often resemble those seen with cardiac tamponade or pericardial constriction.

Low systemic blood pressure is the result of decreased left ventricular filling secondary to diminished right ventricular cardiac output and increased intrapericardial pressure from the dilated right ventricle, which produces, in effect, tamponade of the left ventricle.[48–50] The reverse Bernheim phenomenon (septal bulging into the left ventricle) may also play a role in diminished left ventricular volumes and stroke output. Bradyarrhythmias with loss of an appropriately timed atrial 'kick' also contribute to the decrease in right ventricular function.[51]

Cardiomyopathies/myocarditis

Patients with end-stage dilated cardiomyopathy and markedly depressed left (and often right) ventricular function may develop terminal cardiogenic shock. Left ventricular ejection fraction is usually less than 20 per cent and substantial left ventricular dilatation is usually present. Fulminant acute viral myocarditis can also lead to cardiogenic shock.

Valvular heart disease

Advanced, long-standing valvular heart disease involving one or more valves, stenotic and/or regurgitant, or acute events leading to severe insufficiency can terminate with cardiogenic shock.

Acute aortic or mitral regurgitation is most commonly caused by infectious endocarditis, dissection of the aorta, or spontaneous rupture of a myxomatous valve or chordae tendineae. The left ventricle is not dilated since the regurgitation is acute.[52]

Patients with end-stage aortic or mitral stenosis also develop cardiogenic shock. Individuals with severe aortic stenosis and shock have a small gradient across the aortic valve (usually less than 20–30 mm Hg) and markedly depressed cardiac output and left ventricular ejection fraction. End-stage mitral stenosis leading to cardiogenic shock is associated with marked right ventricular dilatation and severe tricuspid regurgitation.

Myocardial suppression associated with sepsis

It is well recognized that myocardial dysfunction occurs in sepsis,[53–55] contributing directly to patient demise in 20–33 per cent of non-surviving cases. Specific myocardial abnormalities include depression of left and right ventricular ejection fractions, ventricular dilation, and altered Frank–Starling and diastolic pressure–volume relationships.[56–59] These abnormalities typically develop between the first and fourth days after the onset of sepsis and resolve within 5–10 days in surviving patients.

In the early stages of sepsis, cardiac output is usually normal or increased in patients with an adequate volume status; however, in the presence of marked peripheral vasodilation and arteriovenous shunting, a normal or slightly elevated cardiac output may, in fact, be inadequate to meet the overall metabolic demands of the body. Indeed, a cardiac output in excess of 10 L/min may be required in patients with overt septic shock.[59]

'Myocardial depression' implies that the observed decrease in cardiac performance is caused by a decrease in myocardial contractility. However, as previously discussed, cardiac output is influenced by a number of variables in addition to contractility, including preload, afterload, and heart rate.

The findings of a low cardiac output in early studies of sepsis were introduced as evidence for depressed myocardial performance, when in fact the low output probably represented a reduced preload. Once this shortcoming was recognized and adequate volume status was ensured by following pulmonary artery wedge pressure measurements, more than 90 per cent of patients in septic shock were found to have a high cardiac output early in the course of their disease. In the later stages, however, overt myocardial suppression can occur (Figure 7.3).

There is a considerable body of evidence that myocardial performance is depressed in septic shock. Although endotoxin is not a direct myocardial depressant, it appears to provoke the release of a circulating myocardial depressant substance (MDS). The true identity of MDS is still unknown, but possibilities include interleukin-2 and tumor necrosis factor. The myocardial effects of MDS include decreased energy stores, decreased ability to release calcium during contraction, and altered ventricular compliance (possibly secondary to abnormal calcium uptake by the sarcoplasmic reticulum).

Tachyarrhythmias and bradyarrhythmias

Disturbances in cardiac rhythm can lead to: (1) inadequate ventricular diastolic filling (atrial and ventricular tachyarrhythmias); (2) abnormal ventricular contraction patterns resulting from abnormal electrical activation patterns in the ventricle (ventricular tachyarrhythmias); and (3) inadequate heart rate in the face of adequate ventricular function (bradyarrhythmias). Abnormal ventricular function prior to the development of an arrhythmia predisposes to more severe hemodynamic derangement once an arrhythmia develops.

Myocardial depression following cardiopulmonary bypass

Shock following cardiopulmonary bypass is usually multifactorial with both cardiogenic and hypovolemic components. The cardiogenic factors contributing to shock in this setting include arrhythmias, tamponade, myocardial ischemic dysfunction or stunning (from cardioplegia and electrolyte abnormalities), and MI. In general, left ventricular dysfunction predominates in this setting, but right ventricular dysfunction in the face of postoperative pulmonary hypertension may also contribute to the shock syndrome following cardiopulmonary bypass.[60,61]

Pericardial tamponade or constriction

Myocardial function is relatively normal in patients with cardiac tamponade or pericardial constriction. Depressed cardiac output is the result of markedly impaired ventricular diastolic filling secondary to the pericardial abnormality. Severe tamponade and shock can develop within seconds to minutes (myocardial free wall rupture), or it may occur following days or even weeks of subacute, more moderate, restriction of ventricular filling.

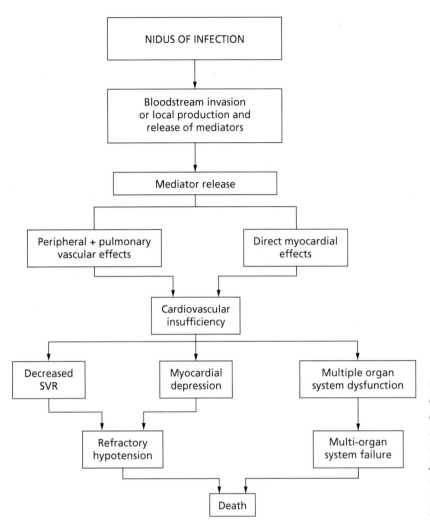

Figure 7.3 *Septic shock is characterized, at least initially, by decreased peripheral vascular resistance and a compensatory increase in cardiac output. Death can result from refractory hypotension, myocardial depression (cytokine-mediated) or multisystem organ failure. SVR = systemic vascular resistance.*

Pulmonary embolism

Massive pulmonary embolism obstructing more than 60 per cent of the pulmonary vascular bed can produce syncope, hypotension, or overt shock. Occasionally, pulmonary embolism presents as cardiogenic shock. The right ventricle fails acutely secondary to a sudden increase in afterload: cardiac output falls and right ventricular filling pressure rises. The increase in right ventricular afterload is the result of mechanical obstruction of the pulmonary arterial bed. Pulmonary arterial and right ventricular systolic pressure typically does not exceed 50–60 mm Hg in individuals with previously normal pulmonary arterial pressure. Left-sided heart pressures are normal or reduced because of inadequate left ventricular filling. Arterial hypoxemia is invariably present. There may be a small to moderate right-to-left shunt of deoxygenated blood through a patent foramen ovale.

Primary pulmonary hypertension/severe pulmonary hypertension

Cardiogenic shock may result from severe, long-standing pulmonary hypertension with marked, chronic right ventricular failure and sudden decompensation. Pulmonary arterial and right ventricular systolic pressure often exceed 80 mm Hg. Left ventricular filling pressures are low to normal. Right-to-left shunting of blood thorough a patent foramen ovale may be present and contribute to chronic hypoxemia.

Coarctation of the aorta

Coarctation of the aorta may cause cardiogenic shock early in life as the ductus arteriosus closes and the left ventricle is unable to adapt to the markedly increased aortic resistance (afterload). In this setting, the left ventricle may fail acutely. Adults with coarctation of the aorta rarely develop cardiogenic shock because they have left ventricular hypertrophy and adequate left ventricular function that is able to maintain peripheral perfusion despite a marked increase in aortic resistance.

Myxoma

Atrial myxomas may suddenly prolapse into the mitral (usual) or tricuspid (rare) valve orifice, totally or near totally obstructing blood flow into the affected ventricle.

Hypertrophic obstructive cardiomyopathy

A rare individual with hypertrophic obstructive cardiomyopathy may develop cardiogenic shock with a sudden increase in left ventricular outflow obstruction. More often, congestive heart failure and shock are the result of severe diastolic dysfunction, progressive left ventricular dilation, and systolic dysfunction or sudden tachyarrhythmias.

Tension pneumothorax

In patients with tension pneumothorax, the great veins within the thorax are subjected to high intrapleural pressure, which, in essence, causes venous collapse and a sudden reduction in ventricular preload. Cardiac output declines precipitously and cardiogenic shock develops.

Vascular causes of shock

Ruptured aortic aneurysms, aortic dissection with aortic valve disruption, or rupture and traumatic perforation of major arteries and veins can each precipitate shock.

PATIENT EVALUATION: AN ETIOLOGY-BASED APPROACH

The initial evaluation of patients with cardiogenic shock must take place swiftly. Important diagnostic benchmarks for establishing a diagnosis and building support for treatment are outlined in Table 7.8. In the process of evaluation the key determinants of systemic blood pressure and myocardial performance must serve as the template for each vital step: stabilization, differential diagnosis, diagnostic testing, and definitive therapy.

Acute myocardial infarction

Patients with acute MI complicated by cardiogenic shock often have features of coronary artery disease and prior cardiac events. They are usually tachycardic ($\geqslant 100$ beats/minute) and display pulmonary rales, S_3 and S_4 gallops, as well as the findings associated with the shock syndrome (peripheral cyanosis; cool, clammy skin; decreased mental status). In patients with large infarctions and extensive left ventricular involvement an anterior injury pattern with ST segment elevation (with or without Q waves) in leads I, AV_L, and V_{1-6} is a common electrocardiographic finding. A complete left or right bundle branch block may also be present. Non-invasive (echocardiography, radionuclide ventriculography) or invasive (contrast ventriculography) studies typically reveal focal wall motion abnormalities and a marked reduction in systolic contractile function. Cardiac output is usually less than 2.0 L/min per m²; pulmonary capillary wedge pressure, a reflection of left ventricular filling pressure, typically exceeds 20 mm Hg.

Patients with cardiogenic shock caused by acute mitral insufficiency or ventricular septal rupture demonstrate all of the findings just described as well as a systolic murmur; however, murmurs may be difficult to appreciate in the presence of profound systemic hypotension and mechanical ventilation. Patients with ventricular septal rupture may also have a palpable precordial thrill. The electrocardiogram (ECG) reveals either an anterior or inferoposterior injury pattern in patients with ventricular septal rupture; 80 per cent of patients with a ruptured papillary muscle and severe mitral regurgitation will have evidence of an inferoposterior infarction. Ventricular septal defects and severe mitral insufficiency can usually be detected with transthoracic echocardiography. Left ventricular systolic function may be mildly or markedly reduced. The cardiac index is low, usually less than 2.0 L/min per m²; left ventricular filling pressures are elevated, usually more than 20 mm Hg; and right ventricular filling pressures may be normal or abnormal.

Individuals with right ventricular infarction in the absence of a mechanical defect usually have distended neck veins, clear lungs, and concomitant bradyarrhythmias or conduction defects. The ECG in these patients invariably reveals an inferoposterior infarction. Non-invasive and invasive tests of cardiac performance typically demonstrate a dilated right ventricle with reduced systolic function. Left ventricular contractility may be normal. The cardiac index is reduced, usually less than 2.0 L/min per m²; left ventricular filling pressures are often normal or only slightly elevated; and right ventricular filling pressures are elevated.

Cardiomyopathies/myocarditis

Patients with idiopathic dilated cardiomyopathy often have a history consistent with chronic heart failure. The physical examination discloses sinus tachycardia, a narrow pulse pressure, jugular venous distension,

Table 7.8 *Diagnostic benchmarks in cardiogenic shock*

	General physical appearance	Signs or history	Jugular venous pressure	Heart sounds	Lung examination	Chest radiograph	Electrocardiography	Other diagnostic tests
Myocardial infarction	Apprehensive Cool, moist skin Agitation	Symptom onset at rest Chest pain Dyspnea Hypotension Tachycardia	↑, ↔	S_3, S_4 gallops ± Holosystolic murmur (papillary muscle dysfunction)	Râles in >50% of lung fields	Pulmonary edema	ST-segment elevation ± Q waves	Elevated creatine kinase Abnormal MB fraction (may not be elevated early) Focal wall motion abnormality on echocardiogram
Ventricular septal rupture	Anxious Diaphoretic	Recent MI (3–5 days)[a] Sudden change in clinical status Chest pain Dyspnea Tachycardia	↑	S_3, S_4 gallops Localized holosystolic murmur (new) Palpable systolic thrill (lower left sternal border)	Râles in >50% of lung fields	Pulmonary edema	Persistent ST-segment elevation Pseudonormalization of T waves	L→R shunt on echocardiogram O_2 saturation 'step-up' Prominent V waves
Mitral insufficiency (acute)	Anxious Diaphoretic	Sudden dyspnea Recent inferior/inferoposterior MI *or* History of mitral valve prolapse *or* History of blunt/penetrating trauma	↑, ↔	S_4 decreased S_3 gallop Holosystolic murmur obscuring S_2 (A_2 component)	Râles in 50% of lung fields	Pulmonary edema	Recent MI Non-specific ST-T wave abnormality	Mitral insufficiency ± flail mitral leaflet on echocardiogram
Right ventricular infarction	Apprehensive Diaphoretic	Chest pain Nausea	↑↑	S_3, S_4 gallops (right sided)	Clear or basilar râles	Clear	Inferior injury pattern with posterior extension ≥0.5 mm ST elevation in V_3R, V_4R Bradyarrhythmias Conduction abnormalities (2°, 3° heart block)	Inferoposterior hypokinesis and right ventricular hypokinesis on echocardiogram
Myocarditis	Apprehensive Diaphoretic	Viral prodrome Progressive shortness of breath Low-grade temperature Narrow pulse pressure	↑	S_3, S_4 gallops	Râles in >50% of lung fields	Pulmonary edema Heart size normal or enlarged	Sinus tachycardia Non-specific ST/T changes Pseudoinfarction pattern Bundle-branch block	Chamber dilation Hypokinesis on echocardiogram
Dilated cardiomyopathy	Diaphoretic Cool Peripheral mottling	History of chronic heart failure Narrow pulse pressure Chronic venous stasis pigmentation-ulceration	↑↑	S_3, S_4 gallops Holosystolic murmur (mitral, tricuspid regurgitation)	Râles in >50% of lung fields	Pulmonary edema Cardiomegaly	Sinus tachycardia/tachyarrhythmias (atrial/ventricular) Low voltage Bundle-branch block Diffuse ST/T-wave changes	Four-chamber dilation on echocardiogram

Condition	Appearance	History/Symptoms	JVP	Heart sounds	Lungs	Chest X-ray	ECG	Other studies
Hypertrophic cardiomyopathy	Anxious, Diaphoretic	History of chest pain, dyspnea, syncope; Family history of sudden death; Apical 'triple' beat; Rapid carotid upstroke	↑,↔ (prominent A wave)	Prominent S4 gallop; Holosystolic blowing murmur at apex; Holosystolic harsh murmur left sternal border (↑ Valsalva)	Râles in >50% of lung fields	Pulmonary edema	Left ventricular hypertrophy; Q waves inferolateral leads	Septal hypertrophy on echocardiogram; Outflow tract obstruction on Doppler studies
Aortic stenosis	Pale, Diaphoretic	Carotid shudder, delayed upstroke; Angina, syncope	↑	S_1 soft; single S_2 (P_2); S_3, S_4 gallops; Harsh, late-peaking systolic murmur (radiation to carotid arteries)	Râles in >50% of lung fields	Pulmonary edema	Left ventricular hypertrophy	Aortic valve thickening; Reduced leaflet motion; Pressure gradient across aortic valve
Aortic insufficiency	Diaphoretic	History of hypertension, endocarditis, or trauma; Chest ± back pain; Dyspnea; Asymmetric blood pressure/pulses; Paralysis/sensory deficits	↑,↔	S_1 soft or absent; S_2 (P_2) prominent; S_3, S_4 gallops; Early, low-pitch diastolic murmur	Râles in >50% of lung fields	Pulmonary edema; 'Calcium' sign	Non-specific ST/T-wave changes	Aortic dissection; Aortic insufficiency; Tranesophogeal echocardiogram
Mitral stenosis	Diaphoretic, Cyanotic	Progressive dyspnea; Frothy blood-tinged sputum; Prior thromboembolism	↑ (prominent A wave)	S_1 prominent or reduced (immobile valve leaflets); P_2 prominent; Opening snap; Diastolic rumbling murmur	Râles in >50% of lung fields	Pulmonary edema; Right ventricular prominence; Left atrial enlargement	Tachyarrythmias (particularly atrial fibrillation); Right-axis deviation; Right ventricular hypertrophy; Atrial enlargement	Calcified, stenotic mitral valve
Pulmonary embolism	Anxious, Cyanotic	Sudden pleuritic chest pain, dyspnea, cough, hemoptysis, or syncope; Risk factors for pulmonary embolism; Tachypnea (>20 breaths/minute)	↑ (prominent A wave)	S_2 (P_2) increased; S_3, S_4 gallops (right sided); Holosystolic murmur (tricuspid regurgitation)	Clear	Oligemia; Elevated hemidiaphragm; Pleural effusion; 'Wedge-shaped' infiltrate; Prominent hilar vessel	S_1, Q_3, T_3 pattern; Nonspecific ST/T-wave changes; Right bundle-branch block	V/Q mismatch; Abnormal pulmonary angiography[b]; Right ventricular prominence on echocardiogram
Cardiac tamponade	Pale, Anxious, Apprehensive	Hypotension; Narrow pulse pressure; Distended neck veins; Pulsus paradoxus	↑↑ (absent Y descent)	Distant (rapid pericardial fluid accumulation); ± Friction rub	Clear	Normal or enlarged cardiac silhouette	Low voltage; T-wave flattening	Pericardial effusion; Right atrial, right ventricular collapse on echocardiogram; Abnormal Doppler flow patterns
Tension pneumothorax	Apprehensive, Cyanotic, Diaphoretic, Subcutaneous emphysema	Tachypnea; Tachycardia	↑	May be distant	Decreased ipsilateral breath sounds	Pneumothorax	Sinus tachycardia	Shift of mediastinal structures (heart, trachea)

[a]May occur earlier (24–48 hours) following thrombolytic therapy. [b]or spiral CT (computed tomography) scan.

L→R = left to right; MI = myocardial infarction; P_2 = pulmonic second heart sound; S_1 = first heart sound; S_2 = second heart sound; S_3 = third heart sound; S_4 = fourth heart sound; ↔ = Normal; ↑ = increased; ↑↑ = markedly increased; MB = myocardial band.

pulmonary rales, S_3 and S_4 gallops, murmurs of mitral and/or tricuspid regurgitation, and peripheral edema. Electrocardiographic findings are usually non-specific, i.e. low-voltage, left bundle branch block, and diffuse ST–T wave changes. Standard cardiac tests including echocardiography and ventriculography demonstrate poor left and often right ventricular systolic performance. The cardiac index is very low (often below 2.0 L/min per m²); left and often right ventricular filling pressures are abnormally high.

Individuals with myocarditis occasionally report the rather sudden onset of heart failure symptoms with or without a prior history of a viral syndrome. Physical findings include sinus tachycardia, narrow pulse pressure, pulmonary rales, S_3 and S_4 gallops, and at times, murmurs of mitral and/or tricuspid regurgitation. Electrocardiographic findings are non-specific. The overall left ventricular systolic function is poor. A myocardial biopsy may disclose inflammatory infiltrates; however, non-specific findings are most commonly observed.

Valvular heart disease

Patients with end-stage mitral insufficiency or aortic insufficiency usually have a history compatible with chronic heart failure. Physical examination and laboratory tests are similar to those described for dilated cardiomyopathy. Atrial fibrillation is a common arrhythmia. The murmurs of mitral and aortic regurgitation, even when associated with hemodynamic compromise, may not be prominent. Patients with aortic stenosis may report angina pectoris, dyspnea on exertion or true syncope. Among these patients the physical findings include sinus tachycardia or atrial fibrillation, a narrow pulse pressure, pulmonary râles, a late-peaking systolic murmur of aortic stenosis, and ventricular gallops (S_3, S_4). The ECG usually demonstrates left ventricular hypertrophy (LVH) with ST-T wave changes or a complete left bundle branch block. Non-invasive and invasive cardiac testing often disclose marked left ventricular hypertrophy with or without and systolic dysfunction as well as a thickened, immobile aortic valve.

Patients with end-stage mitral stenosis also present a history of chronic heart failure. They may report prior episodes of arterial embolism or hemoptysis. The physical findings suggest severe pulmonary hypertension and right ventricular dysfunction: cachexia, irregularly irregular pulse (atrial fibrillation), cyanosis, jugular venous distension, right ventricular heave, an increased pulmonic component of the second heart sound (P_2), right ventricular (right-sided) S_3 and S_4 gallops, hepatomegaly (with or without ascites), and peripheral edema. The murmur of mitral stenosis is often soft or inaudible. Non-invasive and invasive cardiac tests document the presence of severe mitral stenosis.

Sepsis

Patients with sepsis will usually have an associated or antecedent illness predisposing to a blood-borne infection, such as cholecystitis, pyelonephritis, pneumonia, an immunocompromised state, or a prior invasive procedure. These patients usually manifest fever, tachypnea, and sinus tachycardia. Their skin is warm and moist and their pulse is bounding, at least in the initial phase. Other physical findings are related to the underlying illness that is causing sepsis. The ECG demonstrates non-specific findings (e.g. sinus tachycardia and ST-T wave changes). Left ventricular systolic function is initially hyperdynamic by non-invasive and invasive cardiac testing in patients without pre-existing heart disease. The cardiac output is usually normal or elevated; left and right ventricular filling pressures are normal or low. In the later stages, myocardial performance may decline and cause cardiac output to decrease and left ventricular filling pressures to rise.

Tachyarrhythmias and bradyarrhythmias

The diagnosis is rarely in doubt when bradyarrhythmias or tachyarrhythmias lead to hypotension and shock. Accurate, rapid electrocardiographic diagnosis is essential followed by prompt therapy. Therapy should initially be directed at normalizing the heart rate and augmenting stroke volume with volume replacement as needed. Ultimately the etiology of the tachyarrhythmia or bradyarrhythmia must be determined and definitive treatment must be undertaken.

Cardiopulmonary bypass

The unique setting of postbypass cardiogenic shock presents special challenges for diagnosis and management. Left and right ventricular function can be assessed (at the time of surgery) and through hemodynamic monitoring. Transesophageal echocardiography may be useful in determining the adequacy of ventricular systolic performance and diastolic filling as well as valvular function.

Cardiac tamponade/pericardial constriction

The history of individuals with cardiac tamponade is usually dominated by symptoms related to an underlying illness (e.g. malignancy, chest trauma or dissection of the aorta). Physical findings include sinus tachycardia, a narrow pulse pressure, pulsus paradoxus, jugular venous distension, and a small quiet heart (with a traumatic pericardial effusion). The ECG reveals low-voltage and non-specific ST-T changes. Chest roentgenography demonstrates a globular-appearing cardiac silhouette.

Echocardiography is the diagnostic test of choice since it demonstrates the pericardial effusion and its effects on atrial and ventricular filling. Cardiac output is reduced; left and right ventricular filling pressures are moderately elevated and approximately equal (equalization of diastolic pressures).

Patients with constrictive pericarditis usually have a history and physical examination consistent with chronic, severe right ventricular failure. Patients may be cachectic with moderate to large ascitic fluid collections. Jugular and peripheral veins are usually distended; the lungs are clear. Echocardiography, computerized tomography (CT) scanning or magnetic resonance imaging (MRI), and invasive hemodynamic measurements may help distinguish constrictive pericarditis from restrictive cardiomyopathy. The classic 'square root sign' seen on pulmonary catheter tracings in constrictive pericarditis represents a constraint on active filling with a rapid passive filling phase.

Pulmonary embolism

Patients with massive pulmonary embolism present clinically with sudden-onset syncope or overt shock. The history may include an event or disease state that predisposes to deep venous thrombosis. Physical findings include sinus tachycardia, jugular venous distension, clear lungs, and a right ventricular summation (S_3 and S_4) gallop. The ECG may demonstrate right heart strain and the classic S_1–Q_3–T_3 pattern. Echocardiography reveals a dilated right ventricle and normal to hyperdynamic left ventricular function (in the absence of pre-existing heart disease). There is arterial hypoxemia and respiratory alkalosis. The cardiac output is reduced; left ventricular filling pressures are low; right ventricular filling pressures are elevated. A ventilation–perfusion (V/Q) lung scan may demonstrate moderate to large areas of ventilation–perfusion mismatch. Selective pulmonary angiography or a spiral CT scan may be required to confirm the diagnosis.

Pulmonary hypertension

Patients with end-stage pulmonary hypertensive disease and shock have a history compatible with chronic cor-pulmonale, i.e. dyspnea on exertion, fatigue, and peripheral edema. Physical examination often discloses sinus tachycardia, cyanosis, jugular venous distension, clear lungs, right ventricular S_3 and S_4 gallops, ascites, and peripheral edema. Clubbing may be noted if chronic arterial hypoxemia has been present. Non-invasive and invasive cardiac testing demonstrates right ventricular hypertrophy and dilatation along with systolic dysfunction. The cardiac output is reduced; left ventricular filling pressures are normal or low; right ventricular and pulmonary arterial pressures are elevated.

Coarctation of the aorta

Infants with severe coarctation, left ventricular failure, and shock present to the hospital with respiratory distress and cyanosis. Echocardiography usually discloses the coarctation; however, contrast aortography may at times be required to make the diagnosis.

Myxoma

Myxomatous tumors can produce symptoms both at remote sites in the body and directly through obstruction of flow through valves, which include respiratory distress and peripheral cyanosis. Patients may have a past history of dyspnea on exertion or a 'lupus-like' syndrome. Systemic symptoms including generalized malaise, fever, and weight loss may also be present. An initial physical examination may reveal only findings associated with cardiogenic shock; however, a diastolic murmur of mitral or tricuspid stenosis (which may be positional and intermittent) can occasionally be heard. Transthoracic echocardiography is the diagnostic test of choice; however, CT scanning and MRI can be used in the evaluation as well.

Hypertrophic obstructive cardiomyopathy

Severe dynamic obstruction of the left ventricular outflow tract may produce sudden-onset hypotension and cardiogenic shock in a patient with hypertrophic obstructive cardiomyopathy. There is often a prior history of episodic chest discomfort, dyspnea on exertion, and syncope. The physical examination discloses a loud precordial systolic murmur that accentuates with Valsalvae (critically ill patients may not be able to perform this maneuver). The ECG usually reveals left ventricular hypertrophy with associated ST-T wave changes. Q waves in the mid-precordial leads may also be present. Typical echocardiographic features include asymmetric septal hypertrophy, systolic anterior motion of the mitral valve, and accelerated flow in the left ventricular outflow tract.

Tension pneumothorax

Patients with tension pneumothorax usually have a history of trauma, mechanical ventilation or previous spontaneous pneumothorax. Physical findings include sinus tachycardia, tracheal deviation, jugular venous distension, and diminished or absent breath sounds over one or both lungs. The chest x-ray is diagnostic.

Vascular events

Patients with ruptured aortic aneurysms or aortic dissection may complain of severe chest, back, or abdominal pain. Electrocardiographic findings are usually non-specific. In the case of internal hemorrhage, a variety of non-invasive examinations, e.g. transesophageal echocardiography, CT scanning, or invasive tests (e.g. aortography), may be required to make a diagnosis. Hemodynamic monitoring reveals markedly depressed cardiac output and low left and right ventricular filling pressures.

MANAGEMENT OF CARDIOGENIC SHOCK

Patients with cardiogenic shock, particularly if the diagnosis is based on strict clinical and hemodynamic criteria, have an in-hospital mortality rate, when untreated, approaching 80 per cent. Prompt recognition, assessment, and treatment must therefore be undertaken. As with other conditions associated with a poor clinical outcome, initial therapeutic measures may be required for rapid stabilization, allowing specific diagnostic testing and definitive interventions subsequently to take place.

> The management of patients with overt cardiogenic shock is complex, frequently requiring a comprehensive, multidisciplinary approach (Figs 7.4–7.6).

General measures

Patients with cardiogenic shock frequently appear apprehensive and frightened. They also may be in considerable pain. Therefore, assurance from the medical team should be offered and comfort measures provided.

> A rapid assessment of vital signs should be accomplished as well as a brief yet thorough physical examination.

Particular attention must be paid to potential precipitating causes such as tension pneumothorax or cardiac tamponade, for which prompt chest tube placement and pericardiocentesis, respectively, would result in rapid clinical improvement.

> Systemic hypotension must be recognized and treated aggressively with appropriate volume expanders given either alone or in combination with vasopressor agents. In this regard, adequate intravenous access must be secured, at times with central line placement, particularly when profound vasoconstriction limits peripheral venous access.

Initial therapeutic measures also should focus on the respiratory system. Overall adequacy of cardiorespira-

tory function is assessed by arterial blood gas measurements. Arterial hypoxemia (PaO_2 <70 mm Hg), particularly when accompanied by systemic hypotension, limits cardiac performance. In the presence of ventricular compromise, appropriate compensation cannot take place, causing further clinical deterioration.

> Adequate blood and tissue oxygenation, therefore, must receive a high priority in the initial management of patients with cardiogenic shock. Early endotracheal intubation may be required and is recommended in patients with obtundation, moderate to severe hypoxemia accompanied by acid–base disturbances, or other signs of progressive end-organ hypoperfusion.

In many cases, endotracheal intubation is followed by a rapid improvement in clinical status. In patients with cardiogenic shock complicated by ARDS, positive endexpiratory pressure (PEEP) may be required to maximize oxygenation. The use of PEEP, however, can be associated with a decrease in cardiac output; hemodynamic monitoring is suggested.

Prompt correction of arrhythmias and advanced atrioventricular (AV) conduction abnormalities can eliminate primary or, more commonly, secondary contributing factors in cardiogenic shock. Bradyarrhythmias should be treated initially with parasympatholytic agents (e.g. atropine) followed by ventricular pacing (external, transvenous) if necessary.[62]

Intra-arterial monitoring

Direct blood pressure measurement is more accurate than non-invasive, indirect measurement in patients with hemodynamic instability and shock.

> Intra-arterial monitoring allows careful titration of vasoactive drugs and provides immediate access for frequent blood sampling, including blood gas analysis.

The preferred cannulation site is the radial artery; however, other sites (femoral artery, dorsalis pedis artery; brachial artery) also may be used. Potential complications of intra-arterial monitoring include bleeding, thrombosis, embolism, limb ischemia, pseudoaneurysm formation, infection, and peripheral neuropathy.

Hemodynamic monitoring

Pulmonary artery catheterization for hemodynamic monitoring has four primary objectives (Table 7.9):

1 to assess left ventricular and right ventricular function;

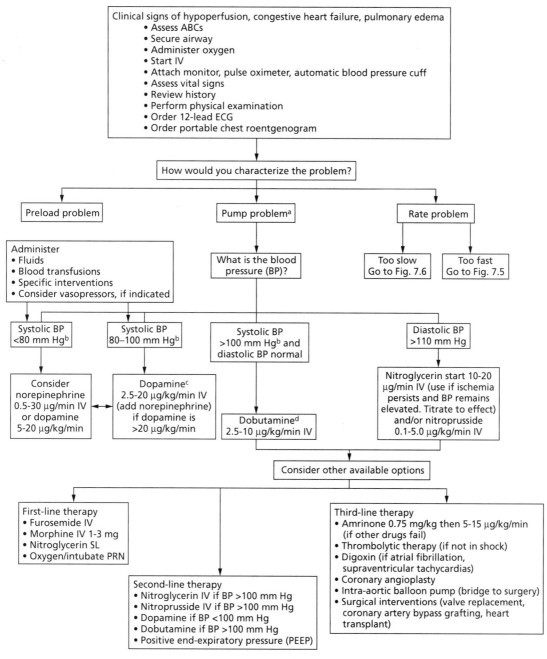

Figure 7.4 *Clinical approach and management of systemic hypotension and overt cardiogenic shock. ECG = electrocardiogram; IV = intravenous.*

2 to assess changes in hemodynamic status;
3 to guide treatment with pharmacologic and non-pharmacologic agents;
4 to gather prognostic information.

The hemodynamic information obtained from pulmonary arterial catheterization can be used directly in both patient management and diagnosis (Table 7.10).

Potential complications of catheterization include balloon rupture, knotting, pulmonary infarction, arterial perforation, thromboembolism, heart block, arrhythmias, myocardial perforation with tamponade, and infection. In addition to the complications just outlined, there is a great deal of debate as to the utility of PA catheters in altering prognosis. Certainly, well-selected patients are essential and the catheters will

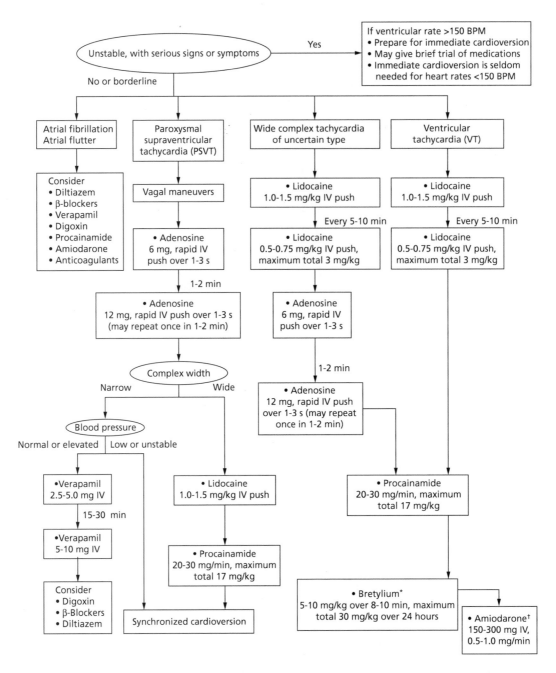

Figure 7.5 *Step-wise approach to tachyarrhythmias associated with hemodynamic compromise. *Seldom used. †Preferred strategy in patients with coronary artery disease and ventricular arrhythmias. BPM = beats/minute; IV = intravenous.*

assist not only in selection but titration of appropriate therapy.[63,64]

Pharmacologic therapy

In the initial stages of evaluation and clinical stabilization, inotropic agents and vasopressors commonly play an important role (Tables 7.11–7.13).

Augmenting systolic function through increased force of contraction as well as increasing afterload and heart rate will all lead to maximized cardiac output and flow. Based on the underlying pathophysiologic mechanism for the patient's hypotension and shock, the appropriate agent can be chosen.

Dopamine is an immediate precursor of norepinephrine. It has both α- and β-adrenergic agonist properties as well as dopaminergic-receptor agonism within the mesenteric and renal vascular beds. At doses required to

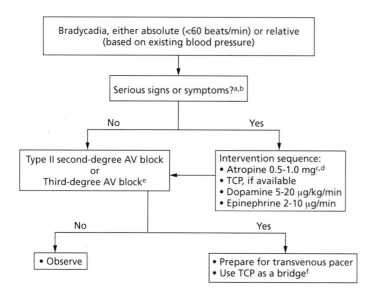

(a) Serious signs or symptoms related to the slow heart rate. Clinical manifestations include:
  • symptoms (chest pain, shortness of breath, decreased level of consciousness)
  • signs (low BP, shock, pulmonary congestion, CHF, myocardial ischemia/infarction).
(b) Do not delay TCP while awaiting IV access or for atropine to take effect if patient is symptomatic.
(c) Denervated transplanted hearts will not respond to atropine. Go at once to pacing, catecholamine infusion, or both.
(d) Atropine should be given in repeat doses at 3-5 min intervals up to total of 0.04 mg/kg. Consider shorter dosing intervals in severe clinical conditions. It has been suggested that atropine should be used with caution in atrioventricular (AV) block at the His-Purkinje level (type II AV block and new third-degree block with wide QRS complexes).
(e) Do not treat third-degree heart block plus ventricular escape beats with lidocaine.
(f) Bridge to transvenous pacer insertion.

Figure 7.6 *Stepwise approach to bradyarrhythmias associated with hemodynamic compromise. TCP = transcutaneous pacing; IV = intravenous; BP = blood pressure; CHF = congestive heart failure.*

Table 7.9 *Hemodynamic parameters in patients with hypotension and shock (guidelines for diagnosis)*

	RA (mm Hg)	RV (mm Hg^a)	PA (mm Hg^a)	PWP (mm Hg)	AO (mm Hg)	CI (L/min per m^2)	SVR (dyne/s per cm^{-5})
Normal	0–6	25/0–6	25/6–12	6–12	120/80	≥2.5	1200–1500
Hypovolemia	0–2	15/0–2	15/2–6	2–6	<90/60	<2.0	>1500
Cardiogenic shock	8	50/8	50/25	25	<90/60	<2.0	>1500
Septic shock							
Early	0–2	25/0–2	25/0–6	0–6	<90/60	>2.5	<1000
Late	0–4	25/4–10	25/4–10	4–10^b	<90/60	<2.0	>1000
Massive PE	8–12	50/12	50/12	<12	<90/60	<2.0	>1200
Tamponade	12–18	30/12–18	30/12–18	12–18	<90/60	<2.0	>1200
RV infarction	12–20	30/12–20	30/12	<12	<90/60	<2.0	>1200
VSR	6	60/6–8	60/25	25	<90/60	<2.0	>1500

^{a}The first value represents the mean value; the second is the range. ^{b}May be higher.

AO = aortic pressure; CI = cardiac index; PA = pulmonary artery; PE = pulmonary embolism; PWP = pulmonary wedge pressure; RA = right atrium; RV = right ventricle; SVR = systemic vascular resistance; VSR = ventricular septal rupture.

increase mean arterial pressure and cardiac output (5–8 µg/kg body weight per minute), heart rate and myocardial oxygen demand may be increased. In the presence of acidemia, higher doses (up to 15 µg/kg body weight per minute) may be required to produce a hemodynamic improvement; at this dose, atrial and ventricular tachyarrhythmias may occur.[65]

Dobutamine is a synthetic derivative of isoproterenol. It increases cardiac output at doses between 2.5 and 5.0 µg/kg/min without significantly increasing either heart rate or myocardial oxygen demand.

Therefore, in the setting of MI complicated by cardiogenic shock, dobutamine is considered the inotropic agent of choice.[66–68]

Norepinephrine is a potent α-receptor agonist (increases peripheral vascular resistance). It exhibits some myocardial β₁-receptor agonism as well. Norepinephrine should be used in patients with hypotension refractory to other inotropic agents.

Table 7.10 *Measurements calculable from hemodynamic data*

$$\text{Cardiac index} = \frac{\text{Cardiac output (L/min)}}{\text{Body surface area (m}^2)}$$

Normal: 2.5–4.5 L/min per m²

$$\text{Mean arterial pressure} = \frac{(2 \times \text{Diastolic}) + \text{Systolic}}{3}$$

Normal: 70–95 mm Hg

$$\text{Systemic vascular resistance} = \frac{\text{MAP} - \text{RAP}}{\text{CO}} \times 80$$

Normal: 1200–1500 dyne/s per cm⁻⁵

CO = cardiac output; MAP = mean arterial pressure; RAP = right arterial pressure.

Table 7.11 *Adrenergic receptor activity of sympathomimetic amines used in the management of patients with hypotension and shock states*

Amine	Alpha (α) (peripheral) stimulation	Beta-1 (β) (cardiac) stimulation	Beta-2 (β) (peripheral) stimulation
Norepinephrine	++++	++++	0
Epinephrine	++++	++++	+
Dopamine[a]	++++	++++	+
Isoproterenol[b]	0	++++	++++
Dobutamine	+	++++	++

[a]Dopamine in low doses (<4 µg/kg per min) has variable effect on α-receptor.
[b]Isoproterenol is rarely used in hemodynamically unstable patients.
+ = mild effect; ++ = moderate effect; ++++ = strong effect; 0 = no effect.

Table 7.12 *Non-cardiac and cardiovascular actions of drugs commonly used in hemodynamically unstable patients*

Drug	Non-cardiac effects	Cardiovascular effects
Alpha-adrenergic agonists Phenylephrine (alpha-1) Methoxamine (alpha-1) Epinephrine (alpha + beta) Norepinephrine (alpha + beta)	Hypertension may result in cerebral hemorrhage; angina; myocardial infarction; headache; inhibits insulin secretion; contracts trigone and sphincter muscles of bladder (may cause urinary retention)	**Alpha-adrenergic effects** Increases systemic vascular resistance (vasoconstriction); decreased mesenteric; cutaneous; renal blood flow; reflex bradycardia; increases myocardial oxygen consumption; may cause myocardial ischemia/infarction
Beta-adrenergic agonists Isoproterenol (beta-1, beta-2) Dobutamine (beta > alpha) Epinephrine (alpha, beta-1, beta-2) Norepinephrine (alpha, beta-2)	Fear; anxiety; restlessness; headache; flushing; nausea; sweating; increases renin secretion; increases glucose output; stimulates glycogenolysis; hyperglycemia; enhances insulin and glucagon secretion; increases lipolysis; decreases circulating potassium; bronchodilation (beta-2); inhibits release of inflammatory mediators from mast cells (beta-2); enhances mucociliary clearance; inhibits uterine tone and contraction (beta-2); relaxes detrusor muscle of bladder (may cause urinary retention); increases white blood cell counts; muscle tremor (beta-2)	**Beta-adrenergic effects** Increases myocardial contractility (beta-1 – positive inotropic effect); increases heart rate (beta-1 – positive chronotropic effect); palpitations; increases cardiac output; increases myocardial oxygen consumption; may precipitate myocardial ischemia; decreases systemic vascular resistance (beta-2); hypotension may occur; arrhythmias may occur; increases automaticity; shortens refractory period of atrioventricular (AV) node; enhances AV and intraventricular conduction

In patients with shock related to sepsis (profound peripheral vascular dilation, reduced SVR), norepinephrine is the drug of choice.

The efficacy of dopamine and dobutamine may decline with long-term administration. Tachyphylaxis may represent a 'down-regulation' of myocardial adrenergic receptors. Phosphodiesterase inhibitors increase cyclic AMP concentrations without relying directly on adrenergic receptors. Amrinone and milrinone have been used successfully in the treatment of cardiogenic shock. It is appropriate to change to one of these agents from dobutamine in patients with cardiomyopathy who no longer demonstrate improved hemodynamics on dobutamine.[69]

Patients with increased left ventricular mass and diastolic dysfunction, hypertensive heart disease, or hypertrophic cardiomyopathy have unique requirements. In fact, inotropic agents may worsen their clinical condi-

Table 7.13 *Drug preparation and dosing guidelines*

Drug	Loading dose	Maintenance dose	Preparation guidelines	Final concentrations	Comments
Amiodarone (150-mg ampl)	150 mg over 5–10 minutes	0.5–1.0 mg/min	300 mg/250 mL D5W	1.2 mg/mL	Use central iv catheter; terminal half-life 18–40 days; asthma exacerbation and AV block may occur. Epinephrine infusion may reverse the effects of the drug on effective refractory period. May potentiate warfarin anticoagulation; may induce digitalis toxicity
Amrinone (100-mg ampl)	0.75 mg/kg (2–3 min)	5–10 μg/kg per min	400 mg/250 mL in 0.9% NaCl	1.6 mg/mL	Infusion solution must not contain dextrose. Do not exceed 10 mg/kg per day. Can induce thrombocytopenia; may potentiate warfarin anticoagulation; hypotension may occur in septic and intravascular volume-depleted patients
Bretylium mesylate (500-mg ampl)	5–10 mg/kg (in 100 mL in 10 min for ventricular tachycardia; same dose intravenous push in ventricular fibrillation	0.5–4.0 mg/min	200 mg/250 mL D5W	8 mg/mL	Maximum loading dose 30 mg/kg; supine and orthostatic hypotension; may exacerbate arrhythmias and underlying hypotension. Intoxication may resemble clinical brain death. Extreme pyrexia may occur
Dobutamine (250-mg ampl)	—	2–20 μg/kg per min (up to 40 μg/kg per min)	500 mg/250 mL D5W	2 mg/mL	Selective inotropic effect; half-life 2–3 mins; hypotension, tachycardia and arrhythmia may occur. Contraindicated in idiopathic hypertrophic subaortic stenosis; use with caution in acute myocardial infarction
Dopamine (100-mg ampl)	—	2–20 μg/kg per min	400 mg/250 mL D5W	1.6 mg/mL	Clinical response is dose-dependent; infusion rate >10 μg/kg per min has predominant alpha-adrenergic effect. Use central iv catheter; may increase diaphragmatic strength and blood flow
Epinephrine (1-mg ampl)	—	0.05–2 μg/kg per min	2 mg/250 mL D5W	8 μg/mL	Dose-dependent pharmacologic effect; use a central iv catheter. Side effects: tachycardia, hypertension. May reverse the effects of quinidine and amiodarone on the effective refractory period. Higher dose may be required in septic patients
Isoproterenol (2-mg ampl)	—	1–10 μg/min	2 mg/250 mL D5W	8 μg/mL	Use with extreme caution in acute myocardial infarction; marked arrhythmogenic effect, tachycardia and hypotension propensity
Lidocaine 1% and 2% solution (100 mL vial)	1 mg/kg	1–4 mg/min	2 g/500 mL D5W or 0.9% NaCl	5 mg/mL	Serum concentrations: 2–6 μg/mL; infusion rate >5 mg/min may lead to seizures, confusion, stupor and negative inotropic effect; half-life prolonged in patients with hepatic dysfunction, CHF, shock, or receiving cimetidine

Table 7.13 *Continued*

Drug	Loading dose	Maintenance dose	Preparation guidelines	Final concentrations	Comments
Milrinone (10-mg ampl)	50 µg/kg (in 10 min)	0.25–1 µg/kg per min	30 mg/250 mL D5W	120 µg/mL	Dose adjustment is necessary in renal failure; may exacerbate ventricular arrhythmias and angina; effective in acute and chronic CHF
Nitroglycerin (5-, 25-, 50-, and 100-mg ampl)	—	5–50 µg/min	100 mg/250 mL D5W or 0.9% NaCl	400 µg/mL	Can use special infusion set. Increase dose 5–10 µg/min every 5–10 min until desirable effect; adverse hemodynamic effects: tachycardia and hypotension; vagal response may require atropine
Nitroprusside (50-mg ampl)	—	0.5–10 µg/kg per min	100 mg/250 mL D5W	400 µg/mL	Infusion precipates in electrolytic solutions and must be protected from light; blood pressure must be monitored to avoid hypotension; during prolonged administration, thyocianate values should be monitored and kept at <10 mg/dL; may induce platelet dysfunction. Do not use if solution is discolored
Norepinephrine (4-mg ampl)	—	2–20 µg/min	8 mg/250 mL D5W	32 µg/mL	Use central iv catheter; potent alpha-adrenergic effect; extravasation associated with local tissue necrosis. Higher dose has been used to achieve desirable hemodynamic effect
Phenylephrine (10-mg ampl)	100–200 µg (in 2–3 min)	2–10 µg/kg per min	30 mg/250 mL D5W	120 µg/mL	Use central iv catheter; variable range of dosage; pure alpha-adrenergic effect; reflex bradycardia
Procainamide (1000-mg ampl)	50–100 mg (every 5 min up to 17 mg/kg)	2–6 mg/min or 0.02–0.08 mg/kg per min	1000 mg/250 mL D5W	4 mg/mL	Negative inotropic effect and afterload reduction; peripheral vasodilation. Contraindicated in torsades de pointes arrhythmia and myasthenia gravis. Elimination half-life of the drug and its metabolite *N*-acetylprocainamide (NAPA) may be increased in renal impairment; both are removed by hemodialysis. Concomitant use of amiodarone may increase NAPA concentrations
Propranalol (1-mg ampl)	1–3 mg	3–8 mg/h	20 mg/250 mL D5W	0.08 mg/mL	Negative chronotropic effect; drug should not be used in patients with asthma. COPD, CHF; may mask symptoms of hypoglycemia

D5W = ampl = ampoule; iv = intravenous; AV = atrioventricular; CHF = congestive heart failure; COPD = chronic obstructive lung disease.

tion. Calcium channel blockers (verapamil, diltiazem) or β-blockers given intravenously may improve ventricular distensibility and diastolic filling. In refractory congestive heart failure accompanied by hypotension, a pure α-agonist, such as phenylephrine hydrochloride, used in combination with supportive care, may be beneficial.

Mechanical support

> *Intra-aortic balloon counterpulsation* (IABP) can provide rapid stabilization of patients with cardiogenic shock, particularly those with global myocardial ischemia or infarction complicated by mechanical defects, such as papillary muscle rupture causing acute, severe mitral regurgitation or a moderate to large ventricular septal defect.

In most instances it can be inserted percutaneously either with or without fluoroscopic guidance, although the latter is preferred. The augmented coronary perfusion pressure during diastole facilitates coronary arterial blood flow. Since the balloon deflates rapidly at the onset of ventricular systole, left ventricular impedance is reduced (decreased afterload). Hemodynamic changes typically include a 10–20 per cent increase in cardiac output, a reduction in systolic and increase in diastolic blood pressures, a diminution in heart rate, and an increase in urine output. In some patients, continued inotropic support is required to maintain an acceptable blood pressure (>90 mm Hg systolic) and cardiac index (>2.2 L/min per m^2) even after IABP insertion.

Intra-aortic balloon counterpulsation was first used in the treatment of cardiogenic shock by Kantrowitz and colleagues in 1968.[70] Clinical improvement occurs in a large percentage (approximately 75 per cent) of patients; however, in-hospital mortality remains high and many patients cannot be removed successfully from mechanical support.[71] Although more powerful circulatory-assist devices providing flow rates of 8–10 L/min have been developed, similar limitations have been recognized with the Hemopump[72,73] and percutaneous cardiopulmonary support system.[74–76] Some patients who do not stabilize with IABP will improve following insertion of the Hemopump.

> Mechanical assistance with these devices, therefore, should be considered in patients with cardiogenic shock who need temporary support while preparation for definitive, corrective intervention is being made. The IABP is contraindicated in patients with severe aortic insufficiency and advanced peripheral vascular disease and should be utilized as a temporizing measure or 'bridge' only.

Coronary angioplasty in patients with cardiogenic shock

Despite significant advances in the treatment of cardiogenic shock, including coronary care unit monitoring, vasopressor and inotropic agents, and circulatory support measures, mortality rates remain unacceptably high.[77] A number of recent studies[78–87] have examined in-hospital and long-term mortality rates in patients who have undergone percutaneous coronary interventions (PCI) in the setting of cardiogenic shock. Although randomized, controlled trials are not available to compare fibrinolytic therapy and PCI directly, these studies suggest a significant improvement in mortality in patients who have undergone PCI. Survival to hospital discharge ranged from 50 to 71 per cent[87] (Table 7.14). A factor common to all studies that have indicated a benefit is successful reperfusion of the infarct-related artery. Bengtson et al.[87] found a mortality rate of 33 per cent in patients with patent infarct-related arteries compared with 75 per cent in those with an occluded vessel and an 84 per cent mortality in patients whose patency status was unknown.

Long-term clinical outcome from prior retrospective studies also suggests a significant improvement in survival rates for patients who underwent successful PCI compared with those who had unsuccessful PCI or when PCI was not attempted. Stack et al.[80] initially reported a 4 per cent mortality rate at 6- and 12-month follow-up in 25 survivors of cardiogenic shock who had successful PCI and survived to hospital discharge. Other studies have reported mortality rates after hospitalization of 11–20 per cent.[83,84,86] Therefore it appears, on the basis of clinical observations, that establishing coronary arterial reperfusion in patients with single-vessel coronary disease, acute MI, and cardiogenic shock may improve both short- and long-term survival.

The clinical outcome among patients with cardiogenic shock and multivessel disease who undergo PCI may not be as promising. Lee et al.[78] reported an 83 per cent mortality rate in patients with multivessel disease, despite successful PCI of the infarct-related coronary artery. However, in a study by Hibbard et al.,[83] 9 of 12 patients with three-vessel coronary disease survived to hospital discharge and 47 per cent were alive at follow-up. Although PCI appears to improve survival in patients with cardiogenic shock even up to 24 hours among patients with multivessel disease,[79] reperfusion in fewer than 6 hours from the onset of symptoms may be a major determining factor.

The use of PCI in patients with prior coronary artery bypass grafting (CABG) and cardiogenic shock was investigated by Kahn et al.[88] In-hospital survival for 9 of 11 patients in shock who underwent successful PCI was 64 per cent, suggesting that coronary angioplasty should be considered in carefully selected patients.

Patients with cardiogenic shock resulting from ischemic papillary muscle dysfunction have also been

Table 7.14 *Coronary angioplasty in patients with cardiogenic shock. (Reproduced with permission from Hochman JS. Cardiogenic shock: can we save the patient? Am Coll Cardiol Educ Highlights 1996; **12**: 1–5.)*

Investigator	Overall survival	PTCA success	Survival– successful PTCA	Survival– unsuccessful PTCA
Brown	43	61	58	18
Disler	59	71	69	20
Eltchaninoff	64	76	76	25
Gacioch and Topol	56	72	78	0
Heuser	70	60	93	25
Hibbard	56	62	71	29
Himbert	22	89	19	50
Laramee	59	86	NA	NA
Lee	50	54	77	18
Lee	55	71	69	20
Meyer	53	88	59	0
Moosvi	53	76	62	22
O'Neill	70	88	75	33
Seydoux	57	85	67	0
Shani	66	67	NA	NA
Verna	86	100	86	100
Yamamoto	38	62	56	10
Total	**54%**	**74%**	**66%**	**19%**

NA = not applicable.

treated successfully with PCI.[89,90] A significant reduction in mitral regurgitation was achieved, enabling resolution of cardiogenic shock and avoiding both valve replacement and long-term anticoagulation.

Experience with newer interventional devices is limited. Smuker *et al.*[91] described a patient in cardiogenic shock who underwent emergency PCI with subsequent abrupt closure and salvage coronary atherectomy. Coronary arterial stenting may play a role in patients with cardiogenic shock and threatened abrupt closure; however, because of the significant amount of thrombus typically present within the infarct-related vessel, there may be some risk. The potential role of new antiplatelet agents in this setting will require investigation. Transluminal extraction catheters (TEC devices) may have a role in patients with acutely occluded saphenous vein bypass grafts; however, in the report by Kahn *et al.*,[88] all vein graft angioplasties were performed using conventional balloon dilation with very high success rates.

In summary, reports thus far are promising and suggest a survival benefit if angioplasty is performed and patency of the infarct-related vessel is achieved. Both short- and long-term survival may be favorably influenced. For this reason, the American Heart Association/American College of Cardiology recommends primary PCI in patients who are within 36 hours of an acute ST segment elevation/bundle branch block MI who develop shock, are less than 75 years old, and revascularization can be performed within 18 hours of shock onset (Class I recommendation).

Surgical intervention

Surgical intervention in the treatment of cardiogenic shock is most successful when mechanical defects, such as acute mitral regurgitation are present. Patients can be stabilized initially with an IABP (or another circulatory-assist device) and inotropic support; however, surgery should not be delayed.

There is substantial evidence that patients with either an isolated mechanical defect or severe coronary artery disease derive the greatest benefit when surgical intervention is undertaken promptly.[92–94] Prompt surgery also may reduce the risks and complications of prolonged end-organ hypoperfusion, such as infections, ARDS, and renal insufficiency. The importance of early cardiovascular support with IABP prior to and following surgery has also been recognized.[95]

A number of uncontrolled, non-randomized studies have been published addressing the efficacy of CABG in patients with acute MI complicated by cardiogenic shock[87,92–103] (Table 7.15). The outcome for these patients correlated significantly with a number of factors, including prior MI, extent of coronary artery disease, left ventricular performance, completeness of revascularization, presence of multisystem organ failure, and the time interval from coronary occlusion to re-establishment of coronary blood flow. Favorable factors included inferior wall MI and revascularization within 16 hours of symptom onset. DeWood *et al.*[97] reported a 62.5 per cent mortality rate in patients with anterior infarction compared

Table 7.15 *Bypass grafting in patients with cardiagenic shock. (Reproduced with permission from Hochman JS. Cardiogenic shock: can we save the patient?* Am Coll Cardiol Educ Highlights *1996;* **12***: 1–5.)*

Investigator	Year	Survival
Dunkman	1972	60
Mundth	1973	39
Miller	1974	42
Willerson	1975	33
Johnson	1977	40
Ehrich	1977	33
Bardet	1977	50
O'Rourke	1979	33
Subramanian	1980	55
DeWood	1980	58
Kirklin	1985	100
Phillips	1986	76
Laks	1986	70
Guyton	1987	78
Bolooki	1989	57
Beyersdorf	1990	45
Bengston	1992	88
Allen	1993	91
Quigley[a]	1993	20
Total (323)	**103/323**	**68%**

[a]Left main stenosis ⩾75%.

with 20 per cent in patients with inferior infarction. Patients surviving to hospital discharge also had a higher long-term mortality with anterior infarction (81.2 *vs* 40 per cent).

A recurring theme in revascularization studies has been the time to reperfusion. In DeWood's study, patients revascularized within 16 hours of the onset of infarction had a mortality rate of 25 per cent, whereas patients revascularized more than 18 hours after symptom onset experienced a mortality rate of 71.4 per cent. This observation is consistent with a critical period for revascularization that can be explained on the basis of improving blood flow to areas of myocardial ischemia (jeopardized but viable) myocardium either adjacent to or remote from the MI. It appears vital therefore to achieve reperfusion as soon as possible.

The available reports of bypass grafting all show significant survival benefits for both short and long term. Without a randomized trial, however, the results are difficult to interpret because of selection bias. Patients undergoing surgery had already survived long enough to be considered operative candidates. Certainly, operative survival rates have continued to improve over time, influenced by better surgical and myocardial preservation techniques.

In the SHOCK Trial,[104] patients receiving aggressive medical therapy (fibrinolytics and IABP) experienced a 56 per cent mortality at 30 days compared with 47 per cent in those who underwent revascularization (PCI or bypass surgery). Although the early differences were not statistically significant, at 6-month follow-up, patients <75 years of age randomized to immediate revascularization had lower mortality rates than those receiving aggressive medical therapy (48 per cent *vs* 69 per cent).

Cardiac transplantation is a surgical option for a small select group of individuals with cardiogenic shock.

> Currently, there are two basic approaches to mechanical circulatory support as a bridge to cardiac transplantation: (1) the total artificial heart; and (2) ventricular-assist devices. Biventricular circulatory support may be particularly beneficial in potential heart transplant candidates with life-threatening refractory ventricular arrhythmias.[105] In select cases, ventricular-assist devices can effectively replace left-sided heart function for prolonged periods of time (weeks to months) until a donor heart can be found.

Fibrinolytic therapy

Clinical experience in trials of coronary fibrinolysis indicate that 2–3 per cent of patients with MI are in shock on hospital arrival, whereas an additional 3–4 per cent have this complication after initial treatment (Table 7.16). Interestingly, a large percentage of patients who have cardiogenic shock are initially classified as Killip Class I or II, suggesting that subsequent events (recurrent ischemia, infarct extension, early infarct expansion) contribute. Predictors of a poor outcome in patients sustaining an acute MI include advanced age, prior infarction, anterior site of infarction, ejection fraction less than 35 per cent, and diabetes mellitus.[106]

Unfortunately, the in-hospital mortality among patients with cardiogenic shock treated with thrombolytic therapy has remained high, paralleling Killip's experience in the prethrombolytic era.[106] The fact

Table 7.16 *Fibrinolytic therapy clinical experience: Killip classification at study entry*

	Killip I	Killip II	Killip III	Killip IV
GISSI-1				
SK	71.2	22.7	3.2	2.5
Placebo	70.1	22.9	4.2	2.3
International study				
SK/aspirin	79.4	16.2	2.7	1.7
tPA/aspirin	79.3	16.9	2.4	1.4
GUSTO-1				
All groups	86.0	12.0	1.0	1.0

GISSI-1 = Gruppo Italiano perlo studio della sopravivenza nell'infarto myiocardico); GUSTO-1 = Global utilization of streptokinase and tPA for occluded coronary arteries; SK = streptokinase; tPA = tissue plasminogen activator.

Table 7.17 *Fibrinolytic therapy clinical experience: mortality according to Killip classification*

| | Mortality (%) | | | |
	Killip I	Killip II	Killip III	Killip IV
GISSI-1				
SK	5.9	16.1	33	69.9
Placebo	7.3	19.9	39	70.1
International study				
SK/aspirin	5.1	17.8	33.3	64.9
tPA/aspirin	4.1	17.7	29.9	78.1
GUSTO-1				
tPA	4.4	13.0	23.3	63.4
SK (subcutaneous heparin)	5.2	15.0	31.0	58.0
SK (intravenous heparin)	4.4	13.0	23.0	63.0
tPA plus SK	5.3	13.8	37.0	56.0

SK = streptokinase; tPA = tissue plasminogen activator.

remains that cardiogenic shock is the strongest independent predictor of mortality after acute MI (Table 7.17).

It is clear from animal experimentation and clinical trials[107] that the beneficial effects of coronary thrombolysis are derived from prompt and complete restoration of coronary arterial blood flow.[108–115] There is some evidence, albeit sparse, that successful reperfusion is also a pivotal factor in the setting of cardiogenic shock.[116,117] This observation is supported by the findings of retrospective studies in patients with shock undergoing coronary angioplasty (outlined in a separate section). A consecutive series of 200 patients with MI complicated by cardiogenic shock in the Duke database identified patency of the infarct-related coronary artery among the most important predictors of in-hospital mortality.[87] Of major concern, however, are the low patency rates experienced by patients with cardiogenic shock after thrombolytic therapy. Experimental data obtained by MRI and by photographing clot dissolution *in vitro* have shown that clots dissolve two orders of magnitude faster when thrombolytic agents are introduced by pressure-induced permeation instead of by diffusion.[118] When coronary perfusion pressure is low, the velocity of thrombolysis is limited by the diffusion constraints of the plasminogen activator itself and by plasmin (the active enzyme).[119] As the concentration profile of diffusing molecules falls exponentially with distance, even high concentrations of thrombolytics would not be expected to fully compensate for slowed transport into a thrombus.

Intraluminal pressure is of particular importance in areas of dynamic coronary arterial stenosis (soft plaque) because it represents the opposing force to both vasoconstriction and passive collapse.[120,121] Perfusion pressure is decreased in patients with cardiogenic shock, favoring

passive collapse of compliant areas and potentially influencing thrombolytic response.[122]

Metabolic factors may also impact the ability of fibrinolytic agents to dissolve an occlusive thrombus. Increased plasma fibrinogen and local thrombin concentrations, common among patients with active coronary artery disease, are associated with formation of thin fibrin strands. In turn, a thrombus composed of thin, tightly packed fibrin strands restricts the transport of plasminogen, plasmin, and plasminogen activators.[123,124] Furthermore, metabolic acidemia may repair the conversion of plasminogen to plasmin by increasing the Michaelis constant and lowering the catalytic rate.[125,126] An 'unfriendly metabolic environment' may limit thrombolysis even if coronary perfusion pressure is increased.

Our group investigated the association between systemic blood pressure and 120-minute angiographic patency in 127 patients with acute MI treated with thrombolytic therapy.[127] By univariate analysis, diastolic blood pressure less than 80 mm Hg at the time of thrombolytic initiation was associated with a reduced angiographic coronary perfusion grade. Significant fluctuations (reductions) in systolic and diastolic blood pressure were also associated with decreased perfusion. However, a multivariate analysis failed to confirm these associations, suggesting that other factors (acting either alone or, more likely, in combination with coronary perfusion pressure) are at play.[128–130]

Benefits of a combined aggressive approach to patients with cardiogenic shock

Although the early administration of fibrinolytic therapy reduces the overall occurrence of cardiogenic shock associated with MI, the ideal management strategy for patients who either present to the hospital with cardiogenic shock or who develop it despite fibrinolysis remains controversial. The data derived from retrospective analysis suggest that mechanical revascularization (predominantly coronary angioplasty) is associated with improved survival, differences in baseline characteristics and selection bias may have influenced the observations.

In GUSTO-1[131] 2200 patients with MI complicated by cardiogenic shock were divided into two management groups. Group 1 had coronary angiography (and revascularization when feasible) within 24 hours of infarction, while Group 2 underwent either late or no angiography. The 30-day mortality was 38 per cent in the 406 patients who underwent early angiography and were referred within 24 hours to coronary angioplasty, bypass surgery or both compared with 62 per cent in the 1794 patients who did not. An aggressive strategy was independently associated with reduced 30-day mortality (odds ratio 0.43). The mortality difference between patients in whom early angiography was and was not performed remained significant at 1 year (44.2 per cent *vs* 66.4 per cent, respectively) (Figure 7.7).

A majority of patients with MI complicated by cardiogenic shock are first evaluated and treated in a community hospital setting. Therapeutic options typically include fibrinolytic therapy or immediate transfer to a tertiary care facility for angiography and revascularization. In a small retrospective study,[132] 46 patients who

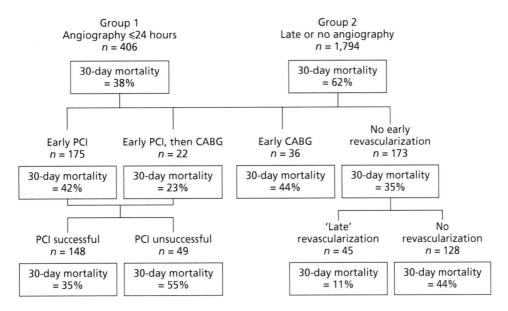

Figure 7.7 *In the GUSTO-1 Study, an aggressive management strategy including angiography and coronary revascularization was associated with a lower 30-day mortality than a more conservative approach in patients with cardiogenic shock. PCI = percutaneous coronary intervention; CABG = coronary artery bypass graft. (Reproduced with permission from Berger et al. for the GUSTO Investigators. Impact of an aggressive invasive catheterization and revascularization strategy on mortality in patients with cardiogenic shock in the Global Utilization of Streptokinase and Tissue plasminogen activator for Occluded coronary arteries (GUSTO-I) Trial. An observational study. Circulation 1997; 96: 122–7.)*

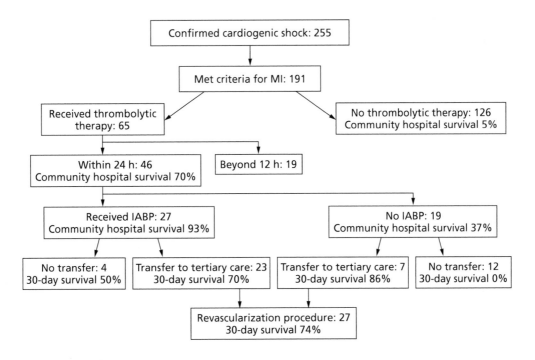

Figure 7.8 *Early treatment including thrombolytics and aortic counterpulsation followed by emergent transfer to a facility capable of urgent coronary revascularization is associated with a comparatively low 30-day mortality. MI = myocardial infarction; IABP = intra-aortic balloon counterpulsation. (Reproduced with permission from Kovack et al. Thrombolysis plus aortic counterpulsation: improved survival in patients who present to community hospitals with cardiogenic shock. J Am Coll Cardiol 1997; 29: 1454–9.)*

received thrombolytics within 12 hours of symptom onset and experienced cardiogenic shock underwent IABP placement ($n = 27$) or did not ($n = 19$). Patients treated with IABP had a community hospital survival of 93 per cent compared with 37 per cent for those in whom it was not placed, and more of them were transferred for revascularization (85 *vs* 37 per cent). Overall hospital and 1-year survival rates were also higher among patients treated with IABP (67 *vs* 32 per cent) (Figure 7.8). Further investigation in the form of randomized clinical trials will be necessary to examine the feasibility and true impact of this strategy.

Cardiogenic shock, regardless of etiology, carries a poor prognosis. In the setting of acute ST segment elevation MI, shock typically developed within 24 hours of the initial event, suggesting that myocardial injury and pump failure are operative. Early diagnosis and reperfusion therapy are the most readily available means to limit infarct size; however, it remains clear that therapies capable of attenuating the hearts' response to injury are needed (Fig. 7.9).

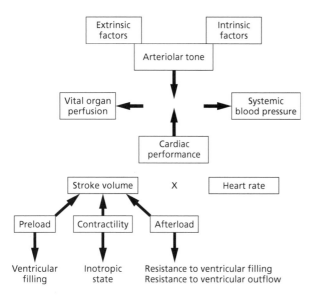

Figure 7.9 *Systemic blood pressure and vital organ perfusion are determined by cardiac performance and peripheral arteriolar tone. The major determinants of cardiac performance are preload, contractility, afterload and heart rate.*

SUMMARY

- Patients with hypotension (mean arterial blood pressure (MAP) <65 mm Hg; relative decrease >30 mm Hg from baseline) most commonly have an impairment in cardiac output and/or peripheral vascular resistance.
- The feature that distinguishes between isolated systemic hypotension and shock is tissue hypoperfusion in the latter.
- The initial management of patients with hypotension and shock must include steps to support systemic blood pressure (and preserve vital organ perfusion).
- Volume replacement, inotropic agents and measures to increase vascular tone represent first-line therapies to achieve patient stabilization. Focused diagnostic testing and definitive interventions should promptly follow initial supportive efforts.
- In myocardial infarction complicated by cardiogenic shock, early and aggressive diagnostic evaluation, reperfusion therapy (predominantly achieved by percutaneous coronary intervention) and surgical correction of mechanical defects represent the standard of care.
- The mortality rate associated with shock states approaches 100 per cent when therapy is delayed or is inadequate.
- Ventricular assist devices as a bridge to heart transplantation should be considered in patients with cardiogenic shock refractory to medical therapy and/or traditional surgical intervention.

REFERENCES

♦ 1. Starling EH. *Linacre lecture on the law of the heart (1915)*. London: Longarans 1918.

2. Green HD. Circulatory systems: physical principals. In: Glasser O, ed. *Medical physics*, Vol. 2. Chicago: Yearbook Publishers, 1950: 228–41.

3. Chien S. Role of the sympathetic nervous system in hemorrhage. *Physiol Rev* 1967; **47**: 214–88.

4. Bond RF, Green HD. Cardiac output redistribution during bilateral common carotid occlusion. *Am J Physiol* 1969; **216**: 393–403.

5. Bereiter DA, Zaid AM, Gann DS. Effect of rate of hemorrhage on sympathoadrenal catecholamine release in cats. *Am J Physiol* 1986; **250**: E69–E75.

6. Davis JO, Freeman RH. Mechanisms regulating renin release. *Physiol Rev* 1976; **56**: 1–56.

7. Abboud FM, Thames MD. Interaction of cardiovascular reflexes in circulatory control. In: *Handbook of physiology: the cardiovascular system. Peripheral circulation and organ blood flow*, Vol. III. Bethesda, MD: American Physiological Society, 1984: section 2, pt 2: 675–753.

8. Liard JF. Vasopressin in cardiovascular control: role of circulating vasopressin. *Clin Sci* 1984; **67**: 473–81.

9. Gann DS, Carlson DE, Byrnes GJ, Pickle JC Jr, Allen-Rowlands CF. Role of solute in the early restitution of blood volume after hemorrhage. *Surgery* 1983; **94**: 439–46.

10. Bond RF, Johnson G III. Vascular adrenergic interactions during hemorrhagic shock. *Fed Proc* 1985; **44**: 281–9.

11. Bond RF, Bond CH, Peissner LC, Manning ES. Prostaglandin modulation of adrenergic vascular control during hemorrhagic shock. *Am J Physiol* 1981; **241**: H85–90.

12. Hift H, Campos HA. Changes in the subcellular distribution of cardiac catecholamines in dogs dying in irreversible hemorrhagic shock. *Nature* 1962; **196**: 678–9.

13. Coleman B, Glaviano VV. Tissue levels of norepinephrine in hemorrhagic shock. *Science* 1962; **139**: 54.

14. Koyama S, Aibiki M, Kanai K, Fujita T, Miyakawa K. Role of the central nervous system in renal nerve activity during prolonged hemorrhagic shock in dogs. *Am J Physiol* 1988; **254**: R761–9.

15. Holaday JW, Faden AI. Naloxone reversal of endotoxin hypotension suggests role of endorphins in shock. *Nature* 1978; **275**: 450–1.

16. Reynolds DG, Gurll NJ, Vargish T, Lechner RB, Faden AI, Holaday JW. Blockade of opiate receptors with naloxone improves survival and cardiac performance in canine endotoxic shock. *Circ Shock* 1980; **7**: 39–48.

17. Schadt JC, Gaddis RR. Endogenous opiate peptides may limit norepinephrine release during hemorrhage. *J Pharmacol Exp Ther* 1985; **232**: 656–60.

18. Carden DL, Smith JK, Zimmerman BJ, Korthuis RJ, Granger DN. Reperfusion injury following circulatory collapse: The role of reactive oxygen metabolites. *J Crit Care* 1989; **4**: 294–307.

♦19. Barroso-Aranda J, Schmid-Schonbein GW, Zweifach BW, Ensler RL. Granulocytes and no-reflow phenomenon in irreversible hemorrhagic shock. *Circ Res* 1988; **63**: 437–47.

20. Barroso-Aranda J, Schmid-Schonbein GW. Transformation of neutrophils as an indicator of irreversibility in hemorrhagic shock. *Am J Physiol* 1989; **257**: H846–52.

21. Hurd TC, Dasmahapatra KS, Rush BF Jr, Machiedo GW. Red blood cell deformability in human and experimental sepsis. *Arch Surg* 1988; **123**: 217–20.

22. Sarnoff SJ, Case RB, Waitag PE, Issacs J. Insufficient coronary flow and myocardial failure as a complicating factor in late hemorrhagic shock. *Am J Physiol* 1954; **176**: 439–44.

23. Horton J, Landreneau R, Tuggle D. Cardiac response to fluid resuscitation from hemorrhagic shock. *Surg Gynecol Obstet* 1985; **160**: 444–52.

24. Lefer AM. Interaction between myocardial depressant factor and vasoactive mediators with ischemia and shock. *Am J Physiol* 1987; **252**: R193–205.

♦25. Parillo JE, Burch C, Shelhamer JH, Parker MM, Natanson C, Schette W. A circulating myocardial depressant substance in humans with septic shock: septic shock patients with a reduced ejection fraction have a circulating factor that depresses in vitro myocardial cell performance. *J Clin Invest* 1985; **76**: 1539–53.

26. Sander-Jensen K, Secher NH, Bie P, Warbers J, Schwartz TN. Vagal slowing of the heart during hemorrhage: observations from twenty consecutive hypotensive patients. *Br Med J* 1986; **295**: 364–6.

○27. Roussos C, Macklem PT. The respiratory muscles. *N Engl J Med* 1982; **307**: 786–97.

28. Rasmussen HH, Ibels LS. Acute renal failure. Multivariate analysis of causes and risk factors. *Am J Med* 1982; **73**: 211–18.

29. Menashe PI, Ross SA, Gottlieb JE. Acquired renal insufficiency in critically ill patients. *Crit Care Med* 1988; **16**: 1106–9.

30. Montgomery A, Hartmann M, Jonsson K, Haglund U. Intramucosal pH measurement with tonometers for detecting gastrointestinal ischemia in porcine hemorrhagic shock. *Circ Shock* 1989; **29**: 319–27.

31. Bulkley GB, Oshima A, Bailey RW. Pathophysiology of hepatic ischemia in cardiogenic shock. *Am J Surg* 1986; **151**: 87–97.

32. Abraham E. Host defense abnormalities after hemorrhage, trauma, and burns. *Crit Care Med* 1989; **17**: 934–39.

33. Abraham E, Freitas AA. Hemorrhage produces abnormalities in lymphocyte function and lymphokine generation. *J Immunol* 1989; **142**: 899–906.

34. Abraham E, Chang Y-H. Cellular and humoral bases of hemorrhage-induced depression of lymphocyte function. *Crit Care Med* 1986; **14**: 81–6.

35. Baker CC, Miller CL, Trunkey DD. Correlation of traumatic shock with immunocompetence and sepsis. *Surg Forum* 1979; **30**: 20–1.

♦36. Goldberg RJ, Gore JM, Alpert JS, *et al.* Cardiogenic shock resulting from acute myocardial infarction: a fourteen year community-wide perspective. *N Engl J Med* 1991; **325**: 1117–22.

○37. Agress CM, Binder MJ. Cardiogenic shock. *Am Heart J* 1957; **54**: 458–77.

38. Kuhn LA. The treatment of cardiogenic shock. Part 1. The nature of cardiogenic shock. *Am Heart J* 1967; **74**: 578–81.

39. Kobayashi M, Niitani H, Hasegawa M, Goto H, Kuwahara K. Effect of medical treatment of acute myocardial infarction in coronary care unit: Study on its effect mainly on the cases with complication. *Jap Circ J* 1984; **48**: 650–8.

40. Jugdutt BI, Warnica JW. Intravenous nitroglycerin therapy to limit myocardial infarct size, expansion, and complications. Effect of timing, dosage and infarct location. *Circulation* 1988; **78**: 906–19.

41. Meinertz T, Kasper W, Schumacher M, Just H, for the APSAC Multicenter Trial Group. The German multicenter trial of anisoylated plasminogen streptokinase activator complex versus heparin for acute myocardial infarction. *Am J Cardiol* 1988; **62**: 347–51.

42. Takano T, Endo T, Saito H, *et al*. Clinical usefulness of intraaortic balloon pumping in acute myocardial infarction complicated with cardiogenic shock, ventricular septal perforation and mitral regurgitation. *Jap Circ J* 1984; **48**: 678–89.

♦43. Page DL, Caulifield JB, Kastor JA, DeSanctis RW, Sanders CA. Myocardial changes associated with cardiogenic shock. *N Engl J Med* 1971; **285**: 133–7.

44. Alonso DR, Scheidt S, Post M, Killip T. Pathophysiology of cardiogenic shock: quantification of myocardial necrosis: clinical, pathologic and electrocardiographic correlation. *Circulation* 1973; **48**: 588–96.

45. Becker RC, Gore JM, Lambrew C, for the National Registry of Myocardial Infarction Investigators. A composite view of cardiac rupture in the United States National Registry of Myocardial Infarction. *J Am Coll Cardiol* 1996; **27**: 1321–6.

46. Holmes DR, Berger PB, Hochman JS, *et al*. Cardiogenic shock in patients with acute ischemic syndromes with and without ST segment elevation. *Circulation* 1999; **100**: 2067–73.

47. Barnard D, Alpert JS. Right ventricular infarction. In: Rippe JM, Alpert JS, eds *Intensive Care Medicine*, 2nd edn. Boston: Little, Brown, 1991: 381–91.

48. Shah PK, Maddahi J, Berman DS, Pichler M, Swan HJ. Scintigraphically detected predominant right ventricular dysfunction in acute myocardial infarction: clinical, hemodynamic correlates and implications for therapy and prognosis. *J Am Coll Cardiol* 1985; **6**: 1264–72.

♦49. Lorrell B, Leinbach RC, Pohost GM, *et al*. Right ventricular infarction: clinical diagnosis and differentiation from cardiac tamponade and pericardial constriction. *Am J Cardiol* 1979; **43**: 465–71.

50. Goldstein JA, Vlahakes GJ, Verrier ED, *et al*. The role of right ventricular systolic dysfunction and elevated intrapericardial pressure in the genesis of low cardiac output in experimental right ventricular infarction. *Circulation* 1982; **65**: 513–22.

51. Love JC, Haffajee CI, Gore JM, Alpert JS. Reversibility of hypotension and shock by atrial or atrioventricular sequential pacing in patients with right ventricular infarction. *Am Heart J* 1984; **108**: 5–13.

52. Benotti JR. Acute aortic insufficiency. In: Dalen JE, Alpert JS, eds *Valvular Heart Disease*, 2nd edn. Boston: Little, Brown, 1987: 319–51.

○53. Voyce SJ, Becker RC. Adaptive and maladaptive cardiovascular responses in human sepsis. *Am Heart J* 1991; **12**: 1441–8.

54. Cunnion RE, Parrillo JE. Myocardial dysfunction in sepsis. *Crit Care Clin* 1989; **5**: 99–118.

55. Parrillo JE, Burch C, Shelhammer JA, Parker MM, Nathanson C, Schuette W. A circulatory myocardial depressant substance in humans with septic shock. *J Clin Invest* 1985; **76**: 1539–53.

56. Parker MM, Shelhamer JH, Backarach SL, Green MV, Natanson C, Frederick TM, Danake BA, Parrillo JE. Profound but reversible myocardial depression in patients with septic shock. *Ann Intern Med* 1984; **100**: 483–9.

57. Parker MM, McCarthy KE, Ognibene FP, Parrillo JE. Right ventricular dysfunction and dilation, similar to left ventricular changes, characterize the cardiac depression of septic shock in humans. *Chest* 1990; **97**: 126–31.

58. Ognibene FP, Parker MM, Natanson C, Shelhamer JH, Parillo JE. Depressed left ventricular performance: response to volume infusion in patients with sepsis and septic shock. *Chest* 1987; **93**: 903–10.

○59. Parillo JE, Parker MM, Natanson C, Suffredini AF, Danner RL, Cunnion RE, Ognibane FP. Septic shock in humans: advances in the understanding of pathogenesis, cardiovascular dysfunction and therapy. *Ann Intern Med* 1990; **113**: 227–42.

60. D'Ambra MN, LaRaia PJ, Philbin DM, Watkins WD, Hilsenberg AD, Buckley MJ. Prostaglandin E₁: a new therapy for refractory right heart failure and pulmonary hypertension after mitral valve replacement. *J Thorac Cardiovasc Surg* 1985; **89**: 567–72.

61. Morel DR, Lowenstein E, Nguyenduy T, *et al*. Acute pulmonary vasoconstriction and thromboxane release during protamine reversal of heparin anticoagulation in awake sheep. Evidence for the role of reactive oxygen metabolites following nonimmunological complement activation. *Circ Res* 1988; **62**: 905–15.

62. Topol EJ, Goldschlager N, Ports TA, *et al*. Hemodynamic benefit of atrial pacing in right ventricular myocardial infarction. *Ann Intern Med* 1982; **96**: 594–7.

63. Forrester JS, Diamond G, Chatterjee K, Swan HJ. Medical therapy of acute myocardial infarction by application of hemodynamic subsets (first of two parts). *N Engl J Med* 1976; **295**: 1356–62.

64. Forrester JS, Diamond G, Chatterjee K, Swan HJC. Medical therapy of acute myocardial infarction by application of hemodynamic subsets (second of two parts). *N Engl J Med* 1976; **295**: 1404–13.

65. Mueller HS, Evans R, Ayres SM. Effect of dopamine on hemodynamics and myocardial metabolism in shock following acute myocardial infarction in man. *Circulation* 1978; **57**: 361–5.

66. Maekawa K, Liang C, Hood WB. Comparison of dobutamine and dopamine in acute myocardial infarction. Effects on systemic hemodynamics, plasma

catecholamines, blood flow and infarct size. *Circulation* 1983; **30**: 371–7.

67. Gillespie TA, Ambos HD, Sobel BE, Roberts R. Effects of dobutamine in patients with acute myocardial infarction. *Am J Cardiol* 1977; **39**: 588–94.

68. Francis GS, Sharma B, Hodges M. Comparative hemodynamic effects of dopamine and dobutamine in patients with acute cardiogenic circulatory collapse. *Am Heart J* 1982; **103**: 995–1000.

69. Klocke RK, Mager G, Kux A, Hopp HW, Hilser HH. Effects of a 24-hour milrinone infusion in patients with severe heart failure and cardiogenic shock as a function of the hemodynamic initial condition. *Am Heart J* 1991; **121**: 1965–73.

70. Kantrowitz A, Tjonneland S, Krakauer JS, Phillips SJ, Freed PS, Butner AN. Mechanical intraaortic cardiac assistance in cardiogenic shock. Hemodynamic effects. *Arch Surg* 1968; **97**: 1000–4.

71. Scheidt S, Wilner G, Mueller H, *et al.* Intra-aortic balloon counterpulsation in cardiogenic shock. *N Engl J Med* 1973; **288**: 979–84.

72. Merhige ME, Smalling RW, Cassidy D, *et al.* Effect of the hemopump left ventricular assist device on regional myocardial perfusion and function: reduction of ischemia during coronary occlusion. *Circulation* 1989; **80**(suppl III): III-158–III-166.

73. Frazier OH, Nakatan T, Duncan JM, Parnis SM, Fuqua SM. Clinical experience with the hemopump. *ASAIO Trans* 1989; **35**: 604–6.

74. Phillips SJ, Ballentine B, Slonine D, *et al.* Percutaneous initiation of cardiopulmonary bypass. *Ann Thorac Surg* 1983; **36**: 223–5.

75. O'Neill P, Menendez T, Hust R, Howell J, Espada R, Pacifico A. Prolonged ventricular fibrillation-salvage using a new percutaneous cardiopulmonary support system. *Am J Cardiol* 1989; **64**: 545.

76. Phillips SJ, Zeff RH, Kongtahworn C, *et al.* Percutaneous cardiopulmonary bypass: application and indication for use. *Ann Thorac Surg* 1989; **47**: 121–3.

77. Hands ME, Rutherford JD, Muller JE, *et al.* The in-hospital development of cardiogenic shock after myocardial infarction: incidence, predictors of occurrence, outcome and prognostic factors. *J Am Coll Cardiol* 1989; **14**: 40–6.

78. Lee L, Bates ER, Pitt B, Walton JA, Laufer N, O'Neill WW. Percutaneous transluminal coronary angioplasty improves survival in acute myocardial infarction complicated by cardiogenic shock. *Circulation* 1988; **78**: 1345–51.

79. Stack RS, O'Connor CM, Mark DB, *et al.* Coronary perfusion during acute myocardial infarction with a combined therapy of coronary angioplasty and high-dose intravenous streptokinase. *Circulation* 1988; **77**: 151–61.

80. Stack RS, Califf RM, Hinohara T, *et al.* Survival and cardiac event rates in the first year after emergency coronary angioplasty for acute myocardial infarction. *J Am Coll Cardiol* 1988; **11**: 1141–9.

81. Brodie BR, Wientraub RA, Stuckey TD, *et al.* Outcomes of direct coronary angioplasty for acute myocardial infarction in candidates and noncandidates for thrombotic therapy. *Am J Cardiol* 1991; **67**: 7–12.

82. Lee L, Erbel R, Brown TM, *et al.* Multicenter registry of angioplasty therapy of cardiogenic shock: initial and long term survival. *J Am Coll Cardiol* 1991; **17**: 599–603.

83. Hibbard MD, Holmes DR Jr, Bailey KR, Reeder GS, Bresnahan JF, Gersh BJ. Percutaneous transluminal coronary angioplasty in patients with cardiogenic shock. *J Am Coll Cardiol* 1992; **19**: 639–46.

84. Gacioch GM, Ellis SG, Lee L, *et al.* Cardiogenic shock complicating acute myocardial infarction: the use of coronary angioplasty and the integration of the new support devices into patient management. *J Am Coll Cardiol* 1992; **19**: 647–53.

85. Moosvi AR, Khaja F, Villanueva L, Gheorghiade M, Douthat L, Goldstein S. Early revascularization improves survival in cardiogenic shock complicating acute myocardial infarction. *J Am Coll Cardiol* 1992; **19**: 907–14.

86. Hochman JS. Cardiogenic shock: can we save the patient? *Am Coll Cardiol Educ Highlights* 1996; **12**: 1–5.

87. Bengston JR, Kaplan AJ, Pieper KS, *et al.* Prognosis in cardiogenic shock after acute myocardial infarction in the interventional era. *J Am Coll Cardiol* 1992; **20**: 1482–9.

88. Kahn JK, Rutherford BD, McConahay DR, *et al.* Usefulness of angioplasty during acute myocardial infarction in patients with prior coronary artery bypass grafting. *Am J Cardiol* 1990; **65**: 698–702.

89. Heuser RR, Maddoux GL, Goss JE, Ramo BW, Raff GL, Shadoff N. Coronary angioplasty for acute mitral regurgitation due to myocardial infarction. A nonsurgical treatment preserving mitral valve integrity. *Ann Intern Med* 1987; **107**: 852–5.

90. Shawl FA, Forman MB, Punja S, Goldbaum TS. Emergent coronary angioplasty in the treatment of acute ischemic mitral regurgitation: long term results in five cases. *J Am Coll Cardiol* 1989; **14**: 986–91.

91. Smucker ML, Sarnat WS, Kil D, Scherb DE, Howard PF. Salvage from cardiogenic shock by atherectomy after failed emergency coronary artery angioplasty. *Cathet Cardiovasc Diagn* 1990; **21**: 23–5.

92. Bert RJ, Selinger SL, Leonard JL, Grunwald RP, O'Grady WP. Immediate coronary artery bypass for acute evolving myocardial infarction. *J Thorac Cardiovasc Surg* 1981; **81**: 493–7.

93. Phillips SJ, Konstahworn C, Skinner JR, Zeff MT. Emergency coronary artery reperfusion: a choice therapy for evolving myocardial infarction. Results in 339 patients. *J Thorac Cardiovasc Surg* 1983; **86**: 679–88.

94. DeWood MA, Notske RN, Hensley GR, *et al*. Intra-aortic balloon counterpulsation with or without reperfusion for myocardial shock. *Circulation* 1980; **61**: 1105–12.

95. Alcan KE, Stertzer SH, Wallsh E, Bruno MS, DePasquale NP. Current status of intraaortic balloon counter-pulsation in critical care cardiology. *Crit Care Med* 1984; **12**: 489–95.

96. Subramanian VA, Roberts AJ, Zema MJ, *et al*. Cardiogenic shock following acute myocardial infarction: late functional results after emergency surgery. *NY State J Med* 1980; **80**: 947–52.

97. DeWood MA, Notske RN, Hensley GR, *et al*. Intra-aortic balloon counterpulsation with and without reperfusion for myocardial infarction shock. *Circulation* 1980; **61**: 1105–12.

98. Berg R Jr, Selinger SL, Leonard JJ, Grunwald RP, O'Grady WP. Immediate coronary artery bypass for acute evolving myocardial infarction. *J Thorac Cardiovasc Surg* 1981; **81**: 493–7.

99. Rosenkranz ER, Buckberg GD, Laks H, Mulder DG. Warm induction of cardioplegia with glutamate-enriched blood in coronary patients with cardiogenic shock who are dependent on inotropic drugs and intra-aortic balloon support. *J Thorac Cardiovasc Surg* 1983; **86**: 507–18.

100. Phillips SJ, Kongtahworn C, Skinner JR, Zeff RH. Emergency coronary artery reperfusion: a choice therapy for evolving myocardial infarction. Results in 339 patients. *J Thorac Cardiovasc Surg* 1983; **86**: 679–88.

101. Laks H, Rosenkranz E, Buckberg GD. Surgical treatment of cardiogenic shock after myocardial infarction. *Circulation* 1986; **74**(suppl III): 11–16.

102. Guyton RA, Arcidi JM Jr, Langford DA, Morris DC, Liberman HA, Hatcher CR Jr. Emergency coronary bypass for cardiogenic shock. *Circulation* 1987; **76**(suppl V): 22–7.

103. Bolooki H. Emergency cardiac procedures in patients in cardiogenic shock due to complications of coronary artery disease. *Circulation* 1989; **79** (suppl I): 137–48.

♦104. Hochman JS, Sleeper LA, Webb JG, *et al*. Early revascularization in acute myocardial infarction complicated by cardiogenic shock. *N Engl J Med* 1999; **341**: 625–34.

105. Joyce LD, Johnson KE, Pierce WS, *et al*. Summary of the world experience with clinical use of total artificial hearts as heart support devices. *J Heart Transplant* 1986; **5**: 229–35.

○106. Killip T, Kimball JT. Treatment of myocardial infarction in a coronary care unit: a two-year experience with 250 patients. *Am J Cardiol* 1967; **20**: 457–64.

107. The GUSTO Investigators. An international randomized trial comparing four thrombolytic strategies for acute myocardial infarction. *N Engl J Med* 1993; **329**: 73–82.

108. Jeremy RW, Hackworthy RA, Bautovich G, Hutton BF, Harris PJ. Infarct artery perfusion and changes in left ventricular volume in the month after acute myocardial infarction. *J Am Coll Cardiol* 1987; **9**: 989–95.

109. Little T, Crenshaw M, Liberman HA, *et al*. Effects of time required for reperfusion (thrombolysis or angioplasty, or both) and location of acute myocardial infarction on left venticular functional reserve capacity several months later. *Am J Cardiol* 1991; **67**: 797–805.

110. Marzoll U, Kleiman NS, Dunn JK, *et al*. Factors determining improvement in left ventricular function after reperfusion therapy for acute myocardial infarction: primacy of baseline ejection fraction. *J Am Coll Cardiol* 1991; **17**: 613–20.

111. Morgan CD, Roberts RS, Haq A, *et al*. Coronary patency, infarct size and left ventricular function after thrombolytic therapy for acute myocardial infarction: results from the Tissue Plasminogen Activator: Toronto (TPAT) placebo-controlled trial. TPAT Study Group. *J Am Coll Cardiol* 1991; **17**: 1451–7.

112. Sheehan FH, Mathey DG, Schofer J, Dodge HT, Bolson EL. Factors that determine recovery of left ventricular function after thrombolysis in patients with acute myocardial infarction. *Circulation* 1985; **71**: 1121–8.

113. Dalen JE, Gore JM, Braunwald E, *et al*. Six- and twelve-month follow up of the phase I Thrombolysis in Myocardial Infarction (TIMI) trial. *Am J Cardiol* 1988; **62**: 179–85.

114. Kennedy JW, Ritchie JL, Davis KB, Stadius ML, Maynard C, Fritz JK. The Western Washington randomized trial of intracoronary streptokinase in acute myocardial infarction. A 12-month follow-up report. *N Engl J Med* 1985; **312**: 1073–8.

♦115. Ohman EM, Califf RM, Topol EJ, *et al*. Consequences of reocclusion after successful reperfusion therapy in acute myocardial infarction. TAMI Study Group. *Circulation* 1990; **82**: 781–91.

116. Mathey DG, Kuck KH, Tilsner V, Krebber HJ, Bleifeld W. Nonsurgical coronary artery recanalization in acute transmural myocardial infarction. *Circulation* 1981; **63**: 489–97.

117. Kennedy JW, Gensini GG, Timmis GC, Maynard C. Acute myocardial infarction treated with intracoronary streptokinase: a report of the Society for Cardiac Angiography. *Am J Cardiol* 1985; **55**: 871–7.

118. Blinc A, Planinsic G, Keber D, *et al*. Dependence of blood clot lysis on the mode of transport of urokinase into the clot: a magnetic resonance imaging study in vitro. *Thromb Haemost* 1990; **65**: 549–52.

119. Zidansek A, Blinc A. The influence of transport parameters and enzyme kinetics of the fibrinolytic system on thrombolysis: mathematical modeling of two idealized cases. *Thromb Haemost* 1991; **65**: 553–9.

120. Li KS, Santamore WP, Morley DL, Tulenko TN. Stenotic amplification of vasoconstriction responses. *Am J Physiol* 1989; **256**: H1044–51.

121. Freedman B, Richmond DR, Kelly DT. Pathophysiology of coronary artery spasm. *Circulation* 1982; **66**: 705–9.

122. Cox RH. Mechanical aspects of large coronary arteries. In: Santamore WP, Bove AA, eds. *Coronary artery disease: etiology, hemodynamic consequences, drug therapy and clinical implications.* Baltimore: Urban & Schwarzenberg, 1982: 19–38.

123. Jones M, Gabriel DA. Influence of the subendothelial basement membrane components on fibrin assembly. *J Biol Chem* 1988; **263**: 7043–8.

124. Carr ME, Powers PL. Effect of glycosaminoglycans on thrombin- and atroxin-induced fibrin assembly and structure. *Thromb Haemost* 1989; **62**: 1057–61.

125. Robbins KC. The human plasma fibrinolytic system: regulation and control. *Molec Cell Biochem* 1978; **20**: 149–57.

126. Wohl RC, Summaria L, Robbins KC. Kinetics of activation of human plasminogen by different activator species at pH 7.4 and 37°C. *J Biol Chem* 1980; **255**: 2005–13.

127. Sabol MB, Luippold RS, Hebert J, *et al.* The association between serial measures of systemic blood pressure and early coronary arterial perfusion status following intravenous thrombolytic therapy. *J Thromb Thrombolysis* 1994; **1**: 79–84.

128. Herlitz J, Harford M, Aune L, Karlsson T. Occurrence of hypotension during streptokinase infusion in suspected acute myocardial infarction, and its relation to prognosis and metoprolol therapy. *Am J Cardiol* 1993; **71**: 1021–4.

129. Prewitt RM, Gu S, Carber PJ, Ducas J. Marked systemic hypotension depresses coronary thrombolysis induced intracoronary administration of recombinant tissue-type plasminogen activator. *J Am Coll Cardiol* 1992; **20**: 1626–33.

130. Prewitt RM, Gu S, Schick U, Ducas J. Intraaortic balloon counterpulsation enhances coronary thrombolysis induced by intravenous administration of a thrombolytic agent. *J Am Coll Cardiol* 1994; **23**: 794–8.

♦131. Berger PB, Holmes DR Jr, Stebbins AL, Bates ER, Califf RM, Topol EJ, for the GUSTO-I Investigators. Impact of an aggressive invasive catheterization and revascularization strategy on mortality in patients with cardiogenic shock in the global utilization of streptokinase and tissue plasminogen activator for occluded coronary arteries (GUSTO-I) Trial. An observational study. *Circulation* 1997; **96**: 122–7.

132. Kovack PJ, Rasak MA, Bates ER, Ohman EM, Stomel RJ. Thrombolysis plus aortic counterpulsation: improved survival in patients who present to community hospitals with cardiogenic shock. *J Am Coll Cardiol* 1997; **29**: 1454–8.

8

Management of complicated myocardial infarction

MAUREEN M BURNS AND RICHARD C BECKER

Coronary arterial occlusion, either partial or complete, occurring at the sites of atheromatous plaque disruption is the prox-imate cause of acute myocardial infarction (MI). Myocardial necrosis follows a critical period of tissue hypoperfusion, set-ting the stage for complications that include ventricular dilation/aneurysm formation, acute free-wall rupture, ventricular septal rupture, papillary muscle rupture, acute/subacute pericarditis, mural thrombosis, systemic thromboembolism and electrical dysrhythmias ranging from sinus bradycardia and complete atrioventricular block to lethal ventricular tachy-cardia/fibrillation. The management of complicated MI begins with a comprehensive understanding of anatomy, physiol-ogy, pathology, and the natural history of coronary arterial thrombosis and myocardial necrosis. Standardized pathways of patient care coupled with knowledge-based awareness provide the necessary means for clinicians rapidly to diagnose and treat life-threatening complications.

INTRODUCTION

Acute coronary syndromes (ACS), including ST segment elevation/bundle branch block myocardial infarction (MI), non-ST segment elevation MI, and unstable angina pectoris are atherothrombotic disorders of the coronary arterial circulatory system. Although the underlying pathoanatomic substrate exhibits features of chronicity, the defining events of plaque disruption, intraluminal thrombosis, and distal embolization are acute. Clinicians involved directly in the management of patients with ACS must be well versed in a broad range of management strategies to rapidly provide the highest level of care and achieve optimal outcomes.

Acute MI is not infrequently complicated by poten-tially lethal events that can be categorized as vascular (recurrent coronary thrombosis or thromboembolism), myocardial or mechanical (ventricular dilation, aneurysm formation, pump failure, ventricular septal rupture, papillary muscle rupture, free wall rupture), pericardial (pericarditis) and electrical (heart block, bradyarrhythmias, tachyarrhythmias) (Table 8.1 and Fig. 8.1). The majority of complications occur within the ini-tial 72 hours of infarction; however, the early risk period extends to include the first 4–6 weeks. This chapter high-lights management strategies for complicated MI.

SUBSTRATE FOR COMPLICATED MYOCARDIAL INFARCTION

Histology and physiology

Acute MI, caused most often by sudden coronary arter-ial thrombosis that impairs myocardial perfusion and less commonly as a result of excessive myocardial oxygen

Table 8.1 *Complications of acute myocardial infarction*

Vascular (coronary) complications
Recurrent ischemia
Recurrent infarction

Myocardial complications
Diastolic dysfunction
Systolic dysfunction
Congestive heart failure
Hypotension/cardiogenic shock
Right ventricular infarction
Ventricular cavity dilation (remodeling)
Aneurysm formation (true, false)

Mechanical complications
Left ventricular free wall rupture with cardiac tamponade
Ventricular septal rupture
Papillary muscle rupture with acute mitral regurgitation

Pericardial complications
Pericarditis
Dressler's syndrome
Pericardial effusion

Thromboembolic complications
Mural thrombosis
Systemic thromboembolism
Deep vein thrombosis
Pulmonary embolism

Electrical complications
Ventricular tachycardia
Ventricular fibrillation
Supraventricular tachyarrhythmias
Bradyarrhythmias
Atrioventricular block (1°, 2°, 3°)

demand, is defined pathologically as an irreversible change or death of an individual cell (myocyte) or, in a majority of cases, group of cells. The necrotic process manifests itself within 6 hours from the onset of myocardial hypoperfusion and is characterized initially by a heavy infiltration of neutrophils that persists for approximately 48 hours. Within 7 days of infarction, the myocardium thins as necrotic tissue is progressively removed by mononuclear cells and phagocytes. Granulation tissue infiltrates the involved region by the second week and virtually covers the involved region by 3–4 weeks. Over time (typically within 12–16 weeks) the zone of infarction contracts to become a thin, white, and firm scar.[1–4]

Inflammatory and cellular responses

The infiltration of inflammatory cells is an immediate response to tissue injury in acute MI and includes neutrophils, lymphocytes, macrophages, and fibroblasts. Collagen degradation is also an early response to myocardial necrosis and involves matrix metalloproteases (MMP) that reside within the myocardium in latent forms.[5–8] The abrupt release of inflammatory mediators and MMPs contribute to coronary arterial thrombosis and plaque instability, respectively, providing, at least in part, one explanation for the heightened propensity for thromboembolic events that persists following the initial event. These same mediators may also play a role in toxic 'localized' apoptosis (programmed myocyte death). The rapid infiltration of inflammatory cells coupled with a significant degree of surrounding

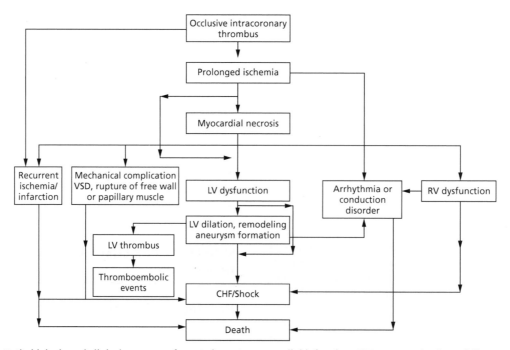

Figure 8.1 *Pathobiologic and clinical sequence of events in acute myocardial infarction. CHF = congestive heart failure; LV = left ventricular; RV = right ventricular; VSD = ventricular septal defect.*

edema creates a profound effect on electrical conduction and refractory periods. Beyond the 'irritability' of necrotic myocardium that can cause automatic ventricular arrhythmias, the differing characteristics of injured and healthy myocardium existing 'side by side' creates 'dispersion of refractoriness' and the substrate for re-entry ventricular arrhythmias, including ventricular tachycardia and ventricular fibrillation. Lastly, collagenase activity within the myocardium, although designed to permit 'rebuilding' of the damaged area, may initially weaken the infarct zone, in increasing the risk of cardiac rupture.

The fibrous stage of wound healing follows the initial inflammatory stage. Increased synthesis of fibrillar type III collagen and, over the subsequent days to weeks, type I collagen provides an organized scaffold for scar development. It is during this stage that most myocardial remodeling takes place, including expansion of the infarct (and non-infarct)-related zones, leading to aneurysm formation and ventricular dilation.

In the final stage, fibrillar fibronectin and collagen are deposited and by 4–6 weeks most of the necrotic myocardium has been removed and replaced by fibrous scar tissue. As with the initial or inflammatory stage, the late scarring stage is characterized by marked heterogeneity of repolarization and refractory periods, creating a permissive environment for malignant arrhythmias.

EARLY RISK CHARACTERIZATION

A vital component of clinical practice and critical care medicine is an ability to anticipate complications either of the MI itself or of its treatment. The development and utilization of risk assessment scales facilitates a response to potentially life-threatening events and represents the logical 'first' step in patient-specific management pathways.

Identification of high-risk patients

EARLY CLINICAL PHASE

Risk stratification tools for patients with ST segment elevation MI have been developed by several experienced clinical trial groups, highlighting the importance of patients demographics, past medical history, clinical features, and the presenting electrocardiogram (ECG). The TIMI (Thrombolysis in Myocardial Infarction) investigators[9] established a risk score that predicted, with considerable accuracy, the occurrence of early morbidity and mortality.

Predictors of early (30-day) mortality were also established by the GUSTO (Global Utilization of Streptokinase and TPA for Occluded coronary arteries) investigators.[10] In a trial including over 40 000 patients

with acute MI, age was identified as the most significant factor, with death rates of 1.1 per cent in the youngest decile (<45 years) and 20.5 per cent in patients >75 years. Overall, five characteristics contained 90 per cent of the prognostic information in the baseline clinical data including age, lower systolic blood pressure, higher Killip Class, elevated heart rate, and anterior site of infarction.

The National Registry of Myocardial Infarction (NRMI) Risk Assessment Assignment was developed as a readily available, bedside clinical 'score card' for rapid triage and management. Predictors of adverse in-hospital clinical outcomes were identified from over 100 000 patients with MI.[11]

PRESENTING SURFACE 12-LEAD ELECTROCARDIOGRAM

The sum of ST segment 'shifts' on the presenting ECG is a reliable marker of infarction size and, as a result, can provide important diagnostic (and prognostic) information. The initial ECG may also contain evidence of a prior MI, identifying patients at increased risk for an early adverse outcome[12] (Fig. 8.2). ST segment area also provides prognostic information.

CARDIAC ENZYME ANALYSIS

Biochemical markers of myocardial necrosis have been used to gauge infarction size and, in general, do provide an estimate of clinical outcome. The alteration of pharmacokinetics, particularly for creatine kinase (CK), following coronary reperfusion has complicated the picture somewhat; however, the 'area under the curve', when calculated correctly does provide prognostic information, but this measurement requires time (serial CK determinations) and effort.

The prognostic value of cardiac specific troponin T (cTNT) and I (cTNI) among patients with unstable angina and non-ST segment elevation MI is recognized; however, data from GUSTO IIA[13] also suggest that an elevated troponin T (>0.1 ng/mL) upon hospital presentation correlates strongly and independently with hospital mortality among patients with ST segment elevation MI.

INFLAMMATORY MARKERS

The measurement of inflammatory markers represents an important tool that links the pathobiologic triad of atherosclerosis, inflammation, and thrombosis. Recent observations with the acute-phase reactant amyloid A protein, in all likelihood will open the door to a variety of new markers that will be used to determine the *activity* of disease and *direct* response to treatment.[14]

RISK FOR STROKE

Stroke is the most feared and devastating complication of fibrinolytic therapy.[15] Overall, 60 per cent of patients

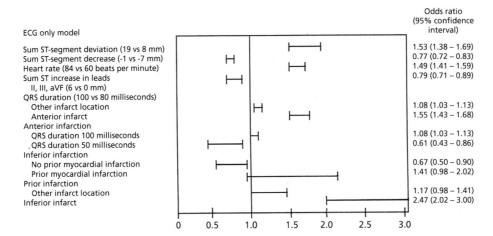

Figure 8.2 *Electrocardiogram (ECG) model to determine risk for 30-day mortality after acute myocardial infarction. The sum of ST segment deviation was the most predictive. (Reproduced with permission from GUSTO-1 Investigators.* JAMA *1998;* **279**: *387–91.)*

Table 8.2 *Risk factors and predictors of hemorrhagic stroke following fibrinolytic therapy: GUSTO-1 trial. (Reproduced with permission from Gore JM.* Circulation *1995* **92**; *2811–18)*

- Advanced age
- Low body weight
- Prior cerebrovascular disease
- Diastolic blood pressure
- History of hypertension (particularly with increased age)
- Combination fibrinolytic therapy (tPA/streptokinase)
- Systolic blood pressure
- Tissue plasminogen activator (tPA) (compared with streptokinase)

GUSTO = Global Utilization of Streptokinase and tPA for Occluded Coronary Arteries: Phase 1 trial.

with hemorrhagic stroke die, while 25 per cent are left with at least a moderate degree of disability (Table 8.2).

NON-ST SEGMENT ELEVATION MI

For nearly two decades the medical community has placed considerable emphasis on the early management of patients with ST segment elevation/bundle branch block MI because of the profound impact of early reperfusion on patient outcome. More recently, it has become clear that patients with non-ST segment elevation MI require careful consideration as well; not solely because of their recognized risk of cardiac events within 6–12 months of discharge, but because a sizeable number of these patients are at increased risk for in-hospital death. It is also conceivable that current efforts in the primary prevention of coronary heart disease and pharmacology-based secondary prevention strategies will 'shift' the clinical expression of disease toward non-ST segment elevation ACS.

A total of 183 113 patients with non-ST segment elevation MI were identified in the National Registry of

Myocardial Infarction (NRMI)-2 database.[16] Risk factors for in-hospital death included advanced age (OR 1.51), female sex (OR 1.20), history of diabetes (OR 1.22), prior congestive heart failure (OR 1.30), and Killip class ≥2 (OR 1.61, 1.94, and 21.4, respectively) (Table 8.3). The similarities in risk profiles for ST segment elevation and non-ST segment elevation MI support aggressive management strategies for high-risk patients regardless of the presenting ECG.

Table 8.3 *Predictors of in-hospital death (after 24 hours) in patients with acute myocardial infarction. (Reproduced with permission from Becker RC et al., for the National Registry of Myocardial Infarction (NRMI-2) participants. Early clinical outcomes and routine management of patients with non-ST segment elevation myocardial infarction: a nationwide perspective.* Arch Intern Med *2001; in press)*

Variable	Odds ratio	95% confidence interval
Aspirin (<24 hours)	0.46	0.43–0.48
Oral β-blocker (<24 hours)	0.59	0.55–0.63
ACE inhibitor (<24 hours)	0.66	0.62–0.71
Normal ECG	0.78	0.70–0.85
ST depression	1.13	1.06–1.20
Prior stroke	1.39	1.29–1.49
Killip class III or IV	8.72	8.56–8.80

ACE = angiotensin-converting enzyme; ECG = electrocardiogram.

CORONARY (VASCULAR) COMPLICATIONS

Recurrent ischemia

Recurrent myocardial ischemia occurs in 15–20 per cent of patients experiencing an acute MI and is typically transient.[17] It does, however, identify patients with the substrate for plaque disruption and thrombosis as well as those with multivessel coronary artery disease and/or a compromised collateral circulation.[18]

Patients with recurrent ischemia can be further stratified according to the extent of ECG changes, hemodynamic stability, and overall clinical status. Three distinct categories of patients have been identified as being at increased risk for postinfarction angina and reinfarction: (1) patients with non-ST segment elevation MI; (2) patients receiving fibrinolytic therapy; and (3) patients with multiple cardiac risk factors.[19] The incidence of postinfarction angina is nearly twice as high after non-ST segment elevation MI (25–35 per cent) than after ST segment elevation or bundle branch block MI (15–20 per cent). Patients treated with fibrinolytics have a 20–30 per cent incidence of recurrent ischemia and a 4–5 per cent incidence of reinfarction even with the concomitant use of aspirin and adjunctive anticoagulant strategies.[20]

MANAGEMENT STRATEGY

Recurrent ischemia must be recognized promptly and managed aggressively. Pain relief is best approached in the context of myocardial oxygen supply and demand. Lowering myocardial oxygen demand can be achieved by decreasing heart rate, inotropic state (using intravenous or oral β-blockers) and/or preload (most commonly with nitrate preparations). Morphine sulfate is also useful in early management. A calcium channel blocker may be added for further heart rate control, prevention of episodic coronary vasospasm, or as an alternative to β-blocker therapy when absolute contraindications exist. Antiplatelet (aspirin ± clopidogrel) therapy should be continued and anticoagulation with intravenous unfractionated heparin or low-molecular-weight heparin (LMWH) instituted (or continued) for patients with ischemic chest pain at rest. Consideration should be given to the addition of an intravenous platelet glycoprotein (GP) IIb/IIIa antagonist.

Anxiolytics such as benzodiazepines can reduce anxiety and provide mild sedation.

The goals of therapy with nitrates, β-blockers and calcium channel blockers are to reduce mean arterial blood pressure and heart rate by approximately 10–20 per cent, but not to a level where coronary arterial perfusion pressure is compromised (mean arterial pressure <70 mm Hg).

In clinically unstable patients with evidence of congestive heart failure, volume status must be assessed carefully and treated appropriately.

If aggressive pharmacologic therapy does not alleviate the myocardial ischemia or if there is concomitant hemodynamic instability, early diagnostic coronary angiography is recommended. Consideration should also be given to inserting an intra-aortic balloon pump to improve myocardial perfusion and serve as a bridge to definitive therapy (revascularization, correction of mechanical defects). Serial ECGs and clinical assessment are recommended to guide optimal management (Fig. 8.3).

Myocardial reinfarction

Reinfarction represents a recurrent atherothrombotic event with subsequent myocardial necrosis. Confirming the diagnosis can be difficult within the initial 24 hours of an index event because serum cardiac markers have not yet returned to a normal range. Thus confirmation must be established in the context of an existing elevation with further (usually two-fold) elevation of cardiac enzymes above a prior level (determined within the past 6 hours). β-Adrenergic blockers have been shown to reduce the risk of reinfarction, whereas fibrinolytic therapy is associated with a slightly increased risk.[21,22] Heart rate-slowing calcium channel blockers reduce the incidence of reinfarction among patients with preserved left ventricular (LV) function after acute MI, whereas the role of unfractionated heparin is controversial.[23]

In contrast, the available data strongly support the ability of LMWH (enoxaparin, dalteparin) and platelet GPIIb/IIIa receptor antagonists to reduce the likelihood of recurrent MI in patients with non-ST segment elevation MI and possibly in ST segment elevation/bundle branch block MI as well.[24,25]

MANAGEMENT STRATEGY

The clinical approach to recurrent MI, as with recurrent myocardial ischemia, is determined by the patients overall clinical status and early indicators of injury (Fig. 8.4).

Coronary angiography and percutaneous coronary interventions

Early recurrent myocardial ischemia, persistent ST segment elevation (>50 per cent of maximal ST segment deviation), hemodynamic instability, and ventricular tachyarrhythmias refractory to antiarrhythmic therapy are indications for early coronary angiography.[26]

The American College of Cardiology/American Heart Association guidelines for coronary angiography and percutaneous coronary interventions (PCI) are outlined in Table 8.4.

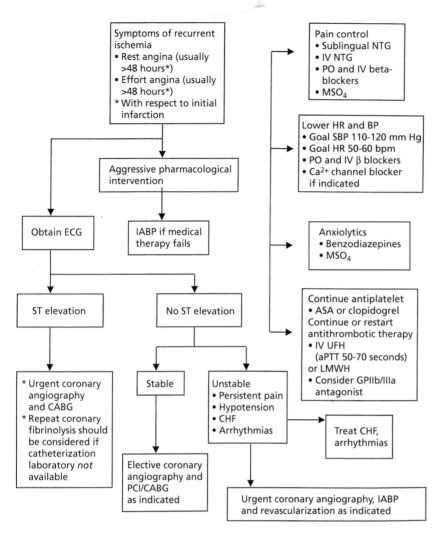

Figure 8.3 *The management of recurrent ischemia is determined by clinical signs and symptoms, electrocardiographic features, hemodynamic status and angiographic findings. aPTT = activated partial thromboplastin time; ASA = aspirin; BP = blood pressure; CABG = coronary artery bypass grafting; CHF = congestive heart failure; ECG = electrocardiogram; HR = heart rate; IABP = intra-aortic balloon pump; IV = intravenous; LMWH = low-molecular-weight heparin; MSO₄ = morphine sulfate; NTG = nitroglycerin; PCI = percutaneous coronary intervention; PO = per os; SBP = systolic blood pressure; UFH = unfractionated heparin.*

Table 8.4 *Early coronary angiography and/or interventional therapy (American College of Cardiology/American Heart Association updated guidelines 1999)*

Class I

1. Patients with persistent or recurrent (stuttering) episodes of symptomatic ischemia, spontaneous or induced, with or without associated ECG changes
2. Presence of shock, severe pulmonary congestion, or continuing hypotension

Class IIa

No recommendation

Class IIb

No recommendation

Class III

This category applies to patients with AMI who:

1. undergo elective angioplasty of a non-infarct-related artery at the time of AMI
2. are beyond 12 hours after onset of symptoms and have no evidence of myocardial ischemia
3. have received fibrinolytic therapy and have no symptoms of myocardial ischemia
4. are eligible for thrombolysis and are undergoing primary angioplasty performed by a low-volume operator in a laboratory without surgical capability

AMI = acute myocardial infarction; ECG = electrocardiogram.

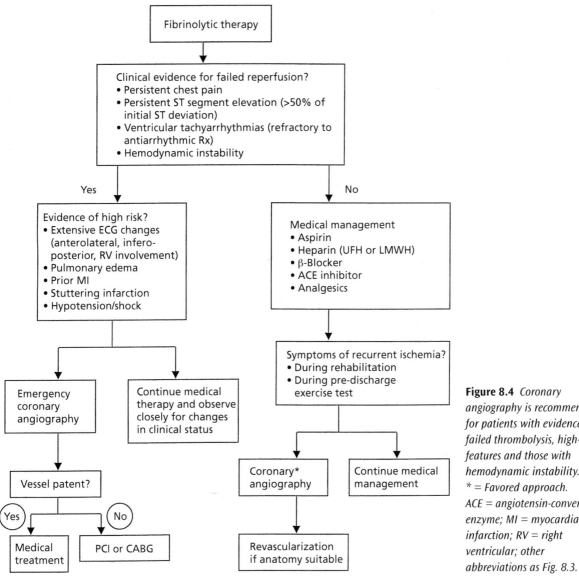

Figure 8.4 *Coronary angiography is recommended for patients with evidence of failed thrombolysis, high-risk features and those with hemodynamic instability.*
* = Favored approach.
ACE = angiotensin-converting enzyme; MI = myocardial infarction; RV = right ventricular; other abbreviations as Fig. 8.3.

Surgical revascularization

Although outcomes following emergent surgical revascularization have improved over time as a result of increasing experience, the application of mechanical, hemodynamic/circulatory support measures, and advanced methods of myocardial protection and anesthetic management, the procedure is typically reserved for a carefully selected subset of patients (Table 8.5).

MYOCARDIAL COMPLICATIONS

Right ventricular infarction

Right ventricular (RV) infarction encompasses a complex spectrum of pathoanatomic and clinical presentations ranging from asymptomatic mild RV dysfunction to overt cardiogenic shock. RV infarction complicates 35–50 per cent of inferior wall infarctions, which, in turn, make up 40–50 per cent of all acute MIs. Right ventricular injury may also accompany an anterior MI. The diagnosis of RV extension is important because of its association with increased morbidity and mortality (25–30 per cent).[27] Only a small percentage (approximately 5 per cent) of patients with acute MI present with isolated RV infarction.

The clinical triad of hypotension, clear lung fields, and increased jugular venous pressure in a patient experiencing an inferior MI strongly supports the diagnosis of RV extension. A right-sided S_3 gallop or Kussmaul's sign (distention of the jugular veins during inspiration) may also be present on physical examination. Other potential clinical features of RV infarction include tricuspid regurgitation, sinoatrial (SA), or atrioventricular (AV) nodal conduction disturbances, and atrioventricular (AV) dissociation. The ECG reveals ST segment elevation of

Table 8.5 *Emergent or urgent coronary artery bypass graft (CABG) surgery (American College of Cardiology/American Heart Association updated guidelines 1999)*

Class I
1. Failed angioplasty with persistent pain or hemodynamic instability in patients with coronary anatomy suitable for surgery
2. AMI with persistent or recurrent ischemia refractory to medical therapy in patients with coronary anatomy suitable for surgery who are not candidates for catheter intervention
3. At the time of surgical repair of postinfarction ventricular septal defect (VSD) or mitral valve insufficiency

Class IIa
1. Cardiogenic shock with coronary anatomy suitable for surgery

Class IIb
1. Failed PCI and small area of myocardium at risk; hemodynamically stable

Class III
1. When the expected surgical mortality rate equals or exceeds the mortality rate associated with appropriate medical therapy

AMI = acute myocardial infarction; PCI = percutaneous coronary intervention.

>0.5 mm in V_4R. A Q wave in this lead is considered a non-specific finding. Other available modalities that can be used to diagnose RV infarction include thallium or sestamibi perfusion imaging, coronary angiography, echocardiography, and hemodynamic measurements with a pulmonary artery catheter.

Complications of acute RV infarction are, in most instances, a manifestation of both LV and RV dysfunction as well as increased parasympathetic tone (Table 8.6). Overt cardiogenic shock, although occurring rarely, is the most serious complication. High-degree AV block is not uncommon and identifies a particularly high-risk patient group. Atrial fibrillation occurs in one-third of patients with RV infarction as a result of concomitant right atrial infarction or dilation due to volume and pressure overload. Other potential complications of RV infarction include ventricular septal rupture (particularly in patients with concomitant transmural posterior septal infarction), RV thrombus formation with subsequent pulmonary embolism, tricuspid regurgitation, and a pericarditis, most likely because of transmural injury involving the thin-walled right ventricle. The development of a right-to-left shunt through a patent foramen ovale is a complication unique to RV infarction

Table 8.6 *Potential complications of right ventricular infarction*

- Cardiogenic shock
- High-degree atrioventricular block
- Atrial fibrillation/atrial flutter
- Ventricular tachycardia/fibrillation
- Ventricular septal rupture
- Right ventricular thrombus with or without pulmonary embolism
- Tricuspid regurgitation
- Pericarditis
- Right-to-left shunt via patent foramen ovale

and should be suspected when severe hypoxia is not responsive to supplemental oxygen therapy.[28]

MANAGEMENT STRATEGY

As with all ST segment elevation infarctions, the initial approach to patients with RV infarction must address the need for early reperfusion therapy directed at limiting infarct size.

Fibrinolytic therapy and primary angioplasty, when successful, improve RV ejection fraction and reduce the incidence of complete heart block.

If hemodynamic compromise is present, measures should be implemented to maintain RV preload, reduce RV afterload, and to support the dysfunctional RV.

The requirement for volume (preload-dependent state) differentiates the treatment of RV infarction from that of 'pure' left ventricular infarction. Volume expansion is the mainstay of therapy, with the goal of maintaining a right atrial or central venous pressure between 12 and 15 mm Hg.

Normal saline given as a bolus of 250–500 mL should be used acutely, with an appreciation that a large volume (5–10 L) of fluid may be required to increase RV filling pressure, left ventricular preload, and cardiac output sufficiently. If volume support does not produce hemodynamic improvement or if features of pulmonary edema emerge, a pulmonary artery catheter may be required to guide further management.

Patients with persistent hypotension (despite volume resuscitation) may benefit from inotropic support with either dobutamine or dopamine. Because of

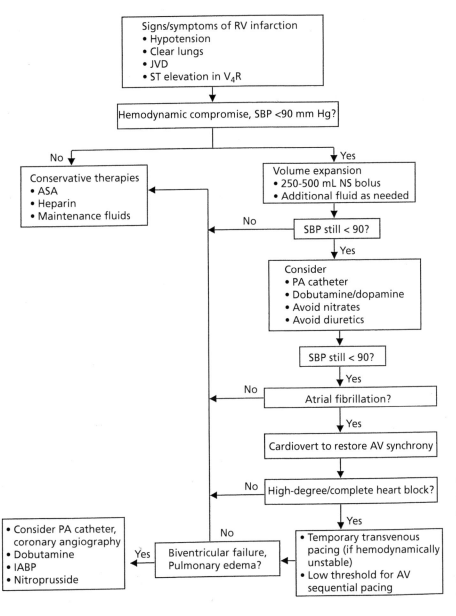

Figure 8.5 *Management algorithm for right ventricular (RV) infarction. ASA = aspirin; AV = atrioventricular; IABP = intra-aortic balloon pump; JVD = jugular venous distension; NS = normal saline; PA = pulmonary artery; SBP = systolic blood pressure.*

their potential to reduce preload, vasodilators including nitroglycerin and morphine sulfate, routinely used in the management of LV infarctions, should be used with great caution in patients with RV infarction. Another crucial factor in sustaining adequate preload is the maintenance of AV synchrony. In patients with high-degree AV block, dual-chamber pacing may be required, particularly if ventricular pacing does not cause an improvement in the patient's overall clinical status.[29]

Atrial fibrillation can cause profound hemodynamic deterioration, necessitating prompt cardioversion.

In patients with biventricular failure, circulatory support using intra-aortic balloon counterpulsation may be required followed by coronary angiography and either percutaneous or surgical intervention as the findings and clinical status dictate (Fig. 8.5).

Left ventricular dysfunction (systolic/diastolic)

The extent of LV compromise correlates directly with the extent of myocardial damage and is a major determinant of clinical outcome. Anterior site of infarction is com-

Table 8.7 *Killip classification of patients with acute myocardial infarction. (Reproduced from Killip T and Kimball JT. Am J Cardiol 1967; **20**: 457)*

Class	Clinical definition	Patients at hospital admission (%)	Mortality[a] (%)
I	No clinical signs of heart failure	30–40	8
II	Râles over ≤50% of lungs, S$_3$ gallop	30–50	30
III	Râles over ≥50% of lungs, pulmonary edema	5–10	44
IV	Cardiogenic shock	10	80–100

[a]Pre-reperfusion/intervention era.

monly associated with extensive LV damage, reduced ventricular performance and reduced survival. The Killip classification separates patients into four distinct groups based on existing clinical signs and symptoms of LV failure. Increasing Killip class represents progressively severe LV compromise and is associated strongly with a poor prognosis (Table 8.7).

The immediate functional consequences of acute myocardial ischemia and infarction include both systolic and diastolic ventricular dysfunction; either may compromise ventricular performance and lead to congestive heart failure. Diastolic dysfunction (impaired ventricular relaxation) occurs uniformly in patients with acute MI, but is clinically evident in only 20–30 per cent of patients. When it does occur, diastolic dysfunction often precedes systolic dysfunction and is the most common cause of congestive failure in the acute phase. Systolic dysfunction, also known as pump failure, is a serious complication of acute MI. The sudden loss of contractile function decreases stroke volume and increases end-systolic volume, end-diastolic volume, and diastolic filling pressure. The clinical manifestations of systolic dysfunction include decreased forward flow (tissue perfusion) and increased backward flow (pulmonary congestion and edema).

The loss of contractile function in the initial minutes to hours of MI is potentially reversible, particularly with successful coronary reperfusion. Myocardial 'stunning' as a cause for systolic dysfunction is also a reversible component of myocardial dysfunction.[30] Stunned myocardium, in some instances, responds to pharmacologic inotropic stimulation.[31]

Hemodynamic instability associated with LV systolic dysfunction is an indication for placement of a pulmonary artery catheter to determine intracardiac pressures, cardiac output, and systemic vascular resistance and to guide patient management. A diagnosis of LV failure is supported by increased pulmonary artery (particularly diastolic) and pulmonary capillary wedge pressures, decreased cardiac index and an elevated systemic vascular resistance.

Cardiogenic shock complicates 5–15 per cent of all infarctions[32] and typically occurs when myocardial necrosis involves ≥40 per cent of the left ventricle.[33] It is the most common cause of in-hospital death among patients with MI and carries a mortality rate approach-ing 80 per cent. Clinically, cardiogenic shock is characterized by hypotension and hypoperfusion of vital organs. Hemodynamic disturbances, as measured by a pulmonary artery catheter, include elevated pulmonary capillary wedge pressure and a markedly reduced cardiac output (Tables 8.8 and 8.9). Complications of acute MI other than severe LV dysfunction may also cause cardiogenic shock, including extensive RV infarction, ventricular septal rupture, papillary muscle rupture or ischemic papillary muscle dysfunction with severe mitral regurgitation, and ventricular free-wall rupture with cardiac tamponade.

Table 8.8 *Signs, symptoms, and common characteristics of cardiogenic shock*

Clinical
Evidence of hypoperfusion
- Cold, clammy, or mottled skin (livedo reticularus)
- Impaired mentation (agitation, obtundation, confusion)
- Oliguria (<30 mL per hour)
Evidence of primary cardiac abnormality

Hemodynamic
Systolic blood pressure <90 mm Hg (mean arterial pressure <65 mm Hg or 20% decrease from baseline)
PCWP ≥20 mm Hg
CI <2.0 L/minutes per m^2

CI = cardiac index; PCWP = pulmonary capillary wedge pressure.

Management strategies

DIASTOLIC DYSFUNCTION

The comprehensive management of LV diastolic dysfunction must concomitantly address ongoing myocardial ischemia and pulmonary congestion. Intravenous furosemide is considered the diuretic of choice for patients not previously receiving diuretics. Larger doses may be required among patients previously on diuretic therapy and for those with compromised renal function. Excessive diuresis should be avoided to prevent hypotension and a decline in coronary arterial perfusion pressure.

β-Blockade is an important treatment consideration in patients with isolated ischemic diastolic dysfunction.

Table 8.9 *Hemodynamic parameters in commonly encountered clinical situations (idealized). (Reproduced with permission from Voyce S.* Intensive care medicine. *Philadelphia: Lippincott–Raven Publishers, 1999; 61.)*

	RA	RV	PA	PCWP	AO	CI	SVR	PVR
Normal	0–6	25/0–6	25/6–12	6–12	130/80	≥2.5	1500	≤250
Hypovolemic shock	0–2	15–20/0–2	15–20/2–6	2–6	≤90/60	<2.0	>1500	≤250
Cardiogenic shock	8	50/8	50/35	35	≤90/60	<2.0	>1500	≤250
Septic shock								
Early[a]	0–2	20–25/0–2	20–25/0–6	0–6	≤90/60	≥2.5	<1500	<250
Late	0–4	25/4–10	25/4–10	4–10	≤90/60	<2.0	>1500	>250
Acute massive pulmonary embolism	8–12	50/12	50/12–15	≤12	≤90/60	<2.0	>1500	>450
Cardiac tamponade	12–18	25/12–18	25/12–18	12–18	≤90/60	<2.0	>1500	≤250
AMI without LVF	0–6	25/0–6	25/12–18	≤18	140/90	≤2.5	1500	≤250
AMI with LVF	0–6	30–40/0–6	30–40/18–25	>18	140/90	<2.0	>1500	>250
Biventricular failure secondary to LVF	>6	50–60/>6	50–60/25	18–25	120/80	~2.0	>1500	>250
RVF secondary to RVI	12–20	30/12–20	30/12	<12	≤90/60	<2.0	>1500	>250
Cor pulmonale	>6	80/>6	80/35	<12	120/80	~2.0	>1500	>400
Idiopathic pulmonary hypertension	0–6	80–100/0–6	80–100/40	<12	100/60	<2.0	>1500	>500
Acute VSR[b]	6	60/6–8	60/35	30	≤90/60	<2.0	>1500	>250

[a]Hemodynamic profile seen in approximately one-third of patients in late septic shock.
[b]Confirmed by appropriate RA–PA oxygen saturation step-up.
RA = right atrium; RV = right ventricle; PA = pulmonary artery; PCWP = pulmonary capillary wedge pressure; AO = aortic; CI = cardiac index; SVR = systemic vascular resistance; PVR = pulmonary vascular resistance; AMI = acute myocardial infarction; LVF = left ventricular failure; RVI = right ventricular infarction; RVF = right ventricular failure; VSR = ventricular septal rupture.

β-Blockers not only reduce myocardial oxygen demand, but also improve LV compliance and reduce LV filling pressures, lessening pulmonary congestion. Caution is recommended when systolic and diastolic dysfunction coexist. In this setting, diuresis should be achieved prior to initiating β-blocker therapy.

Preload and afterload reducing agents are administered to reduce pulmonary venous pressures. Nitroprusside is both an arteriolar dilator and venodilator and, as a result, reduces both afterload and preload. This agent is most useful in situations where ischemic diastolic dysfunction complicates existing systolic dysfunction. Nitroglycerin reduces preload and improves both coronary arterial blood flow and myocardial perfusion. For this reason it is an important therapeutic adjunct in patients with ischemia-mediated congestive heart failure. Because of rapid titratability, intravenous administration is preferred in the intensive care unit setting.

SYSTOLIC DYSFUNCTION

The management of LV systolic dysfunction, when severe, is dictated by specific hemodynamic disturbances as reflected in pulmonary capillary wedge pressure (PCWP), cardiac output (CO), systemic vascular resistance, and systemic blood pressure (BP) readings (Table 8.10). However, in most patients with uncomplicated MI and mild LV failure, invasive hemodynamic monitoring is not required. Frequent assessment of the patient's cardiopulmonary status, mental status, skin and mucous membranes, cardiac rhythm and heart rate, oxygenation and urine output must be undertaken. In most patients

with systolic dysfunction that is mild in severity, conventional therapy with morphine, nasal oxygen, intravenous, oral, or transdermal nitrates, and gentle diuresis will yield clinical improvement.

The initial management of patients with severe congestive heart failure must include a careful evaluation of oxygenation and acid–base balance; occasionally endotracheal intubation with ventilatory support is necessary. In the setting of severe LV dysfunction associated with hypotension, intravenous inotropic agents such as dopamine and dobutamine should be administered. In

Table 8.10 *Indications for hemodynamic monitoring. (American College of Cardiology/American Heart Association guidelines)*

Balloon floatation right-heart catheter monitoring
Class I
1. Severe or progressive CHF or pulmonary edema
2. Cardiogenic shock or progressive hypotension
3. Suspected mechanical complications of acute infarction, i.e. VSD, papillary muscle rupture, or pericardial tamponade

Class IIa
1. Hypotension that does not respond promptly to fluid administration in a patient without pulmonary congestion

Class III
1. Patients with acute infarction without evidence of cardiac or pulmonary complications

CHF = congestive heart failure; VSD = ventricular septal defect.

addition to inotropic support, preload and afterload reduction may be required to augment forward flow and reduce pulmonary congestion. Diuretics and nitrates will diminish pulmonary congestion; however, there may be no overall improvement in CO and, in fact, systemic blood pressure may decrease. Nitroprusside,

through a reduction of both preload and afterload, will commonly increase CO, reduce LV end-diastolic pressure and alleviate pulmonary congestion. In the early hours of acute MI, when ischemia often contributes substantially to LV dysfunction, nitroglycerin represents a preferred agent as it causes a greater degree of venodila-

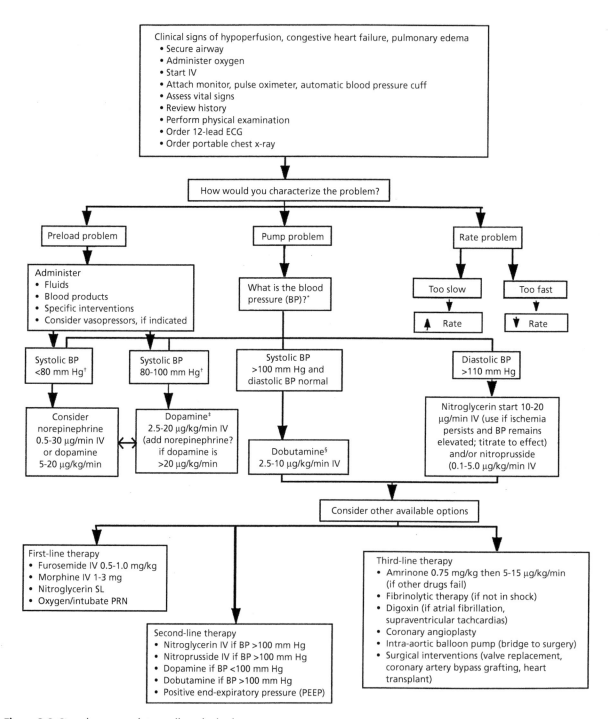

Figure 8.6 *Stepwise approach to cardiogenic shock.*
Base management after this point on invasive hemodynamic monitoring, if possible.
†*Fluid bolus of 250–500 mL normal saline should be tried; if no response, consider sympathomimetics?*
‡*Move to dopamine and stop norepinephrine when BP improves.*
§*Add dopamine when BP improves; cautious use of dobutamine when systolic BP <100 mm Hg.*
BP = blood pressure; ECG = electrocardiogram; IV = intravenous; PRN = as required; SL = sublingual.

tion than does nitroprusside. The phosphodiesterase inhibitors amrinone and milrinone exhibit inotropic and vasodilating properties and, for this reason, should be considered, particularly in patients with reduced LV systolic function who have been treated previously with β-blockers. Inotropic and vasodilator therapies must be carefully titrated to maintain a systemic blood pressure of at least 90 mm Hg (mean arterial pressure ≥70 mm Hg). Once blood pressure has remained stable for 60–90 minutes, diuresis can be initiated safely.

Patients with severe LV dysfunction, depressed CO, elevated LV diastolic pressure, a mean systemic blood pressure <65 mm Hg (or reduced by ≥30 per cent of baseline), and evidence of vital organ hypoperfusion have cardiogenic shock. Hypoxemia is common in this setting and should be corrected using supplemental oxygen with a low threshold for endotracheal intubation in the setting of progressive hemodynamic deterioration and severe acidemia. Although intravenous vasopressors including norepinephrine may be required to achieve a mean systemic blood pressure of 70 mm Hg or greater, mechanical circulatory support is a preferred management adjunct in patients with cardiogenic shock and features of active myocardial ischemia. Early angiography followed by revascularization is a particularly attractive management strategy in patients less than 75 years of age[34] (Fig. 8.6).

MECHANICAL COMPLICATIONS

The most commonly encountered mechanical complications of acute MI include ventricular septal rupture (VSR), left ventricular free wall rupture, mitral valve regurgitation (MR) and left ventricular aneurysm formation. Papillary muscle and chordal rupture (causing acute MR), VSR, and free wall rupture, when they occur, commonly do so suddenly within the first week of infarction, whereas aneurysm formation is more slow and progressive in nature. In general, patients with acute mechanical complications have smaller infarctions than patients who develop pump failure or malignant ventricular arrhythmias.[1] Sudden or rapidly progressive hemodynamic deterioration with systemic hypotension, congestive heart failure, and hypoperfusion should raise suspicion for an acute mechanical defect. The echocardiogram (transthoracic, transesophageal) is an important diagnostic tool that should be used early in the evaluation of patients with suspected mechanical defects (Fig. 8.7).

Ventricular septal rupture

Rupture of the ventricular septum occurs in 2–4 per cent of patients with MI and is responsible for 5 per cent of all in-hospital deaths. Although VSR usually occurs

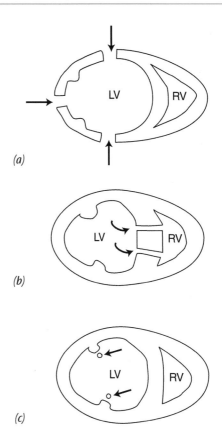

Figure 8.7 *Cardiac rupture, a potentially lethal complication of myocardial infarction, can involve: (a) left ventricular free wall; (b) ventricular septum; or (c) papillary muscle. LV = left ventricle; RV = right ventricle.*

between 3 and 5 days postinfarction, the highest risk is actually within the first 24 hours. Early occurrence is particularly common among patients who have received fibrinolytic therapy. Risk factors for VSR include first infarction, history of hypertension, and female gender. Inferior wall infarction is most often associated with posterior septal rupture, whereas distal septal and apical ruptures are more likely to occur following an anterior site of infarction.

Clinically, acute VSR is characterized by new-onset congestive heart failure in the presence of a new, harsh, holosystolic murmur; however, patients may exhibit a relatively small degree of pulmonary congestion because of left-to-right shunting. The extent of hemodynamic compromise is determined by the combined defect size and reduced ventricular performance. A diagnosis of VSR can be made using Doppler echocardiography or detection of an oxygen saturation 'step-up' between the right atrium and the right ventricle or pulmonary artery during right heart catheterization. An oxygen step-up of greater than 10 per cent indicates a significant left-to-right shunt at the ventricular level.

MANAGEMENT STRATEGY

The immediate supportive treatment of VSR includes intravenous fluid administration and inotropic (dopamine or dobutamine) in combination with afterload reduction using nitroprusside or, more commonly, intra-aortic balloon counterpulsation.

Although surgical repair represents the definitive treatment, operative mortality is high, ranging from 20 to 70 per cent. Preoperative shock and inferoposterior infarction, particularly with RV dysfunction, are risk factors for a poor surgical outcome following surgery.

Emergency repair should be considered when either pulmonary edema or cardiogenic shock is present, but deferred repair may be preferable among hemodynamically stable patients.

Although aggressive and early surgery leads to the highest survival rates, many patients have a complicated postoperative course and prolonged hospital length of stay.[35]

When VSR is suspected, echocardiography with color-flow Doppler imaging should be performed as soon as possible to confirm the diagnosis, establish the coexistence of other cardiac abnormalities (mitral regurgitation, pericardial effusion) and provide estimates of both RV and LV systolic function. If a decision is made to proceed with surgical repair, coronary angiography should be performed in anticipation of concomitant revascularization.

Left ventriculography may not be necessary if echocardiography provides adequate information on LV performance and the existence of concomitant valvular abnormalities.

Left ventricular free-wall rupture

Rupture of the left ventricular free wall occurs in 1–2 per cent of patients, but is responsible for 10–15 per cent of in-hospital deaths. After cardiogenic shock and ventricular arrhythmias, it is the most common cause of early death. In addition, rupture of the LV free wall occurs 8–10 times more frequently than rupture of either a papillary muscle or the ventricular septum. Autopsy series have shown that the lateral wall is the most common site of rupture. Similar to acute VSR, risk factors for free-wall rupture include age >70 years, female gender, hypertension, first MI, and transmural infarction in the absence of collateral vessels.[36,37]

The clinical presentation among patients with ventricular free-wall rupture ranges from sudden hypotension accompanied by electromechanical dissociation (EMD) and death from cardiac tamponade to transient chest discomfort and bradyarrhythmias. The patient frequently develops signs of systemic hypoperfusion, jugular venous distention, pulsus paradoxus, and distant heart sounds. Episodes of chest pain with diaphoresis and nausea can herald subacute or impending free wall rupture. The diagnosis is most often suspected clinically and confirmed by means of echocardiography, pericardiocentesis, or at the time of emergent surgery.

MANAGEMENT STRATEGY

Patients with suspected LV free-wall rupture and systemic hypotension should receive intravenous fluid. A large volume is commonly required to increase ventricular preload and maintain cardiac output. Vasopressor support must follow without delay if the hemodynamic status does not improve. Emergent pericardiocentesis may be a life-saving maneuver in patients with abrupt EMD; however, surgical intervention remains the definitive treatment.[38]

Mitral valve regurgitation

Acute MR is associated with a poor prognosis.[39] With moderate to severe MR, the 1-year survival rate is approximately 50 per cent. Although the diagnosis is typically suggested by the presence of a new holosystolic murmur, up to 50 per cent of the patients with severe MR *do not* have an audible murmur. Because of the frequency of 'silent' MR, the clinician must maintain a high index of suspicion in patients with sudden unexplained hypotension or pulmonary edema.

The papillary muscle is the cardiac structure that ruptures least frequently; however, this event is associated with rapid hemodynamic deterioration because the compromised LV is not able to compensate for an excessive volume load imposed by the incompetent mitral valve. Since the posteromedial papillary muscle receives its blood supply solely from the posterior descending artery (usually as a branch of the right coronary artery), it is prone to ischemia, necrosis, and rupture. The anterolateral papillary muscle has a dual blood supply provided by the left anterior descending and left circumflex coronary arteries and is, therefore, less prone to ischemic dysfunction and injury.

MANAGEMENT STRATEGY

Patients with acute MR causing congestive heart failure or overt cardiogenic shock require hemodynamic monitoring and pharmacologic inotropic/vasopressor therapy. Intra-aortic balloon counterpulsation should be considered for hemodynamic support and to serve as a bridge to coronary angiography and surgical intervention.

Serial echocardiography can be utilized to determine progression and for the purpose of assessing overall LV compensation in relatively stable patients.

> Moderate to severe MR, particularly when unresponsive to pharmacologic and supportive measures, should be addressed surgically;[40] however, concomitant mitral valve replacement (or repair if feasible) and bypass grafting, even in experienced hands, are associated with a high surgical mortality.
>
> The management of patients with mechanical complications of acute MI are summarized in Fig. 8.8.

Left ventricular dilation and aneurysm formation

Infarct 'expansion' occurs acutely (in the first few days following MI) and causes dilation and thinning of the infarcted segment.[41] This event must be distinguished from infarct 'extension' (or reinfarction). Clinically, these two complications of MI may present similarly (electrocardiographic ST segment changes and hemodynamic disturbances); however, infarct expansion is not accompanied by re-elevation of cardiac enzymes as is the case with infarct extension. Infarct expansion usually occurs in the setting of transmural, anterior infarction, is proportional to the size of the MI, and portends a greater likelihood of death.

Left ventricular dilation and remodeling occur more insidiously, and are characterized by a progressive process that begins shortly after the acute event and continues over the subsequent weeks to months. Following acute injury, the ventricle dilates in an effort to maintain cardiac output. Unfortunately, progressive dilation causes increased wall stress, which, in turn, leads to further cavity enlargement, decompensation and impaired performance.

MANAGEMENT STRATEGY

> Efforts to reduce wall stress through reductions in preload and afterload are important. Early treatment with intravenous nitroglycerin and angiotensin converting enzyme (ACE) inhibitors are the most effective, particularly the latter,[42,43] which exerts most of its effects at the tissue level.

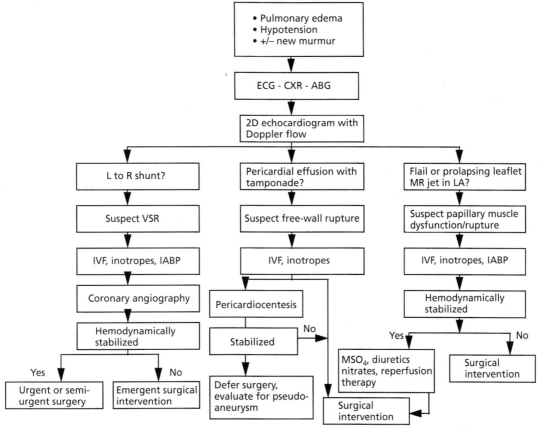

Figure 8.8 *The management of patients with mechanical complications is determined by the site of involvement and the degree of hemodynamic compromise. ABG = arterial blood gas; CXR = chest x-ray; ECG = electrocardiogram; IVF = intravenous fluids; IABP = intra-aortic balloon pump; LA = left atrium; L to R = left to right; MR = mitral regurgitation; MSO₄ = morphine sulfate; VSR = ventricular septal rupture.*

The potential added benefit of combined ACE inhibition and angiotensin II receptor antagonists is under investigation.

At the extreme end of a spectrum that characterizes LV remodeling is aneurysm formation. The prevalence of LV aneurysms following MI, as estimated from postmortem studies, is between 3 and 15 per cent. The location is typically anterior, anteroapical, or apical. Aneurysms may be asymptomatic or associated with angina pectoris, arrhythmias (including malignant ventricular dysrhythmias), cardioembolism and/or congestive heart failure. A diagnosis is most often confirmed by two-dimensional (2D) echocardiography or contrast ventriculography.

> Patients developing ventricular aneurysms should be treated in a manner similar to others with MI (β-blocker, ACE inhibitor, and aspirin therapy). Pharmacologic strategies should not be based solely on the presence of an aneurysm, but according to the presence of congestive heart failure, mural thrombi, and/or life-threatening ventricular arrhythmias. Occasionally, surgical resection is indicated to correct refractory heart failure, recurrent life-threatening arrhythmias and/or recurrent systemic embolization despite anticoagulant therapy.

Aneurysmectomy is usually combined with coronary bypass grafting, and, in patients with concomitant ventricular arrhythmias, the line of resection should be guided by electrophysiologic mapping.

Pseudoaneurysm formation

Pseudoaneurysms are a rare complication of acute MI and, in essence, represent a 'contained rupture' of the ventricular free wall. Clot forms in the pericardial space and an aneurysmal wall consisting of organized thrombus and pericardium prevents hemorrhage within the mediastinum. Unlike a *true* ventricular aneurysm, a pseudoaneurysm (*false* aneurysm) has a narrow base (neck) and the risk of rupture (recurrent rupture) is high. Pseudoaneurysms, which have the potential to expand progressively, are clinically silent in most instances, but may cause congestive heart failure, persistent ST elevation within the region of infarction, or systolic murmurs.[44]

The diagnosis of LV pseudoaneurysm can be established by 2D-echocardiography, ventriculographic radionuclide studies, magnetic resonance imaging, or contrast left ventriculography.

MANAGEMENT STRATEGY

> In addition to the pharmacologic management of congestive heart failure and life-threatening arrhythmias, anticoagulation should be discontinued. Surgical resection with or without bypass grafting is recommended.

PERICARDIAL COMPLICATIONS

Pericarditis

Pericardial inflammation is common following acute MI and typically manifests in either an acute or subacute form. Although pericarditis is currently less common with the advent of reperfusion therapy than it was 2–3 decades ago, it nevertheless must be recognized and diagnosed promptly.

Early postinfarction pericarditis

The most common manifestation of acute pericarditis is chest pain that worsens with inspiration, swallowing, coughing and lying flat, and lessened when the patient sits up and leans forward. Fever, generally less than 38.6°C, can accompany postinfarction pericarditis and typically lasts for several days.[45] A scratchy one-, two- or three-component pericardial friction rub is often appreciated along the left sternal border. Concave upward ST segment elevation in five or more ECG leads supports the diagnosis. Although sinus tachycardia is the most common rhythm abnormality, a wide variety of dysrhythmias, including atrial fibrillation have been described.[46] A pericardial effusion, identified by echocardiography, is not uncommon following MI and its presence or absence neither confirms nor excludes the diagnosis of pericarditis.

MANAGEMENT STRATEGY

> The pain of pericarditis usually responds promptly to aspirin or a non-steroidal anti-inflammatory agent, which should be administered for approximately 5–7 days. Aspirin currently represents the treatment of choice and is given at a dose of 650 mg every 4–6 hours.

Indomethacin also provides effective symptom relief; however, it may cause increased coronary vascular resistance and, in experimental animal models, causes thinning of the infarct zone. Corticosteroids should be avoided whenever possible because of their association with myocardial rupture and recurrent symptoms after discontinuation.

> Anticoagulant therapy, when needed for concomitant thromboembolic disorders (e.g. atrial fibrillation, moral thrombus) must be used cautiously (target activated partial thromboplastin time not to exceed 70 seconds) to minimize the risk of hemorrhagic progression[47] (Table 8.11).

Table 8.11 *Management of early postinfarction pericarditis and Dressler's syndrome*

- Distinguish postinfarction pericarditis from recurrent myocardial ischemia/infarction
- Aspirin, 160–325 mg daily, as high as 650 mg every 4–6 hours if required with decreasing doses as symptoms permit
- Indomethacin, 25–50 mg three times daily, to be used in severe cases
- Morphine sulfate or other oral analgesia for severe pain
- Avoid corticosteroids whenever possible

Post-myocardial infarction syndrome (Dressler's syndrome)

Dressler's syndrome typically occurs between 2 and 12 weeks after the initial event and may follow either ST elevation or non-ST segment elevation MI (although it is rare following the latter). The overall frequency of Dressler's syndrome has diminished substantially over time with the advent of reperfusion therapy.

The clinical features of Dressler's syndrome are fever, pleuritic chest pain, and polyserositis. Pleural and pericardial friction rubs may be appreciated, lasting from several days to weeks. Pericardial and pleural effusions are present in a majority of patients and, although they are typically small, large hemorrhagic effusions have been described. Dressler's syndrome is an immune-mediated phenomenon.

MANAGEMENT STRATEGY

The pharmacologic approach to Dressler's syndrome is similar to that of early postinfarction pericarditis; however, a course of oral corticosteroid therapy is more often needed for complete symptom relief. Nevertheless, treatment should begin with aspirin or non-steroidal anti-inflammatory agents and, if steroids are used, they should be gradually tapered over 1–4 weeks.

Unfortunately, recurrences are common and often require reinstitution of corticosteroids with a more gradual tapering. Drainage procedures may be necessary for large pleural effusions that compromise overall pulmonary performance.

THROMBOEMBOLIC COMPLICATIONS

Thromboembolism is a recognized complication of acute MI, occurring in 5–10 per cent of patients. Both arterial and venous events can occur, with LV mural thrombi accounting for most systemic emboli, and RV or deep vein thrombi serving as a nidus for pulmonary embolism.

Pulmonary embolism

The prevalence of deep vein thrombosis (DVT) among patients with acute MI is reported to be between 18 and 38 per cent.[48] Risk factors in this setting include large infarctions in any location, anterior infarctions, congestive heart failure, and complicated infarctions – each is associated with a systemic inflammatory response, prolonged immobilization, and venous stasis. In addition to traditional risk factors, reduced cardiac output also predisposes to DVT. The diagnosis is particularly challenging in critically ill patients who typically suffer from a variety of active medical problems. Early reports suggested that 10–15 per cent of all patients with DVT experienced a pulmonary embolism and 3–6 per cent had fatal events. More recent estimates are less impressive but still concerning, with rates of 3–5 per cent and 1 per cent respectively.

Early mobilization, as clinical status permits, and prophylactic anticoagulation with LMWH or unfractionated heparin is recommended for all patients experiencing acute MI, particularly those with prior events, medical illnesses concomitant with congestive heart failure (e.g. pneumonia, respiratory failure), or known inherited or acquired thrombophilias. The combined use of pharmacologic and mechanical (e.g. pneumatic compression stockings) should be considered in patients at very high risk for venous thromboembolism.

MANAGEMENT STRATEGIES

Patients with documented venous thromboembolism, in the absence of contraindications, should be treated with systemic anticoagulation, either in the form of unfractionated heparin (activated partial thromboplastin time (aPTT) 60–80 seconds) or LMWH. Those with an absolute contraindication should have an inferior vena caval filter placed. Fibrinolytic therapy with tissue-type plasminogen activator (tPA) is reserved for patients with pulmonary embolism complicated by right heart failure and hypotension.

The benefit derived from thrombolysis among patients with echocardiographic right heart strain (in the absence of hypotension) is under investigation.

Systemic embolism

The prevalence of systemic embolism in patients with MI is of the order of 5 per cent.[49] Emboli to the cerebral, renal, mesenteric, iliofemoral, and/or other arterial beds can occur and typically originate from mural thrombi within the left ventricle.[50] Left atrial appendage thrombi are a potential source of emboli in patients with atrial fibrillation. The predilection of the ventricular apex for thrombus development is due to localized inflammation (from the infarction) and stagnant blood flow. Although depressed LV function and chamber dilation are not absolute prerequisites for thrombus formation, both contribute substantially to the process.[51]

Left ventricular thrombi typically develop with the first three postinfarction days, but can form later (up to 14 days). Systemic embolization occurs, on average, 14 days after infarction and is relatively rare after 6 weeks in the absence of clinical heart failure and LV chamber dilation. The diagnosis is most often made by 2D-echocardiography.

MANAGEMENT STRATEGY

Patients with systemic embolism, particularly those with either a documented cardiac source or high index of suspicion for cardioembolism, should be systemically anticoagulated with unfractionated or LMWH followed by warfarin (target international normalized ratio (INR) 2.5) for 6–12 months. A longer duration of treatment may be indicated for patients with a persistently depressed LV ejection fraction (<30 per cent). Long-term anticoagulation is recommended for patients with chronic atrial fibrillation and those with prior cardioembolism.

ELECTRICAL COMPLICATIONS

Rhythm and conduction disturbances

Abnormalities of cardiac rhythm and conduction are common following MI and can be life-threatening. Prior to hospital arrival, ventricular tachycardia and fibrillation account for a majority of sudden cardiac deaths. Both tachyarrhythmias and bradyarrhythmias are encountered in the hospital phase of acute MI and a majority of patients experience one or more conduction abnormalities (25 per cent) or rhythm disturbances (90 per cent) in the first 24 hours. The etiology of electrical complications is multifactorial and includes myocardial ischemia, necrosis, altered autonomic tone, hypoxia, electrolyte, and acid–base disturbances, and adverse drug effects.

MANAGEMENT STRATEGY

The general goal of therapy in the setting of rhythm and conduction disturbances is to return heart rate and AV synchrony to their normal states (Tables 8.12–8.14).

The use of temporary transvenous pacing in the setting of acute MI is determined by the specific bradyarrhythmia or conduction disturbance, the presence of hemodynamic compromise, and the site of infarction.

Transcutaneous pacing systems are suitable for stable patients judged to be at low to moderate risk for progressive AV block. Transcutaneous modalities are also attractive among patients who have received fibrinolytic therapy within the past 6 hours given their added risk for vascular and hemorrhagic complications.

Recommendations for placement of transcutaneous pacing patches and temporary transvenous pacing wires are detailed in Tables 8.15 and 8.16.

Temporary pacing in the early stages of MI does not automatically translate to a requirement for permanent pacemaker placement. Indications for permanent pacing after acute MI are summarized in Table 8.17.

COMPLICATIONS OF TREATMENT

Hemorrhage

Antithrombotic and fibrinolytic therapy, by design but not by intention, impair both thrombotic potential (a goal of treatment) and hemostatic capacity (an unwanted effect).

Antiplatelet therapy

Bleeding events associated with disorders of primary hemostasis most often involve the skin, joint spaces and mucous membranes; however, the gastrointestinal and genitourinary tracts and central nervous system may occasionally be involved. The severity of bleeding is directly related to the degree of platelet dysfunction, integrity of the vasculature, and status of both the intrinsic and extrinsic coagulation pathways. In general, an isolated platelet defect is rarely the cause of life-threatening hemorrhage.

The template bleeding time has been employed as a general estimate of platelet function; however, it is non-specific and vulnerable to technical errors. Laboratory-based platelet aggregation studies can also be performed if time allows. The evolution of bedside assays and point-of-care platelet aggregometers will provide a readily available means to diagnose platelet abnormalities rapidly, particularly those related to pharmacologic inhibition.

The treatment of bleeding complications is best approached in a targeted, stepwise fashion. The source should be identified, the offending agent discontinued (when feasible), and local measures (manual pressure,

Table 8.12 *Management of ventricular tachycardia/ventricular fibrillation. (American College of Cardiology/American Heart Association guidelines)*

Class I
1. Ventricular fibrillation (VF) should be treated with an unsynchronized electric shock with an initial energy of 200 J; if unsuccessful, a second shock of 200–300 J should be given, and, if necessary, a third shock of 360 J
2. Sustained (more than 30 seconds or causing hemodynamic collapse) polymorphic ventricular tachycardia (VT) should be treated with an unsynchronized electric shock using an initial energy of 200 J; if unsuccessful, a second shock of 200–300 J should be given, and, if necessary, a third shock of 360 J
3. Episodes of sustained monomorphic VT associated with angina, pulmonary edema, or hypotension (blood pressure less than 90 mm Hg) should be treated with a synchronized electric shock of 100 J initial energy. Increasing energies may be used if not initially successful
4. Sustained monomorphic VT not associated with angina, pulmonary edema, or hypotension (blood pressure less than 90 mm Hg) should be treated with one of the following regiments:
   a. Lidocaine: bolus 1.0–1.5 mg/kg. Supplemental boluses of 0.5–0.75 mg/kg every 5–10 minutes to a maximum of 3 mg/kg total loading dose may be given as needed. Loading is followed by infusion of 2–4 mg/minute (30–50 µg/kg per minute)
   b. Procainamide: 20–30 mg/minute loading infusion, up to 12–17 mg/kg. This may be followed by an infusion of 1–4 mg/minute
   c. Amiodarone[a]: 150 mg infused over 10 minutes followed by constant infusion of 1.0 mg/minute for 6 hours and then a maintenance infusion of 0.5 mg/minute
   d. Synchronized electrical cardioversion starting at 50 J (brief anesthesia is necessary)

Class IIa
1. Infusions of antiarrhythmic drugs may be used after an episode of VT/VF but should be discomforted after 6–24 hours and the need for further arrhythmia management assessed
2. Electrolyte and acid-based disturbances should be corrected to prevent recurrent episodes of VF when an initial episode of VF has been treated

Class IIb
1. Drug-refractory polymorphic VT should be managed by aggressive attempts to reduce myocardial ischemia therapies such as β-adrenoceptor blockade, intra-aortic balloon pumping, and emergency PCI/CABG surgery. Amiodarone[a], 150 mg infused over 10 minutes followed by a constant infusion of 1.0 mg/minute for up to 6 hours and then maintenance infusion of 0.5 mg/minute may also be helpful

Class III
1. Treatment of isolated ventricular premature beats, couplets, runs of accelerated idioventricular rhythm, and non-sustained VT
2. Prophylactic administration of antiarrhythmic therapy when using fibrinolytic agents

[a]Amiodarone 300 mg iv push either alone or preceded by vasopressor 40 mg iv may be preferred strategy.
CABG = coronary artery bypass grafting; PCI = percutaneous coronary intervention; VF = ventricular fibrillation; VT = ventricular tachyacardia.

Table 8.13 *Management of atrial fibrillation. (American College of Cardiology/American Heart Association guidelines)*

Class I
1. Electrical cardioversion for patients with severe hemodynamic compromise or intractable ischemia
2. Rapid digitalization to slow a rapid ventricular response and improve left ventricular (LV) function
3. Intravenous β-adrenoceptor blockers to slow rapid ventricular response in patients without clinical LV dysfunction, bronchospastic disease, or atrioventricular block
4. Heparin should be given

Class IIa
1. Either diltiazem or verapamil intravenously to slow a rapid ventricular response if β-adrenoceptor blocking agents are contraindicated or ineffective

Table 8.14 *Management of bradyarrhythmias and heart block. (American College of Cardiology/American Heart Association guidelines)*

Atropine

Class I
1. Symptomatic sinus bradycardia (generally, heart rate less than 50 beats/minute associated with hypotension, ischemia, or escape ventricular arrhythmia)
2. Ventricular asystole
3. Symptomatic atrioventricular (AV) block occurring at the AV nodal level (second-degree type I or third-degree with a narrow-complex escape rhythm)

Class IIa
None

Class III
1. AV block occurring at an infranodal level (usually associated with anterior myocardial infarction with a wide-complex escape rhythm)
2. Asymptomatic sinus bradycardia

Table 8.15 *Indications for temporary pacing. (American College of Cardiology/American Heart Association guidelines)*

Placement of transcutaneous patches and active (demand) transcutaneous pacing

Class I
1. Sinus bradycardia (rate less than 50 beats/minute) with symptoms of hypotension (systolic blood pressure less than 80 mm Hg) unresponsive to drug therapy
2. Mobitz type II second-degree atrioventricular (AV) block
3. Third-degree heart block
4. Bilateral BBB (alternating BBB, or right BBB (RBBB) and alternating left anterior fascicular block (LAFB), left posterior fascicular block (LPFB), irrespective of time onset
5. Newly acquired or age-indeterminate LBBB, LBBB and LAFB, RBBB, and LPFB
6. RBBB or LBBB and first-degree AV block

Class IIa
1. Stable bradycardia (systolic blood pressure greater than 90 mm Hg, no hemodynamic compromise, or compromise responsive to intial drug therapy)

Class IIb
1. Newly acquired or age-determinate first-degree AV block

Class III
1. Uncomplicated myocardial infarction without evidence of conduction disease

BBB = bundle branch block.

suturing) explored first. Thereafter, treatment is dictated by the severity of the event. Platelet transfusions either with or without desamino-8-D-arginine vasopressin (DDAVP) should be given for serious or life-threatening hemorrhage.

Profound thrombocytopenia (platelet counts <2000 per mm) has been observed with the GPIIb/IIIa receptor antagonists. The largest experience is with abciximab. Most patients have responded to discontinuation of the medication and platelet transfusions. Intravenous immunoglobulin and corticosteroid therapy has not impacted the natural history of the acute disorder; however, delayed thrombocytopenia ($\geq$2 weeks after exposure) has been described (after abciximab administration) and may be immune mediated. Accordingly, immunosuppressive therapy and platelet transfusion should be considered. Fibrinogen supplementation with cryoprecipitate or fresh-frozen plasma represents an important first-line treatment when major hemorrhage occurs during administration of the small molecule, competitive inhibitors tirofiban and eptifibatide.

Heparin compounds

Mild to moderate bleeding should initially prompt a reduction in the unfractionated heparin dose (particularly if the aPTT is excessively prolonged) or an interruption of the infusion for a brief period of time (30–60

Table 8.16 *Indications for temporary transvenous pacing. (American College of Cardiology/American Heart Association guidelines)*

Class I
1. Asystole
2. Symptomatic bradycardia (includes sinus bradycardia with hypotension and type I second-degree atrioventricular (AV) block with hypotension not responsive to atropine)
3. Bilateral BBB (alternating BBB or RBBB with alternating LAFB/LPFB) (any age)
4. New or indeterminate-age bifascicular block (RBBB with LAFB or LPFB) with first-degree AV block
5. Mobitz type II second-degree AV block

Class IIa
1. RBBB and LAFB or LPFB (new or indeterminate)
2. RBBB with first-degree AV block
3. LBBB, new or indeterminate
4. Incessant VT, for atrial or ventricular overdriving pacing
5. Recurrent sinus pauses (greater than 3 seconds) not responsive to atropine

Class IIb
1. Bifascicular block of indeterminate age
2. New or age-indeterminate isolated RBBB

Class III
1. First-degree heart block
2. Type I second-degree AV block with normal hemodynamics
3. Accelerated idioventricular rhythm
4. BBB or fascicular block known to exist before acute myocardial infarction

BBB = bundle branch block; LAFB = left anterior fascicular block; LPFB = left posterior fascicular block; RBBB = right bundle branch block.

Table 8.17 *Indications for permanent pacing after myocardial infarction. (American College of Cardiology/American Heart Association guidelines)*

Class I
1. Persistent second-degree atrioventricular (AV) block in the His-Purkinje system with bilateral bundle branch block (BBB) or complete heart block after acute myocardial infarction
2. Transient advanced (second- or third-degree) AV block and associated BBB
3. Symptomatic AV block at any level

Class IIb
1. Persistent advanced (second- or third-degree) block at the AV node level

Class III
1. Transient AV conduction disturbances in the absence of intraventricular conduction defects
2. Transient AV block in the presence of AV block
3. Acquired left anterior fascicular block in the absence of AV block
4. Persistent first-degree AV block in the presence of BBB that is old or age indeterminate

Table 8.18 *Suggested dose of protamine to neutralize anticoagulant effects of enoxaparin[a]*

	Last dose of enoxaparin (1.0 mg/kg)		
	≤8 hours	>8 hours and ≤12 hours	>12 hours
Protamine dose[b]	1 mg protamine per 1 mg enoxaparin	0.5 mg protamine per 1 mg enoxaparin	May not be required

[a]The potentional risk of rapid neutralization must be weighed against the perceived benefit.
[b]Protamine neutralizes the anti-IIa effects of enoxaparin (and other low-molecular-weight heparins). Fresh-frozen plasma may be required in patients with life-threatening hemorrhage.

minutes). More severe hemorrhage may require complete discontinuation or, with life-threatening hemorrhage, neutralization with protamine sulfate (1 mg/100 U heparin administered in the preceding 4 hours). However, in patients with active coronary heart disease, a careful risk–benefit assessment must be undertaken, considering the risks of coronary thrombosis versus those of bleeding. It may be in the patient's best interest to continue systemic anticoagulation, particularly if the bleeding is not serious or life-threatening and can be controlled adequately with local measures (e.g. manual pressure over a site of vascular trauma).

Protamine sulfate (1 mg/100 anti-Xa units) can also be administered to neutralize the anticoagulant effects of low molecular weight heparin. It is important to be aware that the neutralization is incomplete (approximately 60 per cent). Fresh-frozen plasma should be administered in the setting of life-threatening bleeding to correct any residual hemostatic impairment (Table 8.18).

The neutralization of heparinoids (danaparoid sodium) is even more challenging given their long circulating half-life and poor response to protamine. As with LMWH preparations, fresh-frozen plasma should be administered for serious or life-threatening bleeding complications. Plasmapheresis has been used successfully to remove the circulating anticoagulant in several patients following bypass surgery complicated by uncontrolled hemorrhage.

Hirudin and other direct thrombin antagonists

There are no known antidotes for hirudin and other direct thrombin antagonists, creating potentially serious challenges when bleeding occurs. Beyond immediate discontinuation of the drug, fresh-frozen plasma should be considered as a source of clotting factors. Plasmapheresis should be considered for life-threatening hemorrhage.

Warfarin

The anticoagulant effect of warfarin can be reduced or entirely reversed by lowering the dose, discontinuing treatment, administering vitamin K, or replacing the defective coagulation factors with fresh-frozen plasma or prothrombin concentrate. The severity of bleeding and inherent risks of reduced anticoagulation should dictate the course of action (Table 8.19).

Table 8.19 *Management of prolonged international normalized ratio (INR) associated with warfarin therapy[a]*

	<6.0	6.0–10.0	>10.0	>20.0
Clinical profile[a]	No bleeding	No bleeding	No bleeding	No bleeding
Recommended approach	Omit next 1–2 doses of warfarin	Vitamin K 1–2 mg sc ↓ Repeat INR in 8 hours ↓ Consider additional vitamin K	Vitamin K 3 mg sc ↓ Repeat INR in 6 hours ↓ Consider additional vitamin K	Vitamin K 5–10 mg sc ↓ Repeat INR in 6 hours ↓ Consider additional vitamin K

[a]For rapid reversal of anticoagulant effect because of life-threatening hemorrhage, fresh-frozen plasma or prothrombin concentrates should be administered. Concomitant administration of vitamin K (3–5 mg intravenously) should also be considered.
sc = subcutaneously.

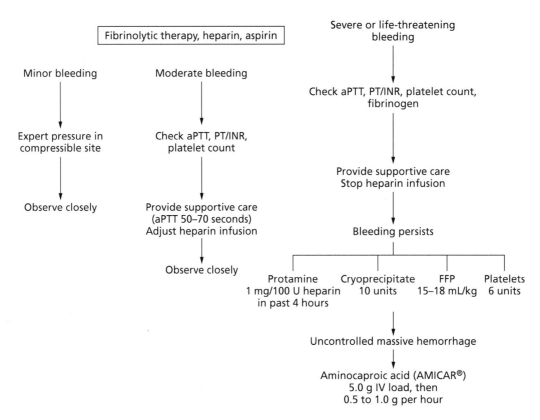

Figure 8.9 *A recommended approach to the management of patients with hemorrhagic complications following fibrinolytic (and adjunctive antithrombotic) therapy. aPTT = activated partial thromboplastin time; FFP = fresh frozen plasma; IV = intravenous; PT/INR = prothrombin time/international normalized ratio.*

Fibrinolytic therapy

Even with careful patient selection and close monitoring, hemorrhage events do occur. Routine management includes volume and blood pressure support as well as a prompt and thorough search for the site of bleeding. Abdominopelvic or head computed tomography scans may be useful in the diagnosis and management of major hemorrhagic events. Life-threatening hemorrhage warrants prompt intervention. Heparin should be discontinued and neutralized with protamine sulfate. Fresh-frozen plasma is an excellent source of Factors V and VIII, α_2-antiplasmin, and plasminogen activator inhibitor. Cryoprecipitate (8–10 U) is the preferred source of fibrinogen (200–250 mg/10–15 mL) and Factor VIII (80 U/10–15 mL). If the platelet count is low (<80 000 per mm³), platelets (6 units random donor) should be given. If indicated, DDAVP (0.3 µg/kg intravenously over 20 minutes) can be used to correct qualitative platelet abnormalities. Persistent and potentially life-threatening hemorrhage unresponsive to standard measures (outlined previously) may require antifibrinolytic therapy. This intervention should be used with

caution because serious thrombotic complications can be precipitated. α-Aminocaproic acid (AMICAR) and tranexamic acid are the most frequently used agents (Fig. 8.9).

SUMMARY

- Myocardial infarction can be complicated in the early or acute phase by vascular (ischemic), myocardial/mechanical, pericardial and electrical events.
- High-risk patients include the following: those with advanced age, prior infarction, anterior site of injury, reduced left ventricular performance, Killip class ≥2, diabetes, and women.
- The management of complicated myocardial infarction is best approached using rapid assessment tools and guidelines developed by the American Heart Association/American College of Cardiology.

REFERENCES

1. Braunwald E. *Heart disease: a textbook of cardiovascular medicine*, Vol. 2. Philadelphia: WB Saunders, 1984: 1262–300.

2. Buja LM, Willerson JT. Clinicopathological correlates of acute ischemic heart disease syndromes. *Am J Cardiol* 1981; **47**: 343–56.

○3. Fishbein MC, Maclean D, Maroko PR. The histopathological evolution of myocardial infarction. *Chest* 1978; **73**: 843–9.

4. Henson DE, Najafi H, Callaghan R, Coogan P, Julian OC, Eisenstein R. Myocardial lesions following open heart surgery. *Arch Pathol* 1969; **88**: 423–30.

5. Tyagi SC, Ratajska A, Weber KT. Myocardial matrix metalloproteinase(s): localization and activation. *Mol Cell Biochem* 1993; **126**: 49–59.

6. Cleutjens JPM, Kandala JC, Guarda E, Guntaka RV, Weber KT. Regulation of collagen degradation in the rat myocardium after infarction. *J Mol Cell Cardiol* 1995; **27**: 1281–92.

7. McCormick RJ, Musch TI, Bergman BC, Thomas DP. Regional differences in LV collagen accumulation and mature cross-linking after myocardial infarction in rats. *Am J Physiol* 1994; **266**: H354–H359.

8. Finesmith TH, Broadley KN, Davidson JM. Fibroblasts from wounds of different stages of repair vary in their ability to contract a collagen gel in response to growth factors. *J Cell Physiol* 1990; **144**: 97–107.

♦9. Mueller HS, Cohen LS, Braunwald E, *et al.*, for the TIMI Investigators. Predictors of early morbidity and mortality after thrombolytic therapy of acute myocardial infarction. Analyses of patient subgroups in the Thrombolysis in Myocardial Infarction (TIMI) Trial, Phase II. *Circulation* 1992; **85**: 1254–64.

♦10. Lee KL, Woodlief LH, Topol EJ, *et al.*, for the GUSTO-1 Investigators. Predictors of 30-day mortality in the era of reperfusion for acute myocardial infarction. Results from an International trial of 41 021 patients. *Circulation* 1995; **91**: 1659–68.

11. Becker RC, Burns M, Gore JM, for the NRMI-2 Investigators. Early assessment and in-hospital management of patients with acute myocardial infarction at increased risk for adverse outcomes: a nationwide perspective of current clinical practice. *Am Heart J* 1998; **135**: 786–96.

12. Hathaway WR, Peterson ED, Wagner GS, for the GUSTO-1 Investigators. Prognostic significance of the initial electrocardiography in patients with acute myocardial infarction. *JAMA* 1998; **279**: 387–91.

♦13. Ohman EM, Armstrong PW, Christenson RH, for the GUSTO IIA Investigators. Cardiac Troponin T levels for risk stratification in acute myocardial ischemia. *N Engl J Med* 1996; **335**: 1333–41.

14. Morrow DA, Rifan N, Antman EM, *et al.* Serum amyloid A protein predicts early mortality in acute coronary syndromes: a TIMI 11A substudy. *J Am Coll Cardiol* 2000; **35**: 358–62.

♦15. Gore JM, Granger CB, Simoons ML, *et al.*, for the GUSTO-1 Investigators. Stroke after thrombolysis. Mortality and functional outcomes in the GUSTO-1 trial. *Circulation* 1995; **92**: 2811–18.

16. Becker RC, Burns M, Every N, *et al.*, for the National Registry of Myocardial Infarction (NRMI-2) participants. Early clinical outcomes and routine management of patients with non-ST segment elevation myocardial infarction: a nationwide perspective. *Arch Intern Med* 2001; in press.

17. TIMI Study Group: Comparison of invasive and conservative strategies after treatment with intravenous tissue plasminogen activator in acute myocardial infarction. Results of the Thrombolysis in Myocardial Infarction (TIMI) Phase II Trial. *N Engl J Med* 1989; **320**: 618.

18. Bosch X, Theroux P, Waters DD, Pelletier GB, Roy D. Early postinfarction ischemia: clinical, angiographic, and prognostic significance. *Circulation* 1987; **5**: 988–95.

19. Gibson RS, Boden WE, Theroux P, *et al.* Diltiazem and reinfarction in patients with non-Q-wave myocardial infarction. Results of a double-blind, randomized, multicenter trial. *N Engl J Med* 1986; **315**: 423–9.

20. Schaer DH, Ross AM, Wasserman AG. Reinfarction, recurrent angina and reocclusion after thrombolytic therapy. *Circulation* 1987; **76**: II–57.

21. ISIS-2 (Second International Study of Infarct Survival) Collaborative Group. Randomized trial of intravenous streptokinase, oral aspirin, both, or neither among 17,187 cases of suspected acute myocardial infarction: ISIS-2. *Lancet* 1988; **2**: 349.

22. Gruppo Italiano per lo Studio della Streptochinasi nell'Infarto Miocardico (GISSI). Effectiveness of intravenous thrombolytic treatment in acute myocardial infarction. *Lancet* 1986; **1**: 397.

♦23. Granger CB, Miller JM, Bovill EG, *et al.* Rebound increase in thrombin generation and activity after cessation of intravenous heparin in patients with acute coronary syndromes. *Circulation* 1995; **91**: 1929–35.

24. Antman EM, for the TIMI 14 investigators. Abciximab facilitates the rate and extent of thrombolysis: results of the TIMI 14 Trial. *Circulation* 1999; **99**: 2720–32.

25. Ross A. Randomized comparison of low molecular weight heparin and unfractionated heparin adjunctive to tPA thrombolysis and aspirin (HART II). *Circulation* 2000; **102**(suppl II): II-600.

26. TIMI Study Group. Comparison of invasive and conservative strategies after treatment with intravenous tissue plasminogen activator in acute myocardial infarction: results of Thrombolysis in Myocardial Infarction (TIMI) Phase 2 Trial. *N Engl J Med* 1989; **320**: 618–27.

27. Zehender M, Kasper W, Kauder E, *et al*. Right ventricular infarction as an independent predictor of prognosis after acute inferior myocardial infarction. *N Engl J Med* 1993; **328**: 981–8.

28. Manno BV, Bemis CE, Carver J, Mintz GS. Right ventricular infarction complicated by right to left shunt. *J Am Coll Cardiol* 1983; **1**: 554–7.

29. Love JC, Haffajee CI, Gore JM, Alpert JS. Reversibility of hypotension and shock by atrial or atrioventricular sequential pacing in patients with right ventricular infarction. *Am Heart J* 1984; **108**: 5–13.

♦30. Braunwald E, Kloner RA. The stunned myocardium: prolonged postischemic ventricular dysfunction. *Circulation* 1982; **66**: 1146.

31. Scott BD, Kerber RE. Clinical and experimental aspects of myocardial stunning. *Prog Cardiovasc Dis* 1992; **35**: 61.

32. Goldberg RJ, Gore JM, Alpert JS, *et al*. Cardiogenic shock resulting from acute myocardial infarction: A fourteen year community-wide perspective. *N Engl J Med* 1991; **325**: 1117–22.

○33. Alonso DR, Scheidt S, Post M, Killip T. Pathophysiology of cardiogenic shock: quantification of myocardial necrosis, clinical, pathologic and electrocardiographic correlations. *Circulation* 1973; **48**: 588–96.

♦34. Hochman JS, Sleeper LA, Webb JG, *et al*. Early revascularization in acute myocardial infarction complicated by cardiogenic shock. *N Engl J Med* 1999; **341**; 625–34.

35. Skillington PD, Davies RH. Luf AJ, *et al*. Surgical treatment for infarct-related ventricular septal defects: improved early results combined with analysis of late functional status. *J Thorac Cardiovasc Surg* 1990; **99**: 798–808.

36. Becker RC, Charlesworth A, Wilcox RG, Hampton J, Skene A, Gore JM, Topol EJ. Cardiac rupture associated with thrombolytic therapy: impact of time to treatment in the Late Assessment of Thrombolytic Efficacy (LATE) Study. *J Am Coll Cardiol* 1995; **25**: 1063–8.

37. Becker RC, Gore JM, Lambrew C, *et al*. A composite view of cardiac rupture in the United States: National Registry of Myocardial Infarction. *J Am Coll Cardiol* 1996; **27**: 1321–6.

38. Becker RC, Hochman JS, Cannon CP, *et al.*, and the TIMI 9 Investigators. Fatal cardiac rupture among patients treated with thrombolytic agents and adjunctive thrombin antagonists. *J Am Coll Cardiol* 1999; **33**: 479–87.

39. Tcheng JE, Jackman JD Jr, Nelson CL, *et al*. Outcome of patients sustaining acute ischemic mitral regurgitation during myocardial infarction. *Ann Intern Med* 1992; **117**: 18–24.

40. Hendren WG, Nemec JJ, Lytle BW, *et al*. Mitral valve repair for ischemic mitral insufficiency. *Ann Thorac Surg* 1991; **52**: 1246–51.

41. Hutchins GM, Bulkley BH. Infarct expansion versus extension: two different complications of acute myocardial infarction. *Am J Cardiol* 1978; **41**: 1127.

42. Pfeffer MA, Braunwald E, Moye LA, *et al*. Effect of captopril on mortality and morbidity in patients with left ventricular dysfunction after myocardial infarction. *N Engl J Med* 1992; **327**: 669.

43. The Acute Infarction Ramipril Efficacy (AIRE) Study Investigators. Effect of ramipril on mortality and morbidity of survivors of acute myocardial infarction with clinical evidence of heart failure. *Lancet* 1993; **342**: 821.

44. Martin RH, Almond CH, Saab S, Watson LE. True and false aneurysms of the left ventricle following myocardial infarction. *Am J Med* 1977; **62**: 418–24.

45. Krainin FM, Flessas AP, Spodick DH. Infarction-associated pericarditis: rarity of diagnostic electrocardiogram. *N Engl J Med* 1984; **311**: 1211–14.

46. Guillevin L, Valere PE. Pericarditis in acute myocardial infarction. *Lancet* 1976; **1**: 429.

47. Guberman BA, Fowler NO, Engel PJ, *et al*. Cardiac tamponade in medical patients. *Circulation* 1981; **64**: 633.

48. Miller RR, Lies JE, Carretta RF, *et al*. Prevention of lower extremity venous thrombus by early mobilization. *Ann Intern Med* 1976; **84**: 700–3.

49. Gueret P, Bubourg O, Ferrier A, *et al*. Effects of full-dose heparin anticoagulation on the development of left ventricular thrombosis in acute myocardial infarction. *J Am Coll Cardiol* 1986; **8**: 419.

50. Weinreich DJ, Burke JF, Pauletto FJ. Left ventricular mural thrombi complicating acute myocardial infarction: Long-term follow-up with serial echocardiography. *Ann Intern Med* 1984; **100**: 789.

51. Keating EC, Gross SA, Schlamowitz RA, *et al*. Mural thrombi in myocardial infarctions: prospective evaluation by two dimensional echocardiography. *Am J Med* 1983; **74**: 989–95.

9

Initial evaluation and management of non-penetrating cardiac trauma

STEPHEN J VOYCE

Although most often associated with serious motor vehicle accidents and chest injury, cardiac trauma may follow seemingly minor events accompanied by acceleration and deceleration of the heart and great vessels. The early manifestations range from superficial myocardial contusion without clinical sequelae to free wall rupture and sudden cardiac death. A high index of suspicion is an important initial step with close monitoring for arrhythmias and change in the hemodynamic status. Prompt surgical intervention is required for patients with cardiac tamponade and/or valvular disruption.

INTRODUCTION

Motor vehicle accidents (MVA) account for upward of 2 000 000 injuries and 55 000 fatalities annually in the USA alone. The incidence of associated cardiac trauma varies from 16 per cent in autopsy series to 76 per cent in clinical series.[1] It must be appreciated, however, that non-penetrating cardiac injuries are the most common unsuspected visceral injury likely to cause death among patients with MVA.[2-4]

PATHOBIOLOGY

The mechanisms most often cited in non-penetrating (blunt) cardiac trauma include rapid deceleration or acceleration, direct trauma, an abrupt rise in intrathoracic or intra-abdominal pressure, and compression of the heart between the sternum and thoracic spine.[5] Non-penetrating cardiac injury occurs most commonly when the driver of a high-speed motor vehicle impacts the steering wheel; however, cardiac trauma has also been described in cases of rapid deceleration from velocities of less than 20 miles/hour. The use of safety belts and low-pressure inflatable air bags reduces the likelihood of non-penetrating cardiac injury in adults.

The spectrum of non-penetrating cardiac injury ranges from mild myocardial contusion to overt myocardial necrosis and fatal rupture. Damage to the cardiac valves and supporting structures, papillary muscle, chordae tendineae, coronary arteries, and pericardium may also occur. A list of potential cardiac injuries is provided in Table 9.1.

Myocardial contusion, by definition, represents an area of identifiable histopathologic changes (myocyte death). The area of contusion resembles a myocardial infarction, although the zone of injury is more sharply defined in the former and is not confined to a specific coronary artery distribution. Subepicardial, subendocardial, or intramyocardial hemorrhage can also be seen along with myocardial cell necrosis and leukocyte infiltration (Figs 9.1 and 9.2 a and b). The overall clinical significance of cardiac injury is determined by the development of associated complications that can include supraventricular and ventricular tachyarrhythmias, valvular dysfunction, or disruption myocardial (free wall, ventricular septal) rupture thromboembolic events, congestive heart failure, ventricular aneurysm formation, and pericarditis (acute, constrictive).[6]

Table 9.1 *The full spectrum of cardiac pathology associated with non-penetrating trauma*

Myocardial injury
Wall motion abnormalities
Aneurysm formation
Free wall rupture
Ventricular septal rupture
Myocardial laceration

Rhythm or conduction disturbances
Atrial tachyarrhythmias
Ventricular tachyarrhythmias
First-, second- or third-degree atrioventricular (AV) block

Valvular injury
Cusp or leaflet tear (mitral, aortic, tricuspid, or pulmonic insufficiency)
Papillary muscle injury (torential mitral insufficiency)

Coronary artery injury
Laceration
Thrombosis
Fistula (A-V or to heart chamber)

Pericardial injury
Rupture or laceration
Hemopericardium (with or without tamponade)
Acute pericarditis
Constrictive pericarditis

AV = arteriovenous.

EARLY DIAGNOSIS

Clinical features

Cardiac injury should be suspected in all patients who have sustained non-penetrating chest trauma, regardless

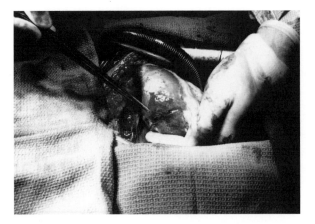

Figure 9.1 *Intraoperative photograph of non-penetrating myocardial injury demonstrating epicardial hemorrhage and laceration (tip of forceps) involving the apex of the left ventricle.*

of the initially perceived severity. In general, myocardial injury is most frequently associated with severe thoracic trauma, but has been reported in the absence of clinically evident external chest injury.[7,8] Snow and colleagues,[9] reported that 73 per cent of patients with necropsy confirmed myocardial damage had externally evident chest trauma; of these, 60 per cent had additional thoracic injuries detected by either physical examination or chest radiography. Although non-penetrating myocardial injury is most commonly the result of a direct blow to the chest from a steering wheel, falls and a variety of sports-related injuries[10] have also been associated with its occurrence. The right ventricle is the chamber most commonly injured because of its vulnerable retrosternal position. In a large autopsy series, Parmley[11] defined the frequency and sites of cardiac injury associated with nonpenetrating chest trauma (Table 9.2).

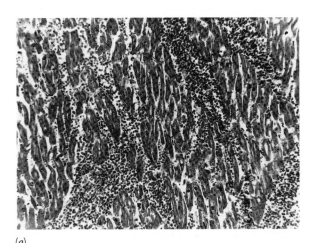

(a)

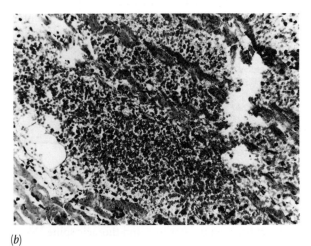

(b)

Figure 9.2 *Photomicrograph of a myocardial contusion (hematoxylin–eosin, ×176.5) demonstrating: (a) a large number of cells crowding the myocardial fibers; and (b) edema, fragmentation and lysis of myocardial fibers. Leukocyte infiltration is also present. (Reproduced with permission from Symbas PN. Traumatic injury of the heart and great vessels, Springfield, IL, Charles C. Thomas Publisher, 1972.)*

Table 9.2 *Cardiac complications reported in a series of 546 autopsy cases following non-penetrating cardiac trauma. (Reproduced with permission of the American Heart Association, Inc. from Parmley CF et al. Non-penetrating traumatic injury of the heart. Circulation 1958; **18**: 371)*

Type and/or site of injury	Number of cases (cardiac only)	Cases (including patients with thoracic aorta rupture)	Total cases
Rupture (cardiac)	273	80	353
Right ventricle	56	10	66
Left ventricle	46	13	59
Right atrium	35	6	41
Left atrium	24	2	26
IV septum	25(20[a])	5(4[a])	30
IA septum	18(10[a])	7(3[a])	25
Multiple chamber ruptures	69	37	106
Myocardial contusion/laceration	105	24	129
Pericardial laceration	18	18	36
Hemopericardium	13	12	25
Valvular laceration/rupture	1(2[b])	0(4[b])	1
Aortic	1(1[b])	0(2[b])	1
Pulmonary	0(4[b])	0	0
Tricuspid	0(8[b])	0	0
Mitral	0(8[b])	0(1[b])	0
Mitral and tricuspid	0(1[b])	0(1[b])	0
Coronary artery laceration rupture	0(7[b])	1(2[b])	1
Papillary muscle rupture laceration/rupture	1(23[b])	0	1
Total	**411**	**135**	**546**

[a] Associated with other sites of cardiac rupture.
[b] Combined with cardiac rupture or other injury.
IV = interventricular; IA = interatrial.

Patients with non-penetrating cardiac trauma complicated by myocardial rupture typically experience rapid hemodynamic decompensation and present to the hospital in extremis (shock). Cardiac rupture is caused either by (1) direct chamber rupture during a vulnerable time in the cardiac cycle, or (2) rapid deceleration of the heart, which rotates anteriorly away from the fixed great vessels.[12] Patients with myocardial rupture also have an incidence of concomitant aortic rupture approaching 20 per cent.[11] Patients with myocardial rupture, if they are to survive, require prompt diagnosis and emergent surgery.

In less severe cases of non-penetrating chest trauma, the decision for hospital admission should be based on the history of injury, associated non-cardiac injuries, and, perhaps most importantly, a high index of clinical suspicion. There are no classic signs or symptoms supporting a diagnosis of myocardial injury, although some patients may complain of an angina-like chest pain (which typically, is not responsive to nitroglycerin). The cardiovascular examination can be entirely normal or, in contrast, reveal evidence of acute valvular dysfunction (mitral insufficiency, aortic insufficiency), congestive heart failure or cardiac tamponade.[13,14]

DIAGNOSTIC EVALUATION

A topic of controversy concerning non-penetrating trauma is the diagnosis of cardiac contusion. The diagnostic tests used most often include surface electrocardiography, serum cardiac enzyme and isoenzyme markers, two-dimensional transthoracic echocardiography (TTE), radionuclide ventriculography (RVG), and radionuclide scanning. Recent additions to the diagnostic armamentarium for cardiac contusion include multiplane transesophageal echocardiography (TEE) and serum levels of cardiac specific troponins (Table 9.3).

Surface electrocardiogram

The electrocardiogram (ECG) is the most widely used non-invasive test for diagnosing myocardial injury. It is readily available and should be obtained in all patients with suspected non-penetrating cardiac injury. In a review of the available literature, Berk[15] reported that 63 per cent of patients with non-penetrating chest trauma exhibited abnormal ECGs, ST and T wave changes were

Table 9.3 *Diagnostic testing in non-penetrating cardiac trauma*

Non-imaging techniques
Electrocardiography (surface 12-lead)
Cardiac isoenzymes
Cardiac troponins

Non-invasive imaging techniques
Chest roentgenography
Radionuclide ventriculography
Technetium pyrophosphate scanning
Antimyosin scanning
2-D transthoracic echocardiography[a]
Transesophageal echocardiography[a]

Invasive techniques
Pulmonary artery catheterization
Cardiac catheterization
Contrast ventriculography

[a]Including Doppler and color-flow imaging.
2-D = two-dimensional.

the most common abnormalities cited. A summary of ECG findings associated with non-penetrating cardiac trauma appears in Table 9.4.

The most common rhythm disturbance following cardiac trauma is sinus tachycardia; however, associated volume depletion from hemorrhage, pain, anxiety, and heightened sympathetic tone make this finding nonspecific. Premature ventricular and atrial contractions are common, as are transient conduction abnormalities. It must be emphasized, however, that the surface ECG is neither a sensitive nor a specific marker of myocardial injury. The sensitivity is limited by left ventricular predominance in determining surface electrical events, frequently masking abnormalities of the more commonly injured right ventricle. The ECG may also be interpreted incorrectly as abnormal in the presence of pre-existing heart disease or when hypoxemia, concomitant pulmonary contusion, electrolyte abnormalities, and acid-based imbalances coexist.

Creatine phosphokinase

Serial measurement of creatine phosphokinase (CK) and its cardiac isoenzyme (CK-MB) have been extrapolated from acute myocardial infarction for diagnostic use in traumatic injury. Serum CK-MB levels typically peak within 24 hours after myocardial cell damage and return to baseline by 72 hours.

The sensitivity and specificity of serial CK-MB measurements in diagnosing traumatic myocardial injury has been studied extensively. Fabian and co-workers[16] found that CK-MB measurements improved the overall sensitivity in detecting myocardial contusion compared with the admission ECG alone. Similarly, Frazee and colleagues[17] reported that an elevated serum CK-MB level (particularly in association with an abnormal two-dimensional transthoracic echocardiogram) yielded important prognostic information. A total serum CK-MB level exceeding two times the upper limit of normal was associated with 100 per cent sensitivity for the development of cardiac complications while a value of less than 200 IU/L had a negative predictive value of 100 per cent.[6]

Despite early support, the routine use of serum CK-MB determinations remains somewhat controversial.[18] Several groups have demonstrated abnormal cardiac wall motion by two-dimensional echocardiography and radionuclide ventriculography in the absence of an elevation of serum CK-MB levels.[19,20] In addition, Ingwall and colleagues[21] demonstrated, by endomyocardial biopsy, negligible CK-MB activity in the muscle of normal ventricles (i.e. patients without coronary artery disease or pressure overload hypertrophy). Therefore, one could conclude that many young, previously healthy patients with non-penetrating myocardial injury may not experience an elevation of CK-MB.

Serum CK-MB levels may be falsely elevated in certain conditions that are unrelated to myocardial damage. For example, non-cardiac crush injuries with total CK values greater than 20 000 IU/L may cause an elevation in the CK-MB fraction. In addition, muscular dystrophies, gas gangrene, Reye's syndrome, Rocky Mountain spotted fever, and tongue trauma are other causes of non-cardiac-related elevations of CK-MB.[21,22] Despite these potential shortcomings, most clinicians obtain serial CK-MB measurements in patients with non-penetrating cardiac trauma. Serum levels should be determined at admission and every 6–8 hours thereafter until levels return to baseline.

Troponins

The troponins (I,C,T) are distinct proteins expressed in cardiac and skeletal muscle.[23] Monoclonal antibodies

Table 9.4 *Electrocardiographic findings in 240 patients with non-penetrating cardiac trauma. (Reproduced with permission from Berk WA. Electrocardiographic findings in non-penetrating chest trauma: a review.* J Emerg Med *1987; 5: 209)*

Total abnormal	63%
ST or T-wave abnormalities	35%
Bundle branch block (total)	10%
RBBB	9%
LBBB	1%
Conduction abnormalities (AV block)	3%
Atrial fibrillation	4%
Myocardial infarction pattern	2%
Sinus bradycardia	2%
Ventricular tachycardia	1%

RBBB = right bundle branch block; LBBB = left bundle branch block; AV = atrioventricular.

techniques to cardiac troponin I (TnI) and T (TnT) have been developed with minimal or no cross-reactivity with skeletal muscle forms.[24,25] The specificity of TnI for cardiac muscle offers a distinct advantage over CK-MB measurement in patients with major skeletal muscle trauma in whom myocardial injury may coexist.

Radionuclide scanning

Radionuclide scanning with technetium-99m pyrophosphate was applied initially to diagnose acute myocardial infarction;[26] however, over the years, it has also been used in the evaluation of traumatic myocardial injury. Although the results of animal studies were promising, subsequent clinical investigations have been disappointing.[19] The overall poor sensitivity of technetium-99m pyrophosphate scanning in post-traumatic myocardial dysfunction may be explained by the following:

1 transmural myocardial injury, an uncommon occurrence in non-penetrating trauma, is more likely to cause a positive scan since a large tissue mass is needed to bind a detectable quantity of tracer; and
2 it is technically difficult to separate the thin-walled right ventricle from the overlying sternum and ribs which also accumulate technetium-99m.[19,26]

Considering these limitations, technetium-99m pyrophosphate scanning cannot be recommended routinely in the diagnostic evaluation of patients with non-penetrating myocardial injury.

Radionuclide ventriculography

Although RVG is somewhat less sensitive for right ventricular as compared with left ventricular abnormalities,[6] it has shown some promise in the clinical evaluation of patients with cardiac trauma. Harley and associates[27] studied 74 patients with blunt chest trauma and detected a 74 per cent incidence of left ventricular wall motion abnormalities, concluding that RVG was a more sensitive diagnostic tool than either surface electrocardiography or serum CK-MB determinations for traumatic myocardial injury. Unfortunately, most medical centers do not offer RVG as a bedside diagnostic test.

Antimyosin scanning

The radionuclide labeled FAB fragment of murine antibody to myosin, antimyosin, has been used to detect, localize, and quantify myocardial necrosis in experimental and clinical myocardial infarction,[28] myocarditis,[29] and cardiac allograft rejection.[29a] When myocyte necrosis occurs, plasma membrane integrity is lost and, as a result, antimyosin is able to diffuse into the cellular compartment where it binds to myosin. Radionuclide labeling of antimyosin with indium-111 or technetium-99m allows gamma camera imaging of damaged regions.

Since myocardial cell damage can occur after non-penetrating cardiac trauma, the use of antimyosin scanning to localize areas of injury is possible. At the UMass-Memorial Medical Center, 17 patients with suspected myocardial injury following non-penetrating chest trauma underwent indium-111 antimyosin scanning, two-dimensional echocardiography, serial ECG analysis, and serum CK-MB determinations. Antimyosin scanning demonstrated focal uptake in only one patient (Fig. 9.3); of interest and clinical relevance, this was the only patient shown to have a focal wall-motion abnormality by two-dimensional echocardiography. Electrocardiographic changes and CK-MB, however, did not correlate with an antimyosin scan evidence of myocardial injury.[30] Although theoretically attractive, antimyosin scanning has not evolved to a point where it has a role in the routine evaluation of patients with non-penetrating cardiac trauma.

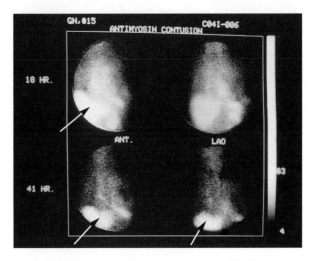

Figure 9.3 *Eighteen- and 41-hour indium-111 antimyosin scans demonstrating uptake of tracer (arrows) in the inferoapical area of the left ventricle, consistent with an area of myocardial contusion. ANT = anterior, LAO = 60° left anterior oblique projections. (Photograph courtesy of JA Leppo, MD, Division of Nuclear Cardiology, UMass-Memorial Medical Center.)*

Two-dimensional transthoracic echocardiography

Two-dimensional echocardiography represents a portable, widely available, and non-invasive means to assess the myocardium, valves and pericardium rapidly following chest trauma. Regional wall motion abnormalities (Fig. 9.4), chamber dilation (Fig. 9.5), aneurysm formation (Fig. 9.6) pericardial effusions, mural thrombi, valvular damage, and intracardiac shunts can be identified readily.[31,32]

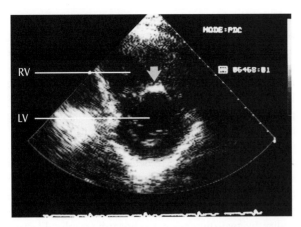

Figure 9.4 *Two-dimensional echocardiogram (parasternal short axis view, systolic frame) performed in a trauma patient demonstrating a septal wall motion abnormality (arrow) and a dilated right ventricle (RV). LV = left ventricle.*

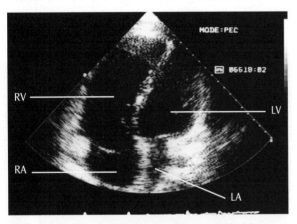

Figure 9.5 *Two-dimensional echocardiogram (apical four-chamber view, end-systolic frame) demonstrating post-traumatic dilation of the right ventricle and right atrium. The arrow demonstrates a thickened flail tricuspid valve chordae. RA = right atrium; RV = right ventricle; LV = left ventricle; LA = left atrium.*

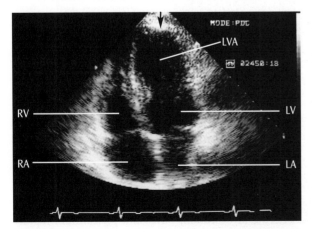

Figure 9.6 *Two-dimensional echocardiogram (apical four-chamber view, end-systolic frame) demonstrating a post-traumatic aneursym of the left ventricle (LVA). An apical mural thrombus is also present (arrow). LV = left ventricle, LA = left atrium, RV = right ventricle, RA = right atrium.*

Frazee and colleagues[17] reported that 23 of 58 (40 per cent) patients with non-penetrating chest trauma and elevated serum CK-MB levels demonstrated wall-motion abnormalities on transthoracic echocardiography. Nine patients (39 per cent) experienced cardiac arrhythmias many of whom required treatment with an antiarrhythmic agent. Similar observations were made by Reif and co-workers,[33] who identified a 26 per cent incidence of cardiac complications among patients with blunt chest trauma and an abnormal echocardiogram, compared with a 1.2 per cent incidence in those with a normal echocardiogram. Reid and colleagues[34] reported echocardiographic abnormalities in 8 of 33 (24 per cent) patients with blunt chest trauma. Although the investigators found that views (windows) were frequently limited by surrounding areas of trauma, they favored routine two-dimensional echocardiography in all patients with an elevated CK-MB level.

In contrast, Fabian and co-workers[16] reported a 19 per cent incidence of echocardiographic abnormalities among patients with chest trauma and either an abnormal ECG or elevated CK-MB level. Furthermore, echocardiography failed to provide added prognostic information. Their experience was shared by Helling and co-workers[35] who were also unable to demonstrate prognostic value for screening echocardiography in patients with chest trauma and suspected non-penetrating cardiac injury. Although one could question the value of routine echocardiography, many published series have been small and confounded by technical limitation.[22]

> Our current practice is to perform echocardiography in patients with persistent hypotension, supraventricular or ventricular tachyarrhythms, heart block, progressive hemodynamic instability, and in those requiring emergent operative intervention.[21]

Transesophageal echocardiography

Transesophageal echocardiography can be performed in critically ill patients,[36] whereas two-dimensional transthoracic echocardiographic imaging is often technically limited by coexisting conditions that adversely influence ultrasound windows and views. Several examples include pneumothorax, subcutaneous or mediastinal emphysema, and chest tubes.

Shapiro and colleagues[37] performed TEE in 19 patients with severe non-penetrating chest trauma. High-quality images were recorded in all patients, revealing abnormalities in 63 per cent that included two cases of aortic injury. Brooks reported findings consistent with myocardial contusion in 26 of 50 patients using TEE as compared with 6 of 50 undergoing standard transthoracic echocardiography.[38] TEE has also been useful in the diagnosis of valvular abnormalities (Fig. 9.7).[39] Traumatic injury of the thoracic aorta can be quickly and safely

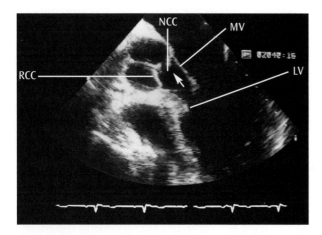

Figure 9.7 *Transesophageal echocardiogram demonstrating post-traumatic rupture of the non-coronary cusp of the aortic valve (arrow). MV = mitral valve; LV = left ventricle; RCC = right coronary cusp; NCC = non-coronary cusp.*

detected by TEE with a high degree of sensitivity and specificity.[40,41]

Pulmonary artery catheterization

Pulmonary artery (PA) catheterization[42] allows rapid determination of hemodynamic parameters and should be considered in patients with systemic hypotension unresponsive to fluid administration, patients with an abnormal two-dimensional echocardiogram requiring non-cardiac surgery, or as a diagnostic aid in patients with a new (or presumably new) heart murmur.

Cardiac catheterization and contrast angiography

Cardiac catheterization and contrast angiography are useful techniques for quantifying intracardiac shunts (Fig. 9.8), assessing the severity of valvular regurgitation, diagnosing coronary artery injuries (Fig. 9.9 a and b), and defining the hemodynamic and anatomical significance of traumatic ventricular aneurysms.

MANAGEMENT

The treatment of traumatic myocardial dysfunction is, in a majority of patients, supportive.

A growing body of evidence suggests that it is possible to identify patients at low risk for cardiac complications following blunt chest injury, i.e. those not requiring hospital admission or telemetry monitoring;[33] however, in many circumstances a monitoring period of 12–24 hours is clinically indicated.[43–45]

Bed rest, continuous cardiac monitoring (telemetry) for arrhythmias, supplemental oxygen, a daily 12-lead ECG, and serial CK-MB (or troponin) determinations are recommended.

The benefit of prophylactic antiarrhythmic therapy has not been established.

If the ECG and serum CK-MB (or troponin) levels remain normal during the initial 24 hours, cardiac

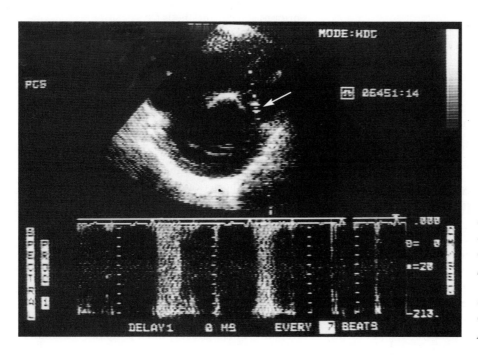

Figure 9.8 *Post-traumatic ventricular septal rupture demonstrated by two-dimensional Doppler echocardiography. The cursor position (arrow) identifies high-velocity pansystolic blood flow (demonstrated by the spectral display in the lower half of the figure).*

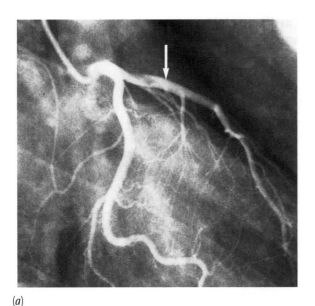

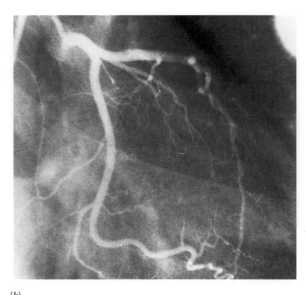

(a)   (b)

Figure 9.9 *(a) Left coronary angiogram (90° left lateral projection) demonstrating an acute thrombus (arrow) in the proximal left anterior descending coronary artery of a 22-year-old patient with mild blunt chest trauma. (b) Six-day follow-up coronary angiogram (90° left lateral projection) demonstrating resolution of the thrombus.*

monitoring can be discontinued.[44] In contrast ECG and/or cardiac marker abnormalities should prompt consideration for additional diagnostic testing and a more prolonged period of cardiac monitoring.[6]

In general, the extent of hemodynamic compromise correlates directly with the amount of myocardial damage; however, low cardiac output states may also be caused by hypovolemia, cardiac tamponade, ventricular septal rupture, or valvular dysfunction. Echocardiography, PA catheterization, or coronary angiography can be used to diagnose these conditions.

Intravenous fluid administration, inotropic support, afterload reduction, and, occasionally, intra-aortic balloon counterpulsation[46] may be required to stabilize a patient's hemodynamic status. If aggressive supportive care is required for stabilization, a thorough diagnostic evaluation should be undertaken to exclude myocardial, valvular, and/or thoracic aorta injury.

Management of patients with non-penetrating trauma requiring general anesthesia

Patients sustaining blunt chest trauma may require emergency surgery to correct non-cardiac injuries. Recent reports have considered the potential risk of myocardial injury among patients undergoing urgent or emergent operations requiring general anesthesia. An increased incidence of perioperative complications,

including hypotension, arrhythmias, and congestive heart failure has been observed. Flancbaum and colleagues[47] reported that 11 of 19 patients with myocardial contusion undergoing general anesthesia required perioperative inotropic support. Similarly, Ross and co-workers[48] found an increased occurrence of perioperative complications in patients with myocardial contusion.

Although not all investigators have observed an increased perioperative risk, most agree that echocardiography and aggressive hemodynamic monitoring should be performed in cardiac trauma patients prior to general anesthesia.[44,48]

Injuries to specific cardiac structures

In addition to myocardial contusion, non-penetrating trauma can cause a variety of cardiac structural abnormalities, including myocardial free wall rupture, ventricular aneurysm formation, interventricular septal rupture, and injuries to the cardiac valves, the coronary arteries, and the pericardium.

Myocardial 'free wall' rupture

Traumatic myocardial rupture is a life-threatening complication that requires immediate intervention.[49]

The combination of sudden hemorrhage, hemopericardium with tamponade, and a profound reduction in left ventricular preload leads to devastating hemodynamic consequences. A study performed at the Shock Trauma Center of the Maryland Institute for Emergency Services[50] underscores the lethal nature of trauma-related myocardial rupture, where, despite emergency surgical intervention, the mortality rate approached 80 per cent. The overall outcome was somewhat better among patients presenting to the emergency department with obtainable vital signs, supporting early and aggressive supportive care.

Ventricular aneurysm formation

Traumatic ventricular aneurysm formation is not a common complication of non-penetrating myocardial injury, but can occur following cardiac contusion or infarction related to traumatic occlusion of the left anterior descending coronary artery[5,51] (Fig. 9.6). The clinical significance of traumatic ventricular aneurysms is determined by associated complication that can include congestive heart failure, ventricular dysrhythmias, thromboembolic events, and rarely, myocardial rupture. The latter is, in most instances, a manifestation of *pseudoaneurysm* formation.

> If a traumatic ventricular aneurysm is suspected by non-invasive testing, cardiac catheterization and contrast ventriculography should be considered. Elective resection of post-traumatic ventricular pseudoaneurysms at 4–8 weeks is recommended when clinically feasible.[5]

Isolated ventricular septal rupture (VSR) is a rare complication of non-penetrating myocardial injury. In a large autopsy series, Parmley and colleagues[11] reported a 5.5 per cent incidence of traumatic VSR; however, VSR was an isolated finding in only 0.9 per cent. The underlying mechanism is, in most instances, thought to be compression of the heart when the ventricles are full and the atrioventricular valves are closed (i.e. late diastole and early systole). Delayed VSR may develop with necrosis of a contused intraventricular septum or when traumatic coronary arterial occlusion causes an anteroseptal myocardial infarction.

Traumatic VSR should be suspected in the presence of either a new systolic murmur or signs of rapidly progressive cardiac decompensation. Doppler color flow echocardiography (transthoracic or TEE) can be used to confirm the diagnosis (Fig. 9.7). VSRs resulting from non-penetrating injury tend to be large and are typically associated with significant myocardial injury. Thus, a marked impairment in overall cardiac performance is common.

> Initial therapy consists of inotropic support and intra-aortic balloon counterpulsation.[52] Cardiac

catheterization and contrast angiography should be performed to determine the overall hemodynamic significance of the intracardiac shunt and to identify associated injuries. Patients with a left-to-right shunt greater than 1.5 to 1 should undergo elective surgical repair, preferably in 4–8 weeks. Immediate repair is necessary in patients with advanced hemodynamic compromise; however, in this setting, a high surgical mortality rate is anticipated.[5]

Valvular injury

Traumatic aortic, mitral, and tricuspid valve dysfunction have been reported following non-penetrating cardiac injury. In general, symptoms are due to acute valvular insufficiency, but may rarely be delayed for several months.[53] Patients typically present with congestive heart failure and on physical examination are found to have a new murmur. The most commonly encountered valvular injury is aortic insufficiency, resulting from a rapid increase in intra-aortic pressure during early diastole. The transvalvular pressure gradient causes rupture at the base of the valve or detaches the commisures, facilitating prolapse (Fig. 9.8). The diagnosis can be confirmed by two-dimensional Doppler color flow echocardiography, TEE, or aortic root angiography.[39]

> If the patient can be medically stabilized, elective surgery should be performed 4–8 weeks later. In hemodynamically unstable situations, however, surgery should not be delayed. Although successful aortic valve repair has been performed,[53] many surgeons advocate valve replacement.[54,55]

Trauma to the mitral valve usually involves the chordae tendinea and the papillary muscles rather than the leaflets themselves. Doppler color flow echocardiography, right heart catheterization[42] or contrast ventriculography can be performed to establish the diagnosis.

> Medical treatment is preferred with surgical intervention reserved for patients with refractory congestive heart failure or hemodynamic instability.

Isolated non-penetrating tricuspid valve injury is rare and, like mitral valve injury, typically involves the supporting structures of the valves rather than the leaflets themselves. Although tricuspid valve injuries do not typically cause symptoms, progressive right heart failure requiring valve repair or replacement has been reported.[56] Injury to the pulmonic valve is rare and frequently accompanies severe chest trauma and injury to the lungs and/or great vessels.

Coronary artery injury

Coronary arterial injury has been reported in patients experiencing non-penetrating chest trauma and most often involves the left anterior descending coronary artery. Patients can present to the hospital with ischemic chest pain, electrocardiographic ST-segment elevation, and elevated serum cardiac enzyme levels. These findings, however, do not distinguish traumatic coronary arterial occlusion from cardiac contusion.

The most common mechanisms cited for traumatic coronary arterial occlusion are: (1) vessel wall disruption with subsequent thrombosis; and (2) external compression by a myocardial hematoma.[5,57,58] The involved artery not uncommonly appears angiographically normal days to months later[42,57] (Fig. 9.9 a and b).

Complications of traumatic coronary arterial injury include ventricular aneurysm formation, VSR, and coronary–cameral fistulas.[5] In the absence of significant extracardiac trauma, emergency coronary angiography followed by mechanical revascularization should be considered.[57–61]

Pericardial injury

Non-penetrating cardiac trauma can cause either acute (3–5 days) or chronic pericarditis. The mechanism of post-traumatic pericarditis developing 4–6 weeks after the initial event is unknown but in many ways is similar to Dressler's syndrome (post-MI pericarditis and post-pericardiotomy syndrome). Signs and symptoms include pleuritic chest pain, fever, ECG changes, and a pericardial friction rub.[2,5] In a majority of cases, clinical improvement follows the institution of anti-inflammatory medications. Cardiac tamponade and chronic constrictive pericarditis are rare complications of post-traumatic pericarditis.

Parmley[8] reported pericardial rupture in 3 per cent of the autopsy cases associated with fatal non-penetrating chest trauma. The primary danger of pericardial rupture is acute cardiac herniation with torsion or constriction of the great vessels. Displacement of the cardiac silhouette on chest x-ray supports the diagnosis. Pericardial rupture is a potentially fatal event with a 63 per cent mortality rate, underscoring the need for accurate diagnosis and urgent surgical correction.[62]

PROGNOSIS AND FOLLOW-UP

The prognosis for patients experiencing an uncomplicated myocardial contusion is excellent. Ventricular wall motion abnormalities seen by two-dimensional echocardiography or RVG typically resolve within 7–10 days, although it occasionally requires several months for complete resolution.[27]

Patients with an abnormal two-dimensional echocardiogram during hospitalization should undergo a follow-up study 6 weeks after discharge. Patients with minimal valvular damage or small intracardiac shunts should have serial two-dimensional echocardiograms until complete resolution or stabilization is confirmed.

Patients with confirmed myocardial contusion in whom ventricular function is not initially compromised or rapidly returns to normal in most cases do not require long-term follow-up care.

SUMMARY

- Non-penetrating cardiac trauma, although most often associated with motor vehicle accidents, can also occur following even seemingly minor blunt chest trauma.
- Pathobiology and clinical expression vary from superficial myocardial contusion to free wall rupture and fatal pericardial tamponade.
- Supraventricular and ventricular tachyarrhythmias, atrioventricular block, valvular disruption, and traumatic coronary arterial occlusion with myocardial infarction can also occur in the early post-traumatic period.
- The late manifestations of non-penetrating cardiac trauma include left or right ventricular aneurysm formation and pericarditis.
- Diagnostic modalities with the greatest overall yield include surface electrocardiography, measurement of serum cardiac markers, echocardiography (transthoracic and/or transesophageal), contrast ventriculography and coronary angiography.
- The initial management of patients with non-penetrating cardiac trauma is predominantly supportive with careful monitoring for dysrhythmias and hemodynamic decompensation.
- Prompt surgical intervention may be life-saving in cases of pericardial tamponade, cardiac rupture, and valvular disruption.

REFERENCES

1. Shackford SR. Blunt chest trauma: the intensivists perspective. *J Intens Care Med* 1986; **1**: 125–36.
○2. Symbas PN. Traumatic heart disease. *Curr Probl Cardiol* 1991; **15**: 539–82.
3. Ivatury RR, Rohman M: The injured heart. *Surg Clin North Am* 1989; **393**: 93–100.

4. Mattox KL, Limacher MC, Feliciano DV, *et al*. Cardiac evaluation following heart injury. *J Trauma* 1985; **25**: 758–65.

5. Chitwood WR, Austin EH. In: Moylan JA, ed. *Cardiac trauma: penetrating and blunt in trauma surgery*. Philadelphia: Lippincott, 1988: 123–81.

6. Kudsk KA, *et al*. Myocardial contusion: diagnosis and management. *Contemp Surg* 1989; **35**: 11–16.

7. Bullock FA, Prothero A, Shaw C, *et al*. Cardiac involvement in seatbelt-related and direct sternal trauma: a prospective study and management implications. *Eur Heart J* 1994; **15**: 1621–7.

8. Santavirta S, Arajarvi E. Ruptures of the heart in seat-belt wearers. *J Trauma* 1992; **32**: 275–9.

○9. Snow N, Richardson JD, Flint LM. Myocardial contusion: implications for patients with multiple traumatic injuries. *Surgery* 1982; **92**: 744–50.

○10. Abrunzo TJ. Commotio cordis: the single most common cause of traumatic death in youth baseball. *AJDC* 1991; **145**: 1279–82.

○11. Parmley LF, Manion WC, Mattingly TW. Nonpenetrating traumatic injury of the heart. *Circulation* 1958; **18**: 371–95.

12. Harmon PK, Trinkle JK. Injury to the heart. In: Moore EE, Mattox KL, eds *Trauma*. Norwalk, CT: Appleton, Century, and Croft, 1986.

13. Hossack KF, Moreno CA, Vanway CW, Burdick DC. Frequency of cardiac contusion in nonpenetrating chest injury. *Am J Cardiol* 1988; **61**: 391–4.

14. Cachecho R, Grindlinger GA, Lee VW. The clinical significance of myocardial contusion. *J Trauma* 1992; **33**: 68–73.

15. Berk WA. ECG findings in nonpenetrating chest trauma: a review. *J Emerg Med* 1987; **5**: 209–15.

○16. Fabian TC, Mangiante EC, Patterson CR, Payne LW, Isaacson ML. Myocardial contusion in blunt trauma: clinical characteristics, means of diagnosis, and implications for patient management. *J Trauma* 1988; **28**: 50–7.

17. Frazee RC, *et al*. Objective evaluation of blunt cardiac trauma. *J Trauma* 1986: **26**: 510–20.

18. Biffl WL, Moore FA, Moore EE, *et al*. Cardiac enzymes are irrelevant in the patient with suspected myocardial contusion. *Am J Surg* 1994; **169**: 523–8.

19. Potkin RT, *et al*. Evaluation and noninvasive tests of cardiac damage in suspected cardiac contusion. *Circulation* 1982; **66**: 627–31.

20. Soutter DI, Rodriquez A. Cardiac contusion: diagnosis and management. *Trauma Quart* 1988; **4**: 16–23.

21. Ingwall JS, Kramer MF, Fifer MA, *et al*. The creatine kinase system in normal and diseased human myocardium. *N Engl J Med* 1985; **313**: 1050–4.

22. Keller KD, Shatney CH. Creatine phosphokinase–MB assays in patients with suspected myocardial contusion: diagnostic test or test of diagnosis? *J Trauma* 1988; **28**: 58–63.

23. Coudrey L. The troponins. *Arch Intern Med*, 1998; **158**: 1173–80.

24. Katus H, Looser S, Hallermayer K, *et al*. Development and in vitro characterization of a new immunoassay of cardiac troponin T. *Clin Chem* 1992; **38**: 386–93.

25. Cummins, B, Auckland ML, Cummins P. Cardiac specific troponin I radioimmune assay in the diagnosis of acute myocardial infarction. *Am Heart J* 1987; **113**: 1333–44.

26. Tenzer ML. The spectrum of myocardial contusion: a review. *J Trauma* 1985; **25**: 620–7.

27. Harley DP, Mena I, Narahara KA, Miranda R, Nelson RJ. Traumatic myocardial dysfunction. *J Thorac Cardiovasc Surg* 1984; **87**: 386–93.

28. Khaw BA, Yasuda T, Gold HK, *et al*. Acute myocardial infarction imaging with indium-111 labeled mono-clonal antimyosin FAB. *J Nucl Med* 1987; **28**: 1671–8.

29. Yasuda T, Palacios IF, Dec GW, *et al*. Indium-111 monoclonal antimyosin antibody imaging in the diagnosis of acute myocarditis. *Circulation* 1987; **76**: 306–11.

29a. First W, Yasuda T, Segall G, *et al*. Noninvasive detection of human cardiac transplant rejection with indium-111 antimyosin (FAB) imaging. *Circulation* 1987; **76**(suppl V): V81–V85.

30. Hendel RC, Cohn S, Aurigemma G, *et al*. Focal myocardial injury following blunt chest trauma: a comparison of indium-111 antimyosin scintigraphy with other noninvasive methods. *Am Heart J* 1992; **123**: 1208–15.

31. Markiewicz W, Best LA, Burstein S, Peleg H. Echocardiographic evaluation after blunt trauma of the chest. *Int J Cardiol* 1985; **8**: 269–74.

32. Karalis DG, Victor MF, Davis GA, *et al*. The role of echocardiography in blunt chest trauma: a transthoracic and transesophageal echocardiographic study. *J Trauma* 1994; **36**: 53–8.

33. Reif J, Justice JL, Olsen WR, Prager RL. Selective monitoring of patients with suspected blunt cardiac injury. *Ann Thorac Surg* 1990; **50**: 530–3.

34. Reid CL, Kawanishi DT, Rahimtoola SH, Chandraratna PA. Chest trauma: evaluation by two dimensional echocardiography. *Am Heart J* 1987; **113**: 971–6.

35. Helling TS, Duke P, Beggs CW, Crouse LJ. A prospective evaluation of 68 patients suffering blunt chest trauma for evidence of cardiac injury. *J Trauma* 1989; **29**: 961–6.

36. Basal RC, Shah PM. Transesophageal echocardiography. *Curr Prob Cardiol* 1990; **15**: 643–720.

37. Shapiro MJ, Yanofsky SD, Trapp J, *et al*. Cardiovascular evaluation in blunt thoracic trauma using transesophageal echocardiography (TEE). *J Trauma* 1991; **31**: 835–40.

○38. Brooks SW, Young JC, Smolik B, *et al*. The use of transesophageal echocardiography in the evaluation of chest trauma. *J Trauma* 1992; **32**: 761–6.

39. Wholey RM, Voyce SJ, Pape LA, *et al*. Aortic valve rupture following nonpenetrating thoracic trauma: diagnosis by transesophageal echocardiography. *J Am Soc Noninvasive Cardiol* 1991; **5**: 372–4.

40. Smith MD, Cassidy JM, Souther S, *et al*. Transesophageal echocardiography in the diagnosis of traumatic rupture of the aorta. *N Engl J Med* 1995; **332**: 356–62.

41. Catoire P, Orliaguet G, Liu M, *et al*. Systematic transesophageal echocardiography for detection of mediastinal lesions in patients with multiple injuries. *J Trauma* 1995; **38**: 96–102.

42. Voyce SJ. Pulmonary artery catheters. In: Irwin RI, Cerra FB, Rippe JM, eds. *Intensive care medicine*. Philadelphia: Lippincott–Raven, 1999: 46–70.

43. Gunnar WP, Martin M, Smith RF, *et al*. The utility of cardiac evaluation in the hemodynamically stable patient with suspected myocardial contusion. *Am Surgeon* 1991; **57**: 373–7.

44. Baxter BT, Moore EE, Moore FA, *et al*. A plea for sensible management of myocardial contusion. *Am J Surg* 1989; **158**: 557–62.

○45. Feghali NT, Prisant LM. Blunt myocardial inury. *Chest* 1995; **108**: 1673–7.

46. Orlando R, Drezner AD. Intra-aortic balloon counterpulsation in blunt cardiac injury. *J Trauma* 1983; **23**: 424–7.

47. Flancbaum L, Wright J, Siegel JH. Emergency surgery in patients with post-traumatic myocardial contusion. *J Trauma* 1986; **26**: 795–802.

48. Ross P, Degutis L, Baker CC. Cardiac contusion. The effects on operative management of the patient with trauma injuries. *Arch Surg* 1989; **124**: 506–7.

49. Kato K, Koshimoto S, Mashiko K, *et al*. Blunt traumatic rupture of the heart: an experience in Tokyo. *J Trauma* 1994; **36**: 859–64.

50. Fulda G, Braithwaite CEM, Rodriguez A, *et al*. Blunt traumatic rupture of the heart and pericardium: a ten-year experience (1979–1989) *J Trauma* 1991; **31**: 167–73.

51. Voyce SJ, Ball SP, Gore JM, *et al*. Angiographically documented thrombotic coronary artery occlusion secondary to mild nonpenetrating thoracic trauma. *Cath Cardiovasc Diagn* 1991; **24**: 179–81.

52. Cowgill LD, Campbell DN, Clarke DR, *et al*. Ventricular septal defect due to nonpenetrating chest trauma: use of intra-aortic balloon pump. *J Trauma* 1987; **27**: 1087–90.

53. Scully RE, Galdabini JJ, McNelly BV. Case records of the Massachusetts General Hospital Case 3-1976. *N Engl J Med* 1976; **294**: 152–8.

54. Kimbler RW, Strokes JP, Bainhorst DA. The surgical treatment of traumatic rupture of the aortic valve: report of a case of blunt chest trauma. *J Trauma* 1977; **17**: 168–70.

55. Devineni R, McKenzie FX. Avulsion of a normal aortic valve cusp due to blunt chest trauma. *J Trauma* 1984; **24**: 910–12.

56. Hilton T, Mezer L, Pearson AC. Delayed rupture of tricuspid papillary muscle following blunt chest trauma. *Am Heart J* 1990; **119**: 1410–12.

57. Gaspard P, Clermont A, Villaro J, Amiel M. Non-arterogenic trauma of the coronary arteries and myocardium: contribution of angiography: report of six cases and literature review. *Cardiovasc Intervent Radiol* 1983; **6**: 20–9.

58. Sigmund M, Nase-Hipmeirer S, Vebis R, Manrath P. Emergency: PTCA for coronary artery occlusion after blunt chest trauma. *Am Heart J* 1990; **119**: 1408–10.

59. Ledley GS, Yazdanfar S, Friedman O, Kotler MN. Acute thrombotic coronary occlusion secondary to chest trauma treated with intracoronary thrombosis. *Am Heart J* 1992; **123**: 518–21.

60. Pifarre R, Grieco J, Garibaldi A, *et al*. Acute coronary artery occlusion secondary to blunt chest trauma. *J Thorac Cardiovasc Surg* 1982; **83**: 122–5.

61. Orhe LE, Gallego FC, Sobrino N, *et al*. Acute myocardial infarction after blunt chest trauma in young people: need for prompt intervention. *Cath Cardiovasc Diagn* 1991; **24**: 182–5.

○62. Fulda G, Rodriguez A, Turney SZ, Cowley RA. Blunt traumatic pericardial rupture – a ten-year experience 1979–1989. *J Cardiovasc Surg* 1990; **31**: 525–30.

10

Management of pulmonary emergencies

NICHOLAS A SMYRNIOS AND BORIS A MURILLO

The respiratory and cardiovascular systems are related in a unique way. Because these systems are interconnected, it is not surprising that cardiovascular physicians will encounter patients with acute respiratory disease in their practice. Some diseases are treated by physicians in both specialties. The symptoms of lung disease (cough, dyspnea, chest pain, hemoptysis, wheeze) are also commonly encountered in the practice of cardiovascular medicine. Some of the causes of cardiovascular disease, most notably cigarette smoking, are also causes of pulmonary disease. Therefore, it is essential that physicians caring for cardiac patients have a sound understanding of the approach to patients with acute pulmonary problems.

STATUS ASTHMATICUS

Epidemiology and pathophysiology

Asthma is defined as being a chronic inflammatory disease of the airways associated with airway obstruction that is often at least partly reversible spontaneously or with treatment, and with airway hyper-responsiveness, and which causes recurrent episodes of wheezing, breathlessness, chest tightness, and coughing.[1] Status asthmaticus is defined as a severe asthma attack that puts the patient at risk for respiratory failure.[2] The prevalence of asthma is estimated at between 5 and 10 per 100. The mortality rate from asthma is calculated as 1.8 per 100 000.

Expiratory airflow obstruction and hyperinflation are the pathophysiologic changes that lead to difficulty with ventilation. These are the result of bronchial hyper-responsiveness and, most importantly, severe inflammation. The majority of patients with acute asthma present with filled, wet airways with eosinophilic bronchitis, edema, sloughing of the mucosa, thickening of the base-ment membrane, smooth muscle hypertrophy, and thick, tenacious mucus plugs that lead to airway obstruction and air trapping. An initial trigger releases inflammatory mediators from epithelial cells, mast cells, and macrophages. The released substances stimulate the infiltration of additional inflammatory cells, such as eosinophils and neutrophils, which perpetuate and exacerbate the tissue damage done, and lead to the pathologic changes seen.[3]

Clinical assessment

Patients in status asthmaticus must be assessed and treatment instituted in prompt fashion. A history of asthma is often, but not invariably, present. A history of previous asthma attacks requiring mechanical ventilation (MV) is particularly ominous. Other important features of past episodes include a history of pneumothorax or pneumomediastinum, hospitalization despite chronic oral steroid use, hypercapnia, psychiatric illness, or medication non-adherence.[2]

The physical examination focuses on detecting signs consistent with a severe attack, and on detecting complications of the attack. For example, it has been observed that patients who assume the upright position also had other findings indicating a severe attack.[4] Other physical examination findings indicative of a severe exacerbation include diaphoresis, use of accessory muscles, altered mental status, and an increased pulsus paradoxus.[5] Physical findings suggestive of complications of asthma include tracheal deviation, asymmetry of breath sounds, hyper-resonance to percussion, subcutaneous emphysema, stridor, and the 'mediastinal crunch'. Of note, it is impossible to describe the severity of an attack based on the intensity of wheezing.

The most important objective testing performed during an attack of status asthmaticus is the quantification of expiratory flow. Changes in peak expiratory flow rate (PEFR) and forced expiratory volume in 1 second (FEV_1) with treatment have both been shown to predict the outcome of an exacerbation and the need for hospital admission.[6,7] Therefore, it is essential that either PEFR or FEV_1 be measured on presentation to medical care and serially thereafter until the attack has resolved.

The other two most commonly obtained tests are the arterial blood gas (ABG) and the chest x-ray (CXR). In general, both of these tests have no role in the routine management of mild to moderately severe attacks of asthma. In severe attacks, the ABG may be useful to measure the presence of elevated levels of P_aCO_2 as an indicator of respiratory failure. The CXR is used during severe attacks to detect complications such as pneumothorax and pneumomediastinum or infiltrates as may be seen in allergic bronchopulmonary aspergillosis or bacterial pneumonia. In milder attacks its use should be reserved for when there is a question about whether asthma is the cause of the patient's symptoms.

Therapy

The goals in managing exacerbations of asthma include:

1 rapid reversal of airflow obstruction and relief of dyspnea;
2 correction of hypoxemia; and
3 prevention of relapse.

The initial management of a mild asthma attack is usually accomplished in the home. The patient should be instructed to take 2–4 puffs of their inhaled beta-2 agonist medication every 20 minutes for up to 1 hour. If they have a good response, including relief of symptoms and return of their PEFR to a stable level of >70 per cent of their baseline, they may continue to administer beta-2 agonist therapy up to every 3 hours as needed for 24–48 hours. Patients whose symptoms persist at rest or with mild exertion, and whose PEFR is between 50 and 70 per cent of baseline should be treated with oral corticosteroids and hourly beta-2 agonist therapy. If the patient fails to improve after 2–6 hours of this regimen or if the PEFR begins at or drops to below 50 per cent of baseline, the patient should seek emergency medical treatment.

> Supplemental oxygen is the first treatment to be administered upon arrival. Oxygen delivered via nasal cannula at 2–4 L/min can relieve symptoms, reverse hypoxemia due to ventilation–perfusion mismatching, and prevent worsening of hypoxia that may be caused by the acute administration of bronchodilating medications.
>
> Inhaled beta-2 adrenergic agonists are the next treatment to be administered. Beta-2 agonists are the bronchodilator drugs of choice because of their rapid onset of action and their large therapeutic window.

Administration of beta-2 agonist medications is equally effective via nebulizer or via metered dose inhaler (MDI) with a spacer device. The MDI method is less expensive. Albuterol is the drug used most commonly, although metaproterenol may also be used.

> Albuterol should be administered as 2.5 mg in 2.5 mL normal saline via a hand-held nebulizer, or as four puffs (0.36 mg per puff) from an MDI every 20–30 minutes for 3–6 doses.

Treatment may need to be adjusted due to side effects such as tremor, cardiac arrhythmia, or hypokalemia. Beyond that point, treatment needs to be titrated to response and side effects.

> Systemic corticosteroids are the cornerstone of the treatment of status asthmaticus because they directly influence airway inflammation.

Prednisone and methylprednisolone are the recommended agents because they have small mineralocorticoid effects.

> Recommendations for dosing in adults are 120–180 mg of prednisone or methylprednisolone in three or four divided doses for 48 hours, then 60–80 mg per day until PEFR reaches > 70 per cent of predicted or personal best.[1]

Ipratropium bromide is an effective bronchodilator that may enhance the bronchodilating effects of beta-2 agonists. Dosing is recommended as 0.5 mg in a nebulizer solution, or 4–8 puffs of a 18 µg/puff MDI every 20 minutes for three doses, then every 2–4 hours as needed. Ipratropium bromide should never be used alone in the treatment of status asthmaticus because it lacks the rapid onset of action seen with albuterol.

Theophylline is a medication that has been used for status asthmaticus for years. At the present time, official recommendations for the treatment of status asthmaticus do not include theophylline. The reason for this is primarily a combination of lack of additional benefit beyond that achieved with inhaled bronchodilators, and the drug's extensive side-effect profile.

Many other non-conventional treatments have been suggested to be beneficial for this group of patients. Among these are intravenous beta-2 agonists, intravenous $MgSO_4$, general anesthesia with halothane and ketamine, and a helium–oxygen mixture. None of these have been demonstrated in a randomized, prospective way to improve outcomes.[8] Therefore, they should not be used unless the patient is failing to respond to conventional therapy.

Should a patient require MV, the appropriate objectives are to decrease minute ventilation and increase expiratory time while accepting hypercapnia. The strategy to accomplish these objectives is called *controlled mechanical hypoventilation with permissive hypercapnia*. This is achieved by reducing the tidal volume and respiratory rate, increasing the peak inspiratory flow rate, and titrating the fraction of inspired oxygen (F_iO_2) to maintain oxygenation in the face of hypercapnia.[9]

Typical *initial* settings are a respiratory rate of 11–14/min, a tidal volume of 6–8 mL/kg ideal body weight, a peak inspiratory flow rate of 80–100 L/min, and an F_iO_2 of 1.0. F_iO_2 is then weaned to the lowest level able to maintain S_aO_2 >0.90.

In managing patients during controlled mechanical hypoventilation with permissive hypercapnia, the minimum 'safe' pH is not known at this time. Three uncontrolled studies have not demonstrated an adverse effect on outcome when pH was allowed to drop as low as 7.0. In addition, there are theoretical disadvantages to the use of sodium bicarbonate such as depression of hemodynamic parameters and paradoxical intracellular acidosis. Therefore, there is no predefined level of pH that must be buffered with exogenous sodium bicarbonate.

Patients receiving MV for status asthmaticus should be monitored for the adequacy of their oxygenation and their risk of barotrauma and hypotension. This involves performing arterial blood gases, pulse oximetry, and monitoring other physiologic indices that predict barotrauma. The most accurate predictor in status asthmaticus is V_{EI}. The V_{EI} is determined by measuring the amount of gas exhaled after a MV tidal breath during a prolonged (60–80 second) apneic period. This measurement can only be made in patients who receive sedation and neuromuscular blocking agents (NMBA) because of the prolonged apneic period needed. A value of ≤20 mL/kg, or ≤1.4 L in a 70 kg adult, appears to be an accurate threshold value for distinguishing between high- and low-risk patients.[10] If V_{EI} is above 20 mL/kg, minute ventilation should be decreased by reducing tidal volume, and if necessary by reducing respiratory rate.

Other related parameters must also be followed while the patient is receiving MV. A CXR should be obtained daily to look for evidence of pneumothorax or pneumomediastinum, pneumonia, or atelectasis. If patients receive intravenous theophylline, they should have a level checked at least once after a steady dose has been established, and thereafter again if signs of toxicity exist. The potassium level must be carefully monitored during therapy for SA. For patients receiving prolonged use of NMBA, it is common practice that they should be monitored with train-of-four nerve stimulation to avoid prolonged paralysis when the drug is withdrawn. This form of monitoring stimulates a peripheral nerve (e.g. the ulnar nerve) four times with a low current electrical impulse and observes the muscle twitches resulting. Two twitches is generally considered to be an adequate level of neuromuscular blockade. Additional doses of NMBA should not be given unless there is evidence of excessive muscle activity.

CHRONIC OBSTRUCTIVE PULMONARY DISEASE

Respiratory failure due to chronic obstructive pulmonary disease (COPD) is the fifth most common cause of death in the USA and leads to 75 000 deaths annually. Many factors have been implicated as causes of acute exacerbations. Viral infections of the respiratory tract are thought to be the most common causes of acute exacerbations. Other possible etiologies include bacterial tracheobronchitis, gastroesophageal reflux disease, aspiration, cardiac arrhythmias, congestive heart failure, cigarette smoking, chest wall injury, pneumonia, sedation, surgery, pneumothorax, and pulmonary embolism.

Diagnosis

Patients experiencing exacerbations of COPD typically present with a pre-existing history of the disease or a long history of cigarette smoking. Symptoms that are often seen at presentation include worsening dyspnea, increased cough with sputum production or change in the amount or color of the sputum, and wheeze.[11] Decreased air movement, expiratory wheezes, and a prolonged expiratory phase are often found on physical examination of the lungs. A patient may be combative, confused, or obtunded due to hypercapnia or hypoxia. Tachypnea, use of the accessory muscles of breathing, and inward movement of the anterior wall of the abdomen during inspiration (*respiratory paradox* or *paradoxical breathing*) are signs of respiratory muscle fatigue.[12–14]

Arterial blood gases may be used to distinguish acute from chronic carbon dioxide retention. To do this, we divide the change in the concentration of hydrogen ions by the change in the partial pressure of carbon dioxide.[15] In practice this is done by subtracting 40 from the most recently measured values for H^+ and P_aCO_2 and placing that number into the fraction below.

$$\Delta H^+/\Delta P_aCO_2 = \begin{cases} 0.8 & = \text{acute} \\ 0.3 & = \text{chronic} \\ >0.3 & \text{but} <0.8 = \text{acute on chronic} \end{cases}$$

The most recent level of H^+ is determined by the following calculation using the most recent ABG values.

$$H^+ = 24 \times (P_aCO_2/HCO_3^-)$$

The most recent level of P_aCO_2 is taken from the ABG.

Indications for hospital and intensive care unit admission

There are no well-validated criteria upon which to base the decision to hospitalize a patient with an exacerbation of COPD. The American Thoracic Society (ATS) used a panel of experts to develop a consensus-derived group of indications.[16] Those indications include the following.

1 An acute exacerbation with dyspnea, cough, or sputum production and at least one of the following: inadequate response to therapy, inability to walk between rooms, inability to eat or sleep, inability to manage at home, high risk co-morbid condition, prolonged course before emergency visit, altered mentation, worsening hypoxemia or hypercapnia.
2 New or worsening cor pulmonale unresponsive to therapy.
3 Planned invasive procedure requiring analgesics or sedatives.
4 Presence of a co-morbid condition that has worsened pulmonary function.

The ATS also established consensus-based indications for admission to an intensive care unit.[16] Those indications are:

1 severe dyspnea that responds inadequately to initial emergency therapy;
2 confusion, lethargy, or respiratory muscle fatigue;
3 severe respiratory acidosis or persistent or worsening hypoxemia; and
4 invasive or non-invasive mechanical ventilation.

Treatment

Treatment can be divided into supportive measures, such as the administration of oxygen or MV when necessary; non-specific therapies such as steroids and bronchodilators; and specific treatments aimed at resolving the cause of the exacerbation, such as antibiotics in the case of a bacterial infection.

Oxygen

> Supplemental oxygen is the single most useful intervention in the treatment of hypoxic respiratory failure.

Oxygen should be administered in sufficient amount to maintain an adequate oxygen content of the blood. This condition is usually thought to be achieved at an oxygen saturation of 90 per cent.

> It is a misconception that is still perpetuated in some educational programs that oxygen is dangerous to COPD patients and its delivery should be restricted to certain amounts. This concept is incorrect and dangerous.

Patients should not be kept hypoxemic for fear of suppressing the respiratory drive. Elevation of the P_aCO_2 is occasionally seen but narcosis is uncommon.[17,18] Elevation in P_aCO_2 is more likely to be due to a change in the dead space volume or a shift of the oxyhemoglobin binding curve rather than decreased respiratory drive.[19]

Bronchodilators

> An inhaled beta-2 agonist is usually the first medication given. Administration of albuterol or other beta-2 agonists by MDI or nebulizer solution appears to be equally effective.[20] The accepted therapeutic equivalent dosages are four puffs of albuterol via MDI or 0.5 mL solution via nebulizer.

Since these drugs exhibit a reduced half-life during exacerbations of COPD, they should be administered up to every 30 minutes until the attack is controlled or side effects become limiting.

> Ipratropium bromide may be used in addition to a beta-2 agonist.

There is evidence to suggest that these two agents act synergistically when used in the chronic setting, although this has not been well established in the acute setting.[21] However, given the long half-life of ipratropium bromide, it is appropriately dosed at 2–8 puffs of an MDI (18 µg per puff) every 6 hours.

Systemic corticosteroids

> Steroids are customarily used in the management of acute exacerbations of COPD, although their effectiveness is not well established. Both oral and intravenous administrations have been used. One prospective, randomized trial using 0.5 mg/kg of

methylprednisolone intravenously every 6 hours showed improvement in FEV_1 in the first 72 hours of treatment.[22]

In addition, a recent trial of oral prednisone in the outpatient management of exacerbations of COPD demonstrated improvements in oxygenation, expiratory flow, and a reduction in treatment failures.[23] Therefore, we customarily use oral prednisone 40–60 mg, tapered over 10–14 days to manage exacerbations in out-patients and methylprednisolone 0.5 mg/kg intravenously every 6 hours for in-patients. In-patients should be discharged with a tapering dose of oral steroids unless a contraindication exists.

Antibiotics

The role of antibiotics in the routine management of exacerbations of COPD has been a controversial issue for many years. Meta-analysis of randomized trials indicated a small advantage to using antibiotic therapy.[24] Any antibiotic used for this purpose should have activity against the primary bacterial pathogens that cause exacerbations of COPD, including *Hemophilus influenzae*, *Streptococcus pneumoniae*, and *Moraxella catarrhalis*. A classification system for acute bronchitis, including acute exacerbations of chronic bronchitis, has been advocated by Grossman.[25] In this scheme, patients with the most substantial risk factors for poor outcome would be treated with oral ciprofloxacin. Unfortunately, a recent comparison of ciprofloxacin with usual care for the treatment of acute exacerbations of chronic bronchitis failed to show statistically significant advantages to the use of ciprofloxacin, although certain trends favored its use.[26] In addition, the studies most often quoted in support of the use of antibiotics reported results from the use of older, less expensive antibiotics.[27] Therefore, until the issue is more clearly resolved, it is likely that a variety of antibiotics will be used for the treatment of acute exacerbations. In making these decisions, the clinician should keep in mind the spectrum of bacteria listed above, patient tolerance, cost, and the lack of a clearly superior choice. Antibiotics used may include amoxicillin–clauvulanate, second- or third-generation cephalosporins, quinolones, macrolides, trimethoprim-sulfa, and tetracyclines. Oral preparations should be used whenever possible.

Theophylline

A double-blind, placebo-controlled trial demonstrated no additional benefit from the use of theophylline over standard therapy but did show increase in adverse effects.[28] Therefore, theophylline is not considered a first-line therapy. Its use should be limited to cases where a systemic route of delivery is considered desirable, or when conventional therapy is failing.

Support of ventilation

A patient may need mechanical support of ventilation when conventional treatment fails to reverse signs of respiratory failure or a patient presents with advanced hypoxic or hypercapnic respiratory failure. The goals of this type of therapy are to rest the respiratory muscles and improve gas exchange to an acceptable level.[16] This may be done either with conventional MV via an endotracheal tube or with non-invasive ventilation. Conventional MV may be done either with assist control, synchronized intermittent mandatory, or pressure support ventilation modes. Minute ventilation should be targeted to maintain the patient's premorbid acid–base status, which may not show normal values of pH and P_aCO_2. The lowest amount of oxygen necessary to maintain an $S_aO_2 > 90$ per cent should be used. Careful attention should be paid to prevent the development of intrinsic PEEP (PEEPi). Techniques used to overcome PEEPi include treating airflow obstruction, reducing the respiratory rate to increase expiratory time, increasing peak flow to increase expiratory time, reducing tidal volume, and applying extrinsic PEEP.

Mechanical support of ventilation may also be done with non-invasive ventilation via a facial or nasal mask. The advantage of this approach is that endotracheal intubation might be avoided. The disadvantage is frequent patient intolerance and the loss of control of the airway.

Studies have shown reductions in the need for intubation, in-hospital mortality, and nosocomial infection rates when the therapy is applied to patients with moderate to severe acute exacerbations of COPD not yet needing intubation.[29,29a]

It is advisable to have a formal policy on the location at which it will be provided, the frequency of monitoring, and indications for advancement to conventional ventilation. It is our bias that non-invasive ventilation for respiratory failure be limited to the intensive care unit.

UPPER AIRWAY OBSTRUCTION

Acute or subacute upper airway obstruction is a serious, potentially fatal condition often confused with asthma or COPD. Although the most common cause appears to be foreign body aspiration, the list of differential diagnoses is broad. Iatrogenic complications resulting in upper airway obstruction have been reported.

Anatomy and physiology of the upper airway

The airway can be divided into three anatomic areas with different physiologic characteristics:

1 the extrathoracic upper airway down to the thoracic inlet;
2 the intrathoracic upper airways including the intrathoracic trachea and bronchi down to the level of the 2 mm airways; and
3 the small airways that are less than 2 mm in diameter.[30]

Upper airway obstructing lesions may be identified by flow-volume loops (Fig. 10.1). If Fig. 10.1a exemplifies a normal flow-volume loop, a variable extrathoracic obstruction typically seen during a maximal inspiratory effort is represented by Fig. 10.1b; a variable intrathoracic obstruction typically observed during a maximal expiratory effort is seen in Fig. 10.1c; a fixed upper airway obstruction seen in both inspiration and expiration is shown in Fig. 10.1d; and small airways obstruction is seen in Figure 10.1e.

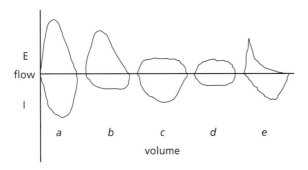

Figure 10.1 *(a) A normal flow-volume loop; (b) a variable extrathoracic obstruction typically seen during a maximal inspiratory effort; (c) a variable intrathoracic obstruction typically observed during a maximal expiratory effort; (d) a fixed upper airway obstruction seen in both inspiration and expiration; (e) a small airways obstruction.*

Differential diagnosis

A complete description of all of the causes of upper airway obstruction is beyond the scope of this chapter. We have limited ourselves to a discussion of the most common causes of this syndrome.

Foreign body aspiration

Aspiration of foreign bodies into the tracheobronchial tree occurs in adults as well as children. One common form in adults is acute food asphyxiation, also called the *café coronary* syndrome.[31] Risk factors for foreign body aspiration are old age, altered consciousness due to alcohol or drugs, poor dentition, Parkinson's disease, and institutionalization.[31] Since the upper airway may also be occluded by extrinsic compression, esophageal foreign bodies can compress the upper airway.[32]

Angioedema

Angioedema is characterized by transient episodes of painless, well-demarcated, non-pitting, asymmetric edema affecting the face, eyelids, lips, tongue, and mucous membranes. Severe upper airway obstruction occurs in about 20 per cent of patients with angioedema.[33,34] Allergic IgE-mediated reactions can have rapid onset of upper airway edema and may be associated with urticaria. Hereditary angioneurotic edema with deficiency of C1 esterase inhibitor may cause upper airway edema that progresses over several hours but typically has no urticaria. Acquired deficiency of C1 esterase inhibitor is seen in association with some hematologic malignancies. Non-IgE-mediated angioedema can be caused by many drugs, including aspirin, non-steroidal anti-inflammatory drugs (NSAIDs), angiotensin-converting enzyme (ACE) inhibitors, morphine, codeine, and iodinated contrast media. Angioedema occurs in 0.1–0.2 per cent of patients on ACE inhibitors, usually within hours of starting therapy, although there are reports of angioedema occurring 3 months or more after drug initiation.[35]

Vocal cord dysfunction syndrome

Patients suffering from vocal cord dysfunction syndrome demonstrate paradoxical movement of their vocal cords in inspiration.[36] The result of this movement is near-complete adduction of the cords during inspiration, leading to dyspnea and wheezing. A helpful indicator in identifying these patients is the absence of an increased alveolar to arterial oxygen tension gradient or $P_{(A-a)}O_2$. This syndrome is thought to be a conversion disorder in response to emotional distress or trauma.[37] These patients may be diagnosed by laryngoscopy performed during an attack. By directly visualizing the unanesthetized cords in an unsedated patient, the physician can see the cords closely during inspiration, thereby confirming the diagnosis.

Supraglottitis

Supraglottitis is an acute infection of the supraglottic region including the arytenoids, epiglottis, aryepiglottic folds, and posterior tongue. Supraglottitis should be suspected when a patient presents with a sore throat which is out of proportion to the severity of the pharyngitis seen. Occasionally respiratory distress, fever, drooling, and muffled voice can be seen. Diagnosis is made by directly visualizing the supraglottic area. Lateral neck radiographs are also helpful in the diagnosis.[38] In addition to *H. influenzae*, other causative organisms include

Streptococcus pneumoniae, group A or F *streptococcus, Staphylococcus aureus, Staphylococcus pyogenes,* and *Streptococcus viridans.*[39]

Ludwig's angina

Ludwig's angina is a cellulitis of the floor of the mouth and submandibular space characterized by bilateral submandibular swelling with posterior and superior displacement of the tongue. Symptoms of respiratory compromise occur in one fourth of patients.[40] The criteria for diagnosis are:

1 bilateral cellulitis without abscess;
2 a gangrenous serosanguinous infiltration with little or no pus;
3 involvement of connective tissues, fascia, and muscles, but not glandular structures; and
4 spread of cellulitis by continuity, not lymphatics.[40,41]

The most common predisposing condition is poor dental hygiene. Eighty-five per cent of patients have either tooth pain or a recent tooth extraction, most commonly the lower second or third molars.[40,42] Symptoms include restricted neck movement with neck swelling, pain, dysphagia, sore throat, drooling, and trismus.[40,41] The tongue is displaced posteriorly and superiorly and may be tender with a 'woody' consistency. Causative organisms include Streptococci, Staphylococci, and anaerobes. More than one organism is isolated in 50 per cent of cases. In patients with no dental source, *H. influenzae* should be considered.

Laryngotracheobronchitis (croup)

Croup is a common respiratory infection of children, with 80 per cent of cases occurring under the age of 4. Up to 15 per cent of children with croup require hospitalization, but fewer than 5 per cent require intubation.[43]

Iatrogenic complications affecting the airways

Endotracheal intubation can cause damage to the glottis, subglottis, and trachea. Estimates of the prevalence of damage to the larynx after intubation range from 63 to 94 per cent.[44,45] The more serious complication of laryngeal stenosis occurs in 6–12 per cent of instances.[45–48] Tracheotomy is associated with stomal stenosis from scarring. In adults, postextubation laryngeal edema occurs in 2–22 per cent of patients.[49–52] The use of low-pressure, high-volume cuffs has decreased the incidence of serious tracheal stenosis.

Despite the established safety record of transtracheal oxygen catheters, there have been reports of tracheal mucoid impactions leading to respiratory compromise.[53]

The overall prevalence of mucous balls is approximately 10 per cent.[53]

Diagnosis

A history of fever and chills, sore throat, frequent throat clearing, difficulty swallowing, recent intubation, weight loss, or voice change is consistent with upper airway obstruction. Similarly, physical findings such as fever, tonsillar exudate, cobblestoned pharyngeal mucosa, goiter, deviated trachea, wheezing, hoarseness, or severe obesity may be invaluable diagnostic clues. When high-pitched wheezing is heard best on inspiration, is loudest over the trachea, and is accentuated by increased flow, then extrathoracic upper airway obstruction should be strongly suspected.[54]

Data suggest that obstruction must narrow the tracheal lumen to less than 8 mm diameter (>80 per cent reduction of the area) before abnormalities can be recognized on a flow–volume loop.[55] Stridor at rest occurs when the lumen is 5 mm or less.[56]

Chest x-rays may identify tracheal deviation, compression, foreign bodies, or vascular abnormalities. Neck films performed with the head in extension during inspiration can be useful in differentiating between laryngotracheitis (croup) and epiglottitis. A lateral view of the neck may be helpful in detecting conditions that reduce the anteroposterior diameter of the airway. Computed tomography (CT) can image the upper airway with high spatial and contrast resolution and evaluate the mediastinum for cases of tumors and other lesions that may compress the airway, but cannot image the trachea along its long axis.[57,58] Magnetic resonance imaging (MRI) is recommended as the preferred technique for imaging the trachea of infants and young children with airway obstruction. Its advantages include multiplanar imaging, lack of ionizing radiation, good resolution without contrast injection, estimation of the length and degree of tracheal occlusions, and evaluation of mediastinal involvement.[58] Finally fiberoptic laryngoscopy and/or bronchoscopy can be used to visualize directly airway structures and obtain tissue for the histologic diagnosis of potentially malignant lesions.

Therapy

Treatments for upper airway obstruction can be divided into general measures designed to ensure patency of the airway, and specific measures aimed at correcting the underlying cause of the obstruction.

GENERAL MEASURES

Intubation and tracheotomy
Artificial airways are commonly used to obtain control of the airway and ensure ventilation.

While endotracheal intubation has traditionally been discouraged in pediatric cases of supraglottitis, it is the initial procedure of choice in most other conditions when the patency of the airway is in doubt.

Care should be taken to adequately ventilate and oxygenate the patient with a bag-valve-mask system prior to the attempt at intubation. The head tilt-chin lift maneuver may be helpful in this regard. An experienced person should be enlisted to perform intubation on patients with upper airway obstruction. An emergency tracheotomy or cricothyrotomy should be performed only as a last resort and only by a physician experienced with these procedures.

Helium–oxygen

A mixture of 80 per cent helium and 20 per cent oxygen, reduces airway resistance to turbulent flow and therefore decreases flow-resistive work. Helium–oxygen works primarily by reducing the Reynold's number, thereby allowing flow to become predominantly laminar.

Compared with turbulent flow, laminar flow allows greater flow rates for a given driving pressure.[59] Helium–oxygen is also available as a mixture of Helium 60 per cent, oxygen 40 per cent.

Racemic epinephrine

Racemic epinephrine administered via a nebulizer is effective in treating croup, with a resultant decrease in morbidity, mortality, and hospital stay.[43] Racemic epinephrine also is used in the empiric treatment of laryngeal edema. The treatments may need to be repeated frequently to avoid reintubation. Racemic epinephrine is usually ineffective and may be deleterious in the treatment of supraglottitis.[60]

Bronchoscopic dilatation

Dilatation of subglottic and tracheal stenosis can be performed with a rigid bronchoscope or by Jackson dilators. This technique is only a palliative measure, and recurrence of symptoms is expected in most patients.[61]

Laser therapy

Laser may be useful in treating malignant tracheobronchial lesions, excising web-like tracheal stenoses, and benign obstructing lesions.[61,62] Neodymium:yttrium-aluminum garnet (Nd-YAG) laser has the advantage of being transmissible through a fiber-optic system. In addition, it exhibits better photocoagulation and control of hemorrhage.

Surgery

Laryngotracheal resection and reconstruction has been used to treat tumors and stenoses of the trachea.[63,64]

SPECIFIC THERAPIES

Foreign body aspiration

The primary therapy for aspiration of a foreign body is removal of the object. Rigid bronchoscopy has a high success rate (98 per cent) for removing aspirated foreign bodies and remains the procedure of choice.[65] Because of the narrow lumen of the fiber-optic scope, its usefulness in removing foreign bodies is limited.

Angioedema

Treatment of hereditary angioneurotic edema consists of securing the airway and administering epinephrine, antihistamines, or corticosteroids. Replenishment of C1 esterase inhibitor with fresh-frozen plasma can be used as therapy of life-threatening angioedema. Replacement therapy with C1 inhibitor concentrate may be effective but is not available in the USA.[66] Both androgenic steroids and epsilon aminocaproic acid have been used for prophylaxis.[66]

Vocal cord dysfunction syndrome

The most important component in the management of vocal cord dysfunction is its recognition. This allows the physician to discontinue non-essential therapies such as steroids. In an acute attack, helium–oxygen mixture may help relieve the obstruction. After the acute attack has passed, the most important treatment is speech therapy with a trained speech pathologist.[67] Patients are taught techniques which will allow them to relax their laryngeal muscles during an attack and hopefully terminate the episode.

Supraglottitis

Treatment of supraglottitis begins with humidification of the air. Cultures of blood and occasionally of the epiglottis should be obtained. Antibiotics should be given intravenously for the first several days and a 10–14-day course completed with oral medication. Cefuroxime, cefotaxime, and ceftriaxone are the agents used most often because they cover the most common pathogens, particularly *H. influenzae*. All adults with supraglottitis should be admitted to an intensive care unit (ICU) for close observation. When conservative measures fail, endotracheal intubation is the procedure of choice. Tracheostomy is an acceptable alternative if intubation is unsuccessful. The use of steroids in supraglottitis is controversial.

Ludwig's angina

Treatment consists of maintaining the airway, antibiotic therapy based on likely organisms, and surgical exploration and drainage. Antibiotics should be given intravenously. Given the increased resistance to penicillin and the superior activity of metronidazole over clindamycin for *ekinella corrodens,* metronidazole should be considered the antibiotic of choice.[68–70] Mortality from Ludwig's angina has decreased from 50 per cent in the pre-antibiotic era to 8.5 per cent today.[40]

Croup

Treatment consists of mist therapy, nebulized racemic epinephrine, and corticosteroids. Results of two meta-analyses support the use of corticosteroids in the treatment of croup.[71,71a] Varying dosages were used in the studies analyzed. These reports indicated a reduction in morbidity, CO-interventions, frequency of intubation, and length of hospital stay.

Iatrogenic complications affecting the airways

There is little prospective information regarding the management of complications of long-term endotracheal intubation. Tracheotomy, laser therapy, and surgical resection of stenotic areas have all been employed. Medical therapy usually consists of removing the offending device whenever possible to relieve pressure on the tissues, and occasionally the administration of systemic corticosteroids. Inhaled steroids have also been used. There is no proven benefit to the use of steroids to prevent post-extubation laryngeal edema in children or adults.[49,51]

ACUTE INHALATION INJURIES

Acute inhalation injuries may result after the exposure to a variety of chemical inhalants. Toxic inhalants can be classified into four categories: (1) smoke inhalation; (2) irritant toxins; (3) asphyxiant toxins; and (4) systemic toxins. Presenting symptoms may vary from mild upper airway irritation to non-cardiogenic pulmonary edema (NCPE) and death. The management of acute inhalation injury presents even greater problems if the offending toxic agent is not known at the time of presentation. Furthermore, there are no large prospective studies of the management of most inhalation injuries. Therefore, recommendations are based on case reports and small series, making their validity questionable.

Smoke inhalation

Approximately 20 per cent of all hospitalized burn patients have smoke inhalation. This accounts for 50–70 per cent of all burn-related deaths.[72] Smoke inhalation causes injury three ways: (1) fire can consume oxygen leading to simple asphyxia; (2) thermal injury of the mucosa of the upper airways leading to upper airway obstruction; and (3) inhalation of toxic gases mixed with the smoke. Gases commonly found in smoke are acrolein, ammonia, chlorine, hydrogen chloride, nitrous dioxide, phosgene, and sulfur dioxide.[73]

The history of smoke inhalation may be obvious or it may be obscured by other features of the history. The physical examination may reveal singed facial hair, hoarseness, stridor, wheezing, and black or carbonaceous sputum.[74] Initial laboratory data should include arterial blood gases, carboxyhemoglobin level, CXR, and plasma cyanide level in cases with lactic acidosis and hypoxemia.[75]

Treatment of smoke inhalation includes supplemental oxygen at an F_iO_2 of 1.0 until carboxyhemoglobin levels are available. Management of carbon monoxide inhalation is discussed below. Bronchodilators and systemic corticosteroids are usually recommended if there are signs of upper airway obstruction. Systemic steroids are not recommended as a prophylactic measure. Since most of these patients have also sustained burns, attention should be paid to maintaining an adequate volume status and hemodynamic monitoring. Patients with significant smoke exposure should be observed for 24 hours because delayed symptoms may occur.

Toxic irritants

Irritant toxins include gases, mists, vapors, fumes, and dusts. Their effects are due in part to particle size and water solubility. Particles with a diameter of greater than 10 μm are usually filtered in the extrathoracic upper airway and therefore exhibit their effects in that area. Smaller particles may penetrate beyond the vocal cords and cause injury in more distal airways. Substances that are highly water soluble will have more effect on the upper airway, while water insoluble substances tend to affect the lower airways and lung parenchyma. High-level acute exposure to some irritants may cause the onset of a syndrome virtually indistinguishable from asthma.[76] This syndrome is treated in a manner identical to asthma. Otherwise, since there are no specific antidotes or treatments for individual substances, the treatment of all irritant exposures involves maintaining adequate oxygenation with supplemental oxygen and MV if necessary. Some common toxic irritants are listed below.

AMMONIA

Ammonia is highly water soluble and has a pungent odor. It is found in fertilizers, refrigerants, and the manufacturing process for dyes, plastics, and explosive. Inhalation of greater than 150 ppm may result in laryngeal edema, tracheitis, bronchoconstriction, mucus hypersecretion, airway obstruction and NCPE.[77–79]

CHLORINE

Chlorine is a dense, heavy, green–yellow gas with intermediate water solubility. Symptoms of exposure may include chest tightness, dyspnea, productive cough, mucosal irritation, bronchospasm, and NCPE. Corticosteroids have been used in cases of severe bronchospasm and airflow obstruction.

HYDROGEN CHLORIDE

Hydrogen chloride may be inhaled from its gaseous phase. It is highly water soluble. It is often found during the manufacturing of dyes, fertilizers, textiles, rubber, and processing of metal ores.[80] Exposure at almost any level may result in mucosal irritation.

OXIDES OF NITROGEN

The most common toxic oxides of nitrogen are nitrogen dioxide and nitrogen tetroxide. These substances have poor solubility in water. Exposure is often a result of exposure to jet fuel, diesel combustion, coal mining, electroplating, acetylene welding, and electroplating. Nitrogen dioxide is the offending agent in Silo-filler's disease.[81]

PHOSGENE

Phosgene (carbonyl chloride) is a poorly water-soluble gas that produces hydrochloric acid and carbon dioxide when it reacts with water in the body. Exposure occurs in the manufacturing of pesticides and dyes, and in occupations such as firefighting, paint stripping, and welding. Chest tightness, dyspnea, and non-productive cough occur several hours after exposure and may progress to NCPE and respiratory failure.[82,83]

SULFUR DIOXIDE

Sulfur dioxide is a highly water-soluble gas found in the smelting of ores, combustion of fossil fuels, paper manufacturing, and winemaking. Low-level exposure results in conjunctival and upper airway irritation and edema. Exposure to concentrations > 50 ppm may cause damage throughout the respiratory tract. Symptoms include cough, mucus secretion, dyspnea, bronchoconstriction, and NCPE.[84,85]

Asphyxiant toxins

Asphyxiant toxins cause adverse effects two ways: (1) by displacing oxygen from the inspired gas; and (2) by blocking oxidative intracellular reactions by binding hemoglobin or blocking cytochrome oxidase function.

CARBON MONOXIDE

Carbon monoxide poisoning causes 3500 deaths in the USA each year. It acts both by displacing oxygen on hemoglobin and by impairing oxidative phosphorylation by binding cytochrome oxidase.[86] Carbon monoxide bound to hemoglobin creates carboxyhemoglobin. Carboxyhemoglobin levels of 10–20 per cent may cause headaches, tinnitus, disinhibition, and nausea; levels between 20 and 40 per cent can cause weakness and depressed mental status; and levels of > 40 per cent may lead to death.

The normal elimination half-life of carbon monoxide at sea level is 4 hours. Supplemental oxygen at F_iO_2 1.0 can reduce the elimination half-life to 80 minutes, while hyperbaric oxygen can reduce it to 25 minutes. Therefore, mild carbon monoxide exposures should be treated with oxygen at F_iO_2 of 1.0, while severe exposures and all patients that present with cardiac or neurologic symptoms should receive hyperbaric oxygen.[87]

METHANE

Methane exposure is seen most often in coal mining. Methane must make up at least 85 per cent of the inspired air to have toxic effects. Treatment includes removal from the exposure area and supplemental oxygen.

HYDROGEN CYANIDE

Exposure to hydrogen cyanide may occur during photographic development, hardening of steel, electroplating, and burning of polyurethane and nitrocellulose. This gas is rapidly absorbed through the skin and the respiratory tract. Exposure to > 50 ppm may result in tachycardia, tachypnea, dizziness, and headache.[88] More intense exposures cause lethargy, seizures, and respiratory failure. A hallmark of hydrogen cyanide exposure is lactic acidosis with an anion gap and hypoxemia that is difficult to correct with high F_iO_2.

Amyl nitrite is an antidote for cyanide toxicity. One amyl nitrite pearl should be inhaled for 30 seconds per minute, with a new pearl every 3–4 minutes until intravenous (iv) access is established. This should be followed by iv sodium nitrite. The dose for adults is 300 mg in 100 mL saline over no less than 5 minutes. Sodium nitrite is then followed by sodium thiosulfate.[89] Adults receive 12.5 g initial dose and 1 g per hour for 24 hours in a continuous infusion. An alternative treatment is hydroxocobalamine.[90]

HYDROGEN SULFIDE

Hydrogen sulfide is produced in volcanic gases, coal mines, natural hot springs, leather tanning, rubber vulcanizing, and during anaerobic degradation of organic material in sewage and petrochemicals. Exposure of < 50 ppm produces irritation of the upper airway and conjunctiva. Exposure to higher concentrations leads to tissue hypoxia. Treatment is similar to that of hydrogen cyanide, with antidotal therapy given with amyl nitrite and sodium nitrite.[91] It is also crucial to provide adequate amounts of supplemental oxygen.

Systemic toxins

The large surface area of the respiratory tract can absorb toxins that have a systemic effect without having any localized pulmonary toxicity. Two examples of this are metal fume fever and polymer fume fever.[92] The pathology and mechanism of injury remain poorly understood. Symptoms of fever, chills, malaise are self-limited and take 24–48 hours to resolve. No specific therapy is available.

ACUTE PULMONARY EMBOLISM

The diagnosis and treatment of pulmonary embolism (PE) remains one of the most difficult challenges in acute pulmonary medicine. Pulmonary embolism has been estimated to be the sole or major contributing cause of death in 15 per cent of all adults dying in acute care hospitals.[93] It has been estimated that venous thromboembolism is clinically suspected over 600 000 times each year in the USA, and that there are 600 000 clinically significant cases of the disease occurring, but that it is diagnosed and treated only 260 000 times each year.[93,94] Only 30 per cent of patients with major PE at autopsy are suspected to have this before death.[95] Despite this, we know from the work of Anderson *et al.* that physicians apply deep venous thrombosis (DVT) prophylaxis in an irregular manner, and that only a minority of patients with indications for prophylaxis actually receive it.[96]

Risk factors

The development of VTE is thought to require the presence of the classic set of conditions known as 'Virchow's triad'. These include stasis, hypercoagulability, and vascular injury. Therefore, risk factors for VTE normally produce at least one or more of the conditions described by Virchow. Table 10.1 lists the generally accepted risk factors for the development of VTE.

Table 10.1 *Risk factors for the development of venous thromboembolism (VTE)*

History of VTE
Immobilization
Recent major surgery
Stroke
Estrogen use
Recent childbirth
Malignancy
Trauma to lower extremities (including fracture of the hip)
Age greater than 40 years
Congestive heart failure
Multiple trauma

In the absence of one of the described risk factors, a history of prior VTE may indicate an inherited disorder of coagulation, the most common of which is the factor V Leiden mutation. In addition, the results of a recent multivariate analysis indicate that obesity, cigarette smoking, and hypertension may also predispose to the development of VTE in women.[97]

Diagnosis

No historical or physical findings are sensitive or specific enough to confirm a diagnosis of PE on their own. Virtually all of the common physical findings in PE (tachypnea, hemoptysis, leg swelling, crackles) are non-specific. On the other hand, most patients with acute PE show one of three syndromes: (1) unexplained dyspnea; (2) pulmonary infarction with pleuritic chest pain and hemoptysis; and (3) circulatory collapse. Among patients who survive long enough to undergo evaluation, the syndrome of pulmonary infarction appears to be the most common.[98] There is no clearly established method to identify which patients with these syndromes warrant further evaluation for PE. The impact of various common tests has been looked at in this regard. Arterial blood gas analysis is typically abnormal, with an elevated alveolar–arterial oxygen tension gradient and respiratory alkalosis.[99] The electrocardiogram (ECG) may show various patterns including sinus tachycardia, an $S_1Q_3T_3$ pattern, anterior T-wave inversion, right bundle branch block, peripheral low voltage, and a pulmonary P wave.[100] The CXR is abnormal in 84 per cent of cases, with findings such as atelectasis, pleural effusion, pleural-based opacity, decreased pulmonary vascularity, and pulmonary edema all being described.[101] However, all of these findings are very non-specific and no formal criteria for their use in the diagnosis of PE have been established. Therefore, the clinical decision-making process of the physician must employ the results of these tests, the presence of risk factors for VTE, and the presence of a typical syndrome of PE in deciding which patients to evaluate for possible PE.

The first test recommended in the specific evaluation of suspected pulmonary embolism is the ventilation–perfusion scan. A six-view scan demonstrating normal or nearly normal perfusion essentially rules out the diagnosis. Multiple segmental or larger perfusion defects without corresponding ventilation defects leads to an interpretation of 'high probability' and make the diagnosis of PE very likely. Any other reading leaves the diagnosis in question. There is a 12–26 per cent likelihood of PE in the 'low probability' group and a 14–33 per cent chance in the 'intermediate' or 'indeterminate' group.[102,103] The fact that there is such an overlap in probability between these two groups makes their distinction clinically irrelevant. Patients in both these categories should proceed to non-invasive evaluation of the proximal deep veins of the legs. The discovery of a DVT by duplex ultrasound of the legs is an indication for anticoagulation. Patients with a negative duplex examination and a low clinical suspicion of PE should probably not have further testing. Patients with a negative duplex examination and a high or uncertain clinical probability of PE are usually sent for pulmonary arteriography. An alternative approach in out-patients with uncertain or high clinical probability would be to perform serial duplex examinations of the lower extremities and to withhold treatment unless a thrombosis of a proximal leg vein is identified. The validity of this approach in critically ill patients is unknown.

Other studies have been advocated for inclusion in the diagnostic approach to PE. Echocardiography, helical CT, the d-dimer test, MRI, and artificial neural networks have all been reported to be effective in certain circumstances. Transesophageal echocardiogram appears to be effective in detecting large thrombi in the main or right pulmonary artery, and in detecting significant right heart dysfunction associated with suspected emboli.[104] Spiral CT may also be useful, with a sensitivity of 87–90 per cent and a specificity approaching 95 per cent.[105,106] However, spiral CT is also more accurate for diagnosing proximal PE and its accuracy decreases as the search moves to the more peripheral arteries. We have developed the practice of using the spiral CT as the first test in patients with COPD and those on mechanical ventilation. Ventilation-perfusion scanning has been found to be less accurate in patients with COPD.[106a] The D-dimer test may help in diagnosing the presence of thrombus in the vasculature, but it cannot localize the thrombus and the assay required is not the same assay available at many institutions today. MRI is currently under investigation for this indication, but its role is yet to be defined. Artificial neural networks are promising for their potential in the long term, but are not yet in use in clinical medicine.

Therapy

Medical and surgical treatments have been used for the treatment of pulmonary embolism.

HEPARIN AND WARFARIN

The standard initial treatment for acute PE is intravenous unfractionated heparin.

An initial bolus of 5000–10 000 units is appropriate, and is often calculated as a weight-based dose with approximately 80 units/kg administered as an iv bolus followed by a maintenance iv drip at approximately 18 units/hour. The usual goal is to achieve an activated partial thromboplastin time (aPTT) > 1.5 × control levels. Alternatively, recent recommendations have advocated maintaining a therapeutic heparin level of 0.2–0.4 μ/mL by protamine titration, or 0.3–0.6 μ/mL by an amidolytic anti-factor Xa assay.[106a]

Since the main problem with iv heparin therapy is the inability to achieve therapeutic levels rapidly leading to recurrence, rather than overdose leading to pathologic bleeding, it is important to check an aPTT 4–6 hours after the bolus administration. The dose of iv heparin

can then be adjusted according to a nomogram such as the one developed by Hull et al.[107]

In the absence of contraindications, warfarin sodium should be begun either simultaneous with heparin or on the second day of heparin therapy.

The duration that heparin should be continued following the initiation of warfarin therapy is not completely agreed upon.[108–110] In some cases a 4–5-day course is adequate, while in cases of major PE, especially those with large residual iliofemoral vein thrombosis, a 7–10-day course has been advocated. Warfarin is given in a dose of 10 mg for the first 2–3 days and then adjusted according to the international normalized ratio (INR). Administration of warfarin with heparin may reduce the amount of heparin necessary to achieve a therapeutic level. Warfarin is continued for at least 3 months for a first episode of VTE, and longer if the risk factor for the development of VTE persists. Low-molecular-weight heparins (LMWH) are also being used increasingly in the management of VTE. The potential advantages of their use include: comparable or superior efficacy; comparable or superior safety; superior bioavailability; convenient administration; lack of need for phlebotomy and laboratory monitoring; and ability to treat many patients at home.[111] However, the clinical superiority of LMWH in treating acute PE has yet to be convincingly demonstrated. This issue is important, given current large differences in the cost of treating patients with LMWH as opposed to unfractionated heparin.

THROMBOLYTIC THERAPY

Streptokinase, urokinase, and tissue plasminogen activator (tPA) have all been used in the treatment of PE. Thrombolytic agents produce more rapid lysis of clots and in some cases may improve right ventricular function more rapidly than heparin. Accepted regimens for the management of PE are shown in Table 10.2.

Table 10.2 *Thrombolytic therapy regimens for the management of pulmonary embolism*

All regimens	Stop heparin and start thrombolytic infusion when activated partial prothrombin time (aPTT) ≤ 1.5 × control
Streptokinase	250 000 IU loading dose; 100 000 IU/hour maintenance dose for 24 hours
tPA	100 mg over 2 hours
All regimens	Restart heparin without a loading dose or with a small loading dose when aPTT or thrombin time is ≤ 1.5 × control.

tPA = tissue plasminogen activator.

An improvement in clinical outcomes using thrombolytic therapy has not been documented in any randomized, prospective trial. A recent retrospective survey suggests that some clinical benefit may exist, but that needs to be further documented.[112] Patients treated with thrombolytic therapy appear to have a higher risk of bleeding complications. Table 10.3 indicates the contraindications to the use of thrombolytic therapy in PE.[113]

Table 10.3 *Contraindications to thrombolytic therapy*[113]

Major internal bleeding in the previous 6 months
Intracranial or intraspinal disease
Operation or biopsy in the preceding 10 days
Hypertension (greater than 200 mm Hg systolic or 110 mm Hg diastolic)
Active infective endocarditis
Pericarditis
Aneurysm (aortic or cerebrovascular)
Presence of a bleeding disorder

At this time, there are no universally accepted guidelines for the use of thrombolytics in the management of acute PE.

> However, many clinicians would favor thrombolysis in cases of major acute PE with syncope or hypotension when none of the contraindications listed in Table 10.3 exist.

Some physicians also advocate the use of thrombolytics, in the absence of contraindications, when there is evidence of severe right ventricular compromise. While there is some preliminary evidence supporting this approach, more work is needed before this can be recommended as a standard of care.[112] In addition, the use of thrombolytics for patients with acute PE and underlying cardiac or respiratory disease has also been proposed, but requires further investigation.

VENA CAVAL INTERRUPTION

Inferior vena cava (IVC) filtering devices are sometimes used to prevent embolization of clot from DVT of the lower extremity.

> The primary indications for the placement of an IVC filter are: (1) the contraindication to anticoagulant therapy or a complication of such therapy; and (2) the failure of anticoagulant therapy despite achieving an adequate anticoagulant level for an adequate period of time.

In the latter circumstance, the recurrence of PE needs to be documented because respiratory symptoms may often be mistaken as recurrent PE in patients receiving anticoagulation.[108] A recent randomized, prospective trial looked at the use of an IVC filter plus heparin versus heparin alone. This study revealed a slight reduction in the rate of subsequent PE over the first 12 days, but no reduction in the overall rate of PE over 2 years, an increase in the rate of development of subsequent DVT, and no change in the mortality rate over 12 days or 2 years.[114] Therefore, the routine use of an IVC filter in that circumstance cannot be recommended. Controversial indications for IVC filter use include: major PE with cardiovascular instability; adjunctive therapy for patients undergoing embolectomy; prophylaxis against PE in patients with exceptionally high risk of VTE when there is a contraindication to anticoagulation; and the presence of a large free-floating caval thrombus. The effectiveness of IVC filters in these circumstances is unproven. In addition, although current filter designs are thought to be safe, some complications, such as venous insufficiency, filter migration, insertion site DVT, and IVC obstruction are still thought to occur in a significant number of patients.[115] Therefore, we would only insert an IVC filter in these circumstances when there is a documented clot in the deep veins of the leg or in the IVC and alternative therapy is deemed to be inadequate.

PULMONARY EMBOLECTOMY

Pulmonary embolectomy is rarely performed. One recent report indicated it was used in only 1.1 per cent of patients with PE and cardiogenic shock or cardiac arrest.[116] Some have speculated that there is no place for embolectomy in the management of PE.[117] Others take a more positive view of its role.[118]

> If it is to be used, the criteria proposed by Weg should be applied to the selection process: (1) angiographically documented massive PE; (2) shock despite heparin therapy and resuscitative efforts; (3) failure or contraindication of thrombolytic therapy; (4) availability of an experienced open heart surgery team.[119]

Even when these criteria are met, the decision must be made on a case by case basis. The mortality for patients who have had a cardiac arrest is as high as 94 per cent in uncontrolled series.[120] Since centers with poor results are unlikely to report case series, even these numbers may exaggerate the success rate. There are no data which prospectively compare the results of embolectomy to alternative treatments.

MASSIVE HEMOPTYSIS

Introduction

Hemoptysis is the expectoration of blood from the airways.[121-126] There is no universally accepted definition of

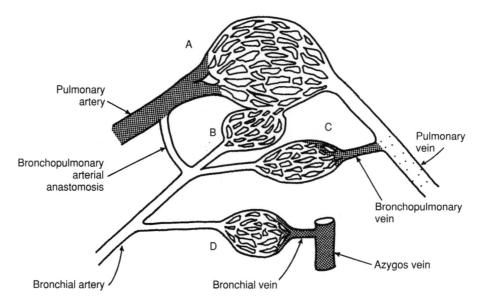

Figure 10.2 *The relationship between the pulmonary and the bronchial circulation. Labels A–D indicate different levels of interrelationship between the pulmonary and bronchial circulations. Area A illustrates the expected communication between the pulmonary artery, capillaries, and pulmonary vein. Area B reveals communication between the bronchial artery and the pulmonary vein through the pulmonary capillaries. Area C demonstrates communication between the bronchial artery and the pulmonary vein through bronchopulmonary capillaries. Area D shows the expected communication between the bronchial artery and the systemic venous circulation through the bronchial capillaries. (Reproduced with permission from Murray JF,* The normal lung *2nd edn, 1986. Philadelphia: W B Saunders Company)*

massive hemoptysis. Therefore, we have elected to define massive hemoptysis as the expectoration of 600 mL of blood from the lower respiratory tract over a 24-hour period. The risk of death from hemoptysis correlates strongly with the amount of blood expectorated, the rate of bleeding, the amount of blood retained within the lungs, and the underlying pulmonary reserve regardless of the cause of bleeding.[121,122,124,127-130]

Anatomy

The lungs are supplied by both the bronchial arterial circulation and the pulmonary circulation (Fig. 10.2). The bronchial circulation acts as a nutritional source for the trachea and major bronchi, esophagus, pericardium, hilar lymph nodes, and visceral pleura.[131] Most individuals have 1 bronchial artery to the right lung originating from the intercostal arteries and 2 bronchial arteries to the left lung originating from the thoracic aorta. In a small percentage of people the anterior spinal artery originates from the bronchial artery.[132] The larger bronchial arteries also have frequent anatomic variants.[132] The bronchial circulation plays an important role in hemoptysis by virtue of its intimate association with the tracheobronchial tree. Because the arterioles are under systemic pressure, they have a tendency to bleed profusely when airways are diseased. In contrast, bleeding originates from a pulmonary artery bed in fewer than 10 per cent of patients with massive hemoptysis.[133-136]

Etiology

Conceptually it is useful to divide causes of hemoptysis into six general categories. A limited number of examples are included here with each category for the sake of illustration:

1. tracheobronchial disorders, such as tracheobronchitis and bronchogenic carcinoma;
2. cardiovascular disorders, such as pulmonary embolism and mitral stenosis;
3. hematologic disorders such as therapy with anticoagulants and disseminated intravascular coagulation;
4. localized pulmonary parenchymal disorders, such as pneumonia or pulmonary tuberculosis;
5. diffuse pulmonary parenchymal diseases such as Goodpasture's syndrome and Wegener's granulomatosis;
6. other causes, including iatrogenic conditions due to bronchoscopy or pulmonary artery catheterization and idiopathic hemoptysis.

Although virtually any cause of hemoptysis may cause massive bleeding, most cases of massive hemoptysis arise from a limited number of causes. The common causes of massive hemoptysis are listed in Table 10.4.

Table 10.4 *Causes of massive hemoptysis*

Lung abscess
Mycetoma
Histoplasmosis
Pulmonary tuberculosis
Bronchogenic carcinoma
Endobronchial metastatic carcinoma
Bronchiectasis
Arteriovenous malformations
Cystic fibrosis
Anticoagulant therapy
Tracheoarterial fistula
Wegener's granulomatosis
Goodpasture's syndrome
Systemic lupus erythematosus
Post-lung biopsy
Pulmonary artery rupture
Chest tube-induced lung injury
Thoracic trauma

Diagnosis

A careful history and physical examination are essential. Important historical points include the patients' age, their history of tobacco use, their history of prior cardiac or pulmonary disease, the presence of hematuria, the duration of hemoptysis, and their travel history. The physical examination is useful in excluding upper airway sources of bleeding. It may also give clues to the presence of underlying cardiac disease, such as mitral stenosis. The presence of clubbing suggests the presence of either a chronic inflammatory disease of the chest, or chronic vascular disease (including cardiac disease) of long standing.

Chest x-rays are also generally obtained. In one series of patients, physical examination and CXR did not produce diagnostic information in 55–60 per cent of patients studied.[137] In another study, 46 per cent of patients had no relevant abnormality detected on the chest film.[138] At present there are no definitive data describing the value of the CXR in massive hemoptysis. Until such information is available, it is conventional to obtain PA and lateral views of the chest in these cases.

Bronchoscopy is considered to be the procedure of choice for the localization of bleeding in patients with massive hemoptysis. Bronchoscopy is able to make a specific diagnosis of diseases of the proximal airway, and is able to localize bleeding to an anatomic location in many other cases. Bronchoscopy performed during an episode of bleeding has a significantly better chance of diagnosing the cause than bronchoscopy performed after the bleeding has stopped. While many surgeons advocate the use of the rigid bronchoscope, many pulmonologists favor the flexible bronchoscope.[121,122,139,140] Advantages of the rigid bronchoscope include better control of the airway and a larger lumen of the scope.

This latter feature provides for better suctioning and allows the introduction of packing materials for treatment.[140] Advantages of the flexible bronchoscope include: (1) no need for general anesthesia; (2) improved access to more peripheral airways; and (3) the procedure can be done in a variety of locations and does not require availability of an operating room. Flexible bronchoscopy for massive hemoptysis should be performed with the patient intubated to control the airway if bleeding becomes overwhelming. In addition, the presence of the endotracheal tube facilitates removal and reintroduction of the bronchoscope if the suction channel becomes obstructed with clotted blood.

Computerized tomography of the chest should be obtained when a strong pretest suspicion of carcinoma is not substantiated by the results of bronchoscopy.[138] In addition, high-resolution CT has largely replaced bronchography and is currently the method of choice for the diagnosis of bronchiectasis. In one study, high-resolution CT was found to be 100 per cent sensitive for cystic and varicose bronchiectasis and 94 per cent sensitive for cylindrical bronchiectasis.[141] Its specificity was 100 per cent regardless of the type of bronchiectasis.[141]

When neither bronchoscopy nor CT can determine a bleeding source, angiography of the pulmonary or the bronchial vessels may be performed. As described above, massive hemoptysis is typically associated with bleeding from the bronchial circulation. However, if pulmonary embolism is a consideration, or if bronchial arteriography fails to demonstrate a site of bleeding, the pulmonary circulation may need to be studied. Limited angiography may be employed if bronchoscopy or CT has been able to localize the bleeding partially to a particular lobe or segment.

Management

The primary goals in the acute management of massive hemoptysis are maintenance of airway patency and control of bleeding. Secondary goals are to determine the site and the cause of the bleeding as well as the patient's ability to withstand surgery, if necessary. Death due to massive hemoptysis is usually a result of asphyxiation and not exsanguination. Therefore, measures aimed at ensuring the adequacy of gas exchange take on primary importance.

GENERAL MEASURES

A patient with massive hemoptysis should be monitored in an ICU. The patient should be evaluated by both a thoracic surgeon and a pulmonary physician soon after presentation. Adequate intravenous access should be ensured by placing at least two large-bore peripheral intravenous lines, or central lines if peripheral access is not available. Blood should be typed and cross-matched and available for transfusion.

Cough suppression and sedation should be avoided since they may result in airway compromise. In addition, anticoagulant medications should be discontinued and their effects reversed pharmacologically, if necessary, except in the special case of hemoptysis due to pulmonary embolism. If the side of the origin of bleeding is known, the patient should be placed in the lateral decubitus position with that side down to prevent flow of blood into the 'good' lung. If bleeding is uncontrollable and has potential to compromise the airway, the patient should be electively intubated with a #8 or larger endotracheal tube. A variety of techniques have been used to try to stop or slow the bleeding. There are no randomized, controlled data to support the use of one method over another. Therefore, only limited recommendations are made here.

EPINEPHRINE

Topical epinephrine has been used in a 1:20 000 concentration to treat hemoptysis after transbronchial biopsy. However, its efficacy as a vasoconstrictive agent in massive hemoptysis is untested.[142]

COLD SALINE

Bronchial lavage with an average of 500 mL normal saline at 4°C by rigid bronchoscopy arrested bleeding due to massive hemoptysis in all 23 patients reported.[143–145]

BALLOON TAMPONADE

Endobronchial balloon tamponade, using balloon-tipped Fogarty catheters has effectively created prolonged periods of stability for patients with massive hemoptysis.[146–148] The balloon must be deflated every 12 hours to avoid necrosis of the bronchial wall.

SINGLE LUNG VENTILATION

Selective lung intubation and unilateral ventilation with a double-lumen endotracheal tube can be used. These tubes should be placed only by experienced operators. The advantage of intubation with a double-lumen tube is that the non-affected lung may be ventilated normally while preventing the overflow of blood from the affected lung. The disadvantage of unilateral ventilation is that right to left shunting through the vessels of the non-ventilated lung may result in worsened hypoxemia.[149] Selective intubation of the right lung also carries the risk of occluding the right upper lobe orifice.

BRONCHIAL ARTERY EMBOLIZATION (BAE)

Occlusion of the offending bronchial artery segment can be highly effective in controlling massive hemoptysis. Reported success rates for this procedure range between 73 and 94 per cent.[150] The most significant complication of BAE is embolization of the spinal artery. This complication has been seen in 5 per cent of cases of BAE.[151] BAE is considered as first-line therapy for patients with massive hemoptysis due to tuberculosis.[150]

PULMONARY ARTERY TAMPONADE

A pulmonary arteriole ruptured by a Swan–Ganz catheter may be isolated from the rest of the pulmonary circulation by the catheter balloon itself. This technique involves deflating the catheter, pulling it back approximately 5 cm and reinflating. The catheter is then allowed to migrate out and occlude the affected segment of vessel. This treatment is a temporizing measure and should be combined with single-lung ventilation and a more definitive long-term treatment. All patients who survive such a complication should have pulmonary arteriography to localize the injury and evaluate for a possible pseudoaneurysm.[152]

ENDOSCOPIC LASER

Laser has been used to stop massive hemoptysis in patients with endobronchial cancers. This has been reported to be successful in 90 per cent of cases, although bleeding typically recurs within a few weeks.[153]

SURGERY

Surgery is used to treat causes of hemoptysis for which there is no alternative treatment, such as a tracheoarterial fistula. In addition, surgery is often used as a nonspecific therapy for massive hemoptysis once the general anatomical location of the bleeding source has been identified. While there have been no randomized trials comparing surgical resection with medical therapy, several consistent findings have emerged from nonrandomized series. Morbidity rates associated with surgical resection range from 23 to 54 per cent. Mortality rates show a similar wide range, from 10 to 50 per cent.[121,126,128] There is an increased risk of respiratory failure in patients with a predicted postoperative FEV_1 of less than 800 mL. Inoperable patients with massive hemoptysis have a higher mortality rate than operable patients whether they are treated medically or surgically.[122,127,128,140,143]

OTHER THERAPIES

Entities such as Goodpasture's syndrome, systemic lupus erythematosis, and Wegener's granulomatosis require specific therapy directed at their pathophysiologic mechanism. Description of these treatments is beyond the scope of this chapter.

ACUTE RESPIRATORY DISTRESS SYNDROME

Ashbaugh *et al.* first described cases of 'acute respiratory distress in adults' in 1967.[154] It is likely that this syndrome was first recognized in the 1960s because advances in medical care allowed for the resuscitation of patients who would previously have died of their initial illness or injury. Although this syndrome was referred to as 'adult respiratory distress syndrome' for several years, the Consensus Committee of the ATS and European Society of Intensive Care Medicine officially recommended a reversion back to the name 'acute respiratory distress syndrome' (ARDS) in recognition of the fact that this same process occurs in children as well as adults.[155]

Etiology

Acute respiratory distress syndrome is normally associated with a predisposing condition. These are divided into *direct* or *indirect* associations (or causes). While the *direct* associations are so named because of the direct contact of a noxious substance with the lung, it has been hard to describe the causative feature of many of the *indirect* causes. The terms *direct* and *indirect* do not in any way describe the strength of the associations. Sepsis, the condition most commonly associated with ARDS, is an *indirect* cause. Table 10.5 is a listing of the conditions associated with ARDS.

Table 10.5 *Conditions associated with the acute respiratory distress syndrome*

Direct association
Aspiration
Near-drowning
Toxic gas inhalation
Pulmonary infection

Indirect association
Sepsis
Shock
Lung trauma
Head trauma
Fat embolism
Burn
Drug ingestion
Pancreatitis
Multiple blood transfusions
Leukoagglutinin reaction
Eclampsia
Air embolism
Amniotic fluid embolism
High altitude
Neurogenic (other than trauma)
Contrast media
Protamine
Diffuse alveolar hemorrhage

Pathology and pathophysiology

The major sites of injury in patients with ARDS are the endothelial and the epithelial barriers. Cytokines such as tumor necrosis factor α (TNF-α) and interleukin 1β (IL-1β) are involved with inciting the inflammatory response that leads to this damage. In the lungs of ARDS patients, the balance between inflammation and anti-inflammatory systems is tipped toward the propagation of inflammation. The pathophysiologic response can be divided into two phases dated from the onset of the inciting event.

The *exudative phase* (days 1–7) consists of interstitial swelling, patchy intra-alveolar edema, alveolar hemorrhage, endothelial cell damage, and basement membrane disruption, all of which contribute to the development of hyaline membranes which line the alveoli of affected areas. This process is heterogeneous and areas of diseased lung sit juxtaposed with relatively preserved areas.

The *fibroproliferative phase* (days 7–14) is the beginning of the repair process in the aftermath of acute injury. Type II alveolar lining cells, which are not terminally differentiated cells that normally serve as surfactant producers, begin to differentiate into Type I cells to repopulate the alveoli. Traditionally, it has been thought that survivors of ARDS separate into two groups during this stage. One group goes on to normal repair of the lungs, while the other group develops fibrosis. Newer information suggests that fibrogenesis may begin at an earlier stage, perhaps as early as 1–2 days after the inciting event.[156] The events that determine which of those groups an individual patient will be in are not known, although medical treatment and iatrogenic injury may play a major role.

These pathologic changes lead to a variety of physiologic abnormalities. Patients exhibit hypoxemia due to right to left shunting that may approach 50 per cent of the cardiac output. Ventilation–perfusion mismatching also plays a role in hypoxemia. There is compensatory hypoxic vasoconstriction and resultant pulmonary hypertension. The dead space to tidal volume ratio may be increased, reducing alveolar ventilation and leading to CO_2 retention in some cases. Total respiratory system static compliance (C_{stat}) is reduced and peak inspiratory and plateau pressures on MV are increased. Oxygen consumption by respiratory muscles increases dramatically. Despite these changes, there is no characteristic hemodynamic pattern associated with ARDS, and the measurements found with pulmonary artery catheterization generally reflect the underlying disease state and the stage of fluid resuscitation.

Clinical features

The clinical features of ARDS reflect the derangements of physiology associated with severe acute lung injury.

The Consensus Committee also developed definitions for acute lung injury and ARDS that reflect the clinical situation. They defined *acute lung injury* as 'a syndrome of inflammation and increased permeability that is associated with a constellation of clinical, radiographic, and physiologic abnormalities that cannot be explained by, but may coexist with, left atrial or pulmonary capillary hypertension'. They defined ARDS as 'the most severe form of acute lung injury'. Tables 10.6 and 10.7 describe the criteria for the diagnosis of ARDS and acute lung injury.

Table 10.6 *Criteria for acute lung injury*

1. Impaired oxygenation – P_aO_2/F_IO_2 ratio $\leqslant$ 300 (whatever the PEEP)
2. Bilateral pulmonary infiltrates on chest x-ray
3. Pulmonary artery occlusion pressure $\leqslant$ 18 mm Hg or no clinical findings suggestive of increased left atrial pressure (congestive heart failure and acute lung injury may coexist, however)

PEEP = positive end-expiratory pressure.

Table 10.7 *Criteria for the acute respiratory distress syndrome*

1. Impaired oxygenation – P_aO_2/F_IO_2 ratio $\leqslant$ 200 (whatever the PEEP)
2. Bilateral pulmonary infiltrates on chest x-ray
3. Pulmonary artery occlusion pressure $\leqslant$ 18 mm Hg or no clinical findings suggestive of increased left atrial pressure (congestive heart failure and acute lung injury may coexist, however)

PEEP = positive end-expiratory pressure.

The most commonly used diagnostic scheme in clinical medicine includes the presence of an associated condition, hypoxemia, bilateral infiltrates, reduced C_{stat}, and no cardiac cause. Lung biopsy is rarely indicated, but when it is performed it shows changes of diffuse alveolar damage, endothelial and epithelial cell necrosis, and hyaline membranes.

Therapy

There is no specific therapy to modify the inflammatory or altered permeability components of ARDS. However, ARDS remains a fertile area of investigation in critical care. Multiple therapies have been tried and failed to show a clinical benefit in the past 15 years. Despite these failures, the mortality rate for patients with ARDS decreased from 60 per cent to approximately 40 per cent in the 1990s.[157,158] It is presumed that improvements in supportive care have led to this improvement in outcome.

Because a large number of therapies have demonstrated advantages in preliminary reports only to fail to show clinical benefits when subjected to more rigorous testing, a great effort is being made to apply the principles of evidence-based medicine rigorously in analyzing and recommending treatments for ARDS. One common approach to evaluating the quality of evidence supporting various interventions in ARDS was proposed by Kollef and Schuster.[159]

QUALITY OF THE EVIDENCE

- Level 1: Randomized, prospective, controlled investigations of ARDS.
- Level 2: Non-randomized, concurrent cohort investigations, historical control investigations, and case series of ARDS.
- Level 3: Randomized prospective controlled trials of sepsis or other conditions with potential application to ARDS.
- Level 4: Case reports of ARDS.

GRADE OF RECOMMENDATION

A: Supported by at least two Level 1 investigations.
B: Supported by one Level 1 investigation.
C: Supported by Level 2 investigations.
D: Supported by Level 3 investigations.
Ungraded: No clinical investigations.

Using these guidelines, the following interventions would receive a recommendation of Grade B or better: (1) early fluid restriction and diuresis;[160] (2) corticosteroids applied during the fibroproliferative phase;[161] and (3) small tidal volumes (6 mL/kg).[161a]

Interventions, such as prone positioning, inverse ratio ventilation, and nitric oxide use are supported by no better than Level 2 studies, and therefore can be given only weak Grade 3 recommendations for use. Some may even suggest that these techniques now deserve a Grade B recommendation *against* their routine use, similar to that earned by high-dose corticosteroid use, prophylactic PEEP, extracorporeal membrane oxygenation, extracorporeal CO_2 removal, high-frequency ventilation, and exogenous surfactant administration. Further use of these latter modalities should be limited to well-constructed clinical trials or cases with significant extenuating circumstances. Finally, interventions, such as prone positioning, application of PEEP just greater than the lower inflection point, nitric oxide, *N*-acetylcysteine, and various substances active on the cytokine cascade of systemic inflammatory response syndrome (SIRS) are in the process of serious investigation and may be available for more definitive recommendations in the near future.

We adhere to strategies employing techniques with the best supporting evidence, as described above. In addition, general lung-protective strategies with application of PEEP and maintenance of lower plateau pressures may be helpful. We avoid excessive reliance on arterial blood gas values and in particular the level of P_aCO_2. We have made some use of prone positioning, despite the lack of randomized prospective trials, because of its low cost and toxicity. This approach allows effective ventilation in all but the most extreme cases. In those cases, when such an approach is clearly failing, we consider using less well-supported therapies that carry a lower cost and toxicity, such as inverse ratio ventilation. Whenever possible, patients and their families should be encouraged to participate in well-designed research protocols of new interventions for ARDS.

DRUG-INDUCED ACUTE RESPIRATORY DISEASE

The lungs manifest toxicity due to medications in a limited number of ways. The spectrum of drug-associated respiratory insufficiency primarily includes: (1) suppression of respiration; (2) bronchospasm; (3) acute pulmonary edema; (4) hypersensitivity pneumonitis; and (5) diffuse alveolar hemorrhage. Since many medications exhibit more than one of these effects, it is difficult to categorize drugs based on the reaction they cause. A list of common drug effects and their treatment is listed below.

CYCLIC ANTIDEPRESSANTS

Cyclic antidepressants account for up to 50 per cent of the drug overdoses in the USA.[162] More than 70% per cent of these patients require MV.[162] Patients exhibit atelectasis, aspiration, and/or suppression of respiratory drive.[162]

ALCOHOL

Alcohol suppresses both hypoxic and hypercapnic respiratory drive. The respiratory depressant effects are first detected at an alcohol level of 100 mg/mL.[163] Aspiration of gastric contents with all of its sequelae also occurs.

SALICYLATES

Salicylates are associated with acute bronchospasm in as many as 20 per cent of asthmatics.[164] In addition, NCPE can be seen in both acute and chronic toxicity, when serum levels are greater than 40-mg/dL.[165] Other nonsteroidal anti-inflammatory drugs can exhibit similar toxicities.

BLEOMYCIN

Some patients develop acute pulmonary insufficiency from either hypersensitivity pneumonitis or acute NCPE.[165–167] Patients who have been given bleomycin within the last 12 months may develop acute NCPE within 24 hours of receiving supplemental oxygen therapy with an $F_iO_2 \geqslant 0.30$.[168,169]

NITROFURANTOIN

Cough, dyspnea, arthralgias, and fever may occur within the first month of therapy with nitrofurantoin.[167] Peripheral eosinophilia and diffuse bilateral infiltrates on CXR are typical.[167] Most patients improve when the drug is withdrawn.

OPIATES

Intravenous heroin use is associated with central respiratory suppression and acute NCPE. Pulmonary edema occurs in up to 90 per cent of patients, although the incidence may be as low as 20 per cent in chronic users.[170] Symptoms usually develop within hours of use, but delay of up to 24 hours has been reported.[171] Patients generally follow one of two courses: rapid resolution over 24–48 hours with full recovery by 7 days, or rapid progression to death.[165,171] Acute pulmonary edema has also been reported after using oral methadone and intravenous naloxone.[170,172]

β-BLOCKERS

Life-threatening bronchospasm has occurred in patients with a history of asthma, family history of asthma, or atopia after systemic or topical ophthalmic β-blocker use.[164]

TOCOLYTICS

Up to 4 per cent of patients develop NCPE following administration of terbutaline, isoxsuprine, or ritodrine used to prevent premature labor. This occurs either prepartum or up to 12 hours postpartum.[173] Symptoms usually resolve within 24 hours.

PROTAMINE

Protamine can cause severe pulmonary edema and bronchospasm usually within 1 hour after the drug is administered.[165,174]

METHOTREXATE

Methotrexate may precipitate an acute interstitial pneumonitis, *Bronchiolitis obliterans* organizing pneumonia (BOOP), and pulmonary fibrosis. Intrathecal administration of methotrexate has been associated with fatal NCPE.[167,175]

NEUROMUSCULAR BLOCKING AGENTS

Neuromuscular blocking agents have been reported to cause bronchospasm due to the release of histamine. However, the most profound effect of neuromuscular blocking agents on the respiratory system is the paralytic effect on the respiratory muscles, which can lead to respiratory failure and death.

DEXTRAN

Intravenous, intrauterine, and intravesicular instillation of low-molecular-weight dextrans have been associated with NCPE.[176–178]

CONTRAST MEDIA

Non-cardiogenic pulmonary edema has been associated with the administration of iv iodinated radiographic contrast media.[179,180] Respiratory failure happens within hours after injection, and may mimic an anaphylactic reaction.

COCAINE

The inhalation of freebase and crack cocaine is associated with an acute pulmonary syndrome characterized by dyspnea, hemoptysis, and diffuse alveolar infiltrates.[181] The spectrum of this illness ranges from transient mild respiratory insufficiency to florid respiratory failure.[181] Other complications from inhalation of cocaine include pneumothorax and pneumomediastinum.[182] Myocardial ischemia may also lead to congestive heart failure.

PHENOTHIAZINES

Pulmonary edema can occur as a sequel to the neuroleptic malignant syndrome secondary to phenothiazine use.[167] This is independent of the total dose and the duration of treatment.

BARBITURATES

Barbiturates cause central nervous system depression resulting in hypercapnic respiratory failure with a normal $P(A–a)O_2$. Pulmonary edema in these patients may be due in part to fluid resuscitation.[170]

TREATMENT

The treatment for virtually all pulmonary toxicity associated with drug ingestion is supportive care. Implicit within that statement is the fact that the offending agent will be withdrawn. Bronchospasm is treated with inhaled beta-2 agonist bronchodilators. There is no known role for systemic corticosteroids in this scenario. The treatment of NCPE is maintenance of blood oxyhemoglobin saturation. When that can be accomplished with supplemental oxygen, that is the treatment of choice. When mechanical ventilation is necessary, the guidelines set out in the section on ARDS apply.

NEAR-DROWNING

In 1994, 3942 people drowned in the USA. Drowning is most common in young children (<5 years) and young adults (15–29 years); among Native Americans and African–Americans; and among males in all groups. *Near-drowning* means 'to survive, at least temporarily, after suffocation by submersion in water'. We estimate the annual incidence of this to be more than 330 000. Over 30 000 of these people would be expected to seek medical attention.

Etiology and pathogenesis

The following factors are associated with an increased risk of drowning and near-drowning.

ALCOHOL

Ethanol use is the major risk factor in immersion accidents. Thirty-seven to 47 per cent of drownings are associated with alcohol consumption.[183–185]

INADEQUATE ADULT SUPERVISION

The backyard pool and family bathtub are common sites of pediatric immersions.[184–186] Inadequate precautions and supervision play a part in many cases.

CHILD ABUSE

One study indicated that 29 per cent of all pediatric near-drownings in bathtubs were purposely caused to inflict harm on the child, while 38 per cent showed evidence of severe neglect.[187]

SEIZURES

The relative risk of immersion injury in children with epilepsy is reported to be 13.8.[188]

BOATING ACCIDENTS

Up to 29 per cent of all drownings occur to boaters.[189] Both alcohol intake and failure to use personal flotation devices contribute to these deaths.[189]

AQUATIC SPORTS

Although the exact number of immersion events associated with the 700 spinal cord injuries caused annually by aquatic sports is not known, it is considered to be substantial.[184]

DRUGS

Central nervous system-active therapeutic drugs are commonly found in the blood of immersion victims. The importance of illegal drugs in causing immersion accidents is not well established.

VOLUNTARY HYPERVENTILATION

Hyperventilation before submersion decreases P_aCO_2 and extends the time that swimmers can function underwater before reaching the point at which they must surface. These persons become hypoxic and lose consciousness before their 'breaking point', because their hypercapnic drive to breathe is circumvented.

Pathophysiology

The drowning sequence begins with a period of panic followed by a vigorous attempt at breath holding. There is a struggle to surface, and gasping may occur. A large amount of water may be swallowed that is eventually regurgitated and often aspirated. Eventually, the breaking point is reached and breath holding is no longer possible. Involuntary breaths are taken, with aspiration of varying amounts of water. Ultimately, the victim becomes unconscious and cardiac arrest occurs.

Survival after extremely long submersion is generally considered possible only when the victim has been submerged in icy water.[190] On the other hand, many deaths from drowning occur not because of inability to float but because of hypothermia caused by exposure to extremely cold water. Mechanisms that protect against hypothermia in a dry environment are not nearly as effective in cold water. Immersion in very cold water can acutely lead to death three ways: (1) a vagally mediated asystolic cardiac arrest may occur (immersion syndrome); (2) hypothermia produces an increased tendency toward malignant arrhythmias separate from this immediate response; and (3) a decrease in core temperature can cause loss of consciousness and subsequent aspiration.

CARDIAC EFFECTS

Heart rate and blood pressure increase immediately after immersion, followed by gradual decreases.[191] Atrial fibrillation and sinus dysrhythmias are common but rarely require therapy.[192] P-R, QRS, and Q-T interval prolongations as well as J-point elevation can be seen.[193,194] The dysrhythmic effects of severe hypothermia are described above. Severe cases result in death due to ventricular fibrillation or asystole. Transient increases in central venous and pulmonary capillary wedge pressures and decreases in cardiac output have been found following experimental near-drowning.[195]

PULMONARY EFFECTS

Freshwater and saltwater solutions cause increases in right to left shunting that result in hypoxemia. Fresh water may inactivate surfactant in the alveoli and lead to NCPE/ARDS. Salt-containing solutions do not inactivate surfactant. Hypertonic sea water may draw fluid from the plasma into the alveoli, causing pulmonary edema despite a decreased intravascular volume.[196] This, combined with ARDS from aspirated gastric contents, causes a clinical scenario similar to that seen with fresh water. Bacterial pneumonia, barotrauma, damage from cardiopulmonary resuscitation (CPR), chemical pneumonitis, centrally mediated apnea, and oxygen toxicity can contribute to respiratory deterioration in the post-resuscitation period.

NEUROLOGICAL EFFECTS

The impact of anoxia is often uncertain because the duration of submersion is unclear, hypothermia may have a direct protective effect on cerebral tissue, and the diving reflex may shunt blood preferentially to the heart and brain. This is more effective in children, whose relatively large surface area and small layer of insulating fat predispose them to rapid cooling. Despite these factors, many near-drowning victims suffer neurologic impairment. Severe anoxic encephalopathy with persistent coma, seizures, delayed language development, spastic quadriplegia, aphasia, cortical blindness, and death have been reported.[186,190,197]

MUSCULOSKELETAL EFFECTS

Children with anoxic encephalopathy due to near-drowning frequently develop musculoskeletal problems due to spasticity.[198] The most common of these are lower extremity contractures, hip subluxation or dislocation, and scoliosis.[198]

SERUM ELECTROLYTES

The actual clinical effect of electrolyte changes is minimal. Humans rarely aspirate enough fluid to cause most of the serious changes seen in experimental situations.[199] The body may rapidly correct the electrolyte changes that do occur.

HEMATOLOGIC EFFECTS

Patients rarely require therapy for anemia. Polymorphonuclear leukocytes are reduced in patients treated with therapeutic hypothermia,[200] and cold water immersion may be associated with increased susceptibility to infection. Disseminated intravascular coagulation (DIC) has been seen complicating freshwater submersions.[201]

RENAL EFFECTS

Acute tubular necrosis, hemoglobinuria, and albuminuria all have been reported as consequences of submersion accidents.[202,203] Diuresis may occur as a result of changes in renal tubular function due to hypothermia.

Diagnosis and clinical presentation

HISTORY AND PHYSICAL EXAMINATION

The minimum history to be obtained includes the patient's age, underlying cardiac, respiratory, or neurologic diseases, and medications used. It is also important to determine the activities precipitating the immersion, the duration of submersion; and the temperature and type of water in which it occurred.

Tachypnea and tachycardia are the most frequent physical findings.[186,199] Patients may be apneic and pulseless. Hypothermia is common. Other physical findings include fever and signs of pulmonary edema.[186] Any physical findings associated with cerebral anoxia or severe hypothermia also may be seen. The physical examination may uncover coexisting injuries that may have caused or resulted from the immersion.

The following classification scale is used to guide the initial neurologic assessment.[204] Category A patients are fully alert within 1 hour of presentation. They uniformly do well neurologically. Category B patients are obtunded and stuporous but arousable at the time of evaluation. Eighty-nine to 100 per cent of these patients survive, and severe permanent neurologic deficit is rare. Category C patients are comatose with abnormal respirations and abnormal response to pain. Category C is further subdivided as: C1 – decorticate posturing; C2 – decerebrate posturing; C3 – flaccid.[205] Category C patients have a much higher mortality, and survivors have a high rate of neurologic dysfunction.

LABORATORY STUDIES

Hemoglobin, hematocrit, and serum electrolytes are usually normal. Arterial blood gas analysis frequently shows metabolic acidosis and hypoxemia. The blood alcohol level, PT, partial thromboplastin time (PTT), serum creatinine, urinalysis, and drug screen are obtained to help determine the cause of the accident and assess for complications of near-drowning. Cervical spine films should be performed whenever there is evidence of trauma. An ECG should be obtained and continuous monitoring performed whenever there is a significant chance of dysrhythmia. Chest x-rays, which are abnormal in up to 80 per cent of victims, are usually obtained.[199]

Therapy

INITIAL RESUSCITATION

Mouth-to-mouth resuscitation of apneic or pulseless victims is begun in the water with careful support of the victim's neck to prevent exacerbation of undiagnosed vertebral injuries.[206] Standard CPR should begin immediately on arrival on shore. The Heimlich maneuver should not be used unless there is suspicion of a foreign body obstructing the airway.[206,207]

Resuscitation must be continued at least until the patient has been rewarmed. In the field, passive external rewarming or inhalation of heated oxygen is used.[208,209] In the hospital, cardiopulmonary bypass should be used in cases of severe hypothermia, especially those with circulatory collapse.[190,209] When this is not possible, rewarming with warmed peritoneal lavage, hemodialysis, or heated oxygen can be attempted.

THERAPY OF THE UNDERLYING CAUSE

Serum alcohol levels and a drug screen can detect potential intoxicants and prompt administration of necessary antidotes or other measures. Anticonvulsants are used in known epileptic patients. If there is any question of possible head or neck trauma, the neck should be immobilized in a brace until cervical spine films are available. Hypoglycemia and severe electrolyte abnormalities can be detected on routine serum testing and corrected rapidly in the emergency department.

TREATMENT OF RESPIRATORY AND OTHER ORGAN FAILURE

The initial management of all pulmonary edema states involves monitoring P_aO_2 and providing supplemental oxygen. The use of nasal continuous positive airway pressure (N-CPAP) may be useful for patients with pulmonary edema.[210] Mechanical ventilation with positive end-expiratory pressure (PEEP) should be instituted if refractory hypoxic or hypercapnic respiratory failure develops.

The goal of MV is to maintain adequate oxygenation while keeping ventilator pressures and volumes at moderate levels. Exogenous surfactant, intravenous steroids, diuretics, and prophylactic antibiotics have all been suggested as potential therapies.[211–213] There is no adequate evidence to support the routine use of any of these therapies.

Serum electrolytes rarely require therapy. The treatment of renal failure in near-drowning focuses on optimizing fluid status and renal blood flow. This may require the placement of a pulmonary artery catheter, and extreme cases may require dialysis.

Lactic acidosis should be corrected by restoration of adequate ventilation and circulation. The cardiac dysrhythmogenic effects of hypothermia are corrected by rewarming. Sinus and atrial dysrhythmias as well as most interval prolongations rarely require additional therapy.[192] Musculoskeletal contractures are treated with casts or splints; subluxed or dislocated hips can be approached with various operative procedures; and scoliosis is treated with bracing or spinal instrumentation.[198]

NEUROLOGIC SALVAGE

Maintaining adequate oxygenation and cerebral blood flow are the central foci of therapy for comatose victims of near-drowning. Measures such as effective MV, vasopressors, and hemodynamic monitoring with careful fluid management have primary importance. Hypothermic patients must be warmed to near-normal core temperature. Seizures should be treated with phenytoin or phenobarbital as required.

PNEUMOTHORAX

Pneumothorax is the accumulation of air or gas in the pleural space.[214] This occurs either due to alveolar rupture, traumatic disruption of the parietal or visceral pleura, gas formation by bacteria, or rupture of the esophagus or trachea. Pneumothorax can be classified into three categories: (1) primary or spontaneous pneumothorax; (2) secondary or complicated pneumothorax; and (3) tension pneumothorax. Since treatment of all three forms is similar, it will be discussed at the end of this section.

Primary pneumothorax

Spontaneous pneumothorax results from the rupture of subpleural blebs smaller than 2 cm diameter that are commonly located in the apices.[215–218] The annual incidence of spontaneous pneumothorax is 1.2 to 7.4 cases per 100 000 population.[219] The male to female ratio is 6:1. There is a well-established relationship between spontaneous pneumothorax and Marfan's syndrome. In addition, one study reported an increase in the incidence of familial pneumothorax in patients with a HLA types A2 and B40.[215,217] Although most patients are cigarette smokers, there is no clearly established association between smoking and the formation of blebs.[215,218]

Chest pain and dyspnea are the most common symptoms, occurring in 90 per cent and 80 per cent of cases respectively.[217] Chest pain is initially sharp and pleuritic, but may become dull and ultimately subside despite the persistence of pneumothorax. Physical examination frequently reveals a mild tachycardia with normal respiratory rate and blood pressure. Hyperinflation, hyperresonance to percussion, decreased breath sounds and tactile fremitus may also be seen. When cyanosis, hypoxia, hypotension, tracheal deviation to the contralateral side, or a heart rate greater than 140 is found, tension pneumothorax should be suspected.

Chest x-ray typically shows both a distinct white line that represents the visceral pleura and absence of lung markings beyond that line. However, occasionally the pleural line may be difficult to see. Displacement of the mediastinum is seen with tension pneumothorax. Whenever possible, studies performed specifically to identify pneumothorax should be done in expiration, since smaller pneumothoraces are better seen with that technique.

Secondary pneumothorax

Chronic obstructive pulmonary disease, MV, and other iatrogenic causes make up the majority of cases of secondary pneumothorax. The etiology of pneumothorax in COPD involves the rupture of a intraparenchymal bleb. Given the low respiratory reserve of this group of patients, the clinical presentation is often dramatic. Chest pain is the most common symptom. When pneumothorax is suspected, or when unexplained chest pain occurs in a patient with COPD, inspiratory and expiratory CXR should be obtained. The presence of a 'concavity' facing the chest wall is suggestive of a peripheral bullae, whereas the presence of a convexity suggests pneumothorax. When this differentiation is not possible, a CT of the chest should be obtained.

Pneumothorax may develop following a medical procedure. The most common procedures involved are central venous catheter placement, percutaneous lung biopsy, pleural biopsy, transbronchial biopsy, thoracentesis, tracheostomy, intercostal nerve block, mediatinoscopy, liver biopsy and cardiopulmonary resuscitation. Symptoms may not occur until the pneumothorax has grown to occupy a large portion of the hemithorax. In addition, symptoms may be delayed up to 24 hours after the procedure is done. Therefore, a CXR should be obtained after these interventions. A tension pneumothorax should be strongly considered when one of these procedures is performed on a patient on MV and the patient subsequently becomes difficult to ventilate.

In addition to its association with procedures performed, pneumothorax is a potentially lethal complication of MV itself. Some of the conditions associated with an increased risk of pneumothorax in ventilated patients are ARDS, COPD, asthma, necrotizing pneumonia, pneumonia, interstitial lung diseases, and right main stem intubation.[214,220–222] Patients may become tachypneic, dyspneic, and experience sudden proportional increase of both the peak and the plateau ventilator pressures with a simultaneous decrease in C_{stat}. On auscultation, the continuous cycling noise from the ventilator may make it difficult to appreciate the difference in air movement between each hemithorax. Plain CXR should be done with the patient in a semierect position and should be compared with old films. A CT of the chest should be obtained when the diagnosis is unclear and if the patient's condition allows it.

Tension pneumothorax

Tension is present when the intrapleural pressure exceeds the atmospheric pressure in both inspiration and expiration. This occurs when the disrupted pleura functions as a one-way valve.[214,215,218] The accumulation of air in the pleural space and the increase in the intrapleural pressure displaces the diaphragm downwards and the mediastinum toward the opposite side. These changes on the mediastinum, great vessels, and heart are responsible for the clinical consequences. Tension pneumothorax is most commonly seen in patients on MV, but may also be seen in patients with blunt or penetrating lung trauma or following a procedure. Dyspnea, tachypnea, tachycardia, diaphoresis, hypotension, cyanosis, distended neck veins, and tracheal deviation to the contralateral side are all physical findings consistent with this condition. Cardiovascular collapse with pulseless electric activity can develop rapidly.[214,218]

Treatment

> Treatment of a pneumothorax not exhibiting tension in a patient not receiving MV is the same regardless of whether it is primary or secondary. Pneumothorax of less than 15 per cent may be managed with observation and supplemental oxygen.

Oxygen is used to enhance the gradient for reabsorption by reducing the partial pressure of nitrogen in the capillary blood. High partial pressures of inspired oxygen are needed to alter the reabsorption rates significantly. Serial CXR should be obtained to detect enlargement, which is indicative of an ongoing air leak.

> If a pneumothorax is greater than 15 per cent, it should be drained either by aspiration or chest tube thoracostomy.

First episodes of primary pneumothorax may be managed best with simple aspiration with little cost or morbidity. A standard thoracentesis kit and three-way stopcock may be used for this procedure. Subsequent episodes, and most moderate- to large-size secondary pneumothoraces usually require more aggressive drainage. Alternatives include use of a narrow drainage catheter with a free-standing low-level suction system or a large tube thoracostomy attached to wall suction.

> Treatment of a tension pneumothorax is a medical emergency. The standard emergency treatment is decompression with a large-bore needle in the second intercostal space at the mid-clavicular line. The needle should be left in place and open to atmospheric pressure until a chest tube is placed.[214,223]

Treatment of recurrent pneumothorax is also a challenge. In an ICU, patients may require several chest tubes to drain the pleura of air completely, if the pleural space is partitioned by scarring. In the subacute setting, it may be necessary to perform either a chemical or mechanical sclerosis of the pleura. Talc and various tetracycline derivatives (doxycycline, minocycline) are the agents of choice. Surgery can be performed either via a thoracoscopic or open approach.

> Indications for surgery include: recurrent primary or secondary pneumothorax despite chemical sclerosis; persistence of an air leak after 5 days of tube drainage; failure of hormonal therapy for catamenial pneumothorax; traumatic rupture of the trachea or esophagus; and failure of a prolonged course of antimycobacterial therapy in patients with tuberculosis.

CLINICAL OVERVIEW

Status asthmaticus

A history of previous asthma attacks requiring mechanical ventilation is particularly ominous. Other important features of past episodes include a history of pneumothorax or pneumomediastinum, hospitalization despite chronic oral steroid use, hypercapnia, psychiatric illness, or medication non-adherence. Physical examination findings indicative of a severe exacerbation include assuming the upright position, diaphoresis, use of accessory muscles, altered mental status, and an increased pulsus paradoxus. Changes in peak expiratory flow rate and forced expiratory volume in 1 second can help predict the need for hospitalization and ICU care.

Supplemental oxygen is the first treatment to be administered upon arrival. Inhaled beta-2 adrenergic agonists administered every 15 minutes are the next treatment. Systemic corticosteroids are the cornerstone of the treatment because they directly influence airway inflammation. Administration of 120–180 mg of prednisone or methylprednisolone in three or four divided doses daily is usually adequate, although doses of methylprednisolone of up to 500 mg daily are sometimes used. Should a patient require MV, the correct approach is to decrease minute ventilation and increase expiratory time while accepting hypercapnia. The most accurate predictor of the appropriateness of MV in status asthmaticus is V_{EI}. If V_{EI} is above 20 mL/kg, minute ventilation should be decreased by reducing tidal volume, and if necessary by reducing respiratory rate.

Exacerbations of chronic obstructive pulmonary disease

Patients experiencing exacerbations of COPD typically present with a pre-existing history of the disease or a long history of cigarette smoking. Symptoms include worsening dyspnea, increased cough with sputum production, or change in the amount or color of the sputum, and wheeze. Tachypnea, use of the accessory muscles of breathing, and respiratory paradox are signs of respiratory muscle fatigue. The $\Delta H^+/\Delta PCO_2$ ratio may be helpful in distinguishing acute from chronic respiratory failure.

The first treatment of an acute exacerbation should be oxygen, administered in sufficient amount to maintain an oxygen saturation of 88–90 per cent. An inhaled beta-2 agonist is usually the first pharmacological treatment given. Administration by MDI or nebulizer solution is equally effective. The accepted therapeutic equivalent dosages are four puffs of albuterol via MDI or 0.5 mL solution via nebulizer administered up to every 30 minutes until the attack is controlled or side effects become limiting. Systemic steroid therapy is also helpful. We customarily use oral prednisone 40–60 mg, tapered over 10–14 days to manage exacerbations in out-patients or methylprednisolone 0.5 mg/kg intravenously every 6 hours for in-patients. Antibiotics used to treat exacerbations of COPD should have activity against *Haemophilus influenzae*, *Streptococcus pneumoniae*, and *Moraxella catarrhalis*. To date no antibiotic has shown clear superiority for this indication. The goals of MV are to rest the respiratory muscles and improve gas exchange to an acceptable level. This may be done either with conventional MV via an endotracheal tube or with non-invasive ventilation. Minute ventilation should be targeted to maintain the patient's premorbid acid base status.

Upper airway obstruction

A history of fever and chills, sore throat, frequent throat clearing, difficulty swallowing, recent intubation, weight loss, or voice change is consistent with upper airway obstruction. Similarly, physical findings, such as fever, tonsillar exudate, cobblestoned pharyngeal mucosa, goiter, deviated trachea, hoarseness, or severe obesity may be invaluable diagnostic clues. Wheezing can be either inspiratory or expiratory with an extrathoracic upper airway obstruction, although inspiratory wheeze is typical. Fiber-optic laryngoscopy and/or bronchoscopy can be used to visualize directly airway structures and obtain tissue for the histologic diagnosis of potentially malignant lesions.

Treatments can be divided into general measures designed to ensure patency of the airway, and specific measures aimed at correcting the underlying cause of the obstruction. Control of the airway with an endotracheal tube or tracheostomy is often necessary. A mixture of helium and oxygen may improve ventilation by reducing airway resistance to turbulent flow and decreasing flow-resistive work. Racemic epinephrine administered via nebulizer is effective in certain circumstances. Corticosteroids, bronchoscopic dilatation, laser therapy, surgery, and various disease specific therapies have all been used.

Acute inhalation injury

Toxic inhalants can be classified into four categories: smoke inhalation, irritant toxins, asphyxiant toxins, and systemic toxins. Presenting symptoms may vary from mild upper airway irritation to NCPE and death.

Treatment of smoke inhalation includes supplemental oxygen at an F_iO_2 of 1.0 until carboxyhemoglobin levels are available. Further oxygen treatment is determined by the severity of carbon monoxide poisoning. Bronchodilators and steroids should be used if there are signs of upper airway obstruction. Patients with significant exposure to smoke should be kept under close observation for 24 hours because delayed symptoms may occur.

Common toxic irritants include ammonia, chlorine, hydrogen chloride, oxides of nitrogen, phosgene, and sulfur dioxide. Since there are no specific antidotes or treatments for individual substances, the treatment of all irritant exposures involves maintaining adequate oxygenation with supplemental oxygen and mechanical ventilation if necessary.

Common asphyxiant toxins include carbon monoxide, methane, hydrogen cyanide, and hydrogen sulfide. Carbon monoxide exposures should be treated with oxygen at F_iO_2 of 1.0 and with hyperbaric oxygen in some cases. Treatment of methane exposure includes supplemental oxygen and removal from the exposure area. Amyl nitrate followed by intravenous sodium nitrite and sodium thiosulfite is an antidote for cyanide toxicity. Treatment of hydrogen sulfide exposure is similar to that of hydrogen cyanide.

The large surface area of the respiratory tract can absorb toxins that have a systemic effect without localized pulmonary toxicity, causing fever, chills, and malaise that take 24–48 hours to resolve. No specific therapy is available.

Acute pulmonary embolism

Most patients with acute PE show one of three syndromes: unexplained dyspnea; pulmonary infarction with pleuritic chest pain and hemoptysis; and circulatory collapse.

All of the common physical findings in PE are non-specific. The first test to be obtained in the evaluation of suspected PE is the ventilation–perfusion scan. A six-view scan demonstrating normal or nearly normal perfusion essentially rules out the diagnosis. Multiple segmental or larger perfusion defects without corresponding ventilation defects (a 'high probability' scan) makes the diagnosis of PE very likely. Any other reading leaves the diagnosis in question. Patients with ventilation–perfusion scan readings other than 'normal', 'near-normal', or 'high probability' should proceed to non-invasive evaluation of the proximal deep veins of the legs. The discovery of a DVT by duplex ultrasound of the legs is an indication for anticoagulation. Patients with a negative duplex examination and a high or uncertain clinical probability of PE are usually sent for pulmonary arteriography, while patients with lower levels of clinical suspicion are sometimes followed with serial duplex examinations of the lower extremities.

The standard initial treatment for acute PE is intravenous unfractionated heparin. An initial bolus of 5000–10 000 units is appropriate, and is often calculated as a weight-based dose with approximately 80 units/kg administered as an iv bolus followed by a maintenance iv drip at approximately 18 units/hour. This is adjusted based on the results of the activated partial thromboplastin time (aPTT), with the goal to achieve an aPTT > 1.5 × control levels. Warfarin sodium should be begun either simultaneous with heparin or on the second day of heparin therapy. Many clinicians would favor thrombolysis with streptokinase, urokinase, or recombinant tissue plasminogen activator (rTPA) in cases of major acute PE with syncope or hypotension when none of the contraindications listed in Table 10.3 exist. The primary indications for the placement of an IVC filter are: (1) the contraindication to anticoagulant therapy or a complication of such therapy; and (2) the failure of anticoagulant therapy despite achieving an adequate anticoagulant level for an adequate period of time. There should be strong evidence of a clot in the deep veins of the lower extremity before an IVC filter is placed. Pulmonary embolectomy is a rarely used treatment that may have a role in the management of an occasional patient in extreme circumstances but is not a standard method of care in any circumstance.

Massive hemoptysis

Massive hemoptysis is the expectoration of 600 mL of blood from the lower respiratory tract over a 24-hour period. Death is usually a result of asphyxiation. Any cause of hemoptysis could potentially cause massive bleeding. Diagnosis usually involves history, physical examination, bronchoscopy, CT scanning, and occasionally angiography. The primary management goals are maintenance of airway patency and control of bleeding. Secondary goals are to determine the site and the cause of the bleeding as well as the patient's ability to withstand surgery if necessary.

Acute respiratory distress syndrome

The criteria for the diagnosis of ARDS include: impaired oxygenation – P_aO_2/F_iO_2 ratio $\leqslant$ 200 (whatever the PEEP); bilateral pulmonary infiltrates on CXR; pulmonary artery occlusion pressure $\leqslant$ 18 mm Hg or no clinical findings suggestive of increased left atrial pressure. ARDS is normally associated with either *direct* or *indirect* predisposing conditions. The pathophysiologic

response can be divided into two phases dated from the onset of the inciting event: the *exudative phase* and the *fibroproliferative phase*.

Multiple therapies have been tried and failed to show a clinical benefit in the past 15 years. Despite these failures, the mortality rate for patients with ARDS has decreased from 60 per cent to approximately 44 per cent in the 1990s. Using an evidenced-based approach to evaluate treatments for ARDS, only early fluid restriction and diuresis, late corticosteroid administration, and small tidal volume ventilation have demonstrated efficacy.

Drug-induced respiratory disease

The spectrum of drug-associated respiratory insufficiency includes suppression of respiration, bronchospasm, acute pulmonary edema, hypersensitivity pneumonitis, and diffuse alveolar hemorrhage. Salicylates, non-steroidal anti-inflammatory drugs, naloxone, amiodarone, beta-blockers, tocolytics, protamine, methotrexate, bleomycin, nitrofurantoin, neuromuscular blockade, dextran, contrast media, cocaine, heroin, methadone, phenothiazines, cyclic antidepressants, and barbiturates are among the drugs implicated most commonly in causing pulmonary disease. Treatment always involves removal of the offending agent and supportive care, sometimes requiring MV.

Near-drowning

Although freshwater and seawater near-drownings cause different clinical pictures in experimental animals, they are difficult to distinguish in humans. In general, patients who aspirate water present with hypoxemia and metabolic acidosis. ARDS and neurological deficits are common.

In hypothermic patients, rewarming methods should be instituted immediately. These include removing wet clothing, covering with warm blankets, infusing warm fluids (37–38°C) intravenously, performing gastrointestinal irrigation with warm fluids, warmed peritoneal dialysis, and cardiopulmonary bypass in severe cases. Therapy for patients with severe hypoxemia includes institution of all the supportive modalities used in ARDS. Abnormalities of multiple organ systems – most commonly metabolic acidosis – should be addressed immediately.

Pneumothorax

Pneumothorax can be classified as primary or spontaneous pneumothorax; secondary or complicated pneumothorax; and tension pneumothorax. Pneumothorax of less than 15 per cent may be managed with observation and supplemental oxygen. Serial CXRs should be obtained to detect enlargement, which is indicative of an ongoing air leak. If a pneumothorax is greater than 15 per cent, it should be drained either by aspiration or chest tube thoracostomy. Moderate to large size secondary pneumothoraces usually require the more aggressive drainage approach. The emergent treatment of a tension pneumothorax is decompression with a large-bore needle in the second intercostal space at the mid-clavicular line. The needle should be left in place and open to atmospheric pressure until a chest tube is placed.

SUMMARY

- The hallmark of therapy for status asthmaticus is anti-inflammatory therapy with corticosteroids. All other modes of therapy are provided to give time for anti-inflammatory therapy to work.
- Treatment of even the most severe exacerbations in patients with advanced chronic obstructive pulmonary disease (COPD) generally results in good outcomes. Mechanical ventilation is not absolutely contraindicated even in severe COPD.
- The key to the management of upper airway obstruction is control of the airway. This may require intubation or tracheostomy, or medical interventions such as helium–oxygen.
- Toxic inhalants can be classified into four categories: smoke inhalation, irritant toxins, asphyxiant toxins, and systemic toxins. Treatment first requires removal from the offending agent.
- The management of acute pulmonary embolism requires an initially high index of suspicion, an organized diagnostic approach, and initiation of treatment as soon as a diagnosis is made.
- Patients with massive hemoptysis should be monitored in an intensive care unit and placed with their good side up to prevent flow of blood from the bleeding to the non-bleeding lung.
- A variety of specific therapies for the acute respiratory distress syndrome (ARDS) have been tried, but none have been clearly proven effective. Improvements in care of patients with ARDS have come through improvements in supportive care.
- The spectrum of drug-associated respiratory insufficiency includes suppression of respiration, bronchospasm, acute pulmonary edema, hypersensitivity pneumonitis, and diffuse alveolar hemorrhage.
- The clinical presentations of freshwater and saltwater near-drowning are nearly identical and do not require significant differences in management.
- The treatment of tension pneumothorax is decompression by needle thoracostomy followed by chest tube placement.

REFERENCES

1. Murphy S, Bleeker ER, Boushey H, and the Second Expert Panel on the Management of Asthma. *Expert Panel Report 2: Guidelines for the diagnosis and management of asthma*. Bethesda, MD: National Institutes of Health, Publication No. 97-4051. April 1997.
2. Corbridge TC, Hall JB. The assessment and management of adults with status asthmaticus. *Am J Resp Crit Care Med* 1995; **151**: 1296–316.
3. Holgate ST, Beasley R, Twentyman OP. The pathogenesis and significance of bronchial hyperresponsiveness in airways disease. *Clin Sci* 1987; **73**: 561–72.
4. Brenner BE, Abraham E, Simon RR. Position and diaphoresis in acute asthma. *Am J Med* 1983; **74**: 1005–9.
5. Knowles G, Clark TJH. Pulsus paradoxus as a valuable sign indicating severity of asthma. *Lancet* 1973; **2**: 1356–9.
6. Rodrigo G, Rodrigo C. Assessment of the patient with acute asthma in the emergency department: a factor analytic study. *Chest* 1993; **104**: 1325–8.
7. Stein LM, Cole RP. Early administration of corticosteroids in emergency room treatment of acute asthma. *Ann Intern Med* 1990; **112**: 822–7.
8. Madison JM, Irwin RS. Heliox for asthma: a trial balloon. *Chest* 1995; **107**: 597–8.
9. Bellomo R, McLaughlin P, Tai E, Parkin G. Asthma requiring mechanical ventilation: a low morbidity approach. *Chest* 1994; **105**: 891–6.
10. Williams TJ, Tuxen DV, Scheinkstel CD, Czarny D, Bowes G. Risk factors for morbidity in mechanically ventilated patients with acute severe asthma. *Am Rev Respir Dis* 1992; **146**: 607–15.
11. Gump DW, Phillips CA, Forsyth BR, *et al*. Role of infection in chronic bronchitis. *Am Rev Respir Dis* 1976; **113**: 465–74.
12. Roussos C, Macklem PT. The respiratory muscles. *N Engl J Med* 1982; **307**: 786–97.
13. Gilbert R, Ashutosh K, Auchincloss JH, *et al*. Prospective study of controlled oxygen therapy: poor prognosis of patients with asynchronous breathing. *Chest* 1977; **71**: 456–62.
14. Cohen CA, Zalgelbaum G, Gross D, *et al*. Clinical manifestations of inspiratory muscle fatigue. *Am J Med* 1982; **73**: 308–16.
15. Demers RR, Irwin RS. Management of hypercapnic respiratory failure: a systematic approach. *Respir Care* 1979; **24**: 328–35.
16. ATS Statement. Standards for the diagnosis and care of patients with chronic obstructive pulmonary disease. *Am J Respir Crit Care Med* 1995; **152**: S78–S121.
17. Bone RC, Pierce AK, Johnson RL Jr. Controlled oxygen administration in acute respiratory failure in chronic

obstructive pulmonary disease: a reappraisal. *Am J Med* 1978; **65**: 896–902.

18. Bone RC. Treatment of respiratory failure due to advanced chronic obstructive pulmonary disease. *Arch Intern Med* 1980; **140**: 1018–21.

19. Aubier M, Murciano D, Fournier M, *et al*. Effects of the administration of O_2 on ventilation and blood gases in patients with chronic obstructive pulmonary disease during acute respiratory failure. *Am Rev Respir Dis* 1980; **122**: 747–54.

20. Berry RB, Shinto RA, Wong FH, *et al*. Nebulizer vs spacer for bronchodilator delivery in patients hospitalized for acute exacerbations of COPD. *Chest* 1989; **96**: 1241–6.

21. Combivent Inhalation Aerosol Study Group. In chronic obstructive pulmonary disease a combination of ipratropium and albuterol is more effective than either agent alone. *Chest* 1994; **105**: 1411–19.

22. Albert RK, Martin TR, Lewis SW. Controlled clinical trial of methylprednisolone in patients with chronic bronchitis and acute respiratory insufficiency. *Ann Intern Med* 1980; **92**: 753–8.

23. Thompson WH, Nielson CP, Carvalho P, Charan NB, Crowley JJ. Controlled trial of oral prednisone in outpatients with acute COPD exacerbation. *Am J Respir Crit Care Med* 1996; **154**: 407–12.

24. Saint S, Vittinghoff E, Grady D. Antibiotics in chronic obstructive pulmonary disease exacerbations. A meta-analysis. *Chest* 1995; **273**: 957–60.

o25. Grossman RF. Guidelines for the treatment of acute exacerbations of chronic bronchitis. *Chest* 1997; **112**: 310S–13S.

26. Grossman R, Mukherjee J, Vaughan D, *et al*. A 1-year community based health economic study of ciprofloxacin vs usual antibiotic treatment in acute exacerbations of chronic bronchitis. *Chest* 1998; **113**: 131–41.

27. Anthonisen NR, Monfreda J, Warren CPW, *et al*. Antibiotic therapy in exacerbations of chronic obstructive pulmonary disease. *Ann Intern Med* 1987; **106**: 196–204.

28. Rice KL, Leatherman JW, Duane PG, *et al*. Aminophylline for acute exacerbations of chronic obstructive pulmonary disease: a controlled trial. *Ann Intern Med* 1982; **97**: 305–9.

29. Plant PK, Owen JL, Elliott MW. Early use of non-invasive ventilation for acute exacerbations of chronic obstructive pulmonary disease on general respiratory wards: a multicentre randomised controlled trial. *Lancet* 2000; **355**: 1931–5.

29a. Girov E, Schortgen F, Delclaux C, Blot F, Lefort Y, Lemaire F, Brochard L. Association of noninvasive ventilation with nosocomial infections and survival in critically ill patients. *JAMA* 2000; **284**: 2361–7.

30. Macklem PT. Airway obstruction and collateral ventilation. *Physiol Rev* 1971; **51**: 368–436.

31. Mittleman RE, Wetli CV. The fatal cafe coronary. Foreign-body airway obstruction. *JAMA* 1982; **247**: 1285–8.

32. Handler SD, Beauregard ME, Canalis RF, *et al*. Unsuspected esophageal foreign bodies in adults with upper airway obstruction. *Chest* 1981; **80**: 234–7.

33. Megerian CA, Arnold JE, Berger M. Angioedema: 5 years' experience, with a review of the disorder's presentation and treatment. *Laryngoscope* 1992; **102**: 256–60.

34. Slater EE, Merrill DD, Guess HA, *et al*. Clinical profile of angioedema associated with angiotensin converting enzyme inhibition. *JAMA* 1988; **260**: 967–70.

35. Israili ZH, Hall WD. Cough and the angioneurotic edema associated with angiotensin-converting enzyme inhibitor therapy. A review of the literature and pathophysiology. *Ann Intern Med* 1992; **117**: 234–42.

36. Christopher KL, Wood RP, Eckert C, Blager FB, Raney RA, Souhrada JF. Vocal-cord dysfunction presenting as asthma. *N Engl J Med* 1983; **308**: 1566–70.

37. Sokol W. Vocal cord dysfunction presenting as asthma. *West J Med* 1993; **158**: 614–15.

38. Jacobs TJ, Irwin RS, Raptopoulos V. Severe upper airway infections. In: Rippe JM, Irwin RS, Fink MP, Cerra FB, eds *Intensive care medicine*, 3rd edn. Boston: Little, Brown and Co., 1996: 883–903.

39. Baxter FJ, Dunn GL. Acute epiglottitis in adults. *Can J Anesthes* 1988; **35**: 428–35.

40. Moreland LW, Corey J, McKenzie R. Ludwig's angina. Report of a case and review of the literature. *Arch Intern Med* 1988; **148**: 461–6.

41. Fritsch DE, Klein DG. Ludwig's angina. *Heart Lung* 1992; **21**: 39–46.

42. Juang YC, Cheng DL, Wang LS, *et al*. Ludwig's angina: an analysis of 14 cases. *Scand J Infect Dis* 1989; **21**: 121–5.

43. Quan L. Diagnosis and treatment of croup. *Am Fam Phys* 1992; **46**: 747–55.

44. Colice GL, Stukel TA, Dain B. Laryngeal complications of prolonged intubation. *Chest* 1989; **966**: 877–84.

45. Kastanos N, Estopa Miro R, Marin Perez A, *et al*. Laryngotracheal injury due to endotracheal intubation: incidence, evolution, and predisposing factors. A prospective long term study. *Crit Care Med* 1983; **11**: 362–7.

46. Elliot CG, Rasmusson BY, Crapo RO. Upper airway obstruction following adult respiratory distress syndrome. An analysis of 30 survivors. *Chest* 1988; **94**: 526–30.

47. Whited RE. A prospective study of laryngotracheal sequelae in long term intubations. *Laryngoscope* 1984; **94**: 367–77.

48. Whited RE. Posterior commissure stenosis post long-term intubation. *Laryngoscope* 1983; **93**: 1314–18.

49. Darmon JY, Rauss A, Dreyfuss D, *et al*. Evaluation of

risk for laryngeal edema after tracheal extubation in adults and its prevention by dexamethasone. *Anesthesiology* 1992; **77**: 245–51.

50. Dixon TC, Sando MJ, Bolton JM, *et al.* A report of 342 cases of prolonged endotracheal intubation. *Med J Aust* 1968; **2**: 529–33.

51. Ho L, Lee JC, Wang JH. Does hydrocortisone prevent post-extubation laryngeal edema in adults. *Chest* 1992; **102**(2 suppl): 184S.

52. Rashkin MC, Davis T. Acute complication of endotracheal intubation. Relationship to reintubation, route, urgency and duration. *Chest* 1986; **89**: 165–7.

53. Christopher KL, Spofford BT, Petrun MD, *et al.* A program for tracheal oxygen delivery: assessment of safety. *Ann Intern Med* 1987; **107**: 802.

54. Kryger M, Bode F, Antic R, Anthonisen N. Diagnosis of obstruction of the upper and central airways. *Am J Med* 1976; **61**: 85–93.

55. Miller RD, Hyatt RE. Obstructing lesions of the larynx and trachea: clinical and physiologic characteristics. *Mayo Clin Proc* 1969; **44**: 145–61.

56. Geffin B, Grillo HC, Cooper JD, *et al.* Stenosis following tracheostomy for respiratory care. *JAMA* 1971; **216**: 1984–8.

57. Davis SD, Maldjian C, Perone RW, *et al.* CT of the airways. *Clin. Imaging* 1990; **14**: 280–300.

58. Sheppard JO, McLoud TC. Imaging the airway. Computed tomography and magnetic resonance imaging. *Clin Chest Med* 1991; **12**: 151–68.

59. Houck JR, Keamy MF III, Madonough JM. Effect of helium concentration on experimental airway obstruction. *Ann Otol Laryngol* 1990; **99**: 556–61.

60. Kissoon N, Mitchell I. Adverse effect of racemic epinephrine in epiglottis. *Pediatr Emerg Care* 1985; **1**: 143–4.

61. Streitz JM, Shapshay SM. Airway injury after tracheotomy and endotracheal intubation. *Surg Clin North Am* 1991; **71**: 1211–30.

62. Shapshay SM, Dumon JF, Beamis JF. Endoscopic treatment of tracheobronchial malignancy. Experience with Nd-YAG and CO$_2$ lasers in 506 operations. *Otolaryngol Head Neck Surg* 1985; **93**: 205–10.

63. Grillo HC, Mathisen DJ. Primary tracheal tumors: treatment and results. *Ann Thorac Surg* 1990; **49**: 69–77.

64. Grillo HC, Mathisen DJ, Wain LC. Laryngotracheal resection and reconstruction for subglottic stenosis. *Ann Thorac Surg* 1992; **53**: 54–63.

65. Black RE, Choi KJ, Syme WC, *et al.* Bronchoscopic removal of aspirated foreign bodies in children. *Am J Surg* 1984; **148**: 778–81.

66. Orfan NA, Kolski GB. Angioedema and C1 inhibitor deficiency. *Ann Allergy* 1992; **69**: 167–72.

67. Newman KB. Vocal cord dysfunction: an asthma mimic. *Pulmonary Perspect* 1993; **10**: 3–5.

68. Chow AW, Roser SM, Brady F. Orofacial odontogenic infections. *Ann Intern Med* 1978; **88**: 392–402.

69. Celikel TH, Mutheswamy PP. Septic pulmonary embolism secondary to internal jugular phlebitis caused by *Ekinella corrodens*. *Am Rev Respir Dis* 1984; **130**: 510–13.

70. Tami TA, Parker GS. *Ekinella corrodens*: an emerging pathogen in head and neck infection. *Arch Otolaryngol Head Neck Surg* 1984; **110**: 752–4.

71. Kairys SW, Olmstead EM, O'Connor GT. Steroid treatment of laryngotracheitis: a meta-analysis of the evidence from randomized trials. *Pediatrics* 1989; **83**: 683–93.

71a. Ausejo M, Saenz A, Pham B, Kellner JD, Johnson DW, Moher D, Klassen TP. The effectiveness of glucocorticoids in treating croup: meta-analysis. *Br Med J* 1999; **319**: 595–600.

72. Pruitt BA, Flemma RJ, DiVincent FC, *et al.* Pulmonary complications in burn patients. *J Thorac Cardiovasc Surg* 1970; **59**: 7–20.

73. Terrill JB, Montgomery RR, Reinhardt CF. Toxic gases from fires. *Science* 1978; **200**: 1343–7.

74. Kinsella J, Carter R, Reid WH, *et al.* Increased airways reactivity after smoke inhalation. *Lancet* 1991; **337**: 595–7.

75. Thom SR. Smoke inhalation. *Emerg Med Clin North Am* 1989; **7**: 371–87.

76. Brooks SM, Weiss MA, Berstein IL. Reactive airways dysfunction syndrome: persistent asthma syndrome after high level irritant exposure. *Chest* 1985; **88**: 376–84.

77. Caplin M. Ammonia gas poisoning. *Lancet* 1941; **2**: 95–6.

78. Montague TJ, MacNeil AR. Mass ammonia inhalation. *Chest* 1980; **77**: 496–8.

79. Close LG, Catlin FI, Cohn AM. Acute and chronic ammonia burns in the respiratory tract. *Arch Otolaryngol* 1980; **106**: 151–8.

80. Dyer RF, Esch VH. Polyvinyl chloride toxicity in fires. *JAMA* 1976; **235**: 393–7.

81. Lowry T, Shuman LM. 'Silo-filler's disease' a syndrome caused by nitrogen dioxide. *JAMA* 1956; **162**: 153–60.

82. Bradley BL, Unger KM. Phosgene inhalation: case report. *Texas Med* 1982; **78**: 51–3.

83. Snyder RW, Mishel HS, Christensen GC. Pulmonary toxicity following exposure to methylene chloride and its combustion product, phosgene. *Chest* 1992; **101**: 860–1.

84. Balmes JR, Fine JM, Sheppard D. Symptomatic bronchoconstriction after short-term inhalation of sulfur dioxide. *Am Rev Respir Dis* 1987; **136**: 1117–21.

85. Charan NB, Myers CG, Lakshminarayan S, *et al.* Pulmonary injuries associated with acute sulfur dioxide inhalation. *Am Rev Respir Dis* 1979; **119**: 555–60.

86. Coburn RF. Mechanism of carbon monoxide toxicity. *Prev Med* 1979; **8**: 310–22.

87. Ilano AL, Raffin TA. Management of carbon monoxide poisoning. *Chest* 1990; **97**: 165–9.

88. Blanc P, Hogan M, Mallin K, *et al*. Cyanide intoxication among silver reclaiming workers. *JAMA* 1985; **253**: 367–71.

89. Graham DL, Laman D, Theodore J, *et al*. Acute cyanide poisoning complicated by lactic acidosis and pulmonary edema. *Arch Intern Med* 1977; **137**: 1051–5.

90. Cottrell JE, Casthely P, Brodie JD, *et al*. Prevention of nitroprusside-induced cyanide toxicity with hydroxcobalamin. *N Engl J Med* 1978; **298**: 809–11.

91. Smith RP, Kruszyna R, Kruszyna H. Management of acute sulfide poisoning. Effects of oxygen, thiosulfate, and nitrite. *Arch Environ Health* 1976; **31**: 166–9.

92. Harris KD. Polymer-fume fever. *Lancet* 1951; **2**: 1008–11.

○93. Dalen JE, Alpert JS. Natural history of pulmonary embolism. *Prog Cardiovasc Dis* 1975; **17**: 259–70.

94. Anderson FA, Wheeler HB. Venous thromboembolism: risk factors and prophylaxis. *Clin Chest Med* 1995; **16**: 235–51.

○95. Goldhaber SZ, Hennekens CH, Evans DA, *et al*. Factors associated with correct antemortem diagnosis of major pulmonary embolism. *Am J Med* 1982; **73**: 822–6.

♦96. Anderson FA, Wheeler HB, Goldberg RJ, Hosmer DW, Forcier A, Patwardhen NA. Physician practices in the prevention of venous thromboembolism. *Ann Intern Med* 1991; **115**: 591–5.

97. Goldhaber SZ, Grodstein F, Stampfer MJ, Manson JE, Colditz GA, Speizer FE, Willett WC, Hennekens CH. A prospective study of risk factors for pulmonary embolism in women. *JAMA* 1997; **277**: 642–5.

98. Stein PD, Henry JW. Clinical characteristics of patients with acute pulmonary embolism stratified according to their presenting syndromes. *Chest* 1997; **112**: 974–9.

99. Santolicandro A, Prediletto R, Fornai E, Formichi B, Begliomini E, Giannella-Neto A, Giuntini C. Mechanisms of hypoxemia and hypocapnia in pulmonary embolism. *Am J Respir Crit Care Med* 1995; **152**: 336–47.

100. Ferrari E, Imbert A, Chevalier T, Mihoubi A, Morand P, Baudouy M. The ECG in pulmonary embolism: predictive value of negative T waves in precordial leads – 80 case reports. *Chest* 1997; **111**: 537–43.

101. Stein PD, Terrin ML, Hales CA, Palevsky HI, Saltzman HA, Thompson BT, Weg JG. Clinical, laboratory, roentgenographic, and electrocardiographic findings in patients with acute pulmonary embolism and no pre-existing cardiac and pulmonary disease. *Chest* 1991; **100**: 598–603.

102. Hull RD, Raskob GE. Low probability lung scan findings: a need for change. *Ann Intern Med* 1991; **114**: 142–3.

103. PIOPED Investigators. Value of ventilation/perfusion scan in acute pulmonary embolism. *JAMA* 1990; **263**: 2753–9.

104. Krivec B, Voga G, Zuran I, Skale R, Pareznik R, Podbregar M, Noc M. Diagnosis and treatment of shock due to massive pulmonary embolism: approach with transesophageal echocardiography and intrapulmonary thrombolysis. *Chest* 1997; **112**: 1310–16.

105. Mayo JR, Remy-Jardin M, Muller N, *et al*. Pulmonary embolism: prospective comparison of spiral CT with ventilation-perfusion scintigraphy. *Radiology* 1997; **205**: 447–52.

106. Pruszczyk P, Torbicki A, Pacho R, Chlebus M, Kuch-Wocial A, Pruszynski B, Gurba H. Noninvasive diagnosis of suspected severe pulmonary embolism: transesophageal echocardiography vs spiral CT. *Chest* 1997; **112**: 722–8.

♦106a. Hartman IJC, Hagen PJ, Melissant CF, Postmus PE, Prins MH. Diagnosing acute pulmonary embolism: effect of chronic obstructive pulmonary disease on the performance of D-Dimer testing, ventilation/perfusion scintigraphy, spiral computed tomographic angiography, and conventional angiograph. *Am J Respir Crit Care Med* 2000; **162**: 2232–7.

106b. Dalen JE, Hirsh J. Fifth ACCP consensus conference on antithrombotic therapy (1998): summary recommendations. *Chest* 1998; **114**(suppl): 439S–769S.

107. Hull R, Raskob G, Rosenbloom D, *et al*. Optimal therapeutic level of heparin therapy in patients with venous thrombosis. *Arch Intern Med* 1992; **152**: 1589–95.

○108. Hirsh J, Hoak J. Management of deep vein thrombosis and pulmonary embolism: a statement for healthcare professionals. *Circulation* 1996; **93**: 2212–45.

109. Hyers TM, Hull RD, Weg JG. Antithrombotic therapy for venous thromboembolic disease. *Chest* 1995; **108**: 335S–51S.

110. Hull RD, Pineo GF. Current concepts of anticoagulation therapy. *Clin Chest Med* 1995; **16**: 269–80.

111. Tapson VF, Hull RD. Management of venous thromboembolic disease: the impact of low molecular weight heparin. *Clin Chest Med* 1995; **16**: 281–94.

112. Konstantinides S, Geibel A, Olschewski M, *et al*. Association between thrombolytic treatment and the prognosis of hemodynamically stable patients with major pulmonary embolism. *Circulation* 1997; **96**: 882–8.

113. Levine MN. Thrombolytic therapy for venous thromboembolism: complications and contraindications. *Clin Chest Med* 1995; **16**: 321–8.

♦114. Decousus H, Leizorvicz A, Parent F, *et al*. A clinical trial of vena cava filters in the prevention of pulmonary embolism with proximal deep vein thrombosis. *N Engl J Med* 1998; **338**: 409–15.

115. Ballew KA, Philbrick JT, Becker DM. Vena cava filter devices. *Clin Chest Med* 1995; **16**: 295–305.

116. Kasper W, Konstantinides S, Geibel A, *et al*. Management strategies and determinants of outcome in acute major pulmonary embolism: results of a multicenter registry. *J Am Coll Cardiol* 1997; **30**: 1165–71.

117. Oakley CM. There is no place for acute pulmonary embolectomy. *Br J Hosp Med* 1989; **41**: 469.

118. Clarke DB. Pulmonary embolectomy has a well defined and valuable place. *Br J Hosp Med* 1989; **41**: 468–9.

119. Weg JG. Pulmonary embolism and deep vein thrombosis. In: Rippe JM, Irvine RS, Fink MP, Cerra FB eds *Intensive care medicine*, 3rd edn. Boston: Little, Brown, and Co., 1996: 660–79.

120. Clarke DB. Pulmonary embolectomy re-evaluated. *Ann Roy Coll Surg Engl* 1981; **63**: 18–24.

121. Bobrowitz ID, Ramakrishna S, Shim YS. Comparison of medical vs. surgical treatment of major hemoptysis. *Arch Intern Med* 1983; **143**: 1343–6.

122. Crocco JA, Rooney JJ, Fankushen DS, *et al*. Massive hemoptysis. *Arch Intern Med* 1968; **121**: 495–8.

123. Jones DK, Davies RJ. Massive hemoptysis: medical management will usually arrest the bleeding. *Br Med J* 1990; **300**: 889–90.

124. Stroller JK. Diagnosis and management of massive hemoptysis: a review. *Respir Care* 1992; **37**: 564–81.

125. Yang CT, Berger HW. Conservative management of life-threatening hemoptysis. *Mt Sinai J Med* 1978; **45**: 329–33.

126. Yeoh CB, Hubaytar RT, Ford JM, *et al*. Treatment of massive hemorrhage in pulmonary tuberculosis. *J Thorac Cardiovasc Surg* 1967; **54**: 503–10.

127. Corey R, Hla KM. Major and massive hemoptysis. Reassessment of conservative management. *Am J Med Sci* 1987; **294**: 301–9.

128. Gourin A, Garzon AA. Operative treatment of massive hemoptysis. *Ann Thorac Surg* 1974; **18**: 52–60.

129. Winter SM, Ingbar DH. Massive hemoptysis: pathogenesis and management. *J Intern Care Med* 1988; **3**: 171–88.

130. Patel U, Pattison CW, Raphael M. Management of massive hemoptysis. *Br J Hosp Med* 1994; **52**: 74–8.

131. Deffebach ME, Charan NB, Lakshminarayan S, *et al*. The bronchial circulation: small but a vital attribute of the lung. *Am Rev Respir Dis* 1987; **135**: 463–81.

132. Uflacker R, Kaemmerer A, Picon PD, *et al*. Bronchial artery embolization in the management of hemoptysis: technical aspects and long-term results. *Radiology* 1985; **157**: 637–44.

133. Keller FS, Rosh J, Loflin TG, *et al*. Nonbronchial systemic collateral arteries: significance in percutaneous embolotherapy for hemoptysis. *Radiology* 1987; **164**: 687–92.

134. Bartter T, Irwin RS, Nash G. Aneurysms of the pulmonary arteries. *Chest* 1988; **94**: 1065–75.

135. Nath H. When does bronchial arterial embolization fail to control hemoptysis?. *Chest* 1990; **97**: 515–16.

136. Remy J, Lematrie L, Lafitte JJ, *et al*. Massive hemoptysis of pulmonary artery origin: diagnosis and treatment. *Am J Radiol* 1984; **143**: 963–9.

137. Pursel SE, Lindskog GE. Hemoptysis: a clinical evaluation of 105 patients examined consecutively on a thoracic surgical service. *Am Rev Respir Dis* 1961; **84**: 329–36.

138. Set PA, Flower CD, Smith IE, *et al*. Hemoptysis: comparative study of the role of CT and fiberoptic bronchoscopy. *Radiology* 1993; **189**: 677–80.

139. Imgrund SP, Goldberg SK, Walkenstein D, *et al*. Clinical diagnosis of massive hemoptysis using the fiberoptic bronchoscope. *Crit Care Med* 1985; **13**: 438–43.

140. Knott-Craig CJ, Oostuizen JG, Rossouw G, *et al*. Management and prognosis of massive hemoptysis. recent experience with 120 patients. *J Thorac Cardiovasc Surg* 1993; **105**: 394–7.

141. Joharjy IA, Bashi SA, Abdullah AK. Value of medium thickness CT in the diagnosis of bronchiectasis. *Am J Roentgenol* 1987; **149**: 1133–7.

142. Zabala DC. Pulmonary hemorrhage in fiberoptic transbronchial biopsy. *Chest* 1976; **70**: 584–8.

143. Conlan AA. Massive hemoptysis- diagnostic and therapeutic implications. *Surg Annu* 1985; **17**: 337–54.

144. Conlan AA, Hurwitz SS. Management of massive hemoptysis with the rigid bronchoscope and cold saline lavage. *Thorax* 1980; **35**: 901–4.

145. Conlan AA, Hurwitz SS, Krige L, *et al*. Massive hemoptysis: review of 123 cases. *J Thorac Cardiovasc Surg* 1983; **85**: 120–4.

146. Feloney JP, Balchum OJ. Repeated massive hemoptysis: successful control using multiple balloon tipped catheters for endobronchial tamponade. *Chest* 1978; **74**: 683–5.

147. Saw EC, Gottlieb LS, Yokohama T, *et al*. Flexible fiberoptic bronchoscopy and endobronchial tamponade in the management of massive hemoptysis. *Chest* 1976; **70**: 589–91.

148. Swersky RB, Chang JB, Wisoff BG, *et al*. Endobronchial balloon tamponade of hemoptysis in patients with cystic fibrosis. *Ann Thorac Surg* 1979; **27**: 262–4.

149. Wood RE, Campbell D, Razzuk MA, *et al*. Surgical advantages of selective unilateral ventilation. *Ann Thorac Surg* 1972; 73–180.

150. Ramakantan R, Bandekar VG, Gandhi MS, *et al*. Massive hemoptysis due to pulmonary tuberculosis: control with bronchial artery embolization. *Radiology* 1996; **200**: 691–4.

151. Thompson AB, Tescheler H, Rennace S. Pathogenesis, evaluation and therapy for massive hemoptysis. *Clin Chest Med* 1992; **13**: 69–81.

152. Bartter T, Irwin RS, Phillips DA, *et al*. Pulmonary artery pseudoaneurysm: a potential complication of pulmonary artery catheterization. *Arch Intern Med* 1988; **148**: 471–3.

153. Clark CP, Jackson KA, Moreland M, *et al*. Bronchoscopic use of the neodymium-yttrium-aluminium-garnet laser for lesions of the trachea and bronchus. *Med J Aust* 1989; **150**: 260–2.

154. Ashbaugh DG, Petty TL, Bigelow DB, *et al*. Acute respiratory distress in adults. *Lancet* 1967; **2**: 319–23.

155. Bernard GR, Artigas A, Brigham KL, *et al*. The American–European Consensus conference on ARDS: definitions, mechanisms, relevant outcomes, and clinical trial coordination. *Am J Respir Crit Care Med* 1994; **149**: 818–24.

156. Deheinzelin D, Jatene FB, Salvida PHN, Brentani RR. Upregulation of collagen messenger RNA expression occurs immediately after lung damage. *Chest* 1997; **112**: 1184–8.

157. Vasilyev S, Schnaap RN, Mortensen JD. Hospital survival rates of patients with acute respiratory failure in modern respiratory intensive care units. *Chest* 1995; **107**: 1083–8.

158. Suchtya MR, Clemmer TP, Orme JF, Morris AH, Elliott CG. Increased survival of ARDS patients with severe hypoxemia (ECMO criteria). *Chest* 1991; **99**: 1417–21.

159. Kollef MH, Schuster DP. The acute respiratory distress syndrome. *N Engl J Med* 1995; **332**: 27–37.

160. Mitchell JP, Schuller D, Calandrino FS, Schuster DP. Improved outcome based on fluid management in critically ill patients requiring pulmonary artery catheterization. *Am Rev Respir Dis* 1992; **145**: 990–8.

161. Meduri GO, Headley S, Golden E, Carson SJ, Umberger RA, Kelso T, Tolley EA. Effect of prolonged methylprednisolone therapy in unresolving acute respiratory distress syndrome: a randomized controlled trial. *JAMA* 1998; **280**: 159–65.

♦161a. Acute Respiratory Distress Syndrome Network. Ventilation with lower tidal volumes for acute lung injury and the acute respiratory distress syndrome. *N Engl J Med* 2000; **342**: 1301–8.

162. Roy TM, Ossorio MA, Cipolla LM, *et al*. Pulmonary complications after tricyclic antidepressant overdose. *Chest* 1989; **96**: 852–6.

163. Aldrich TK, Prezant DJ. Adverse effects of drugs on the respiratory muscles. *Clin Chest Med* 1990; **11**: 177–89.

164. Meeker DP, Wiedemann HP. Drug induced bronchospasm. *Clin Chest Med* 1990; **11**: 163–75.

165. Reed CR, Glauser FL. Drug induced noncardiogenic pulmonary edema. *Chest* 1991; **100**: 1120–4.

166. Holoye PY, Luna MA, Mackay B, Bedrossian CWM. Bleomycin hypersensitivity pneumonitis. *Ann Intern Med* 1978; **88**: 47–9.

167. Cooper LA, White DA, Matthay RA. Drug induced pulmonary disease. Part 1: cytotoxic drugs. *Am Rev Resp Dis* 1986; **133**: 321–40.

168. Rosenow EC III, Myers JL, Swensen SJ, Pisani RJ. Drug induced pulmonary disease: An update. *Chest* 1992; **102**: 239–50.

169. Van Barneveld PWC, Sleijfer DT, Van Der Mark TW, *et al*. Natural course of bleomycin-induced pneumonitis. *Am Rev Resp Dis* 1987; **135**: 48–51.

170. Taviera da Silva AM. Management of respiratory complications. In: Haddad LM, Winchester JF, eds *Clinical management of poisoning and drug overdose*. Philadelphia: WB Saunders, 1990: 198.

171. Heffner JE, Harley RA, Schabel SI. Pulmonary reactions from illicit substance abuse. *Clin Chest Med* 1990; **11**: 151–62.

172. Schwartz JA, Koenigsberg MA. Naloxone induced pulmonary edema. *Ann Emerg Med* 1987; **16**: 1294–6.

173. Pisani RJ, Rosenow EC III. Pulmonary edema associated with tocolytic therapy. *Ann Intern Med* 1989; **110**: 714–18.

174. Holland CL, Singh AK, McMaster RRB, Fang W. Adverse reactions to protamine sulfate following cardiac surgery. *Clin Cardiol* 1984; **7**: 157–62.

175. Hamous JE, Guffy M, Aschebrener CA. Fatal acute respiratory failure following intrathecal methotrexate administration. *Cancer Treat Rep* 1983; **67**: 1025–6.

176. Kaplan AL, Sabin S. Dextran 40: another cause of drug induced noncardiogenic pulmonary edema. *Chest* 1975; **68**: 376–7.

177. Leake JF, Murphy AA, Zacur HA. Noncardiogenic pulmonary edema: a complication of operative hysteroscopy. *Fertil Steril* 1987; **48**: 497–9.

178. Zbella EA, Moise J, Carson SA, *et al*. Noncardiogenic pulmonary edema secondary to intrauterine instillation of 32% dextran 70. *Fertil Steril* 1985; **43**: 479–80.

179. Greganti MA, Flowers WM. Acute pulmonary edema after the administration of contrast media. *Radiology* 1979; **123**: 583–5.

180. Rosenow EC III. Drug-induced pulmonary disease. In: Murray JF, Nadel JA, eds *Textbook of respiratory medicine*. Philadelphia: WB Saunders, 1988: 1681.

181. Forrester JM, Steele AW, Waldrom JA, *et al*. Crack lung: an acute pulmonary syndrome with a spectrum of clinical and histopathologic findings. *Am Rev Resp Dis* 1990; **142**: 462–7.

182. Shesser R, Davis C, Edelstein S. Pneumomediastinum and pneumothorax after inhaling alkaloid cocaine. *Ann Emerg Med* 1982; **10**: 213–15.

183. Plueckhahn VD. Alcohol and accidental drowning: a 25-year study. *Med J Aust* 1984; **141**: 22–5.

184. Centers for Disease Control. Aquatic deaths and injuries: United States. *MMWR* 1982; **31**: 417–19.

185. Pearn JH, Brown J, Wong R, *et al*. Bathtub drownings: report of seven cases. *Pediatrics* 1979; **64**: 68–70.

186. Fandel I, Bancalari E. Near-drowning in children: clinical aspects. *Pediatrics* 1976; **58**: 573–9.

187. Lavelle JM, Shaw KN, Seidl T, Ludwig S. Ten year review of pediatric bathtub near drownings: evaluation for child abuse and neglect. *Ann Emerg Med* 1995; **25**: 344–8.

188. Diekema DS, Quan L, Holt VL. Epilepsy as a risk factor for submersion in children. *Pediatrics* 1993; **91**: 612–16.

189. Dietz PE, Baker S. Drowning. *Am J Public Health* 1974: **64**: 303–12.

190. Bolte RG, Black PG, Bowers RS, *et al*. The use of extracorporeal rewarming in a child submerged for 66 minutes. *JAMA* 1988; **260**: 377–9.

191. Conn AW, Miyasaka K, Katayama M, Fujita M, Orima H, Barker G, Bohn D. A canine study of cold water drowning in fresh versus salt water. *Crit Care Med* 1995; **23**: 2029–37.

192. Gunton RW, Scott JW, Lougheed WM, *et al*. Changes in cardiac rhythm in the form of the electrocardiogram resulting from induced hypothermia in man. *Am Heart J* 1956; **52**: 419–27.

193. Trevino A, Razi B, Beller BM. The characteristic electrocardiogram of accidental hypothermia. *Arch Intern Med* 1971; **127**: 470–3.

194. Vandam LD, Burnap TK. Hypothermia. *N Engl J Med* 1959; **261**: 546–53.

195. Orlowski JP, Abulleil MM, Phillips JM. The hemodynamic and cardiovascular effects of near-drowning in hypotonic, isotonic, hypertonic solutions. *Ann Emerg Med* 1989; **18**: 1044–9.

196. Orlowski JP, Abulliel MM, Phillips JM. Effects of tonicities of saline solutions on pulmonary injury in drowning. *Crit Care Med* 1987; **15**: 126–30.

197. Reilly K, Ozanne A, Murdoch BE, *et al*. Linguistic status subsequent to childhood immersion injury. *Med J Aust* 1988; **148**: 225–8.

198. Abrams RA, Mubarak S. Musculoskeletal consequences of near-drowning in children. *J Pediatr Orthop* 1991; **11**: 168–75.

199. Hasan S, Avery WG, Fabian C, *et al*. Near-drowning in humans: a report of 36 patients. *Chest* 1971; **59**: 191–7.

200. Bohn DJ, Biggar WD, Smith CR, *et al*. Influence of hypothermia, barbiturate therapy, and intracranial pressure monitoring on morbidity and mortality after near-drowning. *Crit Care Med* 1986; **14**: 529–34.

201. Ports TA, Deuel TF. Intravascular coagulation in freshwater submersion: report of three cases. *Ann Intern Med* 1977; **87**: 60–1.

202. Munroe WD. Hemoglobinuria from near-drowning. *J Pediatr* 1964; **64**: 57–62.

203. Grausz H, Amend WJC, Earley LE. Acute renal failure complicating submersion in seawater. *JAMA* 1971; **217**: 207–9.

204. Modell JH, Conn AW. Current neurological considerations in near-drowning. *Can Anaesth Soc J* 1980; **3**: 197–8.

205. Conn A, Montes J, Barker G. Cerebral salvage in near-drowning following neurologic classification by triage. *Can J Anaesth* 1980; **27**: 201–9.

206. Ornato JP. The resuscitation of near-drowning victims. *JAMA* 1986; **256**: 75–7.

207. Rosen P, Stoto M, Harley J. The use of the Heimlich maneuver in near drowning: Institute of Medicine Report. *J Emerg Med* 1995; **13**: 397–405.

208. Hayward JS, Steinman AM. Accidental hypothermia: an experimental study of inhalation rewarming. *Aviat Space Environ Med* 1975; **46**: 1236–40.

209. Wickstrom P, Ruiz E, Lilja GP, *et al*. Accidental hypothermia: core rewarming with partial bypass. *Am J Surg* 1976; **131**: 622–5.

210. Dottorini M, Eslami A, Baglioni S, Fiorenzano G, Todisco T. Nasal continuous positive airway pressure in the treatment of near-drowning in freshwater. *Chest* 1996; **110**: 1122–4.

211. Perez-Benavides F, Riff E, Franks C. Adult respiratory distress syndrome and artificial surfactant replacement in the pediatric patient. *Pediatr Emerg Care* 1995; **11**: 153–5.

212. Calderwood HW, Modell JH, Ruiz BC. The ineffectiveness of steroid therapy for treatment of freshwater near-drowning. *Anesthesiology* 1975; **43**: 642–50.

213. Bernard GR, Luce JM, Sprung CL, *et al*. High dose corticosteroids in patients with the adult respiratory distress syndrome. *N Engl J Med* 1987; **317**: 1565–70.

214. Light RW. Pneumothorax. In: Murray JF, Nadel JA, eds *Textbook of respiratory medicine*. Philadelphia: WB Saunders, 1988: 1745–59.

215. Jenkinson SG. Pneumothorax. *Clin Chest Med* 1985; **6**: 153–61.

216. Kirby TJ, Ginsberg RJ. Management of the pneumothorax and barotrauma. *Clin Chest Med* 1992; **13**: 97–112.

217. O'Neill S. Spontaneous pneumothorax: aeteology, management and complications. *Irish Med J* 1987; **88**: 306–11.

218. Vukich DL. Diseases of the pleural space. *Emerg Med Clin North Am* 1989; **7**: 309–24.

219. Melton LJ, Hepper NG, Offord KP. Incidence of spontaneous pneumothorax in Olmstead County, Minnesota: 1950–1974. *Am Rev Respir Dis* 1979; **120**: 1379–82.

220. Gammon RB, Shin MS, Buchalter SE. Pulmonary barotrauma in mechanical ventilation. *Chest* 1992: **102**: 568–72.

221. Striater RM, Lynch JP. Complications in the ventilated patient. *Clin Chest Med* 1988; **9**: 127–39.

222. Pierrson DJ. Alveolar rupture during mechanical ventilation: role of PEEP, peak airway pressure, and distending volume. *Respir Care* 1988; **33**: 472–84.

223. Symbas PN. Cardiothoracic trauma. *Curr Probl Surg* 1991; **28**: 741–97.

11

Cardiac arrest and sudden cardiac death

ROBERT S MITTLEMAN

Sudden cardiac death remains a significant public health problem worldwide. Since recent studies have confirmed the effectiveness of the implantable defibrillator in treating this problem, this is often the best management, but decision-making remains difficult in many cases. In particular, managing patients with coronary artery disease requires careful individualization for the best treatment.

INTRODUCTION

The management of an aborted episode of sudden cardiac death can be approached in a variety of ways. A simplistic approach would suggest that, if a person has had a cardiac arrest and is fortunate enough to be resuscitated, they are at significant risk of a recurrent event. Since implantable cardioverter defibrillators are now available that are extremely effective in automatically detecting and treating such an event, management might involve nothing more than the insertion of such a device, in many cases a relatively minor operation. In fact, although in many cases decision-making in such a patient can be approached in exactly that way, there is often a great deal of subtlety involved. To appreciate the complexity of the process fully, a thorough understanding of the diagnosis and management of this disorder is necessary.

EPIDEMIOLOGY

Despite the many advances in the management of patients with heart disease, cardiac arrest remains a significant public health problem, resulting in approximately 300 000 deaths per year in the USA.[1] Only 20–30 per cent of such patients are successfully resuscitated and, when that person has significant neurologic recovery, they are very fortunate indeed.[2] Twenty to 25 per cent of these patients have no history of prior cardiac disease.[1] Clearly the best approach to the management of these patients is prevention of the primary event. Although it is beyond the scope of this chapter, the reader should be aware that a considerable amount of work is under way to devise strategies to stratify risk in patients who are known to have cardiac disease. Also of great interest are public health efforts to increase public awareness of the symptoms of acute myocardial infarction and the importance of early access to sophisticated emergency medical care. Such efforts could improve the likelihood of successful resuscitation. There are also efforts under way to increase the use of semiautomatic external defibrillators, with the goal of improving success rates for defibrillation. Unfortunately, there is currently no approach to the prevention of sudden cardiac death in patients without prior history of heart disease, although it would seem likely that risk factor modification for patients prone to the development of coronary artery disease, such as the aggressive treatment of hyperlipidemia, would be of benefit.

PATHOPHYSIOLOGY

Although the pathophysiologic basis of an episode of sudden cardiac death has not been completely defined, there are certain key elements that are largely accepted. In general, a cardiac arrest is felt to occur under most circumstances as a result of an unfortunate coexistence of structural cardiac abnormalities, which are frequently pre-existing, complicated by transient risk factors that act as a trigger to precipitate ventricular fibrillation (Table 11.1). It is hypothesized that the abnormal cardiac substrate predisposes to abnormalities in conduction or repolarization that may support re-entrant arrhythmias and, at a particular time due to ischemia, electrolyte abnormalities, or other causes, ectopy as well as increased cellular excitability combine to either precipitate an episode of ventricular fibrillation directly or a different tachyarrhythmia, which results in hemodynamic instability and therefore a downward spiral toward fibrillation (Fig. 11.1 and Table 11.1).

Certainly coronary disease is the most common factor in sudden cardiac death; most patients who have died suddenly will have significant chronic coronary stenoses in at least one coronary artery, and multivessel disease is not an uncommon occurrence.[3,4] Acute coronary throm-

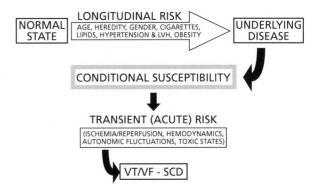

Figure 11.1 *Epidemiology of sudden cardiac death (SCD): long-term risk factors versus transient risk. Longitudinal risk refers to those epidemiological risk factors that predict the evolution of the disease states predisposing to the event (i.e. the conditioning factors). Transient or acute risk refers to those factors that are directly related to electrophysiological instability at a specific point in time. The latter may also be interpreted in terms of individual susceptibility to the adverse influences of the transient risk factor. LVH = left ventricular hypertrophy; VT/VF-SCD = ventricular tachycardia/ventricular fibrillation or sudden cardiac death. (Reproduced with permission of the publisher from Zipes DP, Jalife J, eds* Cardiac electrophysiology: from cell to bedside. *Philadelphia: WB Saunders, 1995: 723–31.)*

Table 11.1 *Etiologic basis and transient risk factors associated with sudden cardiac death. (Adapted from Myerburg RJ, Interian A, Mitrani RM, Kessler KM, Castellanos A. Am J Cardiol 1997; **80**(5B): 10F–19F).*

Structural abnormalities

Coronary heart disease	80%
Acute ischemic events	
Chronic ischemic heart disease	
Cardiomyopathies	10–15%
Dilated cardiomyopathies	
Hypertrophic cardiomyopathies	
Valvular/inflammation/infiltration	±5%
Uncommon, subtle, ill-defined lesions	
e.g. RV dysplasia	
Lesions of molecular structure	?%
e.g. congenital long QT syndromes	
Definable functional abnormalities	

Transient risk factors

Ischemia and reperfusion
   Ischemia ventricular tachycardia/fibrillation
   Initiation of monomorphic VT by ischemia
   Reperfusion arrhythmias
Systemic inciting factors
   Hemodynamic dysfunction
   Hypoxemia, acidosis
   Electrolyte imbalance
Neurophysiologic interactions
   Central and systemic factors
   Local cardiac factors – transmitters/receptors
Toxic cardiac effects
   Idiosyncratic proarrhythmia
   Dose-dependent proarrhythmia
   Transient proarrhythmic risk

RV = right ventricle; VT = ventricular tachycardia.

bosis can also be seen, but it is a less common occurrence.[3,5,6] Healed myocardial infarction or aneurysm is also common, being found in about half of all patients who die suddenly.[7,8] Recent myocardial infarction is seen less commonly, in the order of 20 per cent of the time, and this corresponds well with clinical observations that episodes of aborted sudden cardiac death are associated with an acute myocardial infarction about 20–30 per cent of the time.[1–3,7,8] It is not surprising that patients with coronary artery disease who have a reduced ejection fraction are at increased risk.

Patients with dilated cardiomyopathy without coronary disease are at increased risk of sudden cardiac death, whether due to valvular heart disease, viral myocarditis, alcohol, or other causes.[9,10] The precise pathophysiology may vary in these different conditions. There is no question that congestive heart failure predisposes patients to sudden cardiac death regardless of the etiology, and acute alcohol or drug intoxication, as well as an acute viral myocarditis, can be precipitating factors as well.[9,11–14]

Ventricular hypertrophy is also recognized to be associated with a predisposition to ventricular arrhythmias and sudden cardiac death.[15,16] Certainly patients with hypertrophic cardiomyopathy, either obstructive or non-obstructive, are at increased risk of sudden cardiac death, and there seems to be an association of secondary forms of hypertrophic heart disease with sudden cardiac death as well.[17]

Certain other conditions are also associated with cardiac arrest. Mitral valve prolapse, although a common condition, is usually not associated with life-threatening arrhythmias, but in rare circumstances this can occur.[18] Other uncommon conditions, including the congenital long QT syndrome and the newly recognized Brugada syndrome, although rare, place a person at dramatically increased risk of cardiac arrest, and these etiologies should be considered in patients who present with a cardiac arrest.[19-21]

There are undoubtedly a variety of triggers of cardiac arrest, although it is equally likely that not all of these have been identified. As previously mentioned, severe electrolyte abnormalities can be associated with ventricular arrhythmias, and can place a person at risk. In recent years there has been concern that most antiarrhythmic medications can at least under certain circumstances precipitate an unstable ventricular tachyarrhythmia, which has led to increasing caution about their use, particularly in patients with significant structural heart disease.[22,23] The mechanism by which they promote arrhythmias is most likely by slowing conduction with inadequate prolongation of refractory periods, although this is still under investigation.

Premature ventricular contractions and nonsustained runs of ventricular tachycardia can also promote sustained arrhythmias, either by producing a pause resulting in early afterdepolarization, or by initiating a re-entrant circuit, or by a combination of these two effects. As alluded to earlier, ischemia can promote arrhythmias in a variety of ways, including direct toxic effects (hypoxia, acidosis) resulting in cellular depolarization, the production of reperfusion arrhythmias, as well as other mechanisms.

Congestive heart failure, which will, of course, generally occur in patients with structural heart disease, also will promote the likelihood of an arrest.[9,10] The mechanism for this is unclear. These patients are more likely to have electrolyte abnormalities, ischemia, and hypoxia, but there may be other factors at play as well, such as acute myocardial stretch or neurohumoral factors.

There has recently been a great deal of interest in the importance of autonomic influences on the predisposition to cardiac arrest.[24,25] There also have been reports of stress-related factors being implicated in cardiac arrest.[26] The importance of such factors and the means by which they would be harmful remain undefined.

MANAGEMENT

Historical perspective

Initial studies recognizing the importance of out of hospital cardiac arrest as an important cause of cardiac death and the potential of its prevention occurred more than 20 years ago, with the pioneering studies of Cobb and colleagues.[27] Their work also showed the very high recurrence rate of patients who presented with a cardiac arrest not associated with a myocardial infarction, with a relatively low recurrence when cardiac arrest was associated with an infarction. Antiarrhythmic agents such as quinidine were felt to be effective, but they were initially used in an unguided or empiric fashion.

In the 1980s several studies demonstrated the use of invasive electrophysiologic testing in managing patients who had presented with sustained ventricular tachycardia and ventricular fibrillation.[28-30] The studies reported that patients who presented with life-threatening ventricular arrhythmias could have a similar or even the identical arrhythmia reproducibly produced by programmed ventricular stimulation in the electrophysiology laboratory. They were then treated with antiarrhythmic agents and, if the antiarrhythmic agent was effective in suppressing the inducibility of the arrhythmia in the electrophysiology laboratory, the recurrence rate of the arrhythmia was felt to be low. The result of the programmed stimulation was therefore felt to predict the recurrence of the arrhythmia. This approach gained great popularity and has been in most academic medical centers the preferred management option for the management of an aborted cardiac arrest over a period of 15 years, until the recent dramatic growth in the use of implantable defibrillators.

Also in the 1980s, studies were performed demonstrating that patients with life-threatening ventricular arrhythmias could be managed based on the frequency and type of ventricular ectopy; the investigators once again used this as a surrogate for the spontaneous occurrence of the arrhythmia.[31] Although this approach gained less acceptance than invasive electrophysiologic testing for managing such patients, there was considerable controversy during this era. This controversy prompted the development of the ESVEM (electrophysiologic studies versus electrocardiographic monitoring) study, which was one of the earliest multicenter randomized clinical trials evaluating the management of ventricular tachyarrhythmias.[32,33] In this study, patients who presented with ventricular tachycardia or ventricular fibrillation received an initial invasive electrophysiologic evaluation and a Holter monitor. If they had both inducible ventricular tachycardia and frequent ventricular ectopy by Holter monitor, they were sequentially randomized to a series of six different antiarrhythmic agents, with follow-up testing by either of the two modalities, until the arrhythmia was suppressed. Amiodarone was not one of the drugs tested. The patients were then continued on the antiarrhythmic agent that was defined as successful. Although the study was criticized for slow recruitment and certain other aspects of the study design, the final report surprised many investigators, with the observation that the two techniques produced an equal number of arrhythmia recurrences. Other important observations from the study were a surprisingly high arrhythmia recurrence rate (65 per cent at 3 years follow-up, with a sudden death incidence of 10 per cent and 18 per cent at 1- and 3-year follow-up, respectively) and a dismal rate (<10 per cent) of continuation of antiarrhythmic agents defined as successful during the initial evaluation.

Amiodarone

Amiodarone has also been extensively studied throughout the past two decades for the treatment of ventricular tachyarrhythmias. Several, retrospective, uncontrolled studies reported favorable results of the effectiveness of amiodarone for the control of ventricular tachycardia and fibrillation.[34–36] One randomized trial, the CASCADE study, compared the empiric use of amiodarone to other antiarrhythmic agents guided by Holter or programmed stimulation.[36] The results of this study were questioned by many investigators because of concerns about the protocol structure, including the transition to frequent use of implantable defibrillators during the course of the trial. Nonetheless, amiodarone was shown to produce a lower incidence of recurrent arrhythmias and a lower discharge rate of the implantable defibrillators used in the trial. In addition, in other studies, amiodarone had shown favorable results compared to placebo when used in patients with a history of recent myocardial infarction and frequent but asymptomatic ventricular ectopy.[37]

Implantable cardioverter defibrillators

During the past two decades, as antiarrhythmic agents have been used and extensively studied for the management of ventricular arrhythmias, implantable defibrillators have been used more and more often for the management of this same problem. Initially implants were difficult, requiring a thoracotomy for the insertion of epicardial shocking electrodes, which carried significant morbidity and mortality for this very sick patient population. Nonetheless, even initial reports suggested their very effective prevention of sudden cardiac death, results which have been borne out over the years. Moreover, implantation techniques have improved as a result of improved electrode design, defibrillation waveforms, and electrical components, greatly easing implants and consequently reducing the morbidity of the procedure as well as the expense and the discomfort for the patient. Despite these technical improvements and favorable retrospective reports, defibrillators were not completely accepted as the standard treatment of a cardiac arrest survivor because there were no results of large randomized trials comparing their effectiveness to other methods of treatment.

Recent randomized clinical trials

The disappointing results found in ESVEM for traditional antiarrhythmic agents and the encouraging results found for amiodarone and implantable defibrillators lead to the development of several studies comparing these two methods of treatment, all of which have reported results in recent years.

The AVID (Antiarrhythmics vs Implantable Defibrillator) study was the largest and first to report results, and has had the greatest impact.[38] This study essentially compared the empiric use of amiodarone to the primary use of implantable defibrillators (i.e. without a baseline electrophysiologic study) to treat survivors of cardiac arrest or ventricular tachycardia causing significant hemodynamic compromise. A small number of patients received sotalol as part of the antiarrhythmic limb of the protocol, but the number of patients who received sotalol was small and consequently there was little impact of this drug on the results of the study. The AVID study was stopped prematurely in April 1997 because of improved survival in the patients treated with implantable defibrillators (Fig. 11.2). These patients had a 39 per cent improvement in survival compared to the amiodarone patients after 1 year, and a 31 per cent improvement after 3 years, results which were highly statistically significant. These results were also consistent throughout all patient subsets, with the possible exception of patients with a preserved ejection fraction (Fig. 11.3).

The Canadian Implantable Defibrillator Study (CIDS), which had a protocol that was very similar to

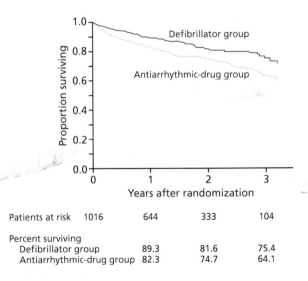

Patients at risk	1016	644	333	104

Percent surviving				
Defibrillator group		89.3	81.6	75.4
Antiarrhythmic-drug group	82.3	74.7	64.1	

Figure 11.2 *Overall survival, unadjusted for baseline characteristics. Survival was better among patients treated with the implantable cardioverter-defibrillator (P<0.02, adjusted for repeated analyses (n = 61)). (Reproduced with permission of the publisher from AVID Investigators: N Engl J Med 1997: 337: 1576–83.)*

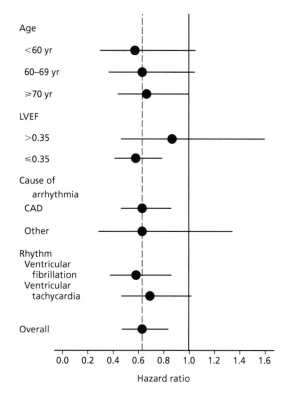

Figure 11.3 *Hazard ratios (and 95 per cent confidence limits) for death from any cause in the defibrillator group as compared with the antiarrhythmic-drug group in prespecified subgroup analyses in the univariate model. No subgroup differed significantly from the entire population. The solid vertical line represents equal effectiveness of the two treatments; points to the left indicate better survival in the defibrillator group, and points to the right better survival in the antiarrhythmic-drug group. The dotted vertical line represents the results for the entire study (hazard ratio = 0.62). LVEF = left ventricular ejection fraction; CAD = coronary artery disease. (Reproduced with permission of the publisher from AVID Investigators.* N Engl J Med *1997:* **337**: *1576–83.)*

AVID, also reported results in 1998.[39] Although these results have not yet been reported in a peer-reviewed journal, this study, which used a smaller patient population than AVID, reported a strong trend toward improved survival in the patients with ICDs that did not achieve statistical significance ($0.1 > P > 0.05$).

The Cardiac Arrest Study of Hamburg (CASH) has reported results in the same time frame.[40] This study examined management of the cardiac arrest survivor with ICDs compared with three other treatments, specifically β-blockers, amiodarone, or the class 1C antiarrhythmic agent propafenone. The propafenone limb of the trial was terminated early because of a worse outcome.[40] Subsequently, the results of the other three limbs have shown nearly identical results with β-blockers compared to amiodarone and, as for CIDS, there was a strong

trend toward improved survival in the ICD limb compared to these two groups.

A meta-analysis combining the results of these three trials has recently been published.[41] These data confirm the consistency of the results from the three trials, and confirm the highly significant benefit of the ICD in comparison to amiodarone. The key finding reported is that the benefit which occurred from the ICD occurred in patients with an ejection fraction less than 35 per cent. The survival with amiodarone was equal to that with the ICD for those patients with an ejection fraction above 35 per cent.

DECISION-MAKING: APPROACH TO THE INDIVIDUAL PATIENT

Acute care

In considering the management of a patient with an aborted episode of sudden cardiac death, there are numerous considerations. First and foremost, it is important to do everything possible to confirm the diagnosis. For these purposes, it is important to remember the definition of a cardiac arrest, which is 'the abrupt cessation of cardiac pump function which may be reversible by a prompt intervention but will lead to death in its absence'.[42] Although there are rare spontaneous reversions, in most cases a patient who develops an arrest associated with ventricular fibrillation will die if defibrillation is not performed. Hence, if a patient had defibrillation performed on the scene, this helps distinguish the condition from spontaneously remitting causes, such as bradyarrhythmias, ventricular tachycardia, or other forms of hemodynamic collapse, which therefore result in syncope. Certainly a recording of a rhythm strip from an external defibrillator or other monitor can help confirm the diagnosis, although artifactual recordings can be mistaken for fibrillation. An experienced nurse, paramedic, or physician on the scene who documents absent pulses is also obviously valuable, although severe hypotension can also result in absent pulses. Under most circumstances, sufficient clinical information is available to confirm the diagnosis but, since there are such critical differences in treatment options based on this fact, it is of the utmost importance to confirm these details to the greatest degree possible prior to proceeding further with the management.

It is now commonly accepted that most patients who suffer a cardiac arrest will do so as a result of ventricular tachycardia or ventricular fibrillation. Nonetheless, bradyarrhythmias can cause an arrest and it has been suggested that, in patients with advanced congestive heart failure, the mechanism of cardiac arrest is more commonly a bradyarrhythmia than for other cardiac patients.[43] On rare occasions a supraventricular tachycardia can lead to a cardiac arrest; this occurs almost exclusively in patients with the Wolfe–Parkinson–White syndrome who have rapid atrial fibrillation.

Evidently the initial priority in managing the survivor of an episode of cardiac arrest is maintaining hemodynamic stability, which may involve ventilatory support, intravenous pressors, invasive hemodynamic monitoring or support, and intravenous antiarrhythmic agents. Although recurrent arrest after initial stabilization can occur, it is far from universal, and it has been estimated that arrhythmias account for no more than 10 per cent of in-hospital deaths.[44]

Nonetheless, frequent ventricular ectopy is common during the first few days after admission, and control of these arrhythmias with intravenous medications is often prudent. Lidocaine remains a reasonable first choice for control of such ectopy. Arrhythmias that are refractory to lidocaine can be treated with any of procainamide, bretylium, or intravenous amiodarone. Usage of intravenous amiodarone is clearly increasing under such circumstances, owing to its efficacy combined with a relatively low side effect profile in randomized comparisons to intravenous bretylium.[45,46] Although I am hesitant to use intravenous amiodarone if a future implantable defibrillator is contemplated due to the interactions between these two treatment modalities, on many occasions control of the spontaneous arrhythmia must take priority.

Convalescent phase

After patients have been stabilized hemodynamically, there is usually a convalescent phase during which the acute interventions and monitoring are gradually withdrawn. My own practice is to withdraw antiarrhythmic medication gradually if the rhythm remains stable over the first 24–48 hours. Over these first few days, serial cardiac enzymes and 12-lead electrocardiograms (ECGs) are also performed to evaluate the possibility of acute myocardial infarction. Frequently, these patients experience aspiration of gastric contents during the arrest, and subsequently develop either a transient pneumonitis or pneumonia requiring antibiotic therapy.

Under most circumstances, a patient who experiences an aborted cardiac arrest will have some degree of anoxic encephalopathy. When this occurs, the degree of impairment can vary from trivial to prolonged coma. This can complicate the evaluation, and it is often wise to obtain neurologic consultation regarding expected long-term neurologic recovery, as this can have a major impact on the approach to therapy.

Even if patients do not show rapid improvement in their neurologic status, considerable late recovery can occur. I have seen cases in which patients have remained comatose for a month or more and have subsequently made very significant recovery, to the point of returning to full-time employment. My own experience is that if patients make significant progress neurologically over the first week, even if they are still severely disoriented, they will usually make a nearly complete recovery over the ensuing months. In these cases, decisions regarding invasive evaluation or defibrillator insertion should be made based on premorbid functional status rather than the current level of neurologic function.

Definitive treatment

As indicated, for patients with a cardiac arrest, it is extremely important to define the nature and severity of existing heart disease. On occasion this can be very straightforward, as patients with a history of cardiovascular disease may have had a recent invasive or non-invasive evaluation. If so, records should be obtained.

It should nonetheless be recognized that there may have been an intervening cardiac event between the last evaluation and the time of admission. For example, occasionally echocardiographic data or data from contrast ventriculography can document a recent myocardial infarction even in cases in which symptomatology is subtle or non-existent. In other cases a patient may have profound acute ischemia, which can result in an arrest without causing a myocardial infarction. This can occur due to coronary spasm, or because of acute occlusion of a bypass graft that supplies a stenosed but patent coronary artery, or alternatively of a native coronary artery, which is also supplied by a patent bypass graft.

In what is possibly a related phenomenon, it is possible to see significant left ventricular dysfunction early after an arrest with significant improvement in ejection fraction noted months later. In these cases, it is difficult to determine whether there has been 'stunning' of the left ventricle without infarction, or alternatively if there has been transient left ventricular dysfunction due to other causes. In any case it is almost always appropriate to re-evaluate left ventricular function either non-invasively or with a cardiac catheterization after a cardiac arrest.

The decision of whether to perform an angiogram after an aborted cardiac arrest should be individualized. In my opinion, if a patient has never had a catheterization, it should be done if a patient has had sustained ventricular tachycardia or fibrillation, as assumptions regarding etiology may prove to be incorrect, and therefore have a significant impact on patient management. In patients who have had a past angiogram and who do not have coronary artery disease, a repeat study would seem to add little that could not be obtained with an echocardiogram.

In patients with a prior catheterization and a history of coronary artery disease, the need for a repeat study should be carefully considered. The additional information which could be gained should be weighed in comparison to the risk of the procedure and the likelihood of the result altering the management. Depending on the anatomy, an evaluation of the ischemic burden may be necessary, using either the traditional radionuclide studies or echocardiography with stress or dobutamine provocation. Sometimes these studies can be used in place of an angiogram; on other occasions, the two techniques yield complementary data.

Once the nature of the underlying heart disease has been defined, decisions can start to be made regarding definitive care. The most immediate question, which generally has been addressed much earlier during the hospitalization, is whether there was a reversible cause. Sometimes this can be obvious, as in the case of a drug overdose, but in other cases there is a great deal of subtlety involved. For example, during the early stages after an arrest, it is not uncommon to find a blood specimen with a low potassium level. However, there are a great many fluid and electrolyte shifts during the early stages after an arrest, and this can be an artifactual or transient phenomenon, which does not reflect the patient's status at the time of the arrest. Other clues must be sought, such as persistent hypokalemia, changes in the ECG that are consistent with the hypothesis, or a history of recent increase in diuretic therapy without augmentation of potassium supplementation.

Myocardial ischemia and sudden cardiac death

The most difficult issue to grapple with in these patients is the relative importance of ischemia. As alluded to earlier, it is generally accepted that arrhythmias occurring in the very early period after a myocardial infarction tend to be generated by an automatic or triggered mechanism, and therefore are not likely to recur after this early period has passed. The mechanism of arrhythmias that occur later after an infarct is more likely to be re-entry, and therefore the arrhythmia is more likely to recur in the future, even with an initiating factor which may be different from that which produced the index event. The dividing line between these two mechanisms is uncertain, but a practical figure is probably about 48 hours.

The decision concerning whether the patient has had a myocardial infarction that is likely to have accounted for the arrhythmia can also be very subtle. Most patients who have had an arrest will have an elevation of cardiac enzymes, so that a relatively small elevation will not be useful. I have seen CPK levels of 700 or higher that I felt were not associated with a myocardial infarction that caused the arrhythmia. Patients will often have ST-T wave changes on their cardiogram after an arrest as well, and it can be unclear whether the arrhythmia caused hemodynamic compromise, which resulted in the ischemia, or instead, if the person developed ischemia that precipitated the arrhythmia.

History can often be helpful. A myocardial infarction (MI) can clearly be diagnosed if a patient comes to the emergency room with symptoms consistent with an acute MI, is in normal sinus rhythm with changes consistent with an acute infarction, and then develops a witnessed, monitored arrest. On the other hand, a patient can develop a rapid ventricular tachycardia, have symptoms consistent with an acute MI as a result of the arrhythmia, and proceed to rapid ventricular fibrillation and hemodynamic collapse prior to the arrival of emergency personnel. If that person is resuscitated and brought in for ongoing care, it can be very hard to discern what was the initiating event. In many cases, it is wise to treat both ischemia and the arrhythmia while acknowledging uncertainty about the precise sequence of events.

In a patient who has demonstrable ischemia without acute infarction, a review of the literature does not lead to any clear-cut guidelines.[47] Multiple retrospective studies have suggested that, when patients who have a cardiac arrest receive coronary artery bypass surgery, their prognosis is good, although these patients often received antiarrhythmic medications or ICDs as ancillary therapy. In one review of 50 patients who presented with a cardiac arrest and had surgically corrected coronary disease, four patients had recurrent arrhythmia and one patient died suddenly.[48] Most of the patients who had inducible polymorphic ventricular tachycardia preoperatively were non-inducible after surgery. However, most of those patients with inducible monomorphic VT (80 per cent) still had inducible tachycardia after surgery, and most of those patients were treated with either antiarrhythmic medication or implantable defibrillator insertion. Although it is not proven, it is assumed that, because these patients have persistent inducible arrhythmias after surgery, they remain at increased risk of recurrent events. There are no prospective studies.

Therefore, the appropriate management is unclear. If the patient has symptoms consistent with angina, it seems reasonable to pursue revascularization aggressively, as this can be life saving. Other cases must be individualized. Decision-making can be difficult as revascularization can be a high-risk procedure, much more risky than a defibrillator insertion. On the other hand, an ischemically mediated episode of ventricular fibrillation may not be terminated successfully by an ICD. To summarize, it seems reasonable to conclude that revascularization is useful therapy but in many cases is not comprehensive.

Invasive electrophysiologic testing

The role for invasive electrophysiologic testing for patients with aborted sudden cardiac death is currently unsettled. As alluded to earlier, although the inducibility of ventricular tachycardia or ventricular fibrillation was previously used to guide antiarrhythmic therapy, recent randomized clinical trial data suggest that the strategy of direct ICD insertion without a prior EP study yields improved survival compared to the empiric use of amiodarone, and the use of class I antiarrhythmic agents for this purpose has fallen out of favor. There is at least one ongoing randomized trial of the use of EP testing prior to ICD implantation to determine the incremental cost and effect on management. At the present time, in patients fitting the AVID entry criteria, the strategy of ICD implantation without an EP study seems reasonable.

Nonetheless, in certain patients, programmed stimulation can be a useful technique. In general, it has been found that 70–80 per cent of patients who present with ventricular fibrillation or cardiac arrest will have a tachycardia inducible. Since ventricular fibrillation appears to be a re-entrant arrhythmia, one would expect a large percentage of these patients to be inducible. Programmed stimulation is performed in a stable patient in a controlled environment, often with significant sedation, and these circumstances clearly do not mimic real-life circumstances in many ways. It is therefore not completely surprising that not all patients are inducible.

Still, the presence of inducible sustained monomorphic ventricular tachycardia does demonstrate that the substrate exists, which could potentially support an unstable arrhythmia. In cases in which circumstances are equivocal, therefore, the inducibility of ventricular tachycardia can yield important decision-making information. It can also be of value in assessing prognosis. It has been demonstrated that patients with a history of cardiac arrest who have inducible tachycardia are at higher risk of recurrence than those who do not.[49] Nonetheless, even those patients who are not inducible remain at significant risk of recurrence compared to the general population, and therefore would still potentially benefit from defibrillator insertion.

PUTTING IT ALL TOGETHER

The initial management of the patient with cardiac arrest is focused on stabilization of the patient, and is not affected in any significant way by the plans for long-term management. If an ICD insertion is considered a possibility, central venous access should be avoided via the left subclavian approach, since this is normally the preferred location for ICD insertion. Very early during hospitalization, bradyarrhythmias should be considered as a possible cause of the cardiac arrest, and a decision should be made regarding whether the patient has had an arrest as a result of a myocardial infarction or if the arrhythmia was the primary event, as these two factors could alter the focus in attempts to stabilize the patient. Analysis of these data will help classify the type of arrhythmic event

and therefore provide the basic data needed for management (Figs 11.4 and 11.5).

Based on randomized clinical trial data, most patients who have an episode of aborted sudden cardiac death and recover reasonable neurologic function should receive an ICD. Since all current ICDs provide pacing for bradyarrhythmias, even if there is uncertainty as to whether the patient has suffered a bradyarrhythmia or tachyarrhythmia, an ICD will deliver appropriate therapy. Since patients who suffer a cardiac arrest tend to be at high risk of recurrence even if they are not inducible, the inducibility of ventricular tachycardia in most cases will not affect the management. Therefore programmed ventricular stimulation should not be considered routine, although in equivocal cases it can be valuable.

Some patients are too ill for an operation, or they may have a prognosis that is limited due to end-stage heart disease or other medical problems. Other patients refuse surgery. In those patients the weight of the evidence supports the use of amiodarone, despite the observation in the CASH study that there was no difference in prognosis between the patients on amiodarone compared to those receiving β-blockers. The use of β-blockers in

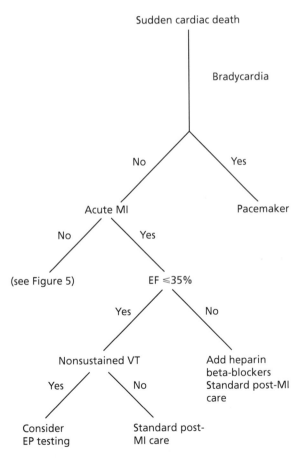

Figure 11.4 *Aborted sudden cardiac death. MI = myocardial infarction. EF = ejection fraction; EP = electrophysiologic; VT = ventricular tachycardia.*

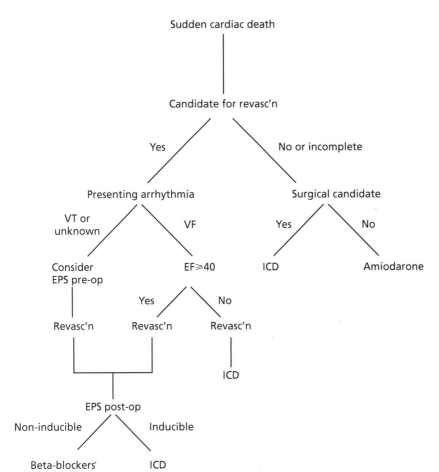

Figure 11.5 *Aborted sudden cardiac death without associated myocardial infarction. EF = ejection fraction; EPS = electrophysiologic testing; ICD = implantable cardioverter defribrillator; VF = ventricular fribillation; VT = ventricular tachycardia.*

addition to amiodarone may be of added benefit, but there is limited information at this time, and brady-arrhythmias can occur with this combination. It is not unreasonable to use both of these medications together if they can be tolerated.

The most problematic management issue is when a patient who has a cardiac arrest also has demonstrable ischemia. It can be difficult to decide whether the patient has had an arrhythmia as a result of an MI. Even when this decision is clear, management decisions often require great judgement, as there can be a wide range of opinions with respect to the management of these patients. Optimally, if there is uncertainty it would be best to treat the patient for both ischemia and the arrhythmia. Surgery can impart significant risk, but on the other hand after surgery an ICD may not be necessary.

As indicated in Fig. 11.5, if the patient has presented with ventricular fibrillation and has a good ejection fraction, revascularization seems desirable. For this patient, an EP study postoperatively can be helpful in deciding on ICD implantation. If the ejection fraction is significantly reduced, the chance of arrhythmia recurrence is higher for a non-inducible patient, and thus ICD

implantation after surgery may be appropriate without the need for an EP study.

If the patient has presented with ventricular tachycardia resulting in severe hemodynamic compromise or an arrest, or the arrhythmia causing the arrest cannot be determined, revascularization is desirable. Since revascularization does not correct the underlying abnormalities of the arrhythmic substrate, most of the time revascularization will not eliminate the potential for sustained ventricular tachycardia postoperatively, and if there is any question evaluation of inducibility postoperatively can be helpful.

If revascularization is not possible, patients should be managed in the same as if they had presented with fibrillation, i.e. with an ICD if they are appropriate candidates.

The value of angioplasty in the treatment of ventricular arrhythmias is unclear. There is no definitive information on the effect of angioplasty on prognosis in patients who present with a cardiac arrest, but since it can provide a degree of ravascularization in many patients, there is surely a role for this procedure in some patients.

Sometimes, despite a careful evaluation of all relevant

data, the circumstances of an arrest remain unclear. Since recent data have shown with a fair amount of consistency that patients with lower ejection fractions are the ones who tend to benefit most from an ICD, increasingly we are more aggressive about ICD implantation in that group of patients. In patients whose ejection fractions are higher, we are more willing to consider other options. As noted earlier, recent data do suggest that amiodarone is equally effective as an ICD if the ejection fraction is greater than 35 per cent. Discussion with the patient and/or family may ultimately be the deciding factor.

CLINICAL OVERVIEW

- Sudden cardiac death remains a significant public health problem, and is the mode of death of a signicant number of patients with heart disease.
- Although implantable defibrillators have had a major impact on the treatment of aborted sudden cardiac death, there remains a great deal of subtlety in deciding on the management in the individual patient.
- A cardiac arrest is felt to occur under most circumstances as a result of an unfortunate coexistence of structural cardiac abnormalities, which are frequently pre-existing, complicated by transient risk factors, which act as a trigger to precipitate vetricular fibrillation. Coronary artery disease remains implicated in the pathophysiology for most patients in the USA.
- The management of an aborted episode of sudden cardiac death and ventricular tachycardia resulting in sudden cardiac death has evolved based on randomized clinical trials demonstrating that implantable cardioverter defibrillator insertion improves survival compared with amiodarone, the most reasonable alternative.
- Initial management is focused on stabilization of the patient and accurate collection of data regarding the circumstances of the arrest. Subsequently diagnostic testing, frequently including cardiac catheterization, is frequently required.
- Most patients who have had an aborted arrest not associated with a myocardial infarction should receive implantable defibrillator insertion if they make a significant neurologic recovery. Revascularization is often appropriate, but decisions must be individualized for the patient.

FUTURE DIRECTIONS

As noted, combined data from the three randomized trials, AVID, CIDS, and CASH, should lead to further insights with respect to which patients would be most likely to benefit from an implantable defibrillator, and in which patients implantation would be cost effective. Currently research efforts seem to be directed toward primary prevention of a cardiac arrest and identification of the patients at highest risk. Many of these studies are looking at reduced ejection fraction, frequent ventricular ectopy, or the presence of congestive heart failure as means of identification of patients at the highest risk of sudden death and consequently implantable defibrillator insertion. This strategy of prevention of a first event of sudden cardiac death is conceptually more appealing than preventing recurrences in patients who have life-threatening arrhythmias and are fortunate enough to be successfully resuscitated.

SUMMARY

- Sudden cardiac death remains a significant public health problem.
- The pathophysiology in most cases involves transient risk factors in conjunction with stuctural cardiac abnormalities.
- Recent randomized clinical trial data (AVID, CIDS, CASH) support the use of implantable cardioverter defibrillators in many patients with ventricular tachycardia and fibrillation.
- The evaluation and treatment of coronary artery disease and ischemia are integral to the management in most cases.
- Management of the individual patient requires detailed assessment of the clinical presentation and underlying heart disease.
- Implantable cardioverter defibrillator insertion is often indicated, but management should be tailored to the individual patient.

REFERENCES

1. Myerburg RJ, Kessler KM, Castellanos A. Sudden cardiac death: epidemiology, transient risk, and intervention assessment. *Ann Intern Med* 1993; **119**: 1187–97.
2. Cobb LA, Weaver WD, Fahrenbrush CE. Community-based interventions for sudden cardiac death: impact, limitations, and charges. *Circulation* 1992; **85**(suppl 1): I-98.
3. Baroldi G, Falzi G, Mariani F. Sudden cardiac death: a post-mortem study in 208 selected cases compared to 97 'control' subjects. *Am Heart J* 1979; **98**: 20–31.
4. Perper JA, Kuller LH, Cooper M. Arteriosclerosis of coronary arteries in sudden, unexpected deaths. *Circulation* 1975; **52**(suppl 3): 27–33.

♦5. Davies MJ, Thomas A. Thrombosis and acute coronary artery lesions in sudden cardiac ischemic death. *N Engl J Med* 1984; **310**: 1137–40.

♦6. Davies MJ, Bland JM, Hangartner JRW, *et al*. Factors influencing the presence or absence of acute coronary artery thrombi in sudden ischaemic death. *Eur Heart J* 1989; **10**: 203–8.

7. Reichenbach DD, Moss NS, Meyer E. Pathology of the heart in sudden cardiac death. *Am J Cardiol* 1977; **39**: 865–72.

8. Newman WP, Tracy RE, Strong JP, *et al*. Pathology of sudden cardiac death. *Ann New Y Acad Sci* 1982; **382**: 39–49.

9. Packer M. Sudden unexpected death in patients with congestive heart failure: a second frontier. *Circulation* 1985; **72**: 681–5.

10. Poll DS, Marchlinski FE, Buxton AE, *et al*. Sustained ventricular tachycardia in patients with idiopathic dilated cardiomyopathy: electrophysiologic testing and lack of response to antiarrhythmic drug therapy. *Circulation* 1984; **70**: 451–6.

11. Surawicz B. Ventricular fibrillation. *J Am Coll Cardiol* 1985; **5**(suppl B): 43–54.

12. Phillips M, Rabinowitz M, Higgins JR, *et al*. Sudden cardiac death in air force recruits. *JAMA* 1986; **256**: 2696–9.

13. Topaz O, Edwards JE. Pathologic features of sudden death in children, adolescents, and young adults. *Chest* 1985; **87**: 476–82.

14. Bhandari AK, Sheinman M. The long QT syndrome. *Mod Concepts Cardiovasc Dis* 1985: **54**: 45.

♦15. Maron BJ, Roberts WC, Epstein SE. Sudden death in hypertrophic cardiomyopathy: a profile of 78 patients. *Circulation* 1982; **65**: 1388–94.

16. Fananapazir L, Epstein SE. Hemodynamic and electrophysiologic evaluation of patients with hypertrophic cardiomyopathy surviving cardiac arrest. *Am J Cardiol* 1991; **67**: 280–7.

17. Messerli FH, Ventura HO, Elizardi DJ, *et al*. Hypertension and sudden death: increased ventricular ectopic activity in left ventricular hypertrophy. *Am J Med* 1984; **77**: 18–22.

18. Chesler E, King RA, Edwards JE. The myxomatous mitral valve and sudden death. *Circulation* 1983; **67**: 632–9.

19. Garza LA, Vick RL, Nora JJ, McNamara DG. Heritable Q-T prolongation without deafness. *Circulation* 1970; **41**: 39–48.

20. Fraser GR, Froggatt P, James TN. Congenital deafness associated with electrocardiographic abnormalities, fainting attacks and sudden death. *Quart J Med* 1964; **33**: 362.

♦21. Brugada J, Brugada R, Brugada P. Right bundle-branch block and ST-segment elevation in leads V1 through V3: a marker for sudden death in patients without demonstrable structural heart disease. *Circulation* 1998; **97**: 457–60.

♦22. Ruskin JN, McGovern B, Garan H, *et al*. Antiarrhythmic drugs: a possible cause of out-of-hospital cardiac arrest. *N Engl J Med* 1983; **309**: 1302–6.

23. Echt DS, Liebson PR, Mitchell LB, *et al*. Mortality and morbidity in patients receiving encainide, flecainide, or placebo: The Cardiac Arrest Suppression Trial. *N Engl J Med* 1991; **324**: 781–8.

24. Bigger JT Jr, Fleiss JL, Steinman RC, Rolnitzky LM, Schneider WJ, Stein PK. RR variability in healthy, middle-aged persons compared with patients with chronic coronary heart disease or recent acute myocardial infarction. *Circulation* 1995; **91**: 1936–43.

25. Bigger JT, Fleiss JL, Rolnitzky LM, Steinman RC. The ability of several short-term measures of RR variability to predict mortality after myocardial infarction. *Circulation* 1993; **88**: 927–34.

26. Engel GL. Psychologic stress, vasodepressor vasovagal syncope, and sudden death. *Ann Intern Med* 1978; **89**: 403–12.

27. Cobb LA, Baum RS, Alvarez H III, Schaffer WA. Resuscitation from out-of-hospital ventricular fibrillation: 4 years follow-up. *Circulation* 1975; **52**(6 suppl): III223–35.

28. Ruskin JN, DiMarco JP, Garan H. Out-of-hospital cardiac arrest: electrophysiologic observations and selection of long-term antiarrhythmic therapy. *N Engl J Med* 1980; **303**: 607–13.

29. Swerdlow CD, Winckle RA, Mason JW. Determinants of survival in patients with ventricular tachycardia. *N Engl J Med* 1983; **308**: 1436–42.

30. Benditt DG, Benson DW Jr, Klein GJ, *et al*. Prevention of recurrent sudden cardiac arrest: role of provocative electrophysiologic testing. *J Am Coll Cardiol* 1983; **2**: 418–25.

○31. Graboys TB, Lown B, Podrid PJ, DeSilva R. Long-term survival of patients with malignant ventricular arrhythmia treated with antiarrhythmic drugs. *Am J Cardiol* 1982; **50**: 437–43.

32. The ESVEM Investigators The ESVEM trial. Electrophysiologic Study Versus Electrocardiographic Monitoring for selection of antiarrhythmic therapy of ventricular tachyarrhythmias. *Circulation* 1989; **79**: 1354–60.

33. Mason JW for the ESVEM investigators. A comparison of electrophysiologic testing with Holter monitoring to predict antiarrhythmic-drug efficacy for ventricular tachyarrhythmias. *N Engl J Med* 1993; **329**: 445–51.

34. Herre JM, Sauve MJ, Malone P, *et al*. Long-term results of amiodarone therapy in patients with recurrent sustained ventricular tachycardia or ventricular fibrillation. *J Am Coll Cardiol* 1989; **13**: 442–9.

35. Greene HL. The efficacy of amiodarone in the treatment of ventricular tachycardia or ventricular fibrillation. *Prog Cardiovasc Dis* 1989; **31**: 319–54.

36. The CASCADE Investigators. Randomized antiarrhythmic drug therapy in survivors of cardiac arrest (the CASCADE Study). *Am J Cardiol* 1993; **72**: 280–7.

37. Burkart F, Pfisterer M, Kiowski W, Follath F, Burckhardt D. Effect of antiarrhythmic therapy on mortality in survivors of myocardial infarction with asymptomatic complex ventricular arrhythmias: Basel Antiarrhythmic Study of Infarct Survival. *J Am Coll Cardiol* 1990; **16**: 1711–18.

♦38. The AVID investigators. A comparison of antiarrhythmic drug therapy with implantable defibrillators in patients resuscitated from near-fatal ventricular arrhythmias. *N Engl J Med* 1997; **337**: 1576–83.

39. Connolly SJ, Gent M, Roberts RS, *et al.* Canadian Implantable Defibrillator Study (CIDS): study design and organization. *Am J Cardiol* 1993; **72**: 103F–8F.

40. Siebels J, Cappato R, Ruppel R, Schneider MA, Kuck KH. Preliminary results of the Cardiac Arrest Study Hamburg (CASH). *Am J Cardiol* 1993; **72**: 109F–13F.

41. Conolly ST, Hallstrom AP, Cappato R, *et al.* Meta-analysis of the implantable cardioverter defibrillator secondary prevention trials. *Eur Heart J* 2000, **15**: 2071–8.

42. Myerburg RJ, Castellanos A. Cardiac arrest and sudden cardiac death. In: Braunwald E, ed. *Heart disease: a textbook of cardiovascular medicine*, 5th edn. Philadelphia: WB Saunders Co., 1997.

43. Luu M, Stevenson WG, Stevenson LW, Baron K, Walden J: Diverse mechanisms of unexpected cardiac arrest in advanced heart failure. *Circulation* 1989; **80**: 1675–80.

44. Thompson RG, Hallstrom AP, Cobb LA. Bystander-initiated cardiopulmonary resuscitation in the management of ventricular fibrillation. *Ann Intern Med* 1979; **90**: 737–40.

45. Kowey PR, Levine JH, Herre JM, *et al.* for the Intravenous Amiodarone Multicenter Investigators Group. Randomized, double-blind comparison of intravenous amiodarone and bretylium in the treatment of patients with recurrent, hemodynamically destabilizing ventricular tachycardia or fibrillation. *Circulation* 1995; **92**: 3255–63.

46. Scheinman MM, Levine JH, Cannom DS, *et al.* for the Intravenous Amiodarone Multicenter Investigators Group. Dose-ranging study of intravenous amiodarone in patients with life-threatening ventricular tachyarrhythmias. *Circulation* 1995; **92**: 3264–72.

47. O'Rourke RA. Role of myocardial revascularization in sudden cardiac death. *Circulation* 1992; **85**(suppl I): I-112–17.

48. Kelly P, Ruskin JN, Vlahakes GJ, Buckley MJ Jr, Freeman CS, Garan H. Surgical coronary revascularization in survivors of prehospital cardiac arrest: its effect on inducible ventricular arrhythmias and long-term survival. *J Am Coll Cardiol* 1990; **15**: 267–73.

49. Poole JE, Mathisen TL, Kudenchuk PJ, McAnulty JH, Swerdlow CD, Bardy GH, Greene HL. Long-term outcome in patients who survive out of hospital ventricular fibrillation and undergo electrophysiologic studies: evaluation by electrophysiologic subgroups. *J Am Coll Cardiol* 1990; **16**: 657–65.

12

The renal–cardiac patient

MARGUERITE A HAWLEY AND DAVID M CLIVE

Cardiac disease causes death in greater than 40 per cent of dialysis patients. The annual cardiovascular mortality is 35 times higher than in the general population. For non-diabetics on dialysis, it is almost 30 times higher. Independent of age, dialysis patients have a high prevalence of atherosclerosis. The high rate of CV disease among patients starting dialysis suggests that the predialysis phase of chronic renal disease is a state of high cardiac risk. Dialysis patients too have a high incidence of the risk factors known to predispose to CV disease in the general population. However, these classic cardiac risk factors are not sufficient to explain the prevalence of CV disease and related death in all age groups in this population. The hemodynamic and metabolic factors characteristic of chronic renal disease must have an impact on increasing CV risk. Alternatively, those patients with known cardiac disease often have their health further compromised by the advent of renal insufficiency. The medical management of these patients is challenging.

INTRODUCTION

Organ system interdependence is a common theme in human physiology. The kidney and heart exert profound influences over each other's functions. It is hardly surprising that clinical renal and cardiac disorders are so often linked. Beyond this physiologic connection, there are also a number of systemic diseases that can affect both the heart and kidneys directly. Table 12.1 lists most of the important cardiorenal syndromes.

Because the entire contents of Table 12.1 are beyond the scope of this text, the present chapter will focus on just two common patterns of association between renal and cardiac disease. The first section will deal with the patient with chronic renal failure who develops cardiac problems. The emphasis in this section will be on dialysis patients. The second section will consider the patient whose primary problem is cardiovascular disease and who then develops acute renal failure as a complication. Although our focus will be on diagnostic and therapeutic strategies, it is impossible to separate these aspects of the syndromes from their pathophysiologic underpinnings.

CARDIOVASCULAR DISEASE IN PATIENTS WITH CHRONIC RENAL FAILURE

In perspective

As the American population ages, the prevalence of chronic renal failure is increasing. More people are 'living long enough' to develop chronic renal failure, and are no longer excluded from dialysis programs solely on the basis of age. The major etiologies of chronic renal failure in this country include hypertension, diabetes mellitus, and glomerular disease. Patients with sufficiently advanced chronic renal failure as to require dialysis or transplantation for maintenance of life are said to have end-stage renal disease. Approximately 300 000 Americans are on some form of maintenance dialysis, and another 100 000 have functioning renal transplants.

The incidence of cardiovascular disease among patients with chronic renal disease is higher than in the population at large. As implied above, the largest growth in the end-stage renal disease (ESRD) population is occurring in the geriatric subset, and atherosclerotic

Table 12.1 *Major cardiorenal syndromes and associations between heart and kidney disease*

Hemodynamic disorders
Low cardiac output with prerenal azotemia
Cardiogenic shock with acute tubular necrosis
Hypertension and hypertensive heart disease

Deposition diseases
Amyloidosis
Fabry's disease

Vascular diseases
Atherosclerosis of coronary and renal arteries
Diabetes mellitus with atherosclerosis and nephropathy
Cardiogenic renal artery thromboembolism

Microvascular diseases
Atheroembolic disease
Thrombotic thrombocytopenic purpura and hemolytic uremic syndrome
Sickle cell disease

Autoimmune disorders
Systemic lupus erythematosus
Systemic vasculitis (polyarteritis nodosa, Wegener's granulomatosis, Takayasu's arteritis)
Progressive systemic sclerosis

Infective endocarditis with glomerulonephritis

Autosomal dominant polycystic kidney disease with associated valvular heart disease

cardiovascular disease (ASCVD) is also prevalent among the elderly. The most common cause of ESRD in the USA is diabetic nephropathy, representing almost one-third of the dialysis population. Clearly, this group is at the highest possible risk for ASCVD. However, across all age strata, renal patients have a high prevalence of ASCVD. Cardiac causes of death collectively account for almost half of all deaths among dialysis patients (Fig. 12.1). Cerebrovascular disease contributes an additional

7 per cent.[1] The consequences of ischemic heart disease are particularly severe in ESRD patients. After stratifying by age, gender, race, and diabetes cardiovascular disease mortality in dialysis patients remains ten to twenty times higher than in the general population. Even in young adults undergoing regular dialysis, coronary artery calcification has been found to be common and progressive. Of sixteen dialysis patients between the ages of 20 and 30 studied, fourteen had coronary artery calcification versus three out of 60 normal subjects.[2] Recent data reveal that mortality following a myocardial infarction among dialysis patients is 59 per cent at 1 year, and almost 90 per cent at 5 years.[3] Another study showed a 1 year mortality overall of 53 per cent.[4] Interestingly, survival of renal transplant recipients after acute myocardial infarction revealed an improved overall 2 year cardiac and all cause mortality rate of approximately 12 and 34 per cent, respectively.[5]

Historical background

The technology for hemodialysis of living organisms has been in existence since the turn of the century. Because of the formidable logistical and technical obstacles, repetitive hemodialysis of humans was not attempted until the 1940s. In the post-World War II era, a wave of pioneering attempts were made to hemodialyze repetitively patients suffering from acute renal failure (ARF). Much of this research took place in clinical trials sponsored by the US military. The goal of translating these gains into sustained, accessible therapy for ESRD remained impractical until two further developments were achieved. In 1962, the shunt was introduced by Dr Belding Scribner as a means of providing reusable vascular access. The arteriovenous fistula followed a few years later. The formidable cost of hemodialysis, and its scarcity as a resource were overcome in 1972 with the assumption of dialysis reimbursement by the Medicare program. The period of the late 1970s and early 1980s

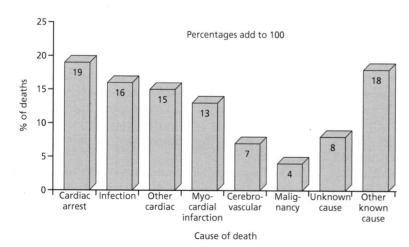

Figure 12.1 *Causes of death among patients with end-stage renal disease aged 45–64 years, 1991–1992. Cardiac causes collectively account for almost half of deaths. (Reproduced with permission from United States Renal Data Service 1995 Annual Report. Am J Kidney Dis 1995; **26**: S85–94.)*

witnessed the evolution and commercial applicability of ambulatory peritoneal dialysis technology. As a result of these achievements, the diagnosis of end-stage renal failure (ESRF) was no longer tantamount to a death sentence. Dialysis and transplantation patients now survive long enough to present medical challenges beyond that of chronic renal failure.

Ischemic heart disease in the ESRD patient: traditional risk factors for coronary atherosclerosis

The risk factors for ASCVD in the population at large are familiar to everyone, and discussed elsewhere in this book. Advanced age and a history of diabetes mellitus clearly increase the risk of cardiac mortality in dialysis patients as in patients without renal disease. However, in several respects, cardiac risk profiles in dialysis patients appear to have distinct features.[6]

DYSLIPIDEMIA

Abnormalities of lipid metabolism are probably more prevalent among patients with renal disease than in the population at large. However, the distribution of dyslipidemias varies among specific renal disease subsets. Table 12.2 summarizes data recently assembled by Kasiske[7] from available studies of lipid levels in renal disease and compared with normative data from the Framingham Offspring Study and NHANES III cohorts. Nephrotic diseases commonly manifest hypercholesterolemia and hypertriglyceridemia. In non-nephrotic renal failure, however, the prevalence of these abnormalities, while high, is closer to that in the general population, and may be influenced by the degree of renal failure, as well the mode of renal replacement therapy in the case of ESRD patients. Hypertriglyceridemia is clearly extremely common among ESRD patients.

The extent to which hyperlipidemia influences the development or progression of ASCVD among renal patients has not been widely studied. Among ESRD patients, as in others, a low serum cholesterol level is associated with a markedly increased mortality. ESRD patients do not demonstrate the familiar 'J-shaped curve' of mortality as a function of serum cholesterol level. High serum cholesterol levels do not exert a significant impact on cardiovascular mortality in this group, rather chronic uremia is confounded by the impact of malnutrition.[8] There may be other factors at play in this set of patients. In uremia, a defect in cholesterol transport has been demonstrated in vitro. There also appears to be a deficiency of lipoprotein lipase which degrades circulating lipoprotein triglyceride.[9] Additionally, lipoprotein (a) has been found by several investigators to be predictive of cardiovascular (CV) disease and death.[10–12] Lipoprotein (a) concentrations are higher in hemodialysis patients compared to normal healthy controls and the high lipoprotein (a) patients were at significantly increased risk for cardiovascular disease and mortality.[11,12]

It may be that selective alteration in lipid subsets influences the development of cardiovascular disease in chronic hemodialysis patients. Oxidized low-density lipoproteins (LDLs) have been shown to be increased more than eight-fold in chronic hemodialysis (HD) patients.[13] These LDLs have been hypothesized to cause endothelial cell damage resulting in smooth muscle cell and fibroblast proliferation and ultimately an expanding atherosclerotic lesion.[14] Because of the rampant nature of ASCVD in the renal disease population, a series of controlled trials analyzing the efficacy of lipid-lowering therapy in preventing this complication may be anticipated.

HYPERTENSION

Hypertension is common in all forms of chronic renal disease. The prevalence of high blood pressure among patients with advanced chronic renal failure (CRF) and ESRD approaches 80 per cent. It is to be remembered that the relationship between renal disease and hyper-

Table 12.2 *Lipoprotein abnormalities by target population (approximate %). (Modified from Kasiske BL. Hyperlipidemia in patients with chronic renal disease. Am J Kidney Dis 1998; 32: S142–56)*

	Total cholesterol (>240 mg/dL)	LDL cholesterol (>130 mg/dL)	HDL cholesterol (<35 mg/dL)	Triglycerides (>200 mg/dL)	L_p (a) (>30 mg/dL)
General population	20	40	15	15	15
CRI with nephrotic syndrome (includes diabetic nephropathy)	90	85	50	60	60
CRI without nephrotic syndrome	30	10	35	40	45
ESRD treated by hemodialysis	20	30	50	45	30
ESRD treated by peritoneal dialysis	25	45	20	50	50
Renal transplant recipients	60	60	15	35	25

LDL = low-density lipoprotein; HDL = high-density lipoprotein; L_p (a) = lipoprotein (a); CRI = chronic renal insufficiency; ESRD = end-stage renal disease.

tension is closely interwoven. Hypertension of all etiologies can lead to renal failure. Conversely, most forms of renal parenchymal and renovascular disease can produce secondary hypertension. The pathogenesis of hypertension caused by chronic renal failure is multifactorial. Extracellular volume expansion plays the major role. Hypertension is not well controlled in the ESRD population. In the HEMO study, the mean predialysis blood pressure (BP), for the first 1000 patients enrolled was 152/82.[15] Suboptimal control is due, in part, to inability to obtain representative BP readings given the large volume fluxes associated with dialysis. In some patients, hypertension appears to be vasoconstrictor mediated, either through overactivity of the renin–angiotensin system, typical of renal vascular diseases, or the autonomic nervous system.[16] Campese and co-workers have marshalled evidence to suggest that renal parenchymal injury may provide an afferent stimulus to the central nervous system, resulting in increased sympathetic outflow, which raises blood pressure.[17]

In the general population, hypertension is a well-described risk factor for cardiovascular morbidity and mortality. Among renal patients, however, the attributive risk of hypertension in cardiovascular morbidity has not been delineated. Hypertension is less closely correlated with mortality in dialysis patients than other variables, such as low serum albumin and increasing age.[8] In some studies, a direct effect of hypertension on cardiovascular mortality has even been found lacking.[18,19] In patients with ESRD the association of BP with mortality appears to be U-shaped, with the excess risk in patients with normal or low BP (<140/90).[20] The increased risk of those with low BP is probably confounded by effects of cardiovascular disease such as poor cardiac output on mortality. While prevailing opinion holds that hypertension poses a major health risk for patients with CRF and ESRD,[21] and should be treated, there are as yet scant data on the impact of such therapy on morbidity and mortality. Furthermore, the extent to which hypertension is associated with cardiovascular complications in ESRD patients may depend, among other things, on their race, socioeconomic status, and their original cause of renal failure.[22] Hypertension probably acts as a co-factor with other pathophysiologic phenomena in the evolution of ASCVD in dialysis patients (Fig. 12.2). That the relationship between ASCVD and hypertension is looser in CRF than in the general population may relate to the fact that, in CRF, hypertension correlates more closely with extracellular volume expansion than with established vascular disease.[23]

Clearly, arterial hypotension augurs poorly in dialysis patients.[8,20,24] Sustained intradialytic hypotension may threaten myocardial perfusion, already at risk. For this reason, efforts to control intradialytic hypotension in patients with known CAD are strongly recommended. On the other hand, chronic hypotension *per*

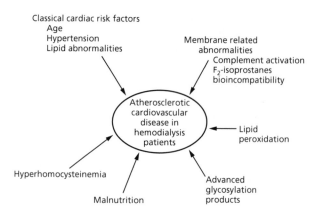

Figure 12.2 *Factors contributing to atherosclerotic cardiovascular disease among end-stage renal disease patients. A relationship between several of these factors and atherosclerotic cardiovascular disease is still purely speculative. (Adapted with permission from Becker RC, et al. Reassessing the cardiac risk profile in chronic hemodialysis patients: a hypothesis on the role of oxidant stress and other non-traditional cardiac risk factors.* J Am Soc Nephrol *1997;* **8:** *482.)*

se may be an epiphenomenon of already poor myocardial function.

HOMOCYSTEINE

Elevated plasma homocysteine levels have relatively recently been added to the list of traditional cardiac risk factors, both in renal failure patients and in the population at large.[25,26] In patients with CRF, the reduced clearance rate of homocysteine, and perhaps other metabolic factors, may account for a high prevalence of hyperhomocysteinemia. ESRD patients who are either heterozygous or homozygous for the 677 C to T substitution mutation of the methylene tetrahydrofolate reductase gene have extemely high homocysteine levels.[27,28] The prevalence of elevated plasma homocysteine is approximately 90 per cent in patients with ESRD versus 5 per cent in the general population and 35 per cent in CAD patients in this group.[29,30] Increased homocysteine levels in the general population appear to be a risk factor for cardiovascular disease.[25,31] Several recent investigations have shown an association between increased homocysteine levels in the dialysis population and their risk for cardiovascular disease and death.[29,31,32] An increase of 1 μmol/L of total homocysteine enhances the relative risk by 1 per cent in end-stage renal disease patients.[33] In the dialysis population supplementation with B complex vitamins has not consistently been shown to significantly lower homocysteine levels unlike in the general population.[34] At this point, the data on any benefit of folic acid supplementation in reducing CVD mortality in the dialysis population is inconclusive.[35]

Other risk factors for ischemic cardiac disease in ESRD patients

The common derangements in calcium and phosphorus balance in chronic renal failure represent another risk factor for coronary disease. Patients manifesting the vicious cycle of phosphate retention, tissue calcium deposition, and secondary hyperparathyroidism develop premature calcification of the coronary arteries, synergizing with the atherosclerotic process and promoting ischemic heart disease.

Hyperparathyroidism is associated with left ventricular hypertrophy (LVH) and increased LV mass index. There may be direct trophic effects on myocardial monocytes and on interstitial fibroblasts. Additionally, cardiac hypertrophy may be related to altered vitamin D status by effects on vascular smooth muscle cell growth and blood pressure. Parathyroid hormone (PTH) and vitamin D are both implicated in BP control. PTH effects on vascular endothelial function and growth may contribute to increased vascular tone and stiffness. Hyperparathyroidism has been implicated in hyperlipidemia with decreased lipoprotein lipase activity as well as insulin resistance.[36]

C-reactive protein (CRP), a marker for systemic inflammation, has recently been shown to be associated with atherothrombosis. Ridker and associates found that the C-reactive protein concentrations of men in the physicians health study predicted their risk of future myocardial infarction (MI) and stroke.[37] Subsequently, Zimmermann and his group looked at serum lipids and acute phase response masters such as CRP in hemodialysis patients. They found that overall mortality, as well as cardiovascular mortality was significantly higher in those patients with elevated CRP.[38]

Hypoalbuminemia has been shown to be predictive of death in dialysis patients. Low serum albumin can be secondary to malnutrition or evidence of inflammation, with elevated CRP and cytokine levels. However, investigators have found that CRP is a significant predictor of cardiovascular mortality and overall mortality in chronic dialysis patients independent of serum albumin levels.[39,40]

Hyaluron is also a marker of inflammatory reactions and has been shown to be markedly elevated in predialysis patients with malnutrition, inflammation and cardiovascular disease. Elevated hyaluron levels were shown to be significantly related to an increased mortality rate independent of CVD, CRP, and age.[41] Inflammation and its associated markers appear to be related to poor cardiovascular outcomes and mortality.

Oxidative stress has also been implicated in the accelerated rate of CVD in hemodialysis patients. Using serum malondialdehyde (MDA) levels as a marker of oxidative stress, investigators found it to be significantly elevated in hemodialysis patients with prevalent CV disease compared to those without. In this population serum MDA rather than lipoprotein or fibrinogen was the single strongest predictor of prevalent CVD.[42,43]

A number of other metabolic and immunologic factors have been seen as possibly contributing to the observed proclivity for ASCVD in hemodialysis patients (see Fig. 12.2). These include advanced glycosylation products, F2-isoprostanes, membrane bioincompatibility and complement activation, and malnutrition.[6] While tenable, a specific pathogenetic role for each of these factors remains purely putative.

Left ventricular hypertrophy and congestive heart failure in ESRD

Left ventricular hypertrophy (LVH) is associated with increased cardiac mortality in patients with ESRD[44,45] and there is a very high prevalence of LVH in this population. In one prospective cohort study, it was found that the risk for LVH was greater for patients with chronic renal insufficiency compared to the general population and varied inversely with the level of renal function.[46] A number of factors may feature in its development (Fig. 12.3). Cardiac ischemia in the absence of major coronary artery occlusive lesions may occur in as many as 27 per cent of ESRD patients, suggesting small-vessel disease.[22] LVH is associated with microanatomical abnormalities of the intramyocardial circulation. Recent studies in a rodent model of CRF indicate that LVH and hypertrophy of ventricular arteriolar smooth muscle can even occur in the absence of hypertension.[47] The adverse impact of hypertension on survival in ESRD is no doubt related to the development of LVH. The presence of LVH may also denote target organ damage in other systems.[48]

Anemia is expected among patients with advanced renal failure, although the advent of recombinant human erythropoietin therapy has helped to mitigate this problem. Anemia may adversely influence the pathophysiology of ischemic heart disease in the ESRD

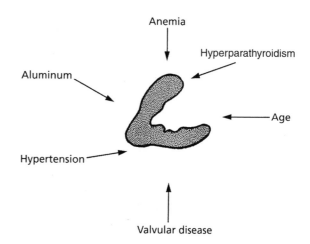

Figure 12.3 *Potential causes of left ventricular hypertrophy in dialysis patients.*

patient in two ways. Obviously, myocardial oxygen delivery is attenuated. In addition, by inducing a hyperdynamic state, it promotes left ventricular hypertrophy.[45,49] A role for calcium and aluminum deposition in the pathogenesis of LVH is also possible.

Valvular heart disease is common in advanced renal failure, particularly premature calcification of the heart valves. This phenomenon has been reported most often in hemodialysis patients, and appears to correlate with length of time since beginning hemodialysis, and with high serum parathyroid hormone levels.[50–52] The most commonly reported lesion is mitral annular calcification, although sclerosis and stenosis of mitral and aortic valves also occur.[50,51] Parathyroid hormone may also induce direct toxic effects on the myocardium.[53]

The inability of patients with chronic renal failure to diurese reliably in response to dietary sodium and water intake renders them prone to symptomatic hypervolemia. Strictly speaking, such episodes should not all be labeled as congestive heart failure, since cardiac function may be normal in patients with pure 'nephrogenic fluid overload'. However, congestive heart failure does have a high incidence and prevalence among ESRD patients, particularly those with older ages, a history of diabetes mellitus, or pre-existing ischemic heart disease as demonstrated in a Canadian multicenter study.[54] In the dialysis population studied only 16 per cent had normal echocardiograms at the start of dialysis. Patients with CHF in this analysis had a median survival of 36 months, 18 months for those developing new-onset CHF on dialysis and 29 months for those with recurrence of pre-existing CHF, as opposed to a median survival of 62 months among patients without CHF.

Several factors, therefore, appear to contribute to the development of hypertrophic myocardial disease in ESRD. Dilated cardiomyopathy also may occur in this population, and appears similarly multifactorial, arising from ischemic disease, chemical imbalances, or myocardial calcium deposition.[55]

Parfrey and colleagues examined the prevalence of myocardial disease by echocardiography in a cross-sectional survey of 128 dialysis patients. Only 23 per cent of these patients had normal studies; 55 per cent had some left ventricular hypertrophy of varying degree, and 19 per cent had evidence of dilated cardiomyopathy. Figure 12.4 represents survival statistics for patients with normal echocardiograms, patients with dilated cardiomyopathy, and the subset of patients with LVH classified as having hypertrophic hyperkinetic myocardia. Approximately two out of three patients in the last category were likely to have had hospital admissions for uncontrolled hypertension or heart failure. Additionally, as can be seen in Fig. 12.4, this group had poorer survival rates than echocardiographically normal dialysis patients or those with dilated ventricles.[44]

Effects of hemodialysis on the cardiovascular system

It is quite common for the arterial blood pressure to decline during a hemodialysis treatment. Frank hypotension, characterized by such symptoms as lightheadedness, cramping, or nausea, occurs in up to 20 per cent of treatments. Although ultrafiltrative fluid removal may contribute to hypotension in dialysis, there is little doubt that other factors are operative (Table 12.3), since many patients tolerate removal of equivalent volumes of fluid by non-dialytic hemofiltration better than removal by dialysis. Acetate-based dialysate solutions may encourage the development of intradialytic hypotension since acetate is a vasodilator, and possibly a direct myocardial suppressant. These solutions are now rarely used.

Autonomic dysfunction, presumably neuropathic in nature, is widespread among ESRD patients,[56] with diabetics being most severely affected. The ability to increase heart rate and contractility in response to baroreceptor stimulation are blunted.[22,56] Additionally,

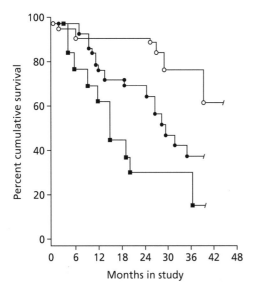

Figure 12.4 *Impact of myocardial disease on survival among hemodialysis (HD) patients.* ○ *= HD patients with normal echocardiograms;* ● *= HD patients with dilated cardiomyopathy;* ■ *= HD patients with hypertrophic, hyperkinetic disease. (Reproduced from Parfrey et al, reference 44, with permission.)*

Table 12.3 *Causes of hypotension during hemodialysis*

Hypovolemia
Autonomic dysfunction
Myocardial ischemia
Rapid osmolar shifts
Intolerance to acetate-based dialysate
Idiosyncratic response to dialyzer membrane

uremic patients may not manifest normal vasomotor responsiveness to adrenergic hormones. It has been suggested that elevated levels of parathyroid hormone, typical of CRF, attenuate the pressor response to exogenous norepinephrine.[57] Autonomic dysfunction may also contribute to the development of arrhythmias during dialysis.[58]

Hypoxemia occurs early during the course of a typical hemodialysis treatment. The fall in the partial pressure of oxygen in arterial blood is usually less than 20 per cent. Dialysis-related hypoxemia is the result of two pathophysiologic processes. Dialysis membranes, particularly the cellulosic types, can activate a cascade of immunologic events, culminating in the release of chemotactic cytokines. These stimulate white cell sequestration in the lungs, impairing transalveolar oxygen diffusion. Diffusive loss of carbon dioxide from the blood during dialysis, particularly when acetate-based dialysate is used, provokes hypoxemia through reduced alveolar ventilation. Although not generally a serious problem, dialysis-induced hypoxemia may be poorly tolerated in unstable patients.

The effects of a hemodialysis treatment on myocardial performance are difficult to predict. In some patients, a reduction in cardiac output is observed, which may reflect myocardial ischemia or volume removal with inadequate cardiac and baroreflex-mediated vasomotor compensation.[22,56] In other patients, stroke volume and ejection fraction may actually increase during hemodialysis. Although this phenomenon has been attributed to removal of unknown myocardial suppressant uremic toxins, which would otherwise promote a so-called 'uremic cardiomyopathy', there is little evidence to support this view. A better explanation for dialysis-induced improvement in myocardial performance is the increase in ionized calcium,[59,60] which attends hemodialysis.

In view of the propensity of hemodialysis to induce hypotension and hypoxemia, and the prevalence among dialysis patients of myocardial perfusion abnormalities, it is not surprising that episodes of myocardial ischemia occur commonly in the dialysis unit. The frequency with which symptomatic anginal episodes occur has not been studied, but they are clearly common. Of particular concern is the prevalence of silent myocardial ischemia, which may approach 40 per cent of hemodialysis patients.[61]

Cardiac diagnosis in patients with chronic renal failure: special considerations

The conventional diagnostic approach to heart disease may be followed in patients with chronic renal failure, but poses a few challenges. First, many end-stage renal disease patients have sufficiently reduced exercise tolerance as to make stress thallium scanning impossible. In these patients, dipyridamole-thallium scanning may offer a suitable alternative, although as illustrated in Table 12.4, studies examining the efficacy of this technique in screening for ischemic heart disease in dialysis patients awaiting renal transplantation indicate that its sensitivity and specificity are lower than in the non-dialysis population.[62-65] Dobutamine echocardiography may be a more accurate method of non-invasive diagnosis in ESRD.[62]

The prevalence of silent myocardial ischemia in the ESRD population is of great consequence in the consideration of candidates for renal transplantation. Transplantation poses the risks of surgery, major postoperative metabolic changes, and immunomodulatory therapy. Furthermore, the difficulties involved in procuring cadaver and living related donor kidneys face the clinician with a blunt reality: donor organs ought not be expended on recipients at high risk for potentially fatal coronary events. de Lemos and Hillis have proposed a systematic approach to screening prospective recipients for CAD.[66] Their recommended algorithm is depicted in Fig. 12.5. The same principles can be applied, at the clinician's judgement, to approaching coronary disease in dialysis patients who are not transplant candidates.

Extra caution is warranted during coronary angiography in renal failure patients. Among all patients undergoing coronary angiography, the risk for radio-contrast nephropathy (RCN) is quite low, probably less than 1 per cent. Of all the reported risk factors for RCN, the best established and most serious is pre-existing renal insufficiency. The worse a patient's renal function, the likelier the development of RCN. Radiocontrast agents, in addition to direct toxic effects to kidney cells, may potentially cause damage via increased formation of reactive oxygen species. Recently, investigators looked to see if treating chronic renal insufficiency patients with the antioxidant acetylcysteine as well as hydration at the

Table 12.4 *Sensitivity and specificity of stress testing for inducible ischemia (%, as compared to coronary arteriography) in the general population and in patients with chronic renal disease. (Reproduced from Murphy SW, et al. Screening and treatment for cardiovascular disease in patients with chronic renal disease. Am J Kidney Dis 1998; **32**: S184–99)*

Method	General population		Chronic renal disease	
	Sensitivity	Specificity	Sensitivity	Specificity
Exercise electrocardiogram	65	85	<50	<50
Dipyridamole radionuclide scan	80	80	40–85	75–80
Dobutamine echocardiography	80	90	70–95	95

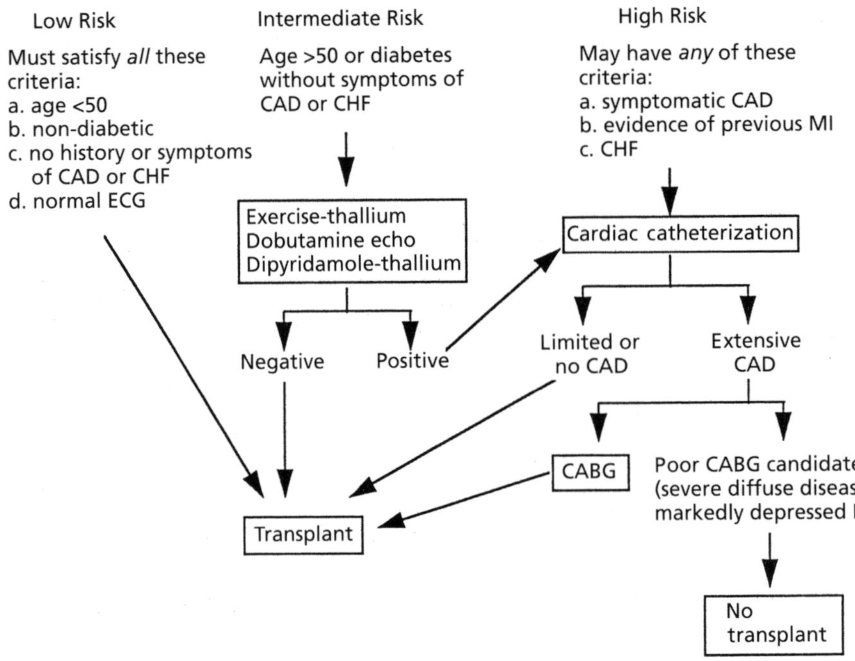

Figure 12.5 *Diagnostic and management algorithm for suspected coronary artery disease in end-stage renal disease patients. The strategy was originally formulated for approaching transplant candidates, but may be modified appropriately for dialysis patients in general. CAD = coronary artery disease; CHF = congestive heart failure; ECG = electrocardiogram; MI = myocardial infarction; CABG = coronary artery bypass graft; LVSF = left ventricular systolic function. (Reproduced with permission from de Lemos JA, Hillis LD. Diagnosis and management of coronary artery disease in patients with end-stage renal disease on hemodialysis. J Am Soc Nephrol 1996; 7: 2044–54.)*

time of computed tomography (CT) with non-ionic contrast prevented a reduction in renal function. In this small study, acetylcysteine and hydration significantly prevented a reduction in renal clearance after CT with non-ionic contrast.[67] These are interesting results that need further study, particularly in those with more advanced renal failure and those receiving ionic as well as larger doses of contrast.

> Prior to catheterization, patients with renal insufficiency should undergo prophylactic hydration with intravenous isotonic saline at a rate appropriate to their measured ability to diurese maximally. Diuretics should not be employed to stimulate the diuresis in this setting, as they may actually heighten the risk of radiocontrast nephropathy.[68] The dose of administered radiocontrast agent should be minimized. Arrangements should be made proactively for dialytic intervention in the event of severe acute-on-chronic renal failure.

The coronary angiographer should also remember that the risk of vascular complications, such as dissection, rupture and atheroembolization, is increased among ESRD patients given their greater prevalence of atherosclerotic and calcific arterial disease.

In patients with ESRD, prophylaxis against radiocontrast nephropathy is obviously no longer an issue. However, the osmolar content of the administered dose of radiocontrast is often enough to cause significant vascular congestion in patients with little or no intrinsic renal function. Hyperkalemia, reflecting the movement of potassium-rich cell water into the vascular compartment in response to the osmotic load, may also occur. These contingencies should be anticipated in the immediate postcatheterization period, and are best managed with dialysis.

Cardiovascular therapeutics in chronic renal failure

The strategic concepts in preventing and treating heart disease in chronic renal failure patients are the same as in others. The key difference relates to the pharmacokinetic alterations of renal failure. Many cardiac drugs are excreted entirely, or in part, via the kidneys. Appropriate modifications of dose or interval are often required.

Some medications may be extracted from the blood during dialysis. This is particularly relevant to hemodialysis patients, in whom dialytic therapy is 'pulsatile' in nature, and drug levels may plummet over a short period of time. Patients receiving readily dialyzable, water-soluble agents such as procainamide or atenolol, should be redosed after hemodialysis. Table 12.5 lists many of the commonly used cardiovascular pharmaceuticals, specifying whether their dose or schedule must be modified according to the patient's level of renal function, or is affected by dialysis.

> Since many patients are prone to hypotension during hemodialysis, it is customary to withhold antihypertensive therapy prior to dialysis. There are exceptions to this: many patients are able to maintain stable blood pressures during treatment even having received their antihypertensives beforehand.

Some patients will experience unacceptable degrees of hypertension in the hours prior to dialysis if their medications are withheld. Still others may suffer an acute hypertensive 'spike' during hemodialysis. This phenomenon, while seemingly paradoxical, probably represents a vasoconstrictor response to dialysis-induced volume contraction.

Because of the complexities that exist in establishing pharmacologic blood pressure control in the ESRD patient, it is prudent for clinicians to monitor the pre- and postdialysis blood pressures of their patients periodically, as well as their running intradialytic blood pressure records. Measurement of blood pressures on non-dialysis days, even with 24-hour monitoring techniques, may be necessary to ensure adequate control throughout the week.

> Control of extracellular volume overload should be viewed as central to the management of hypertension in patients with advanced CRF. Diuretics are generally part of the regimen. In ESRD patients, a target weight, usually called the 'dry weight', should be established. Fluid removal during hemodialysis treatments should be aimed at reaching this weight at the conclusion of each treatment.

Failure to remove enough fluid during dialysis predisposes patients to symptomatic fluid overload or even episodic pulmonary edema between treatments. On the other hand, overzealous fluid removal may render patients hypotensive, and can even trigger seizures, dysequilibrium, or even myocardial ischemia and arrhythmias. Although most clinicians estimate dry weight clinically, more precise techniques are needed.[69] Peritoneal dialysis patients adjust their peritoneal exchange regimen so as to minimize oscillations around their ideal dry weight.

The ability of hemodialysis to cause lability of blood pressure and silent or symptomatic ischemia in susceptible patients poses particular challenges. The routine pharmacologic approaches to this problem, nitrates and ß-blockers may themselves engender a lowering of blood pressure, further complicating the treatment. It may be necessary to titrate these patients' symptoms with small doses of anti-ischemic drugs. Other measures aimed at mitigating the likelihood of intradialytic ischemia should be taken, for example, administering nasal oxygen, and maintaining a hematocrit in the 'target range' (33–36 per cent) using recombinant erythropoietin and, if necessary, periodic transfusion. When angina pectoris develops during a dialysis session, the extracorporeal blood flow rate should be reduced and, if the blood pressure permits, sublingual nitroglycerine given. If symptoms abate, the original treatment plan may be resumed. If the anginal episode proves refractory to these maneuvers, it may be necessary to terminate the treatment.

ESRD patients who, because of cardiac instability, cannot tolerate hemodialysis, may fare better with ambulatory peritoneal dialysis, if they are capable of undertaking this form of self-delivered therapy. The continuous nature of this form of therapy means that the metabolic, osmolar, and volume shifts inherent in dialysis therapy are delivered on a more gradual basis. Although one might, therefore, anticipate more encouraging survival statistics among patients on continuous peritoneal dialysis compared to hemodialysis, various experts have reported the opposite to be true,[70,71] inspiring widespread debate throughout nephrologic circles. A more recent report challenges these findings, and suggests that no differences in relative mortality risk between peritoneal dialysis and hemodialysis can be discerned when comparison cohorts are appropriately adjusted for case-mix differences.[72]

Coronary artery bypass grafting (CABG) is widely performed in patients with ESRD. As in non-ESRD patients, the efficacy of this procedure in relieving symptoms is considerable. Predictably, fluid management is more difficult in dialysis patients in the postcardiac surgery period, and intensive care unit stays are likely to be longer.[73–77] Perioperative mortality rates vary widely among authors, with a range of 0 to over 30 per cent; not surprisingly, mortality is highest among older patients.[73,75] CABG is generally regarded as carrying an acceptable mortality and high likelihood of offering durable symptomatic relief. It appears superior to percutaneous angioplasty in this latter regard.[76] However, long-term survival among hemodialysis patients appears to be reduced compared to otherwise normal patients undergoing CABG.[75,77] These data may reflect differences in the threshold for pursuing surgery between the two groups, with ESRD patients having more severe manifestations of coronary artery disease by the time a surgical approach is undertaken. It has been recommended that CABG be reserved for symptomatic relief in ESRD patients, since data suggesting a beneficial effect on longevity are lacking.[66]

Table 12.5 *Antihypertensive drugs (blood pressure is best guide to dose and intervals)*

Drug	Route of elimination	Normal half-life (h)	Half-life in ESRD (h)	Dose: normal renal function	Renal failure adjustment (GFR mL/min)			Dialysis supplementation	Adverse reactions/comments
Antiadrenergic drugs Peripheral α antagonists									
Prazosin (Minipres)	H	2–3	2–3	1–5 mg bid–tid	>50	None		HEMO: none CAPD: none CAVH: none	May produce profound first dose hypertension
					10–50	None			
					<10	None			
Terazosin (Hytrin)	H	9–12	8–12	1–10 mg qd–bid	>50	None		HEMO: no data CAPD: no data CAVH: no data	
					10–50	None			
					<10	None			
Central α agonists									All agents may cause sedation, dry mouth, sexual dysfunction
Alpha-methyldopa (Aldomet)	R	1.5–6	6–16	250–1000 mg bid–tid	>50	None		HEMO: dose after dialysis CAPD: none CAVH: no data	Orthostatic hypotension Retroperitoneal fibrosis Active metabolites with long $t_{1/2}$
					10–50	q8–12h			
					<10	q12–24h			
Clonidine (Catapres)	R	6–23	39–42	0.1–0.6 mg bid	>50	None		HEMO: none CAPD: none CAVH: no data	Rebound hypertension if drug is abruptly withdrawn
					10–50	None			
					<10	None			
Guanabenz (Wytensin)	H	12–14	?	4–32 mg bid	>50	None		HEMO: no data CAPD: no data CAVH: no data	
					10–50	None			
					<10	None			
Other agents Reserpine (Serpasil)	H	46–168	87–323	100–250 mg qd	>50	None		HEMO: none CAPD: none CAVH: no data	
					10–50	None			
					<10	Avoid			

Angiotensin-converting enzyme (ACE) inhibitors
Monitor renal function in patients with congestive heart failure or possible renovascular hypertension. Hypotensive response in patients taking diuretics. May cause hyperkalemia. Dry cough in 5–10%

Drug	Route of elimination	Normal half-life (h)	Half-life in ESRD (h)	Dose: normal renal function	Renal failure adjustment (GFR mL/min)		Dialysis supplementation	Adverse reactions/comments
Captopril (Captopen)	H/R	1.9	21–32	12.5–50 mg bid–tid	>50	100% q8–12h	HEMO: 25 mg after dialysis CAPD: none CAVH: no data	Rare proteinuria, nephrotic syndrome, dysguesia and granulocytopenia
					10–50	75% q12–18h		
					<10	50% q24h		
Enalapril (Vasotec)	R	11–24	34–60	2.5–20 mg qd–bid	>50	None	HEMO: 20–25% after dialysis CAPD: none CAVH: no data	Enalaprilat, active metabolite formed in the liver
					10–50	50–75%		
					<10	25–50%		
Lisinopril (Prinivil, Zestril)	R	12.6	40–50	5–40 mg qd	>50	None	HEMO: 20% after dialysis CAPD: none CAVH: no data	
					10–50	50–75%		
					<10	25–50%		

β-Adrenergic blockers
Hyperkalemia in ESRD. Hypoglycemia in dialysis patients can occur

Drug	Route of elimination	Normal half-life (h)	Half-life in ESRD (h)	Dose: normal renal function	Renal failure adjustment (GFR mL/min)		Dialysis supplementation	Adverse reactions/comments
Acebutolol (Sectral)	H	7–9	7	200–400 mg qd–bid	>50	None	HEMO: none CAPD: none CAVH: no data	Active metabolites with long half-life
					10–50	50%		
					<10	30–50%		

Drug (Brand)		$t_{1/2}$ Normal	$t_{1/2}$ ESRD	Dose	GFR >50	GFR 10–50	GFR <10	Supplement	Comments
Atenolol (Tenormin)	R	6.7	15–35	50–100 mg qd	None	50% q48h	30–50% q96h	HEMO: none / CAPD: none / CAVH: no data	Accumulates in ESRD
Labetalol (Normodyne, Trandate)	H	3–9	3–9	100–600 mg bid	None	None	None	HEMO: none / CAPD: none / CAVH: no data	
Metoprolol (Lopressor)	H	3.5	2.5–4.5	50–100 mg qd–bid	None	None	None	HEMO: none / CAPD: none / CAVH: no data	
Nadolol (Corgard)	R	19	45	40–320 mg qd	None	50%	25%	HEMO: none / CAPD: none / CAVH: no data	
Penbutolol (Levatol)	H	22	24	20–80 mg qd	None	None	None	HEMO: none / CAPD: none / CAVH: no data	
Pindolol (Visken)	H	2.5–4	3–4	5–20 mg bid	None	None	None	HEMO: none / CAPD: none / CAVH: no data	
Propranolol (Inderal)	H	2–6	1–6	40–160 mg bid	None	None	None	HEMO: none / CAPD: none / CAVH: no data	
Sotalol (Betapace)	R	7.5–15	56	80–160 mg bid	None	30%	15–30%	HEMO: none / CAPD: none / CAVH: no data	
Timolol (Blocadren)	H	2.7	4	10–20 mg bid	None	None	None	HEMO: none / CAPD: none / CAVH: no data	

Direct vasodilators

Commonly cause reflex tachycardia, headache, and edema. May precipitate angina in patients with coronary artery disease.

Drug (Brand)		$t_{1/2}$ Normal	$t_{1/2}$ ESRD	Dose	GFR >50	GFR 10–50	GFR <10	Supplement	Comments
Diazoxide (Hyperstat)	H/R	17–31	30–60	150–300 mg bolus	None	None	None	HEMO: none / CAPD: none / CAVH: NA	Sodium and water retention
Hydralazine (Apresoline)	H	2–4.5	7–16	25–100 mg bid–tid	None	None	q8–16h	HEMO: none / CAPD: none / CAVH: no data	Drug induced lupus at high doses
Minoxidil (Loniten)	H	2.8–4.2	2.8–4.2	2.5–20 mg qd–bid	None	None	None	HEMO: none / CAPD: none / CAVH: no data	
Nitroprusside	H	<10 min	<10 min	0.25–8 µg/kg min by infusion	None	None	None	HEMO: none / CAPD: none / CAVH: no data	Toxic metabolite thiocyanate accumulates causing seizures and coma. Measure thiocyanate levels. Thiocyanate is hemodialyzable

Table 12.5 *(continued)*

Drug	Route of elimination	Normal half-life (h)	Half-life in ESRD (h)	Dose: normal renal function	Renal failure adjustment (GFR mL/min)		Dialysis supplementation	Adverse reactions/comments
Calcium-channel blockers								
May increase serum digoxin level or cause edema, headache, and flushing. Used as antianginal drugs								
Diltiazem (Cardizem)	H	2–8	3–5	30–90 mg tid–qid	>50 10–50 <10	None None None	HEMO: none CAPD: none CAVH: no data	Active metabolites
Nicardipine (Cardene)	H	5	5–7	20–30 mg tid	>50 10–50 <10	None None None	HEMO: none CAPD: none CAVH: no data	
Nifedipine (Procardia, Adalat)	H	4.5–5	5–7	10–30 mg tid–qid	>50 10–50 <10	None None None	HEMO: none CAPD: none CAVH: no data	Protein binding decreased in ESRD
Verapamil (Calan, Isoptin, Verelan)	H	3–7	2.4–4	80–120 mg tid	>50 10–50 <10	None None None	HEMO: none CAPD: none CAVH: no data	
Thiazide and related drugs								Associated with photosensitivity, pancreatitis and interstitial nephritis
Hydrochlorothiazide (Esidrix, Oretic, Hydrodiuril)	R	6–8	12–20	12.5–50 mg qd	>50 10–50 <10	None None Avoid	HEMO: avoid CAPD: avoid CAVH: NA	Ineffective with GFR <30 mL/min
Indapamide (Lozol)	H	14–18	14–18	2.5–5 mg qd	>50 10–50 <10	None None Avoid	HEMO: avoid CAPD: avoid CAVH: NA	Ineffective with GFR <30 mL/min
Metolazone (Zaroxolyn, Diulo)	R	4–20	?	2.5–20 mg qd	>50 10–50 <10	None None Avoid	HEMO: avoid CAPD: avoid CAVH: NA	High doses effective for ESRD
Loop diuretics								Ototoxicity may occur at high doses
Bumetanide (Bumex)	R	1.2–1.5	1.5	1–2 mg q8–12h	>50 10–50 <10	None None None	HEMO: avoid CAPD: avoid CAVH: NA	High doses effective in ESRD, ototoxicity occurs in combination with aminoglycosides
Ethacrynic acid (Edecrin)	H/NR	2–4	?	25–100 mg qd–bid	>50 10–50 <10	None None Avoid	HEMO: none CAPD: none CAVH: NA	Ototoxicity in combination with aminoglycosides
Furosemide (Lasix)	R	0.5–1.1	2–4	20–160 mg bid	>50 10–50 <10	None None None	HEMO: none CAPD: none CAVH: NA	High doses effective in ESRD. Ototoxicity in combination with aminoglycosides

Drug	Route	$t_{1/2}$ Normal	$t_{1/2}$ ESRD	Dose	GFR (mL/min)			Dialysis	Comments
					>50	10–50	<10		
Potassium-sparing diuretics									
Amiloride (Midamor, Moduretic)	R	6–8	10–144	5–10 mg qd	None	50%	Avoid	HEMO: avoid CAPD: avoid CAVH: avoid	Hyperkalemia with GFR <30 mL/min especially in diabetics. Hyperchloremic metabolic acidosis.
Spironolactone (Aldactone, Aldactazide)	H	10–35	10–35	25 mg tid–qid	q6–12h	q12–24h	Avoid	HEMO: avoid CAPD: avoid CAVH: avoid	Hyperkalemia with GFR <30 mL/min especially in diabetics. Active metabolites with long half-life
Triamterene (Dyrenium, Dyazide, Maxide)	H	2–12	10	25–50 mg bid	None	None	Avoid	HEMO: avoid CAPD: avoid CAVH: avoid	Hyperkalemia common with GFR <30 mL/min especially in diabetics. Active metabolites with long half-life
Others									
Acetazolamide (Diamox)	R	1.7–5.8	?	500 mg bid	None	Avoid	Avoid	HEMO: avoid CAPD: avoid CAVH: avoid	Ineffective in ESRD. May potentiate acidosis
Antiarrhythmic drugs									
Class IA									Blood levels most often best guide to therapy
Quinidine	H	6	4–14	200–400 mg q4–6 h	None	None	75%	HEMO: none CAPD: none CAVH: no data	Active metabolite. Increases level of digoxin. Hemodialysis useful in poisoning
Procainamide (Procan)	R	2.5–4.9	5–6	350–400 mg q3–4h	None	q6–12h	Avoid	HEMO: Replace, depending on blood levels CAPD: none CAVH: Replace, depending on blood level	Active metabolite. *N*-acetyl procainamide. Lupus-like syndrome. Hemofiltration useful in poisoning
Disopyramide (Norpace)	R	5–8	10–18	100–200 mg q6h	q8h	q12–24h	q24h	HEMO: none CAPD: none CAVH: no data	V_d decreased in ESRC. Urinary retention
Class IB									
Lidocaine (Xylocaine)	H	2–2.2	1.3–7	50 mg over 2 min, repeat q5 min × 3	None	None	None	HEMO: none CAPD: none CAVH: no data	
Tocainide (Tonocard)	H	14	22–27	200–400 mg q4–6h	None	None	50%	HEMO: none CAPD: none CAVH: no data	
Mexiletene (Mexitil)	H	8–13	16	100–300 mg q6–12h	None	None	50–75%	HEMO: none CAPD: none CAVH: none	
Phenytoin	H	24	24	1000 mg loading dose. Then 400–600 mg/day	None	None	None	HEMO: none CAPD: none CAVH: none	Protein binding decreased and V_d increased in renal failure

Table 12.5 (continued)

Drug	Route of elimination	Normal half-life (h)	Half-life in ESRD (h)	Dose: normal renal function	Renal failure adjustment (GFR mL/min)		Dialysis supplementation	Adverse reactions/comments
Class IC								
Flecainide (Tambocor)	H	12–20	19–26	100–200 mg bid	>50 10–50 <10	None None 50–75%	HEMO: none CAPD: none CAVH: no data	
Encainide	R	2–3	6–9	Withdrawn	>50 10–50 <10	None 75% 50%	HEMO: no data CAPD: no data CAVH: no data	Encephalopathy. Converted to active metabolite $t_{1/2}$ 6h
Propafenone (Rhythmol)	H	5	?	150–300 mg q8h	>50 10–50 <10	None None None	HEMO: none CAPD: none CAVH: none	
Class III								
Sotalol (Betapace)	R	15–17	30–50	80–160 mg bid	>50 10–50 <10	None 80–120 mg q48–72h 80 mg q48–72h	HEMO: none CAPD: none CAVH: no data	
Amiodarone (Cardarone)	H	14–120 d	14–120 d	1200–1600 mg loading dose, then 200–400 mg/day	>50 10–50 <10	None None None	HEMO: none CAPD: none CAVH: no data	Hepatotoxicity. Thyroid dysfunction. Peripheral neuropathy. Pulmonary fibrosis. Increases digoxin plasma levels. Active metabolite
Bretylium (Bretylol)	R	6–14	32	5–30 mg/kg iv loading dose; then 1–2 mg/min iv or 5–10 mg/kg q6–8h	>50 10–50 <10	None q8–12h Avoid	HEMO: 5 mg/kg after dialysis CAPD: no data CAVH: no data	Hypotension due to adrenergic blockade
Cardiac glycosides								
Digitoxin	H	144–200	210	0.1–0.2 mg/day	>50 10–50 <10	None None 50–75%	HEMO: none CAPD: none CAVH: no data	Measure serum levels V_d decreased in uremia
Digoxin	R	36–44	80–120	1–1.5 mg loading dose; 0.25–0.50 mg/day	>50 10–50 <10	None 25–75% q36h 10–25% q48h	HEMO: none CAPD: none CAVH: 0.5 mg q12h	Decrease loading dose by 50% in ESRD. V_d and total body clearance decreased in ESRD
Ouabain	R	21	60–70	0.25 mg loading dose; 0.1 mg q12h	>50 10–50 <10	q12–24h q24–36h q36–48h	HEMO: none CAPD: none CAVH: no data	
Nitrates								
Isosorbide (Isordil)	H	0.15–0.5	4	10–20 mg tid	>50 10–50 <10	None None None	HEMO: none CAPD: none CAVH: no data	
Nitroglycerin (*see* Parenteral cardiac drugs)								

Parenteral drugs for CHF

					GFR (mL/min)				
					>50	10–50	<10		
Direct-acting vasodilators									
Nitroprusside	H	10 min	10 min	0.5–10 µg/kg/min	None	None	None	HEMO: none CAPD: none CAVH: no data	Toxic metabolite, thiocyanate accumulates, causing seizures, coma. Thiocyanate is dialyzable. Measure thiocyanate levels
Nitroglycerin	H	2–4 min	2–4 min	100–200 µg/min	None	None	None	HEMO: no data CAPD: no data CAVH: no data	
Sympathomimetic agents									
Dopamine	H	2–5 min	2–5 min	1–10 µg/kg/min	None	None	None	HEMO: none CAPD: none CAVH: none	
Dobutamine	H	2 min	?	2.5–20 µg/kg/min	None	None	None	HEMO: no data CAPD: no data CAVH: no data	
Phosphodiesterase inhibitors									
Amrinone	H	2.5–8	2.5–8	0.5 mg/kg bolus × 2; 40 µg/kg/min infusion	None	None	50–75%	HEMO: no data CAVH: no data CAVH: no data	Thrombocytopenia. GI upset
Milrinone	R	1	1.5–3	12.5–75 µg/kg (given as 10-mg boluses)	None	None	50–75%	HEMO: no data CAPD: no data CAVH: no data	2.5–15 mg q6h po

GFR = glomerular filtration rate; ESRD = end-stage renal disease; bid = twice a day; tid = three times a day; qd = once a day; CAPD = continuous ambulatory peritoneal dialysis; CAVH = continuous arteriovenous hemofiltration; H/NR = both hepatic and renal; V_d = volume of distribution; (Reproduced with permission from Drug dosing in the ICU in the patient with renal failure. In: Irwin RS, Cerra FB, Rippe JM, eds *Intensive care medicine* 4th edn. Philadelphia: Lippincott-Raven, 1999: 1004–9.)

ACUTE RENAL FAILURE IN THE PATIENT WITH HEART DISEASE

In perspective

The definition of acute renal failure varies among experts. There is little disagreement that ARF implies a rapid deterioration in renal function. Most of the controversy surrounds the extent to which renal function must diminish before the term ARF can be appropriately applied. For the purposes of this chapter, ARF is considered to mean a sudden diminution in renal function from a previously stable baseline level, occurring over a period of hours or days.

It is traditional to categorize ARF by location of the pathophysiologic processes causing it. This approach is not only sensible, but extremely useful as a starting point in diagnosing individual cases of ARF. *Prenal azotemia*, the most common form of ARF, is renal dysfunction brought about by reduced perfusion of otherwise normal kidneys. The physiologic response of the kidney to hypoperfusion is the activation of a series of compensatory processes aimed at maintaining the renal microcirculation, and increasing tubular ion transport so as to preserve the composition of the extracellular space.

In renal azotemia, or *intrinsic ARF*, acute renal failure is caused by diseases of the renal parenchyma itself. These may be toxic, ischemic, or inflammatory in nature. *Postrenal ARF* arises from impedance of urine outflow due to obstructing lesions in the urinary collecting system.

Historical background

Global disasters are responsible for much of what we know about human acute renal failure. Our understanding of clinical ARF stems largely from the experience with post-traumatic cases during the Second World War and Korean conflict. The pathophysiology of ARF continues to unravel gradually in a process deriving directly from the visionary work of the great renal physiologists of the 1930s and 1940s, such as Homer Smith, A.K. Richards, and John P. Peters. With the development of percutaneous renal biopsy in the 1950s, the histopathologic characterization of ARF syndromes was made possible. Despite recent advances in technology for providing dialytic support to patients with ARF, its morbidity and mortality statistics have not changed significantly over the past 20 years. The main thrust of current work is focused upon delineating the cellular and molecular correlates of ARF, and it is hoped that out of this effort will come improved pharmacologic approaches to preventing or ameliorating this important problem.

Prerenal azotemia in cardiac patients

The kidneys are highly vascular organs, with a large metabolic oxygen demand. Their blood flow rate under normal circumstances approaches 25 per cent of the cardiac output. There are three major ways in which blood flow to the kidneys may be reduced. Contraction of the vascular volume, whether as a result of hemorrhage, or loss of fluid from renal, gastrointestinal, or cutaneous routes, may threaten renal perfusion. Diseases in which the flow of blood to the kidneys is compromised not by volume contraction but, rather, by deranged systemic hemodynamics, may also cause prerenal azotemia. In these disorders, such as congestive heart failure and cirrhosis, the patient is said to have a *reduced effective circulatory volume,* even though the actual anatomic blood volume may be normal or increased. Lastly, renal blood flow may be threatened by occlusive lesions in blood vessels proximal to the glomeruli. Renal artery stenosis is the most familiar example of this.

Reductions in renal perfusion are offset by autoregulatory processes. Blood flow into the preglomerular circulation is autoregulated by dilatation of the afferent arterioles, a process which depends largely on prostaglandins. This process is sufficiently effective to afford constancy of renal blood flow to a systolic blood pressure as low as 80 mm Hg. Autoregulation of renal blood flow is hindered by non-steroidal anti-inflammatory drugs that inhibit prostaglandins and thus afferent arteriolar vasodilation.

A separate autoregulatory process maintains glomerular filtration rate (GFR) in these conditions. Autoregulation of glomerular filtration involves constriction of the efferent arteriole, raising the hydrostatic pressure in the glomerular capillary and thereby promoting a higher filtration fraction. Thus, although less blood courses through the glomerulus, a higher fraction of it is converted into filtrate. Constriction of the efferent arteriole is an angiotensin II-dependent process. In patients whose GFR is being maintained by autoregulation, angiotensin-converting enzyme inhibitors may cause ARF.

As shown in Fig. 12.6, raising the filtration fraction in a nephron increases the fractional reabsorption of solute and water from filtrate in the proximal tubule. This proximal tubular avidity is responsible for much of the sodium retention occurring in prerenal azotemia. The reclamation of filtered sodium reaching the distal nephron, stimulated, in part, by aldosterone, is also enhanced. Typically, the urine of patients with prerenal physiology is very low in urine sodium ($\leq$ 20 mEq/L).

Water retention also characterizes prerenal azotemia. The increased proximal fractional reabsorption of filtrate means that less filtrate reaches the diluting segment in the distal nephron where free water is made by reabsorption of solute from the tubular fluid. Vasopressin secretion brought about by volume stimuli in these dis-

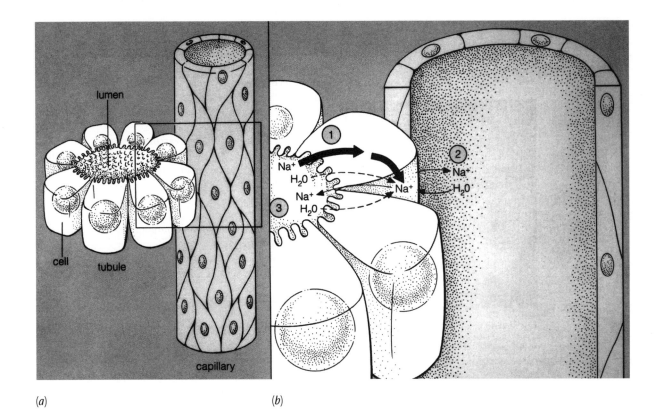

(a)   (b)

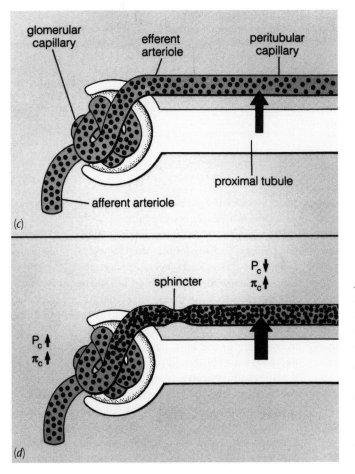

(c)

(d)

Figure 12.6 *Impact of autoregulation of glomerular filtration rate on renal tubular reabsorption. (a and b) Net proximal tubular reabsorption from filtrate represents a balance of reabsorption versus backleak. (c and d) When renal blood flow is reduced, autoregulatory constriction of the efferent arteriole occurs, helping to preserve glomerular filtration rate. The resulting increase in filtration fraction changes Starling forces in peritubular capillary in a manner which favors increased net reabsorption. (Reproduced with permission from Diseases affecting the heart and kidneys. In: Hurst JW, Alpert JS, eds Diagnostic atlas of the heart. New York: Raven Press, 1992.)*

orders, triggers intense water reabsorption from the dilute fluid entering the collecting tubule. Therefore, the urine in prerenal azotemia is generally concentrated ($\geq$ 500 mosmol/kg). Since the reabsorption of water from the urine drives up the sodium concentration, belying the true sodium avidity, the fractional excretion of sodium (FE_{Na}) is a more sensitive indicator of prerenal pathophysiology than the absolute urinary sodium concentration. The FE_{Na} is highly sensitive and specific for detecting reductions in renal blood flow. In the absence of confounding factors, such as hepatic or renovascular disease, diuretic use or metabolic alkalosis, the FE_{Na} actually offers an accurate and non-invasive way of assessing cardiac output.

The avid reabsorption of both sodium and water from nephronal fluid is an adaptive response in hypovolemic conditions. In diseases characterized by a reduced effective circulatory volume, however, this tendency is maladaptive, contributing to the edema and hyponatremia typically encountered in these states.

Because it is generally reversible and often occurs in acute settings, prerenal azotemia is properly grouped with other causes of ARF. In patients with chronically low cardiac output states, however, prerenal azotemia may itself be a chronic condition. In such patients, the conjoint use of diuretics and agents that lower renal perfusion pressure or divert blood from the kidneys, as may some vasodilators, can increase the degree of azotemia.

Intrinsic acute renal failure

A wide variety of renal parenchymal diseases can cause ARF (Table 12.6). The appearance of hematuria, hypertension, and fluid overload in a patient with previously healthy kidneys is called the *acute nephritic syndrome*, and is a presentation of certain forms of glomerulonephritis. In the specific context of patients with heart disease, such presentations are rare. Among cardiac patients, there are two nephritic diseases that deserve special mention: infective endocarditis and postinfectious glomerulonephritis. Immune complex glomerulonephritis may develop in as many as 20 per cent of cases of bacterial endocarditis. This disease can be recognized by the presence of a nephritic urinary sediment (red blood cells, cellular casts) and serologic markers of immune complex activity, specifically a depressed third component of complement. There is no specific therapy other than aggressive treatment of the inciting infection. When ARF is present, the prognosis for return of renal function is variable.

Postinfectious glomerulonephritis can arise in association with impetiginous or cellulitic skin infections, and may occur in patients who develop cutaneous infections at saphenous vein harvest sites following CABG. The serologic and urinary features are as described for endo-

Table 12.6 *Renal parenchymal diseases that may cause acute renal failure*

Acute primary nephritides
Postinfectious glomerulonephritis
Immunoglobulin A nephropathy
Idiopathic crescentic glomerulonephritis

Systemic, autoimmune, and vascular diseases
Systemic vasculitis (Wegener's granulomatosis, polyarteritis nodosa, Henoch–Schonlein purpura, cryoglobulinemia)[a]
Systemic lupus erythematosus
Scleroderma renal crisis
Malignant hypertension
Thrombotic thrombocytopenic purpura and hemolytic–uremic syndrome
Disseminated intravascular coagulation
Goodpasture's syndrome

Acute interstitial nephritis

Acute tubular necrosis and related syndromes
Pigment-related renal failure (myoglobinuria, hemoglobinuria)
Nephrotoxic injury (aminoglycoside, heavy metal, organic solvents, amphoterocin B)
Crystalline micro-obstructive disease (acyclovir, methotrexate, uric acid)
Ischemic acute renal failure

Vasomotor nephropathies
Cyclosporine nephrotoxicity
Radiocontrast nephropathy
Non-steroidal anti-inflammatory drug-associated acute renal failure (ARF)
Hypercalcemia
Hepatorenal syndrome
Angiotensin-converting enzyme inhibitor-associated ARF

[a] These syndromes may induce glomerulonephritis, renal vasculitis, or both.

carditis-associated glomerulonephritis. There is no treatment, but most cases resolve fully.

The most important form of parenchymal ARF in cardiac patients is *acute tubular necrosis* (ATN). This designation has historically been applied to a variety of distinct renal syndromes (Table 12.6) having in common only the facts that the major intrarenal pathogenic locus is the tubules, the urinary sediment often demonstrates the presence of coarse brown granular casts, and the syndromes are, for the most part, reversible. Strictly speaking, the term ATN should probably be reserved for cases of ARF resulting from prolonged renal ischemia or exposure to substances directly toxic to renal tubular cells.

The mechanism by which renal failure occurs in ATN is still controversial. The histopathologic changes, even in cases with severe oliguric ARF, may be quite subtle. The three major historical pathophysiologic constructs of ATN attribute the reduction in renal function respectively to *obstruction* of the tubular lumens by sloughed tubular epithelial cells, intrarenal *vasospasm* without reperfusion, and the tendency of damaged tubular epithelium to allow *backleak* of filtered wastes into the bloodstream. A great deal of experimental data as well as circumstantial clinical observations have been used to corroborate or refute each of these models, and it is likely that each may play a role in the pathogenesis of specific cases of ATN. Current research focuses on events at the cellular and molecular level events in this process. This work has been reviewed.[78]

Renal tubular epithelium loses its normal cellular polarity following ischemia; this is reflected by relocation of transport proteins from the basolateral to the apical membrane surface and dissolution of the cytoskeleton. Loss of intercellular tight junctions accompanies this process, which may damage epithelial integrity and allow backleak of filtered solute wastes into the circulation. The anchoring of cells to the tubular basement membranes is released, and shedding of epithelial cells into tubular lumens occurs, with subsequent formation of obstructive casts. The renal vascular endothelium may also be an important site of tissue injury in ATN. Following a toxic or ischemic insult, endothelial expression of intercellular adhesion molecule 1 (ICAM-1) is increased. This molecule interacts with leuckocyte membrane receptors, promoting leukocyte adhesion at sites of injury.[79] Release of cytokines and activation of phospholipase A_2 with generation of proinflammatory and vasoconstrictive eicosanoids may also occur at these sites.[80] There is evidence to suggest that the ratio of endogenous endothelial vasoconstrictor (endothelin) to vasodilatory nitric oxide may increase in some ATN models.[81,82] Collectively, these events provide an explanation for the reperfusion delay, also called 'no-reflow phenomenon' seen in post-ischemic ATN.

It is often difficult to differentiate ATN from prerenal azotemia, particularly since either can be caused by renal hypoperfusion. The fractional excretion of sodium (FE_{Na}) is particularly useful in this setting. As mentioned, the FE_{Na} is low in prerenal states, with the expected tubular sodium avidity. In ATN, injury to epithelial cells usually impairs their sodium reabsorptive capacity, and a $FE_{Na} > 1$ per cent is expected even in volume-depleted patients. Exceptions are ATN occurring in the presence of severe liver disease, and acute radiocontrast nephropathy. While the latter is often considered under the ATN heading, the fact that a low FE_{Na} is often observed suggests that this may be a pathophysiologically distinct form of ARF (see Table 12.6).

Another lesion which represents an important cause of ARF in hospitalized patients is *acute intersitial nephritis* (AIN). Although this disease can occur as an idiopathic condition or in association with various infections, the vast majority of cases are caused by drugs. AIN is essentially a renal hypersensitivity reaction;

approximately three-quarters of cases demonstrate one or more of the following laboratory findings: peripheral or urinary eosinophilia, or elevated serum immunoglobulin E (IgE) levels. The list of drugs that have been reported to cause AIN is extremely long. The most commonly implicated agents are antibiotics, particularly sulfonamide-like agents, penicillins, and cephalosporins; allopurinol; and other sulfur-containing compounds. The last category applies to several drugs commonly used in cardiovascular medicine including thiazide and loop diuretics, and captopril. Alpha-methyldopa may also provoke this renal lesion.

Postrenal ARF

The most important causes of obstructive uropathy are prostatic bladder outlet obstruction, urinary calculi, malignancies, urinary tract infection, congenital and acquired strictures, bladder dystonia, and trauma. To cause acute renal failure in a patient with two functioning kidneys, an obstruction must either involve both ureters or occur at the bladder outlet. In hospitalized patients, bladder outlet obstructions are fairly common. Patients confined to bedrest, and those receiving anticholinergics or narcotic analgesics may experience impaired bladder emptying, especially if some degree of bladder outlet obstruction were present beforehand. Postrenal causes must be considered in any hospitalized patient developing ARF, particularly if they do not have an indwelling bladder catheter in place.

Diagnosis of ARF in the cardiac patient

Physicians usually recognize ARF based on either of two findings: a fall-off in the urine flow rate, or azotemia on routine blood chemistry studies. Even when closely monitored, urine volume is not a very sensitive indicator in ARF since many cases are non-oliguric or even polyuric.

The historical context in which an acute deterioration in renal function develops may provide important clues to the nature of the specific renal disorder. Daily weight and intake–output records kept in hospitalized patients may help determine whether fluid balance has been inadequate to maintain hydration. Prerenal azotemia, while a form of ARF, evolves gradually in such patients. Patients with prerenal azotemia due to poor myocardial function also lapse relatively slowly into renal failure. The addition of diuretics to the regimen of such a patient can be expected to worsen the azotemia, even though such a maneuver may be medically indicated. Eighty to 90 per cent of cases of ATN can be linked to a discrete triggering event, such as a period of prolonged hypotension, an episode of sepsis, complicated surgery, a sustained arrhythmia, or exposure to a nephrotoxin.

Physical examination should focus on determining

the state of hemodynamic integrity. Is the blood pressure adequate for organ perfusion? Does the patient appear clinically volume depleted? Are the clinical hallmarks of severe left ventricular failure, particularly pulmonary rales and an S_3, present to help substantiate a clinical suspicion of prerenal azotemia due to low cardiac output? The examiner should also remember to look for signs of a distended bladder.

Chemical and microscopic urinalysis are integral parts of the diagnosis of ARF. The characteristic urinary chemical findings (concentrated urine and low FE_{Na}) aid in the recognition of prerenal azotemia, whereas a microscopic examination of the urinary sediment may reveal the muddy brown casts seen in most cases of ATN or the pyuria and eosinophiliuria of AIN.

When the above measures fail to yield a diagnosis, a postrenal cause should be ruled out. Renal sonography is the safest, easiest, and least expensive way to do this (Fig. 12.7).

Prognosis of ARF in cardiac patients

An elevated blood urea nitrogen level (BUN) has negative prognostic impact in the setting of acute myocardial infarction.[83] No recent studies have explored the impact of prerenal azotemia *per se* on cardiac mortality in congestive heart failure. However, recently investigators looked at patients with advanced congestive heart failure (CHF) and questioned whether renal function was a predictor of mortality. They found that GFR was the most powerful predictor of mortality followed by the New York Heart Association functional class. Patients in the lowest quartile of GFR (<44 mL/min) had almost three times the risk of death compared to those in the highest quartile. Moreover, impaired renal function was not related to left ventricular ejection fraction.[84] A reduction in blood flow to the kidneys of sufficient magnitude to cause azotemia is, by definition, one that is severe enough to outweigh the compensatory effects of the autoregulatory mechanisms. This is indicative of a severe derangement in systemic hemodynamics. Indeed, other markers of renal hypoperfusion, e.g. hyponatremia, and hyperreninemia, augur poorly for survival in patients with congestive heart failure.[85] One inference to be drawn from these observations is that a reduction in renal blood flow sufficient to cause prerenal azotemia or frank ATN is a marker of severe ventricular damage, bespeaking an increased probability of cardiac mortality. While this is no doubt true, ARF *per se* may be an independent risk

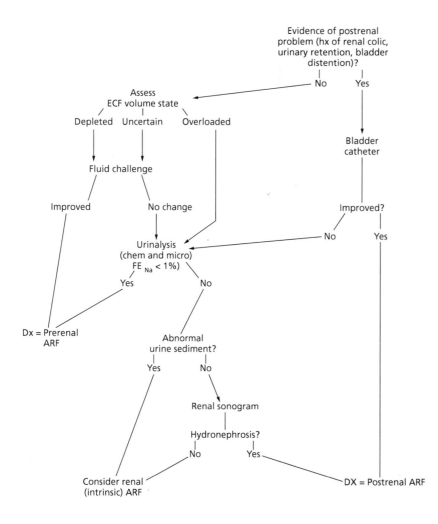

Figure 12.7 *An algorithm for the diagnosis of acute renal failure (ARF). The sequence utilized in this approach is designed to minimize the likelihood of obtaining negative test results. In common practice, it is routine to perform microscopical and chemical urinalysis and a fluid challenge as soon as a patient is found to have oliguria or azotemia. hx = history; ECF = extracellular fluid; dx = diagnosis.*

factor for mortality in hospitalized patients. This possibility is raised by a recent study by Levy and colleagues in which patients developing ARF after routine angiographic procedures had lower survival than equivalently ill patients without this complication.[86] The applicability of this study to other forms of ARF is still unclear.

Treatment of ARF: conservative therapy

Conservative measures utilized in the treatment of ARF have not changed appreciably in the past years. Perhaps the first step that should be taken upon discovering that a patient has newly developed oliguria or azotemia is a fluid challenge. This maneuver has both diagnostic as well as therapeutic value; if volume expansion corrects the disturbance in renal function, the diagnostic suspicion of prerenal azotemia is confirmed. The only reason not to attempt such a fluid challenge is if the patient is clearly fluid overloaded or has signs of pulmonary vascular congestion. In adults, at least one half-liter of isotonic crystalloid should be given, the exact volume and rate of administration to be dictated by the size of the patient and extent of discernible hypovolemia.

Preserving optimal fluid balance in hospitalized patients is integral in the prevention not only of prerenal azotemia, but of toxic and ischemic forms of ATN as well.

> Patients about to undergo radiocontrast procedures, major surgery, administration of nephrotoxic agents such as aminoglycoside antibiotics, or who have sustained major trauma (placing them at risk for myoglobinuric renal failure) should be maintained in a euvolemic and, ideally, diuretic state throughout the period of risk.

It has been suggested, based on studies in the isolated perfused rodent kidney, that pre-emptive use of loop or osmotic diuretics may be prophylactic against ischemic ATN. Morphologic and metabolic studies in this model reveal that the portion of the nephron most susceptible to ischemic injury is the outer stripe of the inner medullary region, an area with a large oxygen requirement based on its high degree of ion transport activity. Diuretics, by blocking this activity, attenuate the degree of ischemic injury to the cells.[87] Although this rationale could apply in clinical situations, it has not yet been proven. As noted earlier, diuretics should be avoided in patients for whom radiocontrast procedures are planned.[68]

Non-oliguric ARF cases generally have a milder, shorter course than cases of oliguric ARF, even though the degree of reduction of the GFR may be equivalent. In one classic study, 84 per cent of oliguric cases of ATN necessitated interim dialysis compared to 28 per cent of non-oliguric patients. Mortality in the oliguric group was twice that of the non-oliguric, and hospital stays

markedly longer.[88] It has been argued that 'converting' oliguric to nonoliguric ARF may improve the outcome, but this, too, is unproven, since the ability of the kidneys to augment urine flow in response to a diuretic may, like non-oliguria, be a favorable prognostic sign in its own right. It is clear that fluid overload is a major cause of morbidity in ARF. Diuretic therapy is a valuable tool in the management of these patients, particularly those whose care obligates the daily delivery of large volumes of fluid for medications and alimentation. Loop diuretics are best for this purpose; the doses may be pushed to maximal levels (e.g. for furosemide, up to 400 mg per day) and may be administered in intravenous boluses or by constant infusion. The co-administration of a thiazide-type agent with a loop diuretic may enhance potency.[89,90]

The use of low-dose dopamine infusion to provoke a diuresis in patients with ARF has been popular among intensivists over the past decade. The efficacy of this approach has recently been called into question,[91] and it is the authors' feeling that the use of low-dose dopamine should be avoided, especially in light of the arrhythmogenic potential of this agent.

In addition to sodium and water overload, other chemical imbalances accompany ARF. Metabolic acidosis arises from reduced filtration of metabolically produced acids, as well as impairment in ammonia production, bicarbonate reabsorption, and hydrogen ion secretion by the renal tubules. Lactic acid production may contribute to acidosis in patients with cardiogenic shock, or following cardiac arrest. It is invariably preferable to correct, if possible, the underlying cause of these acidoses, rather than simply to aim at replacing the base deficit with exogenous sodium bicarbonate. In the case of lactic acidosis, the administration of bicarbonate can actually enhance cellular lactate production.[92]

> Nevertheless, in view of evidence that severe acidemia can compromise cardiac function, it is the authors' practice to give sufficient supplemental bicarbonate to acutely ill cardiac patients with metabolic acidosis in amounts as needed to maintain an arterial blood pH ≥ 7.20 or serum bicarbonate level ≥ 15.

Hyperkalemia remains a leading cause of death in ARF. Since the danger of hyperkalemia resides in its arrhythmogenic potential, it is to be assumed that cardiac patients, particularly in the acute setting, are at greatest risk for such a complication. Cases of hyperkalemia with electrocardiographic signs of cardiac toxicity must be treated as an emergency. The treatment of hyperkalemia in patients receiving cardiac glycosides may induce symptoms of drug toxicity; the clinician must be properly vigilant.

Once a patient is recognized to be suffering from ARF, a review of all medications should be undertaken promptly. The doses of all renally excreted drugs should be adjusted commensurate with the current level of the patient's renal function. The reader is again referred to Table 12.5 for a list of commonly used cardiovascular drugs warranting dose modification in renal failure. All agents with potential adverse effects on the kidney should be eliminated from the pharmaceutical regimen, if possible. This is most important in likely cases of drug-induced ATN and AIN in which drug withdrawal may suffice to resolve the renal problem.

> The management of ongoing prerenal azotemia in patients with chronic left ventricular failure is extremely challenging. Most patients in this category do not become uremic, perhaps because the mortality of heart failure severe enough to cause severe, sustained reductions in GFR is so high. Therapy should be aimed at maximizing renal perfusion. Angiotensin-converting enzyme (ACE) inhibitors may be effective for this purpose, assuming that the heart can respond to afterload reduction with an increase in left ventricular output to the kidneys and that resistance in the afferent (preglomerular) vessels is reduced.

For renal function to be improved, these beneficial hemodynamic effects must outweigh the adverse effects on GFR of efferent arteriolar vasodilation. In some patients with congestive heart failure, this favorable net balance is not achieved, and they may respond to ACE inhibitor therapy with worsened renal function.[93–95] It may be difficult to predict a given patient's response to ACE inhibitors. Diuretics should be used cautiously in patients receiving ACE inhibitors, as overdiuresis of ACE inhibitor-treated patients can provoke severe ARF. Patients unable to tolerate ACE inhibitors due to hyperkalemia or renal dysfunction may fare better on an alternate vasodilator, such as hydralazine.

Renal replacement therapy in ARF

Under the best of circumstances, ARF can be managed conservatively. Occasionally, most often in cases of protracted, oliguric ARF, it will become necessary to invoke dialysis or some related technique of renal replacement therapy.

> The indications for dialysis in ARF include intoxication with a dialyzable drug, hyperkalemia, acidosis, or fluid overload not amenable to medical therapy. Severe uremic manifestations, such as the appearance of a pericardial friction rub or new onset of seizures, are also clear indications to initiate dialysis, although these symptoms may arise from non-uremic causes in intensely ill cardiac patients.

When symptoms are of a more subtle or non-specific nature, such as lethargy, anorexia, and confusion, the timing of dialysis rests more on the clinician's judgement.

Several modalities of renal replacement therapy are routinely employed in the treatment of ARF. *Hemodialysis* is the most familiar of these. Hemodialysis employs a blood pump (the 'dialysis machine') to drive the patient's blood through an extracorporeal circuit, at the center of which is the dialyzer (the 'artificial kidney'). The dialyzer is composed of blood channels bound by a cellulosic or synthetic polymer membrane. The specific permeability characteristics of this membrane, and its surface area, determine its ultrafiltration and clearance characteristics. The most commonly used dialyzers have a hollow-fiber configuration, emulating that of capillaries. These channels are bathed in a physiologic dialysis solution (the 'dialysate'). Solute wastes diffuse across the dialysis membrane from blood to dialysate, a process driven by the concentration gradient between the two compartments. To enhance the gradient, dialysate flow through the dialyzer runs countercurrent to that of the blood. The transmembrane pressure gradient allows ultrafiltration of fluid from blood to dialysate. This gradient is determined by both the blood pressure in the system and the pressure of the dialysate. Ultrafiltration is achieved by applying negative pressure to the dialysate compartment. The current generation of hemodialysis machines afford remarkably precise volumetric control during ultrafiltration.

Hemodialysis is the most rapid and efficient blood purification modality in common use. Barring hypotension, up to 7 L of fluid can be removed during the course of a typical 3–4-hour hemodialysis session. Under steady-state conditions, enough solute waste can be cleared in 10–12 hours of hemodialysis per week to keep a functionally anephric patient free of uremic symptoms. The specifics of hemodialysis prescription will not be considered here. For most patients, intermittent hemodialysis constitutes a safe and effective interim therapy for ARF.

It is possible to utilize the hemodialysis circuit without dialysate to perform a purely ultrafiltrative procedure. This technique is referred to as *hemofiltration*, or *intermittent hemofiltration* to distinguish it from the continuous filtration therapies described below. Removal of solutes occurs only by convection in the ultrafiltrate, proportionate to their concentration in the plasma. Thus, only the volume of the blood is changed, not its chemical composition. Such procedures tend to incite less hypotension in hemodynamically unstable patients than do true dialysis treatments, even when equivalent volumes of fluid are removed.

Continuous renal replacement therapies (CRRT) were first introduced in this country about 15 years ago. These techniques employ artificial membrane filters of extremely high porosity, such that no external pressures need be applied to permit ultrafiltration. In *continuous arteriovenous hemofiltration* or CAVH, no blood pump is used; the movement of blood through the extracorporeal circuit is driven purely by the force of the patient's systole. Blood enters the circuit from an arterial access site, usually the femoral artery, and is returned to a venous site, most likely the adjacent femoral vein. *Continuous venovenous hemofiltration* (CVVH) differs from CAVH in that a double-lumen intravenous catheter provides both the source of blood as well as its return site, necessitating a blood pump to move blood through the circuit. Higher blood flow rates may be reached with CVVH than with CAVH, permitting more aggressive ultrafiltration. Both of these techniques offer the capability of removing large amounts of ultrafiltrate in a relatively gentle, slow, continuous fashion. Since the ultrafiltration rate is determined largely by the patient's blood pressure, the system is, to an extent, self-regulating. Not surprisingly, CAVH and CVVH are often better tolerated than hemodialysis or intermittent hemofiltration in relatively hypotensive patients. The rate of ultrafiltration may easily be adjusted from hour to hour.

Continuous hemofiltration techniques are, like intermittent hemofiltration, purely ultrafiltrative. While useful in conditions of fluid overload, they are less efficient than hemodialysis in treating problems related to solute waste accumulation in ARF, such as hyperkalemia or uremia. Both these treatments may be modified in either of two ways so as to augment solute removal. High-volume continuous hemofiltration means that the ultrafiltration rate is allowed to continue at near-maximal rates (these may approach 500–1000 mL/hour), replacing most of the ultrafiltrate with isotonic crystalloid, such as normal saline, Ringer's lactate, or some other buffered physiologic solution. Thus, waste clearance is achieved by convection, and waste-rich ultrafiltrate is replaced by waste-free fluid. The percentage of ultrafiltrate to be replaced is determined by the desired net rate of fluid removal.

The other modification for enhancing solute clearance in continuous hemofiltration is called hemodiafiltration (CAVH-D or CVVH-D, depending on the fundamental circuit type being used). In these modalities, dialysate is infused into the hemofilter at a constant rate (much more slowly, as a rule, than dialysate flow rates in conventional hemodialysis). This allows for a continuous low rate of dialytic waste transfer and ultrafiltration to occur simultaneously. Continuous hemodiafiltration techniques are gaining increasing popularity as safe, effective methods for treating ARF in critically ill patients. Some experts consider them the treatment of choice for ARF in the intensive care unit.[96–98] The observation that hemofilter membranes are able to clear endotoxin and cytokines raised the possibility of yet another rationale for the use of CRRT in ARF associated with sepsis and the systemic inflammatory response syndrome.[99,100] Unfortunately, this has not yet proven to yield any significant impact on survival.

Both hemodialysis and continuous hemofiltration require vascular access. In ARF, this mandates the placement of indwelling vascular catheters. Both treatment types usually require some degree of anticoagulation to prevent clotting in the system. This is generally accomplished by systemically heparinizing the patient for the duration of the treatment. In the case of patients with problems related to bleeding, it may be possible to minimize or even eliminate the use of heparin, albeit at increased risk of clotted blood lines and filters.

Peritoneal dialysis (PD) utilizes the filtrative properties of the peritoneal membranes in lieu of an artificial membrane filter. Dialysis fluid is instilled into the patient's peritoneal cavity through an indwelling catheter. For this purpose, surgically implanted flexible catheters (like the Tenckhoff catheter) have largely replaced the older rigid catheters placed percutaneously with a stylette. Flexible catheters are physically safer, and have one or more cuffs along their extraperitoneal course to serve as barriers to bacterial ingress. Bedside placement of a rigid catheter is sometimes necessary when the arrangements for surgical placement of a flexible catheter is unsafe or not readily available.

Soluble substance transfer in peritoneal dialysis, like that in hemodialysis, is gradient driven. Increasing the volume of instilled dialysate (the so-called 'dwell volume', usually 1–3 L in an adult patient as size permits) and frequency with which the fluid is exhanged maximize the gradient for waste removal. Since it is not possible to control transmembrane pressures in peritoneal dialysis, ultrafiltration is achieved by using hyperosmolar dialysate solutions. Increasing the concentration of dextrose in these dialysates increases the rate of ultrafiltration. Accordingly, commercially available peritoneal dialysis fluid is available in three 'strengths', 1.5, 2.5, and 4.25 per cent dextrose, respectively. Prescription of the specific dialytic parameters, i.e. the dwell volume, frequency of exchanges, and composition of dialysate, are best left to the nephrologist.

> Although peritoneal dialysis is a time-honored and generally safe technique for treating ARF, its use in this setting is dwindling. Like continuous hemofiltration, it may be better tolerated in hemodynamically tenuous patients than hemodialysis.

PD obviates the need for placement of central venous access, which may be a considerable advantage in patients whose access sites have been exhausted, or are being otherwise used. Should a patient experience hypotension at a given rate of PD-induced ultrafiltration, the dialytic prescription should be adjusted accordingly. Occasionally, the presence of fluid in the abdomen may cause respiratory embarassment, especially in patients with underlying pulmonary disease or coexistent acute respiratory failure. In such a situation, the dwell volume should be reduced, or an alternative form of dialysis selected.

All forms of acute dialysis and hemofiltration are costly and place great demands on nursing care. The decision as to which specific modality to employ should be made mainly on the basis of the individual needs of the patient at hand.

FUTURE DIRECTIONS

Cardiovascular disease in ESRD patients

Over the past 25 years, there has been a transformation in the way maintenance dialysis patients are perceived. ESRD care carries less of a sense of resignation to dreary outcomes and a sense that the patient has 'one foot in the grave'. The approach to cardiovascular risk in ESRD patients emblemizes this transformation. ESRD patients routinely undergo coronary screening, percutaneous angioplasty, and CABG. They should be encouraged to modify cardiovascular risk factors under the expectation that their longevity will be sufficient to make these maneuvers worthwhile. As implied earlier, there is no evidence at this time that cholesterol-lowering diets are indicated in the ESRD dialysis population. Furthermore, dietary interventions are difficult in this group, many of whom already live under the onus of a severely restricted diet while risking malnutrition. It has been suggested that clinical trials of antioxidant therapy, aimed at mitigating the suspected contribution of oxidized lipoprotein products to the atherogenic process, be undertaken in the ESRD patient pool.[6] A recent trial in HD patients suggested a decrease in CV disease end points in those patients receiving vitamin E. Total mortality rates, however, were not different between the vitamin E and placebo treated groups.[101]

The extent to which elevated homocysteine levels enhance cardiovascular risk in ESRD patients, and its specific pathogenetic relationship to coronary artery disease warrant further delineation. B-vitamin and folic acid supplementation can lower homocysteine levels substantially in patients with normal renal function. In ESRD patients, they may lower levels 20–30 per cent, but often fail to achieve normal levels.[102] Nevertheless, evidence of a strong connection between hyperhomocysteinemia and ASCVD is suggested in ESRD, and trials of folic acid–B-vitamin supplementation in selected patients continue to be worthwhile.[34,35] Lastly, the possibility that synthetic, biocompatible hemodialysis membranes pose less of a long-term risk of accelerated atherosclerosis also merits study.[6] An initial review of data culled from the US Renal Data System suggests that deaths due to coronary artery disease are reduced as much as 26 per cent in patients dialyzed using synthetic or modified cellulose membranes versus those dialyzed with conventional unmodified cellulose dialyzers.[103]

Acute renal failure in cardiac patients

Rigorous, controlled trials are overdue to settle the debate as to whether pre-emptive use of loop or osmotic diuretics can protect against ARF in patients at risk, i.e. prior to or at the outset of an ischemic insult. Anti-ICAM 1 antibody appears to prophylax against ATN in animals subjected to ischemia[104] and limited clinical trials have been undertaken. It is likely that the coming years will see clinical trials of agents intended to mitigate the course of ATN. Many of these have been studied experimentally. In clinical ATN, trials of atrial natriuretic factor, which had appeared capable of attenuating established ischemic ATN in animal models, yielded disappointing results.[105] Other agents that may receive similar study are the epidermal, hepatocyte, and insulin-like growth factors,[106,107] endothelin antagonists,[108] and dopamine A-1 receptor agonists.[109]

It has been reported that biocompatible synthetic polymer hemodialysis membranes as opposed to cellulosic membranes for treating ARF may shorten recovery time and be associated with improved morbidity and mortality.[110,111] The authors of these studies theorize that biocompatible membranes induce less cytokine activation, possibly lessening the inherent toxicity of hemodialysis to the kidneys. Many dialysis units are beginning to utilize biocompatible membranes routinely, despite their increased cost, in the treatment of ARF.

Despite the suggestion that continuous renal replacement therapies such as CVVH, CAVH, and their dialytic modifications may be preferable modalities of therapy for critically ill patients with ARF, good data to substantiate this claim are still lacking. This issue would clearly benefit from a large, well-designed, randomized trial.

SUMMARY

- Cardiovascular disease is widespread among patients with chronic renal disease, and represents the leading cause of death among dialysis patients. With the possible exception of hypercholesterolemia, the risk factors are similar to those among non-renal failure patients.
- Most patients with chronic renal disease have hypertension. Although the precise importance of hypertension as a cardiovascular risk factor in this population is not known, vigorous treatment is recommended.
- Homocysteinemia is extremely common in end-stage renal disease (ESRD). Whether treatment of this risk factor will lower cardiovascular morbidity remains to be seen.

- Cardiac ischemia commonly complicates hemodialysis treatments. Silent ischemia occurs in up to 40 per cent of patients during hemodialysis.
- The diagnostic strategy for evaluating coronary artery disease in ESRD patients is the same as for non-renal patients. Thallium myocardial scanning poses particular problems in this group. Special precautions must be observed when subjecting ESRD patients to cardiac catheterization.
- Coronary artery bypass grafting can be performed with acceptable mortality rates in ESRD patients. Effective symptom alleviation is achieved, but evidence of beneficial effects on long-term survival is lacking.
- Acute renal failure in the context of acute myocardial infarction carries a highly adverse impact on survival.
- Chronic prerenal azotemia in patients with congestive heart failure is a poor prognostic sign. Angiotensin-converting enzyme (ACE) inhibitors may be used to improve renal hemodynamics, but may exacerbate prerenal failure in some patients.
- Several choices are available for blood purification in acute renal failure. All are expensive and require intensive nursing-care. Continuous renal replacement therapies such as continuous arteriovenous or venovenous hemodiafiltration may offer selective advantages in very ill cardiac patients.

REFERENCES

1. US Renal Data System. USRDS 1995 Annual Report. *Am J Kidney Dis* 1995; **26**: S85–94.
2. Goodman W, Goldin J, Kuizon B, *et al*. Coronary artery calcification in young adults with end-stage renal disease who are undergoing dialysis. *N Engl J Med* 2000; **342**: 1478–83.
3. Herzog CA, Ma JZ, Collins AJ. Poor long-term survival after acute myocardial infarction among patients on long-term dialysis. *N Engl J Med* 1998; **339**: 799–805.
4. Chertow GM, Normand ST, Silva LR, McNeil BJ. Survival after acute myocardial infarction in patients with end-stage renal disease: results from the Cooperative Cardiovascular project. *Am J Kidney Dis* 2000; **35**: 1044–51.
5. Herzog CA, Ma JZ, Collins AJ. Long term survival of renal transplant recipients in the United States after acute myocardial infarction. *Am J Kidney Dis* 2000; **36**: 145–52.
6. Becker BN, Himmelfarb J, Henrich WL, Hakim RM. Reassessing the cardiac risk profile in chronic hemodialysis patients: a hypothesis on the role of oxidant stress and other non-traditional cardiac risk factors. *J Am Soc Nephrol* 1997; **8**: 475–86.
7. Kasiske BL. Hyperlipidemia in patients with chronic renal disease. *Am J Kidney Dis* 1998; **32**: S142–56.
8. Lowrie EG, Lew NL. Death risk in hemodialysis patients: the predictive value of commonly measured variables and an evaluation of death rate differences between facilities. *Am J Kidney Dis* 1990; **15**: 458–82.
9. Attman P, Samuelsson O, Alaupovic P. Lipoprotein metabolism and renal failure. *Am J Kidney Dis* 1993; **21**: 573–92.
10. Cressman MD, Heyka RJ, Paganini EP, *et al*. Lipoprotein(a) is an independent risk factor for cardiovascular disease in hemodialysis patients. *Circulation* 1992; **86**: 475–82.
11. Ohashi H, Oda H, Ohno M, *et al*. Lipoprotein(a) as a risk factor for coronary artery disease in hemodialysis patients. *Kidney Int* 1999; **56**(suppl. 71): S242–4.
12. Koda Y, Nishi S, Suzuki M, Hirasawa Y. Lipoprotein(a) is a predictor for cardiovascular mortality of hemodialysis patients. *Kidney Int* 1999; **56**(suppl. 71): S251–3.
13. Itabe H, Yamamota H, Imanaka T, *et al*. Sensitive detection of oxidatively modified low density lipoprotein using a monoclonal antibody. *J Lipid Res* 1996; **37**: 45–53.
14. Grainger DJ, Kirschenlohr HL, Metcalfe JC, *et al*. Proliferation of human smooth muscle cells promoted by lipoprotein(a). *Science* 1993; **260**: 1655–8.
15. Rocco M, Benz R, Bukart J, *et al*. Baseline blood pressure in HEMO study participants: an interim report. *J Am Soc Nephrol* 1997; **8**: 1153A.
16. Converse RL Jr, Jacobsen TN, Toto RD, *et al*. Sympathetic overactivity in patients with chronic renal failure. *N Engl J Med* 1992; **327**: 1912–18.
17. Ye S, Ozgur B, Campese VM. Renal afferent impulses, the posterior hypothalamus, and hypertension in rats with chronic renal failure. *Kidney Int* 1997; **51**: 722–7.
18. Salem MM, Bower JD. Hypertension in the hemodialysis population: any relation to one-year survival? *Am J Kidney Dis* 1996; **28**: 737–40.
19. Port FK, Hulbert-Shearon TE, Wolfe RA, *et al*. Predialysis blood pressure and mortality risk in a national sample of maintenance hemodialysis patients. *Am J Kidney Dis* 1999; **33**: 507–17.
20. Zager PG, Nikolic J, Brown RH, *et al*. 'U' curve association of blood pressure and mortality in hemodialysis patients. *Kidney Int* 1998; **54**: 561–9.
21. Mailloux LU, Levey AS. Hypertension in patients with chronic renal disease. *Am J Kidney Dis* 1998; **32**: S120–41.
22. Rostand SG, Brunzell JD, Cannon RO, Victor RG. Cardiovascular complications in renal failure. *J Am Soc Nephrol* 1991; **2**: 1053–62.
23. Salem M. Hypertension in the hemodialysis population? High time for answers. *Am J Kidney Dis* 1999; **33**: 592–4.

24. US Renal Data System. *1993 Annual Data Report.* Bethesda, MD: National Institutes of Health, National Institutes of Diabetes and Digestive and Kidney Disease, 1993.

25. Nygård O, Nordrehaug JE, Refsum H, *et al.* Plasma homocysteine levels and mortality in patients with coronary artery disease. *N Engl J Med* 1997; **337**: 230–6.

26. Chauveau P, Chadefaux B, Coude M, *et al.* Hyperhomocysteinemia, a risk factor for atherosclerosis in chronic uremic patients. *Kidney Int* 1993; **41**: S72–7.

27. Guttormsen AB, Ueland PM, Svarstad E, Refsum H. Kinetic basis of hyperhomocysteinemia in patients with chronic renal failure. *Kidney Int* 1997; **52**: 495–502.

28. Födinger M, Mannhalter C, Wölfl G, *et al.* Mutation (677 C to T) in the methylenetetrahydrofolate reductase gene aggravates hyperhomocysteinemia in hemodialysis patients. *Kidney Int* 1997; **52**: 517–23.

29. Bostom A, Lathrop L. Hyperhomocysteinemia in end-stage renal disease: prevalence, etiology, and potential relationship to arteriosclerotic outcomes. *Kidney Int* 1997; **52**: 10–20.

30. Malinow MR, Sexton G, Averbuch M, *et al.* Hyperhomocysteinemia in daily practice: levels in coronary artery disease. *Coron Art Dis* 1990; **1**: 215–20.

31. Selhub J, Jacques PF, Bostom AG, *et al.* Association between plasma homocysteine concentrations and extracranial carotid-artery stenosis. *N Engl J Med* 1995; **332**: 286–91.

32. Robinson K, Gupta A, Dennis V, Arheart K, *et al.* Hyperhomocysteinemia confers an independent risk of atherosclerosis in end-stage renal disease and is closely linked to plasma folate and pyridoxine concentrations. *Circulation* 1999; **94**: 2743–8.

33. Moustapha A, Naso A, Nahlawi M, *et al.* Prospective study of hyperhomocysteinemia as an adverse cardiovascular risk factor in end-stage renal disease. *Circulation* 1998; **97**: 138–41.

34. Bostom AG, Shemin D, Lapane KL, *et al.* High dose B-vitamin treatment of hyperhomocysteinemia in dialysis patients. *Kidney Int* 1996; **49**: 147–52.

35. Sunder-Plassmann G, Födinger M, Buchmayer H, *et al.* Effect of high dose folic acid on hyperhomocysteinemia in hemodialysis patients. *J Am Soc Nephrol* 2000; **11**: 1106–16.

36. Rostand S, Drüeke T. Parathyroid hormone, vitamin D, and cardiovascular disease in chronic renal failure. *Kidney Int* 1999; **56**: 383–92.

37. Ridker PM, Cushman M, Stampfer MJ, *et al.* Inflammation, aspirin, and the risk of cardiovascular disease in apparently healthy men. *New Engl J Med* 1997; **336**: 973–9.

38. Zimmermann J, Herrlinger S, Pruy A, Metzger T, Wanner C. Inflammation enhances cardiovascular risk and mortality in hemodialysis patients. *Kidney Int* 1999; **55**: 648–58.

39. Yeun JY, Levine RA, Mantadilok V, Kaysen GA. C-reactive protein predicts all-cause and cardiovascular mortality in hemodialysis patients. *Am J Kidney Dis* 2000; **35**: 469–76.

40. Iseki K, Tozawa M, Yoshi S, Fukiyama K. Serum C-reactive protein (CRP) and risk of death in chronic dialysis patients. *Nephrol Dial Transplant* 1999; **14**: 1956–60.

41. Stenvinkel P, Heimburger O, Wang T, *et al.* High serum hyaluron indicates poor survival in renal replacement therapy. *Am J Kidney Dis* 1999; **34**: 1083–8.

42. Boaz M, Matas Z, Biro A, *et al.* Serum malondialdehyde and prevalent cardiovascular disease in hemodialysis. *Kidney Int* 1999; **56**: 1078–83.

43. Boaz M, Matas Z, Biro A, *et al.* Comparison of hemostatic factors and serum malondialdehyde as predictive factors for cardiovascular disease in hemodialysis patients. *Am J Kidney Dis* 1999; **34**: 438–44.

44. Parfrey PS, Griffiths SM, Harnett JD, *et al.* Outcome of congestive heart failure, dilated cardiomyopathy, hypertrophic hyperkinetic disease, and ischemic heart disease in dialysis patients. *Am J Nephrol* 1990; **10**: 213–21.

45. Parfrey PS, Harnett JD, Barre PE. The natural history of myocardial disease in dialysis patients. *J Am Soc Nephrol* 1991; **2**: 2–12.

46. Levin A, Singer J, Thompson CR, *et al.* Prevalent left ventricular hypertrophy in the predialysis population: identifying opportunities for intervention. *Am J Kidney Dis* 1996; **27**: 347–54.

47. Törnig J, Gross M-L, Simonaviciene A, *et al.* Hypertrophy of intramyocardial arteriolar smooth muscle cells in experimental renal failure. *J Am Soc Nephrol* 1999; **10**: 77–83.

48. Topol EJ, Traill TA, Fortuin NJ. Hypertensive hypertrophic cardiomyopathy of the elderly. *N Engl J Med* 1985; **312**: 277–83.

49. Ma KW, Greene EL, Raij L. Cardiovascular risk factors in chronic renal failure and hemodialysis populations. *Am J Kidney Dis* 1992; **19**: 505–13.

50. Straumann E, Meyer B, Misteli M, *et al.* Aortic and mitral valve disease in patients with end stage renal failure on long-term haemodialysis. *Br Heart J* 1992; **67**: 236–9.

51. Stinebaugh J, Lavie CJ, Milani RV, *et al.* Doppler echocardiographic assessment of valvular heart disease in patients requiring hemodialysis for end-stage renal disease. *South Med J* 1995; **88**: 65–71.

52. Mazzaferro S, Coen G, Bandini S, *et al.* Role of aging, chronic renal failure and dialysis in the calcification of the mitral annulus. *Nephrol Dial Transplant* 1993; **8**: 335–40.

53. Smogorzewski M, Massry SG. Uremic cardiomyopathy: role of parathyroid hormone. *Kidney Int* 1997; **52**: S12–14.

54. Harnett JD, Foley RN, Kent GM, *et al.* Congestive heart failure in dialysis patients: prevalence, incidence, prognosis and risk factors. *Kidney Int* 1995; **47**: 884–90.

55. Rostand SG, Sanders C, Kirk KA, Rutsky EA, Fraser RG. Myocardial calcification and cardiac dysfunction in chronic renal failure. *Am J Med* 1988; **85**: 651–7.

56. Daugirdas JT. Dialysis hypotension: a hemodynamic analysis. *Kidney Int* 1991; **39**: 233–46.

57. Iseki K, Massry SG, Campese VM. Evidence for a role of PTH in the reduced pressor response to norepinephrine in chronic renal failure. *Kidney Int* 1985; **28**: 11–15.

58. Jassal SV, Coulshed SJ, Douglas JF, Stout RW. Autonomic neuropathy predisposing to arrhythmias in hemodialysis patients. *Am J Kidney Dis* 1997; **30**: 219–23.

59. Lang RM, Fellner SK, Neumann A, *et al*. Left ventricular contractility varies directly with blood ionized calcium. *Ann Intern Med* 1988; **108**: 524–9.

60. Henrich WL, Hunt JM, Nixon JV. Increased ionized calcium and left ventricular contractility during hemodialysis. *N Engl J Med* 1984; **310**: 19–23.

61. Pochmalicki G, Fouchard JF, Teiger E, *et al*. Frequency of painless myocardial ischemia during hemodialysis in 50 patients with chronic kidney failure. *Arch Malad Coeur Vaiss* 1990; **83**: 1671–5.

62. Murphy SW, Foley RN, Parfrey PS. Screening and treatment for cardiovascular disease in patients with chronic renal disease. *Am J Kidney Dis* 1998; **32**: S184–99.

63. Derfler K, Kletter K, Balcke P, Heinz G, Dudczak R. Predictive value of thallium-201-dipyridamole myocardial stress scintigraphy in chronic hemodialysis patients and transplant recipients. *Clin Nephrol* 1991; **36**: 192–202.

64. Marwick TH, Steinmuller DR, Underwood DA, *et al*. Ineffectiveness of dipyridamole SPECT thallium imaging as a screening technique for coronary artery disease in patients with end-stage renal failure. *Transplantation* 1990; **49**: 100–3.

65. Boudreau RJ, Strony JT, duCret RO, *et al*. Perfusion thallium imaging of type I diabetes patients with end stage renal disease: comparison of oral and intravenous dipyridamole administration. *Radiology* 1990; **175**: 103–5.

66. de Lemos JA, Hillis LD. Diagnosis and management of coronary artery disease in patients with end-stage renal disease on hemodialysis. *J Am Soc Nephrol* 1996; **7**: 2044–54.

67. Tepel M, van der Giet M, Schwarzfeld C, *et al*. Prevention of radiographic-contrast-agent-induced reductions in renal function by acetylcysteine. *N Engl J Med* 2000; **343**: 180–4.

68. Solomon R, Werner C, Mann D, *et al*. Effects of saline, mannitol, and furosemide to prevent acute decreases in renal function induced by radiocontrast agents. *N Engl J Med* 1994; **331**: 1416–20.

69. Jaeger JQ, Mehta RL. Assessment of dry weight in hemodialysis: an overview. *J Am Soc Nephrol* 1999; **10**: 392–403.

70. Bloembergen WE, Port FK, Mauger EA, Wolfe RA. A comparison of mortality between patients treated with hemodialysis and peritoneal dialysis. *J Am Soc Nephrol* 1995; **6**: 177–83.

71. Churchill DN, Thorpe KE, Vonesh EF, Keshaviah PR. Lower probablility of patient survival with continuous peritoneal dialysis in the United States compared with Canada. *J Am Soc Nephrol* 1997; **8**: 965–71.

72. Vonesh EF, Moran J. Mortality in end-stage renal disease: a reassessment of differences between patients treated with hemodialysis and peritoneal dialysis. *J Am Soc Nephrol* 1999; **10**: 354–65.

73. Rostand SG, Kirk KA, Rutsky EA, Pacifico AD. Results of coronary artery bypass grafting in end-stage renal disease. *Am J Kidney Dis* 1988; **12**: 266–70.

74. Opsahl JA, Husebye DG, Helseth HK, Collins AJ. Coronary artery bypass surgery in patients on maintenance dialysis: long-term survival. *Am J Kidney Dis* 1988; **12**: 271–4.

75. Samuels LE, Sharma S, Morris RJ, *et al*. Coronary artery bypass grafting in patients with chronic renal failure: a reappraisal. *J Cardiac Surg* 1996; **11**: 128–33.

76. Rinehart AL, Herzog CA, Collins AJ, *et al*. A comparison of coronary angioplasty and coronary artery bypass grafting outcomes in chronic dialysis patients. *Am J Kidney Dis* 1995; **25**: 281–90.

77. Owen CH, Cummings RG, Sell TL, *et al*. Coronary artery bypass grafting in patients with dialysis-dependent renal failure. *Ann Thorac Surg* 1994; **58**: 1729–33.

78. Thadhani R, Pascual M, Bonventre JV. Acute renal failure. *N Engl J Med* 1996; **334**: 1448–60.

79. Springer TA. Traffic signals for lymphocyte recirculation and leukocyte emigration: the multistep paradigm. *Cell* 1994; **76**: 301–14.

80. Klausner JM, Paerson IS, Goldman G, *et al*. Postischemic renal injury is mediated by neutrophils and leukotrienes. *Am J Physiol* 1989; **256**: F794–802.

81. Brezis M, Heyman SN, Dinour D, *et al*. Role of nitric oxide in renal medullary oxygenation: studies in isolated and intact rat kidneys. *J Clin Invest* 1991; **88**: 390–5.

82. Vetterlein F, Pethö A, Schmidt G. Distribution of capillary blood flow in rat kidney during postischemic renal failure. *Am J Physiol* 1986; **251**: H510–19.

83. Luria MH, Knoke JD, Margolis RM, *et al*. Acute myocardial infarction: prognosis after recovery. *Ann Intern Med* 1976; **85**: 561–5.

84. Hillege H, Girbes A, de Kam P, *et al*. Renal function, neurohormonal activation, and survival in patients with chronic renal failure. *Circulation* 2000; **102**: 203–10.

85. Dzau VJ, Packer M, Lilly LS, *et al*. Prostaglandins in severe congestive heart failure. *N Engl J Med* 1984; **310**: 347–52.

86. Levy EM, Viscoli CM, Horwitz RI. The effect of acute renal failure on mortality. A cohort analysis. *JAMA* 1996; **275**: 1489–94.

87. Brezis M, Rosen S. Hypoxia of the renal medulla – its implications for disease. *N Engl J Med* 1995; **332**: 647–55.

88. Anderson RJ, Linas SL, Berns AS, *et al.* Nonoliguric acute renal failure. *N Engl J Med* 1977; **296**: 1134–8.

89. Fliser D, Schröter M, Neubeck M, Ritz E. Coadministration of thiazides increases the efficacy of loop diuretics even in patients with advanced renal failure. *Kidney Int* 1994; **46**: 482–8.

90. Elllison DH. The physiologic basis of diuretic synergism: its role in treating diuretic resistance. *Ann Intern Med* 1991; **114**: 886–94.

91. Chertow GM, Sayegh MH, Allgren RL, Lazarus JM. Is the administration of dopamine associated with adverse or favorable outcomes in acute renal failure? *Am J Med* 1996; **101**: 49–53.

92. Stacpoole PW. Lactic acidosis: the case against bicarbonate therapy. *Ann Intern Med* 1986; **105**: 276–9.

93. Packer M, Lee WH, Medina N, *et al.* Functional renal insufficiency during long-term therapy with captopril and enalapril in severe chronic heart failure. *Ann Intern Med* 1987; **106**: 346–54.

94. Packer M, Lee WH, Medinca N, Yushak M. Influence of renal function on the hemodynamic and clinical responses to long-term captopril therapy in severe chronic heart failure. *Ann Intern Med* 1986; **104**: 147–54.

95. Badr KF, Ichikawa I. Prerenal failure: a deleterious shift from renal compensation to decompensation. *N Engl J Med* 1988; **319**: 623–9.

96. Ronco C. Continuous renal replacement therapies for the treatment of acute renal failure in intensive care patients. *Clin Nephrol* 1993; **40**: 187–98.

97. Mehta RL. Modalities of dialysis for acute renal failure. *Semin Dialysis* 1996; **9**: 469–75.

98. Clark WR, Mueller BA, Alaka KJ, Macias WL. A comparison of metabolic control by continuous and intermittent therapies in acute renal failure. *J Am Soc Nephrol* 1994; **4**: 1413–20.

99. Goldfarb S, Golper TA. Proinflammatory cytokines and hemofiltration membranes. *J Am Soc Nephrol* 1994; **5**: 228–32.

100. von Bommel EF, Hess CJ, Jutte NH, Zietse R, *et al.* Impact of continuous hemofiltration on cytokines and cytokine inhibitors in oliguric patients suffering from systemic inflammatory response syndrome. *Renal Failure* 1997; **19**: 443–54.

101. Boaz M, Smetana S, Weinstein T, *et al.* Secondary prevention with antioxidants of cardiovascular disease (SPACE): randomised placebo-controlled trial. *Lancet* 2000; **356**: 1213–18.

102. Bostom AG, Lathrop L. Hyperhomocysteinemia in end-stage renal disease: prevalence, etiology, and potential relationship to arteriosclerotic outcomes. *Kidney Int* 1997; **52**: 10–20.

103. Bloembergen WE, Hakim RM, Stannard DC, *et al.* Relationship of dialysis membrane and cause-specific mortality. *Am J Kidney Dis* 1999; **33**: 1–10.

104. Kelly KJ, Williams WW Jr, Colvin RB, Bonventre JV. Antibody to intercellular adhesion molecule 1 protects the kidney against ischemic injury. *Proc Natl Acad Sci USA* 1994; **91**: 812–16.

105. Allgren RL, Marbury TC, Rahman SN, *et al.* Anaritide in acute tubular necrosis. *N Engl J Med* 1997; **336**: 828–34.

106. Hammerman MR, Miller SB. The role of growth factors in preventing acute renal failure. *Semin Dialysis* 1996; **9**: 464–8.

107. Hammerman MR. Potential role of growth factors in the prophylaxis and treatment of acute renal failure. *Kidney Int* 1998; **53**: S19–22.

108. Levin ER. Endothelins. *N Engl J Med* 1995; **333**: 356–63.

109. Singer I, Epstein M. Potential of dopamine A-1 agonists in the management of acute renal failure. *Am J Kidney Dis* 1998; **31**: 743–55.

110. Schiffl H, Lang SM, König A, *et al.* Biocompatible membranes in acute renal failure: prospective case-controlled study. *Lancet* 1994; **344**: 570–2.

111. Hakim RM, Wingard RL, Parker RA. Effect of the dialysis membrane in the treatment of patients with acute renal failure. *N Engl J Med* 1994; **331**: 1338–42.

General cardiology

13

The cardiovascular patient: initial evaluation

JOSEPH S ALPERT AND JOHN A PARASKOS

The key element to obtaining an accurate diagnosis and initiating appropriate therapy is a thorough and carefully performed history and physical examination. Non-invasive and invasive testing are complementary to the history and physical examination, but can never substitute for it. This chapter reviews the essential features of the cardiovascular history and physical examination. Additional advice is given concerning clinical judgment, cost–benefit strategies, and the physician–patient relationship.

CARDIOVASCULAR HISTORY

The history is the most important diagnostic tool. A correct diagnosis can be made in more than 50 per cent of patients after a careful history.[1] The physician should consider both the pathophysiologic disturbance producing the symptoms and the effect these symptoms have on the patient's quality of life. When asking about chest pain, for example, determine the specific quality, frequency, duration, and location of the pain, as well as precipitating factors related to it (e.g. inspiration, positional changes, exertion, or emotional upset). A family history of heart disease, hypertension, diabetes mellitus, sudden death, rheumatic fever, congenital heart lesions, or lipid disorder suggests hereditary predisposition to cardiovascular disease.

The physician should estimate the level of functional disability resulting from cardiac illness. Factors to consider include difficulty in carrying out the tasks of daily living. The level of disability is often expressed in terms of the traditional New York Heart Association Functional Classification, which includes four classes of functional ability/disability[2] (*see* Table 13.1). Newer, more precise classification systems have been developed.[3,4] One such system divides functional class into

Table 13.1 *The New York Heart Association functional classification of heart disease*

Class	Cardiac status	Prognosis
I	Uncompromised	Good
II	Slightly compromised	Good with therapy
III	Moderately compromised	Fair with therapy
IV	Severely compromised	Guarded with therapy

four levels that relate to specific activities and metabolic equivalents (METs) (*see* Table 13.2). Very specific functional status can be obtained by measuring total body oxygen consumption (VO_2) at the peak obtainable exercise level.[5]

SPECIFIC CARDIOVASCULAR SYMPTOMS

Dyspnea

Dyspnea is shortness of breath out of proportion to the level of exertion. The most common causes of dyspnea are left ventricular failure, mitral valve disease, and acute or chronic pulmonary disease, such as chronic obstruc-

Table 13.2 *A functional classification of heart disease.[a] (Adapted from Goldman L, et al. Comparative reproducibility and validity of systems for assessing cardiovascular functional class: advantages of a new specific activity scale. Circulation 1981; **64**: 1227).*

Class	Minutes on treadmill[b]	Specific activity	Metabolic equivalent[c]
I	> 6	Carrying 24 lb object up eight steps	10
		Walking 5 miles	9
		Carrying 80 lb object	8
		Shoveling snow, spading dirt	7
II	3–6	Walking 4 miles/hour	5–6
		Raking, weeding the garden	5–6
		Sexual intercourse	5.0–5.5
		Carrying anything up eight steps	5.0–5.5
III	1–3	Stripping and making bed	4–5
		Pushing power lawn mower	4
		Showering without stopping	3.6–4.2
		Walking 2.5 miles	3.0–3.5
		Dressing without stopping	2.0–2.3
IV	< 1	None of the above	< 2

[a] Based on the patient's ability to meet metabolic demands of selected specific activities.
[b] Bruce protocol.
[c] One metabolic equivalent (MET) represents the energy expended in burning 3.5 mL O_2/kg per minute.

tive pulmonary disease or asthma.[6] Other common causes of dyspnea include pulmonary embolism, interstitial lung disease, and anxiety. Patients with cardiac dyspnea often complain of associated orthopnea or paroxysmal nocturnal dyspnea. It may be difficult to decide whether dyspnea is secondary to heart or to lung disease. Indeed, many patients may have coexisting heart and lung disease, such as chronic obstructive pulmonary disease and coronary artery disease. Information from the patient's history (e.g. previous myocardial infarction or rheumatic fever), physical examination, or laboratory results (e.g. findings on the chest x-ray indicative of severe chronic lung disease) help establish the etiology of dyspnea.[7]

Chest discomfort

Coronary artery disease is the most common serious disease that causes chest discomfort. Decisions about diagnostic testing and patient management depend on estimations of the probability that a patient's chest discomfort is caused by ischemic heart disease. Several useful algorithms are available.[8] For any patient with chest discomfort, the physician should determine the likelihood that the patient is having angina pectoris. Determining factors are central location; radiation to arms, neck, or jaw; and a squeezing pressure character. If the discomfort is anginal and is brought on by a predictable amount of exertion, relieved by rest or nitroglycerin, and severe enough to cause the patient to cease activity, the diagnosis is probably exertional angina. If the pain occurs spontaneously, is less predictably

relieved by rest or nitroglycerin, and is milder, the patient may have atypical angina. If the pain is not anginal, the patient has chest pain not of cardiac origin.[9]

Patients with angina pectoris often complain of a vague, oppressive discomfort in the center of the chest resembling the discomfort associated with indigestion. Unlike indigestion, however, angina pectoris comes with exertion and is relieved by rest. The discomfort of myocardial infarction is usually similar to that associated with angina pectoris, although it is generally more severe and often accompanied by dyspnea, nausea, or diaphoresis. Chest pain associated with pulmonary disorders, such as pneumonia and pulmonary embolism, is usually pleuritic.

Chest wall pain is often confused with angina pectoris. Differences in location, duration, and quality often differentiate chest wall pain from angina pectoris. Pain originating from the distal esophagus (esophageal reflux or spasm) can be similar to the discomfort of angina pectoris. Eating rather than exertion is often the cause of distal esophageal pain. Anxiety, the hyperventilation syndrome, or both are often associated with chest pain that may mimic angina pectoris, although the pain caused by anxiety or hyperventilation is usually sharp and fleeting, or very prolonged and highly localized.

Palpitations

The sensation of an irregular heartbeat is termed palpitation. At times, the patient senses an irregularity in cardiac rhythm (e.g. extrasystoles), and at other times, the patient senses rapid forceful cardiac activity (e.g.

supraventricular tachycardia). Patients may also report that their heart is skipping, fluttering, pounding, or racing.

It is useful to have the patient describe the regularity or irregularity and the approximate rate of the palpitation. Associated light-headedness or syncope should be ascertained. Paroxysmal supraventricular dysrhythmias (e.g. atrial fibrillation) are usually described as sudden in onset and termination. Sinus tachycardia is more gradual in onset and termination. Patients may not sense palpitation during ventricular tachycardia. Rather, they may experience dyspnea, syncope, or severe fatigue. The palpitations sensed during anxiety states may be caused by the patient's heightened awareness of cardiac activity. Normal sinus rhythm or sinus tachycardia is usually present. A routine electrocardiogram or additional testing (i.e. electrocardiographic ambulatory monitoring or exercise testing) may be indicated.

Syncope

Syncope is usually the result of a cardiac or neurologic condition,[10] including seizure disorders, vasodepressor syncope (the simple faint), and cardiac dysrhythmias, such as ventricular tachycardia or complete heart block. Historical points that favor a cardiac origin for syncope include sudden onset without warning, sensation of rapid heart action before loss of consciousness, and lack of an aura or seizure activity, although seizures may occur during dysrhythmias as a result of decreased cerebral perfusion.

Effort syncope occurs in patients with valvular aortic stenosis. Patients with left ventricular outflow obstruction (i.e. hypertrophic cardiomyopathy with subaortic stenosis) may also experience effort syncope. Vasodepressor syncope usually occurs when the patient is physically or emotionally uncomfortable. Associated autonomic nervous symptoms, such as sweating, nausea, and yawning, are often present.

Cough

Cough is more often pulmonary than cardiac in origin (e.g. asthma or pneumonia). However, cough may be a manifestation of pulmonary vascular congestion secondary to left ventricular failure or mitral stenosis. In this setting, cough may be part of the symptom complex of paroxysmal nocturnal dyspnea. Cough secondary to pulmonary vascular congestion is often non-productive. When pulmonary vascular congestion is severe and incipient pulmonary edema develops, small amounts of foamy white sputum may be produced. Occasionally, patients with cardiac disease experience hemoptysis during coughing. Hemoptysis is usually the result of pulmonary disease, such as bronchiectasis or tumor. Cardiovascular etiologies for hemoptysis include pul-

monary embolism, mitral stenosis, and, occasionally, left ventricular failure. Approximately 10 per cent of patients treated with angiotensin-converting enzyme (ACE) inhibitors develop a recurrent, non-productive cough that may prevent them from sleeping.

Peripheral edema

Peripheral edema is often a late finding in patients with left ventricular failure but is more often the result of venous insufficiency. Peripheral edema normally results from right ventricular failure. Elevated jugular venous pressure should be sought on physical examination. Other cardiac causes of peripheral edema include constrictive pericarditis and primary right ventricular failure secondary to pulmonary arterial hypertension. Non-cardiovascular diseases that cause peripheral edema include chronic renal failure, profound hypoalbuminemia, and Cushing's disease.

Cyanosis and clubbing

A level of 5 g/dL or more of unsaturated hemoglobin in the arterial circulation will usually lead to cyanosis. Cyanosis is said to be peripheral (acrocyanosis) when it is seen only in the extremities. Peripheral cyanosis is the result of decreased blood flow to the skin secondary to vasoconstriction. Common causes of peripheral cyanosis include shock and exposure to cold. Peripheral cyanosis is transient and not associated with clubbing of the fingernails.

Central cyanosis involves the entire body and is the result of abnormal saturation of venous blood during its pulmonary transit or right-to-left cardiac shunts. With chronic central cyanosis, fingers and toes are often clubbed. Clubbing may also develop with thoracic tumors or chronic inflammation, and may also be familial and not associated with decreased arterial oxygen saturation.

PHYSICAL EXAMINATION OF THE HEART

Careful physical examination of the heart provides important information about the cardiovascular system. Together with a thorough history, the physical examination provides the initial database and guides further diagnostic tests and therapeutic maneuvers. In many conditions, careful physical examination can yield information as important as that obtained by more complex and costly procedures.

It is also important to recognize the complex interplay between cardiac disease and other systemic illnesses or conditions. A common mistake made by the non-cardiologist is ignoring the cardiac manifestations of a systemic disease process. Conversely, the cardiologist may fail to recognize the systemic nature of a cardiac disease or the effects of cardiac disease on other organ systems. For these reasons every patient suspected of having cardiac abnormalities must be given a thorough physical examination.

OBSERVATIONS, PALPATION, AND PERCUSSION

Jugular venous pulse

Two types of information are obtained from the jugular venous pulse (JVP): the quality of the wave form and the central venous pressure (CVP). The JVP is best observed in the right internal jugular vein. With normal CVP, the JVP is assessed with the patient's trunk raised approximately 30 degrees. With elevated CVP, the patient's trunk must be raised higher, sometimes to as much as 90 degrees. The JVP is accentuated by turning the patient's head away from the examiner and shining a flashlight obliquely across the skin overlying the vein.

Two waves per heartbeat are generally visible in the JVP: the A wave and the V wave. The A wave appears as a brief 'flicker' and represents increased venous pressure resulting from atrial contraction. The V wave is a longer surge that follows the A wave and represents increased venous pressure transmitted during ventricular contraction. The drop in pressure following the A wave is called the X descent, and the fall in pressure after the V wave is denoted as the Y descent. The JVP waves should be timed with simultaneous palpation of the carotid artery. The A wave immediately precedes the carotid pulse; the V wave follows the pulse.

Occasionally, difficulty may be experienced in differentiating venous and arterial pulsations in the neck. Several observations and findings may be helpful: (1) the arterial pulse is more localized and will forcefully strike examining fingers, whereas palpation will often obliterate a venous pulse; (2) compression of the base of the neck will not alter arterial pulses but will obliterate the venous ones; and (3) arterial pulses do not change with patient position while venous pulses will often disappear when the patient assumes an upright posture (either sitting upright or standing). The diagnosis of a variety of pathologic states is assisted by observation of abnormalities in the JVP wave forms (Table 13.3).

Central venous pressure (CVP) can be estimated by observing the vertical distance from the top of the V wave to the right atrium. In the individual at 30° with normal CVP, the V wave rises no more than 1–2 cm above the sternal angle. When the V wave rises to more than halfway to the angle of the jaw in a patient who is not recumbent, elevated CVP is present. In some pathologic conditions (e.g. cardiac tamponade, constrictive pericarditis), CVP may be so high that A and V waves are above the angle of the jaw. In this setting exaggerated X and Y descents may suggest the diagnosis. As a rule of thumb, for a patient sitting upright, a JVP visible at the sternal angle represents a CVP of approximately 10 mm Hg.

During inspiration, the height of the JVP typically declines (although amplitude of the X and Y descents will increase). In certain pathologic conditions, such as chronic constrictive pericarditis and occasionally tricuspid stenosis, congestive heart failure, right ventricular dysfunction, or infarction, the JVP either fails to drop or actually increases with inspiration. This important clinical finding is known as Kussmaul's venous sign.

Arterial pressure pulse

The central arterial pressure pulse is characterized by a rapid rise to a rounded peak with a less rapid decline. Information about the adequacy of ventricular contraction and possible obstruction of the left ventricular outflow tract may be assessed by palpation of the carotid

Table 13.3 *Abnormal jugular venous pulsations*

Finding	Comment/significance
Markedly raised central venous pressure, accentuated X and Y descents	? Cardiac tamponade ? Constrictive pericarditis ? Endocardial fibroelastosis ? Severe right-heart failure
Large A waves	? Pulmonary valvular stenosis ? Hypertension ? Various arrhythmias where atria contract against closed AV valve (e.g. junctional rhythm, AV dissociation)
Absent A wave	Atrial fibrillation
Large V wave	Tricuspid regurgitation

artery. By the time the pulse wave is transmitted to peripheral arteries, much of this initial information is lost.

A variety of pathologic conditions alters the characteristics of the carotid pulse. These conditions, and the corresponding modifications of the carotid pulse, are listed in Table 13.4. In patients with hypertension, simultaneous palpation of radial and femoral arterial pulses helps to rule out coarctation of the aorta.

Precordial palpation

Information concerning the location and quality of the left ventricular impulse is available through precordial palpation. In addition, loud murmurs are usually associated with a palpable thrill.

Palpation is best accomplished using the fingertips, with the patient either supine or in the left lateral decubitus position. Simultaneous auscultation can aid in the timing of events. A list of abnormalities detected by precordial palpation and their significance is found in Table 13.5.

Auscultation

The first heart sound (S1) occurs at the time of closure of the mitral and tricuspid valves. It is probably generated by sudden deceleration of blood caused by the closure of the valves. S1 is frequently split (with mitral closure preceding tricuspid). In some, the split in S1 can be appreciated, but it is of little clinical relevance. More important is variation in intensity of the first sound. S1

Table 13.4 *Abnormalities in the carotid pulse*

Finding	Comment/significance
Pulsus bisferiens (two systolic peaks)	Aortic regurgitation and hypertrophic obstructive cardiomyopathy
Pulsus parvus (small, weak pulse)	Any condition causing diminished left ventricular stroke volume or narrow pulse pressure (hypovolemia, mitral/aortic valve stenosis, restrictive pericarditis, recent myocardial infarction); may also be caused by atherosclerosis of the carotid artery or diseases of the aortic arch
Pulsus tardus (delayed systolic peak of pulse)	Aortic outflow obstruction, e.g. aortic stenosis
Pulsus paradoxus (larger than normal decrease in systolic arterial pressure during inspiration)	Pericardial tamponade, airway obstruction, superior vena caval obstruction; also asthma or chronic obstructive pulmonary disease
Pulsus alternans (consistent alternation in pulse pressure amplitude despite regular rhythm)	Severe left ventricular decompensation for any reason following paroxysmal tachycardia

Table 13.5 *Abnormalities in precordial palpation*

Finding	Comment/significance
Left ventricular thrust	Left ventricular hypertrophy
Displacement of left ventricular pulse downward and to the left	Left ventricular dilatation; left ventricular failure; volume overload (aortic regurgitation or decompensated mitral regurgitation)
Presystolic impulse	Pressure overloaded states (hypertension, aortic stenosis)
Double systolic impulse	Hypertrophic obstructive cardiomyopathy
Systolic bulge (dyskinetic impulse)	Coronary artery disease, recent myocardial infarction (most commonly felt above and medial to the point of maximal impulse)
Parasternal lift	Mitral regurgitation (occurs after the left ventricular apical impulse); right ventricular dilatation (mitral stenosis, pulmonary embolism)
Thrills	Aortic stenosis, pulmonic stenosis; ventricular septal defect, severe mitral regurgitation

varies with the P–R interval of the electrocardiogram (ECG). The shorter the P–R interval, the louder the S1. The best example of S1 variation with P–R interval occurs in complete heart block, in which atrial and ventricular contractions are dissociated.

S1 may be loud and 'snapping' in quality in mitral stenosis, indicating both that the valve is pliable and that it remains wide open at the beginning of isovolumic contraction, closing during the rapid rise of left ventricular pressure. Conversely, a diminished or absent S1 in mitral stenosis suggests a rigidly calcified valve that cannot 'snap' shut.

Other situations in which S1 may be diminished include mitral regurgitation, slow heart rates (long P–R interval), poor sound conduction through the chest wall, and a slow rise of left ventricular pressure. A summary of clinical information derived from variations in S1 is found in Table 13.6.

Table 13.6 *Abnormalities of S1*

Finding	Comment/significance
Loud S1	Short P–R interval
Loud 'snapping' S1	Mitral stenosis (pliable valve)
Variation in intensity of S1	Complete heart block
Diminished intensity of S1	Mitral regurgitation, slow heart rate (long P–R interval), poor conduction of sound through chest wall, slow rise of left ventricular pressure, mitral stenosis (rigidly calcific valve), severe or acute aortic regurgitation

In contrast to S1, in which splitting is less important than changes in intensity, the second heart sound (S2) reveals variations in both splitting and intensity that provide important clinical information. S2 occurs at the time of closure of the aortic and pulmonic valves. In normal circumstances, aortic closure precedes pulmonic closure (A2 followed by P2). Under normal circumstances, the split in S2 is maximal at the end of inspiration and minimal at the end of expiration. This phenomenon reflects an underlying movement of P2 with respect to a relatively constant A2. During inspiration, right ventricular filling increases and P2 is delayed, causing the widely split S2. During expiration, less right ventricular filling occurs and P2 moves towards A2, causing a diminished split in S2. This 'normal splitting' of S2 is invariably present in individuals under 30 years of age, provided heart rates are not fast. It is best appreciated over the 'pulmonic area' and can be heard with either the bell or the diaphragm.

The most common abnormality of S2 is failure of splitting to close at the end of expiration. This 'persistent splitting' occurs for one of these two reasons: P2 is delayed or A2 is early. A split of S2 on expiration may also represent a normal variant. In the latter setting, however, some difference in the degree of splitting should occur between inspiration and expiration.

Persistent splitting of S2 due to delayed P2 is found in four clinical settings: (1) acute right-heart pressure overload (e.g. pulmonary embolism); (2) right bundle branch block; (3) atrial septal defect (ASD); and (4) pulmonic stenosis. In ASD, the splitting usually remains unchanged in inspiration and expiration and is referred to as 'fixed splitting'.

Paradoxical splitting of S2 is said to be present when S2 splits on expiration and closes on inspiration. While persistent splitting is caused by delay in normal closure of the pulmonic valve, paradoxical splitting is most often caused by delayed closure of the aortic valve. This important clinical sign never occurs in the absence of cardiac disease. The most common states in which paradoxical splitting is encountered are aortic stenosis and left bundle branch block. Paradoxical splitting takes place in about 25 per cent of individuals with these conditions.

Paradoxical splitting may occur in patients with coronary artery disease or hypertension or both. In these individuals a closely split S2 may be observed to close to a single sound at mid-inspiration. A similar finding is often made in early stages of aortic stenosis or in incomplete left bundle branch block. Alterations in the intensity of S2 can also yield important clinical information. A2 is frequently decreased in aortic stenosis. The presence of a normal A2 when aortic stenosis is clinically suspected raises the question of outflow obstruction at a site other than the valve. P2 may be augmented in pulmonary hypertension and diminished in pulmonic stenosis. Finally, P2 may appear unusually loud in thin-chested individuals without cardiac disease. A summary of clinical information derived from alterations in S2 is found in Table 13.7.

The third heart sound (S3, or ventricular gallop) is low pitched and best heard at the apex with the stethoscope bell. The S3 is probably the result of rapid filling and stretching of an abnormal left ventricle. Its cadence can be approximated by the word 'luckily' in which the S3 is represented by the 'ly'. An S3 may be heard in any condition resulting in rapid ventricular filling. It is frequently an early sign of left ventricular failure. Third heart sounds may also be present in ASD, mitral or aortic insufficiency, ventricular septal defect, and patent ductus arteriosus. An S3 can also be a normal variant, particularly in young adults. A loud, early diastolic sound is often heard in constrictive pericarditis. This 'pericardial knock' is considered to be an early louder sound than the usual S3.

The fourth heart sound (S4, atrial gallop, presystolic

Table 13.7 *Abnormalities of S2*

Finding	Comment/significance
Abnormalities in timing	
Persistent splitting	Acute right-heart overload (e.g. pulmonary embolism)
	Right bundle branch block
	Atrial septal defect (often widely split and fixed)
	Pulmonic stenosis
Paradoxical splitting	Aortic stenosis
	Left bundle branch block
Closely split with closure at mid-inspiration (variant of paradoxical splitting)	Coronary artery disease
	Hypertension
Abnormalities in intensity	
Increased A2	Hypertension
	Aortic dilatation
Increased P2	Pulmonary hypertension
	Normal finding in thin-chested individual
Decreased A2	Aortic stenosis
Decreased P2	Pulmonic stenosis

gallop) is also the result of altered ventricular compliance. Its cadence has been likened to the word 'appendix' with the S4 represented by the initial soft 'a'. It is a low-pitched sound, best heard with the stethoscope bell. It is loudest at the apex and may be accentuated by placing the patient in the left lateral decubitus position. The presence of an S4 implies effective atrial contraction; it is never heard in atrial fibrillation. An S4 may be heard in any condition causing reduced ventricular compliance: aortic stenosis, systemic or pulmonary hypertension, coronary artery disease, hypertrophic cardiomyopathy, acute mitral regurgitation, and myocardial infarction.

SNAPS, CLICKS, AND OTHER ADVENTITIOUS SOUNDS

An opening snap of the mitral valve is frequently heard in mitral stenosis. The opening snap (OS) arises from the stiff mitral valve's snapping toward the left ventricle in early diastole. The opening snap is best heard in the fourth intercostal space halfway between the apex and the left sternal border. The interval between S2 and the OS is related to the severity of mitral stenosis. The more severe the stenosis, the shorter the S2-OS interval.

Ejection clicks are high-pitched sounds occurring in early systole. They are associated with stenosis of either the aortic or the pulmonic valve, with hypertension or dilatation of either the aorta or the pulmonary artery or both. Aortic clicks are best heard at the apex, while pul-monic clicks are most audible at the left upper sternal border. Pulmonic clicks vary with respiration and are best heard during expiration. Aortic clicks do not vary with respiration.

Mid-systolic clicks often accompanied by a late systolic murmur occur in patients with prolapse of the mitral valve. The clicks may result from sudden tensing of the chordae tendineae or snapping of the prolapsing leaflet. The clicks may be single or multiple, and may occur at any time during systole, although they generally come later than ejection clicks. In contrast to ejection clicks, they are heard best at the lower left sternal border or apex.

MURMURS

Murmurs are extended sounds that are produced by turbulent blood flow. These can be produced by: (1) excessive flow through normal valves or flow through narrowed, i.e. stenotic valves; (2) reguritant flow through incompetent valves; (3) flow through abnormal shunts; (4) normal flow through normal cardiovascular structures, i.e. innocent murmurs. When assessing murmurs the following characteristics need to be noted:

- timing (systolic, diastolic, continuous);
- location of maximal intensity and radiation pattern;
- intensity (Table 13.8);
- pitch and quality;
- response to respiration, position, and other maneuvers.

Table 13.8 *Grading intensity of murmurs*

Grade 1   Soft, barely audible
Grade 2   Soft but easily audible
Grade 3   Medium intensity
Grade 4   Loud intensity
Grade 5   Loud and still audible with rim of stethoscope
Grade 6   Loud and still audible with stethoscope removed
          from skin surface

SYSTOLIC MURMURS

Systolic murmurs are classified according to their time of occurrence, sound quality, and duration. The most fundamental distinction is between systolic ejection murmurs and pansystolic murmurs. Ejection murmurs ordinarily occur in mid-systole. Early and late systolic murmurs also occur and should be distinguished from ejection murmurs. Ejection murmurs begin after S1 and are usually crescendo–decrescendo ('diamond-shaped'), ending before S2. Pansystolic murmurs begin with S1, extend throughout systole, and are characteristically plateau-shaped, i.e. uniform in intensity. Systolic ejection murmurs have been likened to the chug of a steam engine laboring up a hill, while plateau-shaped murmurs have been likened to the high-pitched wail of the engine's whistle (Table 13.9).

Systolic ejection murmurs

Systolic ejection murmurs (SEMs) begin after the semilunar (aortic and pulmonic) valves open at the end of isovolumic systole. Their intensity parallels the amount of blood being ejected through the stenosis, peaking in mid-systole. SEMs arise in the following settings: (1) obstruction to left or right ventricular outflow, as in aortic or pulmonic stenosis; (2) dilatation of the aorta or pulmonary artery distal to the valve; (3) increased rate of ventricular ejection (heart block, fever, anemia, exercise, thyrotoxicosis); and (4) healthy individuals.

Pansystolic murmurs occur when blood flows through a ventricular septal defect, or retrograde through the mitral or tricuspid valve. The even intensity and long duration of these murmurs reflect the large pressure difference across the orifice where the sound originates. The murmur continues as long as pressure in the chamber of origin exceeds that in the recipient chamber.

Early systolic murmurs begin with or shortly after S1 and end by mid-systole. They have been reported in: (1) mitral stenosis probably secondary to coexistent mitral regurgitation; (2) small ventricular septal defects; and (3) individuals without cardiac disease. Late systolic murmurs begin in mid-systole and extend to or through S2. They may be heard in mitral valve prolapse (frequently accompanied by mid-systolic clicks) or coarctation of the aorta.

Systolic murmurs arising from the right side of the heart generally increase with inspiration while those originating on the left side decrease or do not change. Many systolic murmurs are totally innocent (as in pregnant woman, growing children, and individuals with abnormal chest configuration).

Diastolic murmurs

Diastolic murmurs are classified according to their position in diastole as early, mid-, or late. An alternative classification emphasizes etiology: regurgitant murmurs from semilunar insufficiency versus ventricular filling murmurs. Regurgitant murmurs are generally early dias-

Table 13.9 *Systolic murmurs*

Early systolic	Ejection (mid-systolic)	Pansystolic	Late systolic
1. Ventricular septal defect (small)	**Dilatation of vessel** 1. Pulmonary artery dilatation 2. Aortic dilatation	1. Ventricular septal defect 2. Mitral regurgitation 3. Tricuspid regurgitation	1. Mitral valve prolapse 2. Coarctation of the aorta
	Stenosis of value 1. Pulmonic stenosis 2. Aortic stenosis		
	Increased flow across valve 1. Heart block 2. Fever 3. Anemia 4. Exercise 5. Thyrotoxicosis 6. Normal		

Table 13.10 *Diastolic murmurs*

Early diastolic	Mid- and late diastolic
1. Pulmonic regurgitation	1. Mitral stenosis
2. Aortic regurgitation	2. Tricuspid stenosis
	2. Atrial myxoma
	4. Mitral regurgitation
	5. Large left-to-right shunt

tolic, whereas ventricular filling murmurs occur in mid- and late diastole (Table 13.10). Early murmurs begin immediately after S2. The most common causes are aortic or pulmonic valve regurgitation. The murmur is usually high pitched and blowing in quality with a decrescendo configuration. The intensity of the murmur reflects the size of the valvular leak, the acoustic properties of the chest, and the pressure difference across the valve. The distinction between pulmonic and aortic regurgitation may be extremely hard to make and may require echocardiography for definitive determination.

Mid- and late diastolic murmurs

Mid- and late diastolic murmurs are produced by forward flow of blood through the atrioventricular (AV) (mitral and tricuspid) valves. They arise from either augmented blood flow or a stenosed valve. As a rule these murmurs are low pitched and rumbling in quality. They do not begin until the valve from which they originate opens (sometimes with an audible snap) and ventricular pressure has fallen below atrial pressure in early diastole. Conditions in which mid- or late diastolic murmurs may arise include: (1) mitral or tricuspid stenosis; (2) left atrial myxoma; (3) mitral regurgitation (increased flow); and (4) large left-to-right shunts (increased flow).

Continuous murmurs

Murmurs are considered continuous when they are audible throughout all phases of the cardiac cycle. They generally arise when a continuous pressure differential allows blood to flow constantly from a high to a low pressure area, as may occur in a variety of congenital defects, most commonly patent ductus arteriosus, anomalous origin of the left coronary artery, or coronary arteriovenous fistula. Other conditions that may cause continuous murmurs include ruptured aneurysm of a sinus of Valsalva, proximal coronary artery stenosis, and pulmonary artery branch stenosis.

An analogous phenomenon is the venous hum. This continuous, low-pitched murmur results from increased velocity of venous blood flow. It is an innocent finding, usually heard in the lower anterior portion of the neck. Venous hum is accentuated by deep inspiration in most patients and may be obliterated by the Valsalva maneuver or by pressure on the internal jugular vein.

Physiologic and pharmacologic manipulation of heart sounds and murmurs

Various physiologic and pharmacologic maneuvers are available to accentuate heart sounds and murmurs. A partial listing of these maneuvers, together with their physiologic consequences, is found in Table 13.11. Maneuvers that are useful in the analysis of specific murmurs and heart sounds are listed in Table 13.12. Physiologic and pharmacologic manipulations may help untangle difficult problems in differential diagnosis when normal auscultatory findings are ambiguous.

FRICTION RUBS

Friction rubs occur when two serosal surfaces are inflamed and rub against each other. They can occur in pleural, peritoneal, or pericardial surfaces. In the pericardium, they call attention to pericarditis that may be acute or chronic. Pericarditis may be infectious, neoplastic, or immunologic. Characteristically, there are three components to the rub: early systole, early diastole, and presystole. The sounds are rough and are likened to pieces of leather rubbing against each other. They may become louder with positional changes and may be affected by respiration.

CLINICAL JUDGMENT

The combination of knowledge, experience, and common sense enables the physician to recognize many common illnesses. Of course, the experienced physician is aware of the uncertainty involved in making a diagnosis. There is a small but definite probability that a patient does not have a common illness, but rather a serious and complex disease.

Decisions made in an environment fraught with uncertainty should never be considered as objective and incontrovertible facts. Rather, such decisions should be viewed as probability statements (i.e. the favored horse will probably win the race). New information or further examination of existing data may lead to an alteration in the probability statement.

Another aspect of clinical judgment relates to the manner in which the physician approaches the patient. Biased, intellectually arrogant, or unfeeling attitudes on the part of the physician represent an error in clinical judgment, since such attitudes interfere with data collection and appropriate therapy. Clinical judgment usually requires medical knowledge, some experience, common

Table 13.11 *Manipulation of heart sounds and murmurs*

Maneuver	Physiologic consequence	Comment
Physiologic maneuvers		
Respiration	Inspiration: right-heart filling increased, left-heart filling decreased	Right-heart murmurs increased; left-heart murmurs decreased or unchanged
Rapid changes in position (e.g. elevation of legs, standing, squatting)	Changes in right ventricular filling (RV filling increased by lying, leg elevation, or squatting; venous return decreased by standing)	Gallop sounds, murmurs of pulmonic and aortic stenosis, all increased by lying, leg elevation, or squatting; HOCM murmur increased by standing
Valsalva maneuver	Initially causes sharp rise in blood pressure (phase I), then impairs venous return and blood pressure drops (phase II)	During phase II, murmurs of pulmonic and aortic stenosis and mitral regurgitation diminish while murmurs of HOCM increase
Pharmacologic maneuvers		
Phenylephrine	Raised systemic arterial pressure	Murmur of aortic regurgitation and mitral regurgitation increased
Isoproterenol	Increased myocardial contraction	Murmur of HOCM increased
Amyl nitrite	Potent vasodilator; decreased systolic pressure; reflex increase in heart rate	Murmurs of aortic and mitral regurgitation decreased; all ejection murmurs increased; VSD murmur decreased

RV = right ventricular; HOCM = hypertrophic obstructive cardiomyopathy; VSD = ventricular septal defect.

sense, and an awareness of one's own biases. It may also require moral reasoning. Sheehan and his colleagues have been studying determinants of good physician performance. They have found that a highly developed capacity for moral reasoning correlates more strongly with physician performance than do examinations of factual knowledge.[11]

Despite the fact that most physicians like to believe that they are dispassionate and objective with respect to their clinical judgment, it must be acknowledged that we are all prone to subjective forces. Value judgments, prejudices, likes and dislikes all influence clinical judgment at some level. The most one can hope for is to be aware of subjective influences and to attempt to recognize when they are influencing the decision-making process.

Cost–benefit and the differential diagnosis

Another factor that should be considered in the evaluation of a patient's presenting complaint is the ratio of cost to benefit. Cost in this context refers both to economic cost and to pain and suffering. Both entities extract something from the patient: money or physical or psychologic distress. The physician needs to know the potential economic or personal cost of a particular diagnostic test and the likelihood that the test will be definitive in making the diagnosis or changing the treatment. Ideally, an inexpensive and painless test is best; however, the test chosen will depend on risk–benefit as well as cost and discomfort.

The physician should consider whether the results of a given test will alter the patient's therapy or comfort. A test that is not associated with a reasonable likelihood of altering either therapy or patient comfort should not be performed on a patient. It should be stressed that patient comfort has both physical and psychologic or emotional components. Therefore, a test that does not alter therapy, but that confirms a rather benign diagnostic entity and eliminates a frightening one is certainly worth performing.

Another rule of clinical judgment is that it is foolish and wasteful to order two tests that produce the same information. If the physician has obtained an echocardiogram, which allows accurate evaluation of ventricular function, a radionuclide ventriculogram is not needed since the latter test yields information similar to that derived from the echocardiogram. The two tests are (in this instance but not always) redundant. The rational work-up is like a carefully reasoned argument in a debate: it proceeds logically from one point to the next without redundancy or confusion.

Bedside manner

Bedside manner is a term used much more frequently in the first half of the 20th century than the second half. This is because, in the past, bedside manner was all the physician had to offer in many illnesses. In the current high-technology era, more tangible treatment is available, and one rarely hears about bedside manner.

Table 13.12 *Maneuvers for analysis of heart sounds and murmurs. (Adapted from Dohan MC, Criscitiello MG. Physiological and pharmacological manipulations of heart sounds and murmurs.* Mod Concepts Cardiovasc Dis *1970; 39: 121.)*

Condition	Maneuver
Aortic stenosis	Valvular: mid-systolic murmur louder with sudden squatting, leg raising, or amyl nitrite; fades during Valsalva maneuver Hypertropic subvalvular: systolic murmur louder with sitting or squatting, during Valsalva maneuver, or with amyl nitrite; softens with sudden squatting or leg elevation
Aortic regurgitation	Blowing diastolic murmur increases with sudden squatting, fades with amyl nitrite Austin Flint murmur fades with amyl nitrite
Mitral stenosis	Diastolic murmur made louder with tachycardia, exercise, left lateral position, coughing, or amyl nitrite
Mitral regurgitation	Rheumatic systolic murmur louder with sudden squatting, softer with amyl nitrite Mid- to late systolic mitral valve prolapse: late systolic murmur becomes mid- or holosystolic with upright position, with amyl nitrite, and during Valsalva maneuver; mid-systolic click occurs earlier with these maneuvers; murmur fades with lying flat
Pulmonic stenosis	Mid-systolic murmur increases with amyl nitrite, except with marked right ventricular hypertrophy; also may increase with first few beats after Valsalva release
Pulmonic regurgitation	Congenital: early or mid-diastolic murmur (harsh, low-pitched) increases on inspiration and with amyl nitrite Pulmonary hypertensive: high-frequency early diastolic blowing murmur not influenced by respiration; inconstant response to amyl nitrite
Tricuspid stenosis	Mid-diastolic and presystolic murmurs increase during inspiration and with amyl nitrite
Tricuspid regurgitation	Systolic murmur increases during inspiration and with amyl nitrite
Ventricular septal defect	Small defect without pulmonary hypertension: murmur fades with amyl nitrite Large defect with hyperkinetic pulmonary hypertension: murmur louder with amyl nitrite Large defect with severe pulmonary vascular disease: little change with above agents
Gallop rhythm	Ventricular filling sounds: ventricular gallop and atrial gallop are accentuated by lying flat with passive leg raising; decreased by sitting or standing; right-sided gallop sounds usually increased during inspiration, left-sided during expiration Summation gallop may separate into ventricular gallop (S3) and atrial gallop (S4) sounds when heart rate slowed by carotid sinus massage

However, there are some things the physician can do to make his or her visit to the bedside more respectful and more pleasant for the patient. Examples include knocking on the door if it is shut, pulling the curtain or closing the door before beginning an examination, giving a patient time if she or he is in the bathroom at that moment, and apologizing if the visit is at mealtime. All of us can think of other courtesies. In addition, it is nice to sit down on the bed or in a chair, rather than stand at the foot of the bed. Before sitting down on the bed, remember to ask for the patient's permission. It has been shown that patients report more time spent by a physician when she or he sits down, even if the actual time is the same. It is important to greet the patient, perhaps exchange some small talk, and then try to elicit the patient's concerns before proceeding to one's own. Good bedside manner follows if the physician remembers that he or she is visiting a person who is sick in bed, not just seeing a patient.

The physician–patient relationship is fraught with risk for the patient. The physician is in a position to declare sickness or wellness. She or he is also likely to prescribe discomfort or proscribe enjoyment. The patient, aware of these dangers, often faces the physician with a general sense of anxiety, some specific fears, a general type of hostility directed at the physician role, and a pledged resistance to possible unpleasant recommendations. Any one, let alone all, of these attitudes, can complicate the physician's goal of helping to maintain or restore the patient's health. A combination of kindness and respect is helpful in defusing anxiety, allaying fear, converting hostility into trust, and promoting cooperation.

Empathy

Empathy implies the ability to put oneself into the other person's shoes – to feel as well as to grasp intellectually the other person's plight. Empathy should go beyond particular physician–patient encounters to the general role of patient. No one would go to a physician were it not for illness or fear of illness. This immediately places the patient in a dependent role with respect to the physician. The patient's uneasiness about the role and the situation is present by definition. Physician empathy for the patient role should also be there by definition. As a physician explores the patient's health status, it is important to get a feeling for the situation (i.e. to ascertain the emotional as well as the intellectual meaning to the patient of symptoms and signs). Possible treatment plans must be weighed in light of their feasibility for the patient as well as for the physician. During the encounter, the physician should try to change her or his image from one of healer to one of helper, thereby converting an atmosphere of rank and order to one of teamwork. Once a patient senses empathy from the physician, the patient's fears diminish since she or he knows the physician will act to minimize suffering. The physician has many sick patients to worry about. This makes it difficult, but no less important, to remember that, for any one patient, the problem is all-consuming. It is often in the setting of a prolonged problem where no medical solution is available that the physician's empathy is most sought and yet most difficult to give.

It is easy to rejoice with a patient who is recovering from an illness. It is much more difficult to remain faithful to a patient who is not getting well. The frustration of an impasse, the disillusionment of failure, and the indictment accompanying unmet expectations all tend to cause avoidance on the part of the physician. It is easier to be unavailable, or brief, or cool, than to face frustration. Yet if the victories are the physician's, so are the defeats. Empathetic practice is difficult when one is overcommitted and harassed. A great deal of suffering can be caused by placing this human aspect of practice lower in priority than some of the technical aspects. Conversely, a great deal of good can be done by giving patients and families time and concern and by showing empathy. Often, this involves only listening.

Listening skills are important in several different but related ways. Listening is essential in making the correct diagnosis. Listening may be even more important in helping the physician appreciate the meaning of the symptoms or illness to the patient. At times, just being listened to can be therapeutic for the patient. Finally, the listening process may convert a routine or even unpleasant patient into an interesting or appealing one. The more a physician knows about a patient's suffering, the more likely the physician is to feel positively about the patient and, consequently, to have empathy for the patient.

Physician–patient relationship

One of the most important potentially therapeutic or harmful elements existing in clinical medicine is the personal relationship between physician and patient. Before the advent of effective medical and surgical interventions, the only positive therapeutic force that the physician could bring to the patient's bedside was a close, warm, and caring concern for the patient's life. With the advent of efficacious medical and surgical therapy, this positive force has been denigrated by some physicians who refer to it as 'only a placebo effect'.

It may well be that a positive physician–patient relationship involves factors resembling those called into play by administration of a placebo. However, such forces represent potentially powerful therapeutic factors, and, as such, they should never be ignored or denigrated. Why not doubly benefit the patient with both efficacious medicine or surgery and the positive placebo effect of a therapeutic interpersonal relationship?

Central nervous system (CNS) endorphin levels are apparently increased by certain positive interventions such as placebo administration. Endorphins have powerful CNS actions, and their presence in increased amounts following a positive placebo reaction is apparently of considerable benefit to patients with both minor and serious illnesses. Clearly, the clinician should accept all the help he or she can get. The therapeutic effect of a positive physician–patient relationship should not be ignored, even when effective medical–surgical therapy is available.

Patients listen with great care to everything the physician says. Frequently, patients misinterpret direct remarks from the physician or offhand comments made by one physician to another or by the physician to a nurse. It is, therefore, essential for the physician to choose words carefully when speaking to or in front of the patient. Physician behavior even in the vicinity of the patient (i.e. at the next patient's bed or at the door of the patient's room) may have an impact on the patient. The physician must draw on his or her empathetic powers, try to anticipate what words or behavior may be helpful or upsetting, and then attempt to act accordingly.

It has been said, somewhat tongue in cheek, that three essential qualities are required in a physician. In descending order of importance they are: (1) affability, (2) availability, and (3) ability. Although this triplet is meant to be sarcastic rather than realistic, there is more than a modicum of truth involved. However, the order of importance of these qualities is clearly inappropriate and should be: (1) ability, (2) affability, and (3) availability. That a physician must be both intellectually and physically able goes almost without saying. A considerable fund of knowledge, good common sense, and a large store of stamina are prerequisites for most clinicians. Moreover, the clinician should be knowledgeable in social as well as basic science areas: a solid grasp of basic psychology, societal organization, and economics is important in daily clinical work.

Affability implies that the physician has a warm, friendly personality. Such qualities are reassuring to the average patient, who is often highly fearful of contact with the medical profession. Certainly, affability without ability often leads to deception: 'quacks' are usually affable but lack knowledge of medical science. Kindness rather than affability may be a preferable quality for physicians to cultivate. Patients are in an unenviable situation: they are usually fearful, uncomfortable, and weakened from their illness. Kindness in such a setting establishes a strong positive physician–patient relationship, often referred to as the therapeutic partnership.

The third quality appropriate for physicians is availability. The degree to which this characteristic is exercised is often cause for concern for physicians and their families. The nature of clinical medicine makes it a full-time job. Indeed, the more meticulous the care given to each individual patient, the greater the number of hours in each day devoted to patient care. Every physician is aware of friends or colleagues whose personal lives have been destroyed by constant, meticulous, but overzealous attention to patient care. Dedication to patients is an important quality in a physician. Nevertheless, each physician must decide for himself or herself the amount of time that will be dedicated to clinical practice in response to the demands of patient care. Clearly, availability is a two-edged sword. Finally, it should be stressed that physicians need a certain amount of breathing room between themselves and their patients. This allows for objective evaluation of the patient's problems.

SUMMARY

- The cornerstone of good cardiovascular care starts with a thorough history and a careful physical examination.
- Despite recent technological advances, the clinician still needs to assess the patient carefully by listening and observing. A history that is taken with sympathy is also the first step in the therapy of the patient.
- The history and physical examination initiate a physician–patient relationship.
- Careful auscultation in a quiet environment is the most important component of the cardiovascular physical examination. Attention should be paid to the timing, quality, and duration of any murmur that is heard.
- Careful observation and palpation where appropriate of the various venous and arterial pulses is also an important component of the cardiovascular examination.
- Finally, empathy and cultural sensitivity on the part of the physician is of inestimable value in understanding the patient's history and in arriving at an appropriate plan of treatment.

REFERENCES

1. Sandler G. The importance of the history in the medical clinic and the cost of unnecessary tests. *Am Heart J* 1980; **100**: 928–31.
2. Criteria Committee of the New York Heart Association. Major changes made by the Criteria Committee of the New York Heart Association. *Circulation* 1974; **49**: 390.
3. Goldman L, Hashimoto B, Cooks EF, *et al.* Comparative reproducibility and validity of systems for assessing cardiovascular functional class: advantages of a new specific activity scale. *Circulation* 1981; **64**: 1227–34.
4. Campeau L. Grading of angina pectoris (letter). *Circulation* 1976; **54**: 522–3.
5. Wasserman K, Hansen JE, Sue DY, *et al.* Principles of exercise testing and interpretation. Philadelphia: Lea & Febiger, 1987.
6. Manning HL, Schwartzstein RM. Pathophysiology of dyspnea. *N Engl J Med* 1995; **333**: 1547–53.
7. Mulrow CD, Lucey CR, Farnett LE. Discriminating causes of dyspnea through clinical examination. *J Gen Intern Med* 1993; **8**: 383–92.
8. Lee TH, Goldman L. Serum enzyme assays in the diagnosis of acute myocardial infarction. In: Sox HC, ed. *Common diagnostic tests: use and interpretation*, 2nd edn. Philadelphia: American College of Physicians, 1990.
9. Sox HC Jr. Exercise testing in suspected coronary artery disease. *Dis Month* 1985: **31**(12): 1–90.
10. Silver KH, Alpert JS. Syncope. *J Intensive Care Med* 1992; **7**: 138–48.
11. Sheehan TJ, Husted S, Candee D, Cook C, Bargen M. Moral judgment as a predictor of clinical performance. *Eval Health Professions* 1980; **3**: 393–404.

14

Critical pathways for acute coronary syndromes

CHRISTOPHER P CANNON, RAMI ALHARETHI AND PATRICK T O'GARA

'Critical pathways' are standardized protocols for the management for specific disorders that attempt to optimize and streamline patient care. They can be used to reduce hospital length of stay, but also to improve the use of medications and treatments, to increase participation in research protocols, and to reduce the use of unnecessary tests. It is believed that critical pathways can improve the quality and cost effectiveness of patient care.

INTRODUCTION AND HISTORICAL BACKGROUND

What are critical pathways?

'Critical pathways' are standardized protocols for the management of specific disorders that aim to optimize and streamline patient care. Numerous other names have been developed for such programs, including 'clinical pathways' (so as not to suggest to patients that they are in 'critical' condition), or simply 'protocols', such as acute myocardial infarction (MI) protocols used in emergency departments to reduce time to treatment with thrombolysis.[1,2] A broader name of 'disease management' is currently used to denote that these pathways extend beyond the hospital phase of treatment, to optimize medical management over the long term.

Goals of critical pathways

The use of critical pathways is growing rapidly primarily as a means to reduce hospital length of stay. However, several other components can be added to critical pathways, with the overall goal of improving the quality of patient care (Table 14.1). Indeed, physicians involved in developing critical pathways focus on these positive aspects of pathways as a means of utilizing them to advance medical care. These other goals focus on improving the use of medications and treatments, and increasing participation in research protocols. In addition, limitation of unnecessary tests can reduce costs and allow savings to be allocated to other treatments that have been shown to be beneficial. With involvement of physicians in developing these pathways, those responsible for patients can thus control how the patients are managed. It should be noted that data are only beginning to emerge regarding the success of various critical pathways. Indeed, we should remain critical of pathways and monitor their performance to ensure that they meet

Table 14.1 *Goals of critical pathways*

1. Improve patient care *and* decrease costs
2. Increase use of recommended medical therapies, e.g. aspirin for all acute coronary syndromes, reperfusion therapy for ST elevation myocardial infarction)
3. Decrease use of unnecessary tests
4. Decrease hospital length of stay
5. Increase participation in clinical research protocols

the overall goal of reducing costs while improving (or at least maintaining) quality of patient care.

NEED AND RATIONALE FOR CRITICAL PATHWAYS

Underutilization of recommended medications

A major problem in the management of acute coronary syndromes is that a large proportion of patients do not receive recommended medical therapies. For example, aspirin has been shown to be beneficial across the entire spectrum of myocardial ischemia, from primary prevention of MI,[3,4] to prevention of death or MI in unstable angina and acute MI,[5-10] to secondary prevention events.[11,12]

However, in the first National Registry of Myocardial Infarction (NRMI), involving 240 989 patients, among MI patients receiving thrombolytic therapy, only 87 per cent received aspirin. Among patients who did not receive thrombolysis, only 63 per cent were given aspirin.[13] Similarly, in the Cooperative Cardiovascular Project, among patients fully eligible to receive aspirin (i.e. no contraindications to aspirin such as bleeding ulcer), only 80 per cent of patients received the drug.[14] In the GUARANTEE registry of unstable angina patients conducted in 1996, 82 per cent of patients received aspirin.[15] Thus, despite the overwhelming benefits of aspirin (arguably the best studied and most beneficial medication in cardiovascular medicine),[12] a significant minority of patients does not receive this medication. The American Heart Association recently published a Scientific Statement strongly urging physicians to increase the use of aspirin in appropriate patients.[16] Thus, one focus for physicians, hospitals and health-care systems is to increase the use of aspirin.

There are numerous other medications which have been shown to be beneficial in acute coronary syndromes. Both unfractionated and low-molecular-weight heparins have also been shown to reduce death or MI in patients with non-ST segment elevation acute coronary syndromes.[7,17-21] In ST elevation MI, heparin improves infarct-related artery patency following tissue plasminogen activator,[22-24] and the low-molecular-weight heparin enoxaparin has recently been shown in a pilot trial to reduce the incidence of death, MI or recurrent ischemia following thrombolytic therapy.[25]

β-Blockers, nitrates, and calcium channel blockers are useful in patients with acute coronary syndromes (without contraindications).[26,27] Angiotensin-converting enzyme (ACE) inhibitors have been shown to be beneficial in selected patients *post*-MI with either documented left ventricular dysfunction,[28] or congestive heart failure.[29] The Gruppo Italiano per lo Studio della Streptochinasi nell'Infarto Miocardico (GISSI-3), International Study of Infarct Survival Collaborative Group (ISIS-4), and Chinese trials,[30-32] have suggested that the benefit of ACE inhibition may also extend to a much broader group of patients with acute MI.

Unfortunately, not all of these medications are utilized routinely in appropriate patients. In the Thrombolysis in Myocardial Infarction (TIMI) 9 Registry, 91 per cent of patients received heparin, and β-blockers were given to 61 per cent. In patients who developed congestive heart failure or had documented LV dysfunction post-MI, only 39 per cent were treated with ACE inhibitors at hospital discharge. Although these numbers are better than those observed in the NRMI,[13] there remains opportunity for improvement.

The other most notable example of underutilization of medications is thrombolysis. It appears that only 25–30 per cent of all patients with acute MI receive thrombolysis. However, thrombolytic therapy is beneficial only in patients with ST elevation MI.[33-35] We previously conducted the TIMI 9 Registry that tracked all acute MI patients who presented to 20 hospitals in the US and Canada and who presented with ST elevation or new left bundle branch block. Overall, we observed that 69 per cent either received thrombolysis (60 per cent) or underwent primary angioplasty (9 per cent).[36] Of those who presented to the hospital within 12 hours of the onset of pain, 75 per cent received acute reperfusion therapy. Of the 31 per cent of the total group who did not receive reperfusion therapy, delay in presentation explained one-third, another third of them had contraindications to thrombolysis, and the final third had no clear identifiable reason why thrombolysis was not administered. Thus, despite a reasonable percentage of patients receiving reperfusion therapy for ST elevation MI, opportunities for improvement exist, with the ultimate goal of extending the benefits of reperfusion therapy to all patients with ST elevation MI.

Overutilization of cardiac procedures

Another area for potential improvement is in the use of cardiac procedures following admission for acute MI and unstable angina. In acute MI, numerous studies have found wide differences in the use of cardiac procedures but no differences in mortality.[37-43] Such observations have been made comparing hospitals with on-site cardiac catheterization facilities *vs* those without,[37-39] and when comparing patients in Canada *vs* the USA; many fewer procedures are performed in Canada, but overall mortality for patients in the USA and Canada is similar.[40-43] These data suggest that there may be unnecessary procedures performed in some patients.

In order to study this important question, the TIMI Investigators carried out two trials, TIMI IIB in patients with ST elevation MI treated with thrombolytic therapy,[44] and TIMI IIIB in patients with unstable angina and non-ST elevation MI[33] (additional trials are ongoing, e.g. TACTICS-TIMI 18 in patients with unstable angina and non-ST elevation MI).[45]

TIMI IIB

In TIMI IIB, 3339 patients with ST elevation MI were treated with tissue plasminogen activator (tPA), aspirin, and heparin, and were randomized to either an invasive strategy consisting of cardiac catheterization 18–48 hours later followed by percutaneous transluminal coronary angioplasty (PTCA) or bypass surgery if the anatomy was suitable, or to a conservative strategy in which catheterization and PTCA were performed only for recurrent spontaneous ischemia or a positive exercise test.[44,46,47]

Death or recurrent MI through 42 days occurred in 10.9 per cent of patients in the invasive group compared to 9.7 per cent of the conservative group (P = not significant (NS)).[44] Similarly, no difference between the two strategies was observed through 1 year[46] or 3 years of follow-up (21.0 per cent death or reinfarction for the invasive strategy vs 20.0 per cent for the conservative strategy; P = NS).[47] In contrast, the rate of revascularization in the two strategies was vastly different: 72.3 per cent of patients in the invasive strategy underwent PTCA or coronary artery bypass gract (CABG) by 1 year, compared to only 35.5 per cent in the conservative strategy.

Approximately 750 000 patients with acute MI are admitted to acute care hospitals in the USA annually; estimating that one-half have ST segment elevation, the potential cost savings of following a conservative strategy are astounding. Using a rough estimate of $2000 for a diagnostic catheterization and $4000 for a PTCA procedure,[48] this would translate into an annual savings of 1 billion dollars. Even when performing a sensitivity analysis and reducing the cost of the procedures by one-half, the savings of following a conservative strategy still amounts to $500 000 000 annually in the USA. Thus, since both strategies lead to similar long-term outcome, this trial established the 'watchful waiting' approach as the preferred strategy for the management of patients treated with thrombolytic therapy for acute MI.

The findings from TIMI IIB, with the added support of the findings from the 'Should We Intervene Following Thrombosis?' (SWIFT) trial,[49] and other studies,[37–43] lend strong support to the notion that coronary angiography can be reserved for patients who demonstrate recurrent ischemia post-thrombolysis for ST elevation MI. In the current era of cost containment, close scrutiny of the indications for cardiac catheterization, with more strict adherence to its need in patients with documented recurrent ischemia post-MI, may allow reductions in the use of cardiac procedures (and thus costs), without any loss of clinical benefit.

Reducing other cardiac testing

Other areas of potential overutilization of testing also exist, e.g. laboratory tests and echocardiography. Although the performance of myocardial specific troponin assays are prognostically useful in patients with unstable angina, in patients with acute ST elevation MI, it is unnecessary and duplicative to obtain them along with routine creatine kinase-MB (CK-MB) determinations. Echocardiography is used widely to assess left ventricular function post-MI, the most powerful determinant of subsequent prognosis.[50–52] The American College of Cardiology/American Heart Association (ACC/AHA) Acute MI Guidelines recommend that left ventricular function be assessed in all patients.[26] However, a recent study, now validated by three other groups, has shown that several clinical features (non-anterior MI, no prior Q waves, total CK <1000 IU and no evidence of congestive heart failure), can be used to predict normal left ventricular function (ejection fraction $\geq$ 40 per cent) with 97 per cent specificity.[53–55] Thus, for patients with small non-ST elevation MIs, assessment of left ventricular (LV) function via echocardiography or ventriculography may not be necessary, a strategy which could have potential implications for more cost-effective care.

REDUCING HOSPITAL (AND INTENSIVE CARE UNIT) LENGTH OF STAY

Reduction in hospital length of stay has been the driving force behind the creation of critical pathways. As noted in the initial pathways for cardiac surgical patients, early discharge was the main outcome variable.[56] In acute coronary syndromes, length of stay was quite long just 5 years ago. In patients with unstable angina and non-Q-wave MI enrolled in the TIMI IIIB trial, the average length of stay was over 9 days. In the parallel TIMI 3 Registry of patients not entered into the trial, length of stay was also 9 days. Among patients treated with thrombolysis for ST elevation MI, similar observations have been made. In Global Utilization of Streptokinase and TPA for Occluded coronary arteries trial (GUSTO-I), the median length of stay was 9 days.[57] In a follow-up analysis which divided patients into those who had an uncomplicated course (no recurrent ischemia, congestive heart failure, or any other complication) vs any one of these complications, the median length of stay for both groups was 9 days. In the TIMI 9 Registry conducted in 1995, for uncomplicated patients with ST elevation MI the median length of stay was 8 days.[36,58] Thus, it appears that length of stay has historically been long in patients with acute coronary syndromes, and opportunities exist to reduce it safely, especially in low-risk patients.

Identification of low-risk patients

With the benefit of aggressive reperfusion therapy in acute MI, it has been possible to identify patients who are at low risk of subsequent mortality or morbidity.[59] In the TIMI II trial, a group of patients were prespecified as 'low risk' if they had the following characteristics: age <70 years, no prior MI, inferior or lateral MI, normal sinus rhythm, and Killip class 1 at admission.[44] This classification was subsequently validated.[60] Similar observations have been made in the TAMI trials,[61] and more recently in the GUSTO-I trial.[57]

Strategy of early discharge following thrombolysis

Identification of low-risk patients has led to the possibility of early hospital discharge for such uncomplicated patients.[57,61] A pilot trial of such a strategy in 80 patients suggested that hospital stay and costs could be significantly reduced without an increase in morbidity and mortality.[62] However, it should be noted that all patients who received reperfusion therapy also underwent immediate coronary angiography, the information from which was used in the triage of the patients. Such a strategy is not applicable to standard practice.[62] Thus, the strategy of early hospital discharge looks very promising and feasible, but more information is needed to establish it in clinical practice.

Early discharge following primary PTCA

Such a strategy of early hospital discharge for low-risk patients after *primary angioplasty* has recently been reported.[63] The Primary Angioplasty in Myocardial Infarction (PAMI) 2 trial divided patients into low- and high-risk groups based on clinical and angiographic features.[63] The 471 low-risk patients were randomized to a strategy of early discharge or to conventional hospital discharge. Clinical outcomes at 6 months were similar in both groups: mortality 0.8 per cent *vs* 0.4 per cent for early discharge *vs* standard care ($P = 1.0$), unstable angina 10.1 per cent *vs* 12.0 per cent ($P = NS$), recurrent MI 0.8 per cent *vs* 0.4 per cent ($P = NS$), or the combination of death, unstable angina, MI, congestive heart failure or stroke, 15.2 per cent *vs* 17.5 per cent ($P = 0.49$).[63] On the other hand, for the 'critical pathway' group, hospital length of stay was 3 days shorter (4.2 days *vs* 7.1 days, $P = 0.0001$) and hospital costs were lower ($9658 ± $5287 *vs* $11 604 ± 6125, $P = 0.002$).[63] Thus, the strategy of acute catheterization and primary PTCA allowed identification of low-risk patients for whom early discharge was safe, resulting in a substantial reduction in hospital length of stay and cost savings.

Overutilization of intensive care

Overutilization of the intensive and coronary care units (CCU) is another area in which critical pathways may reduce costs. A decade ago, admission to the CCU was standard for all unstable angina and MI (and frequently 'rule out MI') patients.[64,65] Even recently in the multicenter GUARANTEE Registry conducted in the USA in 1996, 40 per cent of patients with unstable angina and non-ST elevation MI were admitted to the CCU.[15] Given that, in the present era, CCU admission is generally recommended for higher risk patients, i.e. those with ST elevation MI and/or hemodynamic compromise or other complications, these current data suggest opportunities may exist for reducing the number of patients admitted to intensive care units.

Methods for critical pathways development

The process of developing a critical pathway first involves defining the problem (Table 14.2). The specific problems in the care of patients with specific diagnoses need to be identified in general (as noted above) in parallel with the prevailing issues at the institutional level. For example, the use of blood tests might be higher than necessary when left to the individual house staff or physicians (e.g. multiple cholesterol measurements during a single hospital stay).

The next step is to establish a task force or committee to create (or adapt) a critical pathway that would include recommended guidelines for patients with specific diagnoses. The third step is to distribute the draft critical pathway(s) to all health care professionals and services who care for patients with those diagnoses, to ensure adequate input from all parties involved. For example, for an unstable angina pathway, one should include members of the cardiology, cardiac surgery, emergency medicine, nursing, the non-invasive laboratory, cardiac rehabilitation, social service, case management, and dietary service. Comments from these parties are then included in the final pathway.

Implementation of the pathway can begin with a 'pilot' and then be available for routine use. The fifth step

Table 14.2 *Steps in developing and implementing critical pathway*

1. Identify problems in patient care
2. Identify task force that develops guidelines for medical care
3. Distribute draft critical pathway to all departments involved
4. Implement the pathway
5. Collect and monitor data on critical pathway performance
6. Modify the pathway as needed to improve performance further

in the process of establishing a critical pathway is to collect and monitor data regarding performance. This could include the number of patients for whom the pathway was used, use of recommended therapy, and the hospital length of stay. The final step is to interpret the initial data and to modify the pathway as needed. These latter three steps collectively consist of the 'continuous quality improvement' that must be ongoing during the implementation of any pathway. In addition, as new therapies become available, the data should be reviewed to determine which steps should be added or modified as part of optimal patient management.

Methods of implementation

Several potential methods of implementation exist. First, one could have voluntary participation in a pathway. Although this appears to be an inefficient means of ensuring participation with a critical pathway, it is frequently all that can be accomplished with limited resources at individual hospitals. The pathway could be sent to physicians and nurses, and presented at staff and house staff meetings. Another means of triggering pathway use is to use reminders via electronic mail messages triggered off by the admission diagnosis, or monthly reminders to physicians and nurses. Another approach is to have independent screening of all admissions, with copies of the pathway placed in the chart. Use of the pathway would be expected to be low with such a voluntary approach. On the other hand, if a pathway becomes implemented in a proportion of patients, that treatment strategy may become the 'standard of care' at a particular hospital, it may not be necessary actually to involve additional personnel to 'implement' a particular pathway.

An alternate approach, which some hospitals have used, is to have a designated case manager to evaluate each patient and to ensure that all steps in the pathway are carried out. Such an approach would be expected to improve the use of the pathway. However, this approach obviously requires additional resources from the hospital or health-care system. The approach used by individual hospitals for specific diagnoses needs to be individualized. However, the pathways reviewed in the literature to date, as well as the examples of specific pathways available on the National Heart Attack Alert Program (NHAAP) web page (http://www.nhlbi.nih.gov/nhlbi/othcomp/opec/nhaap/nhaapage.htm) are provided to facilitate the use of critical pathways and reduce the time and effort needed for hospitals to implement them. The ultimate goal is to improve the care of patients and make such care more cost effective.

'Cardiac checklist'

A very simplified version of a critical pathway is to use a 'cardiac checklist'. While checklists exist for many pur-

poses, including admission tests and procedures, this format can be extended to medical treatments. It is a simple method to ensure that each patient receives all the recommended therapies. Table 14.3 shows a proposed 'Cardiac checklist' for the patient with unstable angina/non-ST elevation MI, which includes aspirin, heparin, or low-molecular-weight heparin, IIb/IIIa inhibitor, β-blockers, heart-rate-lowering calcium antagonists (if needed, and in the absence of congestive heart failure or left ventricular dysfunction), cholesterol-lowering and other risk-factor modifications.

This 'cardiac checklist' could be used in two ways: (1) physicians could keep a copy on a small index card in their pocket – and run down the list when writing admission orders for patients; or (2) it could be used in developing standard orders for an MI patient – either printed order sheets or computerized orders, from which the physician can choose when admitting a patient to the hospital. Such a system has worked well in ensuring extremely high compliance with evidence-based recommendations at Brigham and Women's Hospital (Cannon, unpublished data). In the era of 'scorecard medicine',[66,67] many outside observers such as health maintenance organizations or insurers, tally up the use of recommended medications as quality of care measures; use of a cardiac checklist should allow physicians (and patients) to 'win' the game and improve the quality of care for patients.

Table 14.3 *'Cardiac checklist' for unstable angina and non-ST elevation myocardial infarction*

Medications
1. Aspirin . . . . ☐
2. Heparin / LMWH . . . . ☐
3. IIb/IIIa inhibition . . . . ☐
4. Beta-blockers . . . . ☐
5. Nitrates . . . . ☐
6. ACE inhibitors if low EF/CHF . . . . ☐

Interventions
7. Catheterization/revascularization for recurrent ischemia or high-risk patients . . . . ☐

Secondary prevention
8. Cholesterol – check + Rx as needed . . . . ☐
9. Smoking cessation . . . . ☐
10. Treat other risk factors (hypertension, diabetes) . . . ☐

LMWH = low-molecular-weight heparin; ACE = angiotensin-converting enzymes; EF = ejection fraction; CHF = congestive heart failure; Rx = treatment.

Critical pathways and triage of patients

At many institutions, critical pathways for acute MI and unstable angina have been adopted, with the goals of quickly identifying patients with acute coronary syndromes, rapidly treating with appropriate medications (e.g. anti-ischemic and antithrombotic medications), and to triage the patient to the appropriate level of care.[1,68-71]

BRIGHAM AND WOMEN'S HOSPITAL ACUTE CORONARY SYNDROME PATHWAYS

An overview of our critical pathways for acute coronary syndromes is shown in Fig. 14.1. There are five pathways for the different types of syndromes: two for acute ST elevation MI patients (one for thrombolysis, and one for primary angioplasty) (Fig. 14.2), one for unstable angina and non-ST elevation MI (Fig. 14.3), and two for patients with chest pain of unclear etiology (one 6-hour emergency department-based 'rule out MI' pathway and one 23-hour short stay unit-based pathway) (Fig. 14.4).

ST elevation MI critical pathway

The critical pathway for all acute coronary syndromes begins immediately with the triage nurse who brings patients with chest pain into an 'acute' room of the emergency department (ED). A brief history is obtained and electrocardiogram performed. If ST-segment elevation is present, the patient is immediately evaluated for thrombolysis or primary angioplasty (Fig. 14.2). One critical guideline (based on the importance of time to reperfusion with either thrombolysis or primary PTCA[1,72,73]) is to triage patients to that strategy that will achieve infarct-related artery patency most quickly. During the day, primary angioplasty is the preferred strategy, whereas on nights and weekends, if thrombolysis is preferred, the time necessary to mobilize the catheterization laboratory team is > 90 minutes.

After initial diagnosis, if the patient is eligible, thrombolytic therapy is administered in the ED with a goal of starting the drug in <30 minutes from arrival in the ED.[1]

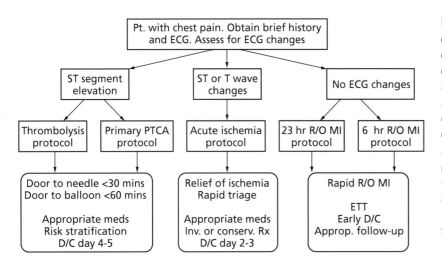

Figure 14.1 *Critical pathways for acute coronary syndromes at Brigham and Women's Hospital (Day 1 = day of admission). Pt = patient; ECG = electrocardiogram; PTCA = percutaneous transluminal coronary angioplasty; R/O MI = rule-out myocardial infarction; D/C = discharge; Rx = treatment. (Reprinted from Cannon CP, O'Gara PT. Critical pathways in acute coronary syndromes. In: Cannon CP, ed. Management of acute coronary syndromes. Totowa: Humana Press, 1999: 611–27.)*

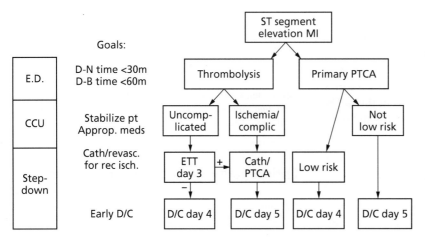

Figure 14.2 *Thrombolysis and primary angioplasty for acute ST elevation myocardial infarction (MI) critical pathways. E.D. = emergency department; D-N time = door-to-needle time; D-B time = door-to-balloon time; PTCA = percutaneous transluminal coronary angioplasty; ETT = exercise tolerance test; D/C = discharge. (Reprinted from Cannon CP, O'Gara PT. Critical pathways in acute coronary syndromes. In: Cannon CP, ed. Management of acute coronary syndromes. Totowa: Humana Press, 1999: 611–27.)*

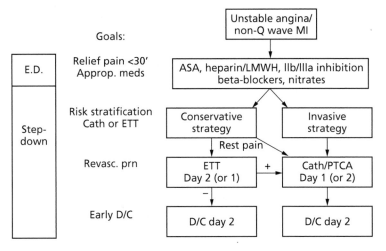

Figure 14.3 *Unstable angina/non-ST elevation myocardial infarction (MI) critical pathway. E.D. = emergency department; ASA = aspirin; LMWH = low-molecular-weight heparin; ETT = exercise tolerance test; PTCA = percutaneous transluminal coronary angioplasty; D/C = discharge; Revasc. prn = revascularization as needed. (Reprinted from Cannon CP, O'Gara PT. Critical pathways in acute coronary syndromes. In: Cannon CP, ed.* Management of acute coronary syndromes. *Totowa: Humana Press, 1999: 611–27.)*

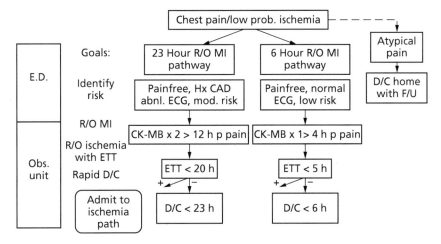

Figure 14.4 *'Rule-out MI' critical pathways. E.D. = emergency department; R/O = rule-out; MI = myocardial infarction; Hx CAD = history of coronary artery disease; ECG = electrocardiogram; D/C = discharge; F/U = follow-up; CK-MB = creatine kinase; ETT = exercise tolerance test. (Reprinted from Cannon CP, O'Gara PT. Critical pathways in acute coronary syndromes. In: Cannon CP, ed.* Management of acute coronary syndromes. *Totowa: Humana Press, 1999: 611–27.)*

The second goal of the pathway (begun in the ED but continued in the CCU) is to treat the patient with all other appropriate medications, such as aspirin, intravenous heparin, anti-ischemic, and cholesterol-lowering medications. The third goal is to ensure that patients are considered for ongoing clinical research trials.

For the thrombolysis pathway, patients are treated in the ED and admitted to the CCU. Low-risk patients are transferred out of the CCU after 24 hours, whereas others are transferred when their condition allows. Risk stratification is the next goal of the pathway. Rescue angioplasty is performed only if patients have evidence of active symptom instability, or ST-segment elevation. Research is ongoing to identify other ECG criteria,[74,75] and serum markers[76,77] to assist in this decision. Otherwise, patients are treated according to the TIMI IIB conservative strategy, with cardiac catheterization performed only if patients have rest ischemia or have evidence of ischemia on a stress test, the latter being performed on hospital day 3 or 4 for low and higher risk patients, respectively. Echocardiography is recommended for most patients, except those with small infe-

rior MIs without complications in whom left ventricular function can be inferred to be normal using a clinical prediction rule.[53]

For the primary angioplasty pathway, the low-risk patients are admitted to the step-down unit in accord with the PAMI-II trial.[63] Primary stenting is common,[78] as is the use of IIb/IIIa inhibition.[79] No additional stress testing is performed except if patients had evidence of significant coronary stenoses other than within the infarct-related artery. Discharge is targeted for hospital day 4 or 5 depending on the extent of infarction.

Unstable angina and non-ST-elevation MI pathway

The pathway for unstable angina and non-ST-elevation MI at Brigham and Women's Hospital emphasizes: (1) early relief of ischemic pain, a symptom which has been found to be a determinant of development of myocardial infarction;[80] (2) administration of antithrombotic and antiischemic therapy; (3) reminders of eligibility criteria for ongoing clinical research trials (e.g. trials of new IIb/IIIa inhibitors or treatment strategy trials); (4) a detailed list of suggested blood tests in an effort to reduce unnecessary tests; (5) the choice of either an early conservative strategy or an early invasive strategy, as used in TIMI IIIB.[68]

Inclusion criteria for the pathway are essentially patients with true unstable angina. This is defined as ischemic pain occurring either at rest or minimal exertion and with an accelerating pattern (i.e. Braunwald Class 1–3 unstable angina).[81] Corroborative information that supports the clinical history is helpful in establishing the diagnosis and identifying higher risk patients:[27] prior history of MI or documented coronary disease by catheterization, or ST- or T-wave changes with the presenting syndrome. ST deviation of ≥ 0.5 mm is used since it appears to have equal prognostic significance as ≥ 1 mm ST depression.[80] Since only a third of patients presenting unstable angina have electrocardiogram (ECG) changes,[80] much of the admission diagnosis relies on the history.

The treatment involves aspirin, heparin, and IIb/IIIa inhibition,[82–84] or consideration of enoxaparin.[21] In addition, β-blockers, nitrates, calcium-channel blockers, if needed, and cholesterol-lowering medications (as guided by prior history or by the admission cholesterol or low-density lipoprotein (LDL) level) are administered.

Tests on admissions

The pathway recommends serial CK-MB determinations for diagnosis of non-ST elevation MI. In addition, a troponin I at entry is measured on admission and every 8 hours for 24 hours. This is very useful in risk-stratifying patients over and above the information available from CK-MB.[85] TACTICS-TIMI 18 recently found that troponin is useful in determining the treatment strategy.[45] Additional blood work is limited in the pathway (to avoid multiple chemistry panels on the same admission). Assessment of LV function with an echocardiogram is generally recommended but can be omitted in patients with known low ejection fraction.

Treatment strategy

Patients are managed by either an early invasive or early conservative strategy, but with the recent TACTICS-TIMI 18 trial showing benefit of the invasive strategy, this is the preferred strategy.

The early invasive strategy involves cardiac catheterization within 18 hours of admission (either the same day or the following morning). Angioplasty (with or without stenting and IIb/IIIa inhibition – used at the discretion of the interventionalist) is carried out immediately. If the patient is referred for CABG, scheduling is arranged as soon as possible. Patients then follow the CABG path-

way, which targets a length of stay of 5 days for uncomplicated patients.

The early conservative strategy involves aggressive medical management and clinical monitoring. If the patient has recurrent ischemic pain, electrocardiograms are performed and, if either the pain is suggestive of ischemia or the ECG changes are present, the patient is referred for catheterization that day. In the absence of recurrent ischemia, an exercise test is performed on the morning of day 2. If negative, the patient is discharged home. If positive for ischemia, the patient undergoes cardiac catheterization that same day. It should also be noted that, because unstable angina can be highly variable in its presentation, exercise testing can sometimes be performed on hospital day 1 in low-risk patients, after approximately 24 hours of optimal medical management.

The overall goal for length of stay with the pathways is 2 days. This includes patients who have angioplasty in the early invasive strategy. If patients fail the early conservative strategy and have an angioplasty on day 2, then their target length of stay will be 3 days. Initial experience with this pathway has shown a reduction in hospital length of stay from a median of 5 days prior to the pathway to 2 days, as well as an improvement in the use of appropriate medications (Cannon, unpublished data). As institutions gain experience with implementation of critical pathways, their impact on care can be assessed more clearly. Nonetheless, they do offer a means of improving care while attempting to control costs.

Secondary prevention and follow-up

Because follow-up is critical in the overall management of all acute coronary syndromes, the primary care physician receives a phone call, a fax summary, or the hospital discharge instructions, a letter from the cardiologist and the hospital discharge summary (the latter three are also sent to other physicians caring for the patient). It provides another opportunity for the cardiologist to justify long-term management with key medications, such as aspirin, β-blockers, and cholesterol-lowering medications.[86,87]

'Rule-out MI pathways'

For the large population of patients without ECG changes, patients are risk stratified. Patients, with clearly atypical pain, not suggestive of ischemia, are discharged home with follow-up from their primary physicians. The remaining patients with pain possibly suggestive of ischemia are observed in the ED. If stable, these patients undergo early exercise testing to determine the presence and extent of ischemia.[69] If positive, the patients are admitted for further evaluation and treatment. If negative, they are discharged home (within 6 hours of ED arrival) with follow-up to their physicians.[69]

We also established a '23-hour rule-out MI' pathway for patients who have chest pain, but who are not clearly 'low-risk' (e.g. patients with prior history of coronary artery disease and new chest pain). In this pathway, patients receive aspirin and β-blockers, have serial CK-MB and admission troponin-I measurements taken, and undergo exercise testing between 12 and 20 hours after presentation. Use of such an approach has reduced the rate of hospital admission for chest pain at our institution, as well as at others.[88]

FUTURE DIRECTIONS

The evolution of critical pathways is just beginning. Evidence is not yet available regarding the usefulness of these pathways in acute coronary syndromes, but research is ongoing to evaluate the outcomes of patients managed with critical pathways. New ways of implementing the pathways will need to be developed, the most promising of which appears to be use of computer technology.

CONCLUSION

The use of critical pathways is rapidly growing. They offer great potential for both reducing hospital length of stay and costs, and improving patient care. Standardized approaches with simple 'checklists' to ensure appropriate medications are being given will be a significant improvement in the care of patients. Improving the administrative links between different departments to make these pathways work may also benefit patient care. After development of pathways, we must monitor their performance to ensure that they meet the overall goal of reducing costs, while improving the quality of patient care. It is our belief that this goal can be achieved.

SUMMARY

- 'Critical pathways' are standardized protocols for the management of specific disorders which aim to optimize and streamline patient care.
- The need and rationale for critical pathways is based on the underutilization of recommended medications and the potential overutilization of cardiac procedures.
- The goals of critical pathways are to: improve care and reduce costs; reduce hospital length of stay; improve the use of guideline-recommended medications and treatments; reduce unnecessary testing; and increase participation in research protocols.

- A 'cardiac checklist' is a simplified version of a critical pathway.
- The methods of creation of critical pathways involve a multidisciplinary approach.
- Examples of the critical pathways used at Brigham and Women's Hospital are detailed in this chapter.

REFERENCES

1. Cannon CP, Antman EM, Walls R, Braunwald E. Time as an adjunctive agent to thrombolytic therapy. *J Thromb Thrombolysis* 1994; **1**: 27–34.
2. National Heart Attack Alert Program Coordinating Committee – 60 Minutes to Treatment Working Group. Emergency department: rapid identification and treatment of patients with acute myocardial infarction. *Ann Emerg Med* 1994; **23**: 311–29.
3. Willard JE, Lange RA, Hillis LD. The use of aspirin in ischemic heart disease. *N Engl J Med* 1992; **327**: 175–81.
4. Steering Committee of the Physicians' Health Study Research Group. Final report on the aspirin component of the ongoing Physicians' Health Study. *N Engl J Med* 1989; **321**: 129–35.
5. Lewis HD, Davis JW, Archibald DG, *et al*. Protective effects of aspirin against acute myocardial infarction and death in men with unstable angina. *N Engl J Med* 1983; **309**: 396–403.
6. Cairns JA, Gent M, Singer J, *et al*. Aspirin, sulfinpyrazone, or both in unstable angina. *N Engl J Med* 1985; **313**: 1369–75.
7. Theroux P, Ouimet H, McCans J, *et al*. Aspirin, heparin or both to treat unstable angina. *N Engl J Med* 1988; **319**: 1105–11.
8. The RISC Group. Risk of myocardial infarction and death during treatment with low dose aspirin and intravenous heparin in men with unstable coronary artery disease. *Lancet* 1990; **336**: 827–30.
9. Roux S, Christeller S, Ludin E. Effects of aspirin on coronary reocclusion and recurrent ischemia after thrombolysis: a meta-analysis. *J Am Coll Cardiol* 1992; **19**: 671–7.
10. ISIS-2 (Second International Study of Infarct Survival) Collaborative Group. Randomised trial of intravenous streptokinase, oral aspirin, both, or neither among 17,187 cases of suspected acute myocardial infarction: ISIS-2. *Lancet* 1988; **2**: 349–60.
11. Klimt CR, Knatterud GL, Stamler J, Meier P, for the PARIS II Investigator Group. Persantine-Aspirin Reinfarction Study. Part II. Secondary coronary prevention with persantine and aspirin. *J Am Coll Cardiol* 1986; **7**: 251–69.
12. Antiplatelet Trialist' Collaboration. Collaborative overview of randomised trials of antiplatelet therapy – I: prevention of death, myocardial infarction and stroke by

prolongued antiplatelet therapy in various categories of patients. *Br Med J* 1994; **308**: 81–106.

13. Rogers WJ, Bowlby LJ, Chandra NC, *et al*. Treatment of myocardial infarction in the United States (1990 to 1993). Observations from the National Registry of Myocardial Infarction. *Circulation* 1994; **90**: 2103–14.

14. Ellerbeck EF, Jencks SF, Radford MJ, *et al*. Quality of care for medicare patients with acute myocardial infarction. A four-state pilot study from the Cooperative Cardiovascular Project. *JAMA* 1995; **273**: 1509–14.

15. Cannon CP, Moliterno DJ, Every N, *et al*. Implementation of AHCPR guidelines for unstable angina in 1996: unfortunate differences between men and women. Results from the multicenter GUARANTEE registry (abstract). *J Am Coll Cardiol* 1997; **29** (suppl A): 217A.

16. Hennekens CH, Dyken ML, Fuster V. Aspirin as a therapeutic agent in cardiovascular disease. A statement for healthcare professionals from the American Heart Association. *Circulation* 1997; **96**: 2751–3.

17. Theroux P, Waters D, Qiu S, McCans J, de Guise P, Juneau M. Aspirin versus heparin to prevent myocardial infarction during the acute phase of unstable angina. *Circulation* 1993; **88**: 2045–8.

18. Cohen M, Adams PC, Parry G, *et al*. Combination antithrombotic therapy in unstable rest angina and non-Q-wave infarction in nonprior aspirin users. Primary end points analysis from the ATACS trial. *Circulation* 1994; **89**: 81–8.

19. Oler A, Whooley MA, Oler J, Grady D. Adding heparin to aspirin reduces the incidence of myocardial infarction and death in patients with unstable angina. A meta-analysis. *JAMA* 1996; **276**: 811–15.

20. FRISC Study Group. Low molecular weight heparin (Fragmin) during instability in coronary artery disease (FRISC). *Lancet* 1996; **347**: 561–8.

21. Cohen M, Demers C, Gurfinkel EP, *et al*. A comparison of low-molecular-weight heparin with unfractionated heparin for unstable coronary artery disease. *N Engl J Med* 1997; **337**: 447–52.

22. Bleich SD, Nichols T, Schumacher RR, Cooke DH, Tate DA, Teichman SL. Effect of heparin on coronary patency after thrombolysis with tissue plasminogen activator in acute myocardial infarction. *Am J Cardiol* 1990; **66**: 1412–17.

23. Hsia J, Hamilton WP, Kleiman N, *et al*. A comparison between heparin and low-dose aspirin as adjunctive therapy with tissue plasminogen activator for acute myocardial infarction. *N Engl J Med* 1990; **323**: 1433–7.

24. de Bono DP, Simoons MI, Tijssen J, *et al*. Effect of early intravenous heparin on coronary patency, infarct size, and bleeding complications after alteplase thrombolysis: results of a randomized double blind European Cooperative Study Group trial. *Br Heart J* 1992; **67**: 122–8.

25. Baird SH, McBride SJ, Trouton TG, Wilson C. Low-molecular-weight heparin versus unfractionated heparin following thrombolysis in myocardial infarction (abstract). *J Am Coll Cardiol* 1998; **31**(suppl A): 191A.

26. Ryan TJ, Anderson JL, Antman EM, *et al*. ACC/AHA guidelines for the management of patients with acute myocardial infarction: a report of the American College of Cardiology/American Heart Association Task Force on Practice Guidelines (Committee on Management of Acute Myocardial Infarction). *J Am Coll Cardiol* 1996; **28**: 1328–428.

27. Braunwald E, Antman EM, Beasley JW, *et al*. ACC/AHA guidelines for the management of patients with unstable angina and non-ST segment elevation myocardial infarction: a report of the American College of Cardiology/American Heart Association Task Force on Practice Guidelines (Committee on the Management of Unstable Angina and Non-ST Segment Elevation Myocardial Infarction). *J Am Coll Cardiol* 2000; **36**: 970–1056.

28. Pfeffer MA, Braunwald E, Moye LA, *et al*. Effect of captopril on mortality and morbidity in patients with left ventricular dysfunction after myocardial infarction. *N Engl J Med* 1992; **327**: 669–77.

29. The Acute Infarction Ramipril Efficacy (AIRE) Study Investigators. Effect of ramipril on mortality and morbidity of survivors of acute myocardial infarction with clinical evidence of heart failure. *Lancet* 1993; **342**: 821–8.

30. Gruppo Italiano per lo Studio della Sopravvivenza nell'Infarto Miocardico. GISSI-3: effect of lisinopril and trasdermal glyceryl trinitrate singly and together on 6-week mortality and ventricular function after acute myocardial infarction. *Lancet* 1994; **343**: 1115–22.

31. ISIS-4 Collaborative Group. ISIS-4: randomized factorial trial assessing early oral captopril, oral mononitrate, and intravenous magnesium sulphate in 58,050 patients with suspected acute myocardial infarction. *Lancet* 1995; **345**: 669–85.

32. Chinese Cardiac Study Collaborative Group. Oral captopril versus placebo among 13,634 patients with suspected myocardial infarction: interim report from the Chinese Cardiac Study(CCS-1). *Lancet* 1995; **345**: 686–7.

33. The TIMI IIIB Investigators. Effects of tissue plasminogen activator and a comparison of early invasive and conservative strategies in unstable angina and non-Q-wave myocardial infarction: results of the TIMI IIIB Trial. *Circulation* 1994; **89**: 1545–56.

34. Fibrinolytic Therapy Trialists' (FTT) Collaborative Group. Indications for fibrinolytic therapy in suspected acute myocardial infarction: collaborative overview of early mortality and major morbidity results from all randomised trials of more than 1000 patients. *Lancet* 1994; **343**: 311–22.

35. Braunwald E, Cannon CP. Non-Q wave and ST segment depression myocardial infarction: is there a role for thrombolytic therapy? (editorial). *J Am Coll Cardiol* 1996; **27**: 1333–4.

36. Cannon CP, Henry TD, Schweiger MJ, *et al*. Current management of ST elevation myocardial infarction and outcome of thrombolytic ineligible patients: results of

the multicenter TIMI 9 Registry (abstract). *J Am Coll Cardiol* 1995; special issue: 231–2A.

37. Every NR, Larson EB, Litwin PE, *et al*. The association between on-site cardiac catheterization facilities and the use of coronary angiography after acute myocardial infarction. *N Engl J Med* 1993; **329**: 546–51.

38. Every NR, Parson LS, Fihn SD, *et al*. Long-term outcome in acute myocardial infarction patients admitted to hospitals with and without on-site cardiac catheterization facilities. *Circulation* 1997; **96**: 1770–5.

39. Blustein J. High-technology cardiac procedures. The impact of service availability on service use in New York State. *JAMA* 1993; **270**: 344–9.

40. Rouleau JL, Moye LA, Pfeffer MA, *et al*. A comparison of management patterns after acute myocardial infarction in Canada and the United States. *N Engl J Med* 1993; **328**: 779–84.

41. Pilote L, Califf RM, Sapp S, *et al*. Regional variation across the United States in the management of acute myocardial infarction. *N Engl J Med* 1995; **333**: 565–72.

42. Mark DB, Naylor CD, Hlatky MA, *et al*. Use of medical resources and quality of life after acute myocardial infarction in Canada and the United States. *N Engl J Med* 1994; **331**: 1130–5.

43. Tu JV, Pashos CL, Naylor D, *et al*. Use of cardiac procedures and outcomes in elderly patients with mycardial infarction in the United States and Canada. *JAMA* 1997; **336**: 1500–5.

44. TIMI Study Group. Comparison of invasive and conservative strategies after treatment with intravenous tissue plasminogen activator in acute myocardial infarction. Results of the Thrombolysis in Myocardial Infarction (TIMI) Phase II Trial. *N Engl J Med* 1989; **320**: 618–27.

45. Cannon CP, Weintraub WS, Demopoulos LA, *et al*. Invasive versus conservative strategies in unstable angina and non-Q wave myocardial infarction following treatment with *tirofiban*: rationale and study design of the international TACTICS-TIMI 18 trial. *Am J Cardiol* 1998; **82**: 731–6.

46. Williams DO, Braunwald E, Knatterud G, *et al*. One-year results of the Thrombolysis in Myocardial Infarction Investigation (TIMI) phase II trial. *Circulation* 1992; **85**: 533–42.

47. Terrin ML, Williams DO, Kleiman NS, *et al*. Two- and three-year results of the Thrombolysis in Myocardial Infarction (TIMI) Phase II clinical trial. *J Am Coll Cardiol* 1993; **22**: 1763–72.

48. Goldman L. Cost-effective strategies in cardiology. In: Braunwald E, ed. *Heart disease. A textbook of cardiovascular medicine*, Vol. 1. Philadelphia: WB Saunders Co., 1992: 1694–707.

49. SWIFT (Should We Intervene Following Thrombolysis?) Trial Study Group. SWIFT trial of delayed elective intervention v. conservative treatment after thrombolysis with anistreplase in acute myocardial infarction. *Br Med J* 1991; **302**: 555–60.

50. Multicenter Postinfarction Research Group. Risk stratification and survival after myocardial infarction. *N Engl J Med* 1983; **309**: 331–6.

51. Zaret BL, Wackers FJT, Terrin ML, *et al*. Value of radionuclide rest and exercise left ventricular ejection fraction in assessing survival of patients after thrombolytic therapy for acute myocardial infarction: results of the Thrombolysis in Myocardial Infarction (TIMI) Phase II study. *J Am Coll Cardiol* 1995; **26**: 73–9.

52. Nicod P, Gilpin E, Dittrich H, *et al*. Influence on prognosis and morbidity of left ventricular ejection fraction with and without signs of left ventricular failure after acute myocardial infarction. *Am J Cardiol* 1988; **61**: 1165–71.

53. Silver MT, Rose GA, Paul SD, O'Donnell CJ, O'Gara PT, Eagle KA. A clinical rule to predict preserved left ventricular ejection fraction in patients after myocardial infarction. *Ann Intern Med* 1994; **121**: 750–6.

54. Tobin K, Stomel R, Harber D, Karavite D, Eagle K. Validation of a clinical prediction rule for predicting left ventricular function post acute myocardial infarction in a community hospital setting (abstract). *J Am Coll Cardiol* 1996; **27**(suppl A): 318A.

55. Krumholtz HM, Howes CJ, Murillo JE, Vaccarino LV, Radford MJ, Ellerbeck EF. Validation of a clinical prediction rule for left ventricular ejection fraction after myocardial infarction in patients ⩾ 65 years old. *Am J Cardiol* 1997; **80**: 11–15.

56. Nickerson NJ, Murphy SF, Kouchoukos NT, Daily BB, Schechtman KB, Davila-Roman VG. Predictors of early discharge after cardiac surgery and its cost-effectiveness (abstract). *J Am Coll Cardiol* 1996; **27**: 264A.

57. Newby LK, Califf RM, for the GUSTO Investigators. Redefining uncomplicated myocardial infarction in the thrombolytic era (abstract). *Circulation* 1994; **90**: I–110.

58. Cannon CP, Antman EM, Gibson CM, Paul SD, Braunwald E. Critical pathway for acute ST segment elevation myocardial infarction: evaluation of the potential impact in the TIMI 9 registry (abstract). *J Am Coll Cardiol* 1998; **31**(suppl A): 192A.

59. Hillis LD, Forman S, Braunwald E, and the Thrombolysis in Myocardial Infarction (TIMI) Phase II Co-Investigators. Risk stratification before thrombolytic therapy in patients with acute myocardial infarction. *J Am Coll Cardiol* 1990; **16**: 313–5.

60. Mueller HS, Cohen LS, Braunwald E, *et al*. Predictors of early morbidity and mortality after thrombolytic therapy of acute myocardial infarction. Analyses of patient subgroups in the Thrombolysis in Myocardial Infarction (TIMI) Trial, Phase II. *Circulation* 1992; **85**: 1254–64.

61. Mark DB, Sigmon K, Topol EJ, *et al*. Identification of acute myocardial infarction patients suitable for early hospital discharge after aggressive interventional therapy. Results from the Thrombolysis and Angioplasty in Acute Myocardial Infarction Registry. *Circulation* 1991; **83**: 1186–93.

62. Topol EJ, Bure K, O'Neill WW, *et al*. A randomized controlled trial of hospital discharge three days after

myocardial infarciton in the era of reperfusion. *N Engl J Med* 1988; **318**: 1083–8.

63. Grines CL, Marsalese DL, Brodie B, *et al*. Safety and cost-effectiveness of early discharge after primary angioplasty in low risk patients with acute myocardial infarction. *J Am Coll Cardiol* 1998; **31**: 967–72.

64. Goldman L, Cook EF, Brand DA, *et al*. A computer protocol to predict myocardial infarction in emergency department patients with chest pain. *N Engl J Med* 1988; **318**: 797–803.

65. Pozen MW, D'Agostino RB, Mitchell JB, *et al*. The usefulness of a predictive instrument to reduce inappropriate admissions to the coronary care unit. *Ann Intern Med* 1980; **92**: 238–42.

66. Topol EJ, Califf RM. Scorecard cardiovascular medicine. Its impact and future directions. *Ann Intern Med* 1994; **120**: 65–70.

67. Topol EJ, Block PC, Holmes DR, Klinke WP, Brinker JA. Readiness for the scorecard era in cardiovascular medicine (editorial). *Am J Cardiol* 1995; **75**: 1170–3.

68. Cannon CP. Optimizing the treatment of unstable angina. *J Thromb Thrombolysis* 1995; **2**: 205–18.

69. Nichol G, Walls R, Goldman L, *et al*. A critical pathway for management of patient with acute chest pain at low risk for myocardial ischemia: recommendations and potential impact. *Ann Intern Med* 1997; **127**: 996–1005.

70. Zalenski RJ, Rydman RJ, McCaren M, *et al*. Feasibility of a rapid diagnostic protocol for an emergency department chest pain unit. *Ann Emerg Med* 1997; **29**: 99–108.

71. Tatum JL, Jesse RL, Kontos MC, *et al*. Comprehensive strategy for the evaluation and triage of the chest pain patient. *Ann Emerg Med* 1997; **29**: 116–25.

72. Cannon CP, Gibson CM, Lambrew CT, *et al*. Relationship of symptom-onset-to-balloon time and door-to-balloon time with mortality in patients undergoing angioplasty for acute myocardial infarction. *JAMA* 2000; **283**: 2941–7.

73. Cannon CP, Braunwald E. Time to reperfusion: the critical modulator in thrombolysis and primary angioplasty. *J Thromb Thrombolysis* 1996; **3**: 109–17.

74. Schroder R, Dissmann R, Bruggemann T, *et al*. Extent of early ST segment elevation resolution: a simple but strong predictor of outcome in patients with acute myocardial infarction. *J Am Coll Cardiol* 1994; **24**: 384–91.

75. Schroder R, Wegscheider K, Schroder K, Dissmann R, Meyer-Sabellek W, for the INJECT Trial Group. Extent of early ST segment elevation resolution: a strong predictor of outcome in patients with acute myocardial infarction and a sensitive measure to compare thrombolytic regimens. A substudy of the International Joint Efficacy Comparison of Thrombolytics (INJECT) trial. *J Am Coll Cardiol* 1995; **26**: 1657–64.

76. Tanasijevic MJ, Cannon CP, Wybenga DR, *et al*. Myoglobin, creatine kinase MB and cardiac troponin-I to assess reperfusion after thrombolysis for acute myocardial infarction: Results from TIMI 10A. *Am Heart J* 1997; **134**: 622–30.

77. Tanasijevic M, Cannon CP, Antman EM, *et al*. Myoglobin, creatine-kinase-MB and cardiac troponin I 60-minute ratios predict infarct-related artery patency after thrombolysis for acute myocardial infarction. Results from the Thrombolysis in Myocardial Infarction Study (TIMI) 10B. *J Am Coll Cardiol* 1999; **34**: 739–47.

78. Stone GW, Brodie BR, Griffin JJ, *et al*. Prospective, multicenter study of the safety and feasibility of primary stenting in acute myocardial infarction: in-hospital and 30-day results of the PAMI Stent pilot trial. *J Am Coll Cardiol* 1998; **31**: 23–30.

79. Brenner SJ, Barr LA, Burchenal JEB, *et al*. Randomized, placebo-controlled trial of platelet IIb/IIIa blockade with primary angioplasty for acute myocardial infarction. *Circulation* 1998; **98**: 734–41.

80. Cannon CP, McCabe CH, Stone PH, *et al*. The electrocardiogram predicts one-year outcome of patients with unstable angina and non-Q wave myocardial infarction: results of the TIMI III Registry ECG Ancillary Study. *J Am Coll Cardiol* 1997; **30**: 133–40.

81. Braunwald E. Unstable angina: a classification. *Circulation* 1989; **80**: 410–14.

82. The Platelet Receptor Inhibition for Ischemic Syndrome Management (PRISM) Study Investigators. A comparison of aspirin plus tirofiban with aspirin plus heparin for unstable angina. *N Engl J Med* 1998; **338**: 1498–505.

83. The Platelet Receptor Inhibition for Ischemic Syndrome Management in Patients Limited by Unstable Signs and Symptoms (PRISM-PLUS) Trial Investigators. Inhibition of the platelet glycoprotein IIb/IIIa receptor with tirofiban in unstable angina and non-Q-wave myocardial infarction. *N Engl J Med* 1998; **338**: 1488–97.

84. The Platelet Glycoprotein IIb/IIIa in Unstable Angina: Receptor Suppression Using Integrilin Therapy (PURSUIT) Trial Investigators. Inhibition of platelet glycoprotein IIb/IIIa with eptifibatide in patients with acute coronary syndromes. *N Engl J Med* 1998; **339**: 436–43.

85. Antman EM, Tanasijevic MJ, Thompson B, *et al*. Cardiac-specific troponin I levels to predict the risk of mortality in patients with acute coronary syndromes. *N Engl J Med* 1996; **335**: 1342–9.

86. Scandinavian Simvastatin Survival Study Group. Randomised trial of cholesterol lowering in 4444 patients with coronary heart disease: the Scandinavian Simvastatin Survival Study (4S). *Lancet* 1994; **344**: 1383–9.

87. Sacks RM, Pfeffer MA, Moye LA, *et al*. The effect of pravastatin on coronary events after myocardial infarction in patients with average cholesterol levels. *N Engl J Med* 1996; **335**: 1001–9.

88. Graff LG, Dallara J, Ross MA, *et al*. Impact on the care of the emergency department chest pain patient from the Chest Pain Evaluation Registry (CHEPER) Study. *Am J Cardiol* 1997; **80**: 563–8.

15

Principles of hematology, hemostasis, and coagulation monitoring in patients with cardiovascular disease

RICHARD C BECKER AND FREDERICK A SPENCER

Patients with cardiovascular disease, particularly those with advanced illness requiring hospitalization not uncommonly have or develop one or more abnormalities that involve circulating blood cells and coagulation proteins. The clinical approach, comprehensive management, and natural history of disease are each influenced strongly by an understanding of pharmacology, available laboratory tests and treatment algorithms.

INTRODUCTION

Hematologic and coagulation abnormalities are common among hospitalized patients with serious cardiac disease, particularly those requiring surgical and other invasive procedures. Their comprehensive assessment and prompt management is vital, yet can challenge even the most astute clinicians for the following reasons: in some instances, the anomaly represents a desired and somewhat predictable response to pharmacologic intervention (e.g. systemic anticoagulation in a patient with active thromboembolic disease). While in other circumstances an inherited (e.g. classic hemophilia) or acquired (e.g. disseminated intravascular coagulation (DIC) in a patient with cardiogenic shock) condition or a complication of treatment (e.g. retroperitoneal hemorrhage associated with excessive anticoagulation) represents the major challenge. Further, it is common for pre-existing and acquired conditions to coexist.

Clinicians involved in the care of critically ill patients with cardiovascular disease must have a solid understanding of *basic hematologic principles, hemostasis and coagulation monitoring* to provide a high level of care. They must also be intimately familiar with antithrombotic therapy, indication for its use, and the treatment of hemorrhagic complications that can occur. This chapter outlines these three important areas, stressing pathobiology, differential diagnosis, and management strategies.

HISTORICAL LANDMARKS

Early observations

The rapid transformation of fluid blood to a gel-like substance (clot) has been a topic of great interest to scientists, physicians, and philosophers dating back to the days of Plato and Aristotle.[1,2] However, it was not until the beginning of the eighteenth century that blood clotting was appreciated as a means to stem blood loss from wounds.[3]

As with other areas of science, the microscope played a pivotal role in our understanding of coagulation. In the mid-seventeenth century, Malpighi separated the individual components of a blood clot into fibers, cells, and serum.[4] The fibers were subsequently found to be derived from a plasma precursor (*fibrinogen*) and given the name *fibrin*. Further developments in the mid-nineteenth century included the recognition of an enzyme (later given the name *thrombin*) that was capable of coagulating fibrinogen.[5]

The thrombin story is particularly interesting and played a prominent role in the evolution of coagulation. In the latter half of the nineteenth century, the scientific community began to appreciate that thrombin could not be a constituent of normal plasma (otherwise clotting would occur continuously and at random).[6] This particular concept was vital to our understanding of the complex 'checks and balances' system of coagulation, where inactive precursors are activated when and where they are needed. It also fostered the important belief that blood contained many if not all the necessary elements for coagulation (circulating predominantly in an inactive form) and serves as the basis for the theory of intrinsic coagulation.

Coagulation cascades

Researchers were able to show that blood coagulated when it came into contact with a foreign surface and that some surfaces were more 'thrombogenic' than others. This con-

cept served as the basis for an expanding knowledge of hereditary disorders of coagulation.[7,8] Developments in our understanding of extrinsic coagulation followed the pioneering work of many bright and insightful investigators,[9–12] all of whom described blood coagulation following the infusion of tissue suspensions (subsequently given the name tissue thromboplastin or *tissue factor*). A revised theory of extrinsic coagulation suggested that an exposed tissue surface (from a damaged blood vessel wall) was capable of stimulating blood clotting. Later discoveries included the direct contribution of *calcium*,[13] *phospholipid* (predominantly from platelet membranes)[14] and other essential components of the *prothrombinase complex* (Factors Va, Xa) to blood coagulation.[15,16]

Platelets

The contribution of *platelets* to the coagulation process can be traced back to the mid-nineteenth century and the original work of Alfred Donné who is believed to have discovered platelets with the help of a newly developed microscope lens (achromatic lens).[17] However, the clinical importance of platelets in normal hemostasis was not appreciated until the end of the nineteenth century when Sir William Osler described platelet aggregation[18] and Hayem cited the importance of platelet plugs in preventing blood loss after tissue injury.[19]

The development of electron microscopy subsequently made it clear that platelets adhered to damaged blood vessels[20] and that platelets could become 'activated' through a variety of pharmacologic (adenosine diphosphate, epinephrine, thrombin) or mechanical stimuli.[21–23]

Fibrinolysis

The inability of blood to coagulate following death was observed centuries ago; possibly as early as the days of Hippocrates.[24] Pioneering work at the end of the eighteenth century described the process of fibrinolysis and a mechanism whereby a circulating precursor (*plasminogen*) generated (with the appropriate stimulus) an active enzyme (*plasmin*) capable of degrading clotted blood.[25,26]

The potential clinical ramifications of fibrinolysis theoretically began with the observations of Gratia in 1921, who observed that clots could be dissolved by staphylococcal extracts.[27] Tillet and Garner later reported that bacteria-free filtrates of β-hemolytic streptococci contained a substance (streptokinase) that was capable of dissolving blood clots.[28] Soon thereafter, the groundbreaking work of Sherry[29] highlighted the use of thrombolytics in man. *Plasminogen activators*, found within many tissues of the body, including vessels themselves, were also discovered[30,31] and have served an important role in understanding natural thromboresistance as well as in the development of potent thrombolytic agents for clinical use in man.

ANEMIA

Anemia is defined as reduction of either the *volume* of red blood cells (hematocrit) or the *concentration* of hemoglobin in a sample of peripheral venous blood when compared with a reference population. By convention, the normal range is defined as including 95 per cent of the reference population. A general classification of anemias is presented in Table 15.1.

Table 15.1 *A functional classification of anemias*

Hypoproliferative anemias
Myelophthisic (infiltrative)
Marrow aplasia
Chronic disease states
Organ failure
    Renal
    Hepatic
    Hypothyroidism
    Hypopituitarism

Hyperproliferative anemias
Hemorrhage (acute blood loss)
Hemolytic
    Primary membrane defects
    Hemoglobinopathies
    Immune hemolysis
    Toxic hemolysis
    Traumatic (microangiopathic) hemolysis
    Hypersplenism

Maturation defects
Hypochromic anemia
Megaloblastic anemia
Myelodysplastic anemia

Dilutional anemia
Pregnancy
Aggressive fluid resuscitation
Massive splenomegaly

Physiologic features

The signs, symptoms, and physiologic effects of anemia are directly proportional to its rate of development. An abrupt loss of 20–30 per cent of the circulating blood volume from acute gastrointestinal hemorrhage will cause systemic hypotension, a fall in cardiac output and, unless supportive measures are provided immediately, circulatory collapse. Patients with underlying coronary artery disease may experience acute myocardial ischemia or infarction (inadequate supply).

The response to chronic anemia is quite different. In most cases, circulating blood volume is maintained as is systemic blood pressure. Cardiac output is increased, allowing the passage of fewer red blood cells through tissues and vital organs more frequently. A reduced affinity of hemoglobin for oxygen (shift of the oxyhemoglobin dissociation curve to the right) coupled with an increased cellular 2,3-diphosphoglycerate concentration increases oxygen delivery at the tissue level by approximately 30 per cent. These latter two compensatory mechanisms are particularly important in patients with compromised left ventricular performance, in whom cardiac output may not increase significantly. In contrast, severe long-standing anemia (hematocrit <20 per cent) may be responsible for high-output congestive heart failure.

Special considerations in hospitalized patients

Blood loss from frequent phlebotomy and invasive procedures, considered collectively, is the most common cause of anemia in hospitalized patients. Both should be considered and thoroughly assessed before other potential etiologies are explored. However, it is important to acknowledge two broad categories of acquired anemia: aplastic anemia and hemolytic anemia. Either can develop swiftly and have a profound impact on overall clinical status.

Aplastic anemia

The term aplasia refers to a condition of bone marrow characterized by a severe reduction or absence of hematopoietic stem cells. In the majority of cases, anemia is also accompanied by leukopenia and thrombocytopenia; however, pure red blood cell aplasia does occur. A general classification of aplasia anemia is presented in Table 15.2. Nearly half of all cases of aplastic anemia are considered idiopathic in origin. The remaining cases are associated with a broad range of drugs, chemicals, toxins, and infectious agents (Table 15.3).

Table 15.2 *General classification of aplastic anemias*

Acquired
Idiopathic
Autoimmune
Drug-related
Toxins
Infectious
Radiation
Pregnancy
Paroxysmal nocturnal
Hemoglobinuria

Other
Familial
Fanconi's anemia
Dyskeratosis congenita

Table 15.3 *Drugs, chemicals, and toxins associated with aplastic anemia (or pancytopenia)*

1. **Antimicrobial agents**
   Penicillin, sulfonamides, cephalosporins, tetracycline derivatives, amphotericin B, chloramphenicol, streptomycin, methicillin

2. **Antineoplastic agents**
   Antimetabolites, alkylating agents, antimitotic agents, radiation (to active marrow sites)

3. **Anticonvulsants**
   Phenytoin, carbamazepine

4. **Oral hypoglycemic agents**
   Chlorpropamide, tolbutamide

5. **Antithyroid drugs**
   Carbimazole, propylthiouracil

6. **Sedatives and tranquilizers**
   Meprobamate, chlordiazepoxide

7. **Antiarrhythmic agents**
   Procainamide, quinidine

8. **Other drugs**
   Furosemide, acetazolamide, heparin, captopril, ticlopidine

9. **Infections**
   Hepatitis, parvovirus, HIV (other viruses)

10. **Toxic chemicals**
    Solvents (benzene, glue, toluene, carbon tetrachloride), bismuth, mercury, arsenic, alcohol

Acquired hemolytic anemias

Hemolytic anemia is characterized by the premature destruction of essentially normal red blood cells from immunologic, physical, or chemical injury (Table 15.4). In disorders of immune-mediated hemolysis, red blood cell destruction is caused by the binding of antibodies, complement components, or both, to the cell's surface membrane. This phenomenon is typically the result of autoimmunization, alloimmunization, or drug exposure.

Immunoglobulin M (IgM) antibodies are agglutinating, complement fixing, and active in cold temperatures. In contrast, most IgG red blood cell antibodies are fully active at 37°C, have minimal agglutinating potential, and have variable complement-fixing activity. The synthesis of polyclonal cold agglutinins increases in response to infections, including mycoplasma, viruses (Epstein–Barr, cytomegalovirus), and protozoa, as well as lymphoproliferative disorders. Nearly 50 per cent of patients with IgG-mediated autoimmune hemolytic anemia have an underlying neoplastic, lymphoproliferative, collagen vascular, or inflammatory condition.

Alloantibodies capable of destroying transfused (but not autologous) red blood cells are most commonly products of immunologic responses to (1) colonizing

Table 15.4 *General classification of acquired hemolytic anemias*

1. Immune
   a. Autoimmune
   b. Alloimmune
   c. Drug-induced
2. Paroxysmal nocturnal hemoglobinuria
3. Toxins/metabolic abnormalities
4. Red cell trauma (microangiopathic)
5. Red cell parasites
6. Sequestrational hemolysis (hypersplenism)

bacteria of the large intestine, or (2) imperfectly matched transfused red blood cells.

Drug-induced hemolysis can be characterized by several distinct mechanisms.

1 *Drug–red blood cell binding.* In this situation, a drug-specific antibody (typically IgG) is produced and attacks the erythrocyte membrane at sites occupied by the offending drug. The cell is then sequestered in the spleen and destroyed by Fc-receptor-bearing macrophages (e.g. penicillin).

2 *Innocent bystander.* Drugs bound by plasma proteins stimulate the production of drug-specific, complement-fixing antibodies. In turn, C3b generated by these complexes covalently binds to red blood cells, activating the terminal C5–C9 attack complex and causing intravascular hemolysis (e.g. quinidine, sulfonamides, and phenothiazines).

3 *Antierythrocyte antibody.* A pure, drug-induced antierythrocyte IgG antibody is rare but can occur (e.g. methyldopa).

A *direct antiglobulin* (Coomb's) test is most frequently used to detect immunoproteins present on the red blood cell membrane. Almost all patients with immune hemolytic anemia exhibit a positive direct Coomb's test. An indirect *antiglobulin* test (indirect Coomb's) detects circulating antibodies capable of attaching to a normal red blood cell. Overall, the direct Coomb's test is more specific for autoimmune processes.

When circulating red blood cells are subjected to excessive mechanical stress, hemolysis can occur. Abnormalities involving the left side of the heart, particularly those characterized by high pressure and shearing stress, are the most common. These include aortic stenosis, aortic insufficiency, and a ruptured sinus of Valsalva aneurysm. Significant red blood cell fragmentation may also occur as a result of traumatic atrioventricular (AV) fistulas or aortofemoral bypass procedures. Hemolysis secondary to mechanical prosthetic heart valves is less common with the development of low-profile prosthetics; however, paravalvular leaks and malfunctioning valves may predispose to hemolysis.

Excessive shearing forces generated in the microvasculature can cause intravascular hemolysis. In a majority of cases, the vessels are either partially occluded by platelet-fibrin thrombi (e.g. DIC) or the vessel wall itself is abnormal (e.g. malignant hypertension, vasculitis). Occasionally a combination of the two coexist (e.g. thrombotic thrombocytopenia purpura, hemolytic uremic syndrome).

A diagnosis of traumatic hemolysis is supported by the presence of fragmented red blood cells (schistocytes) in the peripheral smear. Reticulocytosis (>5.0 per cent), increased serum lactate dehydrogenase (LHD), and decreased haptoglobin are also common. In DIC, thrombocytopenia, prolonged clotting tests, and detectable evidence in plasma of thrombin generation (prothrombin fragment 1.2) or fibrin formation (and subsequent degradation) (D-dimer) may also be present.

POLYCYTHEMIA

Polycythemia is characterized by an increased red blood cell count as measured by the hematocrit, hemoglobin, and absolute erythrocyte mass. A distinction between *absolute* and *relative* polycythemia should be made when evaluating patients with elevated counts. The former refers to conditions in which there is an absolute increase in total red blood cell mass. Absolute polycythemia can further be subcategorized as *primary* or *secondary*, depending on whether the elevation in red blood cell mass is autonomous (primary polycythemia) or under hormonal (erythropoietin) control (secondary polycythemia) (Table 15.5).

The normal red blood cell mass averages 30±3 mL/kg body weight in men and 27±3 mL/kg in women. Generally, as the hematocrit nears 50 per cent, the proportion of patients with an absolute increase in red

blood cell mass increases but does not achieve complete specificity until the hematocrit exceeds 60 per cent.

THROMBOCYTOPENIA

Under normal conditions, platelets circulate in a concentration between 150 000 and 300 000 cells/mm³ for 7±2 days. The splenic pool compromises nearly one-third of the total concentration of blood platelets and is in dynamic equilibrium with the general circulation. Platelets themselves are manufactured in the bone marrow from percussor megakaryocytes; each megakaryocyte produces between 1000 and 1500 platelets in response to existing physiologic requirements.

Thrombocytopenia is defined as a reduction in the circulating platelet count to below 150 000/mm³. The most common mechanisms include: (1) disorders of production; (2) disorders of distribution or dilution; and (3) platelet destruction. On occasion, a combination of abnormalities may coexist. This is not at all uncommon in critically ill patients.

Disorders of platelet production include decreased megakaryocyte synthesis and ineffective platelet production (Table 15.6). A decrease in the number of megakaryocytes is characteristic of some congenital disorders, marrow damage, or bone marrow replacement (fibrosis, tumors, infection). Isolated megakaryocyte hypoplasia has been observed following exposure to drugs, chemicals, and toxins. It has also occurred following infections and in association with collagen vascular disease, particularly systemic lupus erythematosus. As with many cases of aplastic anemia, megakaryocyte hypoplasia is most often idiopathic in origin. Ineffective platelet production is characterized by an increase in bone marrow megakaryocyte mass and a concomitant decrease in circulating platelets. Only a bone marrow examination can distinguish ineffective platelet production from disorders of peripheral destruction. Drug-induced thrombocytopenia is particularly important in clinical practice (Table 15.7).

Table 15.5 *General classification of polycythemias*

1. Absolute polycythemia
   a. Primary: polycythemia rubra vera
   b. Secondary: decreased O₂ transport, appropriate
      erythropoietin stimulation
      Cyanotic congenital heart disease (R-to-L shunts)
      Pulmonary arteriovenous fistula
      High altitude
      Impaired ventilation (chronic lung disease)
   c. Inappropriate erythropoietin stimulation
      Malignancy (lung, kidney, adrenal, liver)
      Benign tumors (Cushing's syndrome,
         pheochromocytoma, cerebellar)
      Renal: cysts, hydronephrosis

2. Relative polycythemia
   Dehydration
   Burns
   Adrenal insufficiency
   Stress (Gaisback's syndrome)

Table 15.6 *Thrombocytopenia: decreased platelet production*

Decreased megakaryocytes
Congenital (Fanconi's anemia, intrauterine infections)
Acquired hypoplasia (chemicals, drugs, infection, alcohol,
   radiation, collagen vascular disease, idiopathic)
Marrow replacement (metastatic malignancy, myeloma,
   leukemia, lymphoma, myelofibrosis)

Ineffective platelet production
Hereditary (autosomal dominant, Wiskott–Aldrich syndrome,
   May–Hegglin anomaly)
Vitamin B₁₂ or folate deficiency
Preleukemia, paroxysmal nocturnal hemoglobinuria

Table 15.7 *Drug-induced thrombocytopenia*

Reduced platelet production
Cytotoxic drugs (alkylating agents, antimetabolites)
Thiazides
Alcohol
Chloramphenicol, phenylbutazone

Immune-mediated or combined (decreased production and destruction)
Antimicrobials (cephalosporins, penicillins, rifampin, sulfonamides)
Cardiac medication (digoxin, quinidine, nitroglycerin, heparin, amrinone, propranolol)
Neuropsychiatric drugs (desipramine, phenothiazine, diphenylhydantoin, carbamazepine)
Antihypertensives/diuretics (thiazides, furosemide, methyldopa)
Anti-inflammatory drugs (aspirin, acetaminophen, gold salts, phenylbutazone)
Oral hypoglycemic agents (chlorpropamide, tolbutamide)
Other: ranitidine, ticlopidine, abciximab (c7E3), and other platelet GPIIb/IIIa antagonists

Disorders of platelet distribution and dilution can be difficult to diagnose with certainty. They include splenic pooling, usually associated with moderate to marked splenomegaly (congestive, infectious, inflammatory, neoplastic), hypothermia (platelet pooling in hepatic sinusoids), and massive blood transfusions, particularly of stored blood (containing non-viable platelets).

In disorders of platelet destruction and consumption, the degree of thrombocytopenia directly correlates with the bone marrow's ability to compensate by producing and releasing new platelets (Table 15.8).

Table 15.8 *Thrombocytopenia: platelet destruction and consumption*

Isolated platelet consumption
Thrombotic thrombocytopenic purpura
Hemolytic–uremic syndrome
Vasculitis
Cardiopulmonary bypass

Immune destruction
Idiopathic
Alloantibodies (post-transfusion)
Drug-induced
Other (infection, malignancy, collagen vascular disease)

Consumption of coagulation factors and platelets
Disseminated intravascular coagulation
Snake venoms
Tissue injury (necrosis, trauma, surgical)
Obstetric complications
Infection (viral, bacteria, rickettsial)
Neoplasms (promyelocytic leukemia, hemangioma)
Thrombolytic agents

DISORDERS OF PLATELET FUNCTION

Platelets are required for primary hemostasis and also to maintain vascular integrity. Qualitative defects in platelet function can be caused by: (1) decreased adhesion; (2) decreased aggregation; (3) reduced thromboxane synthesis; (4) impaired secretion of platelet granule contents; or (5) an inadequate contribution of platelets to blood coagulation. Disorders of platelet function can be classified broadly as congenital (Table 15.9) and acquired (Table 15.10).

Drug-induced abnormalities in platelet function should be considered strongly in patients with bleeding complications despite a normal platelet count. The most common offending agents include (a) aspirin and other nonsteroidal anti-inflammatory agents, (b) antihista-

Table 15.9 *Congenital disorders of platelet function*

Defects in plasma membrane
Bernard–Soulier syndrome (↓ glycoprotein Ib receptors)
Von Willebrand disease
Glanzmann's thrombasthenia (↓ glycoprotein IIb/IIIa receptors)
Primary platelet coagulant defect (platelet factor 3)

Defects in storage organelles
Dense body deficiency
Idiopathic storage pool disease
Wiskott–Aldrich syndrome
Chediak–Higashi syndrome
Thrombocytopenia with absent radii
Alpha-granule deficiency

Thromboxane deficiency
Cyclooxygenase deficiency
Thromboxane synthase deficiency

Other
Ehlers–Danlos syndrome
Marfan's syndrome
Osteogenesis imperfecta

Table 15.10 *Acquired disorders of platelet function*

Uremia
Myeloproliferative diseases
Acute leukemia
Preleukemia states
Dysproteinemias
Liver disease
Circulating fibrin(ogen) degradation products
Drug-induced
Acquired storage pool deficiency
    Autoimmune disorders
    Severe burns
    Cardiopulmonary bypass
    Disseminated intravascular coagulation
    Valvular heart disease

mines, (c) phenothiazines, (d) dextran, (e) heparin, (f) antimicrobial agents (penicillins, cephalosporins), (g) ethanol, and (h) radiographic contrast agents.

THROMBOCYTOSIS

Thrombocytosis refers to an elevation in the platelet count above 400 000/mm³. Three forms have been recognized: (1) *physiologic*; (2) *reactive* (also known as secondary thrombocytosis); and (3) *primary*.

Physiologic thrombocytosis can occur after vigorous physical exertion or stress. Epinephrine administration can elevate the platelet count by 20–30 per cent. In most instances, physiologic thrombocytosis is caused by increased mobilization of platelets rather than increased production. In contrast, reactive thrombocytosis is characterized by accelerated platelet production in response to acute/subacute hemorrhage, acute/chronic inflammation, hemolysis, malignancy, iron deficiency, splenectomy, or prior moderate to severe thrombocytopenia (rebound phenomenon). It is rare for platelet counts to exceed 1 million/mm³. Despite the observed elevation, thrombotic (and hemorrhagic) complications are rare; therefore, treatment should focus on the underlying condition or disorder rather than on the platelet count.

Essential (primary) thrombocythemia is a myeloproliferative disorder characterized by a persistent and marked elevation in platelet count to levels above 1 million/mm³. In essential thrombocythemia, increased platelet production occurs independent of normal regulatory processes; however, other cell lines are unaffected, distinguishing it from polycythemia rubra vera and other myeloproliferative disorders.

LEUKOPENIA

Under normal circumstances the peripheral white blood cell count ranges from 5000 to 10 000/mm³, and includes neutrophils, lymphocytes, monocytes, eosinophils, and basophils. A differential count allows abnormalities of individual components to be determined.

Neutropenia is defined as a peripheral neutrophil count below 2000/mm³. Counts greater than 1000/mm³, under most circumstances, provide adequate protection against infection; however, counts below 500/mm³ are associated with an increased risk of serious infection. A list of conditions and disorders associated with neutropenia is found in Table 15.11.

LEUKOCYTOSIS

White blood cell counts above 11 000/mm³ are common in hospitalized patients. Counts in excess of 25 000/mm³

Table 15.11 *General causes of neutropenia*

Abnormalities of bone marrow
Drugs
- Antiarrhythmics: procainamide, quinidine, propranolol
- Antibiotics: penicillins, sulfonamides, trimethoprim-sulfa, metronidazole
- Phenothiazine: chlorpromazine, prochlorperazine
- Antithyroid agents: methimazole, propylthiouracil
- Antihypertensives: captopril, methyldopa
- Antihistamines: cimetidine, ranitidine
- Anticonvulsants: phenytoin, carbamazepine
- Diuretics: hydrochlorothiazide, acetazolamide
- Cytotoxic agents: hydroxyurea, alkylating agents, antimetabolites
- Other: alcohol, allopurinol, alpha-interferon

Chemicals (arsenic, bismuth, nitrous oxide, benzene)
Radiation
Congenital/hereditary neutropenia
Infection (viral, bacterial)
Infiltrative diseases (metastatic malignancy, fibrosis, CML)
Maturation defects
- Neoplastic (myelodysplastic syndromes, acute non-lymphocytic leukemia)
- Acquired (folic acid/B_{12} deficiency)

Abnormalities in peripheral blood
Shift from circulating to marginated pool
- Hereditary pseudoneutropenia
- Protein calorie malnutrition
- Severe bacterial infections

Sequestration
- Hypersplenism
- Leukoagglutination (complement-mediated)

Abnormalities in extravascular compartment
Destruction (antibody-mediated)
Increased utilization (infection, anaphylaxis)

CML = chronic myelogenous leukemia.

are characterized as a *leukemoid reaction*. Most often, the excess consists predominantly of neutrophils (neutrophilia); however, lymphocytosis, monocytosis, basophilia, and eosinophilia can also occur.

Neutrophilia (>7500/mm³) occurs as a result of changes in the bone marrow, peripheral blood, or extravascular space. Infection and inflammatory states are the most common causes, but many other etiologies exist (Table 15.12).

Lymphocytosis (>5000/mm³) is associated with a variety of infectious (viral, brucellosis, tuberculosis, toxoplasmosis, typhoid fever), malignant (solid tumors, Hodgkin's lymphoma, chronic lymphocytic leukemia, acute lymphocytic leukemia), and endocrine (thyrotoxicosis) diseases.

Monocytosis (>500/mm³) is observed in the following circumstances: infection (brucellosis, tuberculosis, syphilis, bacterial endocarditis, protozoal, fungal), neoplastic disease (Hodgkin's lymphoma, myelomonocytic leukemias), gastrointestinal illness (cirrhosis, ulcerative

Table 15.12 *Common causes of neutrophilia*

Infections
Bacteria
Viruses
Parasites
Fungi

Neoplastic disorders
Pancreas, lung, renal
Metastatic disease to bone marrow
Chronic myeloproliferative disorders
Hodgkin's disease
Acute leukemia

Autoimmune disorders
Vasculitis
Ulcerative colitis
Collagen vascular diseases

Hematologic disorders
Acute hemolysis
Transfusion reactions
Postsplenectomy

Drugs
Corticosteroids
Lithium chloride
Epinephrine
Chemicals
    Venoms (reptiles, insects)
    Ethylene glycol

Trauma
Thermal injury
Crush injuries
Electrical shock

Endocrine disorders
Ketoacidosis
Thyrotoxicosis
Lactic acidosis

Systemic inflammatory reactions

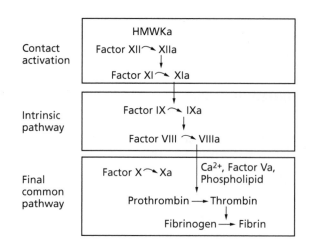

Figure 15.1 *The intrinsic coagulation (pathway) is initiated by contact activation through a series of enzymatic steps involving the activation of coagulation proteins; fibrinogen is converted to fibrin in the final common pathway. HMWKA = high-molecular-weight kininogen.*

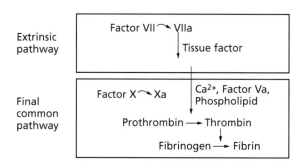

Figure 15.2 *The extrinsic coagulation cascade (pathway) is initiated by tissue factor expression, which combined with Factor VIIa activates the final common pathway and ultimately leads to fibrin generation.*

colitis), drug reactions, and recovery from bone marrow suppression.

Eosinophilia ($>400/\text{mm}^3$) is associated with a wide variety of infectious, allergic, connective tissue, cutaneous, and inflammatory disorders.

Basophilia ($>150/\text{mm}^3$) is relatively uncommon but specific for an underlying abnormality, such as myeloproliferative disorders, or paraneoplastic syndromes.

BLOOD COAGULATION AND HEMOSTASIS

Blood normally circulates through endothelium-lined vessels without appreciable coagulation taking place. Vascular injury triggers the hemostatic process, typically beginning with platelet adherence to damaged or dysfunctional endothelium or exposed subendothelium.

Concomitantly, plasma proteins react with the sub-endothelium, initiating the coagulation cascade (Figs 15.1 and 15.2). In pathologic conditions, platelet-vessel wall (or plaque) interactions initiate local thrombus formation, either causing an immediate impedance to physiologic blood flow or serving as a nidus for subsequent vascular events.

VASCULAR ENDOTHELIUM

The vascular endothelium is structurally simple but functionally complex; more so than previously appreciated. Its integrity is essential for normal vessel responsiveness (vasoconstriction/vasodilation) and thromboresistance. Until recently, the vascular endothelium was thought to represent no more than a protective barrier, separating platelets and the contact-activated coagulation factors from thrombogenic sub-endothelial connective tissues. It is now known that the endothelial lining is, in fact, a multifunctional (multi-dimensional) organ system composed of metabolically active and physiologically responsive component cells. Moreover, we now appreciate that vascular endothelial cells are susceptible to injury (biochemical or mechanical), which may be relevant to certain disease processes such as coronary atherosclerosis.

Structural anatomy

Vascular endothelial cells form a single layer of simple squamous lining cells (0.1–0.5 μm in thickness, and elongated in the long axis of the vessel, thus orienting the cellular longitudinal dimension in the direction of blood flow).

The endothelial cell has three surfaces: non-thrombogenic (luminal), adhesive (subluminal), and cohesive. The *luminal* surface is non-thrombogenic and devoid of any electron-dense connective tissue. It does, however, possess an exterior coat, or glycocalyx, which consists primarily of starches and proteins secreted by the endothelial cells: oligosaccharides, glycoproteins, glyco-lipids, and sialoconugates. Plasma proteins, including lipoprotein lipase, α_2-macroglobulin, antithrombin, heparin cofactor II, albumin, and small amounts of fib-rinogen and fibrin are adsorbed to the luminal surface. The luminal membrane itself adds significantly to the thromboresistant properties by carrying a negative charge that repels similarly charged circulating blood cells.

The *subluminal* (or abluminal) surface adheres to the connective tissue of the subendothelial zone. Small processes penetrate throughout a series of internal layers to form myoendothelial junctions with subjacent smooth muscle cells.

The third surface of the vascular endothelium is *cohesive*, joining endothelial cells to one another by cell junctions of two basic types: occluding (tight) junctions and communicating (gap) junctions. Occluding junctions represent a physical link between two adjoining cells, sealing the intercellular space. The communicating junctions provide the structural substrate for direct two-way communication between cells; they are instrumental in the electronic coupling and intracellular exchange of ions and small metabolites.

Biology

As an active site of protein synthesis, the vascular endothelium may be considered the largest and most productive organ system in the human body. Endothelial cells synthesize, secrete, modify, and regulate connective tissue components, vasodilators, and vasoconstrictors, anticoagulants, procoagulants, fibrinolytic compounds, and prostanoids, each contributing to the maintenance of normal vasomotion, thromboresistance, and physiologic hemostasis (Figs 15.3 and 15.4 a,b).

PROSTACYCLIN

Prostacyclin (PGI$_2$) is a potent vasodilating substance released locally in response to biochemical and mechan-

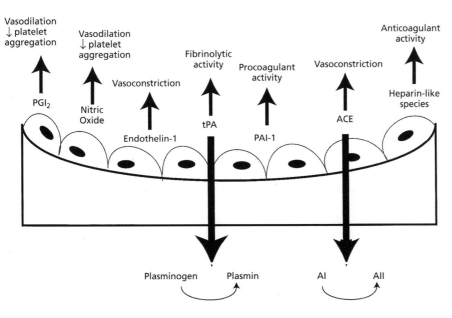

Figure 15.3 *The vascular endothelium is one of the body's most active organs, synthesizing and secreting proteins that are responsible for and that regulate both natural thromboresistance and vasoreactivity. There exists a delicate balance of vascular tone and hemostatic potential.*
PGI$_2$ = prostacyclin; tPA = tissue plasminogen activator; PAI-1 = plasminogen activator inhibitor-1; ACE = angiotensin-converting enzyme; AI = angiotensin I; AII = angiotensin II.

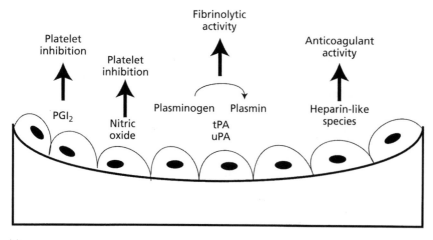

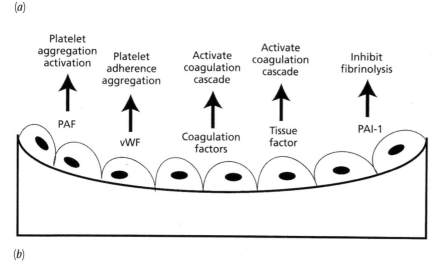

Figure 15.4 *(a) The vascular endothelium normally prevents or limits intravascular thrombosis through the synthesis and secretion of thromboresistant proteins. (b) Damaged or dysfunctional endothelial cells may promote thrombus formation through platelet activation, coagulation, and impaired fibrinolytic activity. PGI$_2$ = prostacyclin; tPA = tissue plasminogen activator; uPA = urokinase-like plasminogen activator; PAF = platelet activating factor; vWF = von Willebrand factor; PAI-1 = plasminogen activator inhibitor-1.*

ical medicators including thromboxane A$_2$, thrombin, bradykinin, histamine, high-density lipoprotein, platelet-derived growth factor, tissue hypoxia, and hemodynamic stress.[32] By increasing intracellular cyclic adenosine monophosphate (cAMP), PGI$_2$ also inhibits platelet aggregation. Furthermore, there is evidence that PGI$_2$ increases the rate of smooth muscle cell cholesterol ester metabolism, suppresses lipid metabolism within macrophages, and inhibits the release of growth factors, which mediate proliferative responses to intravascular shear stress.[33]

NITRIC OXIDE (ENDOTHELIUM-DERIVED RELAXING FACTOR)

Utilizing strips of arteries in organ baths (isolated system), Furchgott and Zawadski[34] discovered that acetylcholine-mediated vasodilation requires an intact vascular endothelium, i.e. it is endothelium dependent. Endothelium-derived relaxing factor (EDRF), recently identified as nitric oxide,[35] is an L-arginine derivative that

relaxes smooth muscles by increasing intracellular cyclic guanosine monophosphate (cAMP). It is released locally in response to a number of mediators, including thrombin, bradykinin, thromboxane A$_2$, histamine, adenine nucleotides, and aggregating platelets. In addition to vasoactive properties, EDRF is also a potent inhibitor of platelet adhesion[36] and aggregation.[37] Moreover, EDRF and PGI$_2$ appear to have synergistic antiaggregatory properties.

ANGIOTENSIN II

Angiotensin II is a potent vasoconstrictor that exerts an important effect on vascular tone.[38] Although the systemic properties of angiotensin II have been known for some time, local synthesis, release, and vascular activity have just recently been appreciated. Angiotensin-converting enzyme (ACE), required for the conversion of angiotensin I to the active peptide angiotensin II, has been isolated from mammalian arteries and veins. While there has been some debate, most studies suggest that

ACE is synthesized within vascular endothelial cells. Moreover, there is mounting evidence that endothelial cells are also capable of producing enzymes other than or in addition to ACE capable of angiotensin II generation.[39]

ENDOTHELIN

The vascular endothelium, in addition to synthesizing vasodilating substances, such as PGI_2 and nitric oxide, also produces vasoconstrictors essential for maintaining vessel tone and responsiveness. Endothelin, a small peptide, has vasoconstricting properties ten times those of angiotensin II.[40] Although three structurally and pharmacologically distinct isopeptides have been isolated and characterized, only endothelin-1 is synthesized by vascular endothelial cells.[41] While a majority of vasoactive mediators are released in surges following local mechanical or biochemical stimulation, endothelin-1 is released slowly and, via specific receptor-mediated mechanisms, activates intracellular protein kinase C,[42] leading to smooth muscle contraction (vasoconstriction).

PLASMINOGEN ACTIVATORS

Vascular endothelial cells synthesize and release activators that are capable of converting plasminogen to the serine protease plasmin, an enzyme that proteolytically degrades fibrin (and fibrinogen). Tissue plasminogen activator and urokinase-type plasminogen activator generate plasmin locally; therefore, fibrinolysis is limited to the immediate local environment. Stimuli for the release of vascular plasminogen activators include epinephrine, thrombin, heparin, interleukin-1, venous occlusion, aggregating platelets, and desamino-8-D-arginine vasopressin (DDAVP).

HEPARIN-LIKE SPECIES

In the past, mast cells were thought to be the only cells capable of synthesizing anticoagulant-active heparin. Investigations performed by Teien,[43] Thomas,[44] and Marcum and Rosenberg[45] have shown, however, that endothelial cells are capable of synthesizing heparin-like molecules, e.g. heparan sulfate, with anticoagulant properties. As a result, it is currently accepted that thromboresistance is mediated, at least in part, through the interaction of heparin-like substances with antithrombin and heparin co-factor II (both located on the endothelial surface), accelerating the neutralization of hemostatic (procoagulant) proteins.

PLATELET-ACTIVATING FACTOR

A lipid capable of inducing platelet aggregation and secretion in a concentration-dependent fashion, platelet-activating factor (PAF) mobilizes platelet surface membrane arachidonic acid, which stimulates thromboxane A_2 synthesis.

TISSUE FACTOR

Tissue factor, also known as tissue thromboplastin, is a lipoprotein present in large quantities in a number of organ systems, including the brain and lung parenchyma. Although tissue factor is, under normal conditions, produced by endothelial cells in small amounts, synthesis can be increased markedly after mechanical or biochemical stimulation, accelerating the activation of Factor X by Factor VIIa.[46,47]

TISSUE FACTOR PATHWAY INHIBITOR

Tissue factor pathway inhibitor (TFPI) I is also located on the endothelial surface. It acts against the combined action of tissue thromboplastin (tissue factor) and Factor VII in the presence of Factor Xa. The proposed mechanism for inhibition of tissue factor-Factor VIIa involves the formation of a quaternary complex with TFPI and Factor X in a two-step reaction: Factor Xa generated by tissue factor–Factor VIIa binds reversibly with TFPI and the binary complex formed binds, in a calcium-dependent manner, to membrane-bound tissue factor–Factor VIIa.[48] In essence, TFPI prevents the extrinsic coagulation cascade from activating the prothrombinase complex; however, it has also be recognized that TFPI inhibits the intrinsic coagulation cascade, supporting the role of tissue factor of Factor VIIa and Factor IX-mediated clotting.[49] Factor IX also impairs TFPI-mediated inhibition or tissue factor–Factor VIIa.

In the presence of glycosaminoglycans, including heparin, heparan sulfate, and dextran sulfate, the inhibiting activity of TFPI is increased.[50]

Tissue factor pathway inhibitor 2

A second human TFPI has recently been identified and characterized.[51] TFPI-2 is found within human umbilical vein endothelial cells, the liver and the placenta and has been shown to inhibit tissue factor–Factor VIIa, kallikrein, Factor XIa, and Factor X activation by Factor IXa.[52] It does not independently (in the absence of heparin) inactivate Factor Xa or thrombin.

ANNEXIN V

Annexins are an interesting family of non-glycosylated proteins that bind to negatively charged phospholipids, including phosphatidylserine and phosphatidylethanolamine.[53] One of the 13 recognized annexins, annexin V, is recognized as a potent endothelial surface anticoagulant based on its ability to displace phospholipid-dependent coagulation factors. It also reduces platelet adhesion.

VON WILLEBRAND FACTOR

Circulating in plasma as a series of self-aggregated structures composed of a single glycoprotein subunit, von Willebrand factor is a vital component of normal hemostasis that mediates both platelet–vessel wall interactions and platelet–platelet interactions.[54]

PLASMINOGEN ACTIVATOR INHIBITOR

Plasminogen activator inhibitor 1 (PAI-1) is a single-chain glycoprotein that forms stable complexes with tissue plasminogen activator and urokinase-type plasminogen activator, inhibiting their fibrinolytic activity.[55] Endothelial cells are able to increase PAI-1 production and do so following administration of exogenous tissue plasminogen activator (tPA), or after direct exposure to platelet lysates or compounds released from activated platelets (epidermal growth factor, transforming growth factor β).[56]

PLATELETS

Despite being simple in appearance, platelets are complex cellular elements with complicated structural and functional characteristics.

Structural anatomy

1 The *peripheral zone* consists of membranes and closely associated structures that provide surfaces for the platelet itself and the tortuous channels of the open canalicular system. The peripheral zone consists of three distinct structural domains: the exterior coat, the unit membrane, and the submembrane region.

The exterior coat, or *glycocalyx*, is rich in glycoproteins (GP). Recent biochemical studies have identified nine distinct glycoproteins: Ia, Ib, Ic, IIa, IIb, IIIa, IV, V, and IX. Many glycoproteins act as receptors for platelet–platelet and platelet–vessel wall interactions (Table 15.13).

The *unit membrane* provides a physiochemical separation between intracellular and extracellular constituents and processes. Important components of the unit membrane include Na^+/K^+, adenosine triphosphatase (ATPase), and other anion or cation pumps that maintain transmembrane ionic gradients.

The *submembrane region* contains a specialized filamentous system similar to actin microfilaments. Functionally submembrane filaments assist circumferential microtubules, maintaining platelet discoid shape, controlling pseudopod extrusion, and interacting with other elements of the platelet contractile mechanism.

Table 15.13 *Platelet surface membrane glycoprotein (GP) receptors*

Receptor	Ligand	Integrin components	Biologic action
GPIa–IIa	Collagen	$\alpha_2\beta_1$	Adhesion
GPIb–IX	Von Willebrand factor	—	Adhesion
GPIc–IIa	Fibronectin	$\alpha_2\beta_1$	Adhesion
GPIIb–IIIa	Collagen	$\alpha_{IIb}\beta_3$	Aggregation
	Fibrinogen		(2° role in adhesion)
	Fibronectin		
	Vitronectin		
	Von Willebrand factor		
GPIV (GPIIIb)	Thrombuspondin	—	Adhesion
	Collagen		
Vitronectin receptor	Vitronectin	$\alpha_v\beta_3$	Adhesion
	Thrombospondin		
VLA-6	Laminin	$\alpha_6\beta_1$	Adhesion

2 The *sol–gel zone* is the matrix of the platelet cytoplasm. It contains several fiber systems in various states of polymerization, maintaining the discoid shape of non-stimulated platelets and providing the intricate contractile system required to initiate shape change, pseudopod extension, internal contraction, and secretion.

3 The *organelle zone* consists of granules, electron-dense bodies, peroxisomes, lysosomes, and mitochondria randomly dispersed in the platelet cytoplasm. It is centrally involved with metabolic processes and also acts as a storage site for enzymes, adenine nucleotides, serotonin, calcium, and a variety of protein constituents.

Membrane systems

The platelet membrane systems include a surface-connected canalicular system, which provides access for plasma-borne substances to the platelet interior and an exit route for products of the release reaction, and a dense tubular system, which acts as a site for calcium sequestration and for storing prostaglandin precursors.

Normal platelet physiology

PLATELET ADHESION

Platelet surface membrane receptors are essential for adhesion. Glycoprotein Ia (GPIa) binds with collagen at low shear rates and may also contribute to platelet adherence in areas of vascular damage. Glycoprotein Ib (GPIb) serves as a binding site for von Willebrand factor, particularly at high shear rates. Glycoprotein IIb/IIIa (GPIIb/IIIa) may also participate in platelet adhesion within areas of high shear rate (Fig. 15.5).

PLATELET AGGREGATION

Activated platelets undergo a progressive change in shape and release calcium from the dense tubular system. Adenosine diphosphate (ADP), serotonin, and thromboxane A_2 are subsequently released, exposing platelet receptors for fibrinogen, the molecular 'glue' for platelet aggregation (Fig. 15.6).

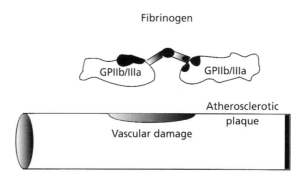

Figure 15.6 *Platelet aggregation is mediated by fibrinogen that binds adjacent platelets via their glycoprotein (GP) IIb/IIIa receptors.*

PLATELET–COAGULATION PROTEIN INTERACTIONS

Beyond their ability to provide coagulation proteins, including Factors II, V, VII, IX, X, XI, and XIII, high-molecular-weight kininogen, and fibrinogen, platelets contain specific receptors for a number of circulating hemostatic proteases and can also trigger contact-activated coagulation. Moreover, platelets provide a protective nidus for activated clotting factors from circulating plasma inhibitors[57] (Fig. 15.7).

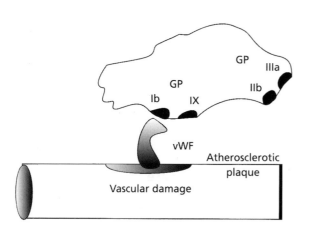

Figure 15.5 *Platelet adhesion occurs at sites of vascular injury and is mediated by von Willebrand factor (vWF) that binds to the platelets surface via the glycoprotein (GP) Ib/IX complex.*

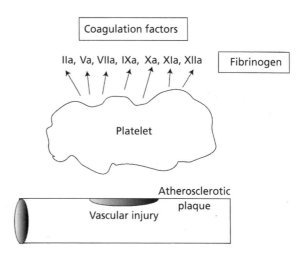

Figure 15.7 *Following platelet adhesion, aggregation, and activation coagulation proteins are expressed on the platelet surface and contribute directly to thrombus growth.*

Platelet–lipid interactions

Hypercholesterolemia has been shown to influence platelet activity. Increased adhesion, aggregation, and serotonin release have been reported,[58] as have increased circulating levels or the potent platelet agonist thromboxane A$_2$[59] and decreased sensitivity to the platelet-inhibiting properties of PGI$_2$. Cholesterol feeding is associated with increased platelet activatability;[60,61] however, a reduction of cholesterol through either dietary or pharmacologic means returns platelet activity to its normal state.[62]

Although the mechanism(s) underlying the relation between serum cholesterol concentration and platelet activity are not fully understood, it has been shown that changes in the cholesterol content of the platelet surface membrane profoundly affect overall membrane fluidity. In turn, fluidity, or the cells' lipid–water interface, influences lipase activity. Therefore, it has been proposed that hypercholesterolemia-mediated increases in the cholesterol content of the platelet surface membrane enhance diglyceride lipase or phospholipase A$_2$ activity (or both), which increases the release of arachidonic acid, the substrate for thromboxane A$_2$ synthesis.[63,64]

Hypercholesterolemia and atherosclerosis impair endothelium-dependent relaxation of major epicardial coronary arteries. Although marked intimal atherosclerosis is frequently observed in these vessels, the endothelium is morphologically intact; however, it fails to release nitric oxide, a potent vasodilator and inhibitor of platelet aggregation.[65,66] It is widely believed, therefore, that hypercholesterolemia in and of itself may directly impair vascular endothelial cell function and enhance platelet–vessel wall interactions prior to the development of overt atherosclerosis.[67]

Platelet–leukocyte interactions

It might be stated that platelets are to thrombosis as leukocytes are to inflammation. However, over the past decade there has been increasing recognition that inflammation and thrombosis are linked at several levels. Study of the modulating effects of neutrophils and platelets on one another became possible with improved methods for the preparation of platelet-free neutrophils and platelet-rich plasma.[68] Early studies focused on the ability of platelets or neutrophils to enhance each other's response to an aggregating agonist. Reintroduction of platelets to a neutrophil preparation increased the neutrophil aggregation response to various chemotactic agents.[69] Similarly reintroduction of activated neutrophils to a platelet preparation caused either direct platelet aggregation or increased the response to various agonists.[70]

Neutrophil-mediated cytotoxicity, oxidant production, lysosome release, and arachidonic acid metabolism are all increased in the presence of platelets.[71] Platelets activated by PAF have increased calcium mobilization and thromboxane b$_2$ release in the presence of activated neutrophils.

The capacity of platelets and leukocytes to modulate one another's activity is potentially explained by one or more mechanisms: (1) release of soluble mediators; (2) metabolism of released mediators; (3) presentation of surface bound mediators; and (4) direct cell adhesion.

INHERITED DISORDERS OF BLOOD COAGULATION

Classic hemophilia

Classic hemophilia, also sometimes referred to as hemophilia A, is a lifelong hemorrhagic disease inherited as a chromosome-linked disorder, and thus limited almost exclusively to males. A coagulant defect in classic hemophilia is the functional deficiency of Factor VIII (antihemophilic factor). The diagnosis is suggested by an abnormally prolonged activated partial thromboplastin time (aPTT) and a normal prothrombin time. The bleeding time is usually normal. These tests allow a semiquantitative estimation of the degree of the coagulant defect, which in most instances parallels the severity of the patient's symptoms. Classic hemophilia must be distinguished from von Willebrand disease (to be discussed in a subsequent section), in which a coagulant deficiency of Factor VIII is coupled with a long bleeding time and impaired aggregation of platelets upon addition of ristocetin to platelet-rich plasma.

Classic hemophilia is the most common genetic (inherited) coagulation defect and has been recorded in all ethnic groups in the world. The overall incidence is approximately 10 persons per 100 000 population.[72]

Christmas disease

Christmas disease, sometimes referred to as hemophilia B, is also a lifelong hemorrhagic disease inherited as a chromosome-linked disorder. The coagulant defect is the functional deficiency of Factor IX. Like classic hemophilia, the diagnosis is suggested by an abnormally prolonged aPTT and a normal prothrombin time.[73]

Von Willebrand disease

The description of a severe bleeding disorder in families by Eric von Willebrand dates back to the mid-1920s[74] and was the first report of a hemorrhagic disorder affecting both sexes. The anomaly was characterized by a prolonged bleeding time despite normal platelet counts and normal clot retraction. Patients with von Willebrand disease have a deficiency of Factor VIII and plasma von Willebrand Factor antigen (VIII: VWF).

TYPE I

Type I von Willebrand disease is the most prevalent variation (70–80 per cent of cases). The plasma levels of both VWF and Factor VIII are moderately decreased (all multimers are present, yet in reduced amounts).

TYPE II

Type II von Willebrand disease, responsible for 20 per cent of cases, is characterized by a qualitative defect in the VWF molecule. This may reduce platelet receptor binding (IIa) or increased binding (IIb), leading to decreased plasma concentrations. Mild to moderate thrombocytopenia is common.

TYPE III

Type III von Willebrand disease is the rarest of all variants and because of very low (or absent) plasma concentrations of both VWF and Factor VIII predisposes to severe or life-threatening spontaneous hemorrhage.

The laboratory evaluation of patient's with suspected von Willebrand disease includes a bleeding time, VIII:C, von Willebrand antigen assay, ristocetin co-factor activity, ristocetin-induced platelet aggregation, and a platelet count. Typically one or more of these tests are abnormal. On rare occasions, the tests are normal in patients with mild disease. It may be necessary in mild cases to repeat the tests several times to establish the diagnosis successfully. It is important to bear in mind that, in most patients with von Willebrand disease, the aPTT is prolonged yet this test may be normal in patients with mild disease who have normal or nearly normal Factor VIII:C. It is also important to recognize that standard aPTT reagents vary in their sensitivity to Factor VIII concentrations.

Hereditary defects of the early intrinsic pathway

Three congenital coagulation defects involving the intrinsic pathway of coagulation are characterized by prolongation of the aPTT in the absence of bleeding. These disorders including Hageman (Factor XII) deficiency, plasma prekallikrein (Fletcher trait) deficiency, and high-molecular-weight kininogen (Fitzgerald trait) deficiency all involve the earliest stages of coagulation. The Hageman trait, inherited as an autosomal recessive defect is the most common cause of a modest prolongation of the aPTT in apparently normal individuals. Plasma prekallikrein deficiency is much more rare. High-molecular-weight kininogen deficiency is the most rare.

Factor XI deficiency

Factor XI deficiency is inherited as an autosomal recessive trait. In most instances bleeding follows moderate to severe trauma or a surgical procedure. The disorder is more common in individuals of Eastern European descent. The aPTT is abnormally prolonged and the prothrombin time is normal. A specific assay (for Factor XI) confirms the diagnosis.

Prothrombin deficiency

Hereditary deficiency (functional) of prothrombin is a rare coagulation defect. It is inherited as an autosomal recessive trait. The diagnosis is suggested by a prolonged prothrombin time and established by specific coagulation factor assays.

Factor VII deficiency

Factor VII deficiency is a rare hereditary coagulation disorder that is inherited as an autosomal recessive trait. The prothrombin time is prolonged and the diagnosis is made by an assay specific for Factor VII. Factor VII deficiency has also been associated with congenital hyperbilirubinemia and Dubin–Johnson syndrome.

Factor V deficiency

Factor V deficiency is a rare hereditary disorder that appears to be transmitted as an autosomal recessive trait. It generally presents as a mild bleeding disorder in childhood. Homozygotes tend to bleed more often and with greater severity. The prothrombin time is prolonged and the diagnosis is confirmed by an assay specific for Factor V.

Factor X deficiency

Factor X deficiency is a rare coagulation abnormality with only a few reported cases. In most patients, coagulation is abnormally prolonged in the presence of Russell's viper venom, which contains an activator of Factor X. This disorder occurs in both sexes and is transmitted as an autosomal recessive trait. Hemorrhagic tendencies are similar to those of classic hemophilia.

Factor XIII deficiency

Factor XIII is the precursor of an enzyme (factor XIIIa) that covalently bonds fibrin monomers. There have been a number of reports of congenital deficiencies, however, the mode of inheritance is still in question. The perponderence of male patients suggests the possibility of a sex-linked disorder. The diagnosis of Factor XIII deficiency is indicated by the solubility of clots in 5 M urea or 1 per cent monocloroacetic acid (which disrupts fibrin that has not been covalently linked). Determination of enzyme levels is now possible using simple rate assays.

COMBINED COAGULATION DEFECTS

Individuals containing 2 or more coagulation factor defects have been described in a wide variety of combinations. Overall, however, these disorders are rare. None of the combined defects with the exception of Factor V/VIII deficiency have been reported in any more than a few families.

Congenital afibrinogenemia

Afibrinogenemia is a rare coagulation disorder that is inherited as an autosomal recessive trait. The abnormality should be considered in the presence of prolonged thrombin time in patients with an unexplained prolongation of the prothrombin and/or partial thromboplastin times. A diagnosis is made by fibrinogen assay.

Hypofibrinogenemia

Congenital hypofibrinogenemia most likely represents the heterozygote state of afibrinogenemia. The concentration of fibrinogen typically ranges from 10 to 50 mg/dL.

Dysfibrinogenemia

Dysfibrinogenemia describes a qualitative defect in the fibrinogen molecule. Many variants have been described, each named for the city in which the defect was first discovered. Bleeding tends to be mild and usually occurs after surgery or trauma. Paradoxically there is also a tendency to thrombosis, perhaps because of the lack of an antithrombotic effect of normal fibrin.

COAGULATION ABNORMALITIES ASSOCIATED WITH CIRCULATING INHIBITORS

Inhibitors against Factors VIII and IX

In a majority of instances, inhibitors against Factors VIII and IX are found in individuals with either classic hemophilia or Christmas disease (as a complication of transfusion therapy). In classic hemophilia, this complication occurs in 5–10 per cent of patients, while in Christmas

disease, it is seen in 1–3 per cent in patients. In both conditions, a majority of antibodies develop in patients with severe disease and very low factor concentrations. Inhibitors are almost all immunoglobulins of the IgG subclass, although a few IgA and IgM inhibitors have been described.

Factor VIII inhibitors have been described in postpartum women and in patients with immunologic disorders (associated with malignancies or drug reactions). However, in rare instances there has been no underlying condition. In almost all cases the inhibitor was discovered because of the onset of bleeding and is almost always IgG. The natural course of the inhibitors is variable.

Acquired Factor IX inhibitors (in the absence of Christmas disease) is a very rare condition. Inhibitors underlying immunologic disorder and/or malignancy should be considered.

Inhibitors against von Willebrand factor

Antibodies directed against the von Willebrand factor portion of Factor VIII:VWF occur in patients with von Willebrand disease as well as in individuals without this disorder. Antibodies are almost always polyclonal IgG. Conditions have been associated with abnormalities in the structure or function in VWF include congenital cardiac defects and acquired valvular disease. There have also been several reported cases of acquired von Willebrand disease associated with hypothyroidism.

Factor V inhibitors

Factor V inhibitors are rare but have been reported in association with antibiotic administration, particularly streptomycin, and other aminoglycosides. Other associated conditions include tuberculosis, pancreatic disease and malignancy. The presence of an inhibitor to Factor V causes prolongation of the prothrombin and partial thromboplastin times. The thrombin time is normal. In most instances the inhibitor is IgG, although IgM and IgA inhibitors have been reported.

Factor VII inhibitors

Acquired Factor VII inhibitors are extremely rare.

Factor X, XI and XII inhibitors

Factor X, XI and XII inhibitors are very rare, although several cases have appeared in the literature. In most cases there is underlying collagen vascular disease, particularly systemic lupus erythematosus.

Inhibitors of prothrombin

Hypoprothrombinemia has been noted in some individuals with systemic lupus erythematosus with a circulating lupus anticoagulant.

Lupus anticoagulants and antiphospholipid antibodies

The term lupus anticoagulant refers to an acquired antibody that prolongs phospholipid-dependent coagulation tests without inhibiting the activity of specific coagulation factors. Thus, the prothrombin time, aPTT, Russell's viper venom time, and one-stage coagulation factor assays (based on these tests) may be abnormal. Prolongation of the aPTT is most common, while prolongation of the prothrombin occurs rarely. Indeed, an abnormality of the latter suggests a presence of hypoprothrombinemia, which may be present in as many as 25 per cent of patients. Despite abnormalities in coagulation tests, these individuals are *not* at risk for hemorrhage. Paradoxically they are at risk for thrombosis.

Acquired disorders of coagulation

Acquired disorders of coagulation are commonly associated with a new condition, disease process, or medication. The coagulation disorder may be due to defective synthesis, increased loss, or the presence of circulating substance (including pharmacologic agents) that interfere with the normal function of one or more vital hemostatic components.

Liver disease

Fibrinogen synthesis is impaired in both acute and chronic liver disease. In addition, the fibrinogen molecule itself is frequently dysfunctional, displaying defective polymerization.[75] The liver is also a primary source of prothrombin and coagulation Factors VII, IX, and X. Vitamin-K-dependent carboxylation, a process occurring in hepatic microsomes, is defective in liver disease, preventing the synthesis of functionally normal coagulation proteins (carboxy forms of Factors II, VII, IX, and X cannot bind calcium and therefore cannot participate in normal hemostasis). Interestingly, defective carboxylation is one of the earliest signs of liver dysfunction. Factor V is partially synthesized by hepatocytes and partially in hepatic reticuloendothelial cells. As a result, low levels of Factor V are found in acute liver failure. Plasminogen and antithrombin levels are also decreased in liver disease. Under normal circumstances the liver metabolizes activated coagulation factors from circulating blood.[76] In addition, it effectively clears both fibrin(ogen) degradation products (FDP) and plasminogen activators. Accordingly, the biochemical environment observed in patients with liver disease is both procoagulant and anticoagulant. However, this unique situation commonly favors anticoagulation. Platelet abnormalities, both qualitative and quantitative, add to the increased bleeding tendency.

Renal disease

Thrombocytopenia is common in renal disease and reflects a combination of reduced production and peripheral consumption. Platelet dysfunction also occurs and is thought to represent a defect in the platelet release reaction.[77] An imbalance between vascular prostacyclin synthesis and platelet thromboxane synthesis may also contribute.[78]

Despite increased fibrinogen and Factor VIII levels in patients with renal disease, prolongation of the prothrombin time (PT) and aPTT is commonly observed, probably from reduced levels of Factors V, VII, and X. Low-grade DIC may also cause reduction in clotting factors through consumption. This may explain, at least in some patients, the elevated FDP concentrations so commonly seen in renal failure. Alternatively, impaired hepatic and renal clearance may be responsible. Antithrombin is reduced in patients with renal disease complicated by nephrotic syndrome.[79] In this situation, patients are at increased risk for venous thromboembolism.

Disseminated intravascular coagulation

Disseminated intravascular coagulation is not a specific disease entity but a complex phenomenon characterized by abnormal bleeding, small-vessel obstruction, tissue necrosis, and end-organ damage. The clinical picture and natural history are quite variable, making diagnosis and treatment difficult. The initial event in DIC is activation of the coagulation cascade. Three major mechanisms may be involved: (1) endothelial injury with activation of the intrinsic pathway; (2) tissue injury with activation of the extrinsic pathway; and (3) direct proteolytic cleavage of Factor X and activation of the prothrombinase complex (Factor Va, Xa, phospholipid, Ca^{2+}), with activation of the coagulation cascade, fibrin is generated. Although it would seem likely that intravascular thrombosis would be the next step, this is not always the case. For reasons that are unclear, the formation of soluble fibrin results in both consumption of coagulation factors (bleeding tendency) and impaired fibrinolysis (thrombotic tendency) (Table 15.14).

Cardiopulmonary bypass

The cardiopulmonary bypass circuit consists of nearly 12 m^2 of synthetic surfaces, including polyvinyl chloride, silicone rubber, polyurethane (flexible tubing), and poly-

Table 15.14 *Conditions and disorders associated with disseminated intravascular coagulation*

Acute
Shock (cardiogenic, septic, neurogenic, anaphylactic, hypovolemic)
Pulmonary embolism
Cardiac arrest
Major trauma
Burns
Hyperthermia
Amnionic fluid embolism

Subacute
Metastatic malignancy
Pancreatic, gastrointestinal, ovarian cancer
Promyelocytic leukemia

Chronic
Liver disease
Collagen vascular disease
Solid tumors
Renal disease
Liver disease

styrene (rigid connectors). In the roller pump, flexible tubing undergoes considerable deformation and the blood is exposed to high shear rates, turbulence, and hydraulic stresses. Additional shear stress is imposed by the heat exchanger, which contains a surface of uncoated or pyrolytic carbon-coated stainless steel. The gas exchange devices, gas interface, and membrane oxygenators impose damaging effects of high shearing stress at both the gas–blood and blood–synthetic membrane interfaces.[80]

Blood coming into direct contact with synthetic surfaces is the proposed mechanism for hemostatic abnormalities observed following cardiopulmonary bypass. Quantitative and qualitative platelet abnormalities occur following platelet activation and release of intracellular granules (acquired storage pool deficiency).[81,82] The reduced platelet count commonly seen is the result of both consumption and hemodilution.[83] Contact activation of the intrinsic coagulation cascade can lead to fibrin formation and consumption of circulation coagulation proteins. Plasmin is generated as well, increasing fibrinolytic potential. For these reasons, adequate systemic anticoagulation is vital during cardiopulmonary bypass.[84]

DISORDERS OF HEMOSTASIS ASSOCIATED WITH ANTITHROMBOTIC THERAPY

Over 50 per cent of bleeding complications occurring in patients with cardiac disease are the result of medical treatment and invasive procedures. As for many patients with advanced cardiac disease treatment with antithrombotic agents and invasive procedures (central line placement, cardiac catheterization, circulatory assist device insertion, coronary angioplasty, bypass grafting) are commonplace, the mechanism of action, pharmacology, biology, monitoring, and management of commonly used pharmacologic agents should be well known to practicing clinicians.

Platelet-inhibiting agents

The participation of platelets in the thrombotic process depends on their ability to adhere to an abnormal surface, to aggregate to form an initial platelet plug, and to activate, thus stimulating further aggregation and triggering the coagulation cascade. Therefore, pharmacologic strategies designed to inhibit platelet activity have focused on these three fundamental mechanisms of action. In addition, the recognition that growth factors released from platelets may influence cellular proliferation and atheroma formation has provided yet another potential target for newer agents[85,86] (Table 15.15).

Agents that inhibit platelet adhesion

In areas of severe coronary arterial narrowing caused by underlying atheroma, plaque rupture, or hemorrhage, platelet adhesion and aggregation are mediated by von Willebrand factor and the platelet receptors GPIb and

Table 15.15 *Platelet antagonists*

Inhibit platelet adhesion
Aurintricardoxylic acid
Von Willebrand factor monoclonal antibody

Inhibit platelet aggregation
Aspirin
Glycoprotein IIb/IIIa receptor antagonists
    Monoclonal antibodies
    RGD peptides
    Non-peptides
Ticlopidine
Clopidogrel
Thromboxane synthetase inhibitors
Thromboxane/endoperoxide receptor inhibitors
Dextran
Nitrate preparations

Inhibit platelet activation
Dipyridamole
Prostaglandin E_1
Prostacyclin
Calcium channel blockers
Purine receptor antagonists
Cilostozol

Inhibit platelet growth factors
Trapidil

GPIIb/IIIa. Monoclonal antibodies to von Willebrand factor[87] and aurintricarboxylic acid,[88] a triphenylmethyl dye compound, inhibit platelets in regions of high shear stress through their binding to von Willebrand factor, preventing its interaction with platelet receptors and damaged or dysfunctional vessel walls. These agents may be useful for short-term therapy. Long-term therapy, however, may be associated with a significant risk of bleeding.

Agents that inhibit platelet aggregation

ASPIRIN

Following oral ingestion, aspirin is rapidly absorbed in the stomach and the duodenum, achieving peak serum levels within 20–30 minutes. Enteric-coated preparations are less well absorbed (unless they are chewed), resulting in a delay in peak serum levels to approximately 60 minutes.

Aspirin irreversibly acetylates cyclooxygenase, impairing prostaglandin metabolism and thromboxane A_2 synthesis. As a result, platelet aggregation in response to collagen, ADP, and thrombin (in low concentrations) is inhibited.[89] Adherence and platelet release, however, are not affected. Because platelets, unlike vascular endothelial cells, lack the synthetic capacity to regenerate cyclooxygenase, aspirin's inhibitory effect persists for the life span of the platelet (7 ± 2 days). The antithrombotic effect of aspirin can be achieved with doses ranging from 160 to 325 mg/day (and possibly lower); therefore, the toxic side effects seen with higher doses can be avoided.[90]

Although non-steroidal anti-inflammatory drugs also inhibit platelet cyclooxygenase, they do so in a reversible manner. In addition, these compounds have not been adequately tested in large randomized clinical trials. Therefore, their use in the prevention or treatment of cardiovascular disease cannot by recommended at this time.

GPIIB/IIIA RECEPTOR ANTAGONISTS

The platelet GPIIB/IIIa receptor is unique in two ways. First, normal platelets have a large number of receptors (~50 000) on their surface. Second, platelet activation exposes the GPIIb/IIIa receptor, leading to platelet aggregation. In essence, all physiologic platelet agonists act by exposing the GPIIb/IIIa receptor (Final Common Pathway).

Monoclonal antibodies to the GPIIb/IIIa receptor have been developed recently. The $F(AB)_2$ fragment of this antibody can completely block *in vitro* platelet aggregation induced by agonists thought to function *in vivo*, even in high concentrations or in combinations.[91]

The ability of GPIIb/IIIa to bind a number of naturally occurring substances has been explained, at least in part, by the fact that it contains a binding site for the tripeptide arginine–glycine–aspartic acid (Arg-Gly-

Asp); therefore, synthetic compounds containing the sequence can inhibit the binding of fibrinogen to GPIIb/IIIa. The RGD (Arg-Gly-Asp), RGDS (Arg-Gly-Asp-Ser), and RGDF (Arg-Gly-Asp-Phe) peptides represent a new class of proteins that inhibit platelet aggregation[92] (Table 15.16).

Table 15.16 *Platelet surface glycoprotein IIb/IIIa receptor antagonists*

Intravenous
Abciximab (ReoPro®)
Lamifiban
Fradafiban
Tirofiban (Aggrastat®)
Eptifibatide (Integrilin®)

Oral
Roxifiban
Xemilofiban (development discontinued)
Orbifiban (development discontinued)
Sibrafiban (development discontinued)

TICLOPIDINE

Ticlopidine is structurally distinct from all other antiplatelet agents. It is a potent inhibitor of platelet aggregation induced by ADP and variably inhibits aggregation provoked by collagen, epinephrine, arachidonic acid, thrombin, and platelet release action and may impair platelet adhesion as well.[93] Structurally similar analogues including clopidogrel have shown some promise[94] and may offer safety advantages (reduced risk of bone marrow suppression and thrombotic thrombocytopenia purpura).

THROMBOXANE SYNTHETASE INHIBITORS

Thromboxane synthetase inhibitors have been developed to suppress platelet thromboxane A_2 synthesis, thereby preventing platelet aggregation.[95,96] Despite their potential beneficial effects, currently available agents have been limited by two factors: incomplete thromboxane A_2 inhibition, and the aggregating potential of endoperoxide intermediates.

INHIBITORS OF THROMBOXANE AND ENDOPEROXIDE RECEPTOR

The potential limitations of thromboxane synthetase inhibitors can, at least theoretically, be managed by inhibiting the receptors for both thromboxane A_2 and the active endoperoxide intermediates. In addition to inhibiting platelet aggregation, the vasoactive effects of thromboxane A_2 can also be blocked.[97]

DEXTRAN

Dextran is a polysaccharide that ranges in molecular weight from 65 000 to 80 000 Da. It has been shown to prolong bleeding time in humans; however, its mechanism of action is unclear. There is evidence suggesting that dextran binds to the platelet surface, altering membrane receptor function and inhibiting platelet aggregation.[98] Decreased levels of the factor VIII:VWF complex have also been reported.[99]

PURINE RECEPTOR ANTAGONISTS

Adenosine diphosphate (ADP)-induced platelet aggregation is mediated by the P_{2T} subtype of purinoceptor, which is unique to platelets and platelet precursor cells, and at which adenosine triphosphate (ATP) is a competitive antagonist. However, ATP is a non-selective P_2-ligand and is metabolically unstable, making it an unsuitable agent for evaluating the contribution of ADP to thrombosis *in vivo*, or as a clinically useful antithrombotic agent. P_{2T} purinoceptor antagonists are both potent and specific *in vitro*. They are also potent *in vivo*, effectively inhibiting platelet accretions in damaged arteries, while causing less bleeding time prolongation than membrane glycoprotein IIb/IIIa antagonists. This may be a significant advantage. Investigation is in progress in the setting of acute coronary syndromes.

Agents that inhibit platelet activation

Cyclic adenosine monophosphate (cAMP) is a major modulator of platelet activation and release. The platelet response to stimulation is inhibited when intracellular cAMP levels are elevated by agents that activate adenylate cyclase (the enzyme that converts ATP to cAMP) or that inhibit phosphodiesterase (the enzyme responsible for cAMP degradation) e.g. Cilostazol.

DIPYRIDAMOLE

Dipyridamole (Persantine®) was first used as an anti-anginal agent because of its vasodilating properties. It was subsequently known to inhibit platelet activation and has been postulated to do so through one or more mechanisms, including inhibition of phosphodiesterase, stimulation and release of endothelial prostacyclin, or inhibiting cellular uptake and metabolism of adenosine, which increases in concentration at the platelet-vessel interface.[100] High concentrations of dipyridamole are required to influence platelet aggregation *in vitro*. It is not surprising, therefore, that the observed effects *in vivo* have been both modest and inconsistent. The combination of aspirin and sustained-release dipyridamole (Aggrenox®) is used in the secondary prevention of stroke.

PROSTAGLANDIN E₁

Prostaglandin E_1 (PGE_1) inhibits platelet activation and aggregation primarily by increasing intracellular cAMP. It may also have the capacity to deaggregate aggregated platelets.[101] The clinical usefulness of PGE_1 is limited by the extensive first-pass metabolism, which takes place in the lungs. Indeed, 70 per cent of the activated compound is eliminated, resulting in extremely low plasma levels. Therefore, direct intravascular infusions are required to achieve therapeutic concentrations.[102]

PROSTACYCLIN

Prostacyclin (PGI_2) is a potent, naturally occurring platelet inhibitor. Its role in the treatment of cardiovascular disease has been limited by its instability in plasma and its propensity to cause systemic hypotension when given in doses required to inhibit platelet activation.[103] In contrast, the prostacyclin analogues iloprost and ciprostene are chemically stable compounds. Because they are both platelet inhibitors, further investigation is in progress.[104]

CALCIUM CHANNEL ANTAGONISTS

Calcium plays a vital role in platelet activation and aggregation. Accordingly, the potential platelet-inhibiting properties of the calcium channel antagonists nifedipine, diltiazem, and verapamil have been investigated. Indeed, each has been shown to inhibit platelet release and aggregation. In addition, diltiazem appears to potentiate the inhibitory effects of aspirin and prevent platelet-activating factor binding.[105,106]

Agents that inhibit growth factors

Platelet-derived growth factor (PDGF) is a potent mitogen and chemoattractant capable of stimulating proliferation of smooth muscle cells and fibroblasts in tissue culture.[107] The *in vitro* and *in vivo* stimulatory effect of PDGF is significantly reduced by Trapidil, a triazolo-pyrimidine derivative that also has vasodilatory and cholesterol-lowering properties.[108]

Anticoagulants

UNFRACTIONATED HEPARIN

The most widely used anticoagulant, heparin, is a heterogenous mucoplysacchoride that accelerates the inhibitory interaction between antithrombin II and several hemostatic proteins, most notably thrombin and Factor X. Following intravenous administration, approximately one-third of circulating heparin molecules bind to antithrombin. The remaining two-thirds have minimal anticoagulant activity A.[109,110]

Heparin is cleared from the circulation through a combination of a rapid saturable mechanism (binding) and a much slower first-order mechanism (renal).[111,112] After its intravenous administration, heparin binds to vascular endothelial cells, macrophages, and plasma proteins (including von Willebrand factor). The latter phenomenon is responsible for the 'heparin resistance' observed in some patients with acute thromboembolic events and subsequent release of acute-phase reactant proteins into the circulation.[113] Because of these complex kinetics, the anticoagulant effect of heparin at therapeutic doses is not linear, although usually both intensity and duration increase as the dose increases. Therefore, the biological half-life of heparin increases from 30 minutes following an intravenous bolus of 25 units/kg to 60 minutes after a dose of 100 units/kg and 150 minutes with a bolus of 400 units/kg.[114]

The anticoagulant effects of heparin are usually monitored with the aPTT, a test sensitive to the inhibitory effects of heparin on thrombin and Factor X. Prior clinical studies have shown convincingly that a therapeutic state of systemic anticoagulation (1.5–2.5 times control) is a prerequisite for patient benefit when heparin is used in the treatment of venous and arterial thromboembolic disorders.[115–117] Because the pharmacokinetics and pharmacodynamics of heparin are complex, frequent monitoring during the course of treatment is required. Unfortunately, the different commercial aPTT reagents vary considerably in their responsiveness to heparin and excessive time delays in the laboratory prevent clinicians from providing optimal care. A preformed study by our group suggested that point-of-care coagulation monitoring could reduce the time needed to achieve a therapeutic state of anticoagulation in heparinized patients

admitted to the coronary care unit with unstable angina, acute myocardial infarction, or pulmonary embolism.[118] A combination of weight-adjusted heparin dose titration and point-of-care coagulation monitoring may represent the ideal management strategy.[119]

The most common side effect of heparin is hemorrhage. Other complications include thrombocytopenia (with or without thrombosis), skin necrosis, alopecia, hypersensitivity reaction, and hypoaldosteronism. The risk of bleeding increases with heparin dose (and anticoagulant effect), age, decreasing body weight, trauma, recent surgery, invasive procedures, and the concomitant use of aspirin.

LOW-MOLECULAR-WEIGHT HEPARINS (LMWHS)

LMWH preparations form a relatively new class of anticoagulants derived from unfractionated heparin (UH) (Table 15.17).[120] They are a mixture of short homogeneous mucopolysaccharide chains, with molecular weights varying from 2000 to 10 000 Da, and a mean molecular weight of 4500–5000 Da. In contrast, UH is a heterogeneous mixture of sulfated polysaccharides ranging in molecular weight from 5000 to 30 000 Da. UH contains both below critical length material (BCLM) and above critical length material (ACLM). The former predominates in LMWH preparations. Accordingly, the anticoagulant properties of LMWH are derived preferentially from their anti-Factor Xa effects, while those of

Table 15.17 *Low-molecular-weight heparin (LMWH) preparations (available or in development)*

Trade name	Manufacturer/supplier	Method of preparation	Chemical change
Ardeparin, Normiflo	Wyeth, Philadelphia PA, USA	Peroxidative cleavage	Generation of labeled glycosidic bonds
Boxol	Rovi, Madrid, Spain	β-elimination or nitrous acid digestion	Formation of anhydromannose (5-member ring)
Enoxaparin/Clexane, Lovenox	Aventis, Pharma, Antony, France	Benzylation followed by alkaline hydrolysis	Introduction of double bond at the end groups
Fluxum	Opocrin, Corlo, Italy	Peroxidative cleavage	Generation of labeled glycosidic bonds
Fragmin, Dalteparin	Kabi, Stockholm, Sweden	Controlled nitrous acid depolymerization	Formation of anhydromannose (5-member ring)
Fraxiparin/Seleparin	Sanofi, Paris, France	Fractionation, optimized nitrous acid depolymerization	Formation of anhydromannose (5-member ring)
Innohep	Dupont, Wilmington, USA	Heparinase digestion	Introduction of double bond at the end groups
Logiparin, Innohep	Novo Nordisk, Copenhagen, Denmark	Heparinase digestion	Introduction of double bond at the end groups
Merckle LMWH	Merckle, Ulm, Germany	Peroxidative cleavage	Generation of labeled glycosidic bonds
Miniparin	Syntex, Buenos Aires, Argentina	Nitrous acid digestion	Formation of anhydromannose (5-member ring)
Reviparin, Clivarin	Knoll AG, Ludwigshafen, Germany	Nitrous acid digestion	Formation of anhydromannose (5-member ring)
Sandoparin, Certoparin	Sandoz AG, Nurenberg, Germany	Isoamyl nitrate digestion	Formation of anhydromannose (5-member ring)

UH are the result of both Factor Xa *and* thrombin inhibition. As with UH, LMWH works by potentiating the effect of antithrombin, a natural plasma inhibitor of coagulation. In contrast to UH, the predominant chains in LMWH preparations are molecules with molecular weight of less than 5400 Da, which do not bind thrombin. This fundamental difference between the two classes of anticoagulants may translate into important differences in safety, bioavailability, and efficacy. Why would a more potent activity against Factor Xa than against thrombin be preferable? Theoretically, inhibition of thrombin *formation* is more effective than attempting to inhibit thrombin activity once the enzyme has already formed.

The bioavailability of LMWH is essentially complete at a broad range of subcutaneous (sc) doses and its plasma half-life is dose independent, with 90 per cent bioavailability at all doses. This is a favorable property compared to the relatively erratic absorption of UH. The half-life of intravenously (iv) administered LMWH is 5–8 hours, again favorable when compared to UH. After sc administration, maximum anti-Factor Xa activity may be present for *up to* 12 hours. Because the elimination of LMWH depends mostly on renal excretion, its biologic half-life is increased in the setting of renal failure. The persistence of anti-Factor Xa activity appears to be vital to its efficacy. In addition, LMWH preparations have lower affinity for plasma proteins, especially acute-phase reactants, resulting in more predictable circulating levels. Finally, unlike UH, LMWH does not bind to macrophages and endothelial cells. Neither LMWH nor UH cross the placental barrier.

In contrast to the uniformity of different preparations of UH with respect to their therapeutic activity, it is important to recognize that each commercial LMWH preparation has distinct pharmacokinetic and probably anticoagulant properties (Table 15.18). The area under the 'concentration versus time' curve increases differently for each LMWH preparation with rising doses, and is also increased differently with repeated doses.

Table 15.18 *Molecular weights and potencies assigned to various low-molecular-weight heparin (LMWH) preparations by the European Pharmacopoeial Forum*

	Molecular weight	AXa (U/mg)	AIIa (U/mg)
Enoxaparin	4300	100–110	25–30
Nadroparin	5200	90–100	25–30
Dalteparin	6300	140–150	60
Certoparin	6000	80–95	30–35
Tinzaparin	6700	80–85	45
Reviparin	3900	130	40
Ardeparin	6500	100	48
Parnaparin	5000	85–90	<30

Axa = anti-Xa; AIIa = anti-IIa.

The only assay sensitive to the anticoagulant activity of LMWH is a chromogenic measurement of Factor Xa activity. This assay is not available in most laboratories, and the need to employ it routinely would make the use of these drugs cumbersome. Other assays for Factor Xa activity are being developed. There are no formal recommendations for the *routine* laboratory monitoring of LMWH at the present time; most authorities agree that it is unnecessary to monitor anticoagulation when using LMWH in standard doses (with the exception of patients experiencing renal failure (creatine clearance <40 mL/min) or those of very low (<50 kg) or very high (>120 kg) body weight). It should be noted, however, that LMWHs do not significantly prolong the aPTT, international normalized ratio (INR), thrombin time, or activated clotting time when administered in currently recommended doses.

Danaparoid sodium

The low-molecular-weight hepainoid, danaparoid (Organan®), is a mixture of non-heparin polysulfated glycosaminoglycans (heparan sulfate, dermatan sulfate, chondroitin sulfate) and low-molecular-weight heparin.[121,122] Its anticoagulant action is characterized predominately by anti-Factor Xa activity. Although related to heparin in structure, danaparoid differs in its degree of sulfation and molecular weight, reducing its potential to produce antiplatelet antibodies. Accordingly, danaparoid has been used in the treatment of heparin-induced thrombocytopenia.[123] Danaparoid sodium is cleared through renal mechanisms and has a long circulatory plasma half-life (approximately 24 hours) of anti-Xa inhibiting activity.

Direct Xa antagonists

Selective inhibitors of factor Xa (oral and intravenous preparation) are in development.

Direct thrombin inhibitors

Direct thrombin inhibitors, including hirudin, hirulog, and argatoban, represent an interesting class of non-antithrombin dependent anticoagulants. Clinical trials to determine their niche in the treatment of thromboembolic disease and for use in percutaneous coronary intervention are ongoing (*see* Chapter 18).

Warfarin

Like heparin, warfarin is a frequently used anticoagulant in clinical practice, particularly among patients with cardiac disease. It is rapidly absorbed from the gastrointestinal tract following oral administration, reaches maximal plasma concentration in 90 minutes, and has a circulating half-life of 36–42 hours. It circulates bound to plasma proteins. The dose–response profile of warfarin differs between individuals and is influenced by both pharmacokinetic and pharmacodynamic factors. Conditions that affect the availability of vitamin K also influence warfarin response (Table 15.19).

The prothrombin time is the method most commonly used for monitoring warfarin therapy. The PT increases in response to depression of three of the four vitamin-K-dependent coagulation proteins – Factors II, VII, and X. At the beginning of warfarin administration, prolongation of the PT primarily reflects Factor VII depression (shortest half-life). During maintenance therapy, the test is sensitive to depressions in Factors II and X as well.

Thromboplastins vary considerably in their responsiveness to depletion of vitamin-K-dependent clotting factors. As a result, PTs determined using different reagents are not interchangeable.[124–126] For this reason, a calibration system known as the international normalized ratio (INR) was adopted by the World Health Organization in 1982 and is currently used to standardize the reporting of prothrombin times. Anticoagulant response to generic warfarin preparations are also variable and introduce yet another potential challenge to monitoring.

Bleeding is the main complication of warfarin therapy. Other complications include skin necrosis, purple-toe syndrome, and microvascular thrombosis in protein C (or rarely protein S)-deficient patients.[127] The risk of bleeding is directly influenced by the intensity of anticoagulant therapy, age, renal insufficiency, and occult disease of the gastrointestinal and genitourinary tracts.

FIBRINOLYTIC AGENTS

The available fibrinolytic agents, including tPA (Alteplase®), TNK-tPA (Tenecteplase®), rPA (Retevase) streptokinase (SK), and anisoylated plasminogen–streptokinase activator complex (APSAC), each convert the inactive proenzyme plasminogen to the active enzyme plasmin, which then is responsible for thrombolysis. The lytic state is characterized by plasmin-mediated degradation of coagulation proteins (Factors V and VIII) and fibrinogen. Fibrin and fibrinogen degradation causes the release of fibrin(ogen) degradation products (FDPs), which are capable of inhibiting thrombin, fibrin monomer polymerization, and platelet aggregation.

Bleeding complications of a serious nature occur in approximately 5 per cent of patients treated with thrombolytic agents. The most feared and devastating complication, intracerebral hemorrhage, occurs in approximately 0.5–0.7 per cent of treated patients. Careful patient screening can minimize the likelihood of hemorrhage (Table 15.20). At the present time, a majority of patients also receive adjuvant treatment with antiplatelet agents (aspirin) and anticoagulants

Table 15.19 *Drugs, conditions and disease states that influence the action of warfarin*

Decreased effect
Impaired absorption of warfarin
    Cholestyramine
Increase metabolic clearance of warfarin
    Ethanol (may also increase effect)
    Rifampin
    Barbiturates
    Carbamazepine
    Hypothyroidism
Increase vitamin K intake (leafy green vegetables, nutritional
    supplements)

Increased effect
Inhibit metabolic clearance of warfarin
    Disulfiram
    Metronidazole
    Amiodarone
    Cimetidine
    Sulfa derivatives
Increase response (direct pharmacodynamic effect)
    Second- and third-generation cephalosporins
    Heparin
    Clofibrate
Unknown mechanisms
    Anabolic steroids
    Isoniazid
    Ketoconazole
    Fluconazole
    Tamoxifen
    Quinidine
    Phenytoin
    Propafenone
Potentiate effect of warfarin
    Low vitamin K intake
    Reduced vitamin K absorption
    Hyperthyroidism
    Liver disease
    Malnutrition (decreased serum albumin)

Table 15.20 *Identifying patients at risk for serious hemorrhage following fibrinolytic therapy*

Patient characteristic/conditions
Bleeding diathesis (congenital or acquired)
Active bleeding (current or within prior 2 months)
Significant trauma (<2 months)
History of cerebrovascular accident, intracranial neoplasm,
    arteriovenous malformation, or aneurysm
Recent major surgery (<4 weeks)
Recent puncture of non-compressible vessel or organ biopsy
    (<7 days)
Pregnancy
Hypertension (>180/110 mm Hg) at any time

(heparin). This practice probably increases the risk of bleeding, particularly if careful monitoring is not carried out during the first 24–48 hours. Hemorrhagic complications including intracranial hemorrhage increase with aPTT values above twice that of controls (Figs 15.8 and 15. 9).

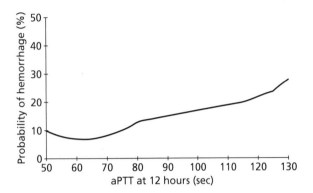

Figure 15.8 *The adjunctive use of anticoagulants in patients receiving fibrinolytic therapy increases the risk of major hemorrhage. The probability of hemorrhage increases steadily with activated partial thromboplastin time (aPTT) values in excess of 70 seconds. (From the TIMI 5 Study, unpublished).*

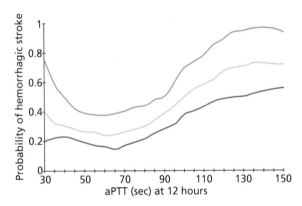

Figure 15.9 *The probability of intracranial hemorrhage increases with activated partial thromboplastin time (aPTT) values in excess of 70 seconds. (From the TIMI 5 Study, unpublished).*

Screening tests for hemostasis

Bleeding in critically ill patients may involve an abnormality of blood vessels, platelets, coagulation, or excessive fibrinolysis. If the bleeding diathesis is inherited, usually only *one* of these components is involved, whereas acquired hemostatic disorders may involve *several* or all components. This is particularly true in the critically ill cardiac patient. The following tests are commonly used to assess the integrity of the hemostatic mechanism.

Bleeding time

The bleeding time has been available for several decades, measuring platelet–vessel wall interactions and formation of a primary hemostatic plug. A prolonged bleeding time, defined as the time between the infliction of a small cut on the forearm to the moment that bleeding stops, occurs when the level of circulation platelets is decreased, the platelets function abnormally, or platelet–vessel wall interactions are abnormal. Although the test provides important information as a screening tool for the early stages of hemostasis, it has been among the most difficult tests to standardize. Indeed, the test is affected by the depth, length, site, and direction of the incision. Automated devices give the most reliable and reproducible results and therefore are used in clinical practice. A normal bleeding time is between 3 and 8 minutes.

Rapid platelet function assay

The rapid platelet function assay (Ultegra®, Accumetrics) is an automated turbidimetric bead agglutination whole blood assay to assess platelet function based upon the ability of activated platelets to bind fibrinogen. Fibrinogen-coated polystyrene microparticles agglutinate in whole blood in proportion to the number of unblocked platelet glycoprotein (GP) IIb/IIIa receptors. The rate of microbead agglutination is more rapid and reproducible if platelets are activated; therefore the reagent iso-TRAP (Thrombin Reception Agonist Peptide) is incorporated into the assay to induce platelet activation without producing fibrin formation. As activated platelets bind and agglutinate fibrinogen-coated beads, there is an increase in light transmittance. The instrument is designed to measure this change in optical signal due to agglutination. Clinical studies employing this technology are in progress. The early experience suggests that patient-to-patient variability in response to fixed, GPIIb/IIIa antagonist dosing can be detected, providing guidance with dose titration and achievement of therapeutic platelet inhibition.[128]

Partial thromboplastin time

The partial thromboplastin time (PTT) measures the intrinsic coagulation cascade. A partial thromboplastin (e.g. cephalin and inosithin) has an activity equivalent to platelet factor 3. They are added to citrated plasma, and the time required to form a clot is measured at 37°C after the addition of calcium. The variability of contact activation of the intrinsic cascade is standardized by the addition of an activator (e.g. kaolin, celite, powdered glass) and referred to as the activated partial thromboplastin time.

The aPTT is prolonged if there is decreased coagulation factor activity or if there is a circulating inhibitor or anticoagulant. Mixing the patient's plasma with normal plasma and repeating the test allows these two mechanisms to be distinguished. If the correction pattern indicates a coagulation factor deficiency, mixing tests can then be performed with artificially depleted plasmas or with patient's plasmas known to be deficient in specific coagulation proteins (Fig. 15.10). The aPTT is the test used most commonly to monitor heparin. The normal range varies between reagents and automated devices; however, it typically is in the range of 25–35 seconds.

Thrombin time

The thrombin time measures the terminal portion of the common coagulation pathway and is determined by adding a solution of thrombin to anticoagulated plasma and performing a clotting time. The thrombin time is particularly sensitive to heparin as well as to low fibrinogen levels, dysfunctional fibrinogen, and the presence of FDPs. If the thrombin time is prolonged and the contribution of heparin is unknown, a reptilase time can be performed. Reptilase (derived from pit viper venom) clots fibrinogen in the presence of heparin. Therefore, the reptilase time will be normal if heparin is responsible for a prolonged thrombin time (or aPTT). In contrast, deficient or dysfunctional fibrinogen, or impaired fibrin monomer polymerization (caused by circulating FDP) will prolong the reptilase time and thrombin time (and occasionally the aPTT as well). A normal thrombin time is between 20 and 30 seconds.

Prothrombin time

The prothrombin time is a measure of clotting initiated by the extrinsic coagulation pathway. The test is performed by adding a thromboplastin (complete) – the equivalent of tissue thromboplastin – to citrated blood and performing a clotting time after the addition of calcium. Like the aPTT, the PT is affected by deficiencies of Factors II, V, and X, and fibrinogen. However, unlike the aPTT, it is also sensitive to deficiencies of Factor VII (the deficiency may be absolute or relative, as is the case with circulating Factor VII inhibitors).

The PT varies with the thromboplastin used. This limitation has been addressed through the adoption of a standardized system (the INR). However, poor-quality thromboplastins (international sensitivity index >1.8) tend to limit the potential benefits of the INR system. A normal INR is between 1.0 and 1.3.

The aPTT, thrombin time, and PT can be used together in clinical practice to investigate unexplained hemorrhagic events (Table 15.21).

Activated clotting time

The activated clotting, or coagulation, time (ACT) is a derivative of the whole blood clotting time used initially in the 1950s to assess coagulation and heparin response. Two commercially available systems are in clinical use – the Medtronic Hemotec ACT (Medtronic Hemotec, Inc., Englewood, CO, USA), and the Hemochron (International Technidyne Corporation, Edison, NJ, USA). The Hemotec device uses a mechanical plunger

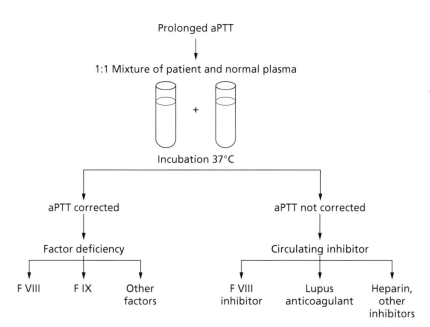

Figure 15.10 *The initial laboratory approach to patients with an unexplained prolongation of the aPTT begins with 'mixing' studies that can distinguish coagulation factor deficiencies from the presence of circulating inhibitors of coagulation factors. aPTT = activated partial thromboplastin time.*

Table 15.21 *Evaluation of bleeding complications and hemostatic abnormalities*

Abnormality	aPTT	Thrombin time	PT
Intrinsic pathway	Prolonged	Normal or mildly prolonged	Normal
Extrinsic pathway	Normal	Normal	Prolonged
Common pathway	Prolonged	Normal or mildly prolonged[a]	Prolonged
Fibrinogen (depletion/dysfunction)	Normal[b]	Prolonged	Normal[b]

[a] Determined by deficient component; thrombin time more sensitive to the terminal portion of common pathway, particularly fibrinogen.
[b] With severe fibrinogen depletion, the aPTT and PT may be prolonged.
aPTT = activated partial thromboplastin time; PT = prothrombin time.

that is dipped in and out of kaolin-activated whole blood samples in cartridges. The device optically senses the time required for the plunger to move through the blood samples. Both high- and low-range cartridges provide an average response of 250 seconds for each unit of heparin/mL of blood. The Hemochron device uses a magnet inside prewarmed glass specimen tubes that contain various activators (diatomaceous earth or glass beads). After whole blood is placed in the tubes, they are rotated inside the device. As blood clots, a magnet is displaced, acting as a proximity switch. The clotting time is derived from the time required to move the magnet a preset distance. High- and low-range cartridges are available for use with the Hemochron device.

The ACT is often used during coronary angioplasty or bypass surgery for heparin monitoring. Extended range aPTT testing may also be used in these settings.

Individual clotting factor assays

Methodologies for individual clotting factor assays are available for their quantification: clot-based, chromogenic utilizing synthetic substrates, and immunologic. Clot-based assays are modifications of aPTT and PT, and are functional assays, which have the advantage that they may be used to detect both quantitative and qualitative defects. Plasma samples deficient in a known single factor, are mixed with the plasma being investigated. If the defects do not match, there will be reciprocal correction of the prolonged clotting time. To quantify a defect, the patient's plasma is mixed in equal volumes with the single factor-deficient plasma, obtained commercially and the resulting clotting time is read against a serially diluted normal control, to obtain the percentage of the decreased factor comparing the clotting times. Using this principle, Factors VII, V, II, and X can be measured by PT-based assays, and Factors VIII , IX, XI, and XII by aPTT-based assays (Fig. 15.11).

The disadvantage of clot-based one-stage assays is that they may give erroneous results when trace amounts of thrombin are present. Lupus inhibitors may also inhibit these assays. More accurate but also more arduous two-stage methods may be employed, since they are less affected by the presence of inhibitors. A radioimmuno-

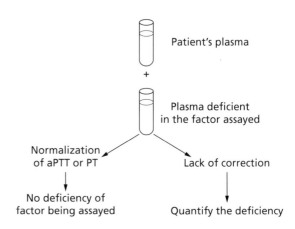

Figure 15.11 *Specific coagulation factor deficiencies can be evaluated and quantified using plasma that is deficient in a particular factor. aPTT = activated partial thromboplastin time; PT = prothrombin time.*

diffusion (RID) kit is available for Factors V, X, and Factor XIII, but it is not practical for a routine laboratory.

Chromogenic assays are available for Factors VIII, VIIa, IX, XIIa, plasmin, antiplasmin, plasminogen, kallikrein, protein C, thrombin, and antithrombin. Since most of the coagulation factors are serine proteases and have the ability to cleave peptide bonds, many of the chromogenic assays are based on the principle that the natural enzyme acts on the multiple cleavage sites available on the synthetic substrate. When coupled with a chromogen or a flourochrome on the carboxyl end, color development can be followed as a reflection of the clotting factor's total activity. Chromogenic assays are easily automated and have greater precision. It should be kept in mind, however, that the enzyme's ability to cleave the synthetic substrate does not necessarily reflect functional activity *in vivo*. They are useful also because deficient plasmas used in clot-based assays may not be available for all factors and there may be some variability in the true deficiency of the missing factor. The chromogenic assays are used most commonly in the evaluation of fibrinolytic pathways, for protein C and for antithrombin III determination.

POINT-OF-CARE COAGULATION MONITORS

The Coagucheck Plus® System (Boehringer Mannheim Diagnostics, Indianapolis, IN), is a battery-powered, portable laser photometer that uses a phospholipid (soybean phosphatide) and an activator of intrinsic coagulation (bovine brain sulfatide) to determine the aPTT. Microliter samples of capillary, arterial, or venous whole blood can be used. In the present study venous samples were used in all cases; however, previous studies at our institution (unpublished data) have shown comparable results with each when meticulous attention to technique is observed.

In brief, a disposable plastic reagent cartridge is inserted into the instrument and allowed to warm. A drop of whole blood is then applied to the application well of the cartridge. The blood is subsequently drawn by capillary action through the reagent chamber, where it mixes with activator and phospholipid. The laser photometer, senses variations in light scatter from red blood flow. The time from blood application to cessation of flow (clotting) is then converted mathematically to a plasma equivalent aPTT. The conversion factor has been established previously by the manufacturer through work performed at the UMASS-Memorial Medical Center (unpublished data) (normal aPTT 31 seconds; range 21–41 seconds). All point-of-care tests in the study were performed by coronary care unit nurses, respiratory therapists or critical care technicians trained and certified by the central laboratory according to current guidelines.[119]

The development of instruments capable of performing Factor Xa-inhibition assays and combined platelet aggregation/coagulation (hemostasis) assessment is ongoing.

TRANSFUSIONS

Blood transfusions are indicated when one or more essential components are deficient and require immediate replacement. The assumption is made that more specific and potentially safer therapy (e.g. iron supplementation) has been considered but precluded because of time and urgency. When blood transfusions are indicated, only the deficient component should be administered.

A standard unit of blood consists of 250 mL of blood mixed with 50–60 mL of a solution containing citrate, glucose, phosphate, and adenine for optimal preservation of red blood cell viability. A majority of anemic patients can be treated with red blood cells supplemented by an electrolyte solution (normal saline, Ringer's lactate) when necessary for blood pressure support. Whole blood replacement is typically reserved for massive hemorrhage complicated by shock.

A variety of red blood cell preparations that are available through most hospital blood banks are listed below.

- *Red blood cells (packed red blood cells)* are the primary treatment for most acute and chronic anemias. Enough plasma is maintained from the original unit to facilitate rapid transfusion when necessary.
- *Leukocyte-poor red blood cells* are available for patients with prior transfusion-related febrile reactions (a majority are caused by alloantibodies reacting to donor leukocytes). Removal of 80–90 per cent of leukocytes is adequate. It is important to realize that the process of removing leukocytes (washing, centrifugation, filtering) also removes some red blood cells, lowering the final hematocrit of the donor unit.
- *Washed red blood cells* are reserved for patients with severe febrile reactions to transfused cells.
- *Frozen red blood cells* can also be used for patients with prior febrile reactions; however, the primary reason to freeze red blood cells is for the purpose of storing (up to 3 years) rare blood types.

Blood compatibility

The surface membrane of all blood cells (and plasma proteins) contain a large number of genetically programmed antigens. Fortunately, many of these antigens are poor immunogens, and therefore, antibody production is minimal. The red blood cell antigens are divided into blood groups, the ABO group being the most important with two antigens: A and B. The second important red blood cell group is Rh (important because one of the antigenic determinants in this group (D) is a very potent antigen). The term Rh-positive indicates the presence of D; Rh-negative indicates its absence (approximately 15 per cent of the population lacks the D antigen).

When a blood transfusion is clinically indicated, the blood bank must type the red blood cells of the patient (recipient) for A, B, and D, and confirm the typing on the donor. Further, tests are performed on the recipient's blood for unexpected antibodies (other than the expected anti-A or anti-B). Cross-matching tests the recipient's serum with red blood cells for the intended donor unit.

Under normal circumstances, transfused cells are the same ABO type as those of the recipient. In urgent situations, incompatible cells may be transfused (type O cells can be given to a recipient of any ABO type; type AB recipients can receive cells of any ABO type). In these situations, only packed red blood cells should be used. A special effort should be made to avoid transfusing Rh-positive cells into Rh-negative female recipients of childbearing potential. Subsequent immunization to the D antigen may cause hemolytic disease of the newborn.

Complications of blood transfusions

Blood transfusions have the potential for a wide variety of complications and side effects. Therefore, it is important in all clinical scenarios to consider the risks and benefits of transfusion carefully (Table 15.22).

Table 15.22 *Potential complications of blood transfusions*

Hemolytic reactions (ABO mismatch)
Febrile reactions
Contaminated blood
  Gram-negative bacilli, *Clostridium*
Non-cardiogenic pulmonary edema
Post-transfusion thrombocytopenia
Disease transmission
  Hepatitis B
  Hepatitis non-A non-B
  Human immunodeficiency virus
  Cytomegalovirus
  Malaria
  Syphilis
Allergic reactions
  Anaphylactic shock
  Urticaria
Air embolism
Congestive heart failure (circulatory overload)
Graft-versus-host disease

CLINICAL APPROACH TO HEMATOLOGIC AND HEMOSTATIC DISORDERS

Anemias: management steps

With acute blood loss, blood pressure support through volume expansion and, if necessary, vasopressor administration is recommended. A prompt and thorough assessment to identify the source (or sources) should be undertaken. The coagulation status and platelet count should also be determined.

Although subacute and chronic anemias often carry less clinical urgency, they nonetheless are frequently of considerable importance, particularly among patients with acute blood loss.

Patients being evaluated for anemia should have a complete blood count, reticulocyte count, and review of the peripheral smear. The erythrocyte mean corpuscular volume (MCV) is a readily available and a useful means to divide anemias into three groups: microcytic (<80 μm^3), normocytic ($80–100$ μm^3), and macrocytic (>100 μm^3).

Several challenges confront the clinician evaluating hospitalized patients. First, many anemias are normocytic,

Table 15.23 *Diagnosing anemias on the basis of mean corpuscular volume (MCV)*

Microcytic (MCV <80 μm^3)	Macrocytic (MCV >100 μm^3)
Iron deficiency	Megaloblastic anemias
Thalassemia	Chemotherapeutic agents[a]
Anemia of chronic disease[a]	Reticulocytosis
Sideroblastic anemia	Aplastic anemias
Erythrocyte fragmentation	Myelodysplastic syndromes
Burns[a]	Aplastic anemias[a]
Hereditary poikilocytosis	Hypothyroidism[a]

[a]MCV may be within the normal range.

necessitating further testing and, second, multiple etiologies, particularly acute on chronic anemia, are common (Table 15.23).

A reticulocyte is a young red blood cell newly released from the bone marrow. The normal reticulocyte circulates for 24 hours before maturing. Because normal red blood cells survive on average for 120 days, the reticulocyte count is typically 1 per cent. As anemia increases the relative concentration of reticulocytes in peripheral blood, the count should always be corrected to a normal hematocrit (45 per cent):

$$\text{Corrected reticulocyte count} = \frac{\text{calculated reticulocyte count} \times (\text{patient's hematocrit})}{45}$$

A marked decrease in reticulocytes (<0.5 per cent) implies primary suppression of the bone marrow. A severe reduction (0.1 per cent) suggests marrow aplasia. Reticulocytosis (>5.0 per cent) is the hallmark of hemolytic anemia.

Information vital to assessing patients with anemia can be obtained from a review of the peripheral blood smear (Table 15.24). A bone marrow examination may be necessary in challenging clinical situations, particularly when a primary blood dyscrasia or infiltrative process (tumor, infection) is a strong consideration.

Polycythemia: management steps

Regardless of the underlying etiology, all disorders characterized by absolute erythrocytosis share common clinical manifestations caused by an expanded blood volume and increased blood viscosity. The expanded blood volume leads to generalized vascular expansion and venous engorgement, while increased viscosity decreases vascular flow rate. The combination greatly increases the risk of thromboembolic events and may also result in both decreased cardiac output and impaired tissue oxygenation.

Table 15.24 *Peripheral blood smear: red blood cell morphologic characteristics and associated anemia*

Red blood cell morphology	Anemia or associated condition
Hypoproliferative anemia	
Normal	Anemia or chronic disease, aplastic anemia
Rouleaux formation	Multiple myeloma
Blast cells	Blood dyscrasias
Nucleated cells	Myelophthisic anemias
Burr cells	Renal failure
Marked poikilocytosis	Myelodysplastic syndrome
Hyperproliferative anemia	
Polychromasia	Hemolysis
Sickle cells	Sickle cell disease
Microspherocytes	Hereditary spherocytosis, autoimmune hemolysis
Bite cells	Oxidant hemolysis
Schistocytes	Microangiopathic hemolysis
Maturation defects	
Microcytes, hypochromia	Iron deficiency
Target cells	Thalassemias
Oval macrocytes	Vitamin B_{12} or folate deficiency

In general, a hematocrit greater than 60 per cent is rarely physiologic, and consideration should be given to therapeutic phlebotomy (target hematocrit 50 per cent) as a means of minimizing the risk of thrombosis and tissue hypoperfusion.

Thrombocytopenia: management steps

A careful history must be taken to identify the time of onset, course, past hemorrhagic complications, a family history of abnormal bleeding tendency, and associated medical illnesses. The hallmark of thrombocytopenia is petechia, most commonly involving the skin and mucous membranes (easily traumatized areas). The stool should be tested for blood and evidence of adenopathy or splenomegaly should be sought.

Several laboratory tests should be ordered, including a complete blood count with differential analysis and a careful review of the peripheral smear (which also allows an assessment of erythrocyte and leukocyte morphology and characteristics).

Spurious thrombocytopenia can occur with cold agglutinins, giant platelets, *in vitro* clotting, and ethylene diamine tetra-acetic acid (EDTA)-induced clumping. The bleeding time is a useful part of the initial assessment of thrombocytopenia; however, it is a measure of both quantitative and qualitative platelet abnormalities. In the presence of normal platelet function, the bleeding time is inversely related to platelet counts between 10 000 and 100 000/mm³.

Coagulation studies, including an aPTT, PT, and thrombin time may be useful when DIC is being considered. A bone marrow examination may be required to assess platelet production (as well as other cell lines). Infiltrative and infectious processes can also be diagnosed using this technique.

In disorders characterized by platelet destruction, laboratory tests can either measure antibody-platelet binding or immune-mediated paraphenomena (lysis, complement fixation, aggregation). As the initial event in immune thrombocytopenia is antibody or immune complex binding, the measurement of platelet-associated IgG is the most commonly used, first-line test. Available assays include inhibition assays, direct binding assays, and immunoprecipitation assays. Unfortunately, platelet-associated IgG is found in many clinical settings manifesting as thrombocytopenia and, therefore, lacks specificity for immune disorders.

Heparin-associated thrombocytopenia is not uncommon in clinical practice. The frequent use of heparin in clinical practice requires a solid understanding of this platelet disorder that can manifest not only as thrombocytopenia and bleeding, but also as life-threatening multiorgan thrombosis. Heparin-induced thrombocytopenia (HIT) and heparin-induced thrombocytopenia with thrombosis syndrome (HITTS) represent an immune-mediated disease spectrum. The currently proposed mechanism is based on the development of an antibody to the heparin-platelet factor 4 (PF4) complex, which is bound to the platelet. The antibody is not heparin-specific and can react with sulfated mucopolysaccharides, including those found on the vascular endothelial surface. Platelet activation and their rapid consumption is responsible for the observed thrombocytopenia, which is typically seen 5 days after heparin exposure. Patients with prior heparin exposure may have 'memory' and develop an accelerated antibody response. Platelet activation may also predispose to thrombosis; however, the occurrence of widespread venous and arterial events suggests a more diffuse vascular abnormality, conceivably immune-mediated.[129]

> The diagnosis of HIT should be suspected in a patient receiving heparin who experiences a 50 per cent decrease in platelet count (from baseline) or a thrombotic event while anticoagulated. Diagnostic tests include a heparin-related platelet aggregation assay and a newly developed ELISA for the heparin-PF4 complex. The management of HIT and HITTS is discussed in greater detail in Chapter 16.

Disorders of platelet function: management steps

The hallmark of qualitative platelet disorders is a prolonged bleeding time in the presence of a normal platelet count. A history of easy bruising, hemorrhage following minor trauma, spontaneous bleeding from mucosal surfaces, and a family history of bleeding are particularly important in congenital disorders. A series of platelet function tests can be performed, including aggregation response to adenosine diphosphate (ADP), collagen, ristocetin, and arachidonic acid. More complex tests are available in experienced laboratories, including assessment of membrane glycoproteins using monoclonal antibodies and flow cytometry, uptake and secretion of serotonin, content and secretion of adenine nucleotides, and structural assessment with electron microscopy.

Thrombocytosis: management steps

Thrombocytosis can give rise to spurious laboratory values. The most common include pseudohyperkalemia, increased lactate dehydrogenase, and falsely elevated acid phosphatase. These abnormalities quickly correct when cell-free plasma is used to perform the tests.

Reactive and secondary forms of thrombocytosis rarely cause hemorrhagic or thrombotic complications. In contrast, essential thrombocythemia is associated with hemorrhage (related to accompanying platelet dysfunction) and thrombosis. The latter can involve both small and large vessels, causing stroke, myocardial infarction, and damage to other major viscera. Overall, thrombotic events are among the leading causes of death in patients with essential thrombocythemia. As the thrombotic diathesis reflects excessive platelet activation, prophylaxis with antiplatelet drugs (aspirin,

dipyridamole) may be beneficial. Plateletpheresis and cytoreduction therapy are indicated in the acute and chronic stages, respectively, if thrombotic events occur in the presence of platelet counts greater than 1 million/mm³. The target goal for maintenance should be 600 000/mm³.

Leukopenia: management steps

Neutropenia occurs in a wide variety of illnesses that often dominate the clinical picture. As previously mentioned, counts below 1000/mm³ are associated with an increased risk of infection. The organs most commonly affected include the lungs, genitourinary tract, and skin. It is important to realize that many of the signs and symptoms of infection (fever, erythema, infiltrates on chest radiography) may be absent. Therefore, with heightened suspicion, immediate treatment should be started. In addition to broad-spectrum antibiotics, some benefit may be derived from the administration of granulocyte colony-stimulating factor.

A careful evaluation of blood counts and the peripheral smear is required in patients with neutropenia. A bone marrow examination may also provide insights through assessment of cellularity and cellular differentiation.

Lymphopenia often represents a response to an underlying disease. Several mechanisms can be involved: (1) suppressed bone marrow production (malnutrition, radiation, viral infection); (2) peripheral destruction (viral infections, autoantibodies); and (3) changes in lymphocyte mobilization (trauma, corticosteroids).

Replacement therapy in individuals with coagulation defects: management steps

Hemostasis can be secured in classic hemophilia and Christmas disease by infusing adequate amounts of *plasma concentrates*.

> The total amount of factor concentrate required depends on the following: (1) baseline level of Factor VIII and/or Factor IX in the patient's plasma; and (2) the integrity of other components of the hemostatic mechanism.

In general terms, 15–20 units/dL is adequate in cases of minor bleeding, about 20–40 units/dL is required for moderate bleeding. The dose can be calculated by multiplying the patients plasma volume in milliliters by the desired increment in units per milliliter. Alternatively, the dose calculation can be made by knowing that each unit of Factor VIII (or IX) per kilogram body weight increases the plasma Factor VIII level (or IX level) by 0.02 units/mL.

CRYOPRECIPITATE

Cryoprecipitate is a starting material for high-purity factor concentrates. After protein contaminants are washed out, cryoprecipitates are redissolved and absorbed. The final product, which may be freeze dried, contains about 500 units of Factor VIII/g protein.

Using monoclonal antibodies, purified Factor VIII can be produced. In addition, identification of the Factor VIII gene has made it possible to clone this coagulation protein in Chinese hamster ovary cell lines, which can then express Factor VIII in culture medium. This highly mature material has a specific activity in the range of 7000 units/mg protein.

Therapy for von Willebrand disease typically includes an infusion of Factor VIII concentrate to normalize both the Factor VIII level and the bleeding time. Infusion of plasma and/or cryoprecipitate seems to be clinically satisfactory and in many patients corrects the bleeding time and the Factor VIII level. Cryoprecipitate corrects the bleeding time for 4 hours after infusion and offers some beneficial effect for up to 20 hours later. Cryoprecipitate is used as replacement therapy: approximately one bag of cryoprecipitate (obtained from a 1500 mL donation) is transfused intravenously per 10 kg body weight/day.

This dose may be necessary on a daily basis for individuals that undergo major surgery or in whom a major bleeding event has occurred. After major surgery, therapy may be required daily for up to 7–10 days. In patients with von Willebrand disease who have circulating antibodies to von Willebrand factor, high-dose intravenous gammaglobulin with or without plasmapheresis may be required. One gram of gammaglobulin per kilogram of body weight is given intravenously on two successive days in patients undergoing surgical procedures. The use of extracorporal absorption is useful for reducing titers of antibodies in individuals with life-threatening bleeding. Plasma change may also be an effective form of therapy.

Prophylactic therapy has been explored because of the potential dangers of transmitting viral disease by infusion of plasma products. Clinical studies have revealed that patients with von Willebrand disease or mild classic hemophilia can benefit from DDAVP administration.

DDAVP increases the Factor VIII: C von Willebrand factor antigen and ristocetin co-factor 3–5-fold over baseline levels. DDAVP has been used to treat mild to moderately severe bleeding, and is a prophylactic form of intervention for patients undergoing surgical procedures. It is commonly given intravenously in a dose of 0.3–0.4 µg/kg over 15–20 minutes.

Patients with coagulation defects undergoing invasive procedures: management steps

Before procedures are performed, the patient's coagulation status should be characterized by means of laboratory testing. These should include prothrombin time, activated prothrombinplastin time, platelet count, bleeding times, and fibrinogen determination. In situations where a fibrinogen defect is suspected, a thrombin time should also be included.

Other studies may apply to a specific diagnosis such as: Factor VIII assay for classic hemophilia; Factor IX assay for hemophilia B; platelet aggregation studies with ristocetin for von Willebrand disease; and determination of thrombin clotting time for dysfibrinogenemia should be performed when appropriate.

For most coagulation abnormalities, a level of at least 30 per cent or preferably 50 per cent of activity is necessary for hemostasis. In classic hemophilia, human Factor VIII should be given preoperatively in a dose of 50 units/kg. Factor VIII levels should be titrated and additional infusions administered as indicated. Sufficient replacement should continue for anywhere from 3 to 7 days postoperatively depending on the surgical procedure and the overall hemostatic challenge. DDAVP should be administered prior to minor surgical procedures in patients with von Willebrand disease, while cryoprecipitate should be utilized for a more extensive procedures.

Once again, the level of Factor VIII and bleeding time should be used to guide therapy. Four to ten units of cryoprecipitate represents a typical starting dose; additional transfusion is determined by the Factor VIII level, normalization of bleeding time and the level of hemostatic control.

Liver disease: management steps

Thrombotic episodes are relatively uncommon among patients with liver disease, despite reductions in antithrombin, plasminogen, and plasminogen activator levels. Instead, hemorrhagic complications predominate the clinical picture. The most common sites of bleeding include the nasopharynx, esophagus, stomach, small intestine, and retroperitoneum.

In acute liver disease, coagulation abnormalities parallel other signs of hepatic damage; in fact, prolongation of standard coagulation tests (PT, aPTT, TT) has prognostic value.

A major challenge confronting the clinician is treatment. Replacement of coagulation factors through fresh-frozen plasma transfusion and vitamin K replacement may reduce the incidence of life-threatening hemorrhage; however, complete correction of the coagulopathy is usually not possible in acute liver failure. Platelet transfusions should also be considered in patients with platelet counts less than 30 000/mm³.

With either acute or chronic liver disease complicated by moderate to severe bleeding, other treatment measures, including endoscopic and surgical, should be considered early given the inherent difficulty in correcting existing coagulation abnormalities.

Renal disease: management steps

Hemorrhage is not an uncommon event among patients with renal disease. In a majority of cases, the skin, mucous membranes, and gastrointestinal tract are the sites of involvement. Occasionally, life-threatening bleeding may occur, particularly in those with both platelet and coagulation abnormalities. In contrast, serious thrombotic (arterial or venous) events have been described in patients with nephrotic syndrome. As a result, these individuals must be approached somewhat differently.

The general approach to bleeding problems in patients with renal insufficiency begins with the correction of underlying metabolic abnormalities. The institution of dialysis in a uremic patient may have an important impact on hemostasis. If the standard coagulation tests (PT, aPTT) are prolonged, vitamin K replacement should be provided, followed by fresh-frozen plasma if the clinical setting so warrants. Platelet transfusions and intravenous DDAVP should also be considered for moderate to severe bleeding complications.

Although the initial approach to bleeding in patients with renal failure begins with hemodialysis or peritoneal dialysis, it is important to recognize, however, that dialysis alone may *not* correct the bleeding tendency.

It has been demonstrated that cryoprecipitate or DDAVP can temporarily correct the bleeding tendency in patients with uremia. Intravenous administration of 10 units of cryoprecipitate leads to shortening of the bleeding time for approximately 18–24 hours that permits major surgical or invasive procedures to be undertaken without excessive blood loss. DDAVP at a dose of 0.3 µg/kg body weight shortens the bleeding time for approximately 4–6 hours.

Repeat infusions of DDAVP may lead to a reduced response. There is increasing evidence that the administration of erythropoietin may also reduce bleeding tendency in patients with renal failure.

Disseminated intravascular coagulation: management steps

The keys to management are diagnosing and treating the underlying disorder (Table 15.25). Antibiotics, volume replacement, inotropic/vasopressor support, and surgical intervention should be applied as indicated without delay. Several laboratory tests should be obtained, including a complete blood count, platelet count, fibrinogen and FDP concentrations, and standard coagulation measurements (PT, aPTT, TT). Other tests such as Bβ-42 (D-dimer), antithrombin, prothrombin fragment 1.2 (F1.2), and fibrinopeptide A concentrations, while helpful at times, lack specificity, are expensive, and are not readily available through non-specialized laboratories.

The specific treatment of DIC is limited but can be broken down into three categories: (1) restoration of hemostasis; (2) thrombosis prevention; and (3) thrombus removal. Transfusion of blood and fresh-frozen plasma may be required to restore blood volume and replace consumed coagulation factors. Cryoprecipitate and platelet transfusions can be used in the presence of severe bleeding; however, the theo-

Table 15.25 *Standard coagulation measurements and laboratory tests in disseminated intravascular coagulation*

Measurement	Acute	Subacute	Chronic
Prothrombin time	↑↑	↑	Normal, ↓, or ↑
Partial thromboplastin time	↑↑	↑	Normal, ↓, or ↑
Thrombin time	↑↑	↑	Normal, ↓, or ↑
Fibrinogen level	↓↓	↓ or normal	Normal, ↓, or ↑
FDP[a] level	↑↑	↑↑	Normal, ↓, or ↑
Platelet count	↓	Variable	Variable
D-dimer	↑↑	↑	↑

[a]Fibrin(ogen) degradation products.

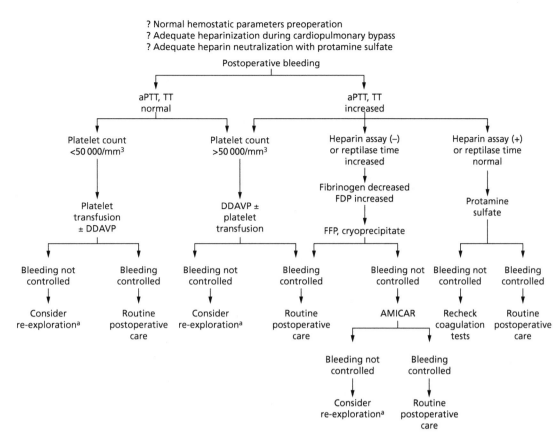

Figure 15.12 *Clinical approach and management of patients with postoperative bleeding.*
[a]Re-exploration for mediastinal/chest tube bleeding.
aPTT = activated partial thromboplastin time; TT = thrombin time; DDAVP = desamino-8-D-arginine vasopressin;
FDP = fibrin(ogen) degradation products; FFP = fresh-frozen plasma; AMICAR = aminocaproic acid.

retical risk of 'fueling the fire' does exist. Low-dose heparin (300–400 units/hour) has been used to prevent microthrombosis in animal models of DIC.

It can be used cautiously in clinical situations where the risk of bleeding is relatively minor compared with the probability of thrombosis. It also should be considered when a thrombotic event (e.g. pulmonary embolism) is the precipitating cause for DIC. In this case, standard heparin doses may be used if clinical bleeding is not evident. However, when bleeding does occur, thrombectomy (surgical, extraction catheter) may be necessary.

Cardiopulmonary bypass: management steps

Bleeding complications following cardiopulmonary bypass require immediate attention. Once the source of bleeding has been identified and local measures have been undertaken, efforts must address the defective hemostatic mechanism. It is important to keep in mind that abnormalities in platelet function, coagulation, and

fibrinolysis almost always coexist. The extent and severity of the acquired coagulopathy may also be augmented by preoperative medical treatment, which for many unstable cardiac patients with coronary artery disease includes heparin, aspirin, and at times, fibrinolytic agents (Fig. 15.12).

Antiplatelet therapy: management steps

Bleeding events associated with disorders of primary hemostasis most often involve the skin and mucous membranes; however, the gastrointestinal and genitourinary tracts may occasionally be involved. The severity of bleeding is directly related to the degree of platelet dysfunction, integrity of the vasculature, and status of the intrinsic/extrinsic coagulation pathways. In general, an isolated platelet defect is rarely the cause of life-threatening hemorrhage.

The template bleeding time can be measured to provide a general estimate of platelet dysfunction; however, it is non-specific and vulnerable to error from variable technique. Platelet aggregation studies can also be performed if time allows.

The treatment of bleeding for the most part is non-specific. As with all hemorrhage, the source should be identified, the offending agent discontinued, and local measures (manual pressure, suturing) explored first. Thereafter, treatment is dictated by the severity of the event. Platelet transfusions either with or without DDAVP should be given for serious or life-threatening bleeding.

Profound thrombocytopenia (platelet counts <2000/mm^3) has been observed with the GPIIb/IIIa antagonists. The largest experience is with abciximab (ReoPro®). Most patients have responded to discontinuation of the medication and platelet transfusions. Intravenous immunoglobulin therapy has had little impact on the syndromes' natural history.

Heparin: management steps

Mild to moderate bleeding can be addressed by reducing the heparin dose (particularly if the aPTT is excessively prolonged) or discontinuing the infusion for a brief period of time (30 minutes). More severe hemorrhage may require complete discontinuation or, with serious life-threatening hemorrhage, neutralization with protamine sulfate (1 mg for every 100 units of heparin administered in the preceding 4 hours).

However, in patients with active coronary heart disease, a careful risk–benefit assessment must be undertaken, considering the risks of coronary thrombosis versus those of bleeding. It may be in the patient's best interest to continue systemic anticoagulation, particularly if the bleeding is not serious/life threatening and can be adequately controlled with local measures (e.g. manual pressure over a site of vascular trauma).

Protamine sulfate (1 mg/100 anti-Xa units administered in the past 6–8 hours) can also be administered to neutralize the anticoagulant effects of LMWH. Unfortunately, the neutralization is incomplete (~60 per cent). Fresh-frozen plasma should be administered in the setting of life-threatening bleeding to correct any residual hemostatic impairment.

Warfarin: management steps

The anticoagulant effect of warfarin can be reduced or entirely reversed by lowering the dose, discontinuing treatment, administering vitamin K, or replacing the defective coagulation factors with fresh-frozen plasma or prothrombin concentrate. The severity of bleeding and inherent risks of reduced anticoagulation should dictate the course of action (Table 15.26).

Fibrinolytic therapy: management steps

Even with careful patient selection and acceptable monitoring, hemorrhagic events do occur.

Routine management includes volume and blood pressure support as well as a prompt and thorough search for the site of bleeding. Abdominopelvic or head computed tomography may be useful in the diagnosis and management of major hemorrhagic events. Life-threatening hemorrhage warrants prompt intervention. Heparin should be discontinued and neutralized with protamine sulfate. Fresh-frozen plasma is an excellent source of Factors V and VIII, α_2-antiplasmin, and plasminogen activator inhibitor. Cryoprecipitate (8–10 units) is the preferred source of fibrinogen (200–250 mg/10–15 mL) and Factor VIII (80 units/10–15 mL). If the platelet

Table 15.26 *Management of prolonged INR associated with warfarin therapy*

	INR			
	<6.0	6.0 – 10.0	>10.0	>20.0
Clinical profile	No bleeding	No bleeding	No bleeding	No bleeding
Recommended approach	Omit next 1–2 doses of warfarin	Vitamin K (1–2 mg sc) ↓ Repeat INR in 8 hours ↓ Consider additional vitamin K	Vitamin K (3 mg sc) ↓ Repeat INR in 6 hours ↓ Consider additional vitamin K	Vitamin K (5–10 mg sc) ↓ Repeat INR in 6 hours ↓ Consider additional vitamin K

INR = international normalized ratio; SC = subcutaneous; iv = intravenous.
Because of life-threatening hemorrhage, fresh-frozen plasma or prothrombin concentrates should be administered. Concomitant administration of vitamin K (3–5 mg iv) should also be considered. IV vitamin K should be considered for a rapid reversal of anticoagulant effect.

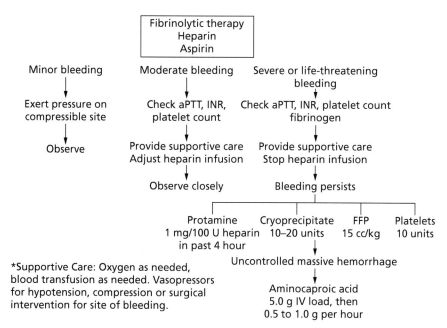

Figure 15.13 *Clinical approach and management of hemorrhage among patients who have received thrombolytic therapy and adjunctive antithrombotic agents. aPTT = activated partial thromboplastin time; INR = international normalized ratio; FFP = fresh-frozen plasma IV = intravenous.*

count is low (<50 000/mm³), platelets (10 units, random donor) should be given. If indicated, DDAVP (0.3 µg/kg iv over 20 minutes) can be used to correct qualitative platelet abnormalities. Persistent and potentially life-threatening hemorrhage unresponsive to standard measures (outlined above) may require antifibrinolytic therapy. This intervention should be used with caution since serious thrombotic complications may be precipitated. Aminocaproic acid and tranexamic acid are the most frequently used agents (Fig. 15.13).

SUMMARY

- Hematologic and coagulation disorders are common in patients with cardiovascular disease and contribute significantly to morbidity and mortality.
- An understanding of basic hematologic principles, hemostasis, and coagulation monitoring are an absolute prerequisite for clinicians committed to achieving the highest possible level of patient care.
- Management algorithms are available for patients with inherited or acquired hemostatic disorders arising from fibrinolytic therapy, anticoagulants, platelet antagonists, and those associated with extracorporeal circulation.

REFERENCES

1. Jewett B, ed. *The dialogues of Plato*, Vol. 3, 3rd edn. New York: Macmillan 1892: 339–543.
2. Lee HDP, translator. *Aristotle: meterologica.* Loeb Classical Library. Cambridge: Harvard University Press, 1952.
3. Petit JL. Dissertation sur la mannière d'arrester le sang dans les hémorragies. *Mem Acad R Sci* 1731; **1**: 85–102.
4. Forester JM, translator. *Malpighi M. De polypo cordis,* 1686. Uppsala: Almquist & Wiksels, 1956.
5. Buchanan A. On the coagulation of the blood and other fibriniferous liquids. *London Med Gaz* 1845; **1**: 617. Reprinted in *J Physiol Lond* 1879–1880; **2**: 158–68.
6. Schmidt A. *Zur Blutleher.* Leipzig: Vogel, 1892.
7. Otto JC. An account of an hemorrhagic disposition existing in certain families. *Med Repository* 1803; **6**: 1–4.
8. Hay J. Account of a remarkable haemorrhagic disposition existing in many individuals of the same family. *N Engl J Med Surg* 1813; **2**: 221–5.
9. Thackrah CT. *An inquiry into the nature and properties of the blood.* London: Cox & Sons, 1819.
10. De Blainville HMD. Injection de matière cérébrale dans les veins. *Gaz Med Paris* 1834; **2**: 524.
11. Howell WH. The nature and action of the thromboplastin (zymoplastic) substance of the tissues. *Am J Physiol* 1912; **31**: 1–21.
12. Mills CA. Chemical nature of tissue coagulants. *J Biol Chem* 1921; **46**: 135–65.
13. Bordet J. The theories of blood coagulation. *Bull Johns Hopkins Hosp* 1921; **32**: 213–18.

14. Chargaff E, Benedich A, Cohen SS. The thromboplastic protein: structure, properties, disintegration. *J Biol Chem* 1944; **156**: 161–78.

15. Quick AJ. *Hemorrhagic diseases*. Philadelphia, Lea & Febiger, 1957.

16. Hougie C, Barrow EM, Graham JB. Stuart clotting defect. I. Segregation of an herediatry hemorrhagic state from the heterogenous group heretofore called 'stable factor' (SPCA, proconvertin, factor VII) deficiency. *J Clin Invest* 1957; **36**: 485–96.

17. Donné A. De l'origine des globules du sang, de leur mode de formation et leur fin. *C R Acad Sci Paris* (abstract) 1842; **14**: 366–8.

18. Osler W. An account of certain organisms occuring in the liquor sanguinis. *Proc Roy Soc* 1874; **22**: 391–8.

19. Hayem G. Sur le méchanisme de l' arrêt des hémorragies. *C R Acad Sci* 1882; **95**: 18–21.

20. Marcus AJ. Platelet function. *N Engl J Med* 1969; **280**: 1213–20, 1278–84, 1330–5.

21. Spaet TH, Zucker MB. Mechanism of platelet plug formation and role of adenosine diphosphate. *Am J Physiol* 1964; **206**: 1267–74.

22. Grette K. Studies on the mechanism of thrombin-catalyzed hemostatic reaction in blood platelets. *Acta Physiol Scan Suppl* 1962; **195**: 1–93.

23. Willis AL, Vane FM, Kuhn DC, *et al.* An endoperoxide aggregator (LASS) formed in platelets in response to thrombotic stimuli. *Prostaglandins* 1974; **8**: 453–507.

24. Konttinen YP. *Fibrinolysis: chemistry, physiology, pathology and clinics*. Tampere: Oy Star Ab, 1968.

25. Christensen LR, MacLeod CM. Proteolytic enzyme of serum: characaterization, activation, and reaction with inhibitors. *J Gen Physiol* 1945; **23**: 559–83.

26. Hedin SG. On the presence of a proteolytic enzyme in the normal serum of the ox. *J Physiol Lond* 1904; **30**: 195–201.

27. Gratia A. Quoted by Kontinnen YP. *Fibrinolysis: chemistry, physiology, pathology and clinics*. Tampere: Oy Star Ab, 1968.

28. Tillet WS, Garner RL. The fibrinolytic activity of hemolytic streptocci. *J Exp Med* 1933; **58**: 484–502.

♦29. Sherry S, Fletcher A. Alkjaersig N. Fibrinolysis and fibrinolytic activity in man. *Physiol Rev* 1959; **39**: 343–81.

30. Macfarlane RG, Pilling J. Fibrinolytic activity of normal urine. *Nature* 1947; **159**: 779.

31. Williams, JRB. The fibrinolytic activity of urine. *Br J Exp Pathol* 1951; **32**: 530–7.

32. Piper P, Vane JR. The release of prostaglandins from the vascular endothelium and other tissues. *Ann New York Acad Sci* 1971; **180**: 363–85.

33. Willis AL, Smith DL, Vigo C, Luge AF. Effects of prostacylin and orally active stable mimetic agent RS-93427–007 on bovine mechanisms of atherogenesis. *Lancet* 1986; **2**: 682–3.

34. Furchgott RF, Zawasdski JV. The obligatory role of endothelial cells in the relaxation of arterial smooth muscle cells by acetylcholine. *Nature* 1980; **228**: 373

35. Palmer RMJ, Fergie AG, Moncada S. Nitric oxide release accounts for the biologic activity of endothelium-derived relaxing factor. *Nature* 1987; **327**: 524–6.

36. Radomski MW, Palmer RM, Moncada S. Endogenous nitric oxide inhibits human platelet adhesion to vascular endothelium. *Lancet* 1987; **1**: 1057–9.

37. Radomski MW, Plamer RM, Mocada S. The antiaggregatory properties of vascular endothelium: interactions between prostacylin and nitric oxide. *Br J Pharmacol* 1987; **92**: 639–46.

38. Heeg E, Meng K. Die wirkung des bradykinins, angiotensis und vasopressins auf verhof appilarmusckel, und isoliert durstromte herzpraprate des meerschweinchens. *Navnyn Schiedebergs Arch Pharmacol* 1965; **250**: 35.

39. Unger TH, Gohlke P, Ganten D, Lang RE. Converting enzyme inhibitors and their effects on the renin-angiotensis system of the blood vessel wall. *J Cardiovasc Pharmacol* 1988; **13**(suppl 3): S8.

40. Simonson MS, Wann S, Mene P, *et al.* Endothelin-1 activates the phosphoinositide cascade in cultured glomerular mesangial cells. *J Cardiovasc Pharmacol* 1989; **13**(suppl 5): S80.

41. Yanagisawa M, Kurihara H, Kimsura S, *et al.* A novel potent vasoconstricter peptide produced by vascular endothelial cells. *Nature* 1988; **332**: 411.

42. Miyanchi T, Tomobe Y, Shiba R, *et al.* Involvement of endothelin in the regulation of human vascular tonus: potent vasoconstrictor effect and existence in endothelial cells. *Circulation* 1990; **81**: 1874.

43. Teien AN, Abildgaard U, Hook M, Lindahl U. The anticoagulant' effect of heparan sulfate and dermatan sulfate. *Thromb Res* 1977; **11**: 107–17.

44. Thomas DP, Merton RE, Barrowcliffe TW, *et al.* Antifactor Xa activity of heparan sulfate and dermatan sulfate. *Thromb Res* 1979; **14**: 501.

♦45. Marcum JA, Rosenberg RD. Heparin-like molecules with anticoagulant activity are synthesized by cultured endothelial cells. *Biochem Biophys Res Commun* 1985; **126**: 365.

46. Maynard JR, Dreyer BE, Stereman MB, Pitlick FA. Tissue factor coagulant activity of cultured human endothelial and smooth muscle cells and fibroblasts. *Blood* 1977; **50**: 387.

47. Stern OM, Bank I, Naworth PP, *et al.* Self regulation of procoagulant events on the endothelial cells surface. *J Exp Med* 1985; **162**: 1223.

48. Broze GJ Jr, Warren LA, Novotny WF, Higuchi DA, Girard TJ, Miletich JP. The lipoprotein-associated coagulation inhibitor that inhibits factor VII–tissue factor complex also inhibits factor Xa; insight into its possible mechanism of acation. *Blood* 1988; **71**: 335–43.

49. van't Veer C, Hackeng TM, Delahaye C, Sixma JJ, Bouma BN. Activated factor X and thrombin

formation triggered by tissue factor on endothelial cell matric in a flow model: effect of the tissue factor pathway inhibitor. *Blood* 1994; **84**: 1132–9.

50. Kaiser B, Hoppensteadt DA, Jeske W, Wun TC, Fareed J. Inhibitory effects of TFPI of thrombin and factor Xa generation in vitro – modulatory action of glycosaminoglycans. *Thromb Res* 1994; **75**: 609–19.

♦51. Sprecher CA, Kisiel W, Mathewes S, Foster DC. Molecular cloning, expression, and partial characterization of a second human tissue-factor-pathway inhibitor. *Proc Natl Acad Sci USA* 1994; **91**: 3353–7.

52. Peterson LC, Sprecher CA, Foster DC, Blumberg H, Hamamoto T, Kisiel W. Inhibitory properties of a novel human Kunitz-type protease inhibitor homologous to tissue factor pathway inhibitor. *Biochemistry* 1996; **35**: 266–72.

53. Tait JF, Gibson D, Fukikawa K. Phospholipid binding properties of human placental anticoagulant protein-I, a member of the lipocortin family. *J Biol Chem* 1989; **264**: 7944–51.

54. Giddings JC. von Willebrand factor – physiology. In: Gimbrone MA Jr, ed. *Vascular endothelium in hemostasis and thrombosis*. New York: Churchill-Livingstone, 1986: 142.

55. Erikson LA, Ginsberg MH, Loskutoff DJ. Detection and partial characaterization of an inhibitor of plasmingoen activator in human platelets. *J Clin Invest* 1984; **74**: 1465–72.

56. Lucore CL, Sobel BE. Interactions of tissue type plasminogen activatior with plasma inhibitors and their pharmacolgic implications. *Circulation* 1988; **77**: 660–9.

○57. Chakrabari R, Hocking ED. Fibrinolytic activity and coronary heart disease. *Lancet* 1968; **1**: 987–90.

58. Zahavi J, Bitteride JD, Jones NAG, *et al*. Enhanced in vitro platelet hyperlipidemia. *Am J Med* 1981; **70**: 59–64.

59. Joist JH, Baker RK, Schonfeld G. Increased in vivo and in vitro platelet function in type II and type IV hyperlipoprotenemia. *Thromb Res* 1974; **15**: 95.

60. Joist JH, Dolezel G, Kinlough-Rathbone RI, Mustard JF. Effect of diet-induced hyperlipidemia on in vitro function of rabbit platelets. *Thromb Res* 1976; **9**: 435–45.

61. Tremoli E, Folco G, Agradi E, Gall C. Platelet thromboxanes and serum cholestrol. *Lancet* 1979; **1**: 107–8.

62. Harker LA, Hazzre W. Platelet kinetic studies in patients with hyperlipoproteinemia: effect of clofibrate therapy. *Circulation* 1979; **60**: 492–7.

63. Worner P, Patscheke H. Hyperactivity by an enhancement of the arachiodonate pathway of platelets treated with cholesterol-rich phospholipid-dispersions. *Thromb Res* 1980; **18**: 439–51.

64. Shattil SJ, Cooper RA. Role of membrane lipid composition organization and fluidity in human platelet function. *Prog Hemost Thromb* 1978; **4**: 59–86.

♦65. Nabel EG, Ganz P, Selwyn AP. Atherosclerosis impairs flow-mediated dilation in human coronary arteries. *Circulation* 1988; **78**(suppl II): II-474.

66. Jayakody L, Sernaratne M, Thompson A, Kapagoda T. Endothelium-dependent relaxation in experimental atherosclerosis in the rabbit. *Circulation Res* 1987; **60**: 251–64.

67. Cohen RA, Zitnay KM, Haudenschild CC, Cunningham LD. Loss of selective endothelial cell vasoactive functions caused by hypercholesterolemia in pig coronary arteries. *Circulation Res* 1988; **63**: 903–10.

68. Redl H, Hammerschmidt ED, Schlag G. Augmentation by platelets of granulocyte aggregation in response to chemotaxins: Studies utilizing an improved cell preparation technique. *Blood* 1983; **61**: 125–31.

69. Boogaerts MA, Vercellotti G, Roelant C, Malbrain S, Verwilghen RL, Jacob HS. Platelets augment granulocyte aggregation and cytotoxicity: undercovering of their effects by improved cell separation techniques using Percoll gradients. *Scand J Haemotol* 1986; **37**: 229–36.

70. De Gaetano G, Evangelist V, Ratjar G, Del Moshio A, Cerletti C. Activated polymorphonuclear leukocytes stimulate platelet function. *Thromb Res* 1990; **11**: 25–32.

71. Oda M, Satouchi K, Yasunage K, Saito K. Polymorphonuclear leukocyte–platelet interactions: acetyglycerol ether phosphocholine-induced platelet activation under stimulation with chemotactic peptide. *J Biochem* 1986; **100**: 1117–23.

♦72. Zimmerman TS, Ratnoff OD, Powell AE. Immunological differentiation of classic hemophilia (factor VIII deficiency) and von Willebrand's disease. *J Clin Invest* 1971; **50**: 244–54.

73. Essien EM. Haemorrhagic disorders. *Clin Haematol* 1981; **10**: 917–32.

74. Von Willebrand EA. *Finska Lakaresallsb Handl* 1926; **68**: 87–112.

75. Mills D, Karpatkin S. The non-plasmin proteolytic origin of human fibrinogen heterogenicity. *Biochem Biophys Acta* 1977; **251**: 121.

76. Spaet TH, Horowitz HI, Franklin DZ, Cintron J, Biezensi JJ. Reticuloendothelial clearance of blood thromboplastin by rats. *Blood* 1961; **17**: 196.

77. Rabiner S. Uremic bleeding. In: Spaet TH, ed. *Progress in thrombosis and hemostasis*, vol 1. New York: Grune & Stratton; 1972: 233.

78. Remuzzi G, Marches D, Livio M, *et al*. Altered platelet and vascular prostaglandin-generation in patients with renal failure and prolonged bleeding time. *Thromb Res* 1978; **13**: 1007–15.

79. Thompson AR. Factor XII and other hemostatic abnormalities in nephrotic syndrome patients. *Thromb Haemost* 1982; **48**: 27–32.

80. Shea MA, Indeglia RA, Dorman FD. The biologic response to pumping blood. *Trans Am Soc Artif Intern Organs* 1967; **13**: 116–23.

81. Salzman EW. Blood platelets and extracorporeal circulation. *Transfusion* 1963; **3**: 274.

82. Friedenberg WR, Myers WO, Plotka ED. Platelet dysfunction associated with cardiopulmonary bypass. *Ann Thorac Surg* 1978; **25**: 298–305.

83. Hope AF, DuPhens A, Lotter MG. Kinetics and sites of sequestration of indium 111-labeled human platelets during cardiopulmonary bypass. *J Thorac Cardiovasc Surg* 1981; **81**: 880–6.

84. Boyd AD, Engelman RM, Beadet RL, Lackner H. Disseminated intravascular coagulation following extracorpeal circulation. *J Thorac Cardiovasc Surg* 1972; **64**: 685–93.

85. Libby P, Warner SJC, Salomon RN, Birinyi LK. Production of platelet-derived growth factor-like mitogen by smooth-muscle cells from human atheroma. *N Engl J Med* 1988; **318**: 1493–7.

86. Williams LT. Signal transduction by the platelet-derived growth factor receptor. *Science* 1989; **243**: 1564–70.

87. Badimon L, Badimon JJ, Chesebro JH, Fuster V. Inhibition of thrombus formation: blockage of adhesive glycoprotein mechanisms versus blockage of the cyclooxygenase pathway. *J Am Coll Cardiol* 1988; **11**(suppl A): 30A(abstract).

88. Strony J, Phillips M, Brands D, *et al*. Aurintricarboxylic acid in canine model of coronary artery thrombosis. *Circulation* 1990; **81**: 1106–14.

89. Cattaneo M, Chahil A, Somers D, *et al*. Effect of aspirin and sodium salicylate on thrombosis, fibrinolysis, prothrombin time, and platelet survival in rabbits with indwelling aortic catheters. *Blood* 1983; **61**: 353–61.

○90. Hirsh J. Progress review: the relationship between dose of aspirin, side effects and antithrombotic effectiveness. *Stroke* 1985; **16**: 1–4.

♦91. Yasuda T, Gold HK, Leinback RC, *et al*. Lysis of plasminogen activator-resistant platelet rich coronary artery thrombus with combined bolus injection of recombinant tissue-type plasminogen activator and antiplatelet GPIIb/IIIa antibody. *J Am Coll Cardiol* 1990; **16**: 1728–35.

92. Musial J, Niewiarowski S, Rucinski B, *et al*. Inhibition of platelet adhesion to surfaces of extracorporeal circuits by disintegrins. RGD-containing peptides from viper venoms. *Circulation* 1990; **82**: 261–73.

93. Saltiel R, Ward A. Ticlopidine: a review of its pharmacodynamics and pharmacokinetic properties and therapeutic efficacy in platelet-dependent disease states. *Drugs* 1987; **34**: 222–62.

♦94. CAPRIE Steering Committee. A randomised, blinded, trial of clopidogrel versus aspirin in patients at risk of ischaemic events (CAPRIE). *Lancet* 1996; **348**: 1329–39.

95. FitzGerald GA, Reilly LA, Pederson AK. The biochemical pharmacology of thromboxane synthase inhibition in man. *Circulation* 1985; **72**: 1194–201.

96. Mullane KM, Fionabaio D. Thromboxane synthetase inhibitors reduce infarct size by a platelet dependent, aspirin-sensitive mechanism. *Circulation Res* 1988; **62**: 668–78.

97. Saussy DL Jr, Mais DE, Knapp DR, Halushka PV. Thromboxane A_2 and prostaglandin endoperoxide receptors in platelets and vascular smooth muscle. *Circulation* 1985; **72**: 1202–7.

98. Evans RJ, Gordon JD. Mechanisms of the antithrombotic actions of dextran. *N Engl J Med* 1974; **290**: 748.

99. Weiss HJ. The effect of clinical dextran on platelet aggregation, adhesion, and ADP release in man: in vivo and in vitro studies. *J Lab Clin Med* 1967; **69**: 37–46.

100. FitzGerald GA. Dipyridamole. *N Engl J Med* 1987; **316**: 1247–57.

101. Emmons RP, Hampton JR, Harrison MJG, *et al*. Effect of prostaglandin E_1 on platelet behavior in vitro and in vivo. *Br Med J* 1967; **2**: 468–72.

102. Treers W, Beythein C, Kupper W, Bliefeld W. Effects of aspirin and prostaglandin E_1 on in vitro thrombolysis and urokinase. *Circulation* 1989; **79**: 1309–14.

103. Weksler BB. Prostaglandins and vascular function. *Circulation* 1984; **70**(suppl III): III-63.

104. Fisher CA, Kappa JR, Sinha AK, *et al*. Comparison of equimolar concentrations of iloprost, prostacyclin, and prostaglandin E_1 on human platelet function. *J Lab Clin Med* 1987; **109**: 184–90.

105. Addonizio VP, Fisher CA, Strauss JF, *et al*. Effects of verapamil and diltiazen on human platelet function. *Am J Physiol* 1986; **250**: H366.

106. Wade PJ, Lunt DO, Lad N, *et al*. Effect of calcium and calcium antagonists on [^{3}H]-PAF-Acether binding to washed human platelets. *Thromb Res* 1986; **41**: 251–62.

107. Fischer-Dzoga K, Kuo YF, Wissler RW. The proliferative effect of platelets and hyperlipidemic serum on stationary primary cultures. *Atherosclerosis* 1983; **47**: 35.

108. Tiell ML, Sussman II, Gordon PB. Suppression of fibroblast proliferation in vitro and of myointimal hyperplasia in vivo by the triazolopyrimadine, trapidil. *Artery* 1983; **12**: 33.

109. Lam LH, Silbert JE, Rosenberg RD. The separation of active and inactive forms of heparin. *Biochem Biophys Res Commun* 1976; **69**: 570–7.

110. Andersson LO, Barrowcliffe TW, Holmer E, Johnson EA, Sims GE. Anticoagulant properties of heparin fractionated by affinity chromatography on matrix-bound antithrombin III and by gel filtration. *Thromb Res* 1976; **9**: 575–83.

♦111. de Swart CA, Nijmeyer B, Roelofs JM, Sixma JJ. Kinetics of intravenously administered heparin in normal humans. *Blood* 1982; **60**: 1251–8.

112. Olsson P, Lagergren H, Ek S. The elimination from plasma of intravenous heparin: an experimental study on dogs and humans. *Acta Med Scand* 1963; **173**: 619.

113. Young E, Prins M, Levine MN, Hirsh J. Heparin binding to plasma proteins, an important mechanism for heparin resistance. *Thromb Haemost* 1992; **67**: 639–43.

114. Bjornsson TD, Wolfram KM, Kitchell BB. Heparin kinetics determined by three assay methods. *Clin Pharmacol Ther* 1982; **31**: 104–13.

115. Hsia J, Hamilton WP, Kleiman N, *et al.* A comparison between heparin and low dose aspirin as adjunctive therapy with tissue plasminogen activator for acute myocardial infarction. *N Engl J Med* 1990; **323**: 1433–7.

116. de Bono DP, Simoons ML, Tijssen J, *et al.* Effect of early intravenous heparin on coronary patency, infarct size and bleeding complications after alteplase thrombolysis: results of a randomized double blind European Cooperative Study Group trial. *Br Heart J* 1992; **67**: 122–8.

117. Hull RD, Raskob GE, Hirsh J, *et al.* Continuous intravenous heparin compared with intermittent subcutaneous heparin in the initial treatment of proximal-vein thrombosis. *N Engl J Med* 1986; **315**: 1109–14.

118. Becker RC, Cyr J, Corrao JM, Ball SP. Bedside coagulation monitoring in heparinized patients with active thromboembolic disease: a coronary care unit experience. *Am Heart J* 1994; **128**: 719–23.

♦119. Becker RC, Ball SP, Borzak S, for the Antithrombotic Therapy Consortium Investigators. A randomized, multicenter trial of weight-adjusted intravenous heparin and point-of-care coagulation monitoring in hospitalized patients with active thromboembolic disease. *Am Heart J* 1998; **137**: 59–71.

○120. Weitz JI. Low molecular weight heparins. *N Engl J Med* 1997; **337**: 688–98.

121. Gent M, Hirsh J, Ginsberg JS, *et al.* Low-molecular-weight heparinoid Orgaran is more effective than aspirin in the prevention of venous thromboembolism after surgery for hip fracture. *Circulation* 1996; **93**: 80–4.

122. deValk HW, Banga JD, Wester JWJ, *et al.* Comparing subcutaneous danaparoid with intravenous unfractionated heparin for the treatment of venous thromboembolism. A randomized controlled trial. *Ann Intern Med* 1995; **123**: 1–9.

123. Magnani HN. Heparin-induced thrombocytopenia (HIT): an overview of 230 patients treated with Orgaran (Org 10172). *Thromb Haemost* 1993; **70**: 554–61.

124. Poller L. Progress in standardization in anticoagulant control. *Hematol Rev* 1987; **1**: 225.

125. Poller L, Taberner DA. Dosage and control of oral anticoagulants: an international collaborative survey. *Br J Haematol* 1982; **51**: 479–85.

126. Bussey HI, Force RW, Bianco TM, Leonard AD. Reliance on prothrombin time ratios causes significant errors in anticoagulation therapy. *Arch Intern Med* 1992; **152**: 278–82.

127. Sallah S, Thomas DP, Roberts HR. Warfarin and heparin-induced skin necrosis and the purple toe syndrome: infrequent complications of anticoagulant treatment. *Thromb Haemost* 1997; **78**: 785–90.

♦128. Kereiakas DJ, Mueller M, Howard W, *et al.* Efficiency of abciximab-induced platelet blockade using a rapid point-of-care assay. *J Thromb Thrombolysis* 1999; **7**: 265–75.

129. Walenga JM, Lewis BE, Hoppensteadt DA, Fareed J, Bakbos M. Management of heparin-induced thrombocytopenia and heparin-induced thrombocytopenia and thrombosis syndrome. *Clin Appl Thromb Hemostas* 1997; **3**: S53–63.

16

Diagnosis and management of inherited and acquired thrombophilias

FREDERICK A SPENCER AND RICHARD C BECKER

Thrombophilia, defined as an inherited or acquired predisposition to unwanted or poorly regulated vascular thrombosis, is responsible for a wide range of venous and arterial events including pulmonary embolism, stroke and myocardial infarction. A rapidly expanding knowledge of vascular biology and genetics has paved the way for diagnostic tests, screening modalities and management strategies that collectively elevate the standard of care for patients at risk for, as well as those with, thromboembolic disorders of the cardiovascular system.

INTRODUCTION

Thromboembolic disease wreaks a devastating toll on humanity whether measured in terms of total mortality, general morbidity, or financial cost. For this reason, the pathophysiology of thrombosis has been intensely studied since the early 1800s. In 1884, Rudolph Virchow first proposed that thrombosis was the end result of three interrelated factors – vascular endothelial *damage, stasis* of blood flow, and *hypercoagulability* of blood. Since then we have come to better understand the delicate equilibrium between blood cells, platelets, coagulant factors, natural inhibitors of coagulation, and the fibrinolytic system. In the last three decades there has been increasing recognition that inherited or acquired defects of these mechanisms can predispose to arterial and venous thrombosis.

The term *thrombophilia* is now applied to all patients with defined familial or acquired disorders of thromboresistance and hemostatic regulation which predispose to thrombosis.[1] While best understood in the context of venous thromboembolism, the contribution of thrombophilias to arterial thrombosis and atherosclerosis are becoming more widely appreciated.

In this chapter we review the inherited and acquired thrombophilias and provide recommendations for practicing clinicians regarding the diagnostic approach and management of these patients.

HISTORICAL LANDMARKS

The first family with antithrombin (AT) (previously referred to as AT III) deficiency was described in 1965;[2] however, it was not until the 1980s with the identification of protein C (PC)[3] and protein S (PS) deficiencies,[4,5] that other causes of inherited thrombophilia were recognized. Despite their recognition and overall importance, together these entities account for less than 10 per cent of cases of recurrent venous thrombosis.[6] Renewed inter-

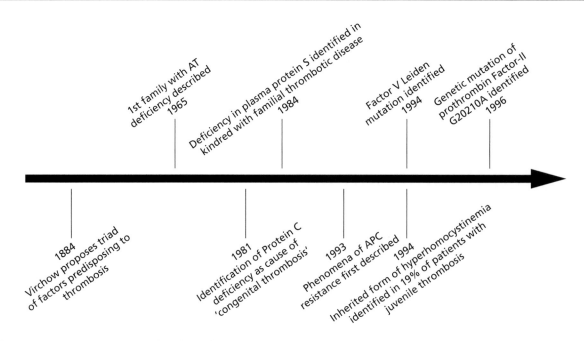

Figure 16.1 *Advances in the detection of inherited thrombophilias. AT = antithrombin; APC = activated protein C.*

est in inherited causes of thrombophilia was sparked by the discovery of activated protein C (APC) resistance by Dahlbäck and colleagues in 1993.[7] Other investigators subsequently reported that between 20–60 per cent of patients with recurrent venous thrombosis have APC resistance.[8–10] In 1994, it was found that 19 per cent of patients with juvenile venous thrombosis had an inherited form of mild hyperhomocystinemia[11] (Fig. 16.1). Finally, a mutation involving a transition of nucleotide 20210 of Factor II (prothrombin) has been identified and recent studies have detected this genotype in up to 18 per cent of patients with venous thrombosis.[12] Thus, in more than 50 per cent of patients with juvenile or idiopathic thrombosis, an inherited thrombophilic condition can now be identified.

In general, defects resulting in deficiencies of or resistance to the natural anticoagulants, i.e. AT, PC, PS deficiency and APC resistance, predispose to venous thromboembolism (deep vein thrombosis, pulmonary embolism). Hyperhomocystinemia and the acquired condition antiphospholipid antibody syndrome are associated with an increased risk of arterial and venous thrombosis.

INHERITED THROMBOPHILIAS – ANTITHROMBIN DEFICIENCY

Antithrombin is a single-chain glycoprotein belonging to the serine protease inhibitor (serpin) super family. It combines with and inactivates thrombin and other coagulation enzymes including Factors Xa, IXa, XIa, and XIIa

(Fig. 16.2). The inhibition of coagulant factors is markedly accelerated by heparin and endogenous heparan sulfate found on the endothelial surface.[13]

In accordance with the classification of other coagulation protein deficiencies, AT deficiency characterized by a reduction in functional activity and protein antigen is called *Type I deficiency*. In *Type II deficiency*, low AT activity occurs in the presence of normal antigen levels, indicating a functional impairment of the protein. Over 100 different mutations resulting in AT deficiency have been identified.[14] Both Type I and Type II AT deficiency are associated with an increased risk of venous thrombosis, but the overall risk within a given kindred (family with the defect) will vary with a specific mutation. Variance in expression is most likely the result of differing AT levels (and activity), concomitant defects (combined thrombophilias) and coexistent risks for thrombosis (pregnancy, inactivity, trauma).[15] Congenital antithrombin deficiency is transmitted in an autosomal dominant pattern. Most homozygotes die *in utero*. A vast majority of affected patients are heterozygotes with AT levels ranging from 40 to 70 per cent of normal.

The prevalence of Type I AT deficiency has been estimated to be approximately 1/2000 to 1/5000,[16–18] while the prevalence of Type II AT deficiency may be much greater (~1/600 to 1/700).[19] In unselected patients with venous thromboembolism the frequency of AT deficiency is 1.1 per cent,[20] while in selected patients it is 2.4 per cent (range 0.5–4.9 per cent)[21–24] (Table 16.1). Patients with inherited AT deficiency are at greater risk for venous thromboembolism than those with protein C or protein S deficiency. In one study up to 85 per cent of patients experienced a thromboembolic event by age

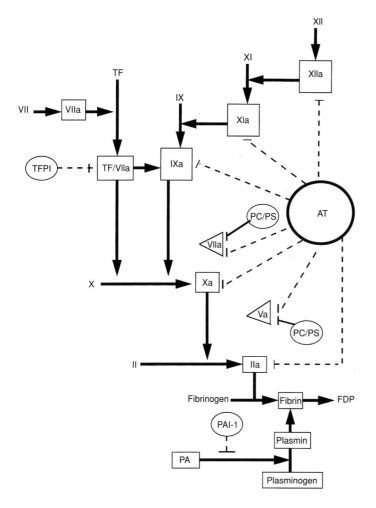

Figure 16.2 *Sites of action of the four major physiologic antithrombotic pathways: antithrombin (AT); protein C/protein S (PC/PS); tissue factor pathway inhibitor (TFPI); fibrinolytic system, consisting of plasminogen, plasminogen activator (PA), and plasmin (PL). TF = tissue factor; FDP = fibrin(ogen) degradation products; – – – – = inhibition.*

50.[25] The frequency of venous thromboembolism is also increased during pregnancy (up to 44 per cent) compared to PC or PS deficiency (10 per cent and 19 per cent, respectively).[26–28]

PROTEIN C DEFICIENCY

Protein C is a vitamin-K-dependent glycoprotein synthesized by the liver. Thrombin complexed to endothelial thrombomodulin cleaves an arginine–leucine bond within PC, causing activation. In turn, APC inactivates Factors Va and XIIIa, thus affecting both the intrinsic and extrinsic coagulation pathways (Fig. 16.2). APC also neutralizes plasminogen activator inhibitor 1 (PAI-1), thus enhancing fibrinolytic activity.[29,30]

A large number of mutations (>160) causing PC deficiency have been identified.[31] The overwhelming majority of defects produce a quantitative (Type I) deficiency, but qualitative (Type II) PC deficiency is recognized as well.[31–33] In almost all cases these defects are transmitted via an autosomal dominant pattern of inheritance.

The frequency of PC deficiency is 3.2 per cent in unselected patients with venous thrombosis[21] and 3.8 per cent (range 1.4–8.6 per cent) in selected patients[34,35] (Table 16.1). Both Type I and Type II PC deficiency predispose to venous thromboembolism and it has been reported that up to 50 per cent of heterozygotes suffer a thrombotic event by age 50. In some severely affected kindreds, 75 per cent will experience one or more events by age 60.[36]

A recent analysis of nearly 10 000 healthy blood donors reported PC deficiency of a frequency of 1/500 to 1/700.[37] Although the prevalence may be overestimated, it remains clear that, in many cases, heterozygous PC deficiency *alone* does not increase thrombotic risk substantially. Differing mutations result in widely different clinical phenotypes and multiple coagulation defects probably contribute as well.[38]

PROTEIN S DEFICIENCY

Protein S, like PC, is a vitamin K-dependent glycoprotein. Approximately 40 per cent of PS circulates in an *active*, or free form, the remaining 60 per cent is *inactive* and circulates bound to C4b-binding protein. Free protein S acts as the principal co-factor of APC and

Table 16.1 *Frequency (%) of inherited thrombophilic syndromes in the general population and in patients with venous thrombosis. (Reproduced with permission from DeStefano V, Finazzi G, Mannucci PM. Inherited thrombophilia: pathogenesis, clinical syndromes and management.* Blood *1996;* **87**: *3531–44)*

Syndrome	General population	Unselected patients with venous thrombosis	Selected patients with venous thrombosis[a]
AT deficiency	0.02–0.17	1.1	0.5–4.9
PC deficiency	0.14–0.5	3.2	1.4–8.6
PS deficiency	—	2.2	1.4–7.5
APC resistance	3.6–6.0	21	10–64

[a]Age <45 years and/or recurrent thrombosis (without obvious precipitant).

increases the protein's affinity for negatively charged phospholipids. The resulting membrane-bound APC–PS complex produces a marked increase in Factor Va and VIIIa inactivation (Fig. 16.2).

Relatively few mutations of the PS gene have been identified, perhaps because of its large size, the existence of many exons, and the presence of a homologous pseudogene.[39] Both Type I and Type II deficiencies have been identified. Type 1 PS deficiency can be further divided into two distinct phenotypes: Type 1a, characterized by a normal level of total PS antigen but a low level of free PS; and Type 1b, characterized by low levels of both total and free PS. It is important to acknowledge that C4b-binding protein is an acute-phase reactant whose concentration is increased in a myriad of inflammatory states. This results in an increase in the bound portion of protein S, which, in turn, lowers the level of free PS. Indeed, up to 20 per cent of hospitalized patients have low free PS levels.[40]

The prevalence of PS deficiency in the general population has been difficult to establish for the reasons stated. A frequency of 2.2 per cent for unselected patients with venous thromboembolism has been reported.[21] For selected patients, a slightly higher prevalence of 3.0 per cent has been reported (range 1.4–7.5 per cent)[21–24] (Table 16.1). As with AT and PC deficiencies, most patients with PS deficiency are at increased risk for venous thromboembolism. Up to 50 per cent of patients with PS deficiency may suffer a first thrombotic event by age 25.[41] Although arterial thrombosis has been reported, a cause–effect relationship is far from established with the exception of paradoxical embolism.[42]

ACTIVATED PROTEIN C RESISTANCE

As previously summarized, thrombin bound to the endothelial cell molecule, thrombomodulin, cleaves protein C causing activation. Activated protein C, through its inactivation of Factors Va and VIIIa, is a critical inhibitor of coagulation. In 1993 Dahlbäck and colleagues introduced the term 'activated protein C resistance' to describe a patient with recurrent thrombosis

whose activated partial thromboplastin time (aPTT) failed to prolong with the addition of activated protein C[7] (Fig. 16.3). Subsequent investigators found that between 20 and 60 per cent of patients with recurrent venous thrombosis displayed the same APC resistance on laboratory testing.[8–10] Furthermore, a familial tendency with an autosomal dominant pattern of inheritance was established.

In 1994 the underlying molecular defect responsible for approximately 90–95 per cent of cases of APC resistance was identified as s single base-pair mutation in the Factor V gene resulting in an Arg[506] to Gln substitution at one of the APC cleavage sites.[43,44]

The mutated Factor V molecule (Factor V Leiden) resists inactivation by APC but can still participate in coagulation. The cause(s) of APC resistance in the remaining 5–10 per cent of cases have not yet been clearly delineated. There have been reports of patients with severely reduced APC-sensitivity ratios consistent with presumed homozygosity for Factor V Leiden who are in fact compound heterozygotes for Factor V Leiden and a Type I quantitative deficiency of Factor V.[44,45]

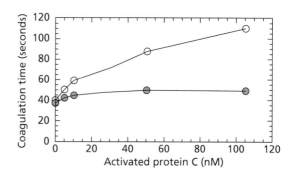

Figure 16.3 *Anticoagulant response to activated protein C (APC). Purified APC was added to normal plasma (○) and plasma from a thrombosis patient with the APC resistance phenotype (●). The coagulation time was measured using a clotting based assay. The APC-resistant patient responds poorly to the added APC. (Reproduced with permission from Hillarp A, Dahlbäck B. New risk factors for thrombosis.* Vessels *1997;* **3**: *4–10.)*

Several investigators have also demonstrated inhibition of APC by antiphospholipid antibodies, suggesting a possible etiology for the increased thrombogenicity seen in patients with antiphospholipid antibody syndrome by virtue of 'acquired APC resistance'.[46–48] It is likely other genetic and acquired causes of APC resistance will be uncovered as work in this area continues.

The Factor V Leiden mutation is present in heterozygous form in approximately 4–6 per cent of the general population.[8,9,49] It is presently felt to be the most prevalent hereditary thrombophilia occurring in 6–33 per cent of consecutive unselected patients with prior venous thromboembolism[8,9,50,51] (Table 16.1). Up to 60 per cent of women who experience venous thromboembolic events during oral contraceptive use are APC resistant.[52] The available evidence suggests that heterozygosity for factor V Leiden is associated with a 3–7-fold increased risk for venous thrombosis.[8,9,49] Thirty per cent of patients will experience an event by 60 years of age. Interestingly, although patients homozygous for Factor V Leiden are at even greater risk for thromboembolism, a full 40 per cent will remain thrombosis-free at age 60,[52] suggesting strongly that additional risk factors are necessary to provoke events in patients with APC resistance.

A proposed link between Factor V Leiden and arterial thrombosis remains controversial. The prevalence of heterozygosity was similar among men in the Physicians Health Study who went on to have myocardial infarctions (6.1 per cent) and strokes (4.3 per cent) to those who remained free of vascular disease (6.0 per cent).[49] However, a recent case control study of young women with myocardial infarction (18–44 years of age) reported a four-fold increased risk for those who carried the Factor V Leiden mutation.[53] The association was confined largely to a subset of women who were active smokers.

FACTOR II (PROTHROMBIN) G20210A

A mutation involving a Gly to Arg substitution within nucleotide 20210 of the Factor II (prothrombin) gene has recently been identified,[12] and may be responsible for up to 18 per cent of selected patients and 6.2 per cent of unselected patients with venous thromboembolism. The calculated relative risk for thrombosis associated with the 20210A allele was 2.8 (95 per cent confidence interval (CI), 1.4–5.6). Even after exclusion of patients with APC resistance and lupus anticoagulants, the unmatched relative risk for thrombosis remained high at 2.7. In this study the prothrombin mutation was associated with an increased prothrombin concentration, suggesting a potential prothrombotic mechanism.

A subsequent review of 99 unselected patients with phlebography verified deep venous thrombosis and 282 controls identified the 20210A allele in 7.1 per cent of the patient group versus 1.8 per cent in the control group.[54] After adjustment for age, sex, and Factor V Leiden carrier status, the relative risk of venous thrombosis was 3.0 (95 per cent CI 1.1–13.2). Of note, is the fact that 2 per cent of the patients were carriers of the Factor V Leiden mutation, therefore 34 per cent of these unselected patients were carriers of an inherited prothrombotic disorder. Further investigation is required to understand the prothrombin mutation and its association with venous thromboembolism. The molecular techniques to detect G20210A are not widely available.

DYSFIBRINOGENEMIAS

Plasma fibrinogen is cleaved by thrombin to form fibrin, which, in turn, spontaneously polymerizes to form a stable, non-soluble fibrin clot. Dysfibrinogen is a structurally or functionally abnormal fibrinogen that can be associated with a propensity toward hemorrhage, thrombosis, or both. Data derived from a meta-analysis of nine studies including a total of 2376 patients with venous thromboembolism revealed a low (0.8 per cent) prevalence of congenital dysfibrinogenemia;[55] however, from a total of 250 cases of congenital dysfibrinogenemia, 20 per cent experienced thromboembolic events (± bleeding), 25 per cent had hemorrhage, and 55 per cent remained asymptomatic. No fewer than 25 distinct mutations of the fibrinogen molecule have been described; however, not all have been linked to an increased thrombotic tendency. For those that have, the risk is not solely fibrinogen-mediated; decreased binding of tissue plasminogen activator (tPA),[56] increased resistance to plasmin,[57] increased capacity to aggregate platelets,[58] and defective binding of thrombin to fibrin[55] may also contribute.

Dysfibrinogenemia should be suspected when a prolonged thrombin time is detected and cannot be explained by heparin administration or fibrinogen consumption. Rarely, a shortened thrombin time may be caused by dysfibrinogenemia.

HYPERHOMOCYSTINEMIA

Homocysteine is a sulfhydryl amino acid derived from the metabolism of methionine which occurs via one of three enzymatic pathways (Fig. 16.4).

1 Remethylation to methionine catalyzed by methionine synthase; the methyl group is donated by methyltetrahydrofolate and cobalamin (Vitamin B_{12}) serves as a co-factor.
2 Remethylation to methionine catalyzed by betaine-homocysteine methyltransferase; betaine is the methyl donor.

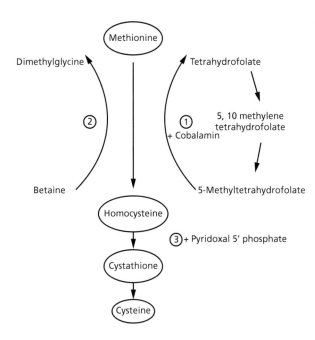

Figure 16.4 *Metabolic pathways for methionine and homocysteine. Cobalamin acts as a co-factor in the reaction catalyzed by methionine synthesis. Pyridoxal 5′-phosphate acts as a co-factor in the reaction catalyzed by cystathionine ß-synthase. 1 = methionine synthase; 2= betaine-homocysteine methyltransferase; 3 = cystathionine ß-synthase.*

3 Trans-sulfuration by cystathionine ß-synthase into cystathionine; pyridoxal-5′-phosphate (vitamin B₆) is the co-factor.

Several inherited or acquired conditions affecting these pathways can result in varying degrees of hyper-homocystinemia, severe (>100 µmol/L), moderate (30–100 µmol/L), and mild (15–30 µmol/L).

Severe homocystinemia is quite rare and caused by either homozygous deficiency of cystathionine ß-syn-thase (90–95 per cent of cases) or inherited defects in the remethylation pathway (5–10 per cent of cases). Affected individuals are afflicted with a variety of neurologic and developmental abnormalities as well as premature vas-cular disease and thromboembolism.[59]

Mild to moderate hyperhomocysteinemia is also caused by a variety of genetic defects. Heterozygous cys-tathionine ß-synthase deficiency has a frequency of 0.4–1.5 per cent within the general population[60] and homozygosity for a thermolabile mutant of methylene tetrahydrofolate reductase is found in ~5 per cent of the general population;[61] both abnormalities are associated with a 50 per cent reduction in enzymatic activity. Phenotypic expression is influenced by other factors; conversely genetically 'normal' individuals may have mild to moderately increased levels of homocysteine from one or more acquired abnormalities.

The most common causes of acquired hyperhomo-cystinemia are nutritional deficiencies of cobalamin (vit-amin B₁₂), folate, or pyridoxine (vitamin B₆) (co-factors for homocysteine metabolism).[62–64] Chronic renal failure and drugs that interfere with folate metabolism (methotrexate, anticonvulsants), cobalamin metabolism (nitrous oxide), or pyridoxine metabolism (theophylline) can cause hyperhomocystinemia.[65] Other factors which may influence homocysteine levels include gender, age, smoking, hypertension, and hypercholesterolemia.

Owing to the relatively large number of potential enzy-matic defects, the variable phenotypic expression, and the influence of acquired factors, the risk of arterial and venous thromboembolism directly attributable to hyper-homocystinemia has been difficult to ascertain. None-theless, *in vitro* studies have provided important information concerning the mechanisms by which homo-cysteine may increase thrombogenicity that include: acti-vation of factor V; interference with PC activation and thrombomodulin expression;[61] inhibition of tPA bind-ing;[66] impaired generation of nitric oxide[67] and prosta-cyclin;[68] induction of tissue factor activity;[69] and suppression of vessel wall heparin sulfate.[70] *In vivo* studies performed in non-human primates have provided evi-dence that homocysteine causes endothelial cell injury, smooth muscle cell proliferation, and intimal thickening.[71]

In the last decade, epidemiologic studies have identi-fied mild to moderate homocystinemia as an indepen-dent risk factor for peripheral arterial disease,[72,73] extracranial carotid artery stenosis,[74] coronary artery dis-ease[75,76] and acute myocardial infarction.[77] Mild to mod-erate homocystinemia has also been associated with an increased risk of venous thromboembolism[12] and recur-rent events following the first.[78,79] The thrombotic mani-festations of hyperhomocystinemia do not differ substantially from those of other thrombophilic dis-orders. In a series of 67 patients with hyperhomocystin-emia,[16] most thrombotic events were associated with other risk factors (oral contraceptives, pregnancy, and immobilization, for example).

ACQUIRED THROMBOPHILIAS

Among the most common acquired factors that predis-pose individuals to thrombosis are the presence of an antiphospholipid antibody and malignancy. Other less common causes include myeloproliferative disorders, the nephrotic syndrome, and paroxysmal nocturnal hemoglobinuria.[80] Iatrogenic etiologies include chemotherapy for cancer,[81] hormonal treatment for infertility,[82] and, perhaps the most common acquired thrombophilia, major surgical procedures.[83]

Antiphospholipid antibody syndrome

Antiphospholipid antibodies (aPLs) are a heterogenous group of circulating serum polyclonal immunoglobulins

(IgG, IgM, IgA, or mixed) directed against negatively charged or neutral phospholipids. Within this group, the lupus anticoagulant (LA) and anticardiolipin antibodies (aCLs) are the most common acquired blood protein defects associated with arterial and venous thrombosis.

Although similar in many ways, aCL thrombosis syndrome and LA thrombosis syndrome are distinct clinical entities – aCL thrombosis syndrome being much more prevalent (about 5:1).[84,85]

The LA was originally identified in patients with systemic lupus erythematosus (SLE). Since then both LA and aCL antibodies have been associated with a variety of autoimmune disorders, malignancies, lymphoproliferative diseases, and viral infections. However, the majority of patients with thrombosis (and one or both of these antibodies) have no underlying clinical condition; they are said to have 'primary antiphospholipid syndrome'.

ANTICARDIOLIPIN ANTIBODY THROMBOSIS SYNDROME

The aCL antibodies are directed primarily against the phospholipids, phosphatidyl serine and phosphatidyl inositol. Unlike the LA they do not prolong any of the phospholipid-dependent anticoagulation tests (aPTT, diluted Russell viper venom time, and/or kaolin clotting time (KCT)).[86–88] Three idiotypes (IgG, IgA and IgM) are currently identified with the solid-phase enzyme-linked immunosorbent assay (ELISA) anticardiolipin assay. This assay is dependent on a plasma co-factor, β_2 glycoprotein I. The *in vivo* significance of this co-factor is unclear.

The mechanism(s) by which the aCL antibodies provoke thrombosis have not been fully elucidated, but there is little doubt that their high affinity for phospholipid is involved. Several potential mechanisms have been proposed:

1 inhibition of prostacyclin release from the endothelium;[89]
2 inhibition of PC activation or PS activity;[90]
3 interference with antithrombin activity;[91]
4 platelet activation;[92]
5 inhibition of pre-kallikrein activation (impaired fibrinolysis);[93]
6 inhibition of plasminogen activator release.[94]

The overall prevalence of aCL antibodies in the general population has not been established; however, a recent study of 1014 medical in-patients identified 72 (7.1 per cent) with at least one idiotype;[95] another study of 552 healthy blood donors identified 64 (15.9 per cent) with either IgG or IgM idiotypes.[96] The prevalence is higher among patients with arterial or venous thromboembolic events. Several studies have reported that an increased proportion of young (<45–50 year) survivors of acute myocardial infarction (MI) have circulating aCL

antibodies,[97–99] and that they are at increased risk for recurrent events. The association of aPLs (including aCLs) and cerebrovascular events is even more impressive. aPL antibodies have been found in 10–46 per cent of stroke patients (depending on study design).[100,101] In the Antiphospholipid Antibodies in Stroke Study Registry, the prevalence was ~10 per cent.[102] In young people the risk of stroke recurrence was eight-fold higher for those with aPLs than for those without. The scope of neurologic manifestations is broad and includes migraine headaches, optic neuritis, Guillain–Barré syndrome, chorea and multi-infarction dementia.

Anticardiolipin antibodies are also associated with venous thromboembolism, most commonly deep venous thrombosis and pulmonary embolism. Thrombosis involving unusual sites has also been reported including intracranial veins, inferior and superior vena cava, and hepatic and portal veins.[103] A wide variety of cutaneous abnormalities have been associated with aCL thrombosis syndrome that include livedo reticularis, vasulitis, Sneddon's syndrome (deep vein thrombosis, cerebrovascular accident, necrotizing purpura), microvascular thrombosis/stasis ulcers, dermal necrosis, acral cyanosis, necrotizing purpura, and cutis marmorata. Moderate to severe thrombocytopenia occurs in 50 per cent of patients with secondary antiphospholipid syndrome and 10 per cent or less of those with the primary disorder.

LUPUS ANTICOAGULANT THROMBOSIS SYNDROME

The LA was originally described in two patients with SLE who were noted to have a prolonged PT and whole blood clotting time.[104] An antiphospholipid antibody with the ability to prolong phospholipid-dependent coagulation tests was eventually identified.[105,106] The term LA is a misnomer stemming from this *in vitro* property. In fact, patients with the LA are at markedly increased risk for thromboembolic disease. Although occasionally associated with arterial thrombosis, the LA more commonly predisposes to venous thrombosis. Like aCL thrombosis syndrome, a wide variety of venous systems may be affected, although deep venous thrombosis (DVT) of the lower extremities and pulmonary embolism (PE) remain the most common manifestations.[107] The prevalence of the LA in the general population has not been clearly defined; however, it has been estimated that 6–8 per cent of otherwise healthy patients with the LA will experience thromboembolism.[107]

MALIGNANCY

It has long been recognized that patients with malignancy are at risk for thromboembolic complications. The overall incidence ranges from 1 to 15 per cent in various clinical series and even higher rates have emerged from autopsy studies.[108,109] Malignancies with the highest rates of thromboembolism include mucin-producing adenocarcinomas of the gastrointestinal tract followed by lung, breast, ovarian, and brain tumors.

The observed propensity for thrombosis among cancer patients is not surprising when one considers the effects of neoplastic tissue on the individual components of Virchow's triad (Fig. 16.5). Venous stasis is common among patients who endure prolonged periods of immobilization compounded by vascular compression from existing tumor burden. There may be direct tumor extension to vascular structures, disrupting normal thromboresistance and exposing tissue factor, a strong procoagulant. It has been demonstrated that ~50 per cent of all cancer patients display abnormalities of routine coagulation parameters,[110,111] including increases in plasma fibrinogen, clotting factors, and platelet count. Increased levels of fibrinopeptide A, a marker of fibrin formation, have been observed in a large proportion of patients with advanced solid tumors.[112] Fibrinopeptide A concentration may also be a marker of disease activity, increasing with malignant recurrence and decreasing with remission.[113] Studies using other biochemical markers of thrombin generation, including F1+2, D-dimers, and thrombin–AT complexes have also been used to document increased coagulation activation in patients with malignancy. Unfortunately, there is considerable variability among patients, precluding a clinically relevant predictive value in individual patients.

There is increasing evidence for the existence of circulating 'hypercoagulable factors' in patients with malignancy. A variety of solid tumors and leukemic cells have been found to express tissue factor, an activator of the extrinsic coagulation cascade.[114–117] A new protein labeled 'cancer procoagulant', capable of directly activating Factor X, has been found in extracts of numerous malignant tissues.[118–120] Interestingly, a sialic acid moiety from mucin (found in adenocarcinomas) has direct Factor X-activating properties as well.[109]

In addition to tumor-derived procoagulant factors, host cells can express procoagulant activity.[109] Monocytes, probably stimulated by tumor-derived chemokines, express tissue factor (TF), other Factor X

activators, fibrinogen, and coagulation protein binding sites. Similarly, platelets and endothelial cells become increasingly procoagulant under the influence of tumor-derived cytokines.[117,121]

Given the strong association between malignancy and venous thrombosis, it follows that thromboembolism may represent the initial clinical manifestation of occult malignancy. Indeed, several studies have shown that patients with venous thromboembolism may be diagnosed with cancer over the subsequent months to years. Three separate studies have compared the occurrence of subsequent cancer (within the next 2 years) in patients presenting with idiopathic DVT versus those with an identifiable risk factor (trauma, prolonged immobilization, known thrombophilia, for example).[122–124] Malignancy was diagnosed at a much higher frequency in the 'idiopathic' group (range 10.5–23 per cent) versus the 'secondary' group (range 1.9–6 per cent). Thus, it is apparent that patients experiencing venous thromboembolism in the absence of a readily defined risk factor should be carefully evaluated for occult malignancy.

> It is generally agreed that *all* patients with venous thromboembolism should have a thorough evaluation that includes past history, family history, physical examination, and routine blood tests. The value of additional studies including serum carcinoembryonic antigen (CEA), serum prostate specific antigen (PSA), mammography, and serial tests for fecal occult blood remains controversial and should be individualized.[109]

Features on presentation that may suggest an occult malignancy include: absence of apparent cause for thromboembolism at time of admission, age >50 years, multiple sites of venous thromboembolism, concurrent venous and arterial thrombosis, thromboembolism resistant to therapy, and the presence of associated paraneoplastic syndromes.[125]

> We currently recommend a careful history and physical examination (including pelvic, breast, and rectal examination) followed by routine blood cell counts (hematocrit, white blood count, platelet count) and chemistries. In patients >50 years of age we also recommend serial (three consecutive days) occult blood testing, prostate examination and PSA (men), and mammography (women) if they have not been performed in the last year. As these tests are performed every 1–2 years following the current standard of care guidelines, we do not feel they incur unnecessary or excessive cost. In smokers, we do suggest performance of a good posterior-anterior (PA) and lateral chest radiograph to screen for lung masses. Additional testing, including endoscopy and computed tomography (CT) imaging, is reserved for patients with positive findings on initial evaluation and/or a high index of suspicion.

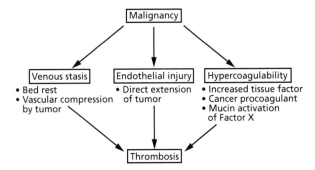

Figure 16.5 *Malignancy increases thrombotic risk via all three components of Virchow's triad.*

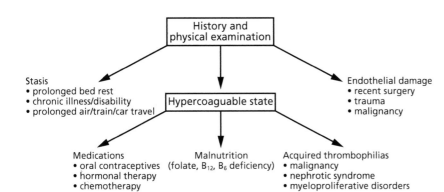

Figure 16.6 *An approach to evaluating patients with thromboembolic disease that is based on Virchow's triad.*

MANAGEMENT OF PATIENTS WITH SUSPECTED THROMBOPHILIC DISORDERS

Initial assessment

All patients with thromboembolism should have a complete history and physical examination with special attention to concomitant clinical disorders that may predispose to a 'hypercoagulable state'. The elements of Virchow's triad can be used as a guide while performing this assessment (Fig. 16.6). A careful medication history should also be conducted. An initial laboratory investigation should include a complete blood count (CBC), smear and an aPTT which may uncover acquired conditions not revealed by the initial history and physical examination (Table 16.2). See the previous section for discussion of appropriate screening for occult malignancy.

Table 16.2 *Initial laboratory testing for patients with thromboembolism. (Adapted with permission from Cavenaugh JD, Colvin BT. Guidelines for the management of thrombophilia.* Postgrad Med J 1996; **72**: 87–94)

Diagnostic test	Finding	Thrombophilic disorder
CBC	Anemia	Paroxysmal nocturnal hemoglobinuria
		Gastrointestinal malignancy
	↑ Hct	Polycythemia
	↑ Platelets	Thrombocythemia
Smear	Macrocytosis	Folate, B_{12} deficiency
aPTT	Increased	Lupus anticoagulant

CBC = complete blood count; aPTT = activated partial thromboplastin time; ↑ = increased; Hct = hematocrit.

Screening for thrombophilia

SELECTION OF PATIENTS

If after the initial evaluation no obvious cause for a thrombotic state has been elucidated, one must decide whether to undertake more detailed (and expensive)

investigations (Fig. 16.7). As of 1990, <10 per cent of cases of idiopathic or recurrent thromboembolism could be attributed to an inherited condition. Accordingly, screening was limited to a selective subset of patients[126] (Table 16.3).

The guidelines recommended by the British Committee for Standards in Hematology represent a reasonable approach to evaluating patients with suspected thrombophilia; however, the discovery and characterization of APC resistance (Factor V Leiden) represents an important advance since these guidelines were first published. Its frequency among patients with thromboembolism may justify routine screening in a broader selection of patients. Furthermore, unlike the other inherited conditions, patients with APC resistance can experience their first thromboembolic event at a relatively old age. Ridker and colleagues recently demonstrated that the risk of venous thromboembolism in heterozygous male carriers of Factor V Leiden increased with age at a rate greater than that in non-carriers.[127] This age-specific incidence rate difference was significant for idiopathic venous thromboembolism, but not for secondary events. It remains to be seen if screening patients older than 45 years of age with idiopathic venous thromboembolism for APC resistance has an important influence on overall management.

Table 16.3 *Individuals in whom screening for inherited/ acquired thrombophilia is recommended*

Venous thromboembolism before age 45
Arterial thromboembolism before age 35
Recurrent spontaneous venous thromboembolism
Thrombosis in unusual site, e.g. mesenteric vein, cerebral sinus
Patients with family history of venous thromboembolism
Relatives of patients with thrombophilic conditions
Skin necrosis, particularly if on warfarin
Unexplained neonatal thrombosis
Recurrent fetal loss
Systemic lupus erythematosus
Unexplained prolongation of activated partial thromboplastin time

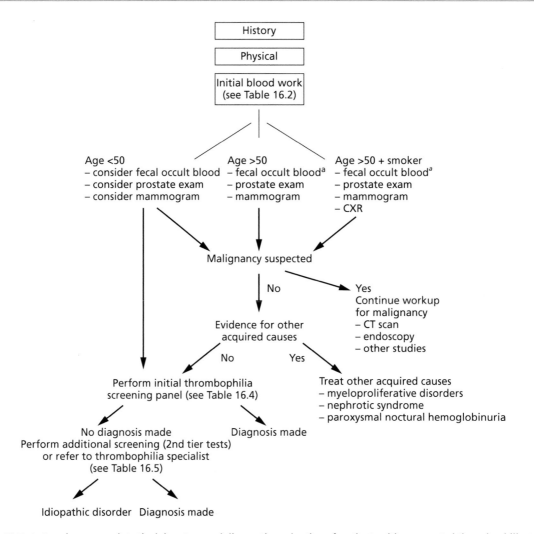

Figure 16.7 *A stepwise approach to the laboratory and diagnostic evaluation of patients with a suspected thrombophilic state.*
[a]Colonoscopy should be undertaken if present. CXR = chest x-ray; CT = computed tomography.

Selection of tests

Once a decision has been made to pursue a diagnosis of inherited or acquired thrombophilia, selection and timing of additional testing must be made carefully to avoid unnecessary cost and potentially misleading results.

According to the British Committee Guidelines, patients with an unexplained venous thromboembolic event who are <45 years of age should undergo the first tier in thrombophilic screening – assays for APC resistance/Factor V Leiden, AT deficiency, protein C deficiency, protein S deficiency, and antiphospholipid antibody syndrome should be performed (Table 16.4). Patients >45 years of age with unexplained venous thrombosis are less likely to have AT/PC/PS deficiency; however, screening for Factor V Leiden and antiphospholipid antibody syndrome is recommended.

Ideally, the tests should be performed prior to initiation of anticoagulant therapy. Heparin can reduce AT antigen

Table 16.4 *Initial laboratory testing for suspected thrombophilia*

Antithrombin activity
Protein C activity
Protein S antigen level
Activated protein C resistance functional assay or Factor V
    Leiden genotype analysis
Lupus anticoagulant screen
Anticardiolipin antibody assay

and activity by 10–15 per cent. Warfarin will reduce both PC and PS levels by 30 per cent due to inhibition of vitamin K-dependent protein synthesis. These tests should be performed prior to or at least 2 weeks after the completion of warfarin therapy to allow for resynthesis of coagulation proteins. Both heparin and warfarin can influence LA assays.

The most commonly used functional assay for APC resistance is an aPTT calculated in the presence and absence of a known concentration of APC. The ratio of the two clotting times normalized against the APC resistance ratios of pooled plasma provide an accurate means to identify patients with APC resistance. Ninety per cent of all patients with a 'positive' functional APC resistance test will have factor V Leiden; the remainder will most likely have one or more alternative mutations of the Factor V gene. Modification of the functional APC resistance test using Factor V-deficient plasma increases the sensitivity and specificity for Factor V Leiden to nearly 100 per cent.[128,129] This modification also allows analysis of samples from patients receiving anticoagulant therapy.

The mutation responsible for Factor V Leiden can be identified directly by genetic analysis (genomic amplification followed by nucleotide sequencing, DNA hybridization, or restriction enzyme fragment analysis). This method of diagnosis has the advantage of not being affected by concomitant coagulation abnormalities or anticoagulant therapy, but is more costly. Genetic testing will also miss the small percentage of patients with APC resistance who do not have Factor V Leiden.

> Patients with venous thromboembolism should be screened for the antiphospholipid antibody syndrome, especially if the first battery of screening tests are negative or if there is clinical evidence for one of the commonly associated diseases (autoimmune disease, malignancy). Young patients with arterial thromboembolism or women with a past history of recurrent miscarriages should also be screened.

Individual idiotypes of aCL antibody can be identified by specific ELISAs. It is now recognized that the aCL antibodies associated with an increased risk of thrombosis require β_2 glycoprotein 1 (a natural anticoagulant) for binding in vitro.[130,131] The role of this co-factor in vivo is still unclear. Non-autoimmune aCL antibodies can develop in the setting of infection; however, they are not dependent on β_2 glycoprotein 1 for binding and carry little risk of thrombosis.[132] It is important to recognize that antibody titers can vary. Therefore, screening should be conducted at least twice, 6–12 weeks apart, to confirm or exclude a diagnosis. An antibody level greater than 40 phospholipid units is considered significant.

The presence of a circulating LA can be identified by prolongation of various in vitro clotting tests. Initially the standard aPTT was used as a screening tool but it was subsequently found to lack sensitivity. Therefore, the diluted Russell viper venom time (dRVVT) is usually performed regardless of the aPTT result.[133] Prolongation of the dRVVT will not correct with the addition of normal plasma in the presence of a LA (in contrast to a clotting factor deficiency). For confirmation, a cephalin neutralization procedure to show the inhibitor is phospholipid dependent can be performed. A third assay, the Kaolin clotting time test, has also be used to detect LA; however, it lacks the sensitivity of the dRVVT.[106] Needless

to say, any functional assay can be influenced by existing coagulation defects or by anticoagulant therapy.

Although little information is available for screening, there is evidence that premature atherosclerosis, arterial thrombosis and venous thromboembolism are linked to mild to moderate hyperhomocystinemia regardless of the underlying enzymatic defect.[72–79] The prevalence of this condition and its relatively simple correction with vitamin supplementation[134] suggests that screening for this disorder may be of utility. Unfortunately, randomized, prospective trials examining morbidity and mortality from thromboembolic disease have not been performed.

> We recommend a fasting plasma homocysteine level in young patients (<50 years) and in older patients without other obvious risk factors.
>
> When the initial tests are unrevealing, yet suspicion remains high for an inherited condition (strong family history, presentation at very young age, recurrent events) additional testing should be performed. The 'second tier' of laboratory evaluation is usually directed towards more rare or newly discovered thrombophilic conditions (Table 16.5). Accordingly, evaluation should take place at an experienced thrombophilia center (Table 16.6).

Table 16.5 *Second tier of laboratory tests for suspected inheritable thrombophilia*

Genetic analysis for prothrombin G20210A
Evaluation for dysfibrinogenemia
Plasminogen/plasminogen activator/plasminogen activator inhibitor levels[a]
Heparin cofactor II levels[a]
Evaluation for thrombomodulin abnormalities[a]

[a]Not clearly established as inheritable causes of thrombophilia.

Management of venous thrombosis

ACUTE

The acute management of venous thromboembolism in patients with an inherited or acquired thrombophilia is similar to other patients without such an underlying predisposition. There are some exceptions.

> In a patient known to be PC or PS deficient (or in whom the suspicion is high), care must be taken to initiate warfarin therapy only after adequate heparinization has been achieved and sustained for 48 hours to prevent warfarin skin necrosis, and a transient prothrombotic state. Patients with AT deficiency may require AT concentrate supplementation to achieve an adequate degree of anticoagulation with

Table 16.6 *Screening for thrombophilic conditions*

Investigation	Type of assay	Indication	Ideal timing of assays	Causes of acquired deficiencies	Comments
AT-III activity	Chromogenic (functional)	Venous thromboembolism	Prior heparinization[a,b]	Heparin, sepsis, acute thrombosis/DIC, liver disease, nephrotic syndrome, estrogens, chemotherapeutic agents (asparaginase)	Detects both Types I and II defects
Protein C activity	Chromogenic (functional)	Venous thromboembolism	Prior initiation of warfarin[a,c]	Warfarin, sepsis, acute thrombosis/DIC, liver disease, chemotherapeutic agents, (asparaginase), vitamin K deficiency	Detects both Types I and II defects
Protein S antigen	ELISA total antigen ELISA free antigen	Venous thromboembolism	Prior initiation of warfarin[a,c]	Warfarin, acute thrombosis/DIC, liver disease, pregnancy, estrogens, chemotherapeutic agents, (asparaginase), inflammation ($\uparrow$ C4b-BP), vitamin $\downarrow$ deficiency	Functional assays give false (+) results in presence of Factor V Leiden
Activated protein C resistance	aPTT assay	Venous thromboembolism Consider in older patients with idiopathic event	Prior heparinization[a,b,c]	Warfarin, acute thrombosis/DIC	90–95 per cent of patients with (+) APC resistance have Factor V Leiden mutation
Factor V Leiden	Genetic analysis	Venous thromboembolism – consider in older patients with idiopathic event	Any time	None	—
Anticardiolipin antibodies	ELISA IgG aCL ELISA IgM aCL	Venous thromboembolism, arterial thromboembolism, pregnancy loss Thrombocytopenia	Any time	See text	
Lupus anticoagulant	Sensitive PTT dRVVT Kaolin clotting time	Venous thromboembolism, arterial thromboembolism, pregnancy loss Thrombocytopenia	Prior warfarin/ heparin[a,b,c]	See text	Heparin and warfarin can prolong clotting assays →false positives
Homocysteine	Plasma chromatography	Arterial thromboembolism, venous thromboembolism Consider screening if other causes ruled out	Improved sensitivity performed after methionine load	Folate deficiency B$_{12}$ deficiency Medications interfering with folate/B$_{12}$ metabolism	

[a] Positive tests done at time of acute presentation should be repeated as out-patient.
[b] Presence of heparin does *not* interfere with some assays; check with laboratory.
[c] Must be performed *prior* to or 2 weeks *after* warfarin therapy.
AT = antithrombin; DIC = disseminated intravascular coagulation; BP = binding protein; aPTT = activated partial thromboplastin time; APC = activated protein C; Ig = immunglobulin; aCL = anticardiolipin antibody; dRVVT = dilute Russel viper venom time; ELISA = enzyme-linked immunosorbent assay; PTT = partial thromboplastin time.

heparin. A non-AT dependent anticoagulant (hirudin for example) is another alternative in this situation and may be preferable.

Duration of therapy

CHRONIC

In the absence of an inherited or acquired thrombophilia, first venous thromboembolic events are commonly treated for 3–6 months. A second event usually mandates 12 months of anticoagulant therapy, while a third may be considered an indication for lifelong treatment. Mounting evidence suggests that patients with idiopathic venous thromboembolism may require longer treatment ($\geq$6 months) than previously recommended.[135]

The management guidelines for patients with known thrombophilic disorders are still in evolution (see Table 16.7 for our current recommendations).

Lifelong anticoagulation is not recommended for most asymptomatic patients with an inherited defect; however, prophylactic therapy should be offered in high-risk situations (e.g. surgery, prolonged immobilization, pregnancy). Asymptomatic women should also be counseled regarding the increased risk of thromboembolism associated with the use of oral contraceptives and estrogen replacement therapy.

Patients with thrombophilic disorders and one or more thromboembolic events represent a challenging subset. Some authorities recommend lifelong therapy, while others do so only after spontaneous events (or recurrence while receiving warfarin). Our practice is to assess each case individually and consider the following:

1 The *severity* of the thromboembolic event. Consider prolonged ($\geq$12 months) or life-long therapy for a patient with a thrombophilic disorder and a single life-threatening event (i.e. a massive pulmonary embolism).
2 The *family history* of thromboembolism. Prophylactic therapy should be considered in asymptomatic patients with affected family members experiencing life-threatening or fatal spontaneous events.
3 The presence of transient or chronic additional *risk factors*. The management of patients with spontaneous events should be more aggressive than those with transient or reversible risk factors.

4 The *thrombophilic* disorder(s) identified:
- AT deficiency is, in general, associated with a greater thrombotic risk than either PC deficiency, PS deficiency, or Factor V Leiden mutation.
- Antiphospholipid antibody syndrome carries a very high risk of a second thrombotic event. Accordingly, lifelong oral anticoagulant therapy after one event should be considered strongly.[136]
- APC resistance (including Factor V Leiden mutation), although clearly associated with increased risk, often does not precipitate a second thromboembolic event in the absence of additional risk factors. Studies to determine the benefit of prolonged therapy are being undertaken (e.g. the PREVENT trial).

Hyperhomocystinemia

Hyperhomocystinemia is associated with an increased risk of premature atherosclerosis, as well as arterial and venous thromboembolism. It has also been demonstrated that vitamin supplementation with folate and B_6 can correct hyperhomocystinemia.[134] Using the known graded effect of plasma homocysteine levels on coronary risk, a meta-analysis of 11 studies estimated that 13 500–50 000 deaths due to coronary artery disease could be avoided by routine fortification of food with folic acid.[137] As previously mentioned, clinical trials assessing the effect of vitamin supplementation (guided or not guided by homocysteine screening) on arterial or venous thromboembolic disease have not been performed.

Patients with hyperhomocystinemia and arterial or venous thromboembolic disease should receive folic acid (1–5 mg/day) and vitamin B_6 (100 μg/day). Cobalamin supplementation (2 μg/day) should also be considered to avoid folic acid refractoriness and to prevent worsening neuropathy in deficient patients.

Antiphospholipid antibody syndrome

Anticoagulant therapy is not recommended for asymptomatic patients with antiphospholipid antibodies. As with other thrombophilias, patients with high titers of aCLs or circulating LA should be counseled on the potential dangers of oral contraceptive use and smoking.

Several retrospective studies have examined anticoagulant strategies for patients with antiphospholipid syndrome following an arterial or venous thromboembolic event. In two of the studies, warfarin was more effective than aspirin in preventing recurrent thrombo-

Table 16.7 *Management of patients with thrombophilic conditions*

Condition	Venous thromboembolism prophylaxis	Acute management	Chronic management	Screen 1° relatives
AT deficiency	Asymptomatic – no (consider high risk kindred) High risk[a] – yes	Heparin→warfarin If resistant to heparin consider AT concentrates or direct thrombin inhibitor[b]	Warfarin INR: 2–3 1st event – 6–12 months 2nd event – life	Yes
PC deficiency	Asymptomatic – no High risk – yes	Heparin→warfarin Hold warfarin until adequate heparinization (risk of warfarin necrosis)	Warfarin INR: 2–3 1st event – 6–12 months 2nd event – life	Yes
PS deficiency	Asymptomatic – no High risk – yes	Heparin→warfarin Hold warfarin until adequate heparinization (risk of warfarin necrosis)	Warfarin INR: 2–3 1st event – 6–12 months 2nd event – life	Yes
APC resistance/Factor V Leiden	Asymptomatic – no High risk – yes	Heparin→warfarin	Warfarin INR: 2–3 1st event – 6 months 2nd event – 12 months → life	Yes
Prothrombin G20210A	Asymptomatic – no High risk – yes	Heparin→warfarin	Warfarin INR: 2–3 1st event – 6 months 2nd event – 12 months → life	Yes
Antiphospholipid Ab syndrome	Asymptomatic – no High risk – yes	Heparin→warfarin Treatment of arterial embolism depends on organ system	Warfarin INR: 3.0–4.0 1st event – life Consider other therapies for recurrent condition (steroids, immunosuppresives)	No

[a] High risk – surgery, prolonged immobilization, pregnancy.
[b] Lepirudin or Argatroban.
AT = antithrombin; INR = international normalized ratio; PC = protein C; PS = protein S; APC = activated protein C; Ab = antibody.

embolism.[138,139] In a third study, treatment with high-intensity warfarin (INR>3.0) (with or without low-dose aspirin) was more effective than low-intensity warfarin;[136] however, bleeding risk is increased as well.[140–142]

> Despite the potential risk, lifelong oral anticoagulant therapy (INR 3–4.5) has been recommended for patients with antiphospholipid syndrome following a thrombotic event.[136]

Numerous other therapies including corticosteroids, immunosuppressives, plasma exchange, and antiplatelet agents have also been attempted with varying success.[143]

> The management of the pregnant patient with antiphospholipid syndrome and recurrent fetal loss represents a major challenge. Initial treatment regimens included prednisone and/or aspirin of varied doses[144–147] with varied success. In the last decade subcutaneous heparin has been used in place of prednisone[148,149] with success. In patients failing therapy with aspirin, prednisone, or heparin (or the combination) intravenous immunoglobulin should be considered.[150,151]

Approach to asymptomatic carriers

The annual incidence of venous thromboembolism is approximately 1 per 1000 in the general population. Because both inherited and acquired conditions influence risk, it has been difficult to define guidelines for screening and management strategies. The Factor V Leiden mutation, present in 5 per cent of healthy caucasians and 30 per cent of unselected patients with venous thromboembolism provides an opportunity to determine the risk of events for asymptomatic carriers of a hereditary thrombophilic condition. The annual incidence of venous thromboembolism in first-degree relatives with Factor V Leiden of a symptomatic carrier is 0.34 per cent (three-fold greater than those without Factor V Leiden). By the sixth decade, 25 per cent of carriers experience a thrombotic event and many do so after exposure to an environmental risk factor such as pregnancy and puerperium (rate ratio 24.7), surgery (rate ratio 16.6), oral contraceptive use (rate ratio 4.9), and immobilization (rate ratio 8.4).[152] Thus, with Factor V Leiden careful observation, counseling, and prophylaxis during high-risk situations is recommended. It is important to recognize that some families are particularly prone to thrombosis (most likely because of combined defects) and, as a result, treatment may be indicated for asymptomatic carriers. A similar approach may be warranted for other hereditary thrombophilias that are highly prothrombotic (e.g. AT deficiency); however, further investigation is needed.

SUMMARY

- The term *thrombophilia* applies to patients with familial or acquired disorders of thromboresistance and hemostatic regulation predisposing to thrombosis.
- In > 50 per cent of patients with juvenile or 'idiopathic' thromboembolism, an inherited condition can be identified.
- Activated protein C resistance (Factor V Leiden mutation) accounts for 20–60 per cent of patients with recurrent venous thrombosis. Other conditions, including protein C, protein S, or antithrombin deficiency are less common. The prothrombin G20210A mutation may be responsible in up to 18 per cent of selected patients.
- Important acquired causes of thrombophilia include malignancy, antiphospholipid antibody syndrome, chemotherapy, surgery, and prolonged immobilization.
- Initial clinical evaluation of all patients presenting with thromboembolism should include a complete history and physical examination.
- Screening for potential thrombophilia conditions in patients whose initial clinical evaluation is unrevealing should include antithrombin activity, protein C activity, protein S antigen, activated protein C resistance, lupus anticoagulant, and anticardiolipin antibodies.
- Thrombophilia tests should ideally be performed at a time remote from the thrombotic event and while the patient is not receiving anticoagulant therapy.

REFERENCES

1. Haemostasis and Thrombosis Task Force. The investigation and management of thrombophilia. In: Roberts B, ed. *Standard haematology practice*. Oxford: Blackwell, 1991: 112–27.
♦2. Egeberg O. Inherited antithrombin deficiency causing thrombophilia. *Thromb Diath Haemorrh* 1965; **13**: 516.
♦3. Griffin J, Evatt B, Zimmerman T, Kleiss A, Wideman C. Deficiency of protein C in congenital thrombotic disease. *J Clin Invest* 1981; **68**: 1370–3.
♦4. Comp P, Esmon C. Recurrent venous thromboembolism in patients with a partial deficiency of protein S. *N Engl J Med* 1984; **311**: 1525–8.
5. Schwarz HP, Fischer M, Hopmeier P, Batard M, Griffin J. Plasma protein S deficiency in familial thrombotic disease. *Blood* 1984; **64**: 1297–300.

6. Allaart CF, Briët E. Familial venous thrombophilia. In: Bloom AL, Forbes CD, Thomas DP, Tuddenham EGD, eds *Haemostasis and thrombosis*, 3rd edn. London: Churchill Livingstone, 1994: 1349.

♦7. Dahlbäck B, Carlsson M, Svensson PJ. Familial thrombophilia due to a previously unrecognized mechanism characterized by poor anticoagulant response to activated protein C: prediction of a cofactor to activated protein C. *Proc Natl Acad Sci USA* 1993; **90**: 1004–8.

8. Koster T, Rosendaal FR, de Ronde H, Briët E, Vandenbroucke JP, Bertina RM. Venous thrombosis due to poor anticoagulant response to activated-protein C: Leiden Thrombophilia Study. *Lancet* 1993; **342**: 1503–6.

9. Svensson PJ, Dahlbäck B. Resistance to activated protein C as a basis for venous thrombosis. *N Engl J Med* 1994; **330**: 517–22.

10. Griffin JHY, Evatt B, Wideman C, Fernandez JA. Anticoagulant protein C pathway defective in majority of thrombophilic patients. *Blood* 1993; **82**: 1989–93.

11. Falcon CR, Cattaneo M, Panzeri D, Martinelli I, Mannucci PM. High prevalence of hyperhomocyst(e)inemia in patients with juvenile venous thrombosis. *Arterioscler Thromb* 1994; **14**: 1080–3.

♦12. Poort SR, Rosendaal FR, Reitsma PH, *et al*. A common genetic variation in the 3-untranslated region of the prothrombin gene is associated with elevated plasma prothrombin levels and an increase in venous thrombosis. *Blood* 1996; **88**: 3698–703.

13. Marcum JA, McKenney JB, Rosenberg RD. Acceleration of thrombin-antithrombin complex formation in rat hindquarters via heparin-like molecules bound to the endothelium. *J Clin Invest* 1984; **74**: 341–50.

14. Cooper DN, Blajchman M, Perry D, Emmerich J, Aiach M. Antithrombin III mutation database: First update. *Thromb Haemost* 1993; **70**: 361–9.

○15. Demers C, Ginsburg JS, Hirsh J, Henderson P, Blajchman MA. Thrombosis in antithrombin-III-deficient persons. Report of a large kindred and literature review. *Ann Intern Med* 1992; **116**: 754–61.

16. De Stefano V, Finazzi G, Mannuccio Mannucci P. Inherited thrombophilia: pathogenesis, clinical syndromes, and management. *Blood* 1996; **87**: 3531–44.

17. Abildgaard U. Antithrombin and related inhibitors of coagulation. In: Poller L, ed. *Recent advances in blood coagulation*. Edinburgh: Churchill Livingstone, 1981: 151–73.

18. Odegard O, Abildgaard U. Antithrombin III: critical review of assay methods: significance of variations in health and disease. *Haemostasis* 1978; **7**: 127.

19. Tait RC, Walker ID, Perry DJ, *et al*. Prevalence of antithrombin III deficiency in the healthy population. *Br J Haematol* 1994; **87**: 106–12.

20. Heijboer H, Brandjes DPM, Buller HR, Sturk A, ten Cate JW. Deficiencies of coagulation-inhibiting and fibrinolytic proteins in outpatients with deep-vein thrombosis. *N Engl J Med* 1990; **323**: 1512–16.

21. Tabernero MD, Tomas JF, Alberca I, Orfao A, Borrasca AL, Vicente V. Incidence and clinical characteristics of hereditary disorders associated with venous thrombosis. *Am J Hematol* 1991; **36**: 249–54.

22. Malm J, Laurell M, Nilsson IM, Dahlbäck B. Thromboembolic disease. Critical evaluation of laboratory investigation. *Thromb Haemost* 1992; **68**: 7–13.

○23. Pabinger I, Brucker S, Kyrle PA, Schneider B, Korninger H, Niessner H, Lechner K. Hereditary deficiency of antithrombin III, protein C and protein S: prevalence in patients with a history of venous thrombosis and criteria for rational patient screening. *Blood Coagul Fibrinolysis* 1992; **3**: 547.

24. Melissari E, Monte G, Lindo VS, *et al*. Congenital thrombophilia among patients with venous thromboembolism. *Blood Coagul Fibrinolysis* 1992; **3**: 749.

25. Thaler E, Lechner K. Antithrombin III deficiency and thromboembolism. *Clin Haematol* 1981; **10**: 369–90.

26. Conrad J, Horellou MH, Van Dreden P, Lecompte T, Samama M. Thrombosis and pregnancy in congenital deficiencies in AT III, protein C or protein S: study of 78 women. *Thromb Haemost* 1990; **63**: 319–20.

○27. DeStefano V, Leone G, Mastrangelo S, *et al*. Thrombosis during pregnancy and surgery in patients with congenital deficiency of antithrombin III, protein C, protein S. *Thromb Haemost* 1994; **71**: 799.

28. Vicente V, Rodriguez C, Soto I, Fernandez M, Moraleda JM. Risk of thrombosis during pregnancy and post-partum in hereditary thrombophilia. *Am J Hematol* 1994; **46**: 151–67.

29. Stenflo J. The biochemistry of protein C. In: Bertina RM, ed. *Protein C and related proteins*. Edinburgh: Churchill Livingstone, 1988: 21–54.

30. deFouw NJ, de Jong YF, Haverkate K, Bertina RM. Activated protein C increases fibrin clot lysis by neutralization of plasminogen activator inhibitor: no evidence for a cofactor role of protein S. *Thromb Haemostas* 1988; **60**: 328–33.

31. Romeo G, Hassan HJ, Staempfli S, *et al*. Hereditary thrombophilia: identification of nonsense and missense mutations in the protein C gene. *Proc Natl Acad Sci USA* 1987; **84**: 2829–32.

32. Reitsma PH, Poort SR, Allaart CF, Briët E, Bertina RM. The spectrum of genetic defects in a panel of 40 Dutch families with symptomatic protein C deficiency type **1**: heterogeneity and founder effects. *Blood* 1991; **78**: 890–4.

33. Bertina RM, Broekmans AW, Krommenhoek van Es C, van Wijngaarden A. The use of a functional and immunologic assay for plasma protein C in the study of the heterogeneity of congenital protein C deficiency. *Thromb Haemost* 1984; **51**: 1–5.

34. Gladson CL, Scharrer I, Hach V, Beck KH, Griffin JH. The frequency of type 1 heterozygous protein S and protein C deficiency in 141 unrelated young patients with venous thrombosis. *Thromb Haemostas* 1988; **59**: 18–22.

35. Broekmans AW, van der Linden IK, Veltkamp JJ, Bertina RM. Prevalence of isolated protein C deficiency in patients with venous thrombotic disease and in the population. *Thromb Haemostas* 1983; **50**: 350.

36. Allaart CF, Poort SR, Rosendaal FR, Reitsma PH, Bertina RM, Briët E. Increased risk of venous thrombosis in carriers of hereditary protein C deficiency defect. *Lancet* 1993; **341**: 134–8.

37. Tait RC, Walker ID, Reitsma PH, *et al*. Prevalence of protein C deficiency in the healthy population. *Thromb Haemost* 1995; **73**: 87–93.

♦38. Miletich JM, Prescott SM, White R, Majerus PW, Bovill EG. Inherited predisposition to thrombosis. *Cell* 1993; **72**: 477–80.

39. Aiach M, Gandrille S, Emmerich J. A review of mutations causing deficiencies of antithrombin, protein C and protein S. *Thromb Haemost* 1995; **74**: 81–89.

40. Cavenagh JD, Colvin BT. Guidelines for the management of thrombophilia. *Postgrad Med J* 1996; **72**: 87–94.

41. Bick RL, Ancypa D. Blood protein defects associated with thrombosis. Thrombosis and hemostasis for the clinical laboratory. *Med Clinics North Am* 1995; **15**: 125–63.

42. Sie P, Boneu B, Bierme R. Arterial thrombosis and protein S deficiency. *Thromb Haemost* 1989; **62**: 1040.

43. Bertina R, Koeleman BPC, Koster T, *et al*. Mutation in blood coagulation factor V associated with resistance to activated protein C. *Nature* 1994; **369**: 64–7.

44. Voorberg J, Roelse J, Koopman R, *et al*. Association of idiopathic venous thromboembolism with single point mutation at Arg^{506} of factor V. *Lancet* 1994; **343**: 1535–6.

45. Guasch JF, Lensen RPM, Bertina RM. Molecular characterization of a type I quantitative factor V deficiency in a thrombosis patient that is 'pseudo homozygous' for activated protein C resistance. *Thromb Haemost* 1997; **77**: 252–7.

46. Marciniak E, Romond EH. Impaired catalytic function of activated protein C: a new in vitro manifestation of lupus anticoagulant. *Blood* 1989; **74**: 2426–32.

47. Malia RG, Kitchen S, Greaves M, Preston FE. Inhibition of activated protein C and its cofactor protein S by antiphospholipid antibodies. *Br J Haematol* 1990; **76**: 101–7.

48. Griffin JH, Heeb MJ, Kojima Y, Fernández JA, Kojima K, Hackeng TM, Greengard JS. Activated protein C resistance: molecular mechanisms. *Thromb Haemost* 1995; **74**: 444–8.

♦49. Ridker PM, Hennekens CH, Lindpaintner K, Stampfer MJ, Eisenberg PR, Miletich JP. Mutation in the gene coding for coagulation factor V and the risk of myocardial infarction, stroke, and venous thrombosis in apparently healthy men. *N Engl J Med* 1995; **332**: 912–17.

50. Greengard JS, Eichinger S, Griffin JH, Bauer KA. Brief report: variability of thrombosis among homozygous siblings with resistance to activated protein C due to an Arg-Gln mutation in the gene for factor V. *N Engl J Med* 1994; **331**: 1559–62.

51. Pickering W, Dixit M, Campbell P, Cohen H. Prevalence of activated protein C resistance and other thrombophilic defects in patients with venous thromboembolism. *Br J Haematol* 1994; **86**(suppl 1): 68.

52. Cumming AM, Fildes S, Pylypczwk CC, *et al*. Low incidence of resistance to activated protein C in patients with venous thrombosis. *Br J Haematol* 1994; **86**(suppl 1): 34.

♦53. Rosendaal FR, Siscovick DS, Schwartz SM, *et al*. Factor V Leiden (resistance to activated protein C) increases the risk of myocardial infarction in young women. *Blood* 1997; **89**: 2817–21.

54. Hillarp A, Zöller B, Svensson PJ, Dahlbäck B. The 20210A allele of the prothrombin gene is a common risk factor among Swedish outpatients with verified deep venous thrombosis. *Thromb Haemost* 1997; **78**: 990–2.

55. Haverkate F, Samama M. Familial dysfibrinogenemia and thrombophilia. Report on a study of the SSC subcommittee on fibrinogen. *Thromb Haemostasis* 1995; **73**: 151–61.

56. Engesser L, Koopman J, de Munk G, *et al*. Fibrinogen Nijmegen: congenital dysfibrinogenemia associated with impaired t-PA mediated plasminogen activation and decreased binding of t-PA. *Thromb Haemost* 1988; **60**: 113–20.

57. Beckmann R. Plasminogen activation by tissue plasminogen activator in the presence of stimulating CNBr fragment FCB-2 of fibrinogen is a two-phase reaction. *J Biol Chem* 1988; **263**: 7167–80.

58. Galanakis DK. Inherited dysfibrinogenemia: emerging abnormal structure associations with pathologic and nonpathologic dysfunctions. *Semin Thromb Hemostasis* 1993; **19**: 386–95.

59. Mudd SH, Levy HL, Skovby F. Disorders of trans-sulfuration. In: Scriver CR, Beaudet AL, Sly WS, Valle D, eds *The metabolic basis of inherited disease*. New York: McGraw-Hill, 1989: 693.

60. Rees MW, Rodgers GM. Homocysteinemia: association of a metabolic disorder with vascular disease and thrombosis. *Thrombos Res* 1993; **71**: 337–59.

61. Cattance M. Hyperhomocysteinaemia. *Vessels* 1997; **3**: 16–21.

62. Selhub J, Jaques PF, Wilson PWF, Rush D, Rosenberg JH. Vitamin status and intake as primary

determinants of homocysteinemia in an elderly population. *JAMA* 1993; **270**: 2693–8.

63. Ubbink JB, van der Merwe A, Delport R, Allen RH, Stabler SP, Riezler R, Vermaak WJH. The effect of a subnormal vitamin B-6 status on homocysteine metabolism. *J Clin Invest* 1996; **98**: 177–84.

64. Joosten E, van den Berg A, Riezler R, Naurath HJ, Lindenbaum J, Stabler SP, Allen RH. Metabolic evidence that deficiencies of vitamin B-12 (cobalamin), folate, and vitamin B-6 occur commonly in elderly people. *Am J Clin Nutr* 1993; **58**: 468–76.

65. McCully KS. Homocysteine and vascular disease. *Nature Med* 1996; **2**: 386–9.

66. Hajjar KA. Homocysteine-induced modulation of tissue plasminogen activator binding to its endothelial cell membrane receptor. *J Clin Invest* 1993; **91**: 2873.

67. Stamler JS, Osborne JA, Jaraki O, Rabban LE, Mullins M, Singel D, Loscalzo J. Adverse vascular effects of homocysteine are modulated by endothelium-derived relaxing factor and related oxides of nitrogen. *J Clin Invest* 1993; **91**: 308–18.

68. Wang J, Dudman NPB, Wilken DEL. Effects of homocysteine and related compounds on prostacyclin production by cultured human vascular endothelial cells. *Thromb Haemost* 1993; **70**: 1047–52.

69. Fryer RH, Wilson BD, Gubler DB, Fitzgerald LA, Rodgers GM. Homocysteine, a risk factor for premature vascular disease and thrombosis, induces tissue factor activity in endothelial cells. *Arterioscler Thromb* 1993; **13**: 1327.

♦70. Nishinaga M, Ozawa T, Shimada K. Homocysteine, a thrombogenic agent, suppresses anticoagulant heparan sulfate expression in cultured porcine aortic endothelial cells. *J Clin Invest* 1993; **92**: 1381.

71. Harker LA, Ross R, Slichter SJ, Scott CR. Homocystine-induced arteriosclerosis: the role of endothelial cell injury and platelet response in its genesis. *J Clin Invest* 1976; **58**: 731.

72. Malinow MR, Kang SS, Taylor LM, *et al*. Prevalence of hyperhomocyst(e)inemia in patients with peripheral arterial occlusive disease. *Circulation* 1989; **79**: 1180–8.

73. Clarke R, Daly L, Robinson K, Naughten E, Cahalane S, Fowler B, Graham I. Hyperhomocystinemia: an independent risk factor for vascular disease. *N Engl J Med* 1991; **324**: 1149–55.

74. Selhub J, Jaques PF, Bostom AG, *et al*. Association between plasma homocysteine concentrations and extracranial carotid–artery stenosis. *N Engl J Med* 1995; **332**: 286–91.

75. Morita H, Taguchi J, Kurihara H, *et al*. Genetic polymorphism of 5,10-methylenetetrahydrofolate reductase (MTHFR) as a risk factor for coronary artery disease. *Circulation* 1997; **95**: 2032–6.

76. Kang SS, Wong PW, Susmano A, Sora J, Norusis M, Ruggie N. Thermolabile methylenetetrahydrofolate reductase: an inherited risk factor for coronary artery disease. *Am J Human Genet* 1991; **48**: 536–45.

♦77. Stampfer MJ, Malinow MR, Willett WC, *et al*. A prospective study of plasma homocyst(e)ine and risk of myocardial infarction in US physicians. *JAMA* 1992; **268**: 877–81.

78. Den Heijer M, Blom HJ, Gerrits WBJ, Rosendaal FR, Haak HL, Wijermans PW, Bos GMJ. Is hyperhomocystinemia a risk factor for venous thrombosis? *Lancet* 1995; **345**: 882.

79. Den Heijer M, Koster T, Blom HJ, *et al*. Hyperhomo-cystinemia as a risk factor for deep vein thrombosis. *N Engl J Med* 1996; **334**: 759–62.

80. Hirsh J, Hoak J. Management of deep vein thrombosis and pulmonary embolism. A statement for healthcare professionals from the Council on Thrombosis (in consultation with the Council on Cardiovascular Radiology), American Heart Association. *Circulation* 1996; **93**: 2212–45.

81. Clarke CS, Otridge BW, Carney DN. Thromboembolism: a complication of weekly chemotherapy in the treatment of non-Hodgkin's lymphoma. *Cancer* 1990; **66**: 2027–30.

82. Benifia JL, Madelenat P. Hyperstimulation ofareienne et risque thrombogène. *Artères Veines* 1990; **8**: 748.

83. Prins MH, Hirsh J. A critical review of the evidence supporting a relationship between impaired fibrinolytic activity and venous thromboembolism. *Arch Intern Med* 1991; **151**: 1721–31.

∘84. Bick RL, Baker WF. Anticardiolipin antibodies and thrombosis. *Hematol Oncol Clin North Am* 1992; **6**: 1287–300.

85. Bick RL. Lupus anticoagulants and anticardiolipin antibodies. *Biomed Prog* 1993; **6**: 35–9.

86. McNeil HP, Chesterman CN, Krilis SA. Anticardiolipin antibodies and lupus anticoagulants comprise separate antibody subgroups with different phospholipid binding characteristics. *Br J Haematol* 1989; **73**: 506–13.

87. Shi BS, Chong BH, Chesterman CN. Beta-2-Glycoprotein I is a requirement for anticardiolipin antibodies binding to activated platelets: differences with lupus anticoagulants. *Blood* 1993; **81**: 1255–62.

88. Ko J, Guaglianone P, Wolin M, Murillo P. Variation in the sensitivity of an activated thromboplastin time reagent to the lupus anticoagulant. *Am J Clin Pathol* 1993; **99**: 333 (abstract).

89. Carreras L, Defreyn GS, Manchin SJ, *et al*. Arterial thrombosis, intrauterine death and 'lupus' anti-coagulant: detection of immunoglobulin interfering with prostacyclin formation. *Lancet* 1981; **1**: 244–6.

90. Cariou R, Tobelem G, Bellucci S. Effect of lupus anticoagulant on antithrombogenic properties of endothelial cells: inhibition of thrombomodulin-dependent protein C activation. *Thromb Haemost* 1988; **60**: 54–8.

91. Cosgriff TM, Martin BA. Low functional and high antigenic antithrombin III level in a patient with the lupus anticoagulant. *Arthritis Rheum* 1981; **24**: 94–6.

92. Khamashta MA, Harris EN, Gharavi AE. Immune mediated mechanism for thrombosis: antiphospholipid antibody binding to platelet membranes. *Ann Rheum Dis* 1988; **47**: 849–53.

93. Sanfellipo MJ, Drayna CJ. Prekallikrein inhibitor associated with the lupus anticoagulant. *Am J Clin Pathol* 1982; **77**: 275–9.

94. Angeles-Cano E, Sultan Y, Clauvel JP. Predisposing factors to thrombosis in systemic lupus erythematosus. Possible relationships to endothelial cell damage. *J Lab Clin Med* 1979; **94**: 312–23.

95. Schved JF, Dupuy-Fons C, Biron C. A perspective epidemiological study on the occurrence of antiphospholipid antibody: the Montpellier Antiphospholipiod (MAP) Study. *Haemostasis* 1994; **24**: 175–82.

96. Vila P, Hernandez MC, Lopez-Fernandez MF. Prevalence, follow-up and clinical significance of the anticardiolipin antibodies in normal subjects. *Thromb Haemost* 1994; **72**: 209–13.

○97. Baker WF, Bick RL. Antiphospholipid antibodies in coronary artery disease. *Semin Thromb Hemost* 1994; **20**: 27–45.

98. Hamsten A, Norberg R, Bjorkholm M. Antibodies to cardiolipin in young survivors of myocardial infarction: an association with recurrent cardiovascular events. *Lancet* 1986; **i**: 113–16.

99. Bick RL, Ismail Y, Baker WF. Coagulation abnormalities in patients with precocious coronary artery thrombosis and patients failing coronary artery bypass grafting and percutaneous transcoronary angioplasty. *Semin Thromb Hemost* 1993; **19**: 411–17.

100. Montalban J, Khamashta M, Davalos A, *et al*. Value of immunologic testing in stroke patients. A prospective multicenter study. *Stroke* 1994; **25**: 2412–15.

101. Brey RL, Hart RG, Sherman DG, Tegeler CH. Antiphospholipid antibodies and cerebral ischemia in young people. *Neurology* 1990; **40**: 1190–6.

102. APASS (The Antiphospholipid Antibodies in Stroke Study) Group. Anticardiolipin antibodies are an independent risk factor for first ischemic stroke. *Neurology* 1993; **43**: 2069–73.

103. Bick RL. Antiphospholipid thrombosis syndromes: etiology, pathophysiology, diagnosis and management. *Int J Hematol* 1997; **65**: 193–213.

104. Conley CL, Hartmann RC. A hemorrhagic disorder caused by circulating anticoagulant in patients with disseminated lupus erythematosus. *J Clin Invest* 1952; **31**: 621–2.

105. Criel A, Collen D, Masson PL. A case of IgM antibodies which inhibit the contact activation of blood coagulation. *Thromb Res* 1978; **12**: 883–92.

○106. Kunkel L. Acquired circulating anticoagulants. *Hematol Oncol Clin North Am* 1992; **6**: 1341–58.

107. Bick RL. Hypercoagulability and thrombosis. *Med Clin North Am* 1994; **78**: 635–66.

108. Minna JD, Bunn PA Jr. Paraneoplastic syndromes. In: De Vita VT Jr, Hellman S, Rosenberg SA, eds *Cancer: principles and practice of oncology*, 3rd edn. Philadelphia: JB Lippincott, 1989: 1920–40.

109. Green KB, Silverstein RL. Hypercoagulability in cancer. *Hematol/Oncol Clinics North Am* 1996; **10**: 499–530.

110. Edwards RL, Rickles FR, Moritz TE, *et al*. Abnormalities of blood coagulation tests in patients with cancer. *Am J Clin Pathol* 1987; **88**: 596–602.

111. Hagedorn AB, Bowie EJ, Elveback LR, Owen CJ. Coagulation abnormalities in patients with inoperable lung cancer. *Mayo Clin Proc* 1974; **49**: 647–53.

112. Rickles FR, Levine M, Edwards RL. Hemostatic alterations in cancer patients. *Cancer Metastas Rev* 1992; **1**: 241.

♦113. Rickles FR, Edwards RL, Barb C, Cronlund M. Abnormalities of blood coagulation in patients with cancer. Fibrinopeptide A generation and tumor growth. *Cancer* 1983; **51**: 301–7.

114. Subcommittee on Haemostasis and Malignancy of the Scientific and Standardization Committee, International Society on Thrombosis and Haemostasis. *Thromb Haemost* 1993; **69**: 205–13.

115. Rao LVM: Tissue factor as a tumor procoagulant. *Cancer Metastas Rev* 1992; **11**: 249.

116. Semeraro N. Differential expression of procoagulant activity in macrophages associated with experimental and human tumors. *Haemostasis* 1988; **18**: 47–54.

117. Bastida E, Ordinas A. Platelet contribution to formation of metastatic foci: The role of cancer cell-induced platelet activation. *Haemostasis* 1988; **18**: 29–36.

118. Falanga A, Alessio MG, Donati MB. A new procoagulant in acute leukemia. *Blood* 1988; **71**: 870–5.

119. Donati MB, Gambacorti PC, Casali B, *et al*. Cancer procoagulant activity in human tumor cells: evidence from melanoma patients. *Cancer Res* 1986; **46**: 6471–4.

120. Falanga A, Gordon SG. Isolation and characterization of cancer procoagulant: a cysteine proteinase from malignant tissue. *Biochemistry* 1985; **24**: 5558–67.

121. Jaffe EA. Biochemistry, immunology, and cell biology of endothelium. In Colman RW, Hirsh J, Marder VJ, Salzman EW, eds *Hemostasis and thrombosis. Basic principles and clinical practice*, 3rd edn. Philadelphia: JB Lippincott, 1994.

122. Prandoni P, Lensing AWA, Buller HR, *et al*. Deep-vein thrombosis and the subsequent incidence of symptomatic malignant disease. *N Engl J Med* 1992; **327**: 1128.

123. Monreal M, Lafoz E, Casals A, *et al*. Occult cancer in patients with deep venous thrombosis: a systematic approach. *Cancer* 1991; **67**: 541–5.

♦124. Aderka D, Brown A, Zelikovski A, Pinkhas J. Idiopathic deep vein thrombosis in an apparently healthy patient as a premonitory sign of occult cancer. *Cancer* 1986; **57**: 1846–9.

125. Naschitz JE, Yeshurun D, Abramson J. Thromboembolism: clues for the presence of occult neoplasia. *Int Angiol* 1989; **8**: 200–5.

126. British Committee for Standards in Haematology. Guidelines on the investigation and mangement of thrombophilia. *J Clin Pathol* 1990; **43**: 703–9.

127. Ridker PM, Glynn RJ, Miletich JP, Goldhaber SZ, Stampfer MJ, Hennekens CH. Age-specific incidence rates of venous thromboembolism among heterozygous carriers of factor V leiden mutation. *Ann Intern Med* **126**: 528–31.

128. Jorquera JI, Montoro JM, Fernandez MA, Aznar JA, Aznar J. Modified test for activated protein C resistance. *Lancet* 1994; **344**: 1162–3.

129. Trossaërt M, Conard J, Horellou MH, *et al.* Modified APC resistance assay for patients on oral anticoagulants. *Lancet* 1994; **344**: 1709.

130. Matsuura E, Igarashi Y, Fujimoto M, *et al.* Anticardiolipin cofactor(s) and differential diagnosis of autoimmune disease. *Lancet* 1990; **1**: 177–8.

♦131. McNeil HP, Simpson RJ, Chesterman CN, *et al.* Antiphospholipid antibodies are directed against a complex antigen that includes a lipid-binding inhibitor: B$_2$-glycoprotein I (apolipoprotein H). *Proc Natl Acad Sci USA* 1990; **87**: 4120–4.

132. Triplett DA, Brandt JT, Musgrave KA, *et al.* The relationship between lupus anticoagulants and antibodies to phospholipid. *JAMA* 1988; **259**: 550–4.

133. Petri M, Nelson L, Weimer F, *et al.* The automated modified Russell viper venom time test for the lupus anticoagulant. *J Rheumatol* 1991; **18**: 1823–5.

134. Brattström L. Vitamins as homocysteine-lowering agents. *J Nutr* 1996; **126**: 1276S–80S.

135. Kearon C, Gent M, Hirsh J *et al.* A comparison of three months of anticoagulation with extended anticoagulation for a first episode of idiopathic venous thromboembolism. *N Engl J Med* 1999; **340**: 901–7.

136. Khamashta MA, Cuadrado MJ, Mujic F, Ta NA, Hunt BJ, Hughes GRV. The management of thrombosis in the antiphospholipid–antibody syndrome. *N Engl J Med* 1995; **332**: 993–7.

137. Boushey CJ, Beresford SAA, Omenn GS, Motulsky AG. A quantitative assessment of plasma homocysteine as a risk factor for vascular disease. Probable benefits of increasing folic acid intakes. *JAMA* 1995; **274**: 1049–57.

138. Rosove MH, Brewer PMC. Antiphospholipid thrombosis: clinical course after the first thrombotic event in 70 patients. *Ann Intern Med* 1992; **117**: 303–8.

139. Derksen RHWM, de Groot PG, Kater L, *et al.* Patients with antiphospholipid antibodies and venous thrombosis should receive long term anticoagulant treatment. *Ann Rheum Dis* 1993; **52**: 689–92.

140. Landefeld CS, Goldman L. Major bleeding in outpatients treated with warfarin: incidence and prediction by factors known at the start of outpatient therapy. *Am J Med* 1989; **87**: 144–52.

141. Fihn SD, McDonell M, Martin D, *et al.* Risk factors for complications of chronic anticoagulation: a multicenter study. *Ann Intern Med* 1993; **118**: 511–20.

142. Gitter MJ, Jaeger TM, Petterson TM, *et al.* Bleeding and thromboembolism during anticoagulant therapy: a population-based study in Rochester, Minnesota. *Mayo Clin Proc* 1995; **70**: 725–33.

143. Babikian VL, Levine SR. Therapeutic considerations for stroke patients with antiphospholipid antibodies. *Stroke* 1992; **23**(suppl I): I-33–7.

144. Lubbe WF, Liggins GC. Lupus anticoagulant and pregnancy. *Am J Obstet Gynecol* 1985; **153**: 322–7.

145. Lubbe WF, Pattison NS. Antiphospholipid antibody syndrome and recurrent fetal loss. *Curr Obstet Gynaecol* 1991; **1**: 196–202.

146. Silver RK, MacGregor SN, Sholl JS, *et al.* Comparative trial of prednisone plus aspirin versus aspirin alone in the treatment of anticardiolipin antibody-positive obstetric patients. *Am J Obstet Gynecol* 1993; **169**: 1411–17.

147. Yoshida A, Morozumi K, Koyama K, *et al.* Prednisolone and aspirin therapy for habitual abortion associated with anti-cardiolipin antibody. *Ryumachi* 1992; **32**: 200–5.

148. Rosove MH, Tabsh K, Wasserstrum N, *et al.* Heparin therapy for pregnant women with lupus anticoagulant or anticardiolipin antibodies. *J Vasc Surg* 1988; **7**: 749–56.

149. Cowchock FS, Reece EA, Balaban D, *et al.* Repeated fetal losses associated with antiphospholipid antibodies: a collaborative randomized trial comparing prednisone with low-dose heparin treatment. *Am J Obstet Gynecol* 1992; **166**: 1318–23.

150. Spinnato JA, Clark AL, Pierangeli SS, *et al.* Intravenous immunoglobulin therapy for the antiphospholipid syndrome in pregnancy. *Am J Obstet Gynecol* 1995; **172**: 690–4.

151. Valensise H, Vaquero E, De Carolis C, *et al.* Normal fetal growth in women with antiphospholipid syndrome treated with high-dose intravenous immunoglobulin (IVIG). *Prenat Diagn* 1995; **15**: 509–17.

152. Lensen RPM, Bertenia RM, de Ronde H, Vandenbrouke JP, Rosendall FR. Venous thrombotic risk in family members of unselected individuals with Factor V Leiden. *Thromb Haemostas* 2000; **83**: 817–21.

17

In-hospital management of antithrombotic therapy: prevention and treatment guidelines

RICHARD C BECKER

Thrombotic disorders of the venous and arterial circulatory system are common in daily clinical practice, particularly for physicians and other health-care providers working in the hospital setting. Considered collectively, thrombotic disorders, including their prevention and treatment, are encountered by almost all surgical and medical disciplines. The development of management guidelines for use on a wide scale represents a vital step toward consistency in practice and a high level of patient care.

INTRODUCTION

A standardized, structured, and easily implemented approach to the management of thromboembolic disease has been recommended as the most efficient and cost-effective means to maintain consistency and achieve a high standard of care among practicing clinicians.

Thrombotic disorders of the venous and arterial circulating systems, considered collectively, represent a leading cause of morbidity, mortality, and health-care expenditures in hospitalized patients. Estimates suggest that there are 1 million myocardial infarctions, 500 000 cases of unstable angina, 2 million strokes, and upward of 250 000 clinically recognized (and an equal number of unrecognized) venous thromboemboli yearly in the USA. The number of individuals at risk for thrombotic events exceeds this already impressive number by, at the very least, 10–20-fold.

Because thromboembolic disease is a concern for a wide variety of health-care professionals, including primary care physicians, cardiologists, hematologists, oncologists, obstetricians, surgeons, pharmacists, physical therapists, and advanced practice nurses, it has assumed a unique and prominent position in hospital-wide prevention and treatment strategies.

Experience gained over the years, coupled with data derived from carefully designed and conducted clinical trials, has fostered the development of practical patient care guidelines. Moreover, the general availability of clinically applicable information provides a level of confidence that can translate to increased awareness and widespread implementation of diagnostic, preventive, and treatment standards.[1,2]

The following chapter provides an abbreviated and structured overview of thromboembolic disease and its management, including diagnostic testing, prevention, and antithrombotic therapy.

ANTITHROMBOTIC THERAPY DURING PREGNANCY

A relative paucity of information derived from randomized clinical trials made it difficult to develop recommendations for anticoagulant therapy during pregnancy. Because it is safer for the fetus, heparin (unfractionated) is often considered the anticoagulant of choice. Experience with low-molecular-weight heparin (LMWH) is increasing and may represent an acceptable alternative. Warfarin use is *not* recommended during the first trimester. The recommendations for antithrombotic therapy during pregnancy listed in Table 17.1 are classified as Grade C (supported only by level III, IV, and V clinical trials).

Traditionally, the risk of deep vein thrombosis is greatest during the third trimester and early postpartum periods; however, events can occur at any time. Several factors are important in the development of venous thromboembolism during pregnancy, including venous stasis from increased venous distensibility, external impingement of the inferior vena cava and iliac veins by the gravid uterus, and a prothrombotic state that, teleologically, is designed to minimize blood loss during delivery.

As in other settings, the clinical diagnosis of deep vein thrombosis (DVT) is unreliable and suspicion must be confirmed by objective testing. Diagnostic approaches to the pregnant patient with suspected DVT and pulmonary embolism (PE) are outlined in Figs 17.1 and 17.2.

PREVENTION OF VENOUS THROMBOEMBOLISM: SURGICAL AND MEDICAL PATIENTS

The risk stratification of patients undergoing surgical procedures and for patients with serious medical illnesses is outlined in Tables 17.2 and 17.3, respectively.

Table 17.1 *Antithrombotic therapy during pregnancy. (Adapted from* Chest *1998;* **114**: *439S–769S.)*

Condition	Therapy
Previous venous thrombosis or PE prior to current pregnancy	Heparin 5000 U every 12 hours or adjusted to yield a heparin level of 0.1–0.2 U/mL throughout pregnancy followed by warfarin (postpartum) for 4–6 weeks.
	or
	Clinical surveillance combined with periodic CUS followed by warfarin (postpartum) for 4–6 weeks
	or
	LMWH
Venous thrombosis or PE during current pregnancy	Heparin in full iv doses for 5–10 days, followed by sc injection every 12 hours to prolong the 6-hour postinjection aPTT into the therapeutic range (2× control) until delivery; warfarin can then be used postpartum
Planning pregnancy in patients who are being treated with long-term oral anticoagulants	Either heparin every 12 hours sc to prolong the 6-hour postinjection aPTT into the therapeutic range (2× control)
	or
	Frequent pregnancy tests and substitute heparin (as above) for warfarin when pregnancy achieved
Mechanical heart valves	Either heparin every 12 hours sc to prolong the 6-hour postinjection aPTT into therapeutic (2× control)
	or
	Adjusted dose sc heparin until the 13th week, warfarin (target INR 2.5–3.0) until the middle of the third trimester, then adjusted dose sc heparin until delivery
APLAs and >1 pregnancy loss	Aspirin (60–150 mg qd) plus heparin (5000 U sc BID)
APLAs and 0 or 1 previous pregnancy loss	Low-dose aspirin during the second and third trimester
APLAs and previous venous thrombosis	Heparin every 12 hours sc to prolong the 6-hour postinjection aPTT into the therapeutic range (2× control)
APLAs without previous venous thrombosis	Either clinical surveillance combined with CUS
	or
	Heparin 5000 U every 12 hours throughout pregnancy

aPTT = activated partial thromboplastin time; APLAs = antiphospholipid antibodies; CUS = compression ultrasonography; LMWH = low-molecular-weight heparin; iv = intravenous; INR = international normalized ratio; PE = pulmonary embolism; SC = subcutaneous.

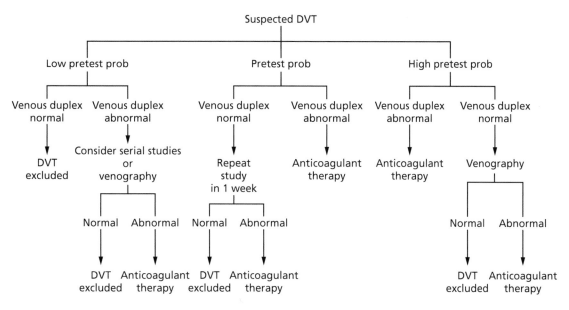

Figure 17.1 *Diagnostic approach to suspected deep venous thrombosis (DVT) during pregnancy. Prob = probability. (UMass-Memorial Anticoagulation Services, 2001.)*

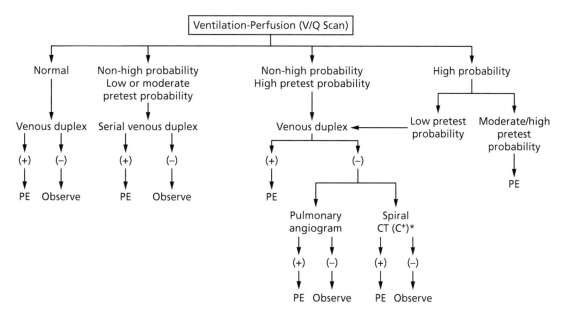

Figure 17.2 *Diagnostic approach to suspected pulmonary embolism (PE) during pregnancy. Pretest probability (increased with)*
- *Respiratory: dyspnea, pleuritic chest pain, O_2 saturation <92% (on room air with suboptimal correction with supplemental O_2), hemoptysis, pleural rub*
- *Risk factors: prior DVT/PE, immobilization, surgery, obesity*

spiral CT of chest with contrast (C^+)

(UMass-Memorial Anticoagulation Services, 2001.)

1 In *low-risk* patients who are younger than 40 years and have no clinical risk factors undergoing general surgery for minor operations, no specific prophylaxis other than early ambulation is recommended.

2 It is recommended that elastic stockings (ES), low-dose (5000 U) heparin (LDH) (given 2 hours before and every 8–12 hours after operation), LMWH (e.g. Enoxaparin 40 mg subcutaneously (sc) 1–2 hours before surgery and daily after surgery), or intermittent pneumatic compression (IPC) be used in *moderate risk* general surgery

Table 17.2 *Classification of venous thrombolism risk in surgical patients. (Adapted from Chest 1998; **114**: 439S–769S.)*

Thromboembolism event	Low risk[a]	Moderate risk[b]	High risk[c]	Very high risk[d]
Calf vein thrombosis (%)	2	10–20	20–40	40–80
Proximal vein thrombosis (%)	0.4	2–4	4–8	10–20
Clinical PE (%)	0.2	1–2	2–4	4–10
Fatal PE (%)	0.002	0.1–0.4	0.4–1.0	1–5
Successful preventive strategies	No specific measures	ES, LDUH (q12h), LMWH or IPC	LDUH (q8h), LMWH or IPC	LMWH, LDUH, oral anticoagulants and IPC

[a]Uncomplicated minor surgery in patients younger than 40 years with no clinical risk factors.
[b]Major surgery in patients older than 40 years with no other clinical risk factors.
[c]Major surgery in patients older than 40 years who have additional risk factors or myocardial infarction.
[d]Major surgery in patients older than 40 years plus previous venous thromboembolic or malignant disease or orthopedic surgery or hip fracture or stroke or spinal cord injury.
PE = pulmonary embolism; ES = elastic stockings; LDUH = low-dose unfractionated heparin; LMWH = low-molecular-weight heparin; IPC = intermittent pneumatic compression.

Table 17.3 *Risk factors for venous thromboembolism in patients with medical illnesses*

Immobilization
Stroke
Myocardial infarction
Serious infection
Respiratory failure
Malignancy
Indwelling venous catheter

patients who are older than 40 years and are undergoing major operations, but who have no additional clinical risk factors for venous thromboembolism. If possible, IPC and ES should be applied during the operation and throughout the postoperative period.

3 It is recommended that LDH (every 8 hours) or LMWH (e.g. Lovenox® 40 mg sc before surgery and daily after surgery) be used in *higher* risk general surgery patients who are older than 40 years, undergoing major operations, and have additional risk factors.

4 In *higher* risk patients (as profiled in recommendation 3) who are prone to wound complications, such as hematomas and infection, IPC would be a good alternative choice for prophylaxis.

5 In *very high risk* general surgery patients with multiple risk factors, it is recommended that effective pharmacologic methods (LDH or LMWH) be combined with IPC. LDH and LMWH therapy should be started preoperatively and continued postoperatively. IPC should also be applied intraoperatively if possible.

6 In selected *very high risk* general surgery patients,

perioperative warfarin (international normalized ratio (INR) 2.0–3.0) therapy may be used.

7 It is recommended that aspirin *not* be used for prophylaxis in general surgery patients.

8 In patients undergoing total hip replacement surgery, postoperative subcutaneous twice-daily fixed-dose unmonitored LMWH (e.g. Lovenox® 30 mg) started 12 hours after surgery, low-intensity (INR 2.0–3.0) oral anticoagulation (started preoperatively or immediately after operation), or adjusted-dose (to maintain activated partial thromboplastin time (aPTT) at the upper limit of normal) unfractionated heparin (started preoperatively) are effective and recommended for routine use. Adjuvant prophylaxis with ES or IPC may provide additional efficacy. Although other agents such as LDH, aspirin, dextran, and IPC reduce the overall incidence of venous thromboembolism, they are less effective and should *not* be used routinely. The optimal duration of prophylaxis is approximately 10–14 days; however, longer periods may offer benefit among high-risk patients.

9 In patients undergoing total knee replacement, postoperative subcutaneous twice-daily fixed-dose unmonitored LMWH (e.g. Lovenox® 30 mg) and warfarin are the most effective pharmacologic prophylactic regimen. IPC is the most effective non-pharmacologic prophylactic regimen and provides a reduction in relative risk comparable to LMWH. The optimal duration of prophylaxis is approximately 10–14 days; however, longer periods may offer benefit among high-risk patients.

10 In patients undergoing hip fracture surgery, either preoperative or early postoperative sc fixed-dose unmonitored LMWH (e.g. Lovenox® 30 mg) or

oral anticoagulation (INR 2.0–3.0) is recommended for routine use. IPC combined with either agent may provide additional benefit.

11 Prophylactic inferior vena cava filter placement should be limited to high-risk patients in whom other forms of anticoagulant-based prophylaxis are *not* feasible due to active bleeding or an anticipated high postoperative bleeding risk.

12 It is recommended that IPC (with or without ES) be used in patients undergoing intracranial neurosurgery. Low-dose unfractionated heparin or LMWH therapy may be acceptable alternatives. IPC and LDH or LMWH may be more effective in combination than individually, and should be considered in high-risk patients.

13 In patients with acute spinal cord injury with paralysis, treatment with LMWH is recommended. LDH, ES, and IPC when used alone, appear ineffective but may be of benefit when used together with LMWH. ES and IPC should be combined when pharmacologic therapy is contraindicated.

14 In trauma patients with an identifiable risk factor, LMWH should be used when feasible. IPC should be used when the risk of bleeding precludes pharmacologic therapy. Serial surveillance venous duplex ultrasonography should be considered among high-risk patients with suboptimal prophylaxis. Inferior vena cava (IVC) filter placement should be considered in the presence of confirmed DVT when anticoagulation is contraindicated.

15 It is recommended that LDH be used in patients with myocardial infarction. Full-dose anticoagulation is also effective. IPC and ES may be useful when heparin therapy is contraindicated.

16 In patients with ischemic stroke and lower extremity paralysis, LDH or LMWH are effective. IPC and ES are also probably effective.

17 In general, medical patients with clinical risk factors for venous thromboembolism, particularly those with congestive heart failure and/or chest infections, LDH or LMWH is effective.

18 It is recommended that warfarin, 1 mg daily, be used in patients with long-term indwelling central vein catheters to prevent axillary–subclavian venous thrombosis.

The issue of clinical superiority between LMWH and unfractionated heparin is important not only because of the universal mission to offer optimal care but because of higher drug costs. At the present time, DVT prophylaxis with LMWH costs approximately $20/day compared with $3–5/day for unfractionated sc heparin. Although the price differential in the USA and other countries will fall as competition increases, the potential financial impact of prophylaxing all patients with LMWH must be

Table 17.4 *Comparative costs^a at the UMass-Memorial Medical Center for thromboembolism prophylaxis. (Information provided by Anticoagulation Task Force, 2001)*

Therapy	Cost ($)
Low-dose heparin (5000 U sc q8h–q12h)	0.58–0.87
Adjusted-dose heparin (25 000 U/day)	5.04
Warfarin (4 mg po/iv)	0.04/3.13
Enoxaparin (30 mg sc bid)	21.88
Dextran (25 mL/hour)	41.50
Pneumatic compression stockings (1× charge)	25.00
Enteric-coated aspirin (325 mg)	0.02

^{a}Costs may vary among hospitals and pharmacies.
SC = subcutaneous; iv = intravenous.

considered by clinicians, pharmacists and administrators (Table 17.4).

ANTITHROMBOTIC THERAPY FOR ESTABLISHED VENOUS THROMBOEMBOLISM

1 Patients with DVT or PE should be treated with intravenous heparin or adjusted-dose sc heparin sufficient to prolong the aPTT to a range that corresponds to a plasma heparin level of 0.2–0.4 U/mL (protamine titration) or 0.3–0.6 U/mL (anti-Xa assay), typically 60–75 seconds.

2 It is recommended that treatment with heparin be continued for 5–10 days and that oral anticoagulation be overlapped with heparin for 4–5 days. For many patients, heparin and warfarin therapy can be started together and heparin therapy discontinued on day 5 or 6 if the INR is therapeutic (for 2 consecutive days). For massive PE or extensive iliofemoral DVT, a longer period of heparin therapy should be considered. IVC filter placement should also be considered in these particular settings.

3 Long-term anticoagulant therapy should be continued for at least 3 months using oral anticoagulants to prolong the INR to a target level of 2.5 (2.0–3.0). When oral anticoagulants are contraindicated or inconvenient, LMWH or adjusted-dose heparin therapy should be given to prolong the aPTT to a time corresponding to a plasma heparin level of 0.3–0.6 anti-Xa U/ml, typically ~60 seconds.

4 Patients with a first DVT or a reversible risk factor should be treated for 3–6 months. Patients with recurrent DVT or a continuing risk factor (e.g. antithrombin deficiency, protein C or S deficiency, malignancy) should be treated indefinitely. The ideal duration of treatment for patients with activated protein C resistance is unknown; however, long-term

therapy is suggested for homozygotes or those with recurrent events.

5   Symptomatic isolated calf DVT should be treated with anticoagulation for 3 months. If for any reason anticoagulation cannot be given, serial non-invasive studies of the lower extremity should be performed (over 7–14 days) to assess for proximal extension (above the popliteal vein) of thrombus.

6   The use of fibrinolytic agents in the treatment of venous thromboembolism must be individualized, but generally is *not* recommended for routine therapy. Patients with hemodynamically compromising PE and massive ileofemoral DVT are most likely to benefit.

7   IVC filter placement is recommended when there is a contraindication or complication of anticoagulant therapy in an individual with, or at very high risk for, DVT or PE. It is also recommended for recurrent thromboembolism that occurs despite adequate (solidly within the target range) anticoagulation, in patients with chronic recurrent embolism with pulmonary hypertension, and during the concurrent performance of surgical pulmonary embolectomy or endarterectomy. When possible, anticoagulation should be given following placement of a vena caval filter in a patient with a lower extremity proximal DVT to reduce the likelihood of chronic venous stasis and postphlebitic syndrome.

8   LMWH preparations (e.g. Lovenox® 1mg/kg sc twice daily) can be used in the treatment of DVT and PE. Home treatment programs are discussed in detail in Chapter 33.

LMWH preparations in the treatment of deep venous thrombosis

Clinical trials have demonstrated comparable efficacy and safety of specific LMWH preparations compared

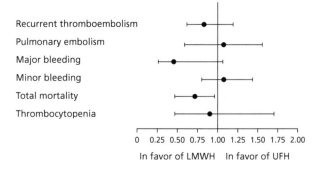

Figure 17.3 *A summary of important end points of clinical trials (presented as odds ratios) comparing low-molecular-weight heparin (LMWH) and unfractionated heparin (UFH) in venous thromboembolism. (Reproduced with permission from Dolovich L, Ginsberg JS. Low molecular weight heparin in the treatment of venous thromboembolism: an updated meta-analysis. Vessels 1997; **3**: 4–11).*

with intravenous unfractionated heparin[3–8] (Table 17.5 and Fig. 17.3). Considerations that are important in choosing the preferred therapeutic approach to DVT are presented in Table 17.6.

Patients with proximal DVT (with or without PE) in whom anticoagulation is either contraindicated or ineffective (i.e. recurrent thrombotic events despite a therapeutic level of anticoagulation) should be considered for IVC interruption. The most common method employed at our institution is transvenous placement of a Greenfield filter.[9]

UNSTABLE ANGINA/NON-ST SEGMENT ELEVATION MYOCARDIAL INFARCTION

Heparin and oral anticoagulants have been used in the treatment of unstable angina and non-ST segment ele-

Table 17.5 *The clinical use of low-molecular-weight heparin (LMWH) preparations in patients at risk for venous thromboembolism. (Information prepared by the Anticoagulation Task Force, 2001)*

Patient groups with strong safety, efficacy and cost–benefit evidence for LMWH
Elective knee replacement
Major trauma
Acute spinal cord injury with lower extremity paralysis
Abdominal surgery for cancer
Trousseau's syndrome (DVT in the setting of cancer)

Patient groups with *insufficient* evidence of clinical advantage for LMWHs
Elective hip replacement: efficacy/safety similar to warfarin, which is less expensive
Hip fracture surgery: efficacy/safety similar to warfarin, which is less expensive
Major general surgery: efficacy/safety similar to low-dose (unfractionated) heparin, which is less expensive
General high-risk medical patients: should receive elastic stockings + low-dose (unfractionated) heparin
Ischemic stroke: efficacy/safety similar to low-dose (unfractionated) heparin, which is less expensive

DVT = deep vein thrombosis.

Table 17.6 *Treatment considerations with low-molecular-weight heparin (LMWH) in established deep vein thrombosis (DVT). (Information prepared by the Anticoagulation Task Force, 2001)[a]*

Agent selection	LMWHs exhibit pharmacodynamic differences. The ratio of anti-Xa to anti-IIa activity, pharmacokinetics, and physiochemical characteristics differ between agents.	These agents (collectively) should not be considered as therapeutically equivalent until more data are available and potency determinations are standardized.
Monitoring	Monitoring anti-Xa activity in patients at high risk for bleeding or rethrombosis.	For the treatment of uncomplicated DVT, LMWHs do not require laboratory monitoring. LMWHs do not affect the aPTT, PT, TT, or ACT.
DVT prophylaxis (for recurrent events)	Following treatment initiation with LMWH, DVT prophylaxis is still required using warfarin or an alternative agent.	As with heparin, conversion to oral warfarin may begin as early as day 1. An overlap of at least 4 days with LMWH and warfarin is required and the INR should be at least 2.0 on 2 consecutive days prior to discontinuing LMWH.
Adverse effects	Bleeding	Protamine only partially reverses and transiently neutralizes the anticoagulant effect of LMWHs.
	Thrombocytopenia (+/− thrombosis)	The incidence of clinically relevant thrombocytopenia is lower than with UFH, but platelet monitoring is still recommended. Patients with documented HIT have a high incidence of cross-reactivity with LMWHs.
Patient factors	Most suitable for patients who are stable, at lower risk for bleeding, and who have no other reason to be in the hospital.	Proper patient selection, education, and follow-up are key elements of a successful outcome. Only one-third to one-half of patients are candidates for home treatment and can be discharged within 24 hours.
Cost issues	Currently the cost of available LMWHs in the treatment of DVT exceeds the cost of unfractionated heparin plus laboratory monitoring.	For in-patient management of acute DVT, standard therapeutic heparin plus monitoring is still cost effective. LMWH is more cost-effective if patient admissions are avoided or patients are discharged early and closely followed.

[a]UMass-Memorial Medical Center.
aPTT = activated partial thromboplastin time; PT = prothrombin time; TT = thrombin time; ACT = activated clotting time; INR = international normalized ratio; UFH = unfractionated heparin; HIT = heparin-induced thrombocytopenia.

vation myocardial infarction (MI) for over three decades.[10–13] The first major clinical trial of anticoagulation was performed by Théroux and colleagues.[14] In their study of 479 patients with unstable angina, benefit (reduced incidence of MI and refractory angina) was observed in patients treated with either aspirin (325 mg twice per day) or intravenous heparin (continuous infusion to maintain the aPTT between 1.5 and 2 times the laboratory control). There was a trend favoring heparin over aspirin. A study by the RISC group[15] subsequently reported that a combination of heparin and aspirin was more beneficial than either agent used alone. The development of more potent platelet antagonists, specifically the platelet surface GPIIb/IIIa inhibitors that include abciximab (ReoPro®), tirofiban (Aggrastat®), and eptifibatide (Integrilin®) may change the treatment of unstable angina and non-ST segment elevation MI. The available data suggest superiority of these agents compared with the combination of unfractionated heparin and aspirin.[16–20] The greatest clinical benefit appears in high-risk patients (refractory angina, postinfarction angina).

In the ESSENCE (Efficacy and Safety of Subcutaneous Enoxaparin in Non Q-wave Coronary Events) trial, the risk of recurrent angina, MI, and death was lower at 14 and 30 days in patients receiving enoxaparin (Lovenox®) 1.0 mg/kg 5c q12h compared to those given iv unfractionated heparin. Major bleeding complications were similar between the two groups.[21] Confirmatory evidence was recently provided in the TIMI 11B trial.[22]

We currently recommend that all patients with unstable angina and non-ST segment elevation MI receive aspirin (160–325 mg), started as soon as possible. Patients with an aspirin allergy should receive ticlopidine, 250 mg twice daily or clopidogrel, 75 mg daily. An initial loading dose of 500 mg and 300 mg, respectively, provides more rapid platelet inhibition. In addition to antiplatelet therapy, anticoagulation with heparin is recommended for patients with ischemic chest pain at rest accompanied by electrocardiographic abnormalities and/or evidence of hemodynamic compromise. Unfractionated heparin should be given intravenously as a bolus, followed by a continuous infusion for a total of 3–5 days. We recommend achieving and maintaining an aPTT of 1.5–2.0 times the laboratory control. Heparin dosing to higher levels of anticoagulation (>2.0 times control) does *not* offer greater benefit but does increase the risk of hemorrhagic complications. LMWH given subcutaneously (e.g. Lovenox® 1.0 mg/kg q12h) is an acceptable alternative and may soon be considered the standard of care. The use of a platelet glycoprotein (GP) IIb/IIIa antagonist should be considered strongly in patients with high-risk features and those undergoing urgent or emergent coronary angioplasty. The combined use of enoxaparin and a GPIIb/IIIa antagonist represents an attractive therapy and experience with this strategy is increasing rapidly. As in other acute clinical settings, when unfractionated heparin is the anticoagulant chosen, we prefer point-of-care coagulation monitoring and a heparin titration nomogram (Table 17.7). Patients treated with enoxaparin in whom coronary angiography or angioplasty is required should be approached somewhat differently (Table 17.8). When intravenous unfractionated heparin is to be discontinued, we recommend downward titration to prevent a *rebound* prothrombotic state. Our current practice is to decrease the heparin infusion by 50 per cent for 12 hours prior to discontinuation. All patients should receive either aspirin or an alternative antiplatelet agent for at least 24 hours prior to heparin discontinuation. Antiplatelet therapy should be continued indefinitely.[23–25] Fibrinolytic therapy is not recommended in the routine care of patients with unstable angina.[26]

Antiplatelet therapy

1 It is strongly recommended that patients with unstable angina or non-ST segment elevation MI be treated with aspirin (160–325 mg/day), commencing as soon as possible after a diagnosis is established and continued indefinitely.
2 It is recommended that patients who have an aspirin allergy be considered for therapy with either ticlopidine (250 mg bid) or clopidogrel (75 mg daily).
3 It is recommended that patients who have contraindications to aspirin, ticlopidine, or clopidogrel receive heparin, followed by warfarin (target INR 3.0; range 2.5–3.5) for a period of several months.

Table 17.7 *Patient-specific heparin dosing nomogram. (Anticoagulation Task Force, 2001)*

aPTT (seconds)	Repeat bolus	Stop infusion	Rate change (U/kg per hour)	Repeat aPTT
<35	60 U/kg	0 min	↑4	6 hours
35–50	30 U/kg	0 min	↑3	6 hours
51–70[a]	0	0 min	No change	6 hours
71–90	0	0 min	↓2	6 hours
>90	0	0 min	↓3	6 hours

Age >65 years: decrease bolus by 10%; decrease/increase infusion by 1 U/kg per hour.
Female sex: decrease bolus by 5%; decrease/increase infusion by 0.5 U/kg per hour.
Height <165 cm: decrease bolus by 2.5%; decrease/increase infusion by 0.25 U/kg per hour.
[a]The target level of anticoagulation should be based on a representative heparin level of 0.3–0.6 U/mL (anti-Xa method).

Table 17.8 *A heparin dosing nomogram for patients with unstable angina/non-ST segment elevation myocardial infarction who have received enoxaparin and subsequently require coronary angiography and/or angioplasty. Time since last dose of enoxaparin (≥1.0 mg/kg sc)*

| | ≤8 hours | | >8 hours | |
	Additional UFH	Sheath removal	Additional UFH	Sheath removal
Diagnostic catheterization	0	>6 hours	2000–3000 U	Immediate
PCI[a] (+ GPIIb/IIIa inhibitor)	0	>6 hours	50–70 U/kg[a] ACT 200 seconds	ACT <160 seconds
PCI (– GPIIb/IIIa inhibitor)	0	>6 hours	70 U/kg[b] ACT 300 seconds	ACT <160 seconds

[a]Low-dose heparin (70 U/kg to target) has been evaluated in clinical trials using abciximab.
[b]Maximum 7000 U.
UFH = unfractionated heparin; PCI = percutaneous coronary intervention; ACT = activated clotting time.

4 GPIIb/IIIa antagonists, particularly as an adjunct to coronary angioplasty should be considered in high-risk patients.

Anticoagulant therapy

1 It is strongly recommended that patients hospitalized with unstable angina or non-ST segment elevation MI should, in addition to aspirin, receive iv unfractionated heparin therapy (60 U/kg iv bolus, initial maintenance 15–18 U/kg per hour, to a target aPTT of 50–70 seconds). The heparin infusion should be maintained for 3–4 days, or until the unstable pain pattern resolves.

2 A shorter duration of treatment may be acceptable if successful revascularization (coronary angioplasty, bypass grafting) is carried out.

3 The combined administration of full-dose unfractionated heparin and GPIIb/IIIa antagonists increases the risk of hemorrhagic complications; however, the benefit outweighs the risk.

4 LMWH (Lovenox® 1mg/kg sc bid) is an acceptable alternative to unfractionated heparin and may soon represent the standard of care.

5 The combined administration of platelet GPIIb/IIIa inhibitors and enoxaparin represents an attractive therapy. Large-scale clinical trials are in progress.

MYOCARDIAL INFARCTION

The use of antithrombotic therapy among patients sustaining MI is based on the established pathobiology, placing intracoronary thrombosis at the forefront. The risk of DVT, PE, and thromboembolic stroke (from left ventricular mural thrombi) in this setting also provides a strong rationale for antithrombotic strategies. Furthermore, the reperfusion era has provided new insights, stressing the importance of thrombin antagonists and platelet inhibitors to reduce coronary arterial reocclusion, recurrent ischemia, reinfarction, and death.

A review of approximately 30 reports on the topic of anticoagulant use in MI indicates that mortality may be reduced by approximately 25 per cent.[27–29] Several studies have also shown that thromboembolic events in high-risk patients (e.g. anterior Q-wave infarction) can be reduced significantly by early institution of anticoagulant therapy with heparin.[30,31]

Cardiac chamber thromboembolism

Left ventricular mural thrombosis is diagnosed either echocardiographically or at the time of the autopsy among patients with MI[32,33] especially in those with anterior infarction involving the ventricular apex.[34–36] In large

clinical trials of anticoagulant therapy, researchers have reported an incidence of cerebral embolism of 2–4 per cent among control patients, frequently causing either severe neurologic deficits or death. Of these trials, two showed a statistically significant reduction in stroke with early anticoagulation, whereas the third trial demonstrated a positive trend.

A meta-analysis performed by Vaitkus and Barnathan[37] supports the findings of three previous studies published in the early 1980s. The odds ratio for systemic embolism in the presence of echocardiographically demonstrated mural thrombus was 5.45 (95 per cent confidence interval (CI) 3.02–9.83). The odds ratio of anticoagulation versus no anticoagulation in preventing embolism was 0.14 (95 per cent CI 0.04–0.52) with an event rate difference of −0.33 (95 per cent CI −0.50 to −0.16). The odds ratio of anticoagulation versus control in preventing mural thrombus formation was 0.32 (95 per cent CI 0.20–0.52) and the event rate difference was −0.19 (95 per cent CI −0.09 to −0.28). A more recent analysis of patients participating in the SAVE (Survival and Ventricular Enlargement)[38] trial suggests that ventricular dysfunction (ejection fraction <35 per cent) increases the likelihood of thromboembolic stroke significantly, with increasing risk as ventricular performance worsens (Fig. 17.4).

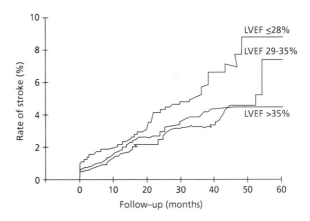

Figure 17.4 *The occurrence of thromboembolic stroke among patients with myocardial infarction according to left ventricular ejection fraction (LVEF). An LVEF below 35 per cent was associated with an increased risk of stroke that persisted over time. (Reproduced with permission from Loh E, et al. Ventricular dysfunction and the risk of stroke after myocardial infarction. N Engl J Med 1997; **336**: 251–7, © 1997 Massachusetts Medical Society. All rights reserved.)*

The available data support the following 4 conclusions:

• Mural thrombosis following acute MI increases the risk of systemic embolism.
• The likelihood of cardioembolic events correlates inversely with left ventricular systolic performance.

- Anticoagulation can reduce mural thrombus formation.
- The risk of systemic embolism can be substantially reduced by anticoagulation.

Heparin therapy

1 It is strongly recommended that every patient with MI receive *not less* than low-dose heparin therapy (7500 U sc every 12 hours) until fully ambulatory unless there is a specific contraindication.
2 It is strongly recommended that patients at increased risk of systemic or pulmonary embolism because of anterior Q-wave infarction, severe left ventricular dysfunction, congestive heart failure (CHF), history of systemic or pulmonary embolism, two-dimensional echocardiographic evidence of mural thrombosis, or atrial fibrillation (AF) receive therapeutic dose heparin (60 U/kg bolus iv, initial maintenance 15–18 U/kg per hour, to a target aPTT of 50–70 seconds), followed by warfarin (target INR 3.0; range 2.5–3.5) for up to 3 months. Warfarin therapy should be maintained long term for chronic AF.
3 The benefit of long-term therapy (>3 months) in patients with MI and a reduced ejection fraction (<35 per cent) is unknown but continued treatment is supported by analyses of non-randomized studies including patients with MI and reduced left ventricular systolic performance.

Antiplatelet therapy

1 It is strongly recommended that all patients with MI receive non-enteric coated aspirin, 160–325 mg, to chew and swallow as soon as possible after clinical impression of evolving MI is formed (whether or not fibrinolytic therapy is to be given). The dose should be repeated daily for an indefinite period (the enteric-coated form may result in fewer gastric side effects with long-term therapy). If the patient is to receive heparin, aspirin should be given conjointly. However, if warfarin therapy is commenced, aspirin therapy should be discontinued (or the dose reduced to 80 mg daily) until the planned course of warfarin is complete. Aspirin can then be restarted (or increased) and maintained indefinitely.
2 Aspirin is recommended for long-term therapy in preference to warfarin because of its simplicity, safety, and low cost. Long-term warfarin therapy is recommended in clinical settings of increased embolic risk (duration 1–3 months following MI or MI complicated by severe left ventricular dysfunction (EF<35 per cent), CHF, previous emboli, or two-dimensional echocardiographic evidence or mural thrombosis. The duration may be indefinite with persistent AF. Patients who have contraindications to aspirin should be considered for long-term therapy with either clopidogrel (75 mg qd) or warfarin (target INR 3.00; range 2.5–3.5) for at least 1–2 years following MI (Fig. 17.5). Because the risk of recurrent events persists, preventive therapy may be required for an indefinite period of time.
3 The combination of aspirin and low-intensity warfarin anticoagulation (INR ≤1.5) does not offer benefit over aspirin alone. The potential benefit of aspirin combined with warfarin given in doses capable of elevating the INR above 1.5 or 2.0 looks promising; however, the risk of hemorrhage is a major limitation.

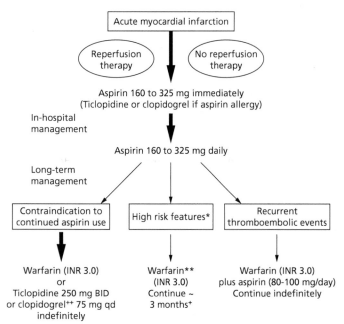

Figure 17.5 *Approach to antithrombotic therapy management in acute myocardial infarction. *Anterior Q-wave infarction, severe left ventricular dysfunction, congestive heart failure, history of systemic or pulmonary embolism, echocardiographic mural thrombosis, and atrial fibrillation. **The aspirin dose should be reduced to 80–160 mg with the initiation of warfarin. ⁺A more prolonged course of treatment may be beneficial and should be considered if one or more high-risk features persist, particularly an ejection fraction <35 per cent. ⁺⁺Clopidogrel may be preferred over ticlopidine for long-term therapy. INR = international normalized ratio.*

4 The long-term benefit of oral GPIIb/IIIa antagonists is unknown and will require further investigation. The findings to date have not been encouraging.

ANTITHROMBOTIC THERAPY: CORONARY FIBRINOLYSIS

The importance of plaque rupture and intraluminal thrombosis was discussed earlier in this chapter. Although fibrinolytic therapy is a mainstay of treatment for patients with ST segment elevation MI (or new bundle branch block), several limitations have been recognized: (1) patency is achieved in only 80–85 per cent of patients; (2) complete perfusion (TIMI grade 3 flow) is achieved in only 50 per cent of patients; and (3) reocclusion occurs in nearly 10 percent of patients within the first 3–4 days of treatment. Anatomically, the post-thrombolytic coronary artery consists of the following components: (1) ruptured/fissured atheromatous plaque; (2) retained mural and intraluminal thrombus; and (3) residual luminal narrowing. Each predisposes to thrombosis and recurrent ischemic events.

While fibrinolytic therapy effectively lyses intracoronary thrombus in a majority of patients, dissolution is rarely complete. In fact, incomplete lysis is the rule rather than the exception. As a result, it is common to have residual thrombus at the original site of plaque rupture.[39–42] There is mounting evidence that the thrombolytic process itself may predispose to thrombus formation. Clot lysis, in essence, re-exposes the original thrombogenic substrate to circulating blood.[43,44] Furthermore, thrombin is released during lysis, stimulating platelets and the coagulation cascade. Factor X may also be activated on the thrombus surface, contributing directly to continued thrombus growth. Beyond the ability to activate and/or release thrombin, fibrinolytic therapy, through the production of plasmin, can directly activate platelets and the intrinsic coagulation cascade. Reperfusion injury of the vascular endothelium and the presence of circulating procoagulant factors may also provoke recurrent cardiac events.

Several recently completed clinical trials have shown that intravenous heparin, dosed sufficiently to elevate the aPTT to at least 1.5 times control, can reduce the incidence of coronary reocclusion among patients given tissue plasminogen activator (tPA). Pooled analyses suggest that mortality may also be reduced, and the findings of GUSTO-I (Global Utilization of Streptokinase and tPA for Occluded Coronary Arteries) strongly support the adjunctive use of intravenous heparin with accelerated tPA and aspirin.[45] The importance of heparin as an adjunct to fibrinolysis with newer tPA molecules (rPA (reteplase), TNK-tPA (tenecteplase)) is unknown; the available evidence suggests that reduced heparin doses (60 U/kg bolus (max. 4000 U); 12 U/kg per hour (max.

1000 U/hour)) may suffice. A reduced requirement for heparin with third-generation fibrinolytics derived from wild-type tPA may be due to increased fibrin specificity (this pertains predominantly to TNK-tPA) and lower concentrations of circulating plasmin. The requirement for heparin may be even less when low-dose fibrinolytics are combined with platelet GPIIb/IIIa antagonists. The target aPTT is 50–70 seconds.

The benefit of adjunctive heparin use among patients treated with streptokinase has been difficult to establish. The available data weigh in favor of heparin administration, although the benefits appear modest. Anticipating that a therapeutic level of anticoagulation must be achieved and maintained to observe benefit, intravenous heparin is the preferred route of administration. In GUSTO-I, intravenous heparin given for at least the initial 48 hours was not associated with an excess of transfusions, major hemorrhagic events, or intracerebral hemorrhage.[21] Pooled data from the GISSI-2/ International Study, the International Study of Infarct Survival (ISIS-3), and GUSTO support adjunctive heparin to reduce in-hospital reinfarction and early mortality. More substantial benefits can be expected in select high-risk groups, including patients with previous MI or large anterior Q-wave infarctions and insulin-requiring diabetics.[46,47]

Little information is available concerning heparin use among patients treated with APSAC (anisoylated plasminogen streptokinase activator complex). As with streptokinase, the benefits are probably modest,[48] and most likely to be manifest in high-risk patients.

In the setting of MI, antiplatelet therapy, primarily with aspirin, has been shown to reduce vascular mortality by one-fourth.[49] In ISIS-2, a 50 per cent reduction in mortality was observed when aspirin, given immediately on hospital presentation, was combined with a fibrinolytic. Recurrent infarction and stroke was also reduced with aspirin administration. Long-term antiplatelet therapy has been (strongly) advocated based on the pooled results of clinical trials[50] (Fig. 17.6).

Anticoagulation therapy as an adjunct to coronary fibrinolysis

1 It is recommended that all patients given tPA (or one of its related derivatives) should also receive unfractionated heparin according to the following regimen:
- 60 U/kg iv bolus (max. 4000 U) at initiation of the tPA infusion, initial maintenance dose 12 U/kg per hour (max. 1000 U/hour), to a target aPTT of 50–70 seconds, maintained for 48 hours.
- Heparin therapy beyond 48 hours should be undertaken *only* in the presence of risk factors for either systemic or venous thromboembolism (anterior MI, CHF, previous emboli, atrial

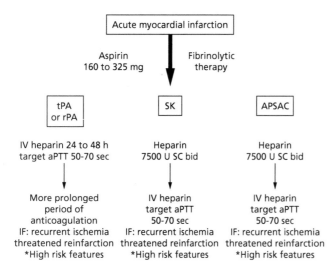

Figure 17.6 *Approach to antithrombotic therapy management in patients with acute myocardial infarction receiving thrombolytic therapy. *High risk for thromboembolism: prior thromboembolism, anterior site of infarction, clinical congestive heart failure, ejection fraction <35 per cent. tPA = tissue plasminogen activator; rPA = recombinant plasminogen activator; SK = streptokinase; APSAC = anisoylated plasminogen streptokinase activator complex; aPTT = activated partial thromboplastin time.*

fibrillation). In high-risk settings the regimen should be sustained or consideration given to subcutaneous administration (initial dose approximately 17 500 U every 12 hours to maintain the aPTT at 1.5–2.0 times control), or conversion to warfarin therapy (target INR 3.0; range 2.5–3.5).

2 It is recommended that patients treated with streptokinase or APSAC receive iv heparin *only* in the presence of high-risk features for systemic or venous thromboembolism (as listed earlier). If given, the following regimen should be followed:

- Measure the aPTT when the indication emerges but not less than 6 hours after beginning the streptokinase or APSAC infusion. If greater than two times control, repeat the aPTT in 2–3 hours. Initiate the heparin infusion when the aPTT is less than two times control. A full heparin bolus may not be required.
- Maintain the aPTT between 50 and 70 seconds as long as the risk of thromboembolism is considered high.
- After 48 hours, consideration may be given to subcutaneous administration (initial dose approximately 17 500 U every 12 hours to maintain the aPTT at 50–70 seconds), or conversion to warfarin therapy.

3 DVT prophylaxis with sc heparin (7500 U bid) is recommended for patients *not* given intravenous heparin.

4 The adjunctive use of LMWH is under investigation.

Percutaneous coronary interventions

1 Pretreatment with aspirin (325 mg) at least 2 hours before coronary angioplasty is recommended to reduce the incidence of early complications.

2 Dipyridamole should *not* be routinely used in patients undergoing coronary angioplasty.

3 Long-term treatment with aspirin (160–325 mg daily) is recommended as secondary prevention against cardiovascular events.

4 For patients who cannot tolerate aspirin, treatment with ticlopidine, 250 mg twice daily or clopidogrel 75 mg qd, is reasonable. It should be started at least 48 hours before elective coronary angioplasty.

5 A bolus and infusion (0.25 mg/kg iv bolus, followed by 10 µg/min for 12 hours) of the GPIIb/IIIa receptor inhibitor abciximab (ReoPro®), or an alternative agent such as tirofiban (Aggrastat®) or eptifibatide (Integrilin®) should be considered in patients at high risk for ischemic complications after coronary angioplasty, particularly those with acute MI, post-MI angina or 'refractory' unstable angina. Abciximab may be the preferred agent in patients with acute coronary syndromes.

6 In high-risk patients given a bolus and an infusion of abciximab, weight-adjusted heparin (70 U/kg iv bolus; max. 7000 U) should be given at the time of intervention.

7 Heparin bolus (70 U/kg; max. 7000 U) should be given prior to coronary angioplasty: additional boluses (20 U/kg) should be administered in dosages sufficient to maintain the activated clotting time (ACT) at 250–300 seconds or more (HemoTec®), and 300–350 seconds or more (if a Hemachron® device is used). Low-dose heparin (to a target ACT of 200–250 seconds) is probably adequate for patients receiving intravenous GPIIb/IIIa antagonists.

8 The use of postprocedural heparin in patients undergoing uncomplicated coronary angioplasty is *not* routinely recommended.

9 The combined administration of LMWH and iv GPIIb/IIIa antagonists is under investigation.

Coronary stents

1 Aspirin (at least 325 mg) should be administered more than 2 hours prior to stent placement. Thereafter, a dose of 160–325 mg/day should be continued indefinitely.
2 Dipyridamole is no longer recommended in patients undergoing stent placement.
3 Dextran 40 appears to provide no incremental benefit over aspirin; therefore, it is not routinely used.
4 Intraprocedural heparin therapy should be given during stent deployment. Heparin can be given using either a non-weight-adjusted or weight-adjusted protocol similar to those used in balloon angioplasty. The latter is preferred.
5 Warfarin (target INR 2.0–2.5) does *not* offer a benefit to antiplatelet therapy even in high-risk patients.
6 The combination of aspirin (325 mg) and ticlopidine (250 mg bid) or clopidogrel (75 mg qd) is the standard of care for patients undergoing coronary stent placement. Ticlopidine or clopidogrel should be continued for the first 30 days.
7 The benefit of long-term treatment with clopidogrel is under investigation.
8 Emerging evidence supports the use of iv GPIIb/IIIa antagonists in patients undergoing coronary stenting.

ATRIAL FIBRILLATION

It is strongly recommended that long-term anticoagulation with warfarin (INR 2.0–3.0) be offered to patients with chronic valvular or non-valvular atrial fibrillation. Patients younger than 65 years *without* organic heart disease (lone atrial fibrillation) do not require anticoagulation. The role of aspirin therapy has not been determined fully; however, it is possible that patients with atrial fibrillation without systemic hypertension (systolic blood pressure <160 mm Hg), left ventricular dysfunction (ejection fraction <40 per cent), clinical congestive heart failure, or previous thromboembolism can be treated with aspirin, 325 mg daily. The combination of moderate intensity warfarin and aspirin is not superior to standard-dose warfarin in high-risk patient groups.[51]

Anticoagulation is not routinely recommended for atrial fibrillation of brief duration (<48 hours) unless there are other features associated with a high risk of thromboembolism (cardiomyopathy, severe left ventricular dysfunction, significant valvular heart disease, or previous thromboembolism). If the duration of atrial fibrillation is unknown, anticoagulation should be instituted unless contraindications exist.

Hospitalized patients with confirmed or suspected atrial fibrillation greater than 48 hours in duration should be anticoagulated with heparin given intravenously to maintain the aPTT between 1.5 and 2.0 times control. If elective chemical or electrical cardioversion is planned, anticoagulation with heparin or warfarin should be continued for 2–3 weeks prior to and 4 weeks after establishing normal sinus rhythm. Anticoagulation with heparin is also recommended for emergency cardioversion, when feasible, if the duration of atrial fibrillation is unknown and additional thromboembolic risk factors are present.

Anticoagulation is *not* routinely recommended for patients with atrial flutter or other atrial tachyarrhythmias, unless they are considered to be at high risk for thromboembolism.

Transesophageal echocardiography

Cardiac causes of stroke (cardioembolism) account for approximately 1 in 5 strokes occurring in the USA. Although transthoracic echocardiography remains the cornerstone of noninvasive diagnostic imaging, transesophageal echocardiography (TEE) is superior for identifying potential sources of emboli, including left arterial and atrial appendage thrombi, valvular vegetations, ascending aortic plaques, and patent foramen ovale (paradoxical embolism).

Although data from large-scale clinical trials are needed to define the role of TEE in dictating specific management recommendations, its diagnostic capabilities remain vital in clinical practice. For example, in the setting of atrial fibrillation accompanied by stroke, atrial thrombi are utilized in nearly half of all patients. Information derived from TEE may influence management among patients with atrial fibrillation (or flutter) scheduled for cardioversion (Fig. 17.7).

Atrial fibrillation

1 It is recommended that long-term warfarin therapy (target INR 2.5; range 2.0–3.0) be considered strongly for all patients older than 65 with AF, and for patients younger than 65 with one or more of the following risk factors: previous transient ischemic attack (TIA) or stroke, systemic hypertension, heart failure, diabetes mellitus, clinical coronary artery disease, mitral stenosis, prosthetic heart valve, or thyrotoxicosis.
2 Patients at low risk and who decline anticoagulants or are considered poor candidates for anticoagulant therapy should be given aspirin 325 mg/day.
3 It is strongly recommended that warfarin (target INR 2.5; range 2.0–3.0) be given for 3 weeks before elective cardioversion of patients who have been in AF for more than 48 hours. Anticoagulants should be continued until normal sinus rhythm has been maintained for at least 4 weeks.

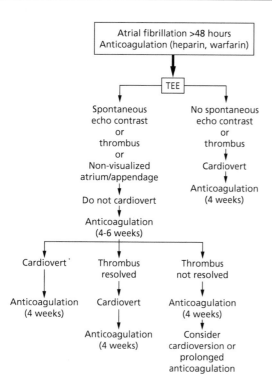

Figure 17.7 *Transesophageal echocardiography (TEE) can be used in the elective management of patients with atrial fibrillation (AF). Clinical trials are being conducted to better define the benefits and clinical indications for this technology. INR = international normalized ratio.*

4 Antithrombotic therapy is not recommended for cardioversion of supraventricular tachycardia or AF of less than 48 hours duration.

5 Consideration should be given to managing atrial flutter in a manner similar to atrial fibrillation, particularly when elective cardioversion is planned or when there is concomitant organic heart disease.

MECHANICAL HEART VALVES

Patients with mechanical heart valves, including Bjork–Shiley, St Judes, Starr–Edwards, and Medtronic–Hall valves, in either the aortic or mitral position should receive long-term (lifelong) anticoagulation with warfarin titrated carefully to an INR of 2.5–3.5. Hemorrhagic complications increase with an INR greater than 4.5 and thromboembolic rates increase with an INR less than 1.8. In high-risk patients, dipyridamole (375–400 mg daily) or aspirin (80–100 mg daily) can be added without increased bleeding complications.[52–55] Higher doses of aspirin are *not* recommended because of the low likelihood of deriving additional benefit and the recognized risk of excessive hemorrhagic events.[56] It must be understood that aspirin or alternative antiplatelet ther-

apy alone does *not* provide adequate protection against thromboembolism.

Patients with mechanical prosthetic valves admitted to the intensive care unit should be anticoagulated with intravenous heparin titrated to an aPTT of 1.5–2.5 times control. Heparin is preferred over warfarin in most instances to allow better control of the state of anticoagulation (Fig. 17.8).

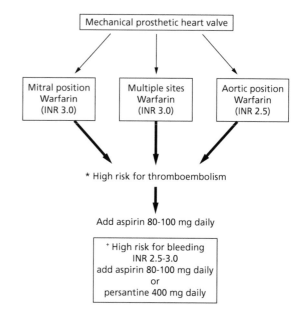

Figure 17.8 *Antithrombotic therapy management strategies for patients with mechanical prosthetic heart valves. *Patients at high risk for thromboembolism (atrial fibrillation, large left atrium (>55 mm), prior or recurrent thromboembolism, and poor left ventricular function) may benefit from more aggressive anticoagulation or the addition of aspirin (80–100 mg daily). ⁺Prior hemorrhagic events requirring hospitalization, surgical intervention, or blood product transfusion. INR = international normalized ratio.*

BIOPROSTHETIC HEART VALVES

Patients with bioprosthetic heart valves, including Hancock and Carpentier–Edwards valves, are less prone to thromboembolism than patients with mechanical prosthetic valves. Despite this recognized advantage, anticoagulation is recommended for at least the first 3 postoperative months. Heparin given intravenously can be used initially, followed by oral warfarin titrated to an INR of 2.0–3.0. Anticoagulation for longer periods may be required in patients at increased risk for thromboembolism (e.g. chronic atrial fibrillation, left ventricular dysfunction, previous thromboembolism)[57] (Fig. 17.9). Low-dose aspirin (162 mg qd) is recommended after the

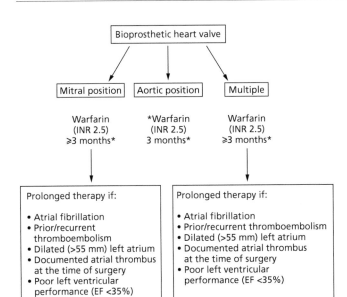

Figure 17.9 *Antithrombotic therapy management strategies for patients with bioprosthetic heart valves. *Aspirin (80 mg qd) is recommended after 3 months in patients at relatively low risk for thromboembolism.*

first 3 months in patients with sinus rhythm and no other risk factors.

PROSTHETIC HEART VALVES

Mechanical prosthetic heart valves

1 It is strongly recommended that all patients with mechanical prosthetic heart valves receive oral anticoagulation with warfarin.
2 Doses of oral anticoagulants that prolong the INR to a target of 2.5 (range 2.0–3.0) are recommended for patients with bileaflet or tilting-disk mechanical prosthetic heart valves. A higher INR (target 3.0) is recommended for patients with caged-ball or caged-disk valves.
3 Patients with tilting-disk or bileaflet mechanical valves in the mitral position and bileaflet aortic valves with AF should receive oral anticoagulants to a target INR of 3.0 (range 2.5–3.5).
4 Patients with caged-ball, caged-disk and/or multiple site mechanical valves should receive oral anticoagulants to a target INR of 3.0 (range 2.5–3.5) and aspirin (80–100 mg daily).
5 Aspirin (80–100 mg/day), in addition to oral anticoagulants, offers additional protection, but with an increased risk of bleeding.
6 Dipyridamole (400 mg/day), in addition to oral anticoagulants, may be considered for additional protection against thromboembolism. In view of the advantageous effects of low-dose aspirin therapy in combination with oral anticoagulants, the indications for dipyridamole are limited.

7 Patients with mechanical prosthetic heart valves who suffer systemic embolism despite adequate therapy with oral anticoagulants should receive aspirin (80–100 mg/day) in addition to oral anticoagulants. Dipyridamole, 400 mg/day, in addition to oral anticoagulation is an alternative.

Bioprosthetic heart valves

1 It is recommended that all patients with bioprosthetic valves in the mitral position be treated for the first 3 months after valve insertion with oral anticoagulatants to an INR of 2.5 (range 2.0–3.0).
2 Anticoagulant therapy in patients with bioprosthetic valves in the aortic position is also recommended for the first 3 months.
3 Patients with bioprosthetic valves (regardless of position) who have atrial fibrillation should be treated with long-term oral anticoagulant therapy in doses sufficient to prolong the INR to a level of 2.5 (range 2.0–3.0).
4 Patients with bioprosthetic valves (regardless of position) who are found to have left atrial thrombus at the time of surgery, should receive long-term oral anticoagulant therapy to a target INR of 2.5 (range 2.0–3.0).
5 Patients with bioprosthetic valves who have a permanent pacemaker are at increased risk for thromboembolism; however, there is *no* evidence that oral anticoagulant therapy is protective (beyond the benefits outlined above).
6 It is recommended that patients with bioprosthetic heart valves who have a history of systemic embolism receive long-term oral anticoagulant therapy (target

INR 2.5) for at least 6–12 months and possibly longer.

7 Among patients with bioprosthetic valves who are in sinus rhythm, long-term therapy with aspirin, 325 mg/day, may offer protection against thromboembolism and is considered optional.

VALVULAR HEART DISEASE

Rheumatic mitral valve disease

1 It is strongly recommended that long-term warfarin therapy sufficient to prolong the INR to a target of 2.5 (range 2.0–3.0) be used in patients with rheumatic mitral valve disease who have either a history of systemic embolism or who have paroxysmal or chronic atrial fibrillation.
2 It is recommended that long-term warfarin therapy (INR 2.5) be considered in patients with rheumatic mitral valve disease and normal sinus rhythm if the left atrial diameter is in excess of 55 mm.
3 It is recommended that, if recurrent systemic embolism occurs despite adequate warfarin therapy, the addition of aspirin (80–100 mg/day) be considered. For patients unable to take aspirin, add dipyridamole 400 mg/day, or clopidogrel 75 mg daily.

Aortic valve disease

It is strongly recommended that long-term antithrombotic therapy *not* be given to patients with aortic valve disease unless they also have concomitant mitral valve disease, AF, or a history of systemic embolism (Fig. 17.10).

Mitral valve prolapse

1 It is strongly recommended that long-term antithrombotic therapy *not* be given to patients with mitral valve prolapse (MVP) who have not experienced systemic embolism, unexplained TIAs or AF.
2 It is recommended that patients with MVP who have documented but unexplained TIAs be treated with long-term low-dose aspirin therapy (160–325 mg/day).
3 It is recommended that patients with MVP who have (1) documented systemic embolism, (2) chronic or paroxysmal AF, or (3) recurrent TIAs despite aspirin therapy be treated with long-term warfarin therapy (INR 2.5).

Mitral annular calcification

1 It is recommended that long-term antithrombotic therapy should *not* be given to patients with mitral annular calcification (MAC) who lack a history of thromboembolism or AF.
2 It is recommended that patients with MAC complicated by (1) systemic embolism or (2) AF should be treated with long-term warfarin therapy (INR 2.5).

Patent foramen ovale and atrial septal aneurysm

1 It is strongly recommended that anticoagulant therapy should *not* be given to patients with either asymptomatic patent foramen ovale (PFO) or atrial septal aneurysm.
2 It is strongly recommended that patients with unexplained systemic embolism or TIAs *and* demonstrable venous thrombosis or pulmonary embolism, *and* either a PFO or atrial septal aneurysm should be treated with long-term warfarin therapy (unless venous interruption or closure of the PFO is considered preferable). In the case of an atrial septal aneurysm, the possibility of both paradoxical embolism and systemic embolism from the arterial side of the aneurysm should be considered in choosing therapy (Fig. 17.11).

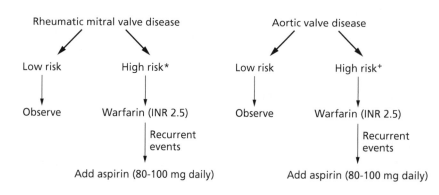

Figure 17.10 *Antithrombotic therapy management strategies for patients with native mitral and aortic valvular heart disease. *Atrial fibrillation, dilated left atrium (>55 mm), prior thromboembolism. +Concomitant mitral valve disease, atrial fibrillation, prior thromboembolism. INR = international normalized ratio.*

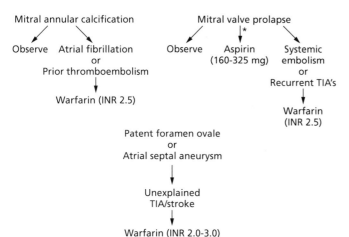

Figure 17.11 *Antithrombotic therapy management strategies for patients with native valvular and atrial septal anomalies. *For unexplained TIAs. TIA = transient ischemic attack; INR = international normalized ratio.*

Infective endocarditis

1 It is strongly recommended that anticoagulant therapy should *not* be given to patients in normal sinus rhythm with uncomplicated infective endocarditis involving a native valve or a bioprosthetic valve.

2 It is recommended that long-term warfarin therapy should be continued when endocarditis occurs in patients with a mechanical prosthetic valve unless there are specific contraindications.

3 The indications for anticoagulant therapy when systemic embolism occurs during the course of infective endocarditis involving either a native or bioprosthetic heart valve are uncertain. The decision should consider co-morbid conditions, including AF, evidence of left atrial thrombus, evidence and size of valvular vegetations, and particularly the success of antibiotic therapy in controlling the infective process.

Non-bacterial thrombotic endocarditis

1 Patients with non-bacterial thrombotic endocarditis (NBTE) and systemic or pulmonary embolism should be treated with heparin.

2 It is recommended that heparin therapy should be considered for patients with disseminated cancer or debilitating disease who are found to have aseptic vegetations on echocardiographic study.

PERIPHERAL VASCULAR DISEASE

The following recommendations are outlined for patients with peripheral vascular disease.

1 Patients who experience arterial thrombi or emboli may benefit from heparin therapy if revascularization is delayed to prevent proximal and distal thrombotic propagation. Heparin therapy followed by oral anticoagulation therapy should be used to prevent recurrent embolism in patients undergoing thromboembolectomy.

2 Selective or intra-arterial fibrinolytic therapy may be considered in patients with acute occlusive disease, provided there is a low risk of myonecrosis developing during the time to achieve revascularization by this method.

3 It is uncertain whether aspirin alone or aspirin combined with dipyridamole will modify the natural history or clinical manifestations of peripheral vascular insufficiency due to arteriosclerosis. However, because these patients are at high risk of future cardiovascular events (stroke and myocardial infarction), they should be given lifelong aspirin therapy (160–325 mg/day) in the absence of contraindications. Clopidogrel (75 mg qd) may offer added benefit in patients with a prior MI.

4 It is recommended that antithrombotic therapy should *not* be used to maintain patency of vascular reconstructions involving high-flow, low-resistance arteries greater than 6 mm in diameter.

5 Aspirin (325 mg/day) may be useful in patients undergoing prosthetic, femoropopliteal bypass operations. Antiplatelet therapy should be initiated preoperatively.

6 In patients undergoing saphenous vein femoropopliteal bypass, aspirin therapy (160–325 mg/day) is recommended to reduce the incidence of myocardial infarction and stroke.

7 Dextran 40 may also be beneficial in the prevention of postoperative thrombosis following lower-extremity vascular reconstructions. However, it should *not* be used routinely because of the serious side effects and cost of dextran therapy.

8 Long-term oral anticoagulation with warfarin (with or without aspirin) is *not* recommended as routine therapy in patients after femoropopliteal bypass and other vascular reconstructions.

CEREBROVASCULAR DISEASE

Guidelines for the treatment of a variety of cerebrovascular conditions are listed below.

Cervical bruits and asymptomatic carotid stenosis

The recommendations for treatment of patients with asymptomatic cervical bruits include control or elimination of vascular risk factors, such as hypertension, smoking, and hyperlipidemia, along with education about the symptoms of TIA and stroke. In addition, patients with an asymptomatic bruit should be given aspirin (325 mg/day) if tolerated. Carotid endarterectomy may be beneficial in patients with asymptomatic bruits in the presence of a stenosis >70 per cent.

Symptomatic carotid stenosis

Symptomatic patients found to have a cervical carotid artery stenosis greater than 70 per cent should be considered as candidates for carotid endarterectomy. The role of carotid endarterectomy in patients with TIA with carotid stenosis in the range of 30–69 per cent is still under investigation.

TIAs and minor ischemic strokes

It is strongly recommended that patients with TIAs be treated initially with aspirin. Aspirin has been established as effective in doses ranging from 75 to 1300 mg/day. While many experts recommend 325 mg/day of aspirin, other authorities believe that the higher doses (975–1300 mg/day) may confer greater benefit. Ticlopidine is more effective than aspirin, but adverse events, including bone marrow suppression and thrombotic thrombocytopenic purpura have been reported with prolonged use. Ticlopidine is also recommended for patients who cannot tolerate aspirin or for patients who experience recurrent ischemic events during aspirin therapy.

Progressive ischemic strokes

Heparin anticoagulation for 3–5 days is reasonable in the setting of progressive ischemic strokes, especially those involving the vertebrobasilar circulation.

Completed thrombotic strokes

Anticoagulant agents are either of no value or harmful to patients with completed strokes. Until more information is available about the toxicity of ticlopidine in general clinical practice, aspirin is recommended; ticlopidine or clopidogrel should be considered for patients who cannot tolerate aspirin or those who develop ischemic symptoms during aspirin therapy.

Acute cardioembolic stroke

It is recommended that heparin administration followed by warfarin therapy, at a dose that prolongs the INR to a target of 2.5 (range 2.0–3.0), be instituted in non-hypertensive patients with small to moderate-sized embolic strokes in whom a computed tomographic (CT) scan obtained 48 hours or more after stroke onset does not reveal spontaneous hemorrhagic transformation.

Anticoagulant therapy should be delayed for 5–14 days in patients with large embolic strokes or uncontrolled hypertension because of the predisposition of these patients to hemorrhagic transformation.

Aortic arch disorders

Patients with cardioembolic events and either mobile aortic athenomas or plaques >4 mm (measured by transesophogeal echocardiography) should receive warfarin (target INR 2.5; range 2.0–3.0).

ANTICOAGULATION BEFORE AND AFTER ELECTIVE SURGERY

Patients requiring warfarin therapy for venous or arterial thromboembolism create a challenge in management when elective surgical procedures are planned. The approach to decision-making is based on the clinicians' ability to determine the risk of thromboembolism on the one hand and hemorrhagic risk on the other. The most common clinical scenarios encountered in daily practice that dictate a need for anticoagulant therapy include atrial fibrillation, venous thromboembolism (DVT, PE), arterial thromboembolism and the presence of a mechanical heart valve.[58]

After warfarin is discontinued, it usually takes between 3 and 4 days for the INR to drop below 1.5 (considered safe for most surgical procedures). After warfarin is restarted, it takes approximately 3 days to reach an INR of 2.0. Thus, the practice of holding warfarin for 4 days before surgery and restarting either the evening of or day after the surgery is associated with a subtherapeutic INR for approximately 2 days.

The estimated rates of thromboembolism associated with acute DVT/PE, recurrent venous thromboembolism, non-valvular atrial fibrillation (with or without prior embolism), mechanical heart valves, and acute arterial embolism are summarized in Table 17.9.

In the setting of acute venous or arterial embolism,

Table 17.9 *Estimated rates of thromboembolism associated with various indications for oral anticoagulation, and the reduction in risk due to anticoagulant therapy. (Reproduced with permission from Kearon C, Hirsh J. Current concepts: management of anticoagulation before and after elective surgery. N Engl J Med 1997; **336**: 1506–11, © 1997 Massachusetts Medical Socity. All rights reserved)*

Indication	Rate without therapy (%)	Risk reduction with therapy (%)
Acute venous thromboembolism		
Month 1	40	80
Month 2 and 3	10	80
Recurrent venous thromboembolism	15	80
Non-valvular atrial fibrillation	5	66
Non-valvular atrial fibrillation and previous embolism	12	66
Mechanical heart valve	8	75
Acute arterial embolism		
Month 1	15	66

the risk of recurrent events is greatest during the first month. Accordingly, patients undergoing surgical procedures should be protected with heparin (intravenous unfractionated or low molecular weight), to be started when the INR drops below 2.0. Typically heparin is discontinued 4–6 hours prior to surgery. In the case of LMWH, the last dose should be given 8–12 hours prior to surgery. Heparin is restarted postoperatively (usually without a bolus) when hemostasis has been achieved and continued until the INR exceeds 2.0 on 2 consecutive days. In the second and third months after venous thromboembolism, preoperative heparin is usually not required; however, it should be used postoperatively given the marked increase in risk of venous thrombosis in the postoperative setting. The risk of embolism in most patients with mechanical heart valves and atrial fibrillation is sufficiently low that routine preoperative heparin administration is not recommended. Venous thromboembolism prophylaxis should be offered and warfarin should be restarted when hemostasis has been achieved.

A recommended approach to anticoagulation prior to and after elective surgery is outlined in Table 17.10. Patients with acute venous or arterial thrombosis in whom surgery must take place within 2 weeks should be considered for IVC filter placement. A similar approach should be taken for patients at high risk for both thrombosis and bleeding.

ANTICOAGULATION IN PATIENTS WITH SUSPECTED HEPARIN-INDUCED THROMBOCYTOPENIA

The diagnosis of immune-mediated heparin-induced thrombocytopenia (HIT) should be suspected in a patient receiving heparin for the first time in whom a greater than 30 per cent reduction in platelet count occurs ≥5 days from the initiation of therapy. Patients exposed to heparin previously may develop thrombocytopenia within hours to days of exposure. The diagnosis of HIT could be confirmed by specific and sensitive tests. The ELISA test appears to have advantages over platelet-based assays.[59] Once the diagnosis of HIT has been confirmed or the suspicion is high in patients requiring anticoagulation, an alternative therapy should be chosen. Cross-reactivity of existing antibodies with LMWH preparations is common (approximately 60–70 per cent) and therefore should not be used. Danaparoid sodium (Orgaran®), a heparinoid comprised of a mixture of low-molecular-weight glycosaminoglycans has been

Table 17.10 *Recommendations for preoperative and postoperative anticoagulation in patients who are taking oral anticoagulants. (Reproduced with permission from Kearon C, Hirsh J. Current concepts: management of anticoagulation before and after elective surgery. N Engl J Med 1997; **336**: 1506–11, © 1997 Massachusetts Medical Society. All rights reserved)*

Indication	Before surgery	After surgery
Acute venous thromboembolism		
Month 1	iv heparin	iv heparin
Month 2 and 3	No change	iv heparin
Recurrent venous thromboembolism	No change	sc heparin
Acute arterial embolism		
Month 1	iv heparin	iv heparin
Mechanical heart valve	No change	sc heparin
Non-valvular atrial fibrillation	No change	sc heparin

used in patients with HIT who require anticoagulation. The recommended dose for full anticoagulation is 2500 U by iv bolus (1250 U if <55 kg; 3750 U if >90 kg body weight) followed by 400 U/h for 4 hours, then 300 U/h for 4 hours, followed by 150–200 U/h to maintain anti-Xa levels of 0.5–0.8 U/ml. There is a cross-reactivity rate of approximately 10 per cent; therefore, a negative *in vitro* platelet aggregation test in response to danaparoid should be considered prior to its use. The direct thrombin antagonist, argatroban (Novastan®), can also be used for anticoagulation in patients with HIT at a dose is 2–10 μg/kg per minute to maintain the aPTT 1.5–2.0 times control.[60] Hirudin is considered in many parts of the world to be the drug of choice for HIT.

QUICK REFERENCE

Therapeutic agents

Warfarin (Tables 17.11–17.13):
- oral anticoagulant, rapidly absorbed from gastrointestinal tract
- half-life 36–42 hours
- inhibits vitamin K-dependent coagulation Factors (II, VII, IX, X).

Unfractionated heparin (UH):
- parenteral anticoagulant (intravenous or subcutaneous administration);
- accelerates inhibitory interaction between antithrombin and coagulation proteins (especially thrombin and Factor Xa).

Fractionated heparin:
- prepared by depolymerization of unfractionated heparin;
- parenteral anticoagulant (iv or sc administration);
- low molecular weight (<4500 Da);
- more predictable bioavailability than UH;
- half-life 2–4 times greater than UH;
- inhibits Factor Xa > IIa.

Aspirin:
- oral antiplatelet agent, inhibits platelet aggregation;
- irreversibly inhibits platelet cyclooxygenase and vascular prostacyclin.

Table 17.11 *Initiation of oral anticoagulation with warfarin*

The dosing of warfarin must be individualized according to the patient's responsiveness to the drug as indicated by the international normalized ratio (INR). Use of a large loading dose may increase the incidence of hemorrhagic and other complications, does not offer more rapid protection against thrombus formation, and is *not* recommended. Low initiation doses are recommended for elderly and/or debilitated patients, and patients with potential for increased sensitivity (responsiveness) to warfarin (see drug interactions with warfarin).

Day 1: Obtain baseline INR.
Begin therapy with warfarin at a dose of 5 mg/day[a] with dosage adjustments based on the results of INR determinations.

For patients on heparin: Because the anticoagulant effect of warfarin is commonly delayed, heparin is administered for rapid anticoagulation. When clinically indicated, conversion to warfarin can begin concomitantly with initiation of heparin therapy. After an overlap of 3–5 days, heparin may be discontinued when a therapeutic INR is achieved.

Day 2: Check INR daily. Adjust warfarin dose based on the results of INR determinations.

Patients stabilized in the therapeutic range: Intervals between subsequent INR determinations should be based upon the clinician's judgement of the patient's reliability, concomitant medications, and response to warfarin to maintain the individual within the therapeutic range. Acceptable intervals for INR determinations are normally 1–4 weeks after a stable dosage has been determined. Most patients are satisfactorily maintained on warfarin at a dose of 2–10 mg daily.

Monitoring – the INR
Because prothrombin time (PT) results are dependent on the thromboplastin reagent used, a system of standardizing the PT in oral anticoagulant therapy was introduced in the World Health Organization in 1983. It is based upon calculation of an INR, which is equivalent to the PT ratio obtained if a sensitive reference thromboplastin is used.

- Thromboplastin sensitivity is determined by the manufacturer and is expressed as an international sensitivity index (ISI).
- The INR can be calculated as: INR = (Observed PT ratio)^{ISI}
- The calculation of the INR from the PT ratio is usually performed in the laboratory.

Reminder
- Be aware of potential drug interactions and other factors that may affect the INR.
- Patient education is an important part of therapy. Effective therapeutic levels with minimal complications are in part dependent upon cooperative and well-instructed patients who communicate effectively with their health care team.

---

[a]Some patients may require a lower initiating dose.

Table 17.12 *Factors that, alone or in combination, may be responsible for increased INR response (potentiate effect of warfarin)*

Exogenous factors
Acetaminophen
Alcohol
Allopurinol
Aminosalicylic acid
Amiodarone HCl
Anabolic sterioids
Anesthetics (inhalational)
Antibiotics
Chenodiol
Chloral hydrate
Chlorpropamide
Chymotrypsin
Cimetidine
Clofibrate
Dextran
Dextrothyroxine
Diazoxide
Diuretics
Disulfiram
Ethacrynic acid
Fluconazole
Fluoroquinolone antibiotics
Glucagon
Hepatotoxic drugs
Influenza virus vaccine
Lovastatin
Mefenamic acid
Methyldopa
Methylphenidate
Metronidazole
Monoamine oxidase inhibitors
Moricizine hydrochloride
Nalidixic acid
NSAIDs
Narcotics (prolonged)
Pentoxifylline
Phenylbutazone
Phenytoin
Propafenone
Pyrazolones
Quinidine
Quinine
Ranitidine
Salicylates
Sulfinpyrazone
Sulfonamides (long acting)
Simvastatin
Tamoxifen
Thyroid drugs
Tolbutamide
Trimethoprim/sulfamethoxazole
Vitamin E
Warfarin overdosage

Also other medications affecting blood elements that may modify hemostatis, dietary deficiencies, prolonged hot weather, unreliable PT determinations, and increased and decreased INR responses have been reported.

INR = international normalized ratio; PT = prothrombin time.

Table 17.13 *Factors that, alone or in combination, may be responsible for decreased INR response (attenuate effect of warfarin)*

Exogenous factors
Adrenocortical steroids
Alcohol
Aminoglutethimide
Diuretics
Antacids
Antihistamines
Antithyroid drugs
Barbiturates
Carbamazepine
Chloral hydrate
Chlordiazepoxide
Cholestyramine
Cyclosporin
Ethchlorvynol
Glutethimide
Griseofulvin
Haloperidol
Meprobamate
Moricizine hydrochloride
Nafcillin
Oral contraceptives
Paraldehyde
Primidone
Rantidine
Rifampin
Sucralfate
Trazodone
Vitamin C
Vitamin K
Warfarin underdosage

Also other medications affecting blood elements that may modify hemostatis, dietary deficiencies, prolonged hot weather, unreliable PT determinations, and increased and decreased INR responses have been reported.

INR = international normalized ratio; PT = prothrombin time.

Platelet glycoprotein (GP) IIb/IIIa antagonists:
- inhibit the platelet surface receptor responsible for fibrinogen binding and platelet aggregation;
- given intravenously for high-risk coronary angioplasty;
- can cause hemorrhage, particularly when used concomitantly with moderate to high doses of unfractionated heparin;
- oral GPIIb/IIIa antagonists are being investigated.

ADP receptor antagonists (ticlopidine, clopidogrel):
- inhibit ADP-mediated platelet aggregation;
- antiplatelet effects observed 2–3 days after therapy initiated;
- more rapid effect if given first as 'loading' dose;
- hepatic metabolism.

Indications for antithrombotic therapy

Prevention of venous thrombosis:
- low-risk general surgery patients – early ambulation;
- moderate-risk general surgery patients – elastic stockings, or intermittent pneumatic compression or low-dose unfractionated heparin (5000 U sc q12h) or LMWH;
- high-risk general surgery patients – low-dose unfractionated heparin (every 8 hours) or LMWH;
- very-high-risk general surgery patients – low-dose unfractionated heparin or LMWH combined with intermittent pneumatic compression.

Treatment of venous thromboembolism:
- intravenous heparin or adjusted-dose subcutaneous heparin sufficient to prolong the aPTT to approximately twice control (~60 seconds);
- treatment with heparin should be continued for 5–10 days; oral anticoagulation should be overlapped with heparin for 3–5 days;
- long-term anticoagulant therapy should be continued for at least 3 months (INR 2.5);
- LMWH may be used in place of unfractionated heparin;
- inferior vena cava interruption is indicated if anticoagulant therapy is contraindicated or ineffective.

Atrial fibrillation. The following conditions increase the risk of stroke:
- increasing age (>65 years);
- previous TIA or stroke;
- hypertension;
- heart failure or clinical coronary artery disease;
- mitral stenosis or prosthetic heart valves;
- diabetes;
- thyrotoxicosis.

Oral anticoagulants (INR 2.5) are indicated in high-risk patients, and aspirin should be used in low-risk patients.

Valvular heart disease
- Rheumatic mitral valve disease:
  - history of systemic embolism of atrial fibrillation: warfarin (INR 2.5);
  - left atrium (LA) diameter >5.5 cm – consider warfarin;
  - recurrent embolism despite warfarin – add ASA (80–100 mg/day);
- Aortic valve disease:
  - history of systemic embolism or atrial fibrillation – warfarin (INR 2.5).
- Mitral valve prolapse:
  - history of TIA – aspirin (160–325 mg/day);
  - history of TIA while on ASA, systemic embolism, or atrial fibrillation – warfarin (INR 2.5);
  - clopidogrel (75 mg qd), if warfarin is contraindicated.
- Mitral annular calcification:
  - history of systemic embolism or atrial fibrillation – warfarin (INR 2.5).

Prosthetic heart valves
- Mechanical prosthetic valves:
  - prophylaxis – warfarin (INR 2.5–3.5); consider addition of aspirin (80–100 mg/day) in high-risk patients;
  - history of systemic embolism – warfarin plus ASA (80–100 mg/day) or warfarin plus dipyridamole (400 mg/day);
  - with infective endocarditis – continue warfarin (INR 3.0).
- Bioprosthetic heart valves:
  - bioprosthetic valve in mitral position – warfarin for 3 months (INR 2.5), then aspirin 80 mg qd;
  - bioprosthetic valve in aortic position – warfarin for 3 months (INR 2.5), then aspirin 80 mg qd;
  - bioprosthetic valve and atrial fibrillation, systemic embolism, or atrial thrombus: warfarin (INR 2.5) indefinitely.

Acute myocardial infarction
- Antiplatelet therapy:
  - non-enteric-coated aspirin (160–325 mg/day) should be given to all patients with suspected acute myocardial infarction;
  - ASA (160–325 mg/day) should be given to all patients for an indefinite period (unless warfarin is used).
- Heparin (unfractionated):
  - patients with MI should receive not less than 7500 U sc bid;
  - patients at high-risk for mural thrombosis, venous thrombosis or systemic embolism should receive full-dose heparin (target aPTT 50–70 sec).
- Warfarin:
  - patients at high risk for mural thrombosis/ systemic embolism should receive warfarin (INR 2.5) for up to 3 months.
- Combination therapy (aspirin/warfarin):
  - there is no clear added benefit to combination therapy.

Coronary bypass grafts
- Aspirin (325 mg/day or higher) started 6 hours after surgery is recommended.
- For patients allergic to aspirin, ticlopidine (250 mg bid) or clopidogrel (75 mg qd) starting 48 hours after surgery is an alternative.

Coronary angioplasty (percutaneous coronary interventions)
- Aspirin (at least 325 mg) should be given 2 or more hours before coronary angioplasty; long-term treatment with aspirin (160–325 mg daily) is recommended as secondary prevention against cardiovascular events.

- Clopidogrel (75 mg qd) is recommended for patients allergic or intolerant to aspirin; it should be started as early as possible prior to elective coronary angioplasty (at least 48 hours before).
- Heparin bolus (70 U/kg; maximum 7000 U) should be given prior to the procedure; additional boluses should be given to maintain ACT >300 seconds (HemoTec® device) or >350 seconds (Hemochron® device) during the procedure.
- The GPIIb/IIIa inhibitor abciximab (ReoPro®) bolus (0.25 mg/kg) and infusion (10 µg/min for 12 hours) or an alternative iv GPIIb/IIIa antagonist should be considered in high-risk patients; in these patients a weight-adjusted nomogram for heparin (70 U/kg to a target ACT of 200–250 seconds) is recommended.

Coronary stents

- Aspirin (at least 325 mg) should be given more than 2 hours prior to the procedure and continued indefinitely thereafter (at a dose of 160–325 mg daily).
- Intraprocedural heparin to maintain ACT at 250–300 seconds (HemoTec® device) or 300–350 seconds (Hemochron® device) is recommended. A lower ACT (200–250 seconds) is recommended when a GPIIb/IIIa antagonist is used.
- Clopidogrel (75 mg qd) should be continued for at least 30 days after stent placement. Initial loading dose 300 mg.

Peripheral vascular disease/surgery

- Aspirin (80–325 mg/day) is recommended for all patients with peripheral vascular disease because of their increased risk of acute MI and stroke.
- Clopidogrel may offer greater benefit among patients with prior MI.
- Aspirin (325 mg/day) ± dipyridamole (75 mg tid) may be useful in patients undergoing femoropopliteal bypass surgery.
- Aspirin (180–1300 mg/day) should be given preoperatively and continued indefinitely among patients undergoing carotid endarterectomy.
- Patients experiencing acute arterial thromboembolism may benefit from heparin; heparin followed by oral anticoagulation should be used to prevent recurrent embolism in patients undergoing thromboembolectomy.

Cerebrovascular disease

- Asymptomatic carotid stenosis/bruit: aspirin (325 mg/day).
- TIA/minor ischemic stroke: aspirin (75–1300 mg/day).
- If aspirin allergy or recurrent TIA on aspirin, then ticlopidine 250 mg bid or clopidogrel 75 mg qd.
- Progressing ischemic stroke: heparin anticoagulation for 3–5 days (CT scan of brain to exclude hemorrhage) is reasonable.

- Completed thrombotic stroke: ASA (325–1300 mg/day), ticlopidine (250 mg bid), or clopidogrel 75 mg qd; some evidence suggests clopidogrel may be the preferred agent.
- Acute cardioembolic stroke: small to moderate sized, no evidence of hemorrhage on CT/magnetic resonance imaging (MRI) performed >48 hours later, non-hypertensive-heparin followed by warfarin (INR 2.5).
- Large embolic stroke or poorly controlled hypertension: delay anticoagulation 5–14 days.
  - AF as presumed source of emboli: Reasonable to initiate warfarin (following CT >48 hours) without initial heparin therapy.
- Fibrinolytic therapy (tPA) should be considered in patients with ischemic stroke presenting within 2–3 hours of symptom onset after careful evaluation. Additional investigation of this therapy is needed to define ideal candidates.

Anticoagulation in patients on warfarin requiring elective surgery

- Careful assessment of thrombotic and hemorrhage risk is essential.
- Preoperative heparin administration is indicated for patients at very high risk for thrombosis (venous or arterial thromboembolism within 1 month).
- Postoperative heparin administration is indicated for patients with moderate to high risk for thrombosis (venous thromboembolism within 2–3 months).

Heparin-induced thrombocytopenia

- Most commonly observed in patients receiving unfractionated heparin for at least 5 days.
- Thrombocytopenia may be accompanied by thrombosis (venous or arterial).
- Treatment includes discontinuation of *all* heparin.
- Alternative therapy (danaparoid sodium, hirudin, argatroban) should be considered for patients requiring anticoagulation.

SUMMARY

- Thrombotic disease of the venous and arterial circulatory systems accounts for a large proportion of hospital admissions and health-care expenditures worldwide.
- The prevention and treatment of deep vein thrombosis, pulmonary embolism, unstable angina, and myocardial infarction is based on antithrombotic therapy directed at platelets and the pathways of coagulation.
- Guidelines for the use of antithrombotic therapies in daily clinical practice have been developed.

- Management guidelines are also available for patients with valvular heart disease, mechanical prostheses, atrial fibrillation, peripheral vascular disease, and cerebrovascular disease.
- Management of patients on warfarin therapy who require elective surgery can be approached logically through an assessment of thrombotic and hemorrhagic risk.
- Heparin-induced thrombocytopenia can be diagnosed clinically with confirmatory support provided by specific assays; alternative anticoagulant treatment options are now available.

REFERENCES

1. Fifth American College of Chest Physicians Consensus Conference on Antithrombotic Therapy. *Chest* 1998; **114**(suppl): 439S–769S.
2. Ryan TJ, Anderson JL, Antman EM, *et al*., and the Task Force Members. ACC/AHA guidelines for the management of patients with acute myocardial infarction. A report of the American College of Cardiology/American Heart Association task force on practice guidelines (committee on management of acute myocardial infarction). *J Am Coll Cardiol* 1996; **28**: 1328–428.
3. Lensing AW, Prins MH, Davidso BL, Hirsh J. Treatment of deep venous thrombosis with low-molecular-weight heparins. A meta-analysis. *Arch Intern Med* 1995; **155**: 601–7.
4. Koopman MM, Prandoni P, Piovella F, *et al*. Treatment of venous thrombosis with intravenous unfractionated heparin administered in the hospital as compared with subcutaneous low-molecular-weight-heparin administered at home. *N Engl J Med* 1996; **334**: 682–7.
5. Levine M, Gent M, Hirsh J, *et al*. A comparison of low-molecular-weight heparin administered primarily at home with unfractionated heparin administered in the hospital for proximal deep-vein thrombosis. *N Engl J Med* 1996; **334**: 677.
6. Hommes DW, Bura A, Mazzolai L, Büller HR, ten Cate JW. Subcutaneous heparin compared with continuous intravenous heparin administration in the initial treatment of deep vein thrombosis. A meta-analysis. *Ann Intern Med* 1992; **116**: 279–84.
7. Simonneu G, Sors H, Charbonnier B, *et al*., for the THÈSÈE Study Group. A comparison of low-molecular-weight-heparin with unfractionated heparin for acute pulmonary embolism. *N Engl J Med* 1997; **337**: 663–9.
8. Büller HR, Gent M, Gallus AS, Ginsbert J, Prins MH, Baildon R, for the Writing Committee of the Columbus Study. Low-molecular-weight-heparin in the treatment of patients with venous thromboembolism. *N Engl J Med* 1997; **337**: 657–62.
9. Greenfield LJ, Michna BA. Twelve year clinical experience with the Greenfield vena cava filter. *Surgery* 1988; **104**: 706.
10. Gifford RH, Feinstein AR. A critique of methodology in studies of anticoagulant therapy for acute myocardial infarction. *N Engl J Med* 1969; **280**: 351.
11. Chapman I. The cause–effect relationship between recent coronary artery occlusion and acute myocardial infarction. *Am Heart J* 1974; **87**: 267.
12. Drapkin A, Merskey C. Anticoagulant therapy after acute myocardial infarction: relation of therapeutic benefit to patient's age, sex, and severity of infarction. *JAMA* 1972; **222**: 541.
13. Telford AM, Wilson C. Trial of heparin versus atenolol in prevention of myocardial infarction in intermediate coronary syndrome. *Lancet* 1981; **1**: 1225.
14. Théroux P, Ouimet H, McCans J, *et al*. Aspirin, heparin, or both to treat acute unstable angina. *N Engl J Med* 1990; **319**: 1105.
15. The RISC Group. Risk of myocardial infarction and death during treatment with lose dose aspirin and intravenous heparin in men with unstable coronary artery disease. *Lancet* 1990; **336**: 827.
16. Coller BS. A new murine monoclonal antibody reports an activation-dependent change in the conformation and/or microenvironment of the platelet glycoprotein IIb/IIIa complex. *J Clin Invest* 1985; **76**: 101–8.
17. Lefkovits J, Plow EF, Topol EJ. Platelet glycoprotein IIb/IIIa receptors in cardiovascular medicine. *N Engl J Med* 1995; **332**: 1553–9.
18. Simoons ML, de Boer MJ, van den Brand MJBM, *et al*., and the European Cooperative Study Group. Randomized trial of a GPIIb/IIIa platelet receptor blocker in refractory unstable angina. *Circulation* 1994; **89**: 596–603.
19. The EPIC Investigators. Use of a monoclonal antibody directed against the platelet glycoprotein IIb/IIIa receptor in high-risk coronary angioplasty. *N Engl J Med* 1994; **330**: 949–55.
20. Schulman SP, Goldschmidt-Clermont PJ, Topol EJ, *et al*. The effects of integrilin, a platelet glycoprotein IIb-IIIa receptor antagonist, in unstable angina: the importance of gender differences in the response to antiplatelet therapy. *Circulation* 1996; **94**: 359–67.
21. Cohen M, Demers C, Gurfinkel E, Turpie AGG, *et al*., for the Efficacy and Safety of subcutaneous Enoxaparin in Non-Q-Wave Coronary Events Study Group. A comparison of low-molecular-weight heparin with unfractionated heparin for unstable coronary artery disease. *N Engl J Med* 1997; **337**: 447–52.
22. Antman EM, McCabe CH, Gurfinkel EP, *et al*. Enoxaparin prevents death and cardiac ischemic events in unstable angina/non-Q wave myocardial infarction: results of the TIMI IIb trial. *Circulation* 1999; **100**: 1593–601.
23. Gold HK, Torres FW, Garadedia HD, *et al*. Evidence for a rebound coagulation phenomenon after cessation of a 4-hour infusion of a specific thrombin inhibitor in

patients with unstable angina pectoris. *J Am Coll Cardiol* 1993; **21**: 1039.

24. Lewis HD, Davis JW, Archibald DG, *et al*. Protective effects of aspirin against acute myocardial infarction and death in men with unstable angina: results of a Veterans' Administration cooperative study. *N Engl J Med* 1983; **309**: 396.

25. Cairns JA, Gent M, Singer J, *et al*. Aspirin, sulfinpyrazone, or both, in unstable angina: results of a Canadian multicenter trial. *N Engl J Med* 1985; **313**: 1369.

26. The TIMI IIIA Investigators. Early effects of tissue type plasminogen activator added to conventional therapy on the culprit coronary lesion in patients presenting with ischemic cardiac pain at rest. *Circulation* 1993; **87**: 38.

27. Report of the 60+ reinfarction study research group: a double-blind trial to assess long term anticoagulant therapy in elderly patients after myocardial infarction. *Lancet* 1980; **2**: 989.

28. Smith P, Areesen H, Holme I. The effect of warfarin on mortality and reinfarction artery myocardial infarction. *N Engl J Med* 1990; **323**: 147.

29. McMahon, S, Collins R, Knight C, *et al*. Reduction in major morbidity and mortality by heparin in acute myocardial infarction (abstract). *Circulation* 1988; **78**(suppl 2): 98.

30. Turpie AGG, Robinson JG, Doyle DJ, *et al*. Comparison of high dose with low dose subcutaneous heparin to prevent left ventricular mural thrombosis in patients with acute transmural anterior myocardial infarction. *N Engl J Med* 1989; **320**: 352.

31. The SCATI (Studio Sulla Calciparina Nell'Angina e Nella Thrombosis Ventriculare Nell'Infarto) Group. Randomized controlled trial of subcutaneous calcium heparin in acute myocardial infarction. *Lancet* 1989; **2**: 182.

32. Tulloch JA, Gilchrist AR. Anticoagulants in treatment of coronary thrombosis. *Br Med J* 1950; **2**: 965–71.

33. Burton CR. Anticoagulant therapy of recent cardiac infarction. *Can Med Assoc J* 1954; **70**: 404–8.

34. Davis MJ, Irelant MA. Effect of early anticoagulation on the frequency of left ventricular thrombi after anterior wall acute myocardial infarction. *Am J Cardiol* 1986; **57**: 1244–7.

35. Arvan S, Boscha K. Prophylactic anticoagulation for left ventricular thrombi after acute myocardial infarction: a prospective randomized trial. *Am Heart J* 1987; **113**: 688–93.

36. Turpie AG, Robinson JG, Doule DJ, *et al*. Comparison of high dose with low dose subcutaneous heparin to prevent left ventricular mural thrombosis in patients with acute transmural anterior myocardial infarction. *N Engl J Med* 1989; **320**: 352–7.

37. Vaitkus PT, Barnathan ES. Embolic potential, prevention and management of mural thrombus complicating anterior myocardial infarction: a meta-analysis. *J Am Coll Cardiol* 1993; **22**: 1004–9.

38. Loh E, St John Sutton M, Wun CC, *et al*. Ventricular dysfunction and the risk of stroke after myocardial infarction. *N Engl J Med* 1997; **336**: 251–7.

39. Ouyang P, Shapiro EP, Gottlieb SO. Thrombolysis in postinfarction angina. *Am J Cardiol* 1991; **68**: 124B.

40. Shapito EP, Brinker JA, Gottlieb SO, *et al*. Intracoronary thrombolysis 3 to 13 days after acute myocardial infarction for post infarction angina pectoris. *Am J Cardiol* 1985; **55**: 1453.

41. Brown BG, Gallery A, Badger RS, *et al*. Incomplete lysis of thrombus in the moderate underlying atherosclerotic lesion during intracoronary infusion of streptokinase for acute myocardial infarction: quantitative angiographic observations. *Circulation* 1986; **73**: 653.

42. Lierde JV, DeGeest H, Verstraete M, van de Werf F. Angiographic assessment of the infarct-related residual coronary stenosis after spontaneous or therapeutic thrombolysis. *J Am Coll Cardiol* 1990; **16**: 1545.

43. Davies MJ. Successful and unsuccessful coronary thrombolysis. *Br Heart J* 1986; **61**: 381.

44. Richardson SG, Callen D, Morton P, *et al*. Pathological changes after intravenous streptokinase treatment in eight patients with acute myocardial infarction. *Br Heart J* 1989; **61**: 390.

45. The GUSTO Investigators. An international randomized trial comparing four thrombolytic strategies for acute myocardial infarction. *N Engl J Med* 1993; **329**: 673.

46. ISIS-3 (Third International Study of Infarct Survival) Collaborative Group. A randomized comparison of streptokinase vs tissue plasminogen activator vs anistreplase and of aspirin plus heparin vs aspirin alone among 41,299 cases of suspected acute myocardial infarction. *Lancet* 1992; **339**: 1.

47. The International Study Group. In hospital mortality and clinical course of 20,9881 patients with suspected acute myocardial infarction randomized between alteplase and streptokinase with or without heparin. *Lancet* 1990; **33**: 71.

48. O'Conner CM, Meese R, Carney R, *et al*. for Duke University Clinical Cardiology Study Group (DUCCS). A randomized trial of intravenous heparin in conjunction with anistreplase (APSAC) in acute myocardial infarction. *J Am Coll Cardiol* 1994; **23**: 11.

49. ISIS-2 (Second International Study of Infarct Survival) Collaborative Group. Randomized trial of intravenous streptokinase, oral aspirin, both or neither among 17,187 cases of suspected acute myocardial infarction. *Lancet* 1988; **2**: 349.

50. Antiplatelet Trialists' Collaboration. Collaborative overview of randomised trials of antiplatelet therapy. I. Prevention of death, myocardial infarction and stroke by prolonged antiplatelet therapy in various categories in patients. *Br Med J* 1994; **308**: 81–106.

51. Stroke Prevention in Atrial Fibrillation Investigators. Adjusted-dose warfarin versus low-intensity, fixed-dose warfarin plus aspirin for high-risk patients with atrial fibrillation: stroke prevention in atrial fibrillation III randomised clinical trial. *Lancet* 1996; **348**: 633–8.

52. Sullivan JM, Harken DE, Gorlin R. Effect of dipyridamole on the incidence of arterial emboli after cardiac valve replacement. *Circulation* 1969; **39–40**(suppl): 1–49.

53. Kasahara T. Clinical effect of dipyridamole ingestion after prosthetic heart valve replacement – especially on the blood coagulation system. *Nippon Kyobu Geka Gakkai Zasshi* 1977; **25**: 1007.

54. Raha SM, Sreeharan N, Joseph A, *et al*. Perspective trial of dipyridamole and warfarin in heart valve patients (abstract). *Act Ther (Brussels)* 1980; **6**: 54.

55. Turpie AGG, Gent M, Laupacis A, *et al*. Reduction in mortality by adding aspirin (100mg) to oral anticoagulants in patients with heart valve replacement (abstract). *J Am Col Cardiol* 1992; (supp A): 103A.

56. Chesbro JH, Fuster V, Elveback LR, *et al*. Trial of combined warfarin plus dipyridamole or aspirin therapy in prosthetic valve replacement: danger of aspirin compared with dipyridamole. *Am J Cardiol* 1983; **51**: 1537.

57. Cohn LH, Allred EN, DiSesa VJ, *et al*. Early and late risk of aortic valve replacement: A 12-year concomitant comparison of the porcine bioprosthetic and tilting disc prosthetic aortic valves. *J Thorac Cardiovasc Surg* 1984; **88**: 695.

58. Kearon C, Hirsh J. Management of anticoagulation before and after elective surgery. *N Engl J Med* 1997; **336**: 1506–11.

59. Amiral J, Bridey F, Wolf M. Antibodies to macromolecular platelet factor 4 heparin complexes in heparin-induced thrombocytopenia: a study of 44 cases. *Thromb Haemostas* 1995; **73**: 21–8.

60. Lewis BE, Walenga JM, Wallis DE. Anticoagulation with Novastan (argatroban) in patients with heparin-induced thrombocytopenia and heparin-induced thrombocytopenia and thrombosis syndrome. *Semin Thromb Haemost* 1997; **23**: 197–202.

18

Fibrinolytics, anticoagulants, and platelet antagonists in clinical practice

RICHARD C BECKER AND LIBERTO PECHET

Venous and arterial thromboembolism are common disorders that share the central pathobiologic scheme of vascular occlusion; however, the inciting sequence of events and natural history differ. Venous thromboembolism is a stasis and activated coagulation factor-mediated process that requires treatment with an anticoagulant. In contrast, arterial thrombosis is initiated by platelet activation and aggregation with subsequent growth determined by contribution of the coagulation cascade. Accordingly, platelet antagonists and anticoagulants are both important for treatment. Whether venous or arterial, thrombus has a supporting framework of fibrin; however, with the latter, fibrin is a predominant component and important target for pharmacologic therapy.

INTRODUCTION

The prevalence and societal impact of atherosclerotic coronary artery disease in general and acute thromboembolic diseases of the venous and arterial circulatory systems in particular has stimulated great enthusiasm for the development of new treatment strategies with the universal goal of reducing morbidity, mortality, and overall health care expenditures. At the forefront of this intensive effort is an understanding among members of the scientific community that *new* is not necessarily *better* and that more potent agents may be accompanied by profound (and potentially dangerous) alterations of physiologic (protective) hemostatic mechanisms.

> Only carefully designed and appropriately powered clinical trials can answer the question of safety and efficacy.

In the past decade there has been a virtual explosion of new information directed at the treatment of acute thromboembolic diseases, accounting for up to 60 per cent of cardiac-based hospital admissions in the USA. Enthusiasm abounds as clinicians become increasingly aware that observations derived from basic and clinical research have found their way into the patient care arena, expanding treatment options and elevating the overall standards of practice.

The following chapter focuses on recent developments in the treatment of thromboembolic diseases and includes discussions on new fibrinolytics, anticoagulants and platelet antagonists.

VASCULAR THROMBOSIS: BASIC PRINCIPLES

Under normal physiologic conditions, blood components do not interact with an intact vascular endothelium. The exposure of circulating blood to disrupted or dysfunctional surfaces initiates a series of complex yet orderly steps that give rise to the rapid deposition of platelets, erythrocytes, leukocytes, and insoluble fibrin, producing a mechanical barrier to blood flow.

In most instances, thrombosis occurring in the arterial system comprises platelets and fibrin in a tightly packed network (white thrombus). In contrast, venous thrombi consist of erythrocytes, leukocytes, and fibrin (red thrombus).

The process of vascular thrombosis, particularly in the arterial system, is dynamic, with clot formation and dissolution occurring simultaneously. The overall extent of thrombosis and ensuing circulatory compromise is therefore determined by the predominant force that 'shifts' this delicate balance in one direction or another. If local stimuli exceed the vessel's own thromboresistant potential, thrombosis will occur. If, on the other hand, the stimulus toward thrombosis is not particularly strong and the intrinsic defenses are intact, clot formation of clinical importance is unlikely. In some circumstances, systemic factors contribute to or magnify local prothrombotic factors, shifting the balance toward thrombosis. A prime example is cigarette smoking. A recent study[1] found that male smokers who died suddenly were as likely to have plaque erosion as they were to have vulnerable plaque rupture underlying coronary thrombi. This pivotal observation confirms prior suspicions that active smokers are at risk for coronary arterial thrombosis even in the absence of advanced plaque development and marked disruption. In other words, smoking is a modest risk factor for atherosclerosis and a very strong risk factor for thrombosis.

Overall, the site, size, and composition of thrombi forming within the arterial and venous circulatory systems is determined by: (1) alterations in blood flow; (2) thrombogenicity of vascular surfaces; (3) the concentration and reactivity of plasma cellular components; and (4) the effectiveness of the physiologic protective mechanism.

FUNDAMENTAL STEPS IN VASCULAR THROMBOSIS

Platelet deposition

Platelets attaching to non-endothelialized or disrupted surfaces undergo adherence by activation and distribution along the involved area and subsequent recruitment to form a rapidly enlarging platelet mass. Under normal physiologic conditions, this represents the primary step in hemostasis. In pathologic thrombosis, however, platelet adherence initiates a process that can escalate to an extent that causes circulatory compromise.

The process of platelet deposition involves: (1) platelet attachment to collagen or exposed surface adhesive proteins; (2) platelet activation and intracellular signaling; (3) the expression of platelet receptors for adhesive proteins; (4) platelet aggregation (to be discussed in greater detail in a later section); and (5) platelet recruitment mediated by thrombin, thromboxane A_2, and adenosine diphosphate (ADP).

Activation of coagulation factors

Thrombin, a pivotal enzyme in both physiolgic hemostasis and pathologic thrombosis, is rapidly generated in response to vascular injury. It also plays a central role in platelet recruitment and the formation of an insoluble fibrin network. The thrombotic process is localized, amplified, and modulated by a series of biochemical reactions driven by the reversible binding of circulating proteins (coagulation factors) to damaged vascular cells, elements of exposed subendothelial connective tissue (especially collagen), platelets (which also express receptor sites for coagulation factors), and macrophages. These events lead to an assembly of enzyme complexes that increases local concentrations of procoagulant material; in this way, a relatively minor initiating stimulus can be greatly amplified to yield a flow-limiting thrombus.

Fibrin formation

The final phase in thrombus formation involves the generation of a stable fibrin network that provides the structural support for the circulating blood's cellular elements and the scaffolding for vascular remodeling. In the process of converting fibrinogen to fibrin monomers, which then polymerize to form soluble fibrin strand, thrombin cleaves two small peptides, fibrinopeptide A and fibrinopeptide B, to form fibrin monomers, which in turn polymerize to form soluble fibrin strands. An orderly assembly, branching, and lateral association of fibrillar strands follows, terminating with Factor XIII-mediated covalent cross-linking to form a mature fibrin network (mature thrombus).

The overall clinical expression of an intravascular thrombotic event is governed by its site, size, and impact on physiologic blood flow. In arterial thrombosis, predominantly platelet driven, activity within an atheromatous plaque is an important determinant of recurrent episodes as well as treatment response. In venous thrombosis, predominantly coagulation factor driven, the local environment (blood flow, local thromboresistant properties) is the critical determinant.

FIBRINOLYTIC AGENTS

In essence, fibrinolytic therapy makes use of the vascular system's native thromboresistant properties by accelerating and amplifying the conversion of an inactive precursor, plasminogen, to the active enzyme plasmin. In turn, plasmin hydrolyzes several key bonds in the fibrin (clot) matrix causing dissolution (lysis). In the setting of acute myocardial infarction or ischemic stroke, blood flow is restored and with it perfusion of vital tissue is achieved.

The ideal fibrinolytic agent should have the following properties. First, it should be fibrin specific, even at doses required to elicit successful thrombolysis at least 90 per cent of the time. The fibrin specificity should be directed at newly formed fibrin (present within pathologic thrombi), while exerting a minimal effect on normal hemostasis. Second, the onset of fibrinolytic activity should be rapid. Third, the circulating half-life should be long enough to permit abbreviated dosing and wide-scale acceptance in clinical practice. Fourth, it should not be antigenic. Lastly, the ideal fibrinolytic agent should be available at a cost that fosters its routine use.

The key components of the vasculatures' intrinsic fibrinolytic system include the following.

Plasminogen

A single-chain glycoprotein consisting of 790 amino acids, plasminogen is converted to plasmin by cleavage of the Arg^{560}–Val^{561} peptide bond. The plasminogen molecule also contains specific lysine binding sites, which mediate its interaction with fibrin and α_2-plasmin inhibitor.

Plasmin

A serine protease with trypsin-like activity, plasmin cleaves lysyl and arginyl bonds of fibrin at two principal sites: (1) the carboxyl terminal portion of α-chain (polar region); and (2) the coiled-coil connectors containing the α-, β- and γ-chains (Fig. 18.1 and Table 18.1).

First-generation agents

STREPTOKINASE

Streptokinase is a non-enzymatic protein produced by β-hemolytic streptococci. It activates the fibrinolytic system indirectly by forming a 1:1 stoichiometric complex with plasminogen, which then activates plasminogen, converting it to the active enzyme plasmin.

UROKINASE

Urokinase is a trypsin-like serine protease composed of two polypeptide chains, connected by a disulfide bridge. It activates plasminogen directly, converting it to the active enzyme plasmin.

Table 18.1 *Physiologic components of the plasma fibrinolytic system*

	Molecular weight	**Activity**
Plasminogen	88 000 (single chain)	Proenzyme form of fibrinolytic enzyme
Plasmin	88 000 (two chain)	Active fibrinolytic enzyme
tPA	70 000 (one/two chain)	Enzyme present in tissues that converts plasminogen to plasmin
UPA	54 000 (two chain)	Plasminogen activator (different from tPA)
α_2PI	70 000 (single chain)	Specific fast-acting inhibitor in plasma
PAI-1	40 000 (single chain)	Fast-acting inhibitor of tPA (and UPA) secreted by endothelial cells

tPA = tissue plasminogen activator; UPA = urokinase plasminogen activator; α_2PI = alpha-2 plasmin inhibitor; PAI-1 = plasminogen activator inhibitor 1.

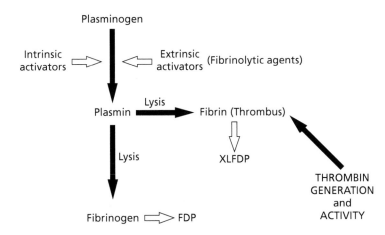

Figure 18.1 *The fibrinolytic system. An inactive enzymatic precursor, plasminogen, is converted by either intrinsic or extrinsic activators to plasmin which, in turn, degrades fibrin. Circulating plasmin can also degrade fibrinogen. XLFDP = cross-linked fibrin degradation products; FDP = fibrinogen degradation products.*

Second-generation agents

APSAC (ANISOLYLATED PLASMINOGEN–STREPTOKINASE ACTIVATOR COMPLEX)

Streptokinase and the plasminogen–streptokinase activator complex are cleared rapidly from the circulation, with half-lives of 15 and 3 minutes, respectively. By temporarily blocking the active center of plasminogen, the plasma half-life can be prolonged substantially. Therefore, acylation of plasminogen (APSAC) protects the molecule from autodigestion and also prevents its inactivation by circulating plasma inhibitors, resulting in a half-life of approximately 100 minutes. These features permit bolus dosing.

scu-PA

scu-PA (single-chain urokinase-like plasminogen activator) is a single-chain glycoprotein containing 411 amino acids, which can be converted to urokinase by hydrolysis of the Lys[148–149] peptide bond. Its fibrin specificity has not been fully characterized; however, the presence of intravascular fibrin, in and of itself, may neutralize a naturally occurring or inducible circulating scu-PA inhibitor.

TISSUE-TYPE PLASMINOGEN ACTIVATOR (tPA)

Native tPA is a serine protease composed of one polypeptide chain containing 527 amino acids. On limited plasmic action, the molecule is converted to a two-chain activator linked by one disulfide bond. This occurs by cleavage of the Arg^{275}–Ile^{276} peptide bond yielding a heavy chain (M_r 31 000) derived from the amino-terminal part of the molecule and a light chain (M_r 28 000) comprising the carboxy-terminal region.

tPA is a poor enzyme in the absence of fibrin; but in fibrin's presence the activation rate of plasminogen is markedly enhanced. This unique property is determined by the increased affinity of fibrin-bound tPA for plasminogen (without a significant influence on the catalytic efficiency of the enzyme). Fibrin increases the local plasminogen concentration by creating an additional interaction between tPA and its substrate. The high affinity of tPA for plasminogen in the presence of fibrin thus allows efficient activation on the fibrin clot, while no efficient plasminogen activation by tPA occurs in plasma.

Third-generation agents

An approach designed to improve fibrinolytic potential involves site-directed mutagenesis to construct fibrin-

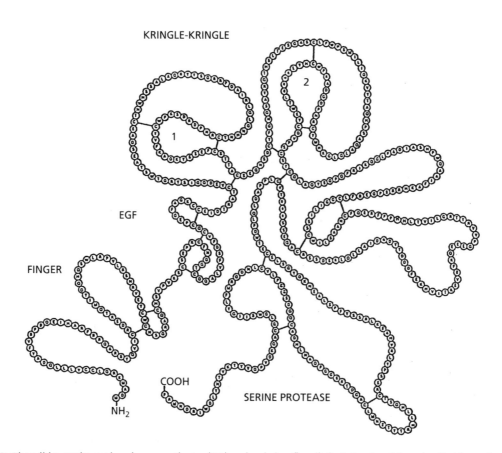

Figure 18.2 *The wild-type tissue plasminogen activator (tPA) molecule has five distinct structural domains that import specific biological properties. EGF = epidermal growth factor.*

olytic molecules either lacking specific structural/functional domains or duplicating specific domains. In this way, the most favorable properties of a given molecule can be used to their fullest potential, such as increasing fibrin specificity or increasing the circulating half-life. Several mutants, hybrids, and variants of existing fibrinolytic agents have been developed and are currently undergoing evaluation.

The wild-type tPA molecule (Fig. 18.2 and Table 18.2) has served as the template for several third-generation molecules with the following distinct goals in mind:

1   more rapid restoration of Thrombolysis in Myocardial Infarction (TIMI) grade 3 (normal) coronary arterial blood flow;
2   restoration of TIMI grade 3 (physiologic) flow in a larger proportion of patients;
3   a longer circulating half-life, permitting bolus administration;
4   a lower risk of major hemorrhage (particularly intracranial hemorrhage);
5   an acceptable cost (promoting wide-scale use).

Table 18.2 *Structure–function relationship of the tPA molecule*

Domain/region	Functional property
Kringle-1	Receptor binding
Kringle-2	Fibrin binding (low affinity)
Fibronectin finger	Fibrin binding (high affinity)
Epidermal growth factor	Hepatic clearance
Protease	Catalytic activity; PAI-1 binding

tPA = tissue plasminogen activator; PAI-1 = plasminogen activator inhibitor-1.

RETEPLASE

Reteplase (rPA) (recombinant plasminogen activator) is a deletion mutant that contains the Kringle-2 and Protease domains of the parent tPA molecule. It has a prolonged half-life (18 minutes) and is given in two abbreviated intravenous infusions (2 minutes) 30 minutes apart. Reteplase is a Food and Drug Administration (FDA) approved fibrinolytic agent for the treatment of acute myocardial infarction and is marketed under the name Retevase®.

Clinical trials

The initial phase II experience with rPA was an open-label, dose-finding study in patients with acute ST segment elevation myocardial infarction (MI).[2] The initial dose (intravenous (iv) bolus) tested in a total of 42 patients, yielded a 90-minute angiographic patency rate of 67 per cent. Employing an increased dose of 15 U (100 patients) the patency rate increased to 76 per cent. With the goal of increasing efficacy even further, the concept

of double-bolus administration was investigated in an additional 50 patients. A regimen consisting of a 10 U bolus followed 30 minutes later by a 5 U bolus yielded a patency rate of 78 per cent.[3]

The 15 U bolus, 10 plus 5 U double-bolus, and a 10 plus 10 U double-bolus regimen of rPA were compared with tPA (alteplase; 100 mg over 3 hours) in RAPID-1 (Reteplase Angiographic Phase II International Dose Finding Trial).[4] The TIMI 3 flow rates at 60 and 90 minutes were 51 *vs* 32.7 per cent (*P*<0.01) and 62.7 *vs* 49.0 per cent (*P*<0.01) for the 10 plus 10 rPA and alteplase-treated patients, respectively (Fig. 18.3). The incidence of hemorrhage did not differ significantly between groups.

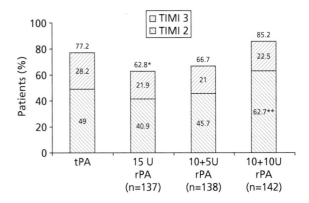

Figure 18.3 *Comparative TIMI 2 and 3 coronary arterial flow rates 90 minutes after treatment initiation among patients with myocardial infarction receiving either tissue-type (tPA) or recombinant plasminogen activator (rPA). *P < 0.01 compared with tPA; **P < 0.05 compared with tPA. (Reproduced with permission from Smalling RW, et al. More rapid, complete, and stable coronary thrombolysis with bolus administration of reteplase compared with alteplase infusion in acute myocardial infarction. Circulation 1995; 91: 2725–32.)*

A second angiographic trial, RAPID-2 (Reteplase versus Alteplase Patency Investigation During Acute MI)[5] compared rPA and accelerated tPA administration (90 minute infusion). The TIMI 3 flow rates at 60 and 90 minutes were 51.2 *vs* 37.4 per cent (*P*=0.03) and 59.9 *vs* 45.2 per cent (*P*=0.01) for rPA- and tPA-treated patients, respectively (Fig. 18.4).

To assess the safety and efficacy of rPA administration, a large-scale comparative, randomized trial with streptokinase was performed. The INJECT (International Joint Efficacy Comparison of Thrombolytics) trial was designed primarily as an equivalency study and indeed failed to identify significant differences between rPA and streptokinase-treated patients in 35-day mortality (primary end point) or the combined end point of death plus disabling stroke (Figs 18.5 and 18.6). The two treatments were associated with similar frequencies of in-

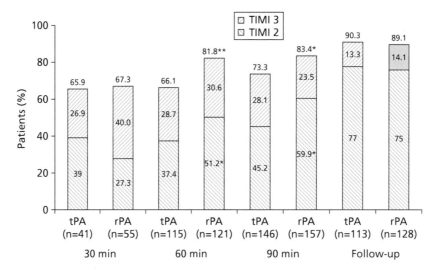

Figure 18.4 *Comparative TIMI 2 and 3 coronary arterial flow rates 30, 60, 90 minutes and 5–14 days (follow-up) after treatment with either tPA or rPA in the RAPID 2 Study. *P < 0.05 rPA vs tPA; **P < 0.01 rPA vs tPA. (Reproduced with permission from Bode C, et al. Randomized comparison of coronary thrombolysis achieved with double bolus reteplase (rPA) and front-loaded 'accelerated' alteplase (rt-PA) in patients with acute myocardial infarction. Circulation 1996; 94: 891–8.)*

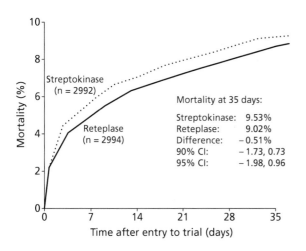

Figure 18.5 *Mortality at 35 days among patients participating in the INJECT Trial. There were no differences between the treatment groups. (Reproduced with permission from INJECT Study Group. Randomized, double-blind comparison of reteplase double-bolus administration with streptokinase in acute myocardial infarction (INJECT): trial to investigate equivalence. Lancet 1995; 346: 329–36.)*

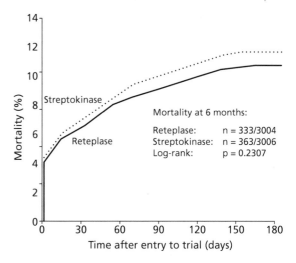

Figure 18.6 *Kaplan–Meier survival curves to 180 days among patients treated with either streptokinase or reteplase in the INJECT Trial. (Reproduced with permission from INJECT Study Group. Randomized double-blind comparison of reteplase double-bolus administration with streptokinase in acute myocardial infarction (INJECT): trial to investigate equivalence. Lancet 1995; 346: 329–36.)*

hospital cardiac events, major hemorrhage and strokes.[6] A strong trend toward improved outcome among rPA-treated patients was observed at 6 months.

GUSTO III was a multicenter, randomized, open-label trial designed to test the primary hypothesis that rPA would significantly reduce 30-day mortality compared with an accelerated tPA infusion in patients with ST segment elevation MI treated within 6 hours from symptom onset.[7] A total of 15 060 patients were enrolled at 822 hospitals in 20 countries. The 30-day mortality was 7.22 per cent (95 per cent confidence interval (CI) 6.5, 7.9) in tPA-treated patients and 7.43 (95 per cent CI 6.9, 7.9) in rPA-treated patients (Fig. 18.7). There were no statistical differences in stroke or death/non-fatal disabling stroke. The incidence of in-hospital cardiogenic shock also did not differ between treatment groups. Several predefined patient subgroups, including those greater than 75 years of age, anterior site of infarc-

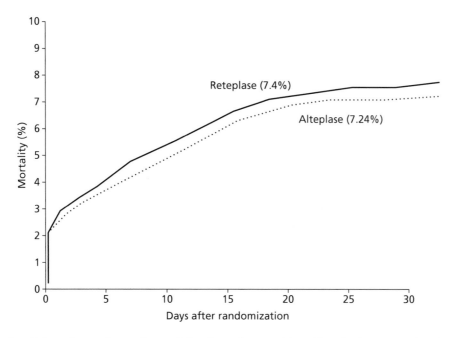

Figure 18.7 *Kaplan–Meier estimate of mortality at 30 days for patients receiving either alteplase or reteplase. (Reproduced with permission from The GUSTO Investigators. A comparison of reteplase with alteplase for acute myocardial infarction.* N Engl J Med *1997;* **337***: 1118–23.)*

tion, and treatment initiated beyond 4 hours from symptom onset, exhibited trends toward improved outcome with tPA compared with rPA.

A trial of prehospital rPA administration is currently being conducted.

TNK-tPA

TNK-tPA is a multiple point mutation of the parent tPA molecule. In its mutant form, T103N, N117Q, KHRR (296–299), AAAA, threonine 103 has been changed to asparagine 103, creating a new glycosylation site (and a longer half-life) (Table 18.3). The change at Asp[117] (to glutamine) also contributes to the molecules prolonged half-life (18 minutes), while the protease sequence change renders TNK-tPA more resistant to plasminogen activator inhibitor 1 (PAI-1).[8]

Clinical trials

The TIMI 10A trial was a phase 1, dose-ranging pilot trial designed to evaluate the pharmacokinetics, safety, and efficacy of TNK-tPA (tenecteplase) in patients (n = 113) with acute ST segment elevation MI presenting to the hospital within 12 hours of symptom onset. TIMI grade 3 flow at 90 minutes was achieved in 57–64 per cent of patients at the 30–50-mg bolus doses (Figs 18.8 and 18.9). A total of seven patients (6.20 per cent) experienced a major hemorrhagic event (vascular access bleeding in six of seven patients).[9]

The TIMI 10B trial[10] was a randomized, phase II trial that evaluated early coronary arterial patency rates with two TNK-tPA doses (30 mg and 40 mg) and an accelerated infusion of tPA. A total of 886 patients with MI presenting to the hospital within 12 hours of symptom

Table 18.3 *Molecular structure of TNK-tPA*

Designation	Substitution	Description
T	T103N	Adds glycosylation site Decreases plasma clearance
N	N117Q	Removes glycosylation site Decreases plasma clearance Increases fibrin binding
K	KHRR (296–299) AAAA	Increases fibrin specificity Increases resistance to PAI-1

tPA = tissue plasminogen activator; T = threonine; N = asparagine; Q = glutamine; K = lysine; H = histidine; R = arginine; A = alanine; PAI-1 = plasminogen activator inhibitor-1.

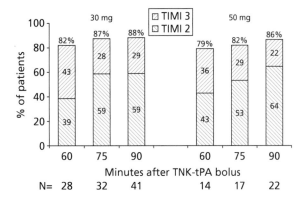

Figure 18.8 *Angiographic TIMI 2 and 3 coronary arterial flow rates at 60, 75, and 90 minutes after the administration of 30 or 50 mg of TNK-tPA. (Reproduced with permission from Cannon CP, McCabe CH, Gibson M, et al., and the TIMI IOA Investigators. TNK-tissue plasminogen activator in acute myocardial infarction. Results of the TIMI IOA dose-ranging trial. Circulation 1997; 95: 351–6.)*

onset were included in the study. A higher TNK-tPA dose (50 mg) yielded an excess number of hemorrhagic events. The 30 mg dose was associated with a signficantly lower rate of TIMI grade 3 flow than was tPA (55 per cent *vs* 63 per cent; *P* < 0.05), and the 40 mg dose was associated with an identical rate, 63 per cent. The 50 mg dose was associated with a slightly higher, but not signif-

icantly different, rate of TIMI grade 3 flow, 66 per cent. The rates of TIMI grades 2 and 3 flow combined did not differ significantly between the groups. A prespecified analysis of weight-based TNK-tPA dosing for corrected TIMI frame count, serious bleeding and intracranial hemorrhage demonstrated a dose response. The lowering of unfractionated heparin dosing led to a reduction in hemorrhagic events for both TNK-tPA and tPA-treated patients.

The ASSENT (ASsesment and Safety and Efficacy of a New Thrombolytic agent) I trial was carried out simultaneously with TIMI 10B and was designed primarily to assess safety. A total of 3325 patients with ST segment elevation MI were enrolled. An intracranial hemorrhage rate of 0.9 per cent was observed with 30 mg TNK-tPA and 0.6 per cent for the 40 mg dose. There were no events in patients given 50 mg TNK-tPA. The unfractionated heparin dose did affect the rate of intracerebral hemorrhage, particularly among patients weighing less than 67 kg. Corresponding 30-day mortality rates for patients receiving 30 or 40 mg were 7.5 per cent and 7.0 per cent, respectively.[11]

The ASSENT II trial was a phase III, randomized, double-blind, international trial designed to demonstrate equivalence in 30-day mortality rates between bolus administration of TNK-tPA (30–50 mg – weight-adjusted dosing) and an accelerated infusion of tPA in patients with ST segment elevation MI (≤6 hours from symptom onset). All patients received aspirin and

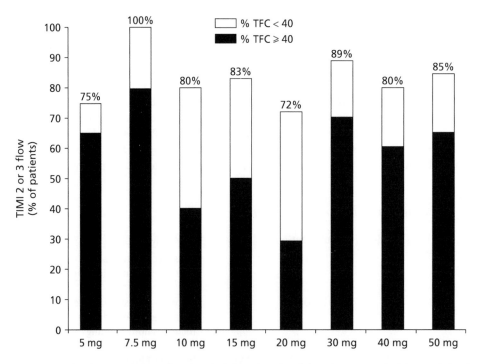

Figure 18.9 *TIMI frame count (TFC) at 90 minutes after the administration of TNK-tPA. (Reproduced with permission from Cannon CP, Gibson CM, McCabe M, et al., for the TIMI 10B Investigators. TNK-tissue plasminogen activator compared with front-loaded alteplase in acute myocardial infarction: results of the TIMI 10B trial. Circulation 1998; 98: 2805–14.)*

unfractionated heparin (aPTT 50–75 seconds). The secondary objectives of the study were to compare the in-hospital rate of death, stroke, intracranial hemorrhage, major bleeding, and non-fatal major cardiac events.

A total of 16 949 patients participated in the trial. Covariate-adjusted 30-day mortality rates were almost identical for the two groups – 6.18 per cent for tenecteplase and 6.15 per cent for alteplase. Rates of intracranial hemorrhage were also similar, 0.93 per cent and 0.94 per cent, respectively; however, fewer non-cerebral hemorrhage complications (26.4 vs 28.9 per cent, P = 0.0003) and less need for blood transfusion (4.25 vs 5.49 per cent, P = 0.0002) occurred with tenecteplase. A lower rate of intracranial hemorrhage was also observed in high-risk patients (women >75 years of age, weight <67 kg) treated with tenecteplase. The 50-mg dose proved to be safe when a strategy of weight-adjusted dosing was employed (50 mg for patients >90 kg)[12] (Fig. 18.10).

The FDA has approved tenecteplase for the treatment of acute ST segment elevation MI.

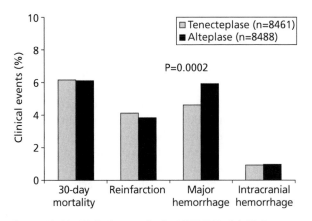

Figure 18.10 *Clinical events in the ASSENT II trial. Major hemorrhage was less likely to occur with tenecteplase than alteplase.*

nPA

nPA is a deletion and point mutant of wild-type tPA. The finger and epidermal growth factor domains have been deleted, and a point mutation within the Kringle-1 domain (Asn[117]→Gln[117]) contributes to the molecules long circulating half-life (30–45 minutes).

Clinical trials

nPA was evaluated in a phase II, randomized, dose-ranging angiographic trial known as In TIME I.[12] A total of 602 patients were enrolled at 77 sites in Europe and North America and received either 15, 30, 60 or 120 kU/kg of nPA or accelerated tPA within 6 hours of symptom onset. The proportion of patients achieving TIMI grade 3 flow increased with an increasing dose of nPA at both 60 and 90 minutes. The proportion of

patients with a patent (TIMI grade 2 or 3) infarct-related coronary artery at 90 minutes was significantly higher in the 120 kU/kg nPA group compared with the tPA group. The rate of TIMI grade 3 flow was also higher. Although a dose-related increase in major hemorrhage was observed with nPA, even at the highest dose (120 kU/kg), the overall rate was comparable to that seen with tPA.

In TIME II was a randomized, double-blind, multi-center trial that determined whether 120 kU/kg single-bolus nPA was at least as effective as 100 mg accelerated tPA in reducing mortality and major morbidity in patients with suspected MI within 6 hours of symptom onset. A total of 15 078 patients entered the trial. Although 30-day mortality rates were similar for tPA- (6.6 per cent) and nPA- (6.7 per cent) treated patients, intracranial hemorrhage occurred in 0.62 per cent and 1.13 per cent, respectively. The intensity of anticoagulation with unfractionated heparin influenced bleeding risk, particularly among older individuals.[13]

Given the worldwide frequency of coronary atherosclerosis and MI, interest in developing new fibrinolytic agents will remain high. In all likelihood, fourth-generation agents will: (1) target pathologic coronary arterial thrombi (minimize hemorrhagic risk); (2) be more enzymatically effective in hostile environments (low blood pressure, acidemia); (3) consist of tPA mutations, chimeras from differing fibrinolytics, and/or combined fibrinolytic-platelet antagonists; and (4) have long circulating plasma half-lives (single bolus dosing compatible).[14–27]

Importance of bolus dosing

A large experience with fibrinolytic therapy has shown that dosing errors, most often the result of complex and prolonged dosing strategies, are associated with higher mortality and intracranial hemorrhage rates. For this reason, the medical field is turning rapidly to fibrinolytic agents that can be given as a single bolus.

NEW ANTICOAGULANTS

The use of anticoagulants in the treatment of thromboembolic disease is based on pathobiologic mechanisms in both venous and arterial thrombosis. Thrombin generation is a pivotal process and serves as the preferred 'target' for evolving treatment strategies. This concept is particularly important in the case of arterial thrombotic disorders (e.g. acute coronary syndromes) for the following reasons:

1 within atherosclerotic plaques, tissue factor mRNA is increased compared with the normal arterial wall[28] and is up-regulated after vascular injury;[29]

2 arterial thrombi express significant Factor Xa and Va activity that is protected from inhibition mediated by

antithrombin-dependent mechanisms.[30]

Furthermore, in most pathologic states, endogenous thrombin-mediated platelet activation precedes the assembly of the prothrombinase complex (platelets provide the Factor Va activity required for full expression).[31,32] Therefore, the absence, attenuation or neutralization of thrombin prevents a critical step in prothrombinase assembly (and arterial thrombus growth).

HEPARIN PREPARATIONS

The anticoagulant heparin is a heterogeneous mixture of polysaccharide chains varying in molecular weight and biological activity. The chain lengths can vary from 5 to 100 or more saccharide units.

The pentasaccharide responsible for heparin–antithrombin binding is a critical part of its biological activity. Heparins containing the pentasaccharide sequence are considered *high-affinity molecules* and catalyze antithrombin-dependent Factor Xa inactivation, but only those containing 18 or more saccharide units are capable of catalyzing thrombin inactivation. In other words, a chain length of 18 saccharide units is required for thrombin inhibition.

Most heparins contain two subfractions. Molecules with chain lengths up to 17 monosaccharide units (1700–5400 Da) catalyze Factor Xa inactivation. Molecules containing chain lengths of 18 saccharide units or larger (>5400 Da) catalyze both Factor Xa and thrombin inactivation. Most unfractionated heparin preparations available for commercial use consist predominantly of long-chain molecules.

Low-molecular-weight heparins

Low-molecular-weight heparins (LMWHs) vary in molecular weight from 2000 to 10 000 Da. As a result, they contain both short and long polysaccharide chains; however, the former predominates in many preparations. In contrast, unfractionated heparin (UFH)

consists almost entirely of long polysaccharide chains. In both UFH and LMWH preparations, less than 40 per cent of the constituent polypeptides contain the pentasaccharide sequence required for high-affinity interactions with antithrombin (Table 18.4).

BIOAVAILABILITY AND PHARMACOKINETICS

The bioavailability of LMWH preparations is essentially complete at a broad range of subcutaneous (sc) doses and its plasma half-life is dose independent, with 90 per cent bioavailability at all doses. This is a favorable property compared to the inconsistent absorption of UFH, which is particularly poor at low doses (commonly employed for prophylaxis). The half-life of intravenously (iv) administered LMWH is 5–8 hours. After sc administration, peak anti-Factor Xa activity is achieved within 3–5 hours with persistent activity for approximately 12 hours. Because the elimination of LMWH depends predominantly on renal excretion, its biologic half-life is increased in the setting of renal failure (creatinine clearance <40 mL/minute). In addition to a prolonged circulating half-life, LMWH preparations have lower affinity for plasma proteins compared with UFH, especially acute-phase reactants, resulting in more predictable pharmacokinetics. Finally, unlike UFH, LMWH does not bind to either macrophages (found with the hepatic and splenic sinusoids) or vascular endothelial cells. Neither LMWH nor UFH cross the placental barrier.

It is important to acknowledge that each commercial LMWH preparation has a distinct pharmacokinetic profile. The area under the concentration versus time curve increases differently for each LMWH preparation with rising doses, and also varies with repeated doses. Enoxaparin reaches peak anti-Factor Xa activity within 3 hours (plasma half-life 129–180 minutes), when administered sc in a dose of 40 mg. In contrast, Dalteparin has a slightly broader molecular weight range resulting in a lower anti-Factor Xa/thrombin ratio (2:1) compared to enoxaparin (2.7:1). It also has a shorter plasma half-life (119–139 minutes) following a 2500 IU administration. Tinzaparin has a molecular weight of 4800 Da, and is 95 per cent bioavailable when injected subcutaneously. At

Table 18.4 *Low-molecular-weight heparins in the prevention and treatment of venous thromboembolism (VTE)*

	Prophylaxis	Indication	Treatment	Indication
Enoxaparin	30 mg q12h; 40 mg qd	Hip, knee, abdominal surgery	1 mg/kg q12h; 1.5 mg/kg qd	VTE
Dalteparin	2500 IU q12h; 5000 IU qd	Hip, abdominal surgery	NA	NA
Tinzaparin	75 U/kg qd	Orthopedic surgery[a]	175 U/kg qd	VTE
Ardeparin	50 U/kg q12h	Orthopedic surgery	130 U/kg q12h	NA

[a]pending FDA approval.
NA = not applicable.

the present time, LMWH preparations are expressed differently, either as anti-Factor Xa units, IU or in milligrams. Standardization will be required to achieve consistency in clinical practice.

CLINICAL EXPERIENCE WITH LMWH

Venous thromboembolism

The prevention of postoperative venous thromboembolism remains an important aspect of daily patient care. The use of low-dose UFH for this purpose has been established and is effective in a majority of patients. However, low-dose UFH alone may be inadequate in high-risk settings.

Approximately 25 studies including a total of 5000 patients undergoing major surgical procedures (abdominal, urologic, vascular, and general) have shown that LMWH is at least as effective as UFH in preventing venous thromboembolism.[33–41] In orthopedic surgery, particularly traumatic hip fracture, LMWH is superior to placebo, superior to fixed-dose UFH, and at least as good as adjusted-dose UFH[42–48] in preventing thromboembolism.

Although the experience is more limited in medical patients, 18 clinical trials, including a total of 2500 LMWH-treated patients have been published, and these trials suggest that it is well tolerated and at least as effective as UFH.[49–58] Over the years, intravenous UFH has been employed in the early treatment of venous thromboembolism; however, LMWH has undergone extensive evaluation. To date, approximately 2000 patients have received either iv or sc LMWH (once- or twice-daily injections) for established DVT.[59–73] Considered collectively,[74] the data suggest strongly that LMWH is at least as effective as UFH in preventing symptomatic recurrent venous thromboembolism and may be associated with less clinically important bleeding (Fig. 18.11). An excep-

tion may be found in patients with malignancy complicated by venous thromboembolism in whom LMWH appears to be particularly beneficial. The cost for in-hospital treatment is essentially the same for UFH and LMWH when all necessary resources are considered; however, hospital stay can be reduced substantially or prevented entirely through the employment of home DVT treatment programs (see Chapter 33).

Arterial thromboembolism

Arterial thromboembolic disorders, including acute coronary syndromes, differ biologically from venous thromboembolic disorders. In the former, platelets are more centrally involved with the secondary contribution of the coagulation cascade, while in the latter coagulation itself is the driving force. Accordingly, treatment strategies have been tailored specifically to biological requirements.

LMWH preparations have been investigated in extracorporeal circuits, including hemodialysis and cardiopulmonary bypass.[75–81] Patients undergoing acute or chronic hemodialysis tolerated the anticoagulant with relatively few occurrences of clotting (within the extracorporeal circuit) or serious bleeding events. Not unexpectedly given their renal clearance, anti-Factor Xa activity accumulated over time.[82] The experience with LMWH in cardiopulmonary bypass has been limited to one open-label study (15 patients). Although bypass was maintained without incident, excessive blood loss was reported despite protamine administration (the anti-Factor Xa activity of LMWH is only partially neutralized by protamine).[83]

There are several reasons why LMWH preparations may offer distinct advantages over UFH in the treatment of coronary arterial thromboembolism. First, Factor X inhibition prevents the generation of thrombin. The ability of LMWH to decrease thrombin generation in

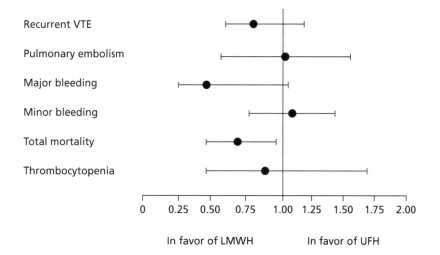

Figure 18.11 *Meta-analysis of venous thromboembolism (VTE) clinical trials comparing low-molecular-weight heparin (LMWH) and unfractionated heparin (UFH). (Reproduced with permission from Lensing AWA, Prins MH, Davidson BL, Hirsh J. Treatment of deep venous thrombosis with low-molecular-weight heparins.* Arch Intern Med *1995;* **155***: 601–7.)*

platelet-rich plasma has been documented.[84] (This is particularly evident in doses of ≥ 1 mg/kg.) Second, thrombin activity can be suppressed by LMWH, even in the presence of activated platelets.[85] Indeed, platelet factor 4 is less likely to inhibit LMWH anticoagulant activity compared with UFH. Further, LMWHs are less likely to activate platelets than UFH.[86,87] Lastly, LMWH anticoagulant activity persists in the presence of acute-phase proteins (histidine-rich glycoproteins, fibronectin, vitronectin, and von Willebrand factor), which exist commonly in acute coronary syndromes.[88] Work in our laboratory suggests that LMWH, in plasma concentrations achieved in patients receiving 1.0–1.5 mg/kg subcutaneously, inhibits platelet-mediated prothrombinase assembly and Factor Xa-mediated thrombin generation more effectively than UFH.[89]

Unstable angina/non-ST segment elevation MI

The original experience with LMWH[90] included 205 patients with unstable angina who were randomized to either aspirin (200 mg daily); aspirin (200 mg daily) plus UFH (5000 U bolus, 400 U/kg per day infusion) or high-dose nadroparin (214 IU/kg twice daily by subcutaneous injection) plus aspirin (200 mg daily). Patients underwent continuous ST-segment monitoring during the first 48 hours of treatment. Overall, 73 per cent of patients receiving LMWH were free from ischemic events, compared with 39 per cent of those receiving UFH and 40 per cent of patients given aspirin alone. There were fewer silent ischemic events in the LMWH group (18 per cent) compared with those receiving unfractionated heparin (29 per cent) or aspirin alone (34 per cent). Recurrent angina occurred in 9, 26, and 19 per cent of patients, respectively, and MIs were not observed in LMWH-treated patients (compared with 1 per cent in the UFH and 6 per cent in the aspirin-alone groups). Major bleeding occurred infrequently in all the treatment groups.

A larger study, FRagmin during InStability in Coronary artery disease (FRISC)-I,[91] included 1506 patients with unstable angina and non-ST segment elevation MI who were randomized to LMWH (dalteparin, Fragmin®, 120 IU/kg body weight sc (maximum 10 000 IU) twice daily for 6 days, then 7500 IU once daily for 35–45 days) or placebo. All patients received aspirin (300 mg first dose, 75 mg daily thereafter). The risk of death or MI was reduced by 63 per cent at day 6. The probability of death, MI and need for revascularization remained lower in the LMWH-treated patients at 40 days; however, little difference between groups was observed beyond the treatment period. A subgroup analysis revealed that the benefit was confined to non-smokers (80 per cent of the total population). Survival analysis revealed a risk of reactivation (recurrent myocardial ischemia) and reinfarction when the dose was reduced (at day 7). At 4–5 months after the completion of treatment, there were no significant differences in the rates of death, new MI, or revascularization.

In the FRIC (FRagmin In unstable Coronary artery disease) Study,[92] 1482 patients with unstable angina and non-ST segment elevation MI were assigned either twice-daily weight-adjusted sc injections of LMWH (dalteparin, Fragmin® 120 IU/kg) or dose-adjusted (target activated partial thromboplastin time (aPTT) 1.5 times the control) iv UFH for 6 days (acute treatment phase). Patients randomized to iv received a continuous infusion for at least 48 hours and were given the option of either continuing the infusion or changing to a sc regimen (12 500 U every 12 hours). In the double-blind comparison that took place from days 6 to 45 (prolonged treatment phase) patients received either LMWH (dalteparin, Fragmin®; 7500 IU sc once daily) or placebo. Aspirin (75–165 mg/day) was started in all patients as early as possible after hospital admission and continued throughout the study. During the first 6 days, the rate of death, recurrent angina and MI was 7.6 per cent in the UFH-treated patients and 9.3 per cent in the LMWH-treated patients (relative risk 1.18; 95 per cent CI 0.84–1.66). Revascularization was required in 5.3 per cent and 4.8 per cent of patients, respectively (relative risk 0.88; 95 per cent CI 0.57–1.35). Between days 6 and 45, the composite end point was reached in 12.3 per cent of patients in both the LMWH and placebo groups. Revascularization procedures were undertaken in 14.2 and 14.3 per cent of patients, respectively.

The ESSENCE (Efficacy and Safety of Subcutaneous Enoxaparin in Non-Q Wave Coronary Events) trial[93] randomly assigned 3171 patients with angina at rest or non-ST segment elevation MI to either LMWH (Enoxaparin, Lovenox® 1 mg/kg sc twice daily) or iv unfractionated heparin (target aPTT 55–85 seconds). Therapy was continued for a minimum of 48 hours (maximum 8 days). All patients received aspirin (100–325 mg daily). The median duration of therapy for both groups was 2.6 days. At 14 days the risk of death, recurrent angina or MI was 16.6 per cent among patients receiving LMWH and 19.8 per cent for patients given iv unfractionated heparin (16 per cent risk reduction). A similar risk reduction (15.0 per cent) for the composite outcome was observed at 30 days (Fig. 18.12). The need for revascularization procedures within the first 30 days was also lower in LMWH-treated patients (27 vs 32.2 per cent).

The TIMI 11B Study, compared enoxaparin and UFH in 3910 patients with unstable angina and non-ST segment elevation MI.[94] The trial design had several unique features compared with ESSENCE. First, enoxaparin therapy was inititated with a 30 mg iv bolus, followed by 1.0 mg/kg sc twice daily. Second, UFH treatment was given according to a weight-adjusted dosing strategy. Lastly, there was an out-of-hospital treatment phase comparing enoxaparin and placebo for approximately 6 weeks. Treatment with enoxaparin was associ-

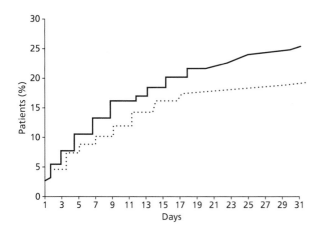

Figure 18.12 *Composite clinical outcome of death, MI, or recurrent angina in patients treated with either unfractionated heparin (——) or enoxaparin (....). (Reproduced with permission from Cohen M, et al., for the ESSENCE Investigators. A comparison of low-molecular-weight heparin with unfractionated heparin for unstable coronary artery disease.* N Engl J Med *1997;* **337***: 447–52.)*

ated with a significant reduction in the composite outcome of death, MI, or urgent revascularization compared with UFH. Although continued treatment beyond the initial hospital phase did not provide added benefit, a meta-analysis of the ESSENCE and TIMI 11B data show conclusively that the likelihood of death or MI at 7, 14, and 43 days is 15–20 per cent lower with enoxaparin than UFH.

The FRAXIS (Fraxiparine in Ischemic Syndromes)[95] study compared the efficacy of nadroparin versus UFH in 3468 patients with non-ST segment elevation ACS. Patients were randomized to either UFH, 6-day treatment with nadroparin (86 IU/kg iv bolus, 86 IU/kg sc twice daily) or 14-day treatment with nadroparin. The combined outcome of cardiovascular death, MI, and recurrent/refractory angina at 14 days occurred in 18.1, 17.8, and 20 per cent of patients, respectively (no significant difference). Hemorrhagic events were more common in patients receiving nadroparin for 14 days.

LMWH-coupled coronary interventions
The FRISC II (FRagmin and fast revascularization during InStability in Coronary artery disease)[96] included 2267 patients with unstable coronary disease who received 5 days of dalteparin (120 IU/kg sc q12h) and were then randomized to either an invasive or conservative treatment strategy. In a separate randomization, patients received either dalteparin (5000 to 7500 IU sc q12h) or placebo injections for 3 months. By 30 days there was a significant reduction in death or MI favoring dalteparin-treated patients (3.1 *vs* 5.9 per cent; *P* = 0.002). The benefit decayed over the next 2 months. An invasive strategy (coronary angiography and revascularization) was asso-

ciated with a significant reduction in death or MI at 6 months compared with ischemia-driven revascularization (9.4 *vs* 12.1 per cent, *P* = 0.03). The mortality rates were 1.9 per cent and 2.9 per cent, respectively.[97]

ST segment elevation MI, conjunctive therapy with fibrinolytics
Rethrombosis of the infarct-related coronary artery after fibrinolysis is a recognized problem and major limitation of current treatment strategies. The effect of LMWH as adjunctive treatment with tPA was investigated in a dog model of electrically induced coronary thrombosis.[98] Reperfusion occurred earlier and was more likely to be sustained in animals receiving LMWH (dalteparin 75 IU/kg over 90 minutes); however, there was evidence of residual luminal thrombosis, even with LMWH administration.

There is a growing but modest experience with LMWH as adjunctive therapy with fibrinolytics in humans. A large-scale clinical trial, Heparins and Reperfusion Therapy (HART-2), addressed the potential benefit of enoxaparin when combined with tPA (accelerated dosing strategy) using early angiographic patency and subsequent reocclusion as clinical end points. A total of 400 patients with ST segment elevation MI received tPA and were then randomized to either enoxaparin (30 mg iv bolus; 1 mg/kg sc q12h for 72 hours) or UFH (target aPTT 2–3 × control). Although the 90-minute angiographic TIMI 3 flow rates were equivalent (47.6 *vs* 52.9 per cent), fewer patients achieving TIMI 3 flow at 90 minutes experienced coronary reocclusion by 7 days in the enoxaparin-treated group (3.1 *vs* 9.1 per cent; *P* = 0.10). Major hemorrhage also occurred with lower frequency in those receiving enoxaparin than UFH.[99]

A study of 103 patients with ST segment elevation MI receiving streptokinase reported that enoxaparin (40 mg sc daily) given for 25 days after discharge reduced the incidence of recurrent cardiac events (MI, unstable angina) without an increased risk of bleeding. The benefit derived from LMWH was greatest among patients with an anterior site of infarction.[100]

A separate study of 300 patients,[101] all of whom received fibrinolytic therapy, compared iv UFH (30 000 units per 24 hours) and enoxaparin (40 mg iv followed by 40 mg sc every 8 hours) for a total of 96 hours. The composite cardiac event rate (death, non-fatal MI, readmission for unstable angina) was lower in LMWH-treated than the iv UFH-treated patients (38 per cent *vs* 55 per cent; *P* = 0.04). The rates of hemorrhage did not differ significantly between the treatment groups.

Undoubtedly, the clinical experience with LMWH and fibrinolytics will need to be investigated in greater detail before any conclusions can be drawn or recommendations for their use can be made. Ongoing large-scale clinical trials of patients with unstable angina/non-ST segment elevation MI will likely provide vital information on dosing; however, only carefully designed studies can determine safety and efficacy. It has become increasingly evident over the past decade that the pathobiology of acute ST segment elevation and non-ST segment elevation MI, although part of a similar spectrum, are unique in their own right.

The available information, based on nearly 15 000 patients with non-ST segment elevation acute coronary syndromes shows that subcutaneous weight-adjusted LMWH is as safe and effective as intravenous UFH. The superiority of enoxaparin in two large-scale clinical trials suggests further that high-risk patient subsets (ST segment shifts, troponin positivity, diabetics) derive added benefit from treatment with LMWH. The logistic ease of administration without a need for coagulation monitoring[102–105] in a majority of patients are attractive features for clinicians in practice (Fig. 18.13).[106]

It does appear, however, that the benefit of LMWH treatment is greatest during the 'active' or 'thrombotic' stage of ACS. With passing time from the acute event, the risk–benefit relationship associated with continued therapy (beyond 30 days) is much less favorable.

Minimizing bleeding risk with LMWH administration

Clinical studies have shown that a bleeding risk *does* exist with LMWH administration particularly when given in high doses.[107–113]

The ability to predict hemorrhagic risk based on plasma anti-Factor Xa activity is an important consideration. In at least three clinical studies,[70,110,111] hemorrhagic events were associated with high plasma activity (steady-state level >0.4 aXa U/mL). The association between plasma anti-Factor Xa activity and hemorrhagic complications has been observed in both prophylaxis and treatment for venous thromboembolism.[114–116]

There is a large experience examining the safety of LMWH among patients with arterial thromboembolism. This body of information is of particular importance given the high frequency of invasive procedures, including cardiac catheterization, coronary angioplasty, and bypass grafting in patients with ACS, as well as the potential use of fibrinolytics upon sudden development of ST segment elevation MI.

The TIMI 11A Study[117] compared the safety and tolerability of enoxaparin in patients with unstable angina and non-ST segment elevation MI. In an initial cohort of 320 patients receiving 1.25 mg/kg every 12 hours, the rate of major bleeding was 7.2 per cent and occurred predominantly at instrumented sites (femoral artery). In a second cohort of 309 patients receiving 1.0 mg/kg every 12 hours, the rate of major hemorrhage was reduced to 2.6 per cent, suggesting that safety may be an issue with higher doses, particularly in patients undergoing invasive procedures.

In ESSENCE,[93] the 30-day incidence of major bleeding complications was 6.5 per cent in the LMWH-treated patients and 7.0 per cent in UFH-treated patients (not statistically different). The overall incidence of bleeding (including ecchymosis at injection sites) was 18.4 per cent and 14.2 per cent, respectively. Similarly, in TIMI 11B[94] the likelihood of major hemorrhage was no higher in enoxaparin-treated patients than in those given UFH. Continued treatment beyond the acute (hospital) phase did increase the incidence of minor hemorrhage.

The safety of LMWH administration, like any other anticoagulant, is strongly influenced by patient selection and clinical judgement. Subjecting patients at high risk for hemorrhage to systemic anticoagulation or using doses beyond those found to be safe in carefully designed clinical trials will have predictable consequences.

Heparinoids

Derivatives of heparin, known as heparinoids, have been under investigation for several decades. *Heparan sulfate*, a glycosaminoglycan, neutralizes both thrombin and Factor Xa. A subfraction of heparan sulfate contains the pentasaccharide sequence, common to UFH and LMWH, that has significant affinity for antithrombin. It has been suggested that heparan sulfate also increases fibrinolytic activity. *Dermatan sulfate* has no affinity for antithrombin; however, it accelerates thrombin inhibition by interacting with heparin co-factor II, another natural inhibitor present in plasma. Interestingly,

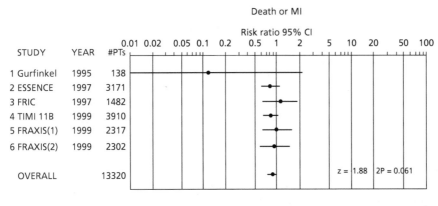

Figure 18.13 *Comparative clinical trials of LMWH and UFH in patients with non-ST segment elevation acute coronary syndromes. LMWH = low-molecular-weight heparin; UFH = unfractionated heparin.*

dermatan sulfate has no effect on ^{45}Ca release from fetal rat calvaria,[118] which may translate to an absence of osteoporosis with long-term administration. In a comparative study, both dermatan and heparan sulfate had relatively weaker antihemostatic effects and greater antithrombotic effects than UFH.[119]

Danaparoid sodium (Orgaran®), a mixture of heparan sulfate (84 per cent), dermatan sulfate (12 per cent) and chondroitin sulfate (4 per cent), is derived from the intestinal mucosa of swine. Danaparoid sodium is a more selective inhibitor of Factor Xa then either UFH or LMWH, with a 28:1 anti-Factor Xa-to-thrombin ratio, and has close to 100 per cent bioavailability following sc administration. Elimination occurs both by renal and non-renal routes with an elimination half-life (24.5 ± 9.6 hours) of anti-Factor Xa activity. Danaparoid sodium administered twice daily by sc route at a dose of 750 anti-Factor Xa units, was found to be safe and to reduce the development of DVT when compared to placebo in patients undergoing elective total hip replacement. Similarly, it was found to be more effective for the prevention of postoperative thromboembolism in patients undergoing surgery for fractured hips, and at least as safe as aspirin.[120] In the *treatment* of venous thromboembolism a significant reduction in recurrence or extension of thrombi was seen in patients receiving a high-dose danaparoid regimen when compared to iv UFH (13 per cent *vs* 28 per cent).[121] Danaparoid, which is free of contaminating heparin, has been shown to have a very low rate of *in vitro* cross-reactivity (~10 per cent) with the serum from patients with heparin-induced thrombocytopenia (HIT), compared with ~75 per cent for LMWH. It has already been used successfully in patients with HIT;[122] however, laboratory testing for cross-reactivity is suggested prior to initiating treatment. There is limited information available concerning the laboratory monitoring of heparinoids or on potential antidotes, although plasmapheresis has been considered the treatment of choice for life-threatening hemorrhage.

DIRECT THROMBIN ANTAGONISTS

Direct thrombin inhibitors have stable anticoagulant activities and predictable pharmacokinetics, they lack a direct effect on platelet function, and have uniformity of composition and activity for each preparation.[123] The largest clinical experience with direct thrombin antagonists has accumulated with hirudin, bivalirudin, and argatroban.

Hirudin and its derivatives

Hirudin is coined from the parapharyngeal gland of the medicinal leech *Hirudo medicinalis*. A number of derivatives and recombinant hirudin preparations have been developed and investigated: hirugen, a synthetic C-terminal peptide fragment of hirudin; bivalirudin, a derivative of hirugen; and the following recombinant preparations: desirudin (CGP 39393), Lepirudin (HBW 023, Refludan®), PEG-hirudin, a chemically defined conjugate of recombinant hirudin (r-hirudin) and two molecules of polyethylene glycol to confer longer duration of action; and albumin r-hirudin fused molecules, again with longer half-lives.

MODE OF ACTION AND PHARMACOKINETICS

Hirudin is a potent direct inhibitor of thrombin that is capable of neutralizing thrombin faster than the physiologic reaction that takes place between thrombin and fibrinogen. This unique property stems from its binding to thrombin's catalytic *and* fibrinogen-binding sites (hirugen and bivalirudin bind only to the fibrinogen-binding site). Hirudin also displaces thrombin from fibrinogen and from its cellular receptors, and inhibits the activation of Factors V, VIII and XIII. It is antithrombin-independent and devoid of anti-Factor Xa activity. Although hirudin does not inhibit other activated clotting factors it does inhibit thrombin-activation of platelets (but not their activation by other agonists). Hirudin's ability to inactivate clot-bound thrombin, contrary to all heparins, may confer an advantage in the *treatment* of thromboembolism.

Hirudin can be administered by either the iv or sc routes. The bioavailability of hirudin after sc injection is 85–90 per cent with peak concentrations reached after 1–2 hours and a terminal half-life of 2–3 hours. After sc injection of 0.1 mg/kg desirudin, the aPTT was prolonged to almost twice its basal value. In subjects administered lepirudin by iv bolus, iv infusion, or sc injection, maximum aPTT prolongations were achieved at 10 minutes, 3–6 hours, and 2–3 hours, respectively. With multiple daily injections, the aPTT returned to normal after 16 hours after the last injection, suggesting that its pharmacodynamic and pharmacokinetic effects are not cumulative. Hirudin is cleared predominantly by the kidneys, dictating dosing adjustments among patients with impaired kidney function.

LABORATORY MONITORING

The potency of hirudin derivatives can be expressed in thrombin inhibitory units (TIU). One TIU inhibits one international unit of thrombin. Within the range of hirudin concentrations achieved in clinical trials, aPTT prologation and hirudin concentration correlated fairly well. As a result, the aPTT is used in clinical practice for dose titration. The activated clotting time (ACT) can also be used in patients undergoing percutaneous coronary interventions and bypass surgery;[124] however, the dose–response is shallow, creating challenges for interventionalists and perfusionists. Ecarin clotting time

(ECT), based on the property of a venom extracted from the snake *Echis carinatus* to convert prothrombin to thrombin, although not widely used, may offer distinct advantages in dose titration because it is much less sensitive to heparin then it is to hirudin and it correlates closely with plasma hirudin concentration. The thrombin time is too sensitive for use in patient care and the prothrombin time is not sensitive enough.

CLINICAL EXPERIENCE

The favorable trends that accompanied hirudin administered adjunctively with either tPA or streptokinase in TIMI 5[125] and TIMI 6,[126] respectively, paved the way for large, phase III clinical trials. Early in the experience, however, it became clear that the combination of fibrinolytic therapy and high-dose hirudin increased hemorrhagic risk. In fact, the TIMI 9A,[127] GUSTO IIA (Table 18.5),[128] and HIT III[129] trials were stopped prematurely because of an unacceptable incidence of serious bleeding.

In TIMI 9B,[130] 3002 patients with acute MI ($\leqslant$12 hours from symptom onset) were treated with aspirin and either accelerated tPA or streptokinase. They were randomized to receive either iv heparin (5000 U bolus, 1000 U/hour infusion) or hirudin (0.1 mg/kg bolus, 0.1 mg/kg per hour infusions) titrated to an aPTT of 55–85 seconds. The primary end point (recurrent MI, death, or the development of severe congestive heart failure or cardiogenic shock) occurred in 11.9 per cent of heparin-

and 12.9 per cent of hirudin-treated patients (P = N.S.). The rate of major and intracranial hemorrhage was similar (5.3 per cent and 0.9 per cent; heparin group) and (4.6 per cent and 0.4 per cent; hirudin group).

In the GUSTO IIb trial,[131] 12 142 patients with acute coronary syndromes were stratified according to the presence of ST segment elevation on the presenting electrocardiogram. Patients with ST segment elevation received reperfusion therapy (fibrinolytics or percutaneous coronary intervention) and either heparin or hirudin (0.1 mg/kg bolus, 0.1 mg/kg per hour infusion). Patients without ST segment elevation (representing a group with unstable angina or non-ST segment elevation MI) received either heparin or hirudin. At 24 hours, the risk of death or MI was lower in hirudin-treated patients (1.3 per cent *vs* 2.1 per cent; P = 0.001). The primary end point of death or non-fatal MI at 30 days was reached in 9.8 per cent of the heparin group and 8.9 per cent of the hirudin group (odds ratio 0.89; P = 0.06) (Fig. 18.14 a, b and c). Hirudin therapy was associated with a higher incidence of moderate bleeding than heparin (8.8 per cent *vs* 7.7 per cent, P = 0.03).

The OASIS-1 (Organization to Assess Strategies for Ischemic Syndromes),[132] included 909 patients with unstable angina or suspected MI without ST segment elevation who were randomized to receive heparin (5000 U bolus, 1000–1200 U/hour infusion), low-dose hirudin (0.2 mg/kg bolus, 0.1 mg/kg per hour infusion) or medium-dose hirudin (0.4 mg/kg bolus, 0.15 mg/kg per hour infusion). At 7 days, 6.5 per cent of patients in the

Table 18.5 *Incidence of hemorrhagic stroke: GUSTO IIA. (Reproduced from The GUSTO Investigators. An international randomized trial compared four thrombolytic strategies for acute myocardial infarction.* N Engl J Med *1993;* **329**: *673–82)*

	Heparin	Hirudin	Corresponding GUSTO 1 data
Total patients, *n*	1291	1273	*a*
Hemorrhagic stroke, *n* (%)	9 (0.7)	17 (1.3)	
95% CI	0.2–1.2	0.7–2.0	
Thrombolytics only*b*			
Patients, *n*	620	644	30 893
Hemorrhagic stroke, *n* (%)	9 (1.5)	14 (2.2)	223 (0.7)
95% CI	0.5–2.4	1.0–3.3	0.6–0.8
Thrombolytic agent tPA			
Patients, *n* (%)	426	460	10 376
Hemorrhagic stroke, *n* (%)	4 (0.9)	8 (1.7)	73 (0.7)
95% CI	0–1.8	0.5–2.9	0.5–0.9
Thrombolytic agent SK			
Patients, *n* (%)	189	189	10 393
Hemorrhagic stroke, *n* (%)	5 (2.7)	6 (3.2)	59 (0.6)
95% CI	0.4–4.9	0.7–5.7	0.4–0.7

*a*Does not apply – all patients received thrombolytics.
*b*The incidence for combined thrombolytics in GUSTO IIa was 1.8% (95% CI, 1.1–2.6).
A limited number of patients in both groups received both tPA and SK.
tPA = tissue plasminogen activator; SK = streptokinase.

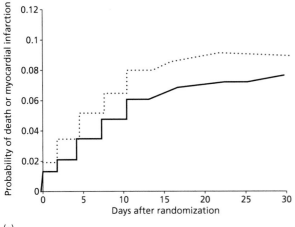

(a)

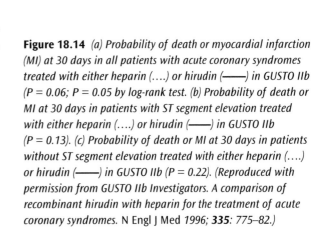

(b)

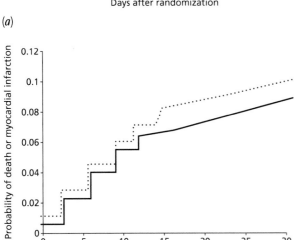

(c)

Figure 18.14 *(a) Probability of death or myocardial infarction (MI) at 30 days in all patients with acute coronary syndromes treated with either heparin (....) or hirudin (———) in GUSTO IIb (P = 0.06; P = 0.05 by log-rank test). (b) Probability of death or MI at 30 days in patients with ST segment elevation treated with either heparin (....) or hirudin (———) in GUSTO IIb (P = 0.13). (c) Probability of death or MI at 30 days in patients without ST segment elevation treated with either heparin (....) or hirudin (———) in GUSTO IIb (P = 0.22). (Reproduced with permission from GUSTO IIb Investigators. A comparison of recombinant hirudin with heparin for the treatment of acute coronary syndromes. N Engl J Med 1996; **335**: 775–82.)*

heparin group, 4.4 per cent of patients in the low-dose hirudin group, and 3.0 per cent (P = 0.047) of patients in the moderate-dose hirudin group suffered MI, death, or refractory angina. The differences between moderate-dose hirudin and heparin persisted at 180 days. A larger trial, OASIS-2, confirmed the early benefit (and safety) of moderate-dose hirudin in patients with unstable angina and non-ST segment elevation MI.[133]

Although the future development and approval of hirudin in acute coronary syndromes are uncertain, its use among patients with heparin-induced thrombocytopenia and as a means to prevent deep venous thrombosis are more secure.

BIVALIRUDIN

The hirudin derivative, bivalirudin, is a 20-amino-acid peptide that inhibits thrombin directly. The efficacy and safety of bivalirudin have been evaluated in several clinical trials of unstable angina, MI, and percutaneous coronary interventions (PCI).[134,135] A total of six trials (5674 patients) represent the randomized, controlled bivalirudin experience in ischemic heart disease. In trials that compared bivalirudin and UFH (4973 patients), the

former was associated with a significant reduction in the composite of death or MI (OR 0.73, 95 per cent CI 0.57–0.95; P = 0.02). There was also a reduction in major hemorrhage.[136] The totality of evidence support consideration of bivalirudin use in patients with coronary artery disease undergoing high-risk PCI.

ARGATROBAN (ARGIDIPIN, NOVASTAN®)

Argatroban belongs to a class of peptidomimetics that also includes inogatran, efegatran and napsagatran. Argatroban has been extensively characterized in both preclinical and clinical investigations. Like hirudin, this agent does not bind appreciably to plasma proteins, does not cause immune-mediated thrombocytopenia, and does not require antithrombin for production of an anticoagulant effect. Argatroban binds clot-bound thrombin and prevents thrombin-mediated platelet activation. It prolongs the prothrombin time (PT), aPTT, and thrombin time in a dose-dependent manner when infused intravenously.

Clinical experience

A trial of 50 patients with heparin-induced thrombocytopenia[137] yielded encouraging results in the setting of PCI. All patients received argatroban at a dose of 350 µg/kg (bolus) and a majority (98 per cent) achieved a successful outcome. In the MINT (Myocardial Infarction with Novastan and TPA) Study[138] low- and high-dose argatroban yielded 90-minute TIMI grade 3 flow rates approaching 60 per cent. The rate of serious hemorrhage was similar to that observed in patients receiving UFH.

Argatroban has been approved by the FDA for use in patients with heparin-induced thrombocytopenia.

PLATELET ANTAGONISTS

Platelet activation can be accomplished via a wide variety of pharmacologic and mechanical mediators and represents an important step toward platelet adhesion and ultimately aggregation. The ability of platelets to adhere (to abnormal surfaces) and aggregate is mediated by surface membrane glycoprotein (GP) receptors (Table 18.6) that can be expressed in greater numbers with platelet activation and serve as potential targets for therapy. The platelet GPIIb/IIIa receptor is of particular interest because of its key role in platelet aggregation.[139–142]

Platelet glycoprotein IIb/IIIa antagonists

The first-generation of platelet GPIIb/IIIa antagonists were murine monoclonal antibodies. Second-generation antibodies lacked the Fc fragment, which was removed to prevent antigenicity, and the Fab fragments were joined with the constant regions of human immunoglobulin forming a chimeric compound designated abciximab or c7E3.

ABCIXIMAB

Abciximab, ReoPro®, is the Fab fragment of the chimeric human–murine monoclonal antibody 7E3. It is produced by continuous perfusion in mammalian cell culture.

Pharmacokinetics

Following intravenous bolus administration, free plasma concentrations of abciximab decrease rapidly with an initial half-life of less than 10 minutes and a second phase half-life of 30 minutes, probably related to rapid binding to the platelet GPIIb/IIIa receptor. Platelet function generally recovers over the course of 48 hours; however, abciximab remains in the circulation up to 10 days in the platelet-bound state. Upon completion of a constant infusion, free plasma concentrations fall rapidly over the next 6 hours then decline at a slower rate.

Pharmacodynamics

Intravenous administration of abciximab in doses ranging from 0.15 mg/kg to 0.3 mg/kg produces a rapid dose-dependent inhibition of platelet function as measured by *ex vivo* platelet aggregation in response to ADP. At the highest dose, 80 per cent of the platelet GPIIb/IIIa receptors are occupied within 2 hours and platelet aggregation, even with 20 mM ADP is completely inhibited. Sustained inhibition is achieved with prolonged infusions (12–24 hours) and low-level receptor blockade is present for up to 10 days following cessation of the infusion. Platelet aggregation in response to 5.0 mM ADP returns to ≥50 per cent of baseline within 24 hours in a majority of cases.

Clinical experience

Following a series of experiments in animals demonstrating superiority over aspirin, and equally promising results in human phase I and II studies, a double-blind placebo-controlled phase III trial, EPIC (Evaluation of

Table 18.6 *Surface membrane glycoprotein (GP) receptors involved with normal platelet physiology*

Receptor	Ligand	Integrin components	Receptors per platelet	Biologic action
GPIa–IIa	Collagen	$\alpha_2\beta_1$	21 000	Adhesion
GPIb–IX	Von Willebrand factor	—	25 000	Adhesion
GPIc–IIa	Fibronectin	$\alpha_2\beta_1$	21 000	Adhesion
GPIIb–IIIa	Collagen	$\alpha_{IIb}\beta_3$	50 000	Aggregation (2° role in adhesion)
	Fibrinogen			
	Fibronectin			
	Vitronectin			
	Von Willebrand factor			
GPIV (GPIIb)	Thrombospondin collagen	—	~100	Adhesion
Vitronectin receptor	Vitronectin Thrombospandin	$\alpha_v\beta_3$	~100	Adhesion
VLA-6	Laminin	$\alpha_6\beta_1$	~100	Adhesion

Table 18.7 *Primary outcome events for patients participating in the EPIC study. (Reproduced with permission from The EPIC Investigators. Use of a monoclonal antibody directed against the platelet glycoprotein IIb/IIIa receptor in high-risk coronary angioplasty.* N Engl J Med *1994;* **330***: 956–61)*

Event	Placebo, n = 696 (%)	c7E3 Fab bolus, n = 695 (%)	c7E3 Fab bolus and infusion n = 708 (%)	P value for dose response
Primary end point	89 (12.8)	79 (11.4)	59 (8.3)	0.009[a]
Components of primary end point				
Death	12 (1.7)	9 (1.3)	12 (1.7)	0.96
Non-fatal myocardial infarction	60 (8.6)	43 (6.2)	37 (5.2)	0.013
Q wave	16 (2.3)	7 (1.0)	6 (0.8)	0.020
Large non-Q wave	28 (4.0)	19 (2.7)	21 (3.0)	0.265
Small non-Q wave	16 (2.3)	17 (2.4)	10 (1.4)	0.239
Emergency PTCA	31 (4.5)	25 (3.6)	6 (0.8)	<0.001
Emergency CABG	25 (3.6)	16 (2.3)	17 (2.4)	0.177
Stent placement	4 (0.6)	12 (1.7)	4 (0.6)	0.98
Balloon-pump insertion	1 (0.1)	1 (0.1)	1 (0.1)	0.99

[a]P = 0.009 for overall test for trend, P = 0.43 for comparison of the placebo group with the group given the bolus only, and P = 0.0088 for comparison of the placebo group with the group given the bolus and infusion.
PTCA = percutaneous transluminal coronary angioplasty or atherectomy; CABG = coronary artery bypass grafting.

c7E3 Fab for the Prevention of Ischemic Complications) was performed.[143] In nearly 2100 patients undergoing either balloon coronary angioplasty or atherectomy who were judged to be at high risk for ischemic (thrombotic) complications, a bolus of c7E3 (0.25 mg/kg) followed by a 12-hour continuous infusion (10 µg/minute) was found to reduce the occurrence of death, MI, or the need for an urgent intervention (repeat PCI, stent placement, balloon pump insertion, or bypass grafting) by 35 per cent (Table 18.7, Fig. 18.15). At 6 months,[144] the absolute

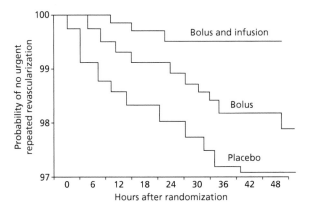

Figure 18.15 *The platelet GPIIb/IIIa receptor antagonist, abciximab, when given as a bolus and 12-hour infusion significantly reduced the need for urgent repeat revascularization in patients undergoing high-risk angioplasty. (Reproduced with permission from The EPIC Investigators. Use of a monoclonal antibody directed against the platelet glycoprotein IIb/IIIa receptor in high-risk coronary angioplasty.* N Engl J Med *1994;* **330***: 956–61.)*

difference in patients with a major ischemic event or elective revascularization was 8.1 per cent comparing patients who received abciximab (bolus plus infusion) with those given placebo (35.1 per cent *vs* 27.0 per cent; 23 per cent reduction) (all patients received aspirin and heparin during the procedure). Further, at 3 years,[145] composite end points occurred in 41.1 per cent of those receiving abciximab bolus plus infusion; 47.4 per cent of those receiving abciximab bolus only; and 47.2 per cent of those receiving placebo. The greatest benefit was observed in patients with refractory angina or evolving MI (Table 18.8).

The EPILOG (Evaluation in PTCA to Improve Long-term Outcome with Abciximab GPIIb/IIIa Blockade) study[146] included 2792 patients undergoing elective or urgent percutaneous coronary revascularization who received either abciximab with standard, weight-adjusted heparin (initial bolus 100 U/kg); abciximab with low-dose, weight-adjusted heparin (initial bolus 70 U/kg); or placebo with standard dose, weight-adjusted heparin. At 30 days the composite event rate was 5.4 per cent, 5.2 per cent, and 11.7 per cent, respectively. The benefit was observed in both high-risk and low-risk patients, suggesting that GPIIb/IIIa blockade has a broad clinical use in reducing ischemic complications associated with coronary revascularization.

The CAPTURE (c7E3 Fab Antiplatelet Therapy in Unstable Refractory Angina) study[147,148] was uniquely designed to assess whether abciximab, given during the 18–24 hours before angioplasty could improve outcome in patients with refractory (myocardial ischemia despite nitrates, heparin, and aspirin) unstable angina. A total of 1265 patients (of 1400 scheduled) were randomly assigned to abciximab or placebo. By 30 days, the

Table 18.8 *Clinical outcomes: death/myocardial infarction/any coronary revascularization: EPIC study. (Reproduced with permission from Topol EJ, et al., for the EPIC Investigator Group. Long-term protection from myocardial ischemic events in a randomized trial of brief integrin B₃ blockade with percutaneous coronary intervention. JAMA 1997; **278**: 479–84)*

End point	Placebo (n = 696)	Bolus (n = 698)	Bolus + infusion (n = 708)	P value[a]	Odds ratio (95% confidence interval)[a]
Composite					
1 year	266 (38.6)	251 (36.3)	216 (30.8)	0.002	0.75 (0.63–0.90)
2 years	290 (42.3)	290 (42.4)	253 (36.3)	0.009	0.80 (0.68–0.95)
3 years	319 (47.2)	321 (47.4)	283 (41.1)	0.009	0.81 (0.69–0.95)
Death					
1 year	31 (4.5)	29 (4.2)	30 (4.2)	0.841	0.95 (0.58–1.57)
2 years	46 (6.6)	40 (5.8)	37 (5.2)	0.277	0.79 (0.51–1.22)
3 years	59 (8.6)	54 (8.0)	47 (6.8)	0.202	0.78 (0.53–1.14)
Myocardial infarction					
1 year	77 (11.2)	62 (9.0)	55 (7.9)	0.032	0.69 (0.49–0.97)
2 years	84 (12.4)	73 (10.8)	64 (9.3)	0.057	0.73 (0.53–1.01)
3 years	91 (13.6)	81 (12.2)	72 (10.7)	0.075	0.76 (0.56–1.03)
Revascularization					
1 year	221 (32.6)	207 (30.4)	178 (25.6)	0.004	0.75 (0.62–0.91)
2 years	242 (36.0)	237 (35.3)	207 (30.2)	0.013	0.79 (0.66–0.95)
3 years	265 (40.1)	256 (38.6)	234 (34.8)	0.021	0.81 (0.68–0.97)

[a]*P* values and odds ratio represent the comparison of bolus + infusion *vs* placebo. All values are numbers of patients (%) except where otherwise indicated.

primary end point (death, MI, urgent revascularization) occurred in 11.3 per cent of abciximab-treated patients and 15.9 per cent of placebo-treated patients ($P = 0.012$). The rate of MI was lower before and during PTCA in those given abciximab.

The RAPPORT (ReoPro in Acute MI and Primary PTCA Organization and Randomized Trial) Study[149] was a randomized, placebo-controlled phase IV trial of patients with ST segment elevation MI. A total of 483 patients were randomized to either ReoPro® (0.25 mg/kg bolus, 0.125 µg/kg per minute to a maximum of 10 µg/minute infusion for 12 hours) or placebo plus standard dose heparin before coronary intervention. The primary end point included the combined incidence of death, MI, and target vessel revascularization. At 30 days there was a non-significant trend favoring ReoPro® (9.9 per cent with placebo *vs* 5.8 per cent with ReoPro®, $P = 0.08$). Patients were significantly less likely to require stent placement, repeated coronary interventions and bypass grafting. The benefits of ReoPro® were maintained at 3 and 6 months. There was a significant increase in hemorrhagic complications with Abciximab that was influenced by heparin dose.

Similar to the RAPPORT trial, the ADMIRAL trial randomized 300 patients with an acute MI to abciximab or placebo prior to PTCA or stent placement.[150] At 24 hours, TIMI 3 flow rates were more frequently seen in the abciximab group (86 *vs* 78 per cent for placebo) and left ventricular ejection fraction was higher (55 *vs* 51 per cent for placebo). At 30 days, the primary end point

(death, recurrent MI, or urgent target vessel revascularization) was lower in the abciximab group (10.7 *vs* 20 per cent for placebo); abciximab favorably affected all the individual components of the end point, but was most evident in reducing the need for revascularization (6 *vs* 14 per cent).

Abciximab may also reduce the incidence of periprocedural MI in patients undergoing elective or urgent intracoronary stent placement. This was addressed in the EPISTENT trial, which randomized 2399 patients undergoing elective or emergent coronary intervention to therapy with stenting alone, stenting plus abciximab, or PTCA plus abciximab.[151] The 30-day and 6-month incidence of the primary end point (death, MI, and need for urgent revascularization) was significantly lower with the use of abciximab (10.8, 5.3, and 6.9 per cent, respectively, and 11.4, 5.6 and 7.8 per cent, respectively), primarily because of a reduced incidence of death and large non-Q wave MI. There was also a significant reduction in late lumen loss and in the need for target vessel revascularization (10.6, 8.7, and 15.4 per cent, respectively) which was primarily seen in diabetic patients. The benefit was similar in those with stable angina or an acute coronary syndrome. At 1 year, the use of adjunctive abciximab was still associated with a significant reduction in mortality (2.4, 1.0, and 2.1 per cent, respectively).

Safety profile

The primary concern for clinicians using antithrombotic therapy is the risk of bleeding. In the EPIC Study[143] major hemorrhage and transfusion requirement was increased two-fold in patients receiving abciximab (bolus plus infusion). The majority of bleeding episodes occurred during bypass surgery at the site of vascular puncture. The bleeding risk was substantially lower in EPILOG[145] when a lower dose of heparin was used and a protocol for vascular access and sheath removal was followed.

Thrombocytopenia, at times profound (1×10^9/L), has been observed within 24 hours of abciximab administration[152] in some cases, and abrupt decrease has occurred within several hours. Accordingly, a platelet count should be checked within 2–4 hours following the initial bolus and daily thereafter (or prior to discharge, whichever is first).

The readministration of GPIIb/IIIa antagonists, evaluated in several large scale registries, appears to be safe; however, patients experiencing thrombocytopenia with an initial treatment should not be re-exposed.

LAMIFIBAN

Lamifiban is part of a new class of GPIIb/IIIa antagonists that lack peptide bonds. The potential advantage of the 'peptidomimetic' inhibitors are their specificity and increased circulating half-life.

Pharmacokinetics
Following intravenous administration, Lamifiban binds minimally to plasma proteins and has a relatively short terminal half-life of 84 minutes.

Pharmacodynamics
Saturation of the platelet GPIIb/IIIa receptor takes place at relatively low concentrations of Lamifiban and ADP-induced aggregation declines to 10 per cent of baseline within 60 minutes of infusion. A return to 50 per cent of baseline occurs within 5–6 hours of discontinuation.

Clinical experience
A pilot study of 365 patients with unstable angina investigated several doses of lamifiban ranging from 150 to 600 μg bolus and 1.0 to 5.0 μg/minute infusion for up to 120 hours.[153] Lamifiban (all doses combined) reduced the risk of death, non-fatal MI, or the need for urgent revascularization (during the infusion period) from 8.1 to 3.3 per cent. At 1 month, death or non-fatal MI occurred in 8.1 per cent of patients given placebo and 2.5 per cent with the two highest doses of lamifiban.

Two large-scale, randomized phase II trials of patients with acute MI receiving fibrinolytics (PARADIGM; Platelet Aggregation Receptor Antagonist Dose Investigation for Reperfusion Gain in Myocardial Infarction) and unstable angina/non-ST segment elevation MI (PARAGON A; Platelet IIb/IIIa Antagonist for the Reduction of Acute Coronary Syndrome Events in a Global Organization Network) have been completed.[154,155] In the former study, encouraging findings concerning coronary arterial reperfusion emerged while the latter failed to document a clear early advantage in favor of lamifiban (with or without heparin). Re-evaluation of the data did identify an early benefit associated with low-dose lamifiban administration in the PARAGON A Study. In addition, a beneficial effect was appreciated at 6-month follow-up. The PARAGON B Study included 5225 patients with non-ST segment elevation ACS. Overall there were no differences in outcome (death, MI, severe recurrent ischemia, hemorrhage) between patients receiving lamifiban (and UFH) and those receiving placebo (UFH).[156]

Safety profile
In the Canadian Lamifiban study,[153] major hemorrhage occurred in 2.9 per cent of patients treated with lamifiban (all in the 4 μg/minute infusion group) and 0.8 per cent of patients treated with placebo. Concomitant heparin administration affected the bleeding rates significantly.

FRADAFIBAN

Fradafiban is a non-peptide mimetic of the arginine–glycine–aspartic acid recognition sequence.[157]

Pharmacokinetics
Following intravenous administration fradafiban reversibly binds to platelet GPIIb/IIIa receptors with a K_d value of 148 nM/L. Both binding and dissociation is rapid (<5 seconds) and reproducible for hours.

Pharmacodynamics
Single doses of 1–15 mg fradafiban administered intravenously to human volunteers produced significant occupancy of the platelet GPIIb/IIIa receptor within 30 minutes. At doses ≥ 3 mg, ADP (20 nM) induced ex vivo platelet aggregation was inhibited completely. The platelet inhibition effect persisted for several hours. Continuous iv infusions reproducibly and reversibly inhibited platelet aggregation in a dose-related manner.[157]

Clinical experience
Phase II and III studies have not been conducted.

LEFRADAFIBAN

Lefradafiban, a prodrug of fradafiban, has been evaluated as an oral platelet GPIIb/IIIa antagonist.

Pharmacokinetics
Fradafiban has limited oral activity because of its high polarity. Esterification of the carboxyl group and acylation of the amino group has yielded a far less polar prodrug, lefradafiban. However, for platelet GPIIb/IIIa receptor inhibition to occur, Lefradafiban must be converted metabolically to fradafiban by esterases (non-cytochrome P450-dependent enzymes).

Pharmacodynamics
Varying doses of lefradafiban, ranging from 10 to 150 mg, have been administered to healthy human

subjects.[157] Although platelet inhibition was not observed with low doses, a 50 mg oral dose inhibited ADP-mediated platelet aggregation by 90 ± 5 per cent at 2 hours, 59 ± 14 per cent at 8 hours, and by <10 per cent at 24 hours following administration. Platelet aggregation was completely inhibited by 75 mg and all higher doses of lefradafiban. Platelet aggregation at 32 and 48 hours did not differ from placebo treatment.

Multiple doses of lefradafiban (25–75 mg three times daily) yielded dose-dependent platelet inhibition. At the 25 mg dose, ADP-mediated platelet aggregation was inhibited by 54 ± 14 per cent at 2 hours on the first day, 69 ± 14 per cent on the second day, and 76 ± 14 per cent on the last day (day 7). Complete suppression of ADP-induced aggregation was observed in both the 50 mg and 75 mg (three times daily) dose groups on all days.

Clinical experience
Phase II and III studies have not been conducted.

TIROFIBAN

Tirofiban (Aggrastat®), a tyrosine derivative with a molecular weight of 495 kDa, is a non-peptide inhibitor of the platelet GPIIb/IIIa receptor.

Pharmacokinetics
Tirofiban, like other non-peptides, mimics the geometric, stereotactic, and change characteristics of the RGD sequence and thus interferes with platelet aggregation.

Pharmacodynamics
Three doses of tirofiban were studied in a phase I study of patients undergoing coronary angioplasty. Patients received one of three graduated regimens of tirofiban intravenously with a bolus dose of 5, 10, and 10 mg/kg and a continuous (16–24 hours) infusion of 0.05, 0.10, and 0.15 µg/kg per minute. A dose-dependent inhibition of *ex vivo* platelet aggregation was observed within minutes of bolus administration and was sustained during the continuous infusion.[158]

Clinical experience
The RESTORE trial (Randomized Efficacy Study of Tirofiban Outcomes and Restenosis)[159] was a randomized, double-blind, placebo-controlled trial of tirofiban in patients undergoing coronary interventions within 72 hours of presenting to the hospital with an acute coronary syndrome.

Patients ($n = 2139$) received tirofiban as a 10 µg/kg intravenous bolus over a 3-minute period and a continuous infusion of 0.15 µg/kg per minute over 36 hours. All patients received unfractionated heparin and aspirin. The primary composite end point (death, MI, angioplasty failure requiring bypass surgery or unplanned stent placement, recurrent ischemia requiring repeat angioplasty) at 30 days was reduced from 12.2 per cent in

the placebo group to 10.3 per cent in the tirofiban group (16 per cent relative reduction). The requirement for urgent or emergent revascularization (bypass or angioplasty) was reduced by 24 per cent and was particularly demonstrable during study drug infusion.

The PRISM (Platelet Receptor Inhibition for Ischemic Syndrome Management) trial included 3231 patients with unstable angina/non-ST segment elevation MI. All patients received aspirin and were randomized to treatment with either heparin or tirofiban, given as a loading dose of 0.6 µg/kg per minute over 30 minutes followed by a maintenance infusion of 0.15 µg/kg per minute for 48 hours (angiography/revascularization was discouraged during the infusion period). The primary composite end point (death, MI, refractory ischemia) at 48 hours was 5.9 per cent in tirofiban-treated patients and 3.8 per cent in placebo (aspirin/heparin) treated patients (risk reduction 36 per cent).[160]

The PRISM PLUS (Platelet Receptor Inhibition for Ischemic Syndrome Management PLUS) trial included 1915 patients with unstable angina and non-ST segment elevation MI who were treated with aspirin and heparin and randomized to either tirofiban (0.4 µg/kg per minute × 30 minutes; then 0.1 µg/kg per minute for a minimum of 48 hours and a maximum of 108 hours) or placebo. Angiography and revascularization were performed at the discretion of the treating physician. Tirofiban-treated patients had a lower composite event rate of 7 days than the placebo group, 12.9 per cent *vs* 17.9 per cent, risk reduction 34 per cent. The benefit was mainly due to a reduction in MI (32 per cent risk reduction) and refractory angina (47 per cent risk reduction). The benefit was maintained at 30 days (23 per cent risk reduction in composite event rate).[161]

Safety profile
In RESTORE,[159] major bleeding occurred in 5.3 per cent of tirofiban-treated patients and 3.7 per cent of placebo-treated patients ($P = 0.096$). Thrombocytopenia was documented in 1.17 per cent and 0.9 per cent of patients, respectively. The overall incidence of major hemorrhage (1.8 per cent) and thrombocytopenia (0.5 per cent) with tirofiban administration was also low in the PRISM-PLUS trial.[161]

EPTIFIBATIDE

Eptifibatide (Integrilin®) is a non-immunogenic cyclic heptapeptide with an active pharmacophore that is derived from the structure of barbourin, a platelet GPIIb/IIIa inhibitor from the venom of the Southeastern pigmy rattlesnake.[162]

Pharmacokinetics
The plasma half-life of Integrilin® is 10–15 minutes and clearance is predominantly renal (75 per cent) and hepatic (25 per cent). The antiplatelet effect has a rapid onset of action and is rapidly reversible.

Pharmacodynamics

In a pilot study of patients undergoing percutaneous coronary interventions,[163] patients were randomized to one of four Integrilin dosing schedules:

1 180 µg/kg bolus, 1.0 µg/kg per minute infusion;
2 135 µg/kg bolus, 0.5 µg/kg per minute infusion;
3 90 µg/kg bolus, 0.75 µg/kg per minute infusion;
4 135 µg/kg bolus, 0.75 µg/kg per minute infusion.

All patients received aspirin and heparin and were continued on study drug for 18–24 hours. The two highest bolus doses produced >80 per cent inhibition of ADP-mediated platelet aggregation within 15 minutes of administration in a majority (>75 per cent) of patients. A constant infusion of 0.75 µg/kg per minute maintained the antiplatelet effect, whereas an infusion of 0.50 µg/kg per minute allowed gradual recovery of platelet function. In all dosing groups, platelet-function returned to >50 per cent of baseline within 4 hours of terminating the infusion. It is important to mention that the use of citrate tubes for sample collection may have overestimated the antiplatelet effects of the doses of eptifibatide studied given the requirement for calcium displacement at RGD binding sites (on the GPIIb/IIIa receptor) prior to adhesive protein binding.

Clinical experience

Unstable angina and non-ST segment elevation MI

Patients ($n = 227$) with unstable angina receiving intravenous heparin and standard therapy were randomized to receive oral aspirin and placebo eptifibatide; placebo aspirin and low-dose eptifibatide (45 µg/kg bolus, 0.5 µg/kg per minute infusion, or placebo aspirin and high-dose eptifibatide (90 µg/kg bolus, 1.0 µg/kg per minute) for 24–72 hours in multicenter pilot study.[164] Patients randomized to high-dose eptifibatide experienced fewer ischemic episodes that were also of shorter duration (by Holter monitoring) than patients receiving aspirin. The overall number of clinical events was small in all treatment groups.

Percutaneous coronary intervention

The IMPACT-II trial (Integrilin to Minimize Platelet Aggregation and Coronary Thrombosis) enrolled 4010 patients undergoing elective, urgent or emergency coronary interventions. Patients were assigned to either placebo, a bolus of 135 µg/kg eptifibatide followed by an infusion of 0.5 µg/kg per minute for 20–24 hours, or 135 µg/kg bolus with a 0.75 µg/kg per minute infusion.[165] The intervention was begun within 60 minutes of study drug administration. By 30 days, the composite end point (death, MI, unplanned revascularization, stent placement for abrupt closure) occurred in 11.4, 9.2 and 9.9 per cent of patients, respectively. On-treatment analysis revealed significant differences in favor of the lower dose eptifibatide group and resulted in relative risk reductions on the order of 25–30 per cent for the composite end

point. Although the benefit of treatment was maintained at 6 months, the differences between groups were not statistically significant. A careful review of the data derived from IMPACT II suggests that the greatest benefit from eptifibatide administration can be expected within the initial 24–72 hours of administration by reducing abrupt vessel closure and other ischemic complications.

ST segment elevation MI

The IMPACT-AMI Study[166] was designed to determine the effect of eptifibatide on coronary arterial patency when used adjunctively with accelerated tPA. A total of 132 patients with MI received tPA, heparin, and aspirin, and were randomized to receive a bolus and continuous infusion of one of six eptifibatide doses or placebo. The doses ranged from 36 to 180 µg/kg (bolus) to 0.2 to 0.75 µg/kg minute (infusion). Study drug was started within 30 minutes of tPA administration and continued for 24 hours. The highest dose eptifibatide groups had more complete reperfusion (TIMI grade 3 flow) and shorter mean time to ST segment recovery then placebo-treated patients. The composite clinical event rate (death, reinfarction, revascularization, heart failure, hypotension, stroke) was relatively high in all groups; 44.8 per cent in eptifibatide-treated patients and 41.8 per cent in placebo-treated patients.

Acute coronary syndromes (without ST segment elevation)

The PURSUIT trial (Platelet Glycoprotein IIb/IIIa in Unstable Angina Receptor Suppression Using Integrilin Therapy)[167] included patients with unstable angina or non-ST segment elevation MI with symptoms within 24 hours and electrocardiographic changes within 12 hours (of ischemia). A total of 10 948 patients were randomized to eptifibatide 180 µg/kg bolus plus 1.3 µg/kg per minute infusion, 180 µg/kg bolus plus 2.0 µg/kg per minute or placebo for up to 3 days (in addition to heparin and aspirin). The 30-day event rate of death or MI was 14.2 per cent with eptifibate and 15.7 per cent with placebo. A reduction in MI and death with eptifibatide was also observed at 96 hours and 7 days.

Safety profile

The large clinical experience with eptifibatide offers a fairly reliable view of its safety profile. In IMPACT-II[165] major bleeding occurred in 4.8 per cent of placebo-treated patient and 5.1 per cent of eptifibatide-treated patients (combined groups). A majority of events (>50 per cent) occurred at vascular puncture sites. Thrombocytopenia (platelet count $<1 \times 10^9/L$) was observed in 2.8 per cent of patients. Severe bleeding complications were not increased with eptifibatide administration in the IMPACT-AMI trial;[166] but were higher (10.6 per cent vs 9.1 per cent) in PURSUIT.[167]

The ESPRIT trial[168] confirmed long-held suspicions that the dose of eptifibatide initially studied in PCI was suboptimal. A total of 200 patients undergoing elective

PCI received either eptifibatide (180 µg/kg bolus; 2 µg/kg per minute infusion; 180 µg/kg bolus 10 minutes after the first bolus), or placebo in combination with UFH and aspirin. There was a 43 per cent reduction in death or MI among eptifibatide-treated patients (8.6 vs 4.9 per cent) compared to those receiving placebo.

ORAL GPIIB/IIIA ANTAGONISTS

The success employed by a majority of iv GPIIb/IIIa antagonists in ACS coupled with the consistent observation that the benefit of treatment wanes over time prompted rapid development of oral antagonists. Despite their ability to inhibit platelet aggregation, an experience that includes nearly 20 000 patients has not shown benefit and, in fact, cardiovascular events and hemorrhage have occurred with increased frequency.[169–174] Efforts to understand the biology of thrombotic events among patients receiving oral GPIIb/IIIa antagonists will likely uncover insights into platelet activation and prothrombotic responses to transient/partial platelet inhibition.

Comparative trials

A 'head-to-head' comparison of two GPIIb/IIIa antagonists was carried out in the target trial (AHA presentation, November 2000). A total of 4750 patients undergoing either elective PCI or iv in the setting of ACS (excluding acute MI) received tirofiban or abciximab. At 30 days the composite outcome of death, nonfatal MI or urgent revascularization occurred in 7.55 per cent of tirofiban-treated patients and 6.0 per cent of abciximab-treated patients (hazard ratio 1.26; $P = 0.03$). Minor bleeding and thrombocytopenia was more common with abciximab.

COMBINED PHARMACOTHERAPIES

Fibrinolytics–GPIIb/IIIa antagonists

Interest among clinicians and investigators to achieve TIMI grade 3 coronary flow more rapidly while reducing hemorrhagic complications has led to the investigation of combined fibrinolytic–GPIIb/IIIa antagonist therapies.

SPEED

SPEED (Strategies for Patency Enhancement in the Emergency Department) randomized 528 patients with acute ST segment elevation MI to reduced dose rPA plus abciximab or abciximab alone. The primary end point was TIMI 3 flow at 60–90 minutes (preintervention). In phase A of the trial, 62 per cent of the abciximab–reteplase (5 + 5U) group achieved TIMI 3 flow compared with 27 per cent of abciximab-alone patients

($P = 0.001$) (Fig. 18.16). In phase B, 54 per cent of the abciximab–reteplase group had TIMI 3 flow at 60–90 minutes compared with 47 per cent in those given reteplase (10 + 10 U) alone ($P = 0.32$). The abciximab–reteplase–UFH (60 U/kg) group had a 61 per cent TIMI 3 flow rate ($P = 0.05$ compared with reteplase alone). Major hemorrhage occurred with greater frequency in combination therapy groups; however, intracranial bleeding was infrequent (two patients given abciximab–reteplase; 1.1 per cent).[175]

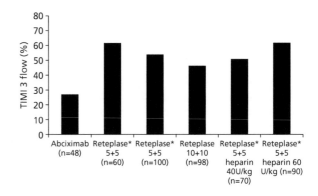

Figure 18.16 *Angiographic TIMI grade 3 flow at 60–90 minutes in patients receiving abciximab and/or reteplase. *Plus abciximab. (Reproduced with permission from the SPEED investigators. Trial of abciximab with and without low-dose reteplase for acute myocardial infarction. Circulation 2000; **101**: 2788–94.)*

TIMI 14

The TIMI 14 trial randomized 888 patients with ST segment elevation MI to either:

1 accelerated tPA (≤100 mg) plus standard dose heparin;
2 abciximab (0.25 mg/kg bolus, 0.125 µg/kg per minute × 12 hours), tPA (20 mg bolus), and low-dose heparin (60 U/kg bolus; 7 U/kg per hour);
3 abciximab, streptokinase (800 000 to 1.5 million units) and low-dose heparin; or
4 abciximab plus low-dose heparin.

TIMI grade 3 flow rates at 90 minutes were 52, 53, 42, and 32 per cent, respectively. A combination of abciximab and tPA (35 mg) yielded a 63 per cent TIMI grade 3 flow rate while a higher dose of tPA (50 mg; 15 mg bolus, 35 mg over 60 minutes) given in combination with abciximab yielded a 90-minute TIMI 3 flow rate of 76 per cent. A higher streptokinase dose 750 000 U and 1.25 million U yielded TIMI 3 grade flow 38 per cent and 48 per cent of the time, respectively.[176] The 50 mg tPA–abciximab strategy was also evaluated in combination with a very low heparin dose (30 U/kg bolus, 4 U/kg per hour), which yielded 60- and 90-minute TIMI flow rates of 68 and 69 per cent, respectively (Fig. 18.17). The

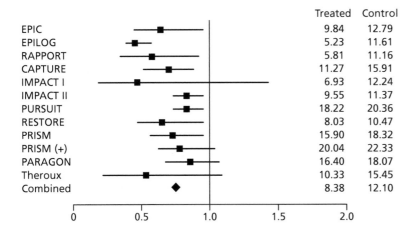

Figure 18.17 *Angiographic TIMI grade 3 flow at 60 and 90 minutes in patients receiving abciximab and/or alteplase. (Reproduced with permission from Antman EM for the TIMI 14 investigators. Abciximab facilitates the rate and extent of thrombolysis. Results of the TIMI 14 trial.* Circulation *1999;* **99***: 2720–32.)*

rates of major hemorrhage were as follows: tPA alone (6 per cent), abciximab alone (3 per cent), streptokinase–abciximab (10 per cent), tPA (50 mg)–abciximab–low-dose heparin (7 per cent), and tPA–abciximab–very-low-dose heparin (1 per cent).

Within the next several years, clinical trials evaluating all combinations of new-generation fibrinolytics and GPIIb/IIIa antagonists (with anticoagulants) will be undertaken. The experience with novel combination therapies suggests strongly that physiologic reperfusion can be achieved more quickly and more often than with traditional pharmacologic modalities.

SK–Eptifibatide

The combined administration of streptokinase (1.5 million U) and eptifibatide has been investigated in a double-blind, placebo-controlled angiographic pilot study of 181 patients. Patients were randomized to either eptifibatide (180 μg/kg bolus) and infusion (0.75, 1.33,

or 2.0 μg/kg per minute for 24 hours) or placebo. TIMI grade 3 flow rates at 90 minutes were 53, 44, 52, and 38 per cent, respectively. There was an increased incidence of bleeding with escalating doses of eptifibatide.[177]

The increased risk of bleeding when streptokinase is combined with platelet GPIIb/IIIa antagonists requires further investigation. Beyond the tendency of streptokinase to induce a systemic fibrinolytic state, the coexistence of a platelet and fibrin(ogen) abnormality may offer insight into the cause of bleeding events in fibrinolytic-treated patients.

Low-molecular-weight heparin–GPIIb/IIIa antagonists

The platelet-dependent and coagulation-dependent phases of arterial thrombosis support combined pharmacotherapies targeting both pivotal components. There is evidence that GPIIb/IIIa antagonists exert a broad range of antithrombotic properties; however, the available data derived from both medically treated patients with ACS and those undergoing PCI[178] suggest strongly that maximum benefit from GPIIb/IIIa treatment requires the conjunctive use of an anticoagulant (Fig. 18.18). Because LMWH preparations offer distinct advantages to UFH, their use in combination with GPIIb/IIIa antagonists is clinically attractive. A series of registries (National Investigators Collaborating on Enoxaparin; NICE) and randomized trials will define the strategy and preferred dosing of combination pharmacotherapies; however, large-scale randomized trials will be required to establish safety and efficacy. It appears likely that LMWH will replace UFH in the management of many arterial thromboembolic disorders.

FUTURE DIRECTIONS

The management of venous and arterial thrombotic disorders is based on pathophysiologic and pathobio-

	Treated	Control
EPIC	9.84	12.79
EPILOG	5.23	11.61
RAPPORT	5.81	11.16
CAPTURE	11.27	15.91
IMPACT I	6.93	12.24
IMPACT II	9.55	11.37
PURSUIT	18.22	20.36
RESTORE	8.03	10.47
PRISM	15.90	18.32
PRISM (+)	20.04	22.33
PARAGON	16.40	18.07
Theroux	10.33	15.45
Combined	8.38	12.10

Figure 18.18 *Odds ratios and 95 per cent confidence intervals for death, MI, or revascularization 30 days after GPIIb/IIIa antagonist treatment compared with placebo. (From Kong D et al. Clinical outcomes of thrombotic agents that block the platelet GPIIb/IIIa integrin in ischemic heart disease.* Circulation *1998;* **98***: 2829–35.)*

logic factors that determine the site, size, and clinical impact of compromised blood flow. The most effective means to combat thrombosis is through prevention; however, for existing clot burden the available pharmacologic strategies include fibrinolysis with third-generation agents, anticoagulants that target one or more coagulation proteins, and platelet antagonists designed to inhibit specific surface receptors that mediate platelet aggregation under various conditions. Mutants of the parent or 'wild-type' tPA molecule that can be administered as a bolus, LMWH preparations with effective factor Xa inhibiting potential, and platelet surface GPIIb/IIIa receptor antagonists meet several of these important prerequisites for benefit. The combined use of pharmacologic agents with the realistic goal of achieving greater overall success is being investigated at a rapid pace and will shape the future of clinical practice.

- The combined administration of compounds that prevent platelet activation and those capable of inhibiting aggregation is particularly attractive as are targeted combination therapies directed at both platelets and the coagulation cascade.

SUMMARY

- Under normal physiologic conditions, cellular components of circulating blood do not interact with the vascular endothelium or vessel wall.
- The exposure of circulating blood to dysfunctional or disrupted surfaces leads to the rapid deposition of platelets, erythrocytes, leukocytes, coagulation proteins and insoluble fibrin.
- Thrombi developing in the arterial circulatory system are composed of platelets and fibrin (white thrombus), while venous thrombi consist of erythrocytes, leukocytes and fibrin (red thrombus).
- Fibrinolytic agents convert an inactive precursor, plasminogen, to an active enzyme plasmin, which in turn, hydrolyzes several key bonds in the fibrin matrix causing dissolution (lysis).
- New (third)-generation fibrinolytic agents, including reteplase (rPA) and tenecteplase (TNK-tPA) have a prolonged circulating half-life, permitting bolus dosing or abbreviated infusions.
- New anticoagulants that are designed to inhibit thrombin or, preferably, coagulation factors more proximally positioned in the coagulation cascade (Factor X, tissue factor-VIIa) include low-molecular-weight heparin preparations, heparinoids, tissue factor pathway inhibitor, and direct thrombin antagonists.
- Platelet inhibition has focused on blocking surface receptors that facilitate platelet aggregation. Several intravenous glycoprotein (GP) IIb/IIIa antagonists have been developed and are being used in clinical practice.

REFERENCES

♦1. Burke AP, Farb A, Malcom GT, Liang Y-H, Smialek J, Virmani R. Coronary risk factors and plaque morphology in men with coronary artery disease who die suddenly. *N Engl J Med* 1997; **336**: 1276–82.

2. Neuhaus KL, von Essen R, Vogt A, *et al*. Dose finding with a novel recombinant plasminogen activator (BM 06.022) in patients with acute myocardial infarction: results of the German Recombinant Plasminogen Activator Study. *J Am Coll Cardiol* 1994; **24**: 55–60.

3. Tebbe U, von Essen R, Smolarz A, *et al*. Open, noncontrolled dose-finding study with a novel recombinant plasminogen activator (BM 06.022) given as a double bolus in patients with acute myocardial infarction. *Am J Cardiol* 1993; **72**: 518–24.

4. Smalling RW, Bode C, Kalbfleisch J, *et al*., and the RAPID Investigators. More rapid, complete, and stable coronary thrombolysis with bolus administration of reteplase compared with alteplase infusion in acute myocardial infarction. *Circulation* 1995; **91**: 2725–32.

♦5. Bode C, Smalling RW, Berg G, *et al*., and the RAPID Investigators. Randomized comparison of coronary thrombolysis achieved with double bolus reteplase (r-PA) and front-loaded 'accelerated' alteplase (rt-PA) in patients with acute myocardial infarction. *Circulation* 1996; **94**: 891–8.

6. INJECT Study Group. Randomized, double-blind comparison of reteplase double-bolus administration with streptokinase in acute myocardial infarction (INJECT): trial to investigate equivalence. *Lancet* 1995; **346**: 329–36.

♦7. The GUSTO III Investigators. A comparison of reteplase with alteplase for acute myocardial infarction. *N Engl J Med* 1997; **337**: 1118–23.

8. Refino CJ, Paoni NF, Keyt BA, *et al*. A variant of tPA (T103N, KHRR-296–299 AAAA) that, by bolus, has increased potency and decreased systemic activation of plasminogen. *Thromb Haemost* 1993; **70**: 313–19.

9. Cannon CP, McCabe CH, Gibson M, *et al*., and the TIMI 10A Investigators. TNK-tissue plasminogen activator in acute myocardial infarction. Results of the TIMI 10A dose-ranging trial. *Circulation* 1997; **95**: 351–6.

♦10. Cannon CP, Gibson CM, McCabe CH, *et al*., for the TIMI 10B Investigators. TNK-tissue plasmingoen activator compared with front loaded alteplase in acute myocardial infarction: results of the TIMI 10B Trial. *Circulation* 1998; **98**: 2805–14.

11. Van de Werf F, Cannon CP, Luyten A, *et al.*, for the ASSENT I Investigators. Safety assessment of single-bolus administration of TNK tissue plasminogen activator in acute myocardial infarction: the ASSENT-1 Trial. *Am Heart J* 1999; **137**: 786–91.

♦12. ASSENT-2 Investigators. Single-bolus tenecteplase compared with front-loaded alteplase in acute myocardial infarction. The ASSENT 2 double blind randomized trial. *Lancet* 1999; **354**: 716–22.

13. Neuhaus K-L, for the In-Time II Investigators. In-Time II Results. *Circulation* 1999; **100**: 574.

14. Lijnen HR, Stassen JM, Vanlinthout I, *et al.* Comparative fibrinolytic properties of staphylokinase and streptokinase in animal models of venous thrombosis. *Thromb Haemost* 1991; **66**: 468–73.

15. Collen D, Bernaerts R, Declerck P, *et al.* Recombinant staphylokinase variants with altered immunoreactivity. I: construction and characterization. *Circulation* 1996; **94**: 197–206.

16. Vanderschueren S, Barrios L, Kerdsinchai P, *et al.*, for the STAR Trial Group. A randomized trial of recombinant staphylokinase versus alteplase for coronary artery patency in acute myocardial infarction. *Circulation* 1995; **92**: 2044–9.

○17. Pannekoek H, de Vries C, Van Zonnerveld A-J. Mutants of human tissue-plasminogen activator (tPA): structural aspects and functional properties. *Fibrinolysis* 1988; **2**: 123–32.

18. Marx G. Divalent cations induce protofibril gelation. *Am J Hematol* 1988; **27**: 104–9.

19. Stewart UA, Bradley MS, Johnson Jr CS. Transport of probe molecules through fibrin gels as observed by means of holographic relaxation methods. *Biopolymers* 1988; **27**: 173–85.

20. Blomback B, Okada M. Fibrin gel structure and clotting time. *Thromb Res* 1982; **25**: 51–70.

21. Carr ME, Powers PL. Effect of glycosaminoglycans on thrombin- and atroxin-induced fibrin assembly and structure. *Thromb Haemost* 1989; **62**: 1057–61.

22. Bale MD, Westrick LG, Mosher DF. Incorporation of thrombospondin into fibrin clots. *J Biol Chem* 1985; **260**: 7502–8.

23. Sabovic M, Lijnen HR, Keber D, Collen D. Effect of retraction on the lysis of human clots with fibrin specific and nonfibrin specific plasminogen activators. *Thromb Haemost* 1989; **62**: 1083–7.

24. Wohl RC, Summaria L, Robbins KC. Kinetics of activation of human plasminogen by different activator species at pH 7.4 and 37°C. *J Biol Chem* 1980; **255**: 2005–13.

25. Schafer AI, Mars AK, Ware JA, Johnson PC, Rittenhouse SE, Salzman EW. Platelet protein phosphorylation, elevation of cytosolic calcium, and inositol phospholipid breakdown in platelet activation induced by plasma. *J Clin Invest* 1986; **78**: 73–9.

26. Greenberg JP, Packham MA, Guccione MA, Rand ML, Reimers H-J, Mustard JF. Survival of rabbit platelets treated in vitro with chymotrypsin, plasmin, trypsin and neuramidase. *Blood* 1979; **53**: 916–27.

♦27. Eisenberg R, Sherman L, Rich M, *et al.* Importance of continued activation of thrombin reflected by fibrinopeptide A to the efficacy of thrombolysis. *J Am Coll Cardiol* 1986; **7**: 1255–62.

28. Wilcox JN, Smith KM, Schwartz SM, Gordon D. Localization of tissue factor in the normal vessel wall and in the atherosclerotic plaque. *Proc Natl Acad Sci USA* 1989; **86**: 2839–43.

29. Drake TA, Morrissey JH, Edgington TS. Selective cellular expression of tissue factor in human tissues. *Am J Pathol* 1989; **134**: 1087–97.

30. Teitel JM, Rosenberg RD. Protection of factor Xa from neutralization by heparin-antithrombin complex. *J Clin Invest* 1983; **71**: 1383–91.

31. Miletich JP, Jackson CM, Majerus PW. Properties of the factor Xa binding site on platelets. *J Biol Chem* 1978; **253**: 6908–16.

♦32. Mann KG, Nesheim ME, Church WR, Haley P, Krishnaswamy S. Surface-dependent reactions of the vitamin K-dependent enzyme complexes. *Blood* 1990; **76**: 1–16.

33. Kakkar VV, Murray WJH. Efficacy and safety of low molecular weight heparin (CY216) in prevention postoperative venous thromboembolism: a co-operative study. *Br J Surg* 1985; **72**: 786–91.

34. Koller M, Schoch U, Buchmann P, Largiader F, Von Felten A, Frick PG. Low molecular weight heparin (KABI-2165) as thromboprophylaxis in elective visceral surgery. A randomized double-blind study versus unfractionated heparin. *Thromb Haemost* 1986; **56**: 243–6.

35. Schmidt-Huebner U, Bunte H, Freise G, *et al.* Clinical efficacy of low molecular weight heparin in postoperative thrombosis prophylaxis. *Klin Wochenschr* 1984; **62**: 349–53.

36. Cade JF, Wood M, Magnani HN, Westlake GW. Early clinical experience of a new heparinoid, ORG 10172, in prevention of deep venous thrombosis. *Thromb Res* 1987; **45**: 497–503.

37. Grunebaum L, Fricker JP, Wiesel ML, Vergnes Y, Cazenave JP, Barbier P, Kher A. Efficacy and safety of a low molecular weight heparin in prophylaxis of postoperative vein thrombosis after gynecologic surgery. *Thromb Haemost* 1987; **1**(suppl): 420a.

38. Briel RC, Hermann P, Hermann C, Doller P. Low molecular weight heparin (fragmin) prophylaxis after gynecologic surgery. *Thromb Haemost* 1987; **1**(suppl): 424A.

39. Le Gagneux F, Steg A, Le Guillov M. Subcutaneous enoxaparin versus placebo for preventing deep vein thrombosis after transurethral prostatectomy. *Thromb Haemost* 1987; **1**(suppl): 413A.

40. ten Cate H, Henny CP, ten Cate JW, Buller HR, Dabhoiwala NF. Randomized double-blind, placebo controlled safety study of low molecular weight

heparinoid in patients undergoing transurethral resection of the prostate. *Thromb Haemost* 1987; **54**: 92–6.

41. Samama M, Bernard P, Bonnardot JP, Combe-Tamzali S, Lanson Y, Tissot E, on behalf of the participants of the Groupe d'Etude de l'Enoxaparine (GENOX) multicentric trial. Low molecular weight heparin compared with unfractionated heparin in prevention of postoperative thrombosis. *Br J Surg* 1988; **75**: 128–31.

42. Turpie AGG, Levine MN, Hirsh J, *et al.* A randomized controlled trial of a low molecular weight heparin (enoxaparine) to prevent deep vein thrombosis in patients undergoing elective hip surgery. *N Engl J Med* 1986; **315**: 925–9.

43. Le Balch T, Landais A, Butel J, Weill D, Pascariello JC, Planes A. Enoxaparin (Lovenox®), versus standard heparin in prophylaxis of deep vein thrombosis after total hip replacement. *Thromb Haemost* 1987; **1**(suppl): 892A.

44. Potron G, Barre J, Droulle C, Bauduillard JC, Barbier P, Kher A. Thrombosis prophylaxis with low molecular weight heparin (KABI 2165) and calcium heparin in patients with total hip replacement. *Thromb Haemost* 1987; **1**(suppl): 421A.

45. Planes A, Vochelle N, Mansat C. Prevention of deep vein thrombosis after total hip replacement by enoxaparine: one daily injection of 40 mg versus two daily injections of 20 mg. *Thromb Haemost* 1987; **1**(suppl): 415A.

46. Breyer HG, Rahmarzdet R, Bacher P, Werner B. LMW-heparin versus heparin-DHE in orthopaedic surgery. *Thromb Haemost* 1987; **1**(suppl): 890A.

47. Barsotti J, Dabo B, Andrew J, Alison D, Leroy J, Delahousse B. Prevention of deep vein thrombosis by enoxaparine after surgery for fracture of femoral neck. Once daily injection of 40 mg versus two daily injections of 20 mg. *Thromb Haemost* 1987; **1**(suppl): 891A.

48. Planes A, Vochelle N, Ferru J, Przyrowski D, Clerc J, Fagola M, Planes M. Enoxaparine low molecular weight heparin: Its use in the prevention of deep venous thrombosis following total hip replacement. *Haemostasis* 1986; **16**: 152–8.

49. Dahan R, Houlbert D, Caulin C, *et al.* Prevention of deep vein thrombosis in elderly medical inpatients by a low molecular weight heparin: a randomized double-blind trial. *Haemostasis* 1986; **16**: 159–64.

50. Aquino JP, Gambier A, Durcros JJ. Prevention of thromboembolic accidents in elderly subjects with Fraxiparine®. In: Bounameaux H, Samama M, ten Cate JW, eds *Fraxiparin Second International Symposium Recent Pharmacological and Clinical Data.* Stuttgart: Schattauer, 1990: 51–4.

51. Turpie AGG, Hirsh J, Jay RM, *et al.* Double-blind randomized trial of ORG 10172 low-molecular-weight

heparinoid in prevention of deep-vein thrombosis in thrombotic stroke. *Lancet* 1987; **11**: 523–6.

52. Green D, Lee MY, Lim AC, *et al.* Prevention of thromboembolism after spinal cord injury using low-molecular-weight heparin. *Ann Intern Med* 1990; **113**: 571–4.

53. Sandset PM, Dahl T, Stiris M, Rostad B, Scheel B, Abildgaard U. A double-blind and randomized placebo controlled trial of low molecular weight heparin once daily to prevent deep vein thrombosis in acute ischemic stroke. *Semin Thromb Hemost* 1990; **16**(suppl): 25–33.

54. Yelnik A, Dizien O, Bussel B, Schouman-Claeys E, Frija G, Pannier S, Held JP. Systematic lower limb phlebography in acute spinal cord injury in 147 patients. *Paraplegia* 1991; **29**: 253–60.

55. Turpie AGG, Gent M, Côte R, *et al.* A low-molecular-weight heparinoid compared with unfractionated heparin in the prevention of deep vein thrombosis in patients with acute ischemic stroke. A randomized, double-blind study. *Ann Intern Med* 1992; **117**: 353–7.

56. Harenberg J, Kallenbach B, Martin U, Dempfle CE, Zimmermann R, Kübler W, Heene DL. Randomized controlled study of heparin in low molecular weight heparin for prevention of deep-vein thrombosis in medical patients. *Thromb Res* 1990; **59**: 639–50.

57. Scala P-J, Thiollet M, Midavaine M, Kher A, Funck-Brentano C, Jaillon P, Robert A, Valty J. Deep venous thrombosis and left ventricular thrombosis prophylaxis by low molecular weight heparin in acute myocardial infarction. *Haemostasis* 199; **20**: 368–9.

58. Nesvold A, Kontny F, Abildgaard U, Dale J. Safety of high doses of low molecular weight heparin (Fragmin) in acute myocardial infarction. A dose-finding study. *Thromb Res* 1991; **64**: 579–87.

59. Bratt G, Törnebohm E, Granquist S, Aberg W, Lockner D. A comparison between low molecular weight heparin (KABI 2165) and standard heparin in the intravenous treatment of deep venous thrombosis. *Thromb Haemost* 1985; **54**: 813–17.

60. Hull RD, Raskob GE, Pineo GF, *et al.* Subcutaneous low-molecular-weight heparin compared with continuous intravenous heparin in the treatment of proximal-vein thrombosis. *N Engl J Med* 1992; **236**: 975–82.

61. Vogel G, Machulik M. Efficacy and safety of a low molecular weight heparin (LMW-heparin Sandoz) in patients with deep vein thrombosis. *Thromb Haemost* 1987; **59**: 120.

62. Albada J, Nieuwenhuis HK, Sixma JJ. Treatment of venous thromboembolism with low molecular weight heparin (Fragmin). *Circulation* 1989; **80**: 935–40.

63. Bratt G, Aberg W, Johannsson M, Törnebohm E, Granquist S, Lockner D. Two daily subcutaneous injections of Fragmin as compared with intravenous standard heparin in the treatment of deep venous thrombosis (DVT). *Thromb Haemost* 1990; **64**: 506–10.

64. Harenberg J, Huck K, Bratsch H, *et al*. Therapeutic application of subcutaneous low-molecular-weight heparin in acute venous thrombosis. *Haemostasis* 1990; **20**: 205–19.

65. Duroux P. A randomized trial of subcutaneous low molecular weight heparin (CY 216) compared with intravenous unfractionated heparin in the treatment of deep vein thrombosis. A collaborative European multicentre study. *Thromb Haemost* 1991; **65**: 251–6.

66. Prandoni P, Lensing AWA, Büller HR, *et al*. Comparison of subcutaneous low-molecular-weight heparin with intravenous standard heparin in proximal deep-vein thrombosis. *Lancet* 1992; **339**: 441–5.

67. Holm HA, Ly B, Handeland GF, *et al*. Subcutaneous heparin treatment of deep venous thrombosis: a comparison of unfractionated with low molecular weight heparin. *Haemostasis* 1986; **16**: 30–7.

68. Lopaciuk S, Meissner AJ, Filipecki S, *et al*. Subcutaneous low molecular weight heparin versus subcutaneous unfractionated heparin in the treatment of deep vein thrombosis: a Polish multicenter trial. *Thromb Haemost* 1992; **68**: 14–18.

69. Holmström M, Berglund M-C, Granquist S, Bratt G, Torneböhm E, Lockner D. Fragmin once or twice daily subcutaneously in the treatment of deep venous thrombosis of the leg. *Thromb Res* 1992; **67**: 49–55.

70. Théry C, Simonneau G, Meyer G, *et al*. Randomized trial of subcutaneous low-molecular-weight heparin CY 216 (Fraxiparin) compared with intravenous unfractionated heparin in the curative treatment of submassive pulmonary embolism. A dose-ranging study. *Circulation* 1992; **85**: 1380–9.

71. Lockner D, Johansson M, Aberg W, Bratt G, Granquist S. Fragmin (Kabi) subcutaneously once or twice daily in the treatment of deep venous thrombosis (DVT). *Thromb Haemost* 1989; **62**: 526.

72. A Collaborative European Multicentre Study. A randomized trial of subcutaneous low molecular weight heparin (CY 216) compared with intravenous unfractionated heparin in the treatment of deep vein thrombosis. *Thromb Haemost* 1991; **65**: 251–6.

73. Simonneau G, Charbonnier B, Decousus H, *et al*. Subcutaneous low-molecular-weight heparin compared with continuous intravenous unfractionated heparin in the treatment of proximal deep vein thrombosis. *Arch Intern Med* 1993; **153**: 1541–6.

74. Lensing AWA, Prins MH, Davidson BL, Hirsh J. Treatment of deep venous thrombosis with low-molecular-weight heparins. *Arch Intern Med* 1995; **155**: 601–7.

75. Renaud H, Morinière P, Dieval J, *et al*. Low molecular weight heparin in haemodialysis and haemofiltration – comparison with unfractionated heparin. *Proc EDTA-ERA* 1984; **21**: 276–80.

76. Hory B, Cachoux A, Saunier F, *et al*. Comparative study of heparin and a very low molecular-weight heparin in hemodialysis in chronic renal insufficiency. *Presse Med* 1987; **16**: 955–8.

77. Dieval J, Morinière P, Bayrou B, Roussel B, Fournier A, Delobel J. In: Breddin K, Fareed J, Samam M, eds *Fraxiparin, First International Symposium*. Stuttgart: Schattauer, 1989: 169.

78. Grau E, Sigüenza F, Maduell F, Linares M, Angels Olaso M, Martinez R, Caridad A. Low molecular weight heparin (CY-216) versus unfractionated heparin in chronic hemodialysis. *Nephron* 1992; **62**: 13–17.

79. Briquel ME, Kessler M, André E, Cao Huu T, Alexandre P, Renoult E, Jonon B. Is enoxaparine (PK 10169) a good anticoagulant for chronic hemodialysis? *J Mal Vasc* 1987; **12**(suppl B): 111–13.

80. Dechelette E, Pouzol P, Jurkovitz C, Kuentz F, Polack B, Cuzin E, Woler M. The use of enoxaparine for anticoagulation in extracorporeal circulation in hemodialysis at high risk for hemorrhage. *J Mal Vasc* 1987; **12**(suppl B): 105–7.

81. Dueber HJ, Schulz W. Reduced lipid concentrations during four years of dialysis with low molecular-weight heparin. *Kidney Int* 1991; **40**: 496–500.

82. Dieval J, Morinière P, Roussel B, Bayrou B, Fournier A, Delobel J. Anticoagulation in hemodialysis sessions with a low molecular weight heparin (CY 222). *J Mal Vasc* 1987; **12**: 114–18.

83. Massonnet-Castel S, Pelissier E, Bara L, *et al*. Partial reversal of low molecular weight heparin (PK 10169) and anti-Xa activity by protamine sulfate. *Haemostasis* 1986; **16**: 139–46.

♦84. Bendetowicz AV, Kai H, Knebel R, Caplain H, Hemker HC, Lindhout T, Béguin S. The effect of subcutaneous injection of unfractionated and low molecular weight heparin on thrombin generation in platelet rich plasma – a study in human volunteers. *Thromb Haemost* 1994; **72**: 705–12.

85. Melandri G, Semprini F, Cervi V, Candiotti N, Branzi A, Palazzini E, Magnani B. Comparison of the efficacy of low molecular weight heparin (parnaparin) with that of unfractionated heparin in the presence of activated platelets in healthy subjects. *Am J Cardiol* 1993; **72**: 450–4.

86. Dehmer GJ, Fisher M, Tate DA, Teo S, Bonnem EM. Reversal of heparin anticoagulation by recombinant platelet factor 4 in humans. *Circulation* 1995; **91**: 2188–94.

87. Landolfi R, de Candia E, Rocca B, Ciabattoni G, Antinori A, Masetti R, Patrono C. Effects of unfractionated and low molecular weight heparins on platelet thromboxane biosynthesis 'in vivo'. *Thromb Haemost* 1994; **72**: 942–6.

88. Young E, Walls P, Holloway S, Weitz J, Hirsh J. Ex vivo and in vitro evidence that low molecular weight heparin exhibits less binding to plasma proteins than unfractionated heparin. *Thromb Haemost* 1994; **71**: 300–4.

♦89. Spencer FA, Ball SP, Zhang Q, Liv L, Benoit S, Becker RC. Enoxaparin, a low molecular weight heparin, inhibits prothrombinase assembly and activity by Factor Xa neutralization. *J Thromb Thrombolysis* 2000; **9**: 223–9.

♦90. Gurfinkel EP, Manos EJ, Mejail RI, *et al*. Low molecular weight heparin versus regular heparin or aspirin in the treatment of unstable angina and silent ischemia. *J Am Coll Cardiol* 1995; **26**: 313–18.

91. The FRISC Study Group. Low molecular weight heparin during instability in coronary artery disease. *Lancet* 1996; **347**: 561–8.

92. Klein W, Buchwald A, Hillis SE, *et al*. Comparison of low molecular weight heparin with unfractionated heparin acutely and with placebo for 6 weeks in the management of unstable coronary artery disease. Fragmin in Unstable Coronary Artery Disease Study (FRIC). *Circulation* 1997; **96**: 61–8.

♦93. Cohen M, Demers C, Gurfinkel EP, for the ESSENCE Investigators. A comparison of low-molecular weight heparin with unfractionated heparin for unstable coronary artery disease. *N Engl J Med* 1997; **337**: 447–52.

♦94. Antman E, for the TIMI 11B Investigators. Enoxaparin prevents death and cardiac ischemic events in unstable angina, non-Q wave MI: results of the TIMI IIB Trial. *Circulation* 1999; **100**: 1593–601.

95. The FRAX.I.S study group. Comparison of two treatment durations (6 days and 14 days) of a low molecular weight heparin with a 6 day treatment of unfractionated heparin in the initial management of unstable angina or non-Q wave myocardial infarction: FRAX.I.S *Eur Heart J* 1999; **20**: 1553–62.

♦96. FRISC II Investigators. Prolonged low molecular mass heparin (dalteparin) in unstable coronary artery disease: a prospective randomized multicenter trial. *Lancet* 1999; **354**: 701–7.

97. FRISC II Investigators. Invasive compared with non-invasive treatment in unstable coronary artery disease: FRISC II prospective randomized multicenter trial. *Lancet* 1999; **354**: 708–15.

98. Nicolini FA, Nichols WW, Saldeen TGP, Khan S, Mehta JL. Adjunctive therapy with low molecular weight heparin and recombinant tPA causes sustained reflow in canine coronary thrombosis. *Am Heart J* 1992; **124**: 280–8.

99. HART II Study.

100. Glick A, Laniado S, Keren G. Low molecular weight heparin after acute MI can prevent recurrence of acute cardiac events after thrombolytic treatment. Presented at the *American Heart Association Meetings*, Orlando, FL, November 9–13, 1997.

101. Wilson C, Baird S, Trouton T. Enoxaparin versus unfractionated heparin after thrombolysis for acute myocardial infarction. Presented at the *American Heart Association Meetings*, Orlando, FL, November 9–13, 1997.

102. Alhenc-Gelas M, Jestin-Le Guernic C, Vitoux JF, *et al*. Adjusted versus fixed doses of the low molecular weight heparin fragmin in the treatment of deep venous thrombosis. *Thromb Haemost* 1994; **71**: 698–702.

103. Bara L, Billaud E, Gramond G, Kher A, Samama M. Comparative pharmacokinetics of a low molecular weight heparin (PK 10169) and unfractionated heparin after intravenous and subcutaneous administration. *Thromb Res* 1985; **39**: 631–6.

104. Handeland GF, Abildgaard U, Holm HA, Arnesen KE. Dose adjusted heparin treatment of deep venous thrombosis: a comparison of unfractionated and low molecular weight heparin. *Eur J Clin Pharmacol* 1990; **39**: 107–12.

105. Bratt G, Tornebohm E, Granqvist S, Aberq W, Lockner D. A comparison between low molecular weight heparin (Kabi 2165) and standard heparin in the intravenous treatment of deep venous thrombosis. *Thromb Haemost* 1989; **59**: 813–17.

106. Nguyen M-TL, Spencer FA. Low molecular weight heparin versus unfractionated heparin in acute coronary syndromes: a meta-analysis. *J Thromb Thrombolysis* 2001: In press.

107. Palm M, Mattsson C, Magnus Svahn C, Weber M. Bleeding times in rats treatment with heparin, heparin fragments of high and low anticoagulant activity and chemically modified heparin fragments of low anticoagulant activity. *Thromb Haemost* 1990; **64**: 127–32.

108. Carter CJ, Kelton JG, Hirsh J, Cerskus A, Santos AV, Gent M. The relationship between the hemorrhagic and antithrombotic properties of low molecular weight heparin in rabbits. *Blood* 1982; **59**: 1239–45.

109. Peyrou V, Lormeau JC, Caranobe C, *et al*. Pharmacological properties of CY 216 and of its ACLM and BCLM components in the rabbit. *Thromb Haemost* 1994; **72**: 268–74.

110. Koller M, Schoch U, Buchmann P, Largiader F, Fon Felten A, Frieck PG. Low molecular weight heparin (Kabi 2165) as thromboprophylaxis in elective visceral surgery. A randomized, double-blind study versus unfractionated heparin. *Thromb Haemost* 1986; **56**: 243–6.

111. Bergqvist D, Burmark US, Frisell J, Lindblad B, Risberg B, Torngren S, Walling G. Low molecular weight heparin once daily compared with conventional low-dose heparin twice daily. A prospective double-blind multicentre trial on prevention of postoperative thrombosis. *Br J Surg* 1986; **73**: 204–8.

112. Samama M, Bernard P, Bonnardot JP, Combe-Tamzali S, Lanson Y, Tissot E. Low molecular weight heparin compared with unfractionated heparin in prevention of post operative thrombosis. *Br J Surg* 1988; **75**: 128–31.

♦113. Nieuwenhuis K, Albada J, Banga JD, Sixma JJ. Identification of risk factors for bleeding during treatment of acute venous thromboembolism with heparin or low molecular weight heparin. *Blood* 1991; **78**: 2337–43.

114. Anderson DR, O'Brien BJ, Levine MN, Roberts R, Wells PS, Hirsh J. Efficacy and cost of low-molecular-weight heparin compared with standard multicentre trial on prevention of postoperative thrombosis. *Br J Surg* 1986; **73**: 204–8.

115. Hemker H, Béguin S, Bendetowicz A, Wielders S. The determination of the levels of unfractionated heparin and low molecular weight heparins in plasma: their effect on thrombin mediated feedback reactions in vivo. Preliminary results after subcutaneous injection. *Haemostasis* 1991; **21**: 258–72.

116. De Swart CAM, Nijmeyer B, Roelofs JMM, Sixma JJ. Kinetics of intravenously administered heparin in normal humans. *Blood* 1982; **60**: 1251–8.

117. The TIMI 11A Investigators. Dose ranging trial of enoxaparin for unstable angina: results of TIMI 11A. *J Am Coll Cardiol* 1997; **29**: 1474–82.

118. Shaughnessy SG, Young E, Deschamps P, Hirsh J. The effects of low molecular weight heparin and standard heparin on calcium loss from fetal rat calvaria. *Blood* 1995; **86**: 1368–73.

119. Hoppenstead D, Racanelli A, Walenga JM, Fareed J. Comparative antithrombotic and hemorrhagic effects of dermatan sulfate, heparan sulfate, and heparin. *Semin Thromb Hemost* 1989; **15**: 378–85.

120. Gent M, Hirsh J, Ginsberg JS, *et al*. Low-molecular-weight heparinoid Orgaran is more effective than aspirin in the prevention of venous thromboembolism after surgery for hip fracture. *Circulation* 1996; **93**: 80–4.

121. de Valk HW, Banga JD, Wester JWJ, *et al*. Comparing subcutaneous danaparoid with intravenous unfractionated heparin for the treatment of venous thromboembolism. A randomized controlled trial. *Ann Intern Med* 1995; **123**: 1–9.

122. Magnani HN. Heparin-induced thrombocytopenia (HIT): an overview of 230 patients treated with orgaran (Org 10172). *Thromb Haemost* 1993; **70**: 554–61.

123. Callas D, Fareed J. Comparative pharmacology of site directed antithrombin agents. Implication in drug development. *Thromb Haemost* 1995; **74**: 473–81.

124. Potzsch B, Madlener K, Seelig C, *et al*. Monitoring of r-hirudin anticoagulation during cardiopulmonary bypass – assessment of the whole blood ecarin clotting time. *Thromb Haemost* 1997; **77**: 920–5.

125. Cannon CP, McCabe CH, Henry TD, *et al*. A pilot trial of recombinant desulfatohirudin compared with heparin in conjunction with tissue-type plasminogen activator and aspirin for acute myocardial infarction: results of the Thrombolysis In Myocardial Infarction (TIMI) 5 Trial. *J Am Coll Cardiol* 1994; **23**: 993–1003.

126. Lee LV, McCabe CH, Antman EM, *et al*. Initial experience with hirudin and streptokinase in acute myocardial infarction: results of the TIMI 6 trial. *Am J Cardiol* 1995; **75**: 7–13.

♦127. Antman E, for the TIMI 9A Investigators. Hirudin in acute myocardial infarction: safety report from the Thrombolysis and Thrombin Inhibition in Myocardial Infarction (TIMI) 9 A Trial. *Circulation* 1994; **90**: 1624–30.

♦128. The GUSTO Investigators. An international randomized trial comparing four thrombolytic strategies for acute myocardial infarction. *N Engl J Med* 1993; **329**: 673–82.

129. Neuhaus K-L, v Essen R, Tebbe U, *et al*. Safety observations from the pilot phase of the randomized r-Hirudin for Improvement of Thrombolysis (HIT-III) study. *Circulation* 1994; **90**: 1638–42.

♦130. TIMI 9B Investigators. Hirudin in acute myocardial infarction. Thrombolysis and thrombin inhibition in myocardial infarction (TIMI) 9B trial. *Circulation* 1996; **94**: 911–21.

♦131. GUSTO IIb Investigators. A comparison of recombinant hirudin with heparin for the treatment of acute coronary syndromes. *N Engl J Med* 1996; **335**: 775–82.

132. OASIS Investigators. Comparison of the effects of two doses of recombinant hirudin compared with heparin in patients with acute myocardial ischemia without ST elevation. A pilot study. *Circulation* 1997; **96**: 769–77.

133. Anand SS, Yusuf S, Pogue J, Weitz JI, Flather M. Long-term oral anticoagulant therapy in patients with unstable angina or suspected non-Q-wave myocardial infarction: Organization to Assess Strategies for Ischemic Syndromes (OASIS) pilot study results. *Circulation* 1998; **98**: 1064–70.

134. Fuchs J, Cannon CP, for the TIMI 7 Investigators. Hirulog in the treatment of unstable angina: results of the Thrombin Inhibition in Myocardial Ischemia (TIMI 7) trial. *Circulation* 1995; **92**: 727–33.

♦135. Bittl JA, S Trony J, Brinker JA, *et al*., for the Hirulog Angioplasty Study Investigators. Treatment with Bivalirudin (hirulog) as compared with heparin during coronary angioplasty for unstable or postinfarction angina. *N Engl J Med* 1995; **333**: 764–9.

136. Kong DF, Topol EJ, Bittl JA, *et al*. Clinical outcomes of bivalirudin for ischemic heart disease. *Circulation* 1999; **100**: 2049–53.

137. Lewis BE, Matthas W, Grassman JD, *et al*. Results of phase 2/3 trial of argatroban anticoagulation during PTCA of patients with heparin-induced thrombocytopenia (HIT). *Circulation* 1997; **96**: I-217 (abstract).

138. Jang I-K. A randomized study of argatroban vs heparin as adjunctive therapy to tissue plasminogen activator in acute myocardial infarction: MINT (Myocardial Infarction with Novastan and tPA) study. *Circulation* 1997; **96**: I-331 (abstract).

139. Hynes RO. Integrins: a family of cell surface receptors. *Cell* 1987; **48**: 549–54.

○140. Plow EF, Ginsberg MH. Cellular adhesion: GPIIb/IIIa as a prototypic adhesion receptor. *Prog Hemostas Thromb* 1989; **9**: 117–56.

○141. Hynes RO. Integrins: versatility, modulation, and signaling in cell adhesion. *Cell* 1992; **69**: 11–25.

142. Albelda SM, Buck CA. Integrins and other cell adhesion molecules. *FASEB J* 1990; **4**: 2868–80.

♦143. The EPIC Investigators. Use of a monoclonal antibody directed against the platelet glycoprotein IIb/IIIa receptor in high-risk coronary angioplasty. *N Engl J Med* 1994; **330**: 956–61.

144. Topol EJ, Califf RM, Weisman HF, *et al.*, on behalf of the EPIC Investigators. Randomized trial of coronary intervention with antibody against platelet IIb/IIIa integrin for reduction of clinical restenosis: results at six months. *Lancet* 1994; **343**: 881–6.

145. Topol EJ, Ferguson JJ, Weisman HF, *et al.*, for the EPIC Investigator Group. Long-term protection from myocardial ischemic events in a randomized trial of brief integrin B₃ blockade with percutaneous coronary intervention. *JAMA* 1997; **278**: 479–84.

♦146. The EPILOG Investigators. Platelet glycoprotein IIb/IIIa receptor blockade and low-dose heparin during percutaneous coronary revascularization. *N Engl J Med* 1997; **336**: 1689–96.

147. Simoons ML, Jan de Boer M, van den Brand MJBM, *et al.*, and the European Cooperative Study Group. Randomized trial of a GPIIb/IIIa platelet receptor blocker in refractory unstable angina. *Circulation* 1994; **89**: 596–603.

♦148. The CAPTURE Investigators. Randomized placebo-controlled trial of abciximab before and during coronary intervention in refractory unstable angina: the CAPTURE study. *Lancet* 1997; **349**: 1429–35.

149. Brenner ST, Barr LA, Burchemal JE, *et al.*, for the RAPPORT Investigators. Randomized, placebo-controlled trial of platelet GPIIb/IIIa blockade with primary angioplasty for acute myocardial infarction. *Circulation* 1998; **98**: 734–41.

150. Morris DC. Results from late-breaking clinical trial sessions at ACCIS '99 and ACC '99. American College of Cardiology. *J Am Coll Cardiol* 1999; **34**: 1.

151. Lincoff AM, Califf RM, Moliterno DJ, *et al.*, for the Evaluation of Platelet IIb/IIIa Inhibition in Stenting Investigators. Complementary clinical benefits of coronary-artery stenting and blockade of platelet glycoprotein IIb/IIIa receptors. *N Engl J Med* 1999; **341**: 319.

♦152. Berkowitz SD, Harrington RA, Rund MM, Tcheng JE. Acute profound thrombocytopenia after c7E3 Fab (Abciximab) therapy. *Circulation* 1997; **95**: 809–13.

153. Théroux P, Kouz S, Roy L, *et al.*, on behalf of the investigators. Platelet membrane receptor glycoprotein IIb/IIIa antagonism in unstable angina. The Canadian Lamifiban Study. *Circulation* 1996; **94**: 899–905.

154. The PARADIGM Investigators. Combined fibrinolysis with the GPIIb/IIIa inhibitor lamifiban: results of the PARADIGM trial. *J Am Coll Cardiol* 1998; **32**: 2003–10.

155. The PARAGON Investigators. International, randomized, controlled trial of lamifiban (a platelet glycoprotein IIb/IIIa inhibitor), heparin, or both in unstable angina. *Circulation* 1998; **97**: 2386–2396.

156. Paragon B Trial. Late breaking clinical trials. American College of Cardiology Meetings. Orlando, FL, 2001.

157. Müller TH, Weisenberger H, Brickl R, Narjes H, Himmelsbach F, Krause J. Profound and sustained inhibition of platelet aggregation by fradafiban, a nonpeptide platelet glycoprotein IIb/IIIa antagonist, and its orally active prodrug, Lefradafiban, in men. *Circulation* 1997; **96**: 1130–8.

158. Kereiakes DJ, Kleiman NS, Ambrose J, *et al.* Randomized, double-blind, placebo-controlled dose-ranging study of tirofiban (MK-383) platelet IIb/IIIa blockade in high risk patients undergoing coronary angioplasty. *J Am Coll Cardiol* 1996; **27**: 536–42.

159. The RESTORE Investigators. Effects of platelet glycoprotein IIb/IIIa blockade with tirofiban on adverse cardiac events in patients with unstable angina or acute myocardial infarction undergoing coronary angioplasty. *Circulation* 1997; **96**: 1445–53.

♦160. The PRISM Study Investigators. A comparison of aspirin plus tirofiban with aspirin plus heparin for unstable angina. *N Engl J Med* 1998; **338**: 1498–505.

161. The PRISM-Plus Study Investigators. Inhibition of the platelet glycoprotein IIb/IIIa receptor with tirofiban in unstable angina and non-Q-wave myocardial infarction. *N Engl J Med* 1998; **338**: 1488–97.

162. Phillips DR, Scarborough RM. Clinical pharmacology of eptifibatide. *Am J Cardiol* 1997; **80**: 11B–20B.

163. Harrington RA, Kleiman NS, Kottke-Marchant K, *et al.* Immediate and reversible platelet inhibition after intravenous administration of a peptide glycoprotein IIb/IIIa inhibitor during percutaneous coronary intervention. *Am J Cardiol* 1995; **76**: 1222–7.

164. Schulman SP, Goldschmidt-Clermont PJ, Topol EJ, *et al.* Effects of integrilin, a platelet glycoprotein IIb/IIIa receptor antagonist, in unstable angina. A randomized multicenter trial. *Circulation* 1996; **94**: 2083–9.

165. The IMPACT-II Investigators. Randomized placebo-controlled trial of effect of eptifibatide on complications of percutaneous coronary intervention: IMPACT-II. *Lancet* 1997; **349**: 1422–8.

166. Ohman EM, Kleiman NS, Gacioch G, *et al.*, for the IMPACT-AMI Investigators. Combined accelerated tissue-plasminogen activator and platelet glycoprotein IIb/IIIa integrin receptor blockade with integrilin in acute myocardial infarction. Results of a randomized, placebo-controlled, dose-ranging trial. *Circulation* 1997; **95**: 846–54.

167. The Platelet Glycoprotein IIb/IIIa in Unstable Angina Receptor Suppression using Integrilin Therapy Trial

Investigators. Inhibition of platelet glycoprotein IIb/IIIa with eptifibatide in patients with acute coronary syndromes. *N Engl J Med* 1998; **339**: 436–43.

168. The ESPRIT Investigators. Novel dosing regimen of eptifibatide in planned coronary stent implantation: a randomized, placebo-controlled trial. *Lancet* 2000; **356**: 2037–44.

169. Szalony JA, Haas NF, Salyers AK, Taite BB, Nicholson NS, Mehrotra DV, Feigen LP. Extended inhibition of platelet aggregation with the orally active platelet inhibitor SC-54684A. *Circulation* 1995; **91**: 411–16.

170. Kereiakes DJ, Kleiman N, Ferguson JJ, *et al.* Sustained platelet glycoprotein IIb/IIIa blockade with oral Xemilofiban in 170 patients after coronary stent deployment. *Circulation* 1997; **96**: 1117–21.

171. Kereiakes DJ, Runyon JP, Kleiman NS, Higby NA, Anderson LC, Hantsbarger G, McDonald S, Anders RJ. Differential dose-response to oral Xemilofiban after antecedent intravenous abciximab. Administration for complex coronary intervention. *Circulation* 1996; **94**: 906–10.

172. Kereiakes DJ, Kleiman NS, Ferguson JJ, for the ORBIT Investigators. Pharmacodynamic efficacy, clinical safety, and outcomes following prolonged platelet glycoprotein IIb/IIIa receptor blockade with oral Xemilofiban: results of a multicenter placebo-controlled randomized trial. *Circulation* 1998; **98**: 1268–78.

173. Cannon CP, McCabe CH, Borzak S, for the TIMI 12 Investigators. A randomized trial of an oral platelet glycoprotein IIb/IIIa antagonist, sibrafiban, in patients post an acute coronary syndrome: results of the TIMI 12 trial. *Circulation* 1998: **97**: 340–9.

♦174. Cannon CP, McCabe CH, Wilcox RG, *et al.*, for the OPUS-TIMI 16 Investigators. Oral glycoprotein IIb/IIIa inhibition with Orbofiban in patients with unstable coronary syndromes. *Circulation* 2000; **102**: 149–56.

♦175. Strategies for patency enhancement in the emergency department (SPEED) group. Trial of Abciximab with and without low-dose reteplase for acute myocardial infarction. *Circulation* 2000; **101**: 2788–94.

♦176. Antman EM for the TIMI 14 Investigators. Abciximab facilitates the rate and extent of thrombolysis. Results of the TIMI 14 Trial. *Circulation* 1999; **99**: 2720–32.

177. Simoons ML. *George Washington Symposium*, Orlando, FL, November 1997.

○178. Kong DF, Califf RM, Miller DP, *et al.* Clinical outcomes of therapeutic agents that block the platelet GPIIb/IIIa integrin in ischemic heart disease. *Circulation* 1998; **98**: 2829–35.

19

Evaluation and management of patients with heart failure in clinical practice

THEO E MEYER, EUGENE S CHUNG AND WILLIAM H GAASCH

Heart failure (HF) is a major and escalating health problem. The medical management of these patients requires: (1) the search for reversible causes of heart failure; (2) an appreciation of the differences between systolic and diastolic heart failure; and (3) expertise in pharmacological and non-pharmacological interventions that have been shown to be beneficial in terms of attenuating the progression of heart failure and those that are useful to improve the symptomatic state of these patients.

INTRODUCTION

Definition and classification of heart failure

Heart failure is a clinical syndrome caused by a wide variety of disorders that include valvular, myocardial, pericardial, and other non-cardiac diseases. The clinical syndrome of heart failure is characterized by signs and symptoms of either intravascular and interstitial fluid overload, including shortness of breath, rales and edema, or fatigue and decreased exercise tolerance, or the combination of these symptoms. In this chapter the phrase 'heart failure' is preferred over the commonly used 'congestive heart failure' since many patients with heart failure do not have congestive symptoms. The definition of heart failure is problematic. The syndrome of heart failure has on occasion very little to do with a failing heart, as for example when the 'failure' is secondary to volume overload from a large arteriovenous fistula or severe anemia. However, heart failure for the most part represents a constellation of signs associated with abnormal cardiac

function and a morbid progression of the underlying cardiac disease. For the purposes of clarity, the terms and clinical heart failure syndromes that are used throughout this chapter are defined in Table 19.1.

Prevalence and incidence

Over the past decade, heart failure has become a major and escalating health problem in the USA and other industrialized societies, particularly those with aging populations. It is estimated that heart failure afflicts 1.5 per cent of the adult population in the USA and it is the principal cause for hospital admissions in the elderly.[3,4] The prevalence of heart failure is reported to rise from 0.8 per cent at age 50–59 years to 9.1 per cent at age 80–89 years, approximately doubling with each decade of age.[5] Data from the Framingham study showed that the incidence of heart failure also increased dramatically with age. The annual incidence increased from 3 cases/1000 in men aged 50–59 years of age to 22 cases/1000 in those aged 80–89 years of age.[6] The inci-

Table 19.1 *Terms used to define heart failure syndromes*

Asymptomatic left ventricular dysfunction

This clinical state is present when asymptomatic patients have moderately or severely impaired left ventricular systolic function (ejection fraction ⩽ 35–40%)

Diastolic dysfunction

Failure of the heart to fill at low diastolic pressures (i.e. ⩽ 8 mm Hg for the right ventricle and ⩽ 12 mm Hg for the left ventricle)[1,2]

Systolic dysfunction

Failure of the ventricles to eject blood into the great vessels under sufficient systolic pressure (⩾ 15 mm Hg for the right ventricle and ⩾ 90 mmHg for the left ventricle)[1,2]

Diastolic heart failure

Pulmonary and/or systemic congestion in the absence of significant systolic dysfunction (ejection fraction ⩾ 40%)

Systolic heart failure

Systemic hypoperfusion associated with structural heart disease in the absence of hypovolemia or sepsis (ejection fraction usually ⩽ 40%)

Acute heart failure

Clinical syndrome characterized by the sudden onset of pulmonary congestion in association with reduced organ perfusion

Chronic heart failure

Clinical syndrome in which structural heart disease produces a constellation of secondary changes (not always congestion) in other organs, leading to symptoms and exercise limitation

Etiology of heart failure

Among 652 subjects in the Framingham Heart study who developed heart failure during the follow-up period, hypertension and coronary disease were the two most common pre-existing conditions.[6] Seventy per cent of men and 78 per cent of women had antecedent diagnosis of hypertension, while 40 per cent of both men and women had a prior history of both hypertension and coronary disease. Prevalent coronary disease was less common in women than in men. A list of the etiologies of heart failure encountered in the Framingham study and other large treatment trials are shown in Table 19.2.

Table 19.2 *Etiologies of heart failure*

Etiology	Patients (%)
Ischemic	50.3
Non-ischemic	49.7
Etiology uncertain	13.3
Etiology provided	36.4
Idiopathic	18.2
Valvular	4.0
Hypertensive	3.8
Ethanol	1.8
Viral	0.4
Postpartum	0.4
Amyloidosis	0.1
Other	7.6

Hospitalization rates

Hospital discharges associated with heart failure in the USA have increased dramatically over time, increasing the clinical and public health burden from this condition. The number of hospital discharges in which heart failure was the first listed diagnosis in 1993 (over 875 000 admissions) was almost five times greater than it was 25 years earlier, a sentinel point in time at which death rates from coronary heart disease in the USA began to exhibit a dramatic decline which has continued to the present.[7] Despite the limited availability of comparative data from other population settings, in Scotland, hospital discharges for heart failure as a principal diagnosis increased by nearly two-thirds in men and by more than one-half in women between 1980 and 1990.[8]

Repeat hospitalizations for patients with heart failure are a relatively frequent occurrence within a short period of time following hospital discharge. The rate of hospitalizations have not changed over the last 16 years. In 1982, the 6-month readmission rate was 36 per cent and in 1993 the admission rate was 31 per cent. Recent data suggest that the readmission rate amongst Medicare recipients may even be higher; approaching almost 40 per cent within 6 months of discharge.[9]

dence in men was higher than in women. Similar to the changes in prevalence, the incidence of heart failure doubled with each decade of age. Extrapolation of the annual incidence from the Framingham study to the population of the USA yields an estimate of 465 000 new cases per year.

Risk factors for the development of heart failure

Data from the Framingham study showed that in younger men and women, aged 35–64 years, hypertension was associated with a 3–4-fold increase in the incidence of heart failure, diabetes with a 4–8-fold increase and electrocardiographic evidence of left ventricular (LV) hypertrophy with 13–15-fold increase.[6] In men and women older than 65 years of age, the relative risks for heart failure associated with hypertension, diabetes, electrocardiographic evidence of LV hypertrophy were slightly less than those of younger men, but the excess risks were higher. Left ventricular hypertrophy was associated with increased incidence of heart failure, even after adjusting for blood pressure.

Economic costs

There are considerable costs associated with the diagnosis and treatment of heart failure. In 1991, Medicare alone paid over 5.5 billion dollars for hospital admissions for patients with a principal diagnosis of heart failure, a total that not only exceeded the cost of hospitalizations for myocardial infarctions, but was twice the Medicare hospital expenditure for all forms of cancer.[10] In the USA, the total direct economic costs devoted to the management of heart failure is estimated to exceed 10 billion dollars based on hospitalizations for this condition, physicians' office visits, nursing home costs, and treatment modalities annually. The economic burden of heart failure has been calculated to consume approximately 1 per cent of the national health care budgets of countries in Europe.[11] About 75 per cent of the cost is attributable to the high rate of readmissions and the long hospital stay of patients with heart failure. It is estimated that about half of the cost can be saved through prudent outpatient management of heart failure.

Prognosis of heart failure

Data from population-based studies suggest that the survival rates of heart failure remain poor. In the Framingham study, the median survival time was 1.7 years for men and 3.2 years for women.[6] After 5 years, only 25 per cent of men and 38 per cent of women remained alive, and these figures fell to 11 per cent and 21 per cent respectively, after 10 years. In the Rochester Epidemiology project, the 3-month and 1-year survival rates among newly diagnosed cases of heart failure were 75 per cent and 65 per cent, respectively;[12] relatively similar survival rates have been seen for patients with heart failure in the Framingham study.

PATHOPHYSIOLOGY OF HEART FAILURE

It falls outside the scope of this chapter to provide a detailed review of the pathophysiological mechanisms that underlie the development and progression of heart failure. The reader is referred to earlier reviews on this topic.[13–17] However, as a basis for the subsequent discussions on the timing of pharmacological interventions and the assessment of asymptomatic and symptomatic heart failure, it is relevant to review certain pathophysiological concepts regarding the progression of myocardial dysfunction and the factors that contribute to exercise limitation in patients with chronic heart failure.

Chamber remodeling

Cardiac chambers can alter their size and geometry in response to chronic changes in hemodynamic load.

Longstanding pressure overload, as a consequence of either significant aortic stenosis or hypertension, or prolonged volume overload, as for example from chronic mitral regurgitation, lead to remodeling of the LV chamber. The chamber remodels in direct relation to the imposed hemodynamic burden. A specific type of remodeling can occur as a result of myocardial infarction. These and other patterns of geometric remodeling are shown in Fig. 19.1.

During pressure overload, the left ventricle remodels initially by hypertrophic growth, characterized by concentric remodeling, in which increased mass is out of proportion to chamber volume. This response appears to be regulated in part by increased myocardial angiotensin converting enzyme (ACE) activity, and may be modified by ACE inhibitors. Over a period of time the chamber decompensates and dilates and fails. ACE inhibitors may attenuate the progression of LV chamber dysfunction. With volume overload, secondary to longstanding valvular regurgitant lesions, the increase in LV mass is due to an increase in chamber volume out of proportion to increase in wall thickness (eccentric hypertrophy). Similar to pressure overload, progression is characterized by further dilatation and decreased chamber performance. In general, surgical correction of the underlying lesion may attenuate progression of volume overload hypertrophy. Ventricular remodeling after myocardial infarction is characterized by early infarct area expansion and thinning followed by non-ischemic regional dilatation. As before, the natural history of these hearts is to dilate further with eventual decreased non-ischemic regional shortening and consequent chamber dysfunction. ACE inhibitors attenuate ventricular remodeling in this setting.

Remodeling in response to pathological conditions can initially be considered to be adaptive, but over a period of time these changes become maladaptive[18] and eventually progress to chamber and myocardial dysfunction, usually with significant ventricular enlargement.

Impaired exercise tolerance

Structural changes in the heart are of paramount importance in generating the clinical disorder. However, the changes in extracardiac systems such as sympathoexcitation,[19–22] activation of the renin angiotensin system[23,24] and other neurohumoral factors,[24] and abnormalities of peripheral blood flow[25–27] and skeletal muscle metabolism and function,[28–31] contribute to the progression and exercise limitation of this syndrome.

CLINICAL PRESENTATION OF HEART FAILURE

The onset and severity of symptoms are variable, and depend importantly on the nature of the underlying car-

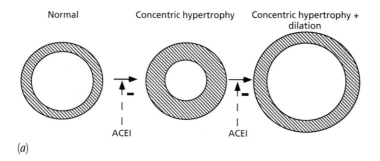

(a)

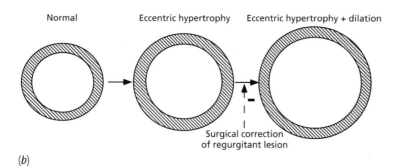

(b)

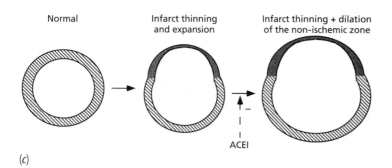

(c)

Figure 19.1 *Schematic representation of the patterns of ventricular remodeling in response to: (a) pressure overload, (b) volume overload, and (c) secondary to myocardial infarction. ACEI = angiotensin-converting enzyme inhibitor; — = attenuation of remodeling.*

diac disease and the rate at which the syndrome develops (Fig. 19.2). A large proportion of patients with damaged or dysfunctional hearts are asymptomatic since the transition to myocardial failure is fairly slow. The following discussion will briefly review the clinical presentation of specific chronic heart failure syndromes. The evaluation and treatment of acute heart failure is discussed elsewhere.

Chronic heart failure

Patients with chronic heart failure invariably have large hearts with markedly impaired systolic function and typically complain of symptoms of shortness of breath and fatigue during exercise, and as a consequence have markedly reduced exercise capacity. These and other related manifestations of chronic heart failure are briefly discussed in the following section and are listed in Tables 19.3 and 19.4.

SYMPTOMS

Breathlessness is one of the prominent manifestations of heart failure and may present with exertional dyspnea, orthopnea, paroxysmal nocturnal dyspnea, dyspnea at rest or acute pulmonary edema. Dyspnea defined as an exaggerated uncomfortable awareness of breathing may be manifest during moderate physical activity or in patients with advanced disease, with mild exertion. In its severest form, the patient complains of shortness of breath at rest. A manifestation of dyspnea at rest is orthopnea, defined as breathlessness that develops in the recumbent position and is relieved by sitting upright or standing. Another manifestation of shortness of breath at rest is paroxysmal nocturnal dyspnea. This symptom usually begins 2–4 hours after the onset of sleep and is associated with marked dyspnea followed by coughing, wheezing, and sweating. As with orthopnea, this symptom is relieved by sitting upright and getting out of bed. Intuitively, all these aforementioned symptoms may

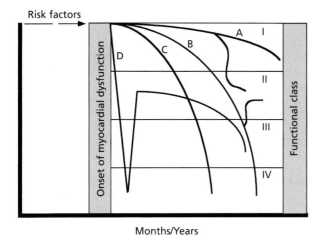

Figure 19.2 *This schematic representation depicts the variability in the natural history of heart failure. The onset of myocardial dysfunction is usually preceded by a period when the patient was exposed to risk factors for coronary disease (the most common cause of heart failure in Western societies). Four theoretical courses are shown (A–D). The onset of heart failure may be slow (A) or rapid (D), and patients may improve with aggressive medical treatment (B and D) or have an acute exacerbation (A) (secondary to precipitating factors such as an arrhythmia).*

simply reflect varying degrees of pulmonary congestion, but recent evidence suggests exertional dyspnea may be related more to abnormalities of the periphery, analogous to a deconditoned state,[30] while the symptoms of orthopnea and paroxysmal nocturnal dyspnea are more likely to reflect the presence or development of interstitial pulmonary edema. Whereas a dry, irritating, spasmodic and nocturnal cough, also indicative of pulmonary venous hypertension, is common, the symptoms of orthopnea and paroxysmal nocturnal dyspnea are relatively uncommon.

Another universal manifestation of chronic heart failure is a reduction in exercise capacity due to either the development of breathlessness, as discussed before, or muscle fatigue or both. Although not specific for heart failure, fatigue is a prominent symptom in patients with chronic heart failure, limiting physical activity and impairing quality of life. Although the underlying mechanisms are not clearly identified, recent evidence suggests that similar to exertional dyspnea, alterations associated with peripheral adaptation in heart failure appear to play an important role, including impaired peripheral perfusion during exercise, reduced oxidative capacity of skeletal muscle, impaired muscle strength, and possibly reflex mechanisms associated with alterations in the metabolism of skeletal muscle.[31,32]

Varying degrees of fluid retention marks the onset of the congestive phase of heart failure. Over time the retention of sodium leads to peripheral edema, hepatomegaly with ascites, increased circulating blood

Table 19.3 *Symptoms of chronic heart failure*

	Severity		
	Asymptomatic/mild	Moderate	Severe/advanced
Physical activity[a]	No symptoms or dyspnea and fatigue with ordinary activity	Dyspena and fatigue with less than ordinary activity	Largely restricted to activities at rest
Systemic	No symptoms or mild ankle swelling	Ankle swelling Right hypochondrial discomfort	Ankle and/or abdominal swelling Upper abdominal pain Nausea Weight loss
Respiratory	No symptoms or mild cough	Cough Orthopnea	Cough Dyspnea at rest Orthopnea Paroxysmal nocturnal dyspnea
Renal	No symptoms	Nocturia	Nocturia Oliguria Anuria
Neuropsychiatric	No symptoms	Anxiety Insomnia Bad dreams Depression	Anxiety Insomnia Bad dreams Depression Impaired memory
Other		Impotence	Impotence

[a] The activities of daily living provide the best index of the severity of heart failure.

Table 19.4 *Physical findings in patients with chronic heart failure*

	Severity		
	Asymptomatic/mild	Moderate	Severe/advanced
General appearance	No distress at rest Mild ankle swelling	No distress at rest Ankle edema	Anxious Distressed Malar flush Cyanosis Cachexia Jaundice Ankle edema
Respiratory	Normal	Rales over lung bases	Rales over lung bases Wheezes and/or coarse crackles Signs of a pleural effusion Cheyne–Stokes breathing
Abdominal	Normal	Mild hepatomegaly	Hepatojugular reflux Hepatomegaly Ascites

Cardiac	Normal or:
	  Cardiomegaly
	  Third and/or fourth heart sounds
	  Mitral regurgitant murmur
	  Tricuspid regurgitant murmur
		Rarely normal
		Regular or irregular rhythm
		Elevated venous pressure
		Cardiomegaly
		Third and/or fourth heart sounds
		Mitral regurgitant murmur
		Tricuspid regurgitant murmur
			Cold extremities
			Regular or irregular rhythm
			Decreased pulse volume
			Pulsus alternans
			Elevated venous pressure
			Cardiomegaly
			Third and/or fourth heart sounds
			Mitral regurgitant murmur
			Tricuspid regurgitant murmur

Neurologic		Confusion	Confusion Delirium Psychosis

volume with elevated filling pressures. Persistent venous congestion results in hepatic swelling, may manifest as right hypochondrial tenderness. With severe hepatic congestion the patient may, in addition to upper abdominal pain, complain of nausea. Also, a patient with mild to moderate heart failure may present with nocturia, which is largely due to the improved renal perfusion in the recumbent position at night.

Elderly patients with heart failure may initially present with a number of neurological symptoms, including confusion, headaches, insomnia, bad dreams, anxiety, disorientation and impaired memory.

Patients with less severe degrees of heart failure may be asymptomatic or only have mild symptoms. These may include fatigue or dyspnea with ordinary physical activity without symptoms at rest.

PHYSICAL FINDINGS

The careful and skillful detection of overt and subtle physical signs of cardiac disease may be diagnostic of heart failure in a patient with compatible symptoms. In general, physical signs are not highly sensitive or specific for detecting heart failure. An elevated jugular venous pressure, the presence of a third heart sound and a later-

ally displaced apex beat are the most specific of the physical findings, whereas pulmonary rales and pedal edema are relatively non-specific signs.

ASSESSMENT OF ASYMPTOMATIC LEFT VENTRICULAR DYSFUNCTION AND HEART FAILURE

A schematic outline of the steps (goals) that are required to assess a patient adequately with suspected LV dysfunction and heart failure is shown in Table 19.5.

Recognition of asymptomatic and symptomatic LV dysfunction

It is now well recognized that patients with LV dysfunction can be asymptomatic for long periods of time prior to the development of overt heart failure.[33] Based on the strong evidence that the early treatment with ACE inhibitors delay and even prevent the progression to heart failure,[34–49] there is a more compelling reason to identify the asymptomatic or minimally symptomatic patient with LV dysfunction. The recognition of asymp-

Table 19.5 *Objectives when evaluating a patient with left ventricular dysfunction or heart failure*

Identify the patient with asymptomatic LV dysfunction
Establish whether the signs and symptoms are consistent with the clinical syndrome of heart failure
Define the predominant hemodynamic abnormality
Determine the stage of severity of heart failure
Identify the etiology of the underlying cardiac condition
Identify precipitating factors
Assess the overall prognosis

Table 19.6 *Clinical indicators of left ventricular dysfunction in an asymptomatic patient*

History
Alcohol or cocaine abuse
Prior myocardial infarction(s)
Prior chemotherapy
Longstanding hypertension
Family history of heart failure

Physical signs
Resting tachycardia
Abnormal apical impulse
Third and/or fourth heart sound
New mitral regurgitant murmur

Electrocardiographic findings
Evidence of extensive ischemic myocardial injury
Electrocardiogram repolarization abnormalities and/or left bundle branch block
Atrial fibrillation or other arrhythmia

Chest x-ray
Increased cardiothoracic ratio
Apical redistribution of pulmonary blood flow

tomatic patients with LV dysfunction and those with mild to moderate heart failure are problematic. In one report, 20 per cent of patients with reduced ejection fractions met no criteria for heart failure.[49] In addition, other data suggest that few patients with ejection fractions of 30 per cent or less had exertional dyspnea.[50,51] The recognition of patients with asymptomatic LV dysfunction or mild symptoms of chronic heart failure is further complicated by the reality that many of the signs and symptoms of chronic heart failure may also occur in other conditions, such as obesity and chronic non-cardiac diseases. The simplest approach to this problem is to have a high index of suspicion when an asymptomatic patient is encountered with certain physical signs, and radiological and electrocardiographic abnormalities. The clinical findings that would alert one to suspect LV dysfunction are listed in Table 19.6. Moreover, in many elderly patients the diagnosis of early or even more advanced heart failure may not be made since these patients often lead a fairly sedentary life due to their age and other debilitating non-cardiac problems.

In contrast to asymptomatic LV dysfunction, the identification of moderate to severe heart failure is far less problematic, especially when a patient presents with the triad of fluid retention, exertional dyspnea and fatigue, and an enlarged heart. However, it is important to stress that symptoms of fluid retention (i.e. congested state) do not necessarily indicate heart failure. For example, 40 per cent of patients diagnosed as having heart failure on the grounds of pedal edema are wrongly diagnosed.[52] In addition, exertional dyspnea or fatigue may be due to heart failure, although it could also be due to a range of other conditions, all of which should be considered before attributing these symptoms to heart failure. These conditions include, amongst others, pulmonary embolism, pneumonia, chronic obstructive lung disease, asthma, pulmonary fibrosis, pleural effusion, anemia, hyperthyroidism, and musculoskeletal disorders. In order to overcome the lack of accuracy in diagnosing heart failure, clinical criteria (Framingham[53] and Boston[54]) have been developed to improve and standardize the recognition of this syndrome. Although these criteria are useful in standardizing the diagnosis in clinical treatment trials and epidemiological surveys, the utility

of these criteria to establish the diagnosis of mild to moderate heart failure in the primary health care setting is questionable. In a recent study from Finland, a high false-positive rate was found when primary care physicians based the diagnosis of heart failure on the Boston criteria, especially in obese women.[51]

An outline of the diagnostic approach to recognize patients with asymptomatic LV dysfunction or heart failure of varying severity is summarized in Fig. 19.3. This outline represents an integrative approach to recognize patients with asymptomatic LV dysfunction and heart failure. The history, physical, electrocardiographic, and chest x-ray findings are used together with echocardiographic findings, where appropriate, to diagnose asymptomatic LV dysfunction or the clinical syndrome of heart failure.

The diagnosis of the heart failure syndrome may be obvious when a patient, in whom non-cardiac causes for the symptoms have been excluded, has symptoms, physical signs, electrocardiogram (ECG), and chest x-ray findings that are consistent with heart failure. Under these circumstances no further tests are needed to diagnose this condition. However, echocardiographic information may well be needed later on to define the etiology and severity of LV dysfunction (*see* Fig. 19.4). An echocardiogram should be obtained when there is uncertainty about the diagnosis. Significant LV systolic (ejection fraction (EF) <40 per cent) or diastolic dysfunction (EF >40 per cent; presence of Doppler LV filling abnormalities and/or left ventricular hypertrophy (LVH)) together with compatible symptoms and signs, is likely to be consistent with the diagnosis of heart failure.

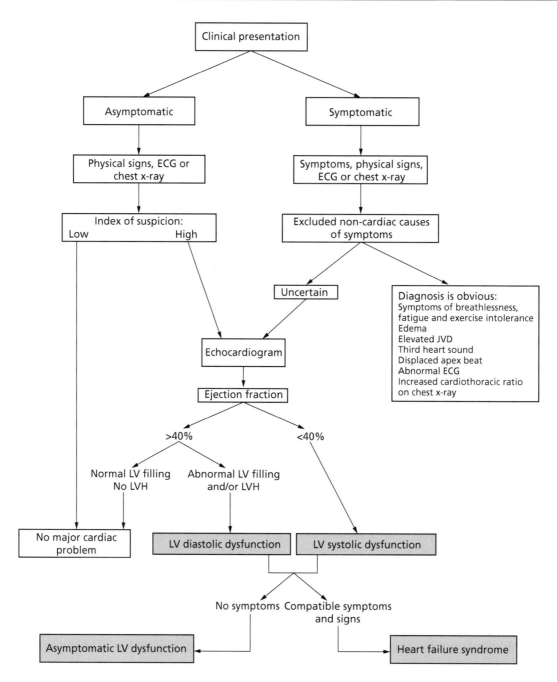

Figure 19.3 *Summary of an integrative approach to recognize patients with asymptomatic left ventricular (LV) dysfunction and heart failure. ECG = electrocardiogram; JVD = jugular venous distension; LVH = left ventricular hypertrophy.*

The diagnosis of asymptomatic LV dysfunction is based on the recognition of patients at risk for abnormal cardiac function. An echocardiogram should be obtained when there is a high index of suspicion (defined as two or more of the 14 clinical indicators listed in Table 19.6) of LV dysfunction. When there is a straightforward explanation (low index of suspicion) for the abnormal physical or ECG findings (for example, a third heart sound in a young person may be an entirely normal finding, or if there are electrolyte abnormalities that may explain the abnormal ECG), no further tests are required.

Recognition of specific heart failure syndromes

PREDOMINANT RIGHT-SIDED HEART FAILURE

Predominant right-sided failure (Table 19.7) may result from dysfunctional right ventricular (RV) myocardium, excessive RV afterload or preload, restriction to RV filling, or a combination of these. The clinical signs of right heart failure are more or less similar regardless of the etiology, and are manifested by elevated filling pressures

Table 19.7 *Clinical characteristics of common right-sided failure syndromes*

Etiology	Clinical features	ECG findings	Echocardiographic features
Acute			

RV infarction[a]	Hypotension
	Kussmaul's sign
		Inferior MI
		ST elevation in
		  right-sided leads
			Inferior wall motion abnormality
			RV dilation and decreased
			  systolic function

Acute pulmonary
  embolism
	Acute dyspnea
	Borderline hemodynamics
	Hypoxia
		Sinus tachycardia
		Acute RV strain
		S_1, Q_3, T_3
			RV dilation and decreased
			  systolic dysfunction
			Flattening of the interventricular
			  septum

Cardiac tamponade	Venous pulse: prominent
	  X′ descent
	Hypotension
	Pulsus paradoxus
		Sinus tachycardia
		Low voltage and varies
		  with respiration
			Moderate to large pericardial
			  effusion
			RV, RA, and LA collapse

Chronic			

Cor pulmonale[a]
  COPD and restrictive
    lung disease
  PTED and PPH
  Eisenmenger syndrome
	History: smoking,
	  recurrent emboli,
	  congenital disease
	Cyanosis, plethora
	TR murmur, loud P_2
		Right axis
		RV strain
		p-pulmonale
			RV dilation and decreased
			  systolic dysfunction
			Flattening of the interventricular
			  septum

LV systolic dysfunction[a]	LV apex displaced
	S_3, MR murmur
	  abnormalities
		LBBB
		Diffuse T wave
		Restrictive mitral filling
		  pattern
			Dilated, poorly contractile LV
			Varying degrees of MR

Mitral valve disease	Characteristic murmurs Loud P_2	RV strain p-mitrale	Stenotic or regurgitant mitral valve Large LA Dilated RV
Tricuspid regurgitation	Venous pulse: prominent CV wave	RA enlargement	Abnormal tricuspid valve Dilated RA, RV Normal RV systolic function

Constrictive pericarditis	Prominent X′ and Y
	  descents
	Kussmaul's sign
	Pericardial knock
	X-ray: calcified
	  pericardium
		Diffuse T-wave inversion	Small RV and LV, but large atria
			Restrictive mitral filling pattern
			Abnormal hepatic vein flow

This table highlights clinical aspects that may be useful in identifying the specific cause of predominant right-sided failure. It is assumed that all patients will present varying degrees of jugular venous distension and peripheral edema.

[a]Most common causes of right-sided failure.

COPD = chronic obstructive pulmonary disease; ECG = electrocardiogram; LA = left atrium; LBBB = left bundle branch block; LV = left ventricle; LVH = left ventricular hypertrophy; MI = myocardial infarction; MR = mitral regurgitation; P_2 = pulmonary component of the second heart sound; PPH = primary pulmonary hypertension; PTED = pulmonary thromboembolic disease; RA = right atrium; RV = right ventricle; S_3 = third heart sound; TR = tricuspid regurgitation.

and decreased right-sided output, the extent of which depends on the rate at which the right-sided failure develops. Acute or recent-onset right-sided failure, secondary to either RV infarction, acute severe pulmonary embolism or cardiac tamponade is usually characterized by elevated jugular venous pressure and a depressed cardiac output. Owing to the acute nature of these conditions, as a rule they are not associated with a generalized edematous state. In contrast, marked fluid retention as manifested by peripheral edema, visceromegaly and ascites are more consistent with chronic right-sided failure. The most common cause of right-sided failure, however, is advanced LV systolic dysfunction, and the second most common cause is cor pulmonale secondary

to chronic lung disease. The recognition of certain causes of right-sided failure is important because the management differs considerably from that of predominant left-sided failure. For example, the treatment of right-sided failure secondary to chronic obstructive pulmonary disease should be directed towards maximizing oxygenation, whereas right-sided failure due to LV dysfunction is usually managed by diuretics, ACE inhibitors, digitalis, and afterload reducing agents.

HIGH-OUTPUT HEART FAILURE

On occasion, the clinical picture of heart failure is characterized by a high-output state resulting from decreased peripheral resistance, and is clinically manifested by tachycardia, bounding pulses, warm periphery, pistol-shot femoral pulses, a third heart sound, and varying degrees of fluid retention. Identifying this syndrome is important in that many of the conditions associated with high-output heart failure are reversible (Table 19.8). Certain conditions associated with increased cardiac output, such as anemia, rarely cause heart failure, and when failure is apparent, it is likely that abnormal hemodynamics is superimposed on an underlying cardiac abnormality, such as valvular heart disease or myocardial dysfunction.

RECOGNITION OF DIASTOLIC HEART FAILURE

The symptoms of heart failure may present in the absence of LV systolic dysfunction.[54–65] This syndrome has been termed diastolic heart failure (Table 19.1) and the prevalence of this condition varies from 13 to 74 per cent.[55] It is frequently due to coronary disease or LV hypertrophy, and it is especially common in the elderly.[61,62] In patients with heart failure who were less than 65 years of age, diastolic heart failure was found in approximately 10 per cent compared to 30–35 per cent of patients 65 years of age and older.[55] Its prevalence exceeds 50 per cent in patients over the age of 80 years.[62]

The symptoms of diastolic heart failure are largely indistinguishable from those of heart failure due to impaired systolic function. However, it is most prevalent in elderly females,[65] who are most likely to present with acute pulmonary edema as the initial manifestation of heart failure. Several factors should alert the clinician to suspect underlying diastolic dysfunction including a history of hypertension, the physical findings of a sustained apical impulse with a brisk carotid upstroke and ejection systolic murmur audible over the base of the heart, an apical fourth heart sound, the electrocardiographic finding of LV hypertrophy, and evidence of pulmonary congestion without cardiomegaly on chest x-ray. The diagnosis of diastolic heart failure is usually confirmed by non-invasive tests, such as echocardiography, and when indicated, by cardiac catheterization techniques.

Etiologic considerations

AN APPROACH TO EVALUATE A PATIENT WITH NEW-ONSET HEART FAILURE

The initial evaluation of patients with new-onset heart failure should be approached in a stepwise fashion. First, as outlined in Fig. 19.3, confirm that the constellation of symptoms and signs are compatible with diagnosis of heart failure. Once there is reasonable certainty that the clinical findings are consistent with heart failure, further diagnostic testing is indicated to: (1) establish the primary cardiac pathology; (2) evaluate the extent of extracardiac (e.g. renal) involvement; (3) identify disease states that are amenable to specific interventions and (4) evaluate and recognize factors that are likely to have contributed or will conceivably contribute to the development and progression of heart failure.

The Agency for Health Care Policy and Research[66,67] and American College of Cardiology/American Heart Association Task Force on Evaluation and Management of Heart Failure[68] have made several recommendations

Table 19.8 *High output heart failure syndromes: clinical characteristics, pathophysiological mechanisms and diagnostic tests*

Etiology	Clinical features	Pathophysiological mechanisms	Diagnostic tests
Chronic anemia	Pale appearance When failure present, search for underlying cardiac pathology	Decreased O_2 carrying capacity, blood viscosity and peripheral vascular resistance, with augmented venous return	Markedly decreased hemoglobin and hematocrit
Arteriovenous fistula or other conditions that produce arteriovenous shunting Paget's disease Hepatic disease	Continuous murmur over fistula or arteriovenous malformation Branham's sign[a]	Decreased peripheral vascular resistance, increased preload	Ultrasound and/or angiography
Beri-beri	Alcohol abuse Peripheral neuritis	Thiamine deficiency leading to autonomic dysfunction Other mechanisms as above	Low blood thiamine levels and erythrocyte transketolase activity
Hyperthyroidism	Atrial arrhythmias Enlarged thyroid Elderly patient Seek underlying cardiac disease	Decreased peripheral vascular resistance, increased preload	Thyroid function tests

[a] Branham's sign: slowing of the heart after manual compression of the fistula.

for diagnostic testing in patients with stable heart failure due to LV systolic dysfunction (Table 19.9). These recommendations are divided into those tests that should be done routinely in all patients with new-onset heart failure as well as the tests that may be helpful in selected patients. Figure 19.4 provides a logical and cost-effective outline of the diagnostic steps (detailed below) that are needed to assess patients adequately that present with new-onset heart failure. This approach relies on the clinical judgment of the physician and the ability to integrate clinical data with the echocardiographic findings.

Step 1: Once there is certainty about the diagnosis of the clinical syndrome of heart failure, the next step is to characterize the predominant hemodynamic abnormality. Two-dimensional echocardiography provides the most straightforward approach to identify whether heart failure is due to LV systolic dysfunction (ejection fraction ≤40 per cent) or LV diastolic dysfunction (ejection fraction >40 per cent), or valvular heart disease (often associated with LV systolic and/or diastolic dysfunction).

Step 2: The next important step is identify whether LV systolic or diastolic dysfunction is due to an ischemic etiology. In many instances an ischemic etiology is self-evident, as for example in patients with ECG manifestations of an extensive anterior myocardial infarction (definite ischemic etiology). A non-ischemic cause of the LV dysfunction may be equally apparent, for instance in patients with adriamycin cardiotoxicity or where ischemia would be extremely unlikely, such as in a young person (definite non-ischemic etiology). When it is not clear whether ischemia caused or contributed to LV dysfunction (uncertain etiology), stress imaging (thallium scintigraphy or pharmacological stress testing) may help clarify this issue.

Step 3: The next important step is to establish whether LV dysfunction can be completely or partially reversed. Further testing is contingent on whether the patient would be a suitable candidate for revascularization procedures or not. Cardiac catheterization is indicated when reversible ischemia is obvious from the history or ECG changes (definite), whereas stress imaging is indicated when uncertainty exists. Also, reversible causes of a non-ischemic cardiomyopathy should be excluded (*see* Table 19.10). Further tests are indicated when reversible causes are possible, as for example in patients with suspected hemochromatosis (i.e. serum ferritin).

COMMON ERRORS IN THE DIAGNOSIS AND EVALUATION OF HEART FAILURE

The Agency for Health Care Policy and Research[66] has identified several aspects about the diagnosis and evaluation of heart failure patients in the community that are not optimal. These are:

- patients with symptoms suggestive of heart failure are often not thoroughly evaluated to rule out non-cardiac causes before treatment for heart failure is started;

Table 19.9 *Recommended diagnostic and other tests for the evaluation of heart failure*

Test/procedure	AHCPR All patients	AHCPR Selected patients	ACC/AHA All patients	ACC/AHA Selected patients	Rationale (narrow differential diagnosis for HF and /or identify factors that contibute to HF)
Laboratory tests					
CBC	+	−	+	−	Detect anemia, a contributing factor to HF
Electrolytes	+	−	+	−	Detect electrolyte disturbances
Urea/Cr	+	−	+	−	Assess renal function, guide to treatment
Albumin	+	−	+	−	Exclude hypoalbuminemia as a cause of edema
LFTs	+	−	+	−	Assess liver function
$Ca^{2+}/Mg^{2+}/PO_4^-$	−	+	+	−	Detect electrolyte disturbances
Urinalysis	+	−	+	−	Exclude nephrotic syndrome
T_4/TSH	−	+	−	+	Detect occult hyperthyroidism in the elderly and in patients with atrial fibrillation
Other routine tests					
ECG, chest x-ray	+	+	+	−	Establish recent infarction, detect pneumonia
Echo-Doppler	+	+	+	−	Detect valvular and wall motion abnormalities
Stress test with imaging	−	+	−	+	Assess extent of ischemia
Ambulatory ECG	−	+	−	+	Assess cause of syncope
Endomyocardial biopsy	−	+	−	+	Diagnose infiltrative disorders (i.e. hemochromatosis)
Measurement of exercise capacity	−	+	−	+	Assess functional status

Recommended routine diagnostic tests for patients with stable heart failure according to the Agency for Health Care Policy and Research[66] (AHCPR) and American College of Cardiology/American Heart Association (ACC/AHA) Task Force on Evaluation and Management of Heart Failure.[68] + = tests that should be done routinely; − = tests that should not be done routinely; CBC = complete blood count; Cr = creatinine; ECG = electrocardiogram; HF = heart failure; LFTs = liver function tests; T_4 = thyroxine; TSH = thyroid-stimulating hormone.

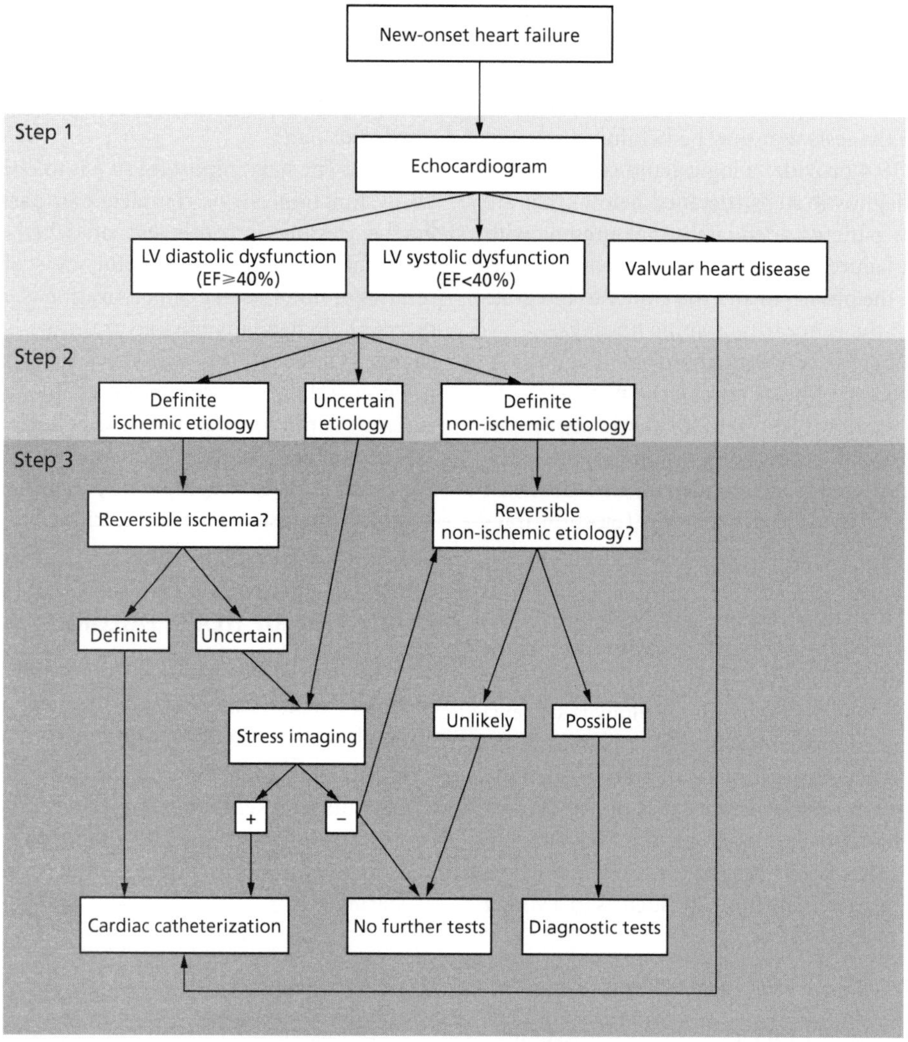

Figure 19.4 *A stepwise approach to establishing the etiology of the underlying cardiac pathology and to identify reversible and contributing factors in patients with new-onset heart failure (see text for details). LV = left ventricular; EF = ejection fraction.*

- symptoms of heart failure may be attributable to chronic lung disease and treated inappropriately;
- reversible causes of heart failure are not always identified, or when identified, they may be undertreated;
- patients with peripheral edema may be inappropriately labeled as having heart failure when there is another cause for edema;
- an initial measurement of LV function is not always obtained;
- concurrent angina or other evidence of ischemia is not always properly evaluated.

PRECIPITATING CAUSES OF HEART FAILURE

These factors can be defined as those factors that may precipitate decompensation in patients with underlying cardiac disease, but are unlikely to cause cardiac decom-

pensation in patients with normal hearts. Identifying the precipitating causes of the decompensation has obvious therapeutic implications. A list of the more common precipitating factors are shown in Table 19.11. Most of the cardiac arrhythmias that can worsen the hemodynamic and clinical status of patients with heart failure are supraventricular in origin. These tachyarrhythmias reduce the time available for filling, an event that is particularly deleterious in patients with impaired ventricular relaxation. Moreover, tachycardia increases myocardial oxygen consumption and decreases the time available for myocardial perfusion, and thus may exacerbate myocardial ischemia. Mild ischemia that ordinarily may not have a major hemodynamic effect may precipitate acute pulmonary edema in elderly patients with left ventricular hypertrophy secondary to hypertension or in patients with compromised ventricular function (e.g. prior myocardial infarction). Ischemia may manifest as

Table 19.10 *Reversible myocardial dysfunction: causes, clinical features, and treatment*

Etiology	Clinical features	Treatment
Ischemic	Angina, ischemic ECG, and stress imaging scans	Revascularization
Toxins		
Alcohol	History of alcoholism, ↑MCV, ↑GGT	Abstinence
Anthracyclines	Recent chemotherapy	Termination of treatment
Cocaine	Use of cocaine, hyperadrenergic state	Abstinence
Endotoxic sepsis	Gram-negative sepsis	Transient, treat bacteremia
Infections		
Viral	Recent viral illness, myopericarditis	Supportive treatment only
Lyme disease	Conduction abn, skin and joint involvement	Usually resolves within 6 months
Toxoplasmosis	AIDS, lymphadenopathy	Antibiotics
Mycoplasma	Pneumonia, cold, agglutinins	Antibiotics
Metabolic		
Hypocalcemia	Hypoparathyroidism, ↑Q-T interval	Calcium and parathyroid hormone
Hypophosphatemia	Alcoholism, hyperalimentation, recovery of DKA	Phosphate
Uremia	Renal failure	Dialysis
Endocrinopathies		
Hyperthyroidism	Hyperthyroid state, elderly patient	Antithyroid drugs, I$_2$, or surgery
Pheochromocytoma	Hyperadrenergic state, hypertension	Tumor excision
Acromegaly	Typical acromegalic features	Surgery or radiation
Infiltrative disorders		
Hemochromatosis	Bronze diabetic, cirrhosis, ↑serum ferritin,	Chelation therapy, phlebotomy
Sarcoid	Skin and lung manifestations, conduction abn	Steroids
Nutritional deficiencies		
Beri-beri	Alcohol abuse, polyneuropathy	Thiamine
Carnitine deficiency	Inherited progressive skeletal myopathy	Carnitine
Selenium	Occurs mainly in China	Selenium
Miscellaneous		
Tachycardia-induced	Incessant SVT or AF with ↑ ventricular response	β-blockers, ablation
Peripartum CMO	Within 6 months of delivery	Spontaneous recovery

Abn = abnormalities; AF = atrial fibrillation; CMO = cardiomyopathy; DKA = diabetic ketoacidosis; ECG = electrocardiogram GGT = gamma glutamyl transferase; I$_2$ = iodine; MCV = mean corpuscular volume; SVT = supraventricular tachycardia; ↑ = increased.

episodes of typical angina or may occur without symptoms. Several commonly used medications, such as non-steroidal anti-inflammatory drugs, antiarrhythmic drugs, calcium-channel blocking and β-adrenergic blocking agents, may exacerbate the symptoms of heart failure in patients with severe LV systolic dysfunction.

Severity and prognosis of heart failure

An important component of the initial evaluation is to assess the severity of heart failure since this will determine both overall prognosis and the initial and long-term treatment strategies. Assessment of the severity further enables one to identify high-risk patients who might derive benefit from more aggressive medical or surgical therapy. In addition, it is useful to document the extent of functional impairment during the first encounter with the patient so that it may be used as a reference for subsequent assessments.

SEVERITY OF FUNCTIONAL IMPAIRMENT

The severity of symptoms is an important indicator of overall morbidity and mortality. The most widely utilized symptom scale is the New York Heart Association (NYHA) functional classification[69] (Table 19.12), but its accuracy and reproducibility is limited. For example, the NYHA classification is not predictive of the degree of LV dysfunction or of the exercise capacity.[70–72] Nevertheless, it is still a useful crude index of the patient's perception of their functional impairment. An accurate assessment of the activities of daily living may be the best barometer of the degree of functional impairment in any particular patient. Several tools, of which the *Minnesota Living with Heart Failure questionnaire*[73] is the most widely used, have been developed to measure the 'quality of life' of heart failure patients. These tools are more useful in research settings than in the clinical management of patients.

Exercise testing with measurement of peak oxygen

Table 19.11 *Precipitating causes of heart failure*

1. Dietary indiscretion
2. Excessive postoperative fluid administration
3. Non-compliance to medical regimen
4. Worsening renal failure
5. Anemia
6. Systemic infection
7. Pulmonary embolism
8. Myocardial ischemia
9. Tachyarrhymia and bradyarrhythmia
10. Electrolyte disturbances
11. Hyperthyroidism and hypothyroidism
12. Cardiodepressant drugs and other drugs that may worsen heart failure:
    - Anti-inflammatory drugs: steroids, non-steroidal anti-inflammatory agents.
    - Anti-arrhythmic drugs: Disopyramide, Flecainide, Encainide, Mexilitine, Tocainide, Procainamide, Lidocaine
    - Calcium-channel blockers: Verapamil, Diltiazem, Nifedipine
    - β-Blocking agents

consumption is widely accepted as the best index of the severity of heart failure. Maximum oxygen consumption has shown not only to be an independent predictor of mortality in large treatment trials[71] but it has become a valuable tool to determine the need and timing of cardiac transplantation.[74] However, such testing is not routinely available in an outpatient setting and it is probably not needed in the vast majority of patients. A useful and simple measure of the severity of heart failure is the 6-minute walk test.[75] This test can be safely done in the outpatient setting and has been shown in clinical trials to predict mortality and morbidity.[76]

Table 19.12 *New York Heart Association classification of heart failure*

Class I	*No limitations*: ordinary physical activity does not cause undue fatigue, dyspnea, or palpitation
Class II	*Slight limitation of physical activity*: comfortable at rest but ordinary physical activities lead to fatigue, shortness of breath, or palpitations
Class III	*Marked limitation of physical activity*: although patients are comfortable at rest, less than ordinary activity will lead to symptoms
Class IV	*Inability to engage in any physical activity without discomfort*: symptoms are present at rest

FACTORS THAT PREDICT SURVIVAL IN PATIENTS WITH HEART FAILURE

In addition to functional disability of patients with heart failure, several other factors appear to be predictive of

increased mortality. Table 19.13 provides a list of the cardiac and non-cardiac factors that affect survival.

MANAGEMENT OF PATIENTS WITH HEART FAILURE

Historical perspectives

Early treatments for marked congestion included therapies such as leeches and subcutaneous Southey's tubes. These measures were moderately successful at relieving edema but were cumbersome and complicated by a high incidence of skin infections. Diuretic treatment evolved from the discovery in 1920 that sulfonamides possess diuretic actions, to the effects of mercurial agents in 1949 and the renal effects of thiazides in 1958. More potent loop diuretics were developed in the 1960s. Vasodilator treatment for heart failure was introduced in the 1950s but the survival benefit of these agents were only demonstrated in large clinical trials in the mid-1980s. In 1987, ACE inhibitors were shown for the first time to reduce mortality in patients with advanced heart failure. Although the benefits of digoxin was recognized by Withering in 1785, it was only in 1996 that this agent was shown in a large randomized trial to be safe and useful in the treatment of heart failure. More recently, β-blockers were shown to benefit patients with moderate to severe heart failure.

Management options in heart failure

NON-PHARMACOLOGICAL MANAGEMENT OF HEART FAILURE

The non-pharmacological non-surgical management of heart failure consists of identification and avoidance of factors that are likely to contribute to the progression of LV dysfunction, and implementation of measures that may reduce symptoms, improve quality of life, reduce the psychological burden of patients and family members having to deal with the consequences of heart failure, and enhance the effectiveness of drug therapy. Several interventions have been proposed to achieve these objectives and these are listed in Table 19.14. Studies of other chronic illnesses such as diabetes and asthma support the notion that many of these measures reduce morbidity and are cost effective.[87,88]

PHARMACOLOGICAL TREATMENT OF HEART FAILURE

The drugs that are routinely used in the treatment of heart failure are listed in Table 19.15.[89] Several other and newer agents have also been shown in well-designed prospective trials to either improve survival or to relieve symptoms in patients with heart failure (Table 19.16).

Table 19.13 *Factors that affect survival in patients with heart failure*

Factors	Comments
Subtypes of heart failure	
Ischemic *vs* non-ischemic[69]	Ischemic LV dysfunction is associated with a higher mortality than non-ischemic LV dysfunction
Systolic *vs* diastolic heart failure[77,78]	Systolic dysfunction is associated with a worse long-term survival than diastolic dysfunction
Systolic and diastolic dysfunction[79]	Diastolic dysfunction coexistent with impaired systolic function worsens survival
Demographic factors	
Age[80]	Risk of death in patients 64 years and older at 1 year is 1.5× greater than those under 64 years of age
Race[81]	African Americans have about 1.5–2.0-fold higher mortality risk when diagnosed with heart failure than whites
Hemodynamic parameters	
LV ejection fraction[71]	The mortality risk related to depressed ejection fraction (EF) is markedly increased for each decrement of the EF under 30 per cent
RV ejection fraction[82]	RV ejection fraction as measured by radionucleotide techniques appears to be directly related to survival in patients with NYHA class II and IV heart failure
Symptoms and functional impairment	
NYHA classification[69]	Survival is inversely related to NYHA class
Peak O_2 consumption[74]	Peak O_2 consumption of < 14 mL/kg per minute predicts a high 1-year mortality, independent of ejection fraction
6-minute walk test[76]	A total distance <305 m was associated with annual mortality of 11% *vs* 4% in patients who could walk for >443 m
Electrolytes	
Sodium[83]	A sodium concentration of < 130 mEq/L was shown to be associated with survival rate of less than 20% compared to nearly 50% for those with a sodium level of over 130 mEq/L
Arrhythmias	
Non-sustained ventricular tachycardia (NSVT)[84–86]	Two studies have shown prospectively that NSVT is an independent risk factor for sudden death in patients with heart failure
Comorbid conditions associated with increased mortality	
Hepatic dysfunction	
Renal dysfunction	
Hypertension	
Diabetes	
Pulmonary hypertension	

LV = Left ventricular; RV = right ventricular; NYHA = New York Heart Association.

The pharmacological treatment according to the functional class of heart failure is listed in Table 19.17.

ACE inhibitors

The angiotensin-converting enzyme is identical to kininase II, the enzyme responsible for the degradation of kinins. Thus, the primary actions of ACE inhibitors are to inhibit the production of angiotensin II and the degradation of kinins.[90] As a result, ACE inhibition causes peripheral vasodilation not only by blocking the formation of angiotensin II but also by enhancing kinin-mediated prostaglandin synthesis. Recent work further suggests that ACE inhibition may affect the course of heart failure by improving diastolic function,[91] preventing progressive loss of myocardial cells,[92] and attenuating ventricular remodeling in response to pressure overload[93,94] or secondary to ischemic injury.[95] These actions of ACE inhibitors have translated into an improved survival in a broad spectrum of patients with myocardial infarction and heart failure, ranging from those who are asymptomatic with LV dysfunction to those who are symptomatic with advanced heart failure[34–45] (*see* Table 19.18). In addition, ACE inhibitors improve functional status in patients with heart failure, with 40–80 per cent of patients showing improvement in NYHA functional class.[96–99] It should be recognized, however, that improve-

Table 19.14 *Non-pharmacological interventions in the treatment of heart failure*

Interventions	Objectives	Implementation and guidelines
General	Smoking cessation Vaccinations against influenza and pneumococcal disease	Motivational and behavioral modifying techniques may be required
Regular exercise	Increased physical activity Physical conditioning Reduce risk factors for CAD Lose weight if patient is obese	Encourage exercise; unless unstable HF Walking programs: aim to double distance in 2 weeks[a] Tailored exercise training programs[a] Avoid isometric exercise
Dietary interventions	Alcohol restriction (<2 oz/day) Salt restriction (*see* Table 19.15) Fluid restriction (if required) Low-fat, low-cholesterol diet when there are risk factors for CAD Vitamin supplementation if indicated	Refer to dietitian, clinical nurse specialist, or nurse practitioner for dietary education and counseling Fluid restriction is not advisable unless there is hyponatremia
Self-care strategies and patient education	To achieve an understanding of the nature of HF, the reason for symptoms, what symptoms can be expected, the rationale behind the use of medications and the anticipated side-effects To formulate with patient and family members the actions desired surrounding the need for advanced care Able to self-monitor symptoms and body weight Clarify the patient's and care giver's responsibilities Treatment plan of what to do if symptoms worsen	Three or four educational sessions may be needed Provide patient with literature Group sessions may be helpful Direct patient to community resources Obtain advance directives from patient and family Provide patient with a logbook to record weights and symptoms Frequent telephone contact may improve compliance and motivation Referral to nurse-run HF program with emphasis on education and self-management if time requirements prevents the practitioner from implementing these strategies

[a]Insufficient evidence at present to recommend routine use of supervised exercise programs.
CAD = coronary artery disease; HF = heart failure.

ment in exercise tolerance does not occur immediately after initiating therapy with an ACE inhibitor, despite improvements in hemodynamics. Rather, it increases slowly, with the maximum benefit appearing after 3–6 months.[100,101] All patients with heart failure should therefore be considered for such treatment even if they are asymptomatic. Of note is that the clinical, hemodynamic, and prognostic benefits of ACE inhibitors appear to be attenuated by the co-administration of aspirin,[102,103] which blocks kinin-mediated prostaglandin synthesis. It is not yet known whether aspirin should be discontinued or the dose reduced when given with an ACE inhibitor. All ACE inhibitors are similar in their therapeutic profile. However, when ACE inhibitor treatment is initiated in severe heart failure, the shorter acting inhibitor, captopril, is preferred since it is less likely to be associated with prolonged hypotension and renal dysfunction than longer acting agents.[104]

An outline of how to initiate therapy with an ACE inhibitor is provided in Fig. 19.5.

First it should be established whether there are any clear contraindications to initiating an ACE inhibitor, which may include bilateral renal artery stenosis and advanced renal failure (creatinine (Cr) > 3.5 mg/dL). If the renal function is acceptable (Cr $\leq$ 1.5 mg/dL) and there is low risk for first-dose hypotension, an ACE inhibitor could be initiated at the doses outlined.

If after 1 week the dose was well tolerated in terms of blood pressure, creatinine and K+, then the medications could be increased to the desired target doses (*see* Table 19.15) within 2–3 weeks. However, when the risk of first-dose hypotension is increased (hypovolemia, pre-renal azotemia, metabolic alkalosis, advanced LV dysfunction and patients aged 75 years and older), diuretics should be decreased before 6.25 mg of captopril is given as an initial test dose. If this is tolerated (after 2 hours), then the dose of captopril or a long-acting ACE inhibitor could be doubled and continued for a week as before, but

Table 19.15 *Drugs routinely used in the treatment of chronic stable heart failure*

Drug Name	Dose (mg)	Frq	Target dose	Dose adjustments	Drug interactions	Adverse effects	Contraindications
ACE inhibitors				• Initiate with a low dose (e.g. 12.5 mg of captopril or 2.5 mg of enalapril) and then ↑ to target range within 1–4 weeks • Start at lower dose if Na$^+$ <135 mmol/L • Discontinue with progressive azotemia or intolerable cough • See Fig. 19.8	• Reduce diuretic dose if BUN and Cr ↑ • ACEI + K$^+$-sparing diuretics may ↑↑ K$^+$ • ASA or NSAID may counteract the beneficial effects of ACEI[89,90] • ACEI + vasodilators may cause hypotension	• Dizziness (3.3%) • Headache (5%) • Agranulocytosis[a] • ↑ BUN and Cr • Angioedema[a] • Nausea (1.4%) • ↑K$^+$ (1%) • Cough (1.9–3.4%)	• Pregnancy • Renal artery stenosis • Prior ACEI anaphylaxis • Severe renal impairment • K$^+$>5.5 mmol/L
Captopril	6.25–150	3×/day	50 mg TID				
Enalapril	2.5–20	2×/day	10 mg BID				
Lisinopril	2.5–40	1×/day	—				
Ramipril	2.5–10	1–2×/day	5 mg BID				
Quinapril	5–20	1×/day	—				
Zofenopril[b]	—	—	30 mg BID				
Trandopril[b]	—	—	4 mg QD				
β-Blocking agents				See Fig. 19.7	• Worsening heart failure administered with calcium antagonists • Hypotension when given with other vasodilators	• Fatigue • Worsening heart failure • Worsening asthma • Bradycardia • Hypotension	• Asthma • Heart block and bradycardia • Unstable heart failure
Carvedilol	3.125–50	2×/day	25 mg BID				
Metoprolol CR/XL	25–200	2×/day	150–200 mg QD				
Diuretics				• A thiazide 2–3×/week may be adequate in certain patients • ↓ dose when starting ACEI • ↓ dose when ↑ in BUN and Cr • A flexible program is useful if ↑↑ doses are needed • Refractory fluid retention may require IV loop diuretics • Combination of synergistic diuretics is more effective than ↑↑ doses of loop diuretics • See Fig. 19.9	• As above with ACEI • Aminoglycosides: ↑ risk of ototoxicity • Anticoagulants: ↑ effects • Lithium: ↑ concentrations • Probenecid: ↓ action of loop diuretics • Digoxin: ↑ risk of arrhythmias	• Anorexia, nausea, diarrhea, pancreatitis • Hearing impairment • ↑ BUN, Cr • ↓↑K$^+$, Mg^{++} • Urticaria, pruritus, photosensitivity, Stevens–Johnson's syndrome • Aplastic anemia, leukopenia, thrombocytopenia • ↑ uric acid, glucose • Gynecomastia	• Anuria • Allergy to sulfonamides
Thiazide							
HTZ	25–50	1×/day	As needed				
Chlothalidone	25–100	1×/day	As needed				
Metolazone[c]	2.5–10	1–2×/day	As needed				
Loop							
Furosemide	20–200	1–2×/day	As needed				
Bumetanide	0.5–4	1–2×/day	As needed				
Ethacrynic acid	50–200	1–2×/day	As needed				
Torsemide	5–100	1×/day	As needed				
K$^+$-sparing							
Trimaterene	50–100	1–2×/day	As needed				
Amiloride	5–10	1×/day	As needed				
Spironolactone	25–100	1–2×/day	As needed				

Table 19.15 (continued)

Drug Name	Dose (mg)	Frq	Target dose	Dose adjustments	Drug interactions	Adverse effects	Contraindications
Digitalis Digoxin	0.125–0.375	Varies	—	• Discontinue or adjust dose if: • ↑ serum digoxin levels • ↓ renal function • Symptoms of toxicity • Conduction abnormalities • Ventricular arrhythmias	• ↑ levels: (1) ↓ renal + non-renal clearance: amiodarone, verapamil, diltiazem, spironolactone, quinidine; (2) other mechanisms: propafenone, tetracycline, erythromycin, tiapamil, nicardipine • ↓ levels: antacids, neomycin, phenytoin, cholestyramine	• Cardiotoxicity • Nausea, vomiting • Confusion • Anorexia, psychosis • Visual disturbances • Gynecomastia • Thrombocytopenia	• Certain pre-excitation states • A-V block • Cor pulmonale (relative) • Hypertrophic obstructive cardiomyopathy

^aRare complications; ^bnot approved by the FDA in the USA for the treatment of heart failure; ^cthiazide-like diuretic; ↓ = decreased; ↑ = increased.

ACEI = angiotensin converting enzyme inhibitor; ASA = aspirin; BID = twice a day; BUN = blood urea nitrogen; Cr = creatine; Frq = frequency; HTZ = hydrochlorothiazide; IV = intravenous; NSAID = non-steroidal anti-inflammation drug; QD = once a day; TID = 3× per day.

Table 19.16 *Other drugs used in the treatment of chronic stable heart failure*^a

Drug Name	Dose (mg)	Frq	Target dose	Dose adjustments	Drug interactions	Adverse effects	Contraindications
Hydralazine^b	40–400	3–4×/day	50 mg QD	• Initiate at a dose of 25 mg TID and increase to 75 mg TID. Then change to QD. Patients with severe heart failure, advanced age or low BP start with 10 mg TID • ↓ dose when patient complains of headaches and dizziness • ↓ dose with severe renal failure	• Hypotension when given with other anti-hypertensive agents	• Dizziness • Headache • Edema • Lupus syndrome • Tachycardia	• Aortic or mitral stenosis • Myocardial ischemia
ISDN	5–40	4×/day	40 mg TID	• Start with 10 mg TID and increase weekly to 40 mg TID	• Hypotension when given with other anti-hypertensive agents	• Hypotension • Headaches • Flushing	• Hypertrophic cardiomyopathy
Losartan	25–50	1×/day	50 mg QD	Start with 25 mg QD	• No significant drug interactions	• Angioedema • Musculoskeletal: cramps, myalgias • ↑ BUN and Cr • ↑ K⁺	• Hypersensitivity to losartan

^a Abbreviations as in Table 19.15.

^b Not approved by the FDA in the USA for the treatment of heart failure. ISDN = isosorbide dinitrate; QD = once a day.

Table 19.17 *Standard pharmacological treatment according to the functional class of heart failure*

	Asymptomatic	FC I	FC II	FC III	FC IV
ACEI	+	+	+	+	+
β-Blockers	–	–	+	+	–
Spironolactone	–	–	–	+	+
Digoxin	–	–	+	+	+
Diuretics	–	–	+	+	+

FC = functional class; + = indicated; - = not indicated.

Table 19.18 *Beneficial effects of ACE inhibitors in heart failure and LV dysfunction after myocardial infarction: data from large trials*

Acronym	Year	Agent (target dose)	Patient profile	Number of patients	End points: % reductions in Hospitalizations for HF (95% CI)	All-cause mortality (95% CI)
Consensus I[34]	1987	Enalapril (10 mg BID)	NYHA IV	253	40% (NP)	40% (NP)
SOLVD[38] (Treatment)	1991	Enalapril (10 mg BID)	NYHA II–III EF ≤35%	2569	26% (18–34%)	16% (5–26%)
SOLVD[39] (Prevention)/	1992	Enalapril (10 mg BID)	NYHA I EF ≤35%	4228	20% (9–30%)[a]	12% (−3–26%) (P<0.12)
SAVE[35]	1992	Captopril (50 mg TID)	Post-MI patients EF <40%	2231	22% (4–37%)	19% (3–32%)
AIRE[40]	1993	Ramipril (5 mg BID)	Post-MI patients with HF	2006	NP	27% (11–40%)
TRACE[41]	1995	Trandalopril (4 mg QD)	Post-MI patients EF ≤35%	1749	29% (11–44%)	22% (9–33%)
SMILE[42]	1995	Zofenopril (30 mg BID)	Acute anterior MI	1556	46% (11–71%)	29% (6–51%)

The trials listed here pertain only to those that examined the effect of ACE inhibitors on patients with LV dysfunction post-myocardial infarction (MI) and those with asymptomatic LV dysfunction, and mild to severe heart failure.
[a]The data showed for the SOLVD prevention study does not give hospitalization rates for heart failure but rather the reduction in the risk of death or the development of heart failure.
ACE = angiotensin-converting enzyme; BID = twice daily; CI = confidence interval; EF = ejection fraction; HF = heart failure; LV = left ventricular; NP = not provided; NYHA = New York Heart Association; TID = three times daily.

if this dose is not well tolerated, diuretic dosages should be decreased further and/or (other) vasodilators discontinued so that the patient could be rechallenged with captopril at a later stage (Fig. 19.5, arrowed by broken lines). Should this fail again, an angiotensin II receptor blocker or hydralazine in combination with isosorbide dinitrate (HYD/ISDN) appear to be reasonable alternatives. When hyperkalemia develops as a result of an ACE inhibitor, therapy should be changed to HYD/ISDN. With moderate renal impairment the same protocol should be followed as outlined for the patient at increased risk of hypotension, but if there is severe renal impairment (Cr = 2.6–3.5 mg/dL), the patient should be admitted to hospital and started on captopril 6.25 mg qd. In the event that this dose is not tolerated after 2 hours, the same steps as before could be taken. However, if the ACE inhibitor is tolerated, captopril 6.25 mg qd should be continued for 3 days. The ACEI should be replaced by HYD/ISDN should the Cr increase by more than 0.5 mg/dL after 3 days of treatment, but if the Cr

increased by less than 0.5 mg/dL, a lower dose of an ACE inhibitor may be acceptable for chronic therapy.

Angiotensin receptor blockers

Losartan, the commercially available angiotensin-2 receptor blocker, has been shown to have favorable hemodynamic effects in chronic heart failure. The recently completed ELITE II trial showed that losartan was not superior to captopril in patients 60 years and older with NYHA class II–IV heart failure and ejection fractions of ≤ 40 per cent.[104a] Until more is known about these agents, it would seem reasonable to reserve these agents for those patients that are intolerant of ACE inhibitors.

β-Adrenergic blockers

Controlled clinical trials have shown that β-blockers can produce hemodynamic and symptomatic improvement in chronic heart failure, but until recently the effect of these drugs on survival was not established.[105–111] These agents were considered for the most part to be experi-

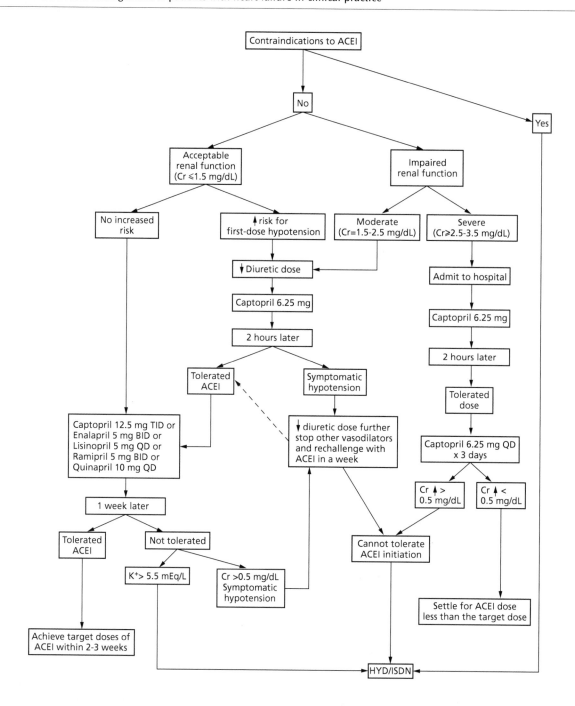

Figure 19.5 *This flow diagram represents the steps that are recommended when initiating an ACE inhibitor (ACEI). BID = twice daily; Cr = creatinine; HYD/ISDN = hydralazine in combination with isosorbide dinitrate; QD = once a day; TID = three times daily.*

mental, but promising therapy for heart failure. However, there is now strong evidence that β-blockers combined with digoxin, diuretics, and an ACE inhibitor may reduce the risk of death as well as the risk of hospitalization for worsening heart failure. Carvedilol, a new class of non-selective β-blocker with vasodilating as well as antioxidant properties, was shown in a randomized trial of 1094 patients with chronic heart failure to decrease mortality by 65 per cent (95 per cent confidence interval (CI): 39–80 per cent).[112] In addition, when com-

pared with placebo, carvedilol therapy was accompanied by a 27 per cent reduction in the risk of hospitalization for cardiovascular causes. The effects of carvedilol on morbidity and mortality was equally apparent for both ischemic and non-ischemic causes of LV dysfunction. Extended release was also shown in a recent randomized trial to improve survival in patients with chronic heart failure.[113]

Selection of patients for β-blocker therapy remains difficult and there are no comparative data between the β-blockers to select one over the other. Although many patients may show transient worsening of symptoms and require increased diuretic therapy and/or a decrease in the dose of the ACE inhibitor during the first 2–4 weeks of treatment, symptomatic benefits usually appear after about 6–8 weeks.

The steps that are required to initiate these agents in heart failure are shown in Fig. 19.6. Any health care professional who plans to initiate a β-blocker in a patient with symptomatic heart failure should have a clear understanding of the commitment that is required to start these agents in patients in whom symptoms may

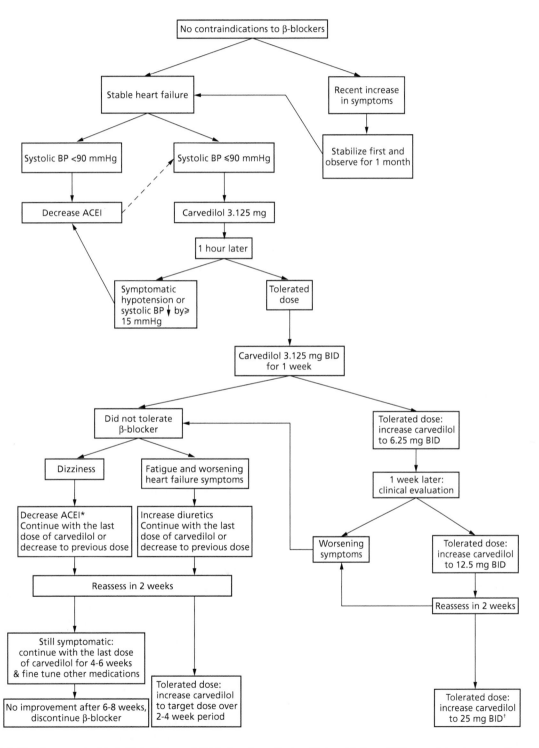

Figure 19.6 *The steps required to initiate the use of β-blockers in patients with heart failure. ACEI = angiotensin-converting enzyme inhibitor; BID = twice daily; BP = blood pressure; * or other vasodilators; † increase dose to 50 mg BID if patient weighs more than 100 kg. Metroprolol may be substituted for carvedilol in this scheme.*

actually worsen before they improve. In general, most patients will tolerate the initiation of a β-blocker if the dose is increased over a 6–8 week period. Although the flow diagram in Fig. 19.6 represents the steps that allow the safe initiation of carvedilol, it is equally applicable to metoprolol.

> If there are no apparent contraindications to β-blockers (asthma, NYHA class IV heart failure, heart block or symptomatic bradycardia) but the systolic blood pressure (BP) is < 90 mm Hg, the dose ACE inhibitor or other vasodilator should be decreased before initiating carvedilol. If the BP is ⩾ 90 mm Hg, however, start carvedilol, at a test dose of 3.125 mg. The patient should then be observed for 1 hour for any changes in BP and heart rate.

If the patient becomes hypotensive or symptomatic with a low BP, the same steps (decreasing ACE inhibitor) as before should be taken before attempting a second test dose. When the test dose is tolerated, carvedilol should be continued at a dose of 3.125 mg twice a day for 1 week after which the patient should be reassessed. If after a week the patient complains of dizziness and the BP is lower than before, the dose of ACEI or other vasodilators may have to be decreased. If the patient complains of fatigue, and there are symptoms and signs of worsening heart failure, the diuretic dosages may have to be increased. At this point up-titration of the dose should only be undertaken when the patient feels better. Furthermore, the carvedilol dose can either be kept at the same level or may be decreased for a while until the patient feels better. If at the higher doses the patient becomes symptomatic (again or for the first time), the same steps as before should be followed. The patient should be assessed every 2 weeks and, if symptoms persist, a lower dose of carvedilol could be continued for another 4–6 weeks. In the event that, after 6–8 weeks of treatment, the patient still feels worse than before the β-blocker was started, then this agent should be discontinued. However, if the patient tolerates the up-titration phase, then carvedilol should be increased to the target dose of 25 mg twice daily.

Diuretics

These agents are extremely effective in the symptomatic treatment of heart failure when there is evidence of a congestive state. Four main principles underlie their use in heart failure:

- use in moderation and avoid excessive doses of any single drug;
- make use of synergism between different classes of drugs, especially when there is apparent tolerance to loop diuretics;
- monitor electrolytes, avoid uremia, hyponatremia, hypokalemia, hypomagnesemia;
- use in combination with an ACE inhibitor unless not tolerated.

The frequency with which electrolytes should be monitored during the treatment with diuretics is dependent on the strength of the diuretics prescribed, the extent of diuresis required, the pharmacological actions of the agent chosen and the underlying renal function. Biochemical studies once or twice weekly will usually suffice in a majority of patients until the electrolytes are stable and/or the patient is on a stable dose. Thereafter, electrolytes should be checked every time a higher dose of the existing diuretic is prescribed or a new agent is added. Table 19.19 provides recommendations for the most appropriate diuretic regimen for varying degrees of fluid retention.

Digoxin

Although the efficacy of digitalis in patients with heart failure and atrial fibrillation has long been established, its value in patients with heart failure and sinus rhythm has often been questioned. In the 1980s, reports of some large-scale trials indicated that digoxin, with or without vasodilators or ACE inhibitors, reduced signs and symptoms of congestive heart failure and improved exercise tolerance.[114–117] This beneficial influence was mainly found in patients with advanced heart failure and dilated ventricles,[116] whereas the effect in those with mild disease appeared to be less pronounced. In the last few years, new data have shown that digoxin may also have clinical value in mild heart failure, either when used in combination with other drugs or when administered alone.[115] The large-scale survival trial by the Digitalis Investigators Group (DIG) has shown that although digoxin has a neutral effect on total mortality during long-term treatment, it reduces the number of hospital admissions and deaths due to worsening heart failure.[118] This trial further showed there was greater benefit at the lower range of ejection fractions and in the patients with a non-ischemic etiology than in those with ischemic etiology for heart failure. There was also a trend toward more benefit in patients with NYHA class III and IV symptoms compared with those with milder symptoms.

> Based on these findings, digoxin should be initiated with ACE inhibitors and diuretics in patients with moderate and severe heart failure. Loading doses of digoxin are not generally needed. In the presence of normal renal function, the typical doses of 0.25 mg daily may be instituted.[66]

On the whole, the dosing schedule followed by the DIG study represents a rational approach[118] and a summary of this schedule has been published.[119] Usually after a week of treatment a steady state is reached, the patient should then be questioned for symptoms of toxicity, and an ECG, serum digoxin level, serum electrolytes, blood urea nitrogen (BUN) and creatinine obtained.

Table 19.19 *Diuretic regimen for fluid overload states*

Extent of fluid overload	Diuretic	Dose	Site of action	Comments
Asymptomatic LV dysfunction or the absence of congestion	Nil			
Mild fluid retention	HCTZ	25–50 mg QD (3 × /week may suffice)	Distal convulated tubule	Dietary Na+ should not exceed 2 g/day
Moderate fluid retention	Furosemide **or** bumetanide	20–40 mg QD 0.5–1 mg QD	Ascending limb of loop of Henle	As above Elderly patients may be started on 10 mg of furosemide Provide guidance about the timing of the dose when patients complain of urinary incontinence
Severe fluid retention or fluid retention not responding to low-dose loop diuretics	Furosemide **or** bumetanide	40–80 mg BID 1–2 mg BID	As above	As above K+ depletion more likely at the higher doses
Fluid retention refractory to high oral doses of loop diuretics alone	Furosemide and HCTZ **or** bumetanide and HCTZ	80–120 mg BID 25–50 mg QD 2–4 mg BID 25–50 mg BID	Loop of Henle and distal tubule	As above Exclude progressive renal failure Improve cardiac output GI absorption may be decreased If the addition of HCTZ does not produce adequate diuresis, consider MTZ 2.5 mg QD (K+ depletion is a major problem)
Fluid retention refractory to the combination of a loop diuretic and a thiazide (including MTZ)	Furosemide and MTZ and Spironolactone	80–120 mg BID 5 mg QD 25 mg BID	As above	As above Monitor K+ if spironolactone given with ACEI
Acute pulmonary edema or marked edema (anasarca)	Furosemide	IV 40–80 mg (as needed)	As above	

ACEI = angiotensin-converting enzyme inhibitor; GI = gastrointestinal; HCTZ = hydrochlorothiazide; IV = intravenous; LV = left ventricular; MTZ = metolazone; QD = once daily.

Other vasodilators

Apart from certain exceptions, direct-acting vasodilator drugs are not generally regarded as first-line therapy for long-term management of heart failure. These exceptions are heart failure complicated by valvular insufficiency or intolerance to ACE inhibitors. Of the vasodilators, nitrates and hydralazine are the most commonly used in this setting. This practice is based on the data from the V-HeFt I trial that showed that the combination isosorbide dinitrate–hydralazine improves survival and the symptoms of heart failure.[120] Nitrates have not been approved by the US Food and Drug Administration, but there is evidence that it may be useful in a number of clinical scenarios in heart failure. For example, nitrates may be first-line therapy when heart failure is complicated by or attributed to myocardial ischemia.

Hydralazine in combination with isosorbide dinitrate is usually well tolerated in the majority of patients with symptomatic heart failure and may be used as an alternative in patients with contraindications or intolerance to ACE inhibitors.

It may be further useful in patients who remain symptomatic on ACE inhibitors, although no controlled trials with this combination of drugs have been performed. However, side effects may cause a significant proportion of the patients to discontinue one or both of these medications. The dosing schedule and a list of the adverse effects of these agents are provided in Table 19.16.

Calcium-channel blockers

The negative inotropic effects of first-generation calcium antagonists have led to a strong recommendation against their use in heart failure. The second-generation calcium antagonists, however, such as felodipine and amlodipine, produce peripheral vasodilation without associated negative inotropic effects. These calcium blockers were recently evaluated in two controlled trials to assess whether they provide additional hemodynamic and survival benefit to patients already on ACE inhibitors. Amlodipine was shown to improve angina and heart failure symptoms without increasing mortality in patients with underlying ischemic heart disease.[121] Felodipine likewise showed no adverse effects on survival in patients with ischemic heart disease and heart failure.[122] These agents may therefore be useful for patients with heart failure and angina-like symptoms not controlled with nitrates or β-blockers.

Anticoagulant therapy

Based on the lack of data and the findings from the two Veterans Administration Heart Failure trials[123] that reported an embolic complication rate of below 2.5 per cent per 100 patients years, the Agency for Health Care Policy and Research[66,67] does not recommend routine anticoagulation in patients with heart failure unless there is history of recent pulmonary or systemic embolism, recent atrial fibrillation, or mobile LV thrombi. It is further recommended that the prothrombin ratio should be between 1.2 and 1.8 times each individual laboratory control time (international normalized ratio (INR) of 2–3). Older individuals with a decreased ejection fraction after a myocardial infarction deserve special mention since these patients have a substantial risk of stroke up to 5 years after the acute event.[124] Anticoagulant therapy may have a protective effect against stroke after myocardial infarction in this subset of patients.

SURGICAL OPTIONS FOR HEART FAILURE

Although this chapter deals primarily with the medical management of patients with heart failure, it should be recognized that certain patients may derive survival and symptomatic benefit from timely surgical interventions. The major surgically remediable causes of chronic heart failure include ischemic LV dysfunction, LV aneurysm, and valvular heart disease. Despite the lack of randomized clinical trials, it has become increasingly clear that carefully selected patients undergoing coronary artery bypass grafting with ejection fractions below 20 per cent show improvements in mortality and symptom class.[125–128] Thus, even in the absence of angina and an ejection fraction below 20 per cent, there is a compelling reason to evaluate all patients with suspected underlying coronary disease for ischemia.

> Consideration should be given to cardiac transplantation in patients with severe limitation despite aggressive medical therapy.

More information about heart transplantation can be obtained from a recent publication of the American College of Cardiology and American Heart Association on the selection and prioritization of patients for this procedure.[129]

Management of specific heart failure syndromes

GOALS OF THERAPY

The principal objectives of treatment in patients with heart failure are to enhance quality and duration of life and to attenuate, prevent, or actually reverse the progression of LV dysfunction. The relative importance of these therapeutic goals will vary depending on the clinical stage of heart failure. As heart failure progresses from the asymptomatic to the severe state, the focus of management shifts from interventions that halt or reverse LV dysfunction to treatments that are also aimed at relieving symptoms and preventing complications. To achieve these objectives, the management of heart failure is based on three principles: the removal and amelioration of the underlying cause; the removal and treatment of the precipitating causes; and the containment of the heart failure syndrome.[87]

ASYMPTOMATIC AND SYMPTOMATIC LV SYSTOLIC DYSFUNCTION

The therapy of asymptomatic LV dysfunction is principally directed towards amelioration of the underlying cause and prevention of the progression of disease. Treatment may differ somewhat depending on the underlying cause. ACE inhibitors form the basis of the pharmacological therapy of these patients with either ischemic or non-ischemic LV dysfunction. Large clinical trials have consistently shown a reduction of about 20 per cent in all-cause mortality when ACE inhibitors were given to postmyocardial infarction patients with LV dysfunction.[34,35,40–42] The weight of evidence further supports the early (within the first day) judicious use of an ACE inhibitor in acute myocardial infarction and continued long-term use in those with depressed LV function.[42,130] Patients with significant LV dysfunction after myocardial infarction may derive additional benefit from β-blockers. Collective data from over 10 000 patients have shown that β-blockers given at discharge after myocardial infarction results in a highly significant reduction in mortality, especially in those patients with pump failure during the hospital admission.[131]

> The management of patients with symptomatic LV dysfunction is based on the same principles as those without symptoms, but the focus of pharmacological treatment now shifts to agents that are useful in containing the heart failure syndrome (Table 19.20).

The initial treatment will vary depending on the severity of the heart failure symptoms. Sodium restriction in combination with a diuretic and an ACE inhibitor usually suffice in a patient who complains of difficulty with ordinary physical activity and who on physical examination has signs of congestion. When a patient presents with more advanced symptoms, the addition of digoxin is indicated. The vast majority of symptomatic patients can be adequately managed with the combination of an ACE inhibitor, a diuretic, and digoxin. In general, mild symptomatic deterioration in many patients is inevitable, requiring frequent adjustments to their medications. 'Fine-tuning' of the drug regimen is frequently required in diabetics and older patients due to coexistent coronary disease and/or decreased drug clearance. In patients with severe, diffuse coronary disease and heart failure, as often found in diabetics, excessive vasodilator treatment may lead to a low central aortic pressure and, as a consequence, to decreased myocardial perfusion and ischemia, especially during upright physical activity. Under these circumstances it is prudent to keep the systolic pressure at $\geq$ 95 mm Hg.

In view of the data on the beneficial effects of β-blockers in heart failure,[115–121] it could be argued that all patients with less than advanced heart failure should receive these agents.

In many instances the addition of a β-blocker to the standard treatment regimen of heart failure is likely to provide further improvements in symptoms and survival. Health care professionals that have limited experience with these agents in heart failure should refer patients who may derive benefit from β-blockers to centers that have experience with the use of these medications.

REFRACTORY SYMPTOMATIC LV SYSTOLIC DYSFUNCTION

The evaluation and management of patients that remain symptomatic despite treatment with an ACE inhibitor, a diuretic and digoxin, will first require an assessment of whether other conditions or contributing factors are responsible for the refractory symptoms before further treatment is initiated.

The approach and treatment of refractory heart failure are summarized in Fig. 19.7. This flow diagram represents the steps that are recommended when a patient remains symptomatic despite treatment with ACE inhibitors, β-blockers diuretics and digoxin. The first step is to assess whether other conditions or contributing factors are responsible for the refractory symptoms. These may include drug-related complications, such as digitalis toxicity, electrolyte disturbances and/or hypovolemia, and symptoms that may be attributable to coexistent disease, such as chronic lung, liver, or renal disease. Once these conditions are excluded, the next step is to establish whether the patient is compliant with their medications

and/or salt restriction. It is often helpful to discuss this issue with the spouse or caregiver. If the patient is not compliant, referral to a nurse-run heart failure program may be helpful. Should the patient be compliant, one must now determine whether the patient is on the optimal dose of an ACE inhibitor and a β-blocker (see Table 19.15). If not, the dose should be adjusted accordingly. However, if despite optimal ACE inhibitor and β-blocker doses the patient is still symptomatic, one should establish whether there are any contributing factors that may be reversed or treated, such as atrial fibrillation, ischemia, anemia, or hyperthyroidism (see Table 19.11). These should be treated before further adjustments in medicines are introduced. If on the other hand no such factors can be identified, further management can be based on whether there are physical signs of congestion.

When congestion is apparent despite diuretic treatment, a more aggressive diuretic regimen is appropriate (see Table 19.19), but if fluid retention is not obvious, further treatment may be initiated based on the serum creatinine.

If the creatinine is $\leq$ 2.5 mg/dL, then a therapeutic trial of diuretics is appropriate, but if the creatinine is >2.5 mg/dL, consideration should be given to the combination of hydralazine and isosorbide dinitrate (HYD/ISDN). Admission to hospital with invasive hemodynamic monitoring and inotropic support is advisable when there is evidence of a low output state (deteriorating renal function). Also, during the phase when patients do not respond to conventional treatment, serious consideration should be given at any time to whether the patient may benefit from heart transplantation and a timely referral to a transplant center is desirable.

The role of intermittent infusion of positive inotropic agents for refractory heart failure deserves special mention. Uncontrolled observational studies have shown that this form of treatment improves the NYHA class, increases exercise tolerance, and reduces the frequency of hospital readmissions.[132–136] However, this treatment is associated with an increased mortality, primarily due to an increase in the incidence of sudden death.[137] Thus, although the short-term use of this approach may have beneficial effects, this therapy should be undertaken cautiously – if at all.

DIASTOLIC HEART FAILURE

Medical management of diastolic heart failure differs from that caused by LV systolic dysfunction.

The approach to treatment is based on the following principles: (1) determine and treat the underlying cause (e.g. ischemia and hypertension); (2) restore sinus rhythm when appropriate; (3) relieve venous congestion; and (4) promote relative bradycardia.

Table 19.20 *Outline of management strategies for asymptomatic and symptomatic left ventricular systolic dysfunction*

			Heart failure syndromes			
Goals	Intervention	Measures	Asymp LVD	Mild-Mod HF	Mod-Sev HF	Advanced HF
Removal and amelioration of the underlying cause	1. Surgical options	Assess whether patients may benefit from revascularization	+++	+++	+++	+
		Remediable surgery (i.e. valvular)	+++	+++	+++	+
	2. Non-surgical options	Treat reversible causes (i.e. phlebotomy for hemochromatosis or ablation for tachycardia-induced cardiomyopathy)	+++	+++	+++	++
	3. Modify disease progression	Modify risk factors for CAD	+++	+++	+++	++
		ACE inhibitor	+++	+++	+++	+++
Removal and treatment of the precipitating causes (*see* Table 19.11)	Identify precipitating factors	Eliminate and/or treat these factors		+++	+++	+++
Containment of HF syndrome	1. Non-pharmacological (*see* Table 19.14)	General	++	+++	+++	++
		Regular exercise	+	++	++	++
		Dietary interventions	+	++	+++	+++
		Self-care strategies	+	++	+++	+++
	2. Pharmacological	ACE inhibitor	+++	+++	+++	+++
		β-Blockers		+	++	++
		Diuretics		++	+++	+++
		Digoxin		+	++	+++
		Hyd/ISDN			+	++
		IV inotropes				+
	3. Surgical	Heart transplant				++

ACE = angiotensin-converting enzyme; Asymp = asymptomatic; CAD = coronary artery disease; HF = heart failure; Hyd/ISDN = hydralazine and isosorbide nitrate; IV = intravenous; LVD = left ventricular dysfunction; Mod = moderate; Sev = severe; + = may be useful; ++ = definitely useful; +++ = should always be considered.

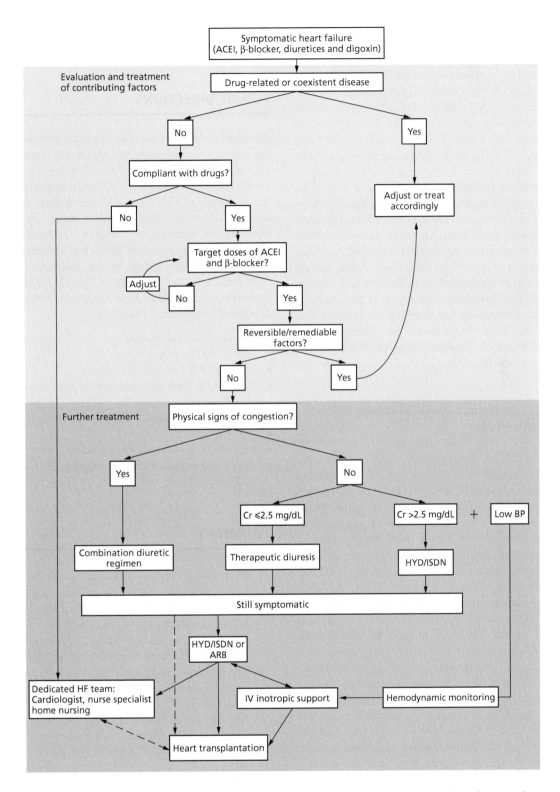

Figure 19.7 *The steps recommended when a patient remains symptomatic despite treatment with angiotensin-converting enzyme inhibitor (ACEI), β-blockers, diuretics, and digoxin. ARB = angiotensin receptor blocker; BP = blood pressure; Cr = creatinine; HF = heart failure; HYD/ISDN = hydralazine and isosorbide dinitrate; IV = intravenous.*

The most effective treatment of diastolic heart failure is to address the underlying cause. In this regard, ischemia should always be suspected, especially in the elderly. No drug currently exists that has been shown to improve isolated ventricular diastolic function effectively. The American College of Cardiology/American Heart Association Task Force on Evaluation and Management of Heart Failure[68] recommends only nitrates and diuretics in the treatment of symptomatic diastolic heart failure; neither agent affects diastolic function. When prescribing these agents it should be understood that a small change in central blood volume will result in a substantial decrease in LV filling pressure in patients with a stiff heart. Aggressive diuresis or veno-dilatation may result in hypotension and cautious administration of lower than usual doses of diuretics are advisable. Other agents such as β-blockers and calcium antagonists may have theoretical appeal in the treatment of diastolic dysfunction, but there is little evidence that these agents improve symptoms or exercise capacity.[68,138,139] For a more detailed review on this topic, the reader is referred elsewhere.[1]

Strategies to reduce hospital readmissions and length of stay

Repeat hospitalizations for patients with heart failure are a relatively frequent occurrence within a short period of time following hospital discharge. In one recent study,[140] the 3-month readmission rate was reported to be approximately 42 per cent, while a study from Connecticut found that slightly more than two out of every five elderly Medicare beneficiaries were readmitted to the hospital at least once in the 6-month period following the index admission for heart failure.[9] An additional one-sixth of patients were readmitted two or more times to Connecticut hospitals over this relatively short follow-up period. The medical costs of readmissions alone are likely to contribute to more than 50 per cent of the total cost of treating heart failure. Another key determinant of hospital cost is the hospital length of stay.

There may be several reasons for the high readmission rates. For example, in community hospitals in Canada during 1992 and 1993, only slightly more than half (53 per cent) of patients hospitalized with heart failure received ACE inhibitors during their acute hospitalization.[141] Moreover, this agent was used significantly less often in women and patients 70 years and older. In addition, poor patient adherence to pharmacological and dietary therapy is a common cause of readmission for heart failure.[142,143]

In recent times several strategies have been employed to manage heart failure better, including a multidisciplinary approach,[140] disease management programs,[144] and the addition of nurse practitioners to assist in managing patients.[145] It is clear that programs that focus on patient education, self-monitoring strategies, and frequent telephone contact with the patients are likely to be cost-effective at improving patients outcomes with heart failure.

FUTURE DIRECTIONS

Although a great deal of progress has been made in treating patients with heart failure, much still remains to be accomplished. After many years of debate, the place of chronic positive inotropic agents has been clarified. With the exception of digitalis, such agents have been consistently shown to be associated with an unfavorable outcome. In contrast, the ongoing research on the disease-modifying effects of β-blockers is likely to result in a better understanding of the mechanism(s) that contribute to the progression of LV dysfunction. Furthermore, many new treatments are currently being developed or evaluated, including:

- vasopeptidase inhibition;
- new β-blocking agents;
- blockers of the endothelin system;
- angiotensin II receptor blockers in patients on ACE inhibitors;
- inhibitors of cytokine pathways;
- gene therapy;
- continuous positive airway pressure;
- ventricular volume reduction surgery (Battista or Pott's procedure).

SUMMARY

- Heart failure (HF) is a major and escalating health problem. Repeat hospitalizations approach 40 per cent within 6 months of discharge. Almost half of all patients who present with HF symptoms have left ventricular (LV) ejection fractions in the near-normal range (diastolic HF).
- The diagnostic work-up of patients with new-onset HF should include the search for reversible causes of HF.
- Angiotensin-converting enzyme (ACE) inhibitors should be provided to all asymptomatic or symptomatic patients with LV systolic dysfunction.
- β-Blockade reduces mortality as well as the risk of hospitalization for worsening HF. Initiation of these agents in HF requires patience and the careful selection of patients with stable HF.
- Angiotensin II receptor blockade should be reserved for patients who are intolerant of ACE inhibitors.
- Digoxin is safe and is best reserved for patients with moderate and severe HF.

- Diuretics are given to alleviate the symptoms of congestion. Combining different classes of diuretics are often effective for refractory congestion.
- Amlodipine or hydralazine in combination with isosorbide dinitrate may be used as an alternative in patients with contraindications or intolerance to ACE inhibitors.
- Patient outcomes have been favorably modified by patient education, self-monitoring strategies, and frequent telephone contact.

REFERENCES

1. Gaasch WH, Blaustein AS, LeWinter MM. Heart failure and clinical disorders of left ventricular diastolic function. In: Gaasch WH, LeWinter MM, eds *Left ventricular diastolic dysfunction and heart failure.* Philadelphia: Lea & Febiger, 1994: 245–58.
2. Grossman W. Congestive heart failure: role of systolic and diastolic dysfunction. In: Gwathmey JK, Briggs GM, Allen PD, eds *Heart failure, basic science and clinical aspects.* New York: Marcel Dekker, Inc., 1993: 1–9.
3. US Department of Health and Human Services. *Morbidity and mortality chartbook on cardiovascular, lung and blood diseases, 1990 and 1994.* Bethesda, MD: National Institutes of Health, National Heart, Lung and Blood Institute, 1990, 1994.
4. Garg R, Packer M, Pitt B, Yusuf S. Heart failure in the 1990's: evolution of a major public health problem in preventive medicine. *J Am Coll Cardiol* 1993; **22**: 3A–5A.
5. Schocken DD, Arrieta MI, Leaverton PE, Ross EA. Prevalence and mortality rate of congestive heart failure in the United States. *J Am Coll Cardiol* 1992; **20**: 301–6.
6. Ho KK, Pinsky JL, Kannel WB, Levy D. The epidemiology of heart failure: the Framingham Study. *J Am Coll Cardiol* 1993; **22** (4 suppl A): 6A–13A.
7. National Center for Health Statistics. *National hospital discharge survey.* Vital and Health Statistics, Series 13, 1990. Hyattsville, MD: National Center for Health Statistics.
8. McMurray J, McDonagh T, Morrison CE, Dargie HJ. Trends in hospitalization for heart failure in Scotland 1980–1990. *Eur Heart J* 1993; **14**: 1158–62.
9. Krumholz HM, Parent EM, Tu N, *et al.* Readmission after hospitalization for congestive heart failure among medicare beneficiaries. *Arch Intern Med* 1997; **157**: 99–104.
10. O'Connell JB, Bristow MR. Economic impact of heart failure in the United States: a time for a different approach. *J Heart Lung Transplant* 1994; **154**: 1143–9.
11. Eriksson H. Heart failure: a growing health care problem. *J Intern Med* 1995; **237**: 135–41.
12. Rodeheffer RJ, Jacobsen SJ, Gersh BJ, *et al.* The incidence and prevalence of congestive heart failure in Rochester, Minnesota. *Mayo Clin Proc* 1993; **68**: 1143–50.
13. Packer M. New concepts in the pathophysiology of heart failure: beneficial and deleterious interaction of endogenous haemodynamic and neurohormonal mechanisms. *J Intern Med* 1996; **239**: 327–33.
14. Wagoner LE, Walsh RA. The cellular pathophysiology of progression to heart failure. *Curr Opin Cardiol* 1996; **11**: 237–44.
15. Poole-Wilson PA. Relation of pathophysiologic mechanisms to outcome in heart failure. *J Am Coll Cardiol* 1993; **22**: 22–9A.
16. Eichhorn EJ, Bristow MR. Medical therapy can improve the biological properties of the chronically failing heart. A new era in the treatment of heart failure. *Circulation* 1996; **94**: 2285–96.
17. Colluci WS, Braunwald E. *Atlas of heart diseases, heart failure: cardiac function and dysfunction.* Philadelphia: Mosby, 1995.
18. Katz AM. The cardiomyopathy of overload: an unnatural growth response in the hypertrophied heart. *Ann Intern Med* 1994; **121**: 363–71.
19. Eisenhofer G, Friberg P, Rundqvist B, *et al.* Cardiac sympathetic nerve function in congestive heart failure. *Circulation* 1996; **93**: 1667–76.
20. Benedict CR, Shelton B, Johnstone DE, *et al.* Prognostic significance of plasma norepinephrine in patients with asymptomatic left ventricular dysfunction. SOLVD Investigators. *Circulation* 1996; **94**: 690–7.
21. Rundqvist B, Elam M, Bergmann-Sverrisdottir Y, Eisenhofer G, Friberg P. Increased cardiac adrenergic drive precedes generalized sympathetic activation in human heart failure. *Circulation* 1997; **95**: 169–75.
22. Packer M. Neurohumoral interactions and adaptations in congestive heart failure. *Circulation* 1988; **77**: 721–30.
23. Dzau VJ. Tissue renin-angiotensin system in myocardial hypertrophy and failure. *Arch Intern Med* 1993; **153**: 937–42.
24. Francis GS, Benedict C, Johnstone DE, *et al.* Comparison of neuroendocrine activation in patients with left ventricular dysfunction with and without congestive heart failure. A substudy of the Studies of Left Ventricular Dysfunction (SOLVD). *Circulation* 1990; **82**: 1724–9.
25. Kubo SH, Rector TS, Bank AJ, Williams RE, Heifetz SM. Endothelium-dependent vasodilation is attenuated in patients with heart failure. *Circulation* 1991; **84**: 1589–96.
26. Katz SD. The role of endothelium-derived vasoactive substances in the pathophysiology of exercise intolerance in patients with congestive heart failure. *Prog Cardiovasc Dis* 1995; **38**: 23–50.

27. Katz SD, Krum H, Khan T, Knecht M. Exercise-induced vasodilation in forearm circulation of normal subjects and patients with congestive heart failure: role of endothelium-derived nitric oxide. *J Am Coll Cardiol* 1996; **28**: 585–90.

28. Minotti JR, Johnson EC, Hudson TL, *et al*. Skeletal muscle response to exercise training in congestive heart failure. *J Clin Invest* 1990; **86**: 751–8.

29. Minotti JR, Christoph I, Oka R, Weiner MW, Wells L, Massie BM. Impaired skeletal muscle function in patients with congestive heart failure. Relationship to systemic exercise performance. *J Clin Invest* 1991; **88**: 2077–82.

30. Clark AL, Poole-Wilson PA, Coats AJ. Exercise limitation in chronic heart failure: central role of the periphery. *J Am Coll Cardiol* 1996; **28**: 1092–102.

31. Piepoli M, Clark AL, Volterrani M, Adamopoulos S, Sleight P, Coats AJ. Contribution of muscle afferents to the hemodynamic, autonomic, and ventilatory responses to exercise in patients with chronic heart failure: effects of physical training. *Circulation* 1996; **93**: 940–52.

32. Drexler H, Coats AJ. Explaining fatigue in congestive heart failure. *Annu Rev Med* 1996; **47**: 241–56.

33. Konstam MA, Kronenberg MW, Rousseau MF, *et al*. Effects of the angiotensin converting enzyme inhibitor enalapril on the long-term progression of left ventricular dilatation in patients with asymptomatic systolic dysfunction. SOLVD (Studies of Left Ventricular Dysfunction) Investigators. *Circulation* 1993; **88**: 2277–83.

34. The Consensus Trial Study Group. Effects of enalapril on mortality in severe congestive heart failure. Results of the Cooperative North Scandinavian Enalapril Survival Study (CONSENSUS). *N Engl J Med* 1987; **316**: 1429–35.

35. Pfeffer MA, Braunwald E, Moyé LA, *et al*. Effect of captopril on mortality and morbidity in patients with left ventricular dysfunction after myocardial infarction. Results of the survival and ventricular enlargement trial. The SAVE Investigators. *N Engl J Med* 1992; **327**: 669–77.

36. Pfeffer MA. Mechanistic lessons from the SAVE Study. Survival and ventricular enlargement. *Am J Hypertens* 1994; **7**: 106–11S.

37. St John Sutton M, Pfeffer MA, Plappert T, *et al*. Quantitative two-dimensional echocardiographic measurements are major predictors of adverse cardiovascular events after acute myocardial infarction. The protective effects of captopril. *Circulation* 1994; **89**: 68–75.

38. The SOLVD Investigators. Effect of enalapril on survival in patients with reduced left ventricular ejection fractions and congestive heart failure. *N Engl J Med* 1991; **325**: 293–302.

39. The SOLVD Investigators. Effect of enalapril on mortality and the development of heart failure in asymptomatic patients with reduced left ventricular ejection fractions. *N Engl J Med* 1992; **327**: 685–91.

40. The Acute Infarction Ramipril Efficacy (AIRE). Study investigators effect of ramipril on mortality and morbidity of survivors of acute myocardial infarction with clinical evidence of heart failure. *Lancet* 1993; **342**: 821–8.

41. Kober L, Torp-Pedersen C, Carlsen JE, *et al*. A clinical trial of the angiotensin-converting-enzyme inhibitor trandolapril in patients with left ventricular dysfunction after myocardial infarction. *N Engl J Med* 1995; **333**: 1670–6.

42. Ambrosioni E, Borghi C, Magnani B. The effect of the angiotensin-converting-enzyme inhibitor zofenopril on mortality and morbidity after anterior myocardial infarction. The Survival of Myocardial Infarction Long-Term Evaluation (SMILE) Study Investigators. *N Engl J Med* 1995; **332**: 80–5.

43. Borghi C, Ambrosioni E, Magnani B. Effects of the early administration of zofenopril on onset and progression of congestive heart failure in patients with anterior wall acute myocardial infarction. The SMILE Study Investigators. Survival of Myocardial Infarction Long-term Evaluation. *Am J Cardiol* 1996; **78**: 317–22.

44. Gruppo Italiano per lo Studio della Sopravvivenza nell'infarto Miocardico (GISSI-3). Effects of lisinopril and transdermal glyceryl trinitrate singly and together on 6-week mortality and ventricular function after acute myocardial infarction. *Lancet* 1994; **343**: 1115–22.

45. Fourth International Study of Infarct Survival (ISIS-4). A randomised factorial trial assessing early oral captopril, oral mononitrate, and intravenous magnesium sulphate in 58,050 patients with suspected acute myocardial infarction. *Lancet* 1995; **345**: 669–85.

46. Pitt B. Use of converting enzyme inhibitors in patients with asymptomatic left ventricular dysfunction. *J Am Coll Cardiol* 1993; **22**: 158–61A.

47. Gaasch WH. Diagnosis and treatment of heart failure based on left ventricular systolic or diastolic dysfunction. *JAMA* 1994; **271**: 1276–80.

48. Braunwald E. ACE inhibitors: a cornerstone of the treatment of heart failure. *N Engl J Med* 1991; **325**: 351–3.

49. Marantz PR, Tobin JN, Wassertheil-Smoller S, *et al*. The relationship between left ventricular systolic function and congestive heart failure diagnosed by clinical criteria. *Circulation* 1988; **77**: 607–12.

50. Mattleman SJ, Hakki AH, Iskandrian AS, Segal BL, Kane SA. Reliability of bedside evaluation in determining left ventricular function: correlation with left ventricular ejection fraction determined by ventriculography. *J Am Coll Cardiol* 1983; **1**: 417–20.

51. Remes J, Miettinen H, Reunanen A, Pyörälä K. Validity of clinical diagnosis of heart failure in primary health care. *Eur Heart J* 1991; **12**: 315–21.

52. Wheeldon NM, McDonald TM, Flucker CJ, *et al.* Echocardiography in chronic heart failure in the community. *Q J Med* 1993; **86**: 17–23.

53. Kannel WM, Belanger AJ. Epidemiology of heart failure. *Am Heart J* 1991; **121**: 951–7.

54. Ikram H. Identifying the patient with heart failure. *J Int Med Res* 1995; **23**: 139–53.

55. Vasan RS, Benjamin E, Levy D. Prevalence, clinical features and prognosis of diastolic heart failure: an epidemiologic perspective. *J Am Coll Cardiol* 1995; **26**: 1565–74.

56. Cregler LL, Georgiou D, Sosa I. Left ventricular diastolic dysfunction in patients with congestive heart failure. *J Natl Med Assoc* 1991; **83**: 49–52.

57. Warren SE, Grossman W. Diastolic left ventricular dysfunction – significance for differential diagnosis and therapy of heart failure in the aged. Prognosis in heart failure: is systolic or diastolic dysfunction more important? *Herz* 1991; **16**: 324–9.

58. Bonow RO, Udelson JE. Left ventricular diastolic dysfunction as a cause of congestive heart failure. Mechanisms and management. *Ann Intern Med* 1992; **117**: 502–10.

59. Grossman W. Diastolic dysfunction and congestive heart failure. *Circulation* 1990; **81**(suppl III): 1–7.

60. Lorell BH. Significance of diastolic dysfunction of the heart. *Annu Rev Med* 1991; **42**: 411–36.

61. Gaasch WH. Congestive heart failure in patients with normal left ventricular systolic function: a manifestation of diastolic dysfunction. *Herz* 1991; **16**: 22–32.

62. Gaasch WH. Diagnosis and treatment of heart failure based on left ventricular systolic or diastolic dysfunction. *JAMA* 1994; **271**: 1276–80.

63. Litwin SE, Grossman W. Diastolic dysfunction as a cause of heart failure. *J Am Coll Cardiol* 1993; **22**: 49–55A.

64. Federmann M, Hess OM. Differentiation between systolic and diastolic dysfunction. *Eur Heart J* 1994; **15**: 2–6.

65. Topol EJ, Traill TA, Fortuin NJ. Hypertensive hypertrophic cardiomyopathy of the elderly. *N Engl J Med* 1985; **312**: 277–83.

66. Konstam M, Dracup K, Baker D, *et al. Heart failure: evaluation and care of patients with left ventricular systolic dysfunction.* Clinical Practice Guideline Number 11 (amended) AHCPR Publication no. 94–0612. Rockville, MD: Agency for Health Care Policy and Research and the National Heart, Lung, and Blood Institute, Public Health Service, US Department of Health and Human Services. June 1994.

67. Rodeheffer R. Initial evaluation. In: Kasper EK, ed. *Heart failure, evaluation and care of patients with left ventricular systolic dysunction: commentary on the Agency for Health Care Policy and Research Clinical Practice guidelines # 11.* New York, Chapman & Hall, 1996; 23–36.

68. American College of Cardiology/American Heart Association Committee on Evaluation and Management of Heart Failure. Guidelines for the evaluation and management of heart failure. *J Am Coll Cardiol* 1995; **26**: 1376–98.

69. Braunwald E, Colucci WS, Grossman W. Clinical aspects of heart failure: high output heart failure; pulmonary edema. In: Braunwald E, ed. *Heart disease: a textbook of cardiovascular medicine*, 5th edn. Philadelphia: WB Saunders Co, 1997; 445–70.

70. Smith RF, Johnson G, Ziesche S, Bhat G, Blankenship K, Cohn JN. Functional capacity in heart failure. Comparison of methods for assessment and their relation to other indexes of heart failure. The V-HeFT VA Cooperative Studies Group. *Circulation* 1993; **87**(suppl VI): 88–93.

71. Cohn JN, Johnson GR, Shabetai R, *et al.* Ejection fraction, peak exercise oxygen consumption, cardiothoracic ratio, ventricular arrhythmias, and plasma norepinephrine as determinants of prognosis in heart failure. The V-HeFT VA Cooperative Studies Group. *Circulation* 1993; **87**(suppl VI): 5–16.

72. Goldman S, Johnson G, Cohn JN, Cintron G, Smith R, Francis G. Mechanism of death in heart failure. The Vasodilator-Heart Failure Trials. The V-HeFT VA Cooperative Studies Group. *Circulation* 1993; **87**(suppl VI): 24–31.

73. Rector TS, Cohn JN. Assessment of patient outcome with the Minnesota Living with Heart Failure questionnaire: reliability and validity during a randomized, double-blind, placebo-controlled trial of pimobendan. Pimobendan Multicenter Research Group. *Am Heart J* 1992; **124**: 1017–25.

74. Mancini DM, Eisen H, Kussmaul W, Mull R, Edmunds LH Jr, Wilson JR. Value of peak exercise oxygen consumption for optimal timing of cardiac transplantation in ambulatory patients with heart failure. *Circulation* 1991; **83**: 778–86.

75. Lipkin DP, Scriven AJ, Crake T, Poole-Wilson PA. Six minute walking test for assessing exercise capacity in chronic heart failure. *Br Med J* 1986; **292**: 653–5.

76. Bittner V, Weiner DH, Yusuf S, *et al.* Prediction of mortality and morbidity with a 6-minute walk test in patients with left ventricular dysfunction. SOLVD Investigators. *JAMA* 1993; **270**: 1702–7.

77. Itoh A, Saito M, Haze K, Hiramori K, Kasagi F. Prognosis of patients with congestive heart failure: its determinants in various heart diseases in Japan. *Intern Med* 1992; **31**: 304–9.

78. Setaro JF, Soufer R, Remetz MS, Perlmutter RA, Zaret BL. Long-term outcome in patients with congestive heart failure and intact systolic left ventricular performance. *Am J Cardiol* 1992; **69**: 1212–16.

79. Xie GY, Berk MR, Smith MD, Gurley JC, DeMaria AN. Prognostic value of Doppler transmitral flow patterns in patients with congestive heart failure. *J Am Coll Cardiol* 1994; **24**: 132–9.

80. Bourassa MG, Gurné O, Bangdiwala SI, *et al.* Natural history and patterns of current practice in heart failure. The Studies of Left Ventricular Dysfunction (SOLVD) Investigators. *J Am Coll Cardiol* 1993; **22**(suppl A): 14–19A.

81. Massachusetts Medical Society. Mortality from congestive heart failure – United States, 1980–1990. *MMWR* 1994; **43**: 77.

82. Di Salvo TG, Mathier M, Semigran MJ, Dec GW. Preserved right ventricular ejection fraction predicts exercise capacity and survival in advanced heart failure. *J Am Coll Cardiol* 1995; **25**: 1143–53.

83. Lee WH, Packer M. Prognostic importance of serum sodium concentration and its modification by converting-enzyme inhibition in patients with severe chronic heart failure. *Circulation* 1986; **73**: 257–67.

84. Just H, Drexler H, Taylor SH, Siegrist J, Schulgen G, Schumacher M. Captopril versus digoxin in patients with coronary artery disease and mild heart failure. A prospective, double-blind, placebo-controlled multicenter study. The CADS Study Group. *Herz* 1993; **18**(suppl 1): 436–43.

85. Doval HC, Nul DR, Grancelli HO, Perrone SV, Bortman GR, Curiel R. Randomised trial of low-dose amiodarone in severe congestive heart failure. Grupo de Estudio de la Sobrevida en la Insuficiencia Cardiaca en Argentina (GESICA). *Lancet* 1994; **344**: 493–8.

86. Doval HC, Nul DR, Grancelli HO, *et al.* Nonsustained ventricular tachycardia in severe heart failure. Independent marker of increased mortality due to sudden death. GESICA-GEMA Investigators. *Circulation* 1996; **94**: 3198–203.

87. Bolton MB, Tilley B, Kuder J, Reeves T, Schultz LR. The cost and effectiveness of an education program for adults who have asthma. *J Gen Intern Med* 1991; **6**: 401–7.

88. Glasgow RE, Osteen VL. Evaluating diabetes education. Are we measuring the most important outcomes? *Diabetes Care* 1992; **15**: 1423–32.

89. Smith TW, Kelly RA, Stevenson LW, Braunwald E. Management of heart failure. In: Braunwald E, ed. *Heart disease: a textbook of cardiovascular medicine*, 5th edn. Philadelphia: WB Saunders Co, 1997; 492–514.

90. Mullane KM, Moncada S. Prostacyclin mediates the potentiated hypotensive effect of bradykinin following captopril treatment. *Eur J Pharmacol* 1980; **66**: 355–65.

91. Anning PB, Grocott-Mason RM, Lewis MJ, Shah AM. Enhancement of left ventricular relaxation in the isolated heart by an angiotensin converting enzyme inhibitor. *Circulation* 1995; **90**: 2760–5.

92. McDonald KM, Mock J, D'Aloia A, *et al.* Bradykinin antagonism inhibits the antigrowth effect of converting enzyme inhibition in the dog myocardium after discrete myocardial necrosis. *Circulation* 1995; **91**: 2043–8.

93. Schunkert H, Jackson B, Tang SS, *et al.* Distribution and functional significance of cardiac angiotensin converting enzyme in hypertrophied rat hearts. *Circulation* 1993; **87**: 1328–39.

94. Litwin SE, Katz SE, Weinberg EO, Lorell BH, Aurigemma GP, Douglas PS. Serial echocardiographic-Doppler assessment of left ventricular geometry and function in rats with pressure-overload hypertrophy. Chronic angiotensin-converting enzyme inhibition attenuates the transition to heart failure. *Circulation* 1995; **91**: 2642–54.

95. Pfeffer JM, Pfeffer MA, Braunwald E. Influence of chronic captopril therapy on the infarcted left ventricle of the rat. *Circ Res* 1985; **57**: 84–95.

96. Sharpe DN, Murphy J, Coxon R, Hannan SF. Enalapril in patients with chronic heart failure: a placebo controlled, randomized double blind study. *Circulation* 1984; **70**: 271–8.

97. Franciosa JA, Wilen MM, Jordan RA. Effects of enalapril, a new angiotensin-converting enzyme inhibitor, in a controlled trial in heart failure. *J Am Coll Cardiol* 1985; **5**: 101–7.

98. McGrath BP, Arnolda L, Matthews PG, *et al.* Controlled trial of enalapril in congestive cardiac failure. *Br Heart J* 1985; **54**: 405–14.

99. Riegger GA. The effects of quinapril on exercise tolerance in patients with mild to moderate heart failure. *Eur Heart J* 1991; **12**: 705–11.

100. Kramer BL, Massie BM, Topic N. Controlled trial of captopril in chronic heart failure: a rest and exercise hemodynamic study. *Circulation* 1983; **67**: 807–16.

101. Drexler H, Banhardt U, Meinherz T, Wollschläger H, Lehmann M, Just H. Contrasting peripheral short-term and long-term effects of converting enzyme inhibition in patients with congestive heart failure: a double blind, placebo-controlled trial. *Circulation* 1989; **79**: 491–502.

102. Hall D, Zeitler H, Rudolph W. Counteraction of the vasodilator effects of enalapril by aspirin in severe heart failure. *J Am Coll Cardiol* 1992; **20**: 1549–55.

103. Nguyen KN, Aursnes I, Kjekshus J. Interaction between enalapril and aspirin on mortality after acute myocardial infarction: subgroup analysis of the Cooperative New Scandinavian Enalapril Survival Study II (CONSENSUS II). *Am J Cardiol* 1997; **79**: 115–19.

104. Packer M, Lee WH, Yushak M, Medina R. Comparison of captopril and enalapril in patients with severe chronic heart failure. *N Engl J Med* 1986; **315**: 847–53.

104a. Pitt B, Poole-Wilson PA, Segal R, *et al.* Effect of losartan compared to captopril on mortality in patients with symptomatic heart failure: randomised trial-the losartan Heart Failure Survival Study ELITE II). *Lancet* 2000; **355**: 1582–7.

105. Andersson B, Caidahl K, di Lenarda A, *et al.* Changes in early and late diastolic filling patterns induced by long-term adrenergic beta-blockade in patients with idiopathic dilated cardiomyopathy. *Circulation* 1996; **94**: 673–82.

106. Eichhorn EJ, Heesch CM, Risser RC, Marcoux L, Hatfield B. Predictors of systolic and diastolic improvement in patients with dilated cardiomyopathy treated with metoprolol. *J Am Coll Cardiol* 1995; **25**: 154–62.

107. Waagstein F, Caidahl K, Wallentin I, Bergh CH, Hjalmarson A. Long-term beta-blockade in dilated cardiomyopathy. Effects of short- and long-term metoprolol treatment followed by withdrawal and readministration of metoprolol. *Circulation* 1989; **80**: 551–63.

108. Heilbrunn SM, Shah P, Bristow MR, Valantine HA, Ginsburg R, Fowler MB. Increased beta-receptor density and improved hemodynamic response to catecholamine stimulation during long-term metoprolol therapy in heart failure from dilated cardiomyopathy. *Circulation* 1989; **79**: 483–90.

109. Waagstein F, Bristow MR, Swedberg K, *et al*. Beneficial effects of metoprolol in idiopathic dilated cardiomyopathy. Metoprolol in Dilated Cardiomyopathy (MDC) Trial Study Group. *Lancet* 1993; **342**: 1441–6.

110. Eichhorn EJ, Bedotto JB, Malloy CR, *et al*. Effect of beta-adrenergic blockade on myocardial function and energetics in congestive heart failure. Improvements in hemodynamic, contractile, and diastolic performance with bucindolol. *Circulation* 1990; **82**: 473–83.

111. CIBIS Investigators and Committees. A randomized trial of beta-blockade in heart failure. The Cardiac Insufficiency Bisoprolol Study (CIBIS). *Circulation* 1994; **90**: 1765–73.

112. Packer M, Bristow MR, Cohn JN, *et al*. The effect of carvedilol on morbidity and mortality in patients with chronic heart failure. US Carvedilol Heart Failure Study Group. *N Engl J Med* 1996; **334**: 1349–55.

113. MERIT-HF study group. Effect of metoprolol CR/XL in chronic heart failure: Metoprolol CR/XL Intervention Trial in Congestive Heart Failure (MERIT-HF). *Lancet* 1999; **353**: 2001–7.

114. Jaeschke R, Oxman AD, Guyatt GH. To what extent do congestive heart failure patients in sinus rhythm benefit from digoxin therapy? A systematic overview and meta-analysis. *Am J Med* 1990; **88**: 279–86.

115. The Captopril–Digoxin Multicenter Research Group. Comparative effects of therapy with captopril and digoxin in patients with mild to moderate heart failure *JAMA* 1988; **259**: 539–44.

116. Lee DCS, Johnson RA, Bingham JB, *et al*. Heart failure in outpatients. A randomized trial of digoxin versus placebo. *N Engl J Med* 1982; **306**: 699–705.

117. Packer M, Gheorghiade M, Young JB, *et al*. Withdrawal of digoxin from patients with chronic heart failure treated with angiotensin-converting-enzyme inhibitors. RADIANCE Study. *N Engl J Med* 1993; **329**: 1–7.

118. The Digitalis Investigation Group. The effect of digoxin on mortality and morbidity in patients with heart failure. *N Engl J Med* 1997; **336**: 525–33.

119. Cohn J. The management of chronic heart failure. *N Engl J Med* 1996; **335**: 490–8.

120. Cohn JN, Archibald DG, Ziesche S, *et al*. Effect of vasodilator therapy on mortality in chronic congestive heart failure. Results of a Veterans Administration Cooperative Study. *N Engl J Med* 1986; **314**: 1547–52.

121. Packer M, O'Connor CM, Ghali JK, *et al*. Effect of amlodipine on morbidity and mortality in severe chronic heart failure. Prospective Randomized Amlodipine Survival Evaluation Study Group. *N Engl J Med* 1996; **335**: 1107–14.

122. Cohn J, Ziesche SM, Loos LE, *et al*. Effect of felodipine on short-term exercise capacity and long-term mortality in heart failure: results of V-HeFT III. *Circulation* 1995; **92**(suppl 1): I–143 (abstract).

123. Dunkman WB, Johnson GR, Carson PE, Bhat G, Farrell L, Cohn JN. Incidence of thromboembolic events in congestive heart failure. The V-HeFT VA Cooperative Studies Group. *Circulation* 1993; **87**: VI94–101.

124. Loh E, Sutton MS, Wun CC, *et al*. Ventricular dysfunction and the risk of stroke after myocardial infarction. *N Engl J Med* 1997; **336**: 251–7.

125. Kron IL, Flanagan TL, Blackbourne LH, Schroeder RA, Nolan SP. Coronary revascularization rather than cardiac transplantation for chronic ischemic cardiomyopathy. *Ann Thorac Surg* 1989; **210**: 348–52.

126. Lansman SL, Cohen M, Galla JD, *et al*. Coronary bypass with ejection fraction of 0.20 or less using centrigrade cardioplegia long-term follow-up. *Ann Thorac Surg* 1993; **56**: 480–5.

127. Dreyfus G, Duboc D, Blasco A, *et al*. Coronary surgery can be an alternative to heart transplantation in selected patients with end-stage ischemic heart disease. *Eur J Cardiothorac Surg* 1993; **7**: 482–7.

128. Luciani GB, Faggian G, Razzolini R, Livi U, Bortolotti U, Mazzucco A. Severe ischemic left ventricular failure; coronary operation or heart transplantation? *Ann Thorac Surg* 1993; **55**: 719–23.

129. Mudge GH, Goldstein S, Addonizio LJ, *et al*. 24th Bethesda Conference: Cardiac transplanation. Task Force 3: Recipient guidelines/prioritization. *J Am Coll Cardiol* 1993; **22**: 21–31.

130. Pfeffer MA, Greaves SC, Arnold JM, *et al*. Early versus delayed angiotensin-converting enzyme inhibition therapy in acute myocardial infarction. The healing and early afterload reducing therapy trial *Circulation* 1997; **95**: 2643–51.

131. Beta-Blocker Pooling Project Research Group. The Beta-Blocker Pooling Project (BBPP): subgroup findings from randomized trials in post infarction patients. *Eur Heart J* 1988; **9**: 8–16.

132. Roffman DS, Applefeld MM, Grove WR, *et al*. Intermittent dobutamine hydrochloride infusions in outpatients with chronic congestive heart failure. *Clin Pharm* 1985; **4**(2): 195–9.

133. Adamopoulos S, Piepoli M, Qiang F, *et al*. Effects of pulsed beta-stimulant therapy on beta-adrenoceptors

and chronotropic responsiveness in chronic heart failure *Lancet* 1995; **345**: 344–9.

134. Roffman DS, Applefeld MM, Grove WR, *et al*. Intermittent dobutamine hydrochloride infusions in outpatients with chronic congestive heart failure. *Clin Pharm* 1985; **4**: 195–9.

135. Thomas RL, Watson D, Marshall LE. Review of intermittent dobutamine infusions for congestive cardiomyopathy. *Pharmacotherapy* 1987; **7**: 47–53.

136. Levinoff Roth S, Moe G. Intermittent intravenous amrinone infusion: a potentially cost-effective mode of treatment of patients with refractory heart failure. *Can J Cardiol* 1993; **93**: 231–7.

137. Krell MJ, Kline EM, Bates ER, *et al*. Intermittent, ambulatory dobutamine infusions in patients with severe congestive heart failure. *Am Heart J* 1986; **112**: 787–91.

138. Vasan R, Benjamin EJ, Levy D. Congestive heart failure with normal left ventricular systolic function. *Arch Intern Med* 1996; **156**: 146–57.

139. Shah PM, Pai RG. Diastolic heart failure. *Curr Probl Cardiol* 1992; **17**: 781–868.

140. Rich MW, Beckham V, Wittenberg C, *et al*. A multidisciplinary intervention to prevent the readmission of elderly patients with congestive heart failure. *N Engl J Med* 1995; **333**: 1190–5.

141. Clinical Quality Improvement Network Investigators. Mortality risk and patterns of practice in 4606 acute care patients with congestive heart failure. The relative importance of age, sex and medical therapy. *Arch Intern Med* 1996; **156**: 1669–73.

142. Ghali JK, Kadakia S, Cooper R, Ferlinz J. Precipitating factors leading to decompensation of heart failure. Traits among urban blacks. *Arch Intern Med* 1988; **148**: 2013–16.

143. Vinson JM, Rich MW, Sperry JC, Shah AS, McNamara T. Early readmission of elderly patients with congestive heart failure. *J Am Geriatr Soc* 1990; **38**: 1290–5.

144. Block L, Fredericks LA, Moore B, Wilker J. The design and implementation of a disease management program for congestive heart failure at a community hospital. *Congest Heart Failure* 1997; July/August: 2237.

145. West JA, Miller NH, Parker KM, *et al*. A comprehensive management system for heart failure improves clinical outcomes and reduces medical resource utilization. *Am J Cardiol* 1997; **79**: 58–63.

20

Atrial fibrillation: current management

EDWARD P GERSTENFELD AND ROBERT S MITTLEMAN

Atrial fibrillation is the most common supraventricular arrhythmia. Patients with atrial fibrillation may develop fatigue, shortness of breath, palpitations, and wortst of all, stroke. Management should be directed toward controlling the ventricular response, anticoagulation to prevent stroke, and, if indicated, cardioversion and maintenance of sinus rhythm. Advances in our understanding of the mechanism underlying atrial fibrillation is leading to the development of new therapies aimed at treating the underlying pathophysiology.

INTRODUCTION

Atrial fibrillation (AF) is the most common supraventricular arrhythmia, affecting approximately 2.5 million people in the USA. The incidence rises with increasing age, affecting approximately 6 per cent of patients over age 65.[1,2] The rapid ventricular response and loss of atrial contraction can cause dyspnea, palpitations, and worsen symptoms of heart failure. Stasis of blood in the atria with thrombus formation leads to an average stroke risk of 4.5 per cent per year without anticoagulation[3]. In the Framingham study, the overall mortality of patients with chronic AF was twice that of the general population.[1]

In contrast to coronary artery disease, there are few large randomized trials of patients with AF on which to base clinical decisions. There has recently been an explosion of interest in AF in the scientific community, and several important clinical trials are now under way. Promising new therapies including implantable atrial defibrillators to convert AF to sinus rhythm automatically or under patient control, and catheter-based Maze procedures for definitive cure are now on the horizon. Until these become available, however, management of patients with AF will depend on knowledge of the existing data and good clinical judgment.

HISTORICAL LANDMARKS AND DEVELOPMENT

Atrial fibrillation has puzzled physicians for centuries. In the second century AD, Galen[4] described a case of a patient with complete irregularity of the pulse and progressive dyspnea. He wondered 'how anyone with such a pulse could still be alive'. This may be the first reported case of AF complicating mitral stenosis. Withering[5] first described the use of digitalis leaf to treat patients with an irregular pulse and 'dropsy of the chest' in 1785. Many of the patients he described probably had AF. Until this century, patients with an irregular heart rate and dyspnea were often diagnosed with the clinical syndrome of *pulsus irregularis perpetuus*; however the causes of the rapid irregular pulse were unknown.

Hoffa and Ludwig[6] first described fibrillation in the ventricle in 1850 and AF was first described in the laboratory by Vulpian[6] in 1874. During experiments involving atrial electrical stimulation, he noted that the atrial muscle would sometimes continue to 'quiver' after electrical stimulation had ceased. Vulpian described this phenomenon as *mouvement fibrillaire*, and coined the term fibrillation. Early investigators never considered that this laboratory anomaly had a clinical manifestation. Cushny[7] first suggested a connection between AF seen in the laboratory and the clinical syndrome of *pulsus irregularis*, but was largely ignored. Sir Thomas Lewis,[8] followed shortly by Rothberg and Winterberg,[6] finally proved this connection in 1908. They used tracings from Einthoven's newly developed electrocardiogram to demonstrate that patients with this condition had the usual discrete atrial depolarization replaced by a fibrillating baseline reminiscent of experimental AF.

Early scientists first proposed that the mechanism of AF was due to an ectopic focus that fired at such a fast rate that homogeneous atrial conduction could not occur, and fibrillatory conduction resulted.[9] Gordon Moe[10] proposed an alternative mechanism in 1969 based on earlier experiments performed by Mayer,[11] Mines,[12] and Garrey.[13] He suggested that AF consisted of multiple re-entrant wavelets of electrical activity wandering over the surface of the atrium and interacting in a self-sustaining manner. This 'multiple wavelet hypothesis' was later confirmed by Allessie[14] in 1982 using multiple electrodes to map atrial activation during AF. More recently, Haissaguerre[14a] demonstrated in humans that paroxysmal AF is often triggered by atrial premature beats, usually originating in the pulmonary veins. Ablation of these trigger sites cured AF in some patients. This has led to our current understanding that AF is often triggered by premature beats originating in the pulmonary veins, and once initiated it is perpetuated by the interaction of multiple wandering wavelets. All these patients are currently grouped under a single diagnosis of AF based on the surface electrocardiogram (ECG). The ability to stratify patients based on particular subtypes of AF will likely help guide more specific treatment in the future.

DIAGNOSIS

The symptoms of AF are variable, depending on the ventricular rate and underlying heart disease. Some patients are asymptomatic. Palpitations or an irregular pulse are often noted. The increased ventricular rate can lead to angina in patients with coronary artery disease. The loss of atrial contraction along with the increased ventricular rate can lead to worsening symptoms of congestive heart failure. The hemodynamic compromise is often worse in patients with disorders reliant on the atrial component of ventricular filling, such as dilated and hypertrophic cardiomyopathies and aortic stenosis.

On clinical examination the pulse is completely irregular. The intensity of the peripheral pulse and the first heart sound varies with each beat, depending on the ventricular filling time. Physical examination should be directed at finding a possible cause of the atrial fibrillation, such as murmurs indicative of valvular disease, a pericardial friction rub, or signs of hyperthyroidism.

Electrocardiographically, atrial activity is irregular in both timing and morphology at a rate of 350–600 beats/minute. The ventricular response is 'irregularly irregular', with a variable rate that depends on the conduction time through the atrioventricular (AV) node. In untreated patients with normal AV node function, the ventricular rate is usually 120–180 beats/minute (Fig. 20.1).

Independent risk factors for developing AF identified in the Framingham Heart Study[15] are shown in Table 20.1. Many other risk factors have been described, including pericarditis/myocarditis, hyperthyroidism, alcohol use ('holiday heart'), pulmonary disease (pulmonary embolism or chronic obstructive pulmonary disease), and hyperthyroidism. Although AF may complicate an acute myocardial infarction because of left ventricular dysfunction and volume overload of the left atrium, ischemia itself is only rarely a cause of AF. Initial laboratory data should exclude electrolyte abnormalities and hyperthyroidism. A transthoracic echocardiogram is usually performed on an elective basis to assess left atrial size and left ventricular function, two indices helpful in guiding management.

Table 20.1 *Independent risk factors for atrial fibrillation. (Reprinted from Benjamin et al., Independent risk factors for atrial fibrillation in a population-based cohort. The Framingham Heart Study. JAMA 1994; **271**: 840–4)*

Risk factor	Relative risk
Congestive heart failure	4.5
Age (per decade)	2.1
Valve disease	1.8
Hypertension	1.5
Myocardial infarction	1.4
Diabetes mellitus	1.4

MANAGEMENT

The management of patients with AF should always address three areas: control of the ventricular rate, anticoagulation, and consideration of cardioversion/maintenance of sinus rhythm.[16]

For an individual patient presenting with new-onset AF, several treatment options are available: immediate chemical or electrical cardioversion; ventricular rate control and anticoagulation only; ventricular rate control and anticoagulation with delayed cardioversion in 3–4 weeks; or early transesophageal echocardiography (TEE)-guided cardioversion. Given the bewildering array of options, treatment needs to be tailored to the individual patient based on symptoms, hemodynamic tolerance, time of AF onset, and underlying heart disease.

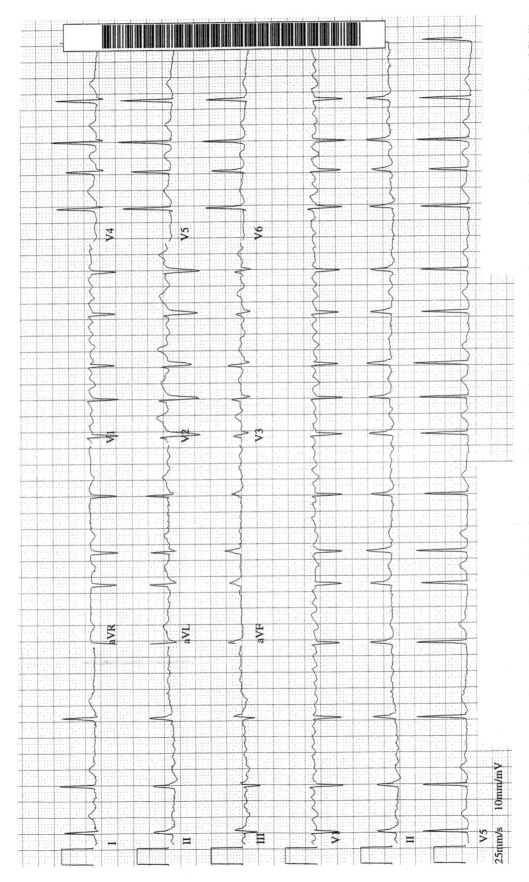

Figure 20.1 A typical 12-lead electrocardiogram of a patient in atrial fibrillation. The usual discrete atrial depolarizations in sinus rhythm are replaced by a baseline consisting of fibrillatory waves that are irregular in timing and morphology. The ventricular response is irregularly irregular. There are ST changes in the lateral leads which may be due to digoxin effect.

Immediate symptom relief should be the first priority. Most patients who present with new-onset AF without symptoms of angina or congestive heart failure can be started on an oral medical regimen after initial evaluation and treatment in the clinic or emergency room. Patients with prolonged chest pain, congestive heart failure, or a difficult to control ventricular rate may need to be admitted to the hospital to initiate treatment. In addition, patients with rheumatic mitral stenosis, severe left ventricular dysfunction, or a history of a prior stroke or transient ischemic attack (TIA) should be admitted for heparinization. Approximately 70 per cent of patients who present with recent onset AF (< 72 hours) will revert spontaneously to sinus rhythm in the next 24 hours.[17]

Ventricular rate control

Patients with AF often have a rapid ventricular rate at rest, an exaggerated heart rate response to exercise, and a decreased cardiac output compared to patients in sinus rhythm.[18] This often leads to palpitations, fatigue, dyspnea, and decreased exercise tolerance. Three classes of drugs can be used to slow the ventricular response to AF by prolonging refractoriness in the AV node. These include digitalis preparations, β-blockers, and calcium-channel blockers. A complete list of available drugs, dosages, and routes of administration is given in Table 20.2.

DRUGS USED FOR VENTRICULAR RATE CONTROL

Digitalis preparations, primarily digoxin, were the first drugs described to slow the ventricular response to AF. Digoxin slows ventricular rate by enhancing vagal tone, thereby lengthening the refractory period of the atrioventricular node.[19] Its onset of action is relatively slow, and its effects are minimal during stress or exercise.[20] A large randomized trial of long-term digoxin used in patients with congestive heart failure demonstrated a neutral effect on overall mortality.[21] Digoxin is renally excreted and therefore contraindicated in renal failure. Digoxin toxicity can cause nausea, anorexia, confusion, and both bradyarrhythmias and tachyarrhythmias.

β-Blockers slow the ventricular rate by competitively inhibiting the binding of catecholamines to β-adrenergic receptors. This makes them an ideal agent for control of ventricular rate during times of stress, or in patients whose paroxysms in AF are preceded by an increase in heart rate. β-Blockers decrease the ventricular response to AF both at rest and with exercise, although studies suggest that exercise tolerance may be reduced.[22] β-Blockers also exert negative inotropy and can precipitate congestive heart failure acutely in patients with depressed left ventricular function. In addition, they can cause bronchoconstriction and should be used cautiously in patients with reactive airways diseases.

Calcium-channel antagonists block the slow calcium channels, leading to a decrease in ventricular rate by slowing conduction in the AV node. They are well tolerated and the onset of action is rapid. The ventricular rate is decreased both at rest and with exercise, and exercise tolerance may improve in some patients.[23] Calcium-channel blockers can worsen symptoms of congestive heart failure and can cause sinus bradycardia or AV block.

ACUTE THERAPY

For symptomatic patients with acute-onset AF and a rapid ventricular rate who present to the emergency ward, an intravenous medication may be used to decrease the ventricular rate. Intravenous administration of β-blocker, diltiazem, or verapamil are all effective in patients without heart failure.[24,25] For patients with poor left ventricular function or borderline systolic blood pressure, intravenous digoxin should be used, even though the onset of action is relatively slow. Patients who develop hemodynamic compromise should undergo immediate synchronized cardioversion.

CHRONIC THERAPY

Most patients can be treated with oral drug therapy. The choice of drug for chronic therapy must be tailored to the individual patient.

> Owing to its slow onset of action, narrow therapeutic index, and lack of effectiveness during times of exertion or stress, digoxin should no longer be considered the first-line drug for ventricular rate control in patients with preserved left ventricular function.[26]

Patients with coronary artery disease or previous myocardial infarction should be treated with β-blockers to limit heart rate during exercise. Young, active patients or patients with pulmonary disease often respond well to calcium-channel blockers.[27] If either calcium-channel blockers or β-blockers alone are not effective in controlling ventricular rate, the addition of digoxin often has synergistic effects.[28,29] Digoxin is still the initial drug of choice in patients with AF and reduced left ventricular function. The addition of a low-dose β-blocker may sometimes be needed in these patients to control the ventricular rate during exercise. A suggested algorithm is outlined in Fig. 20.2.

The ideal measure of 'adequate' ventricular rate control is unclear. Symptom relief should be the primary objective. For patients with persistent symptoms of exertional dyspnea or palpitations, or patients with coronary ischemia, more objective measures of heart rate control during exercise may be warranted. A single resting apical pulse during an office visit is often misleading. An easy and inexpensive method of assessing heart rate with exercise is to recheck the pulse after the patient has walked up and down a flight of stairs. A dramatic increase in heart

Table 20.2 Drugs for controlling ventricular response to atrial fibrillation. (*Reproduced from Gerstenfeld EP, Beaudette SP, Mittleman RS. Supraventricular tachycardias. In: Irwin RS, Cerra FB, Rippe JM, eds Intensive care medicine, 4th edn. Philadelphia: Lippincott–Raven, 1999*)

Drug	Most commonly used dosage	Half-life	Route of elimination	Major adverse effects	Comments
Digoxin	IV loading: 1 mg over 24 hours po: 0.125–0.5 mg/day	36–48 hours	Renal	Fatigue, nausea, visual disturbances, arrhythmias	Adjust maintenance dose in renal failure
Propranolol	IV: 1–3 mg po: 10–80 mg q6hr po: 80–160 mg qd (long acting)	4–6 hours	Hepatic	CHF, bronchospasm, SA and AV block, hypotension, masks hypoglycemia, depression	Non-selective β-receptor blocker
Metoprolol	IV: 5 mg q5min (to 15 mg) po: 25–100 mg q12hr po: 50–200 mg qd (long acting)	3–7 hours	Hepatic	See propranolol	β_1-selective
Esmolol	IV loading: 500 μg/kg over 1 minute, then 25 μg/kg per minute; increase by 25–50 μg/kg per minute q4min to desired effect	9 minutes	Erythrocytes	See propranolol	β_1-selective. Very short half-life
Verapamil	IV bolus: 0.10–0.15 mg/kg po: 40–120 mg q8hr po: 120–360 mg qd (long acting)	3–7 hours	Hepatic	Hypotension, bradycardia, AV block, CHF, constipation	Increases digoxin levels
Diltiazem	IV bolus: 0.25 mg/kg; 0.35 mg/kg if ineffective IV maintenance: 10–20 mg/hour po: 30–120 mg q8hr po: 120–360 mg qd (long acting)	4–5 hours	Hepatic	Hypotension, bradycardia, AV block, CHF	

AV = atrioventricular; CHF = congestive heart failure; IV = intravenous; po = per os; SA = sinoatrial.

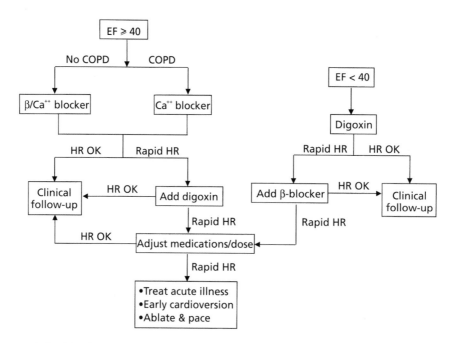

Figure 20.2 *A suggested algorithm for managing ventricular rate in patients with atrial fibrillation. Patients with preserved left ventricular function are initially treated with a β-receptor or calcium (CA⁺⁺)-channel blocker, while patients with impaired left ventricular function are treated with digoxin. Patients with chronic obstructive pulmonary disease (COPD) or asthma may not tolerate β-receptor blockers. 'Ablate & Pace' refers to ablation of the atrioventricular node and placement of a permanent ventricular pacemaker. EF = ejection fraction (%); HR = heart rate.*

rate indicates poor heart rate control. A 24-hour Holter monitor is often useful in documenting heart rate variation during the patient's typical daily activities. A useful guideline is that the mean heart rate should not be above 100 beats/minute for any consecutive hour, and that the mean heart rate over 24 hours should be less than 80 beats/minute. Alternatively, a treadmill exercise test is often performed to exclude coronary artery disease. Any patient who achieves 85 per cent predicted heart rate during stage I of a standard Bruce protocol does not have adequate heart rate control.

Some patients continue to have poor rate control despite multiple medications. Often, a change of medication may help. For example, a patient on a calcium-channel blocker may respond better to a β-blocker, or a patient on diltiazem will often respond better to verapamil. Patients who are ill will often remain tachycardic until the underlying disease process is treated. Sometimes, the only way to maintain adequate rate control is early cardioversion and maintenance of sinus rhythm. Under these circumstances, it is often necessary to use an antiarrhythmic agent to assist in cardioversion and maintenance of sinus rhythm. If all else fails, consider referral to an electrophysiologist for AV node ablation and pacemaker placement. When this procedure is performed, there is often a significant improvement in symptoms and left ventricular function with return of a regular ventricular rate and elimination

of the need for multiple medications for rate control.[30] However, anticoagulation is still needed to prevent thromboembolism if the patient remains in AF.

Anticoagulation

The most feared complication of AF is stroke. Anticoagulation with warfarin can significantly ameliorate this risk. Five large prospective randomized trials comparing warfarin and placebo in patients with non-valvular AF have been performed: the Danish Atrial Fibrillation Aspirin Anticoagulation Trial (AFASAK),[31] Boston Area Anticoagulation Trial for Atrial Fibrillation (BAATAF),[32] Canadian Atrial Fibrillation Anticoagulation trial (CAFA),[33] Stroke Prevention in Atrial Fibrillation trials (SPAF),[34,35] and the Stroke Prevention in Nonrheumatic Atrial Fibrillation Trial (SPINAF).[36] A pooled analysis performed by the principal investigators of each trial identified four important clinical risk factors for thromboembolism (Table 20.3).[37] In addition, several echocardiographic risk factors have been identified (Table 20.3).[38]

Overall, the incidence of stroke in the placebo group was 4.5 per cent per year. This was effectively reduced to an incidence of 1.5 per cent per year with warfarin. The results of the pooled analysis of the anticoagulation trials, stratified by age, are shown in Table 20.4.

Table 20.3 *Independent risk factors for thromboembolism. (Reprinted from [a]Benjamin et al., Independent risk factors for atrial fibrillation in a population-based cohort. The Framingham Heart Study. JAMA 1994; **271**: 840–4; [b]The Stroke Prevention in Atrial Fibrillation Investigators. Predictors for thromboembolism in atrial fibrillation: II. Echocardiographic features of patients at risk. Ann Intern Med 1992; **116**: 6–12)*

Clinical risk factors[a]	Relative risk	Echocardiographic risk factors[b]	Relative risk
Prior stroke or TIA	2.5	Left ventricular dysfunction	4.5
Diabetes mellitus	2	Increased left atrial size	2.1
Hypertension	1.6		
Age	1.4		

TIA = transient ischemic attack.

All patients over age 65, or with at least one other risk factor for thromboembolism, benefited from anticoagulation with warfarin. All patients with AF due to rheumatic valvular disease, regardless of age, are also at high risk of stroke and should be anticoagulated with warfarin.

Patients with 'lone AF' can often provide a challenge to the physician. These patients are less than 65 years of age, have no underlying heart disease by history and echocardiography, and no risk factors for thromboembolism. In the pooled analysis performed by the AF anticoagulation investigators, no strokes occurred in the 112 patients under age 60 with 'lone' AF. A natural history study by Kopecky and colleagues[39] was equally optimistic, with a cumulative stroke incidence of 1.5 per cent over 15 years, and no strokes occurring in patients under age 60. Although the risk of stroke is slightly higher in patients age 60–65 years of age with no underlying heart disease, the pooled analysis did not reveal any benefit in treating this subgroup of patients with warfarin (Table 20.4). Therefore, it is reasonable to treat such patients

under the age of 65 with documented 'lone AF' with aspirin or nothing.

The decision of whether or not to anticoagulate the small subgroup of patients age 65–75 with no risk factors for thromboembolism can also be difficult. As can be seen in the pooled analysis (Table 20.4), the risk in this group is not small (4.3 per cent) and can be significantly reduced with warfarin. The subgroup of patients in this age range with no angina or heart failure in addition to the absence of the independent clinical risk factors for stroke (Table 20.3), had a low risk of stroke (<2 per cent) in the pooled analysis. The observational SPAF III registry[40] prospectively followed patients who were excluded from the randomized SPAF III trial because they were felt to be at low risk of stroke (women age <75 years, no history of stroke or congestive heart failure, and no current systolic hypertension) and were treated with 325 mg/day of aspirin alone. The overall rate of primary events (stroke or systemic embolism) was 2.2 per cent per year; however, patients with a history of treated hypertension had a significantly higher stroke rate (3.6 per cent per year) than patients with no history of hypertension (1.1 per cent per year). Therefore, aspirin treat-

Table 20.4 *Annual event rates by age groups and risk factors (total patients: placebo 1802 vs warfarin 1889). (Reproduced with permission from Atrial Fibrillation Investigators. Risk factors for stroke and efficacy of antithrombotic therapy in atrial analysis of pooled data from five randomized trials. Arch Intern Med 1994; **154**: 1449)*

Risk category	Placebo			Warfarin		
	Per cent[a]	Number of events	Event rate (95% CI)	Per cent[a]	Number of events	Event rate (95% CI)
Age < 65 years						
No risk factors	15	3	1.0 (0.3–3.1)	17	3	1.0 (0.3–3.0)
One or more risk factors	17	16	4.9 (3.0–8.1)	17	6	1.7 (0.8–3.9)
Age 65–75 years						
No risk factors	20	16	4.3 (2.7–7.1)	20	4	1.1 (0.4–2.8)
One or more risk factors	27	27	5.7 (3.9–8.3)	27	7	1.7 (0.9–3.4)
Age > 75 years						
No risk factors	11	6	3.5 (1.6–7.7)	11	3	1.7 (0.5–5.2)
One or more risk factors	9	13	8.1 (4.7–13.9)	9	2	1.2 (0.3–5.0)

[a]Per cent refers to the percentage of patients in each risk category.
CI = confidence interval.

ment is a reasonable alternative to warfarin in patients less than 75 years of age with no evidence of structural heart disease and no risk factors for thromboembolism, including treated hypertension. However, since there are no data from a large randomized trial in this small subgroup of patients, we continue to offer warfarin anticoagulation to these patients after a detailed discussion of the risks and benefits.

There is a justifiable concern about the excess bleeding risk from warfarin, especially among the elderly. This concern was increased by the SPAF II trial, which found that the excess risk of bleeding from warfarin outweighed the advantage of stroke reduction in the elderly when compared to aspirin. These concerns are largely unfounded provided that anticoagulation status is monitored systematically. The SPAF trials used a goal prothrombin time (PT) of 1.2–1.8 times control for patients on warfarin, a level that corresponds to an international normalized ratio (INR) of 2–4.5. It has clearly been documented that an INR over 3 significantly increases bleeding risk, especially in the elderly.[41] The pooled analysis of the five randomized trials found a non-significant excess bleeding risk of 0.3 per cent in patients on warfarin, and a non-significant excess risk of intracranial hemorrhage of only 0.2 per cent. In addition, the risk of stroke clearly increases with age. A patient over the age of 75 in AF with only one risk factor for thromboembolism has a stroke risk of 8 per cent per year, and if there has been a previous stroke or TIA within 6 months, as high as 12 per cent per year. Therefore, the risk–benefit ratio in most elderly patients with AF is in favor of anticoagulation with warfarin.

The data on the effectiveness of aspirin for the prevention of stroke are less clear. SPAF II is the only trial that demonstrated an effect of aspirin on stroke prevention, a significant risk reduction of 44 per cent. AFASAK found no significant benefit of aspirin compared to placebo. The European Atrial Fibrillation Trial (EAFT),[42] a secondary prevention trial, found no benefit of aspirin in preventing a second thromboembolism. SPAF III[43] compared combined treatment with 325 mg of aspirin and low-dose warfarin versus traditional dose-adjusted warfarin to an INR of 2–3 in patients at high risk for stroke. The trial was terminated prematurely because the incidence of stroke in the combined treatment arm was 8.3 per cent, compared to 1.8 per cent in patients on warfarin. As mentioned above, the SPAF III registry did not find an increased risk of stroke among patients at low risk for thromboembolism treated with aspirin. Until the benefit of aspirin for preventing thromboembolism is clarified, aspirin should only be considered in patients at risk of stroke who have a strong contraindication to warfarin, or in the small subgroup of patients under age 75 with no structural heart disease.

The optimal range of anticoagulation has also been carefully studied. An INR below 2 substantially increases the risk of stroke. Patients with an INR of 1.7 have twice the stroke risk, and patients with an INR of 1.5 have three times the risk of stroke compared to patients with an INR between 2 and 3.[44] 'Low dose' anticoagulation is therefore not a viable treatment option. An INR above 4 substantially increases the risk of bleeding. An INR between 2 and 3 should therefore be the goal in all patients being treated with warfarin for AF. In the pooled analysis mentioned above, eight of the 27 strokes occurred in patients who were not taking warfarin as prescribed. Anticoagulation clinics can be extremely helpful in maintaining the INR in the therapeutic range, removing the burden of anticoagulation from the physician, and preventing excess bleeding events.[45]

A cost-effectiveness analysis of anticoagulation for AF was performed by Eckman and Pauker.[46] Comparing warfarin anticoagulation with a strategy of no anticoagulation, they found anticoagulation with warfarin cost only $1712 per quality adjusted life-year gained. This is extremely inexpensive compared to the cost effectiveness of other common preventive treatments, such as treating hypertension ($17 493–$34 165)[47,48] or hyperlipidemia ($50 510).[48] Because the true benefit of aspirin in reducing stroke is unknown, the true cost effectiveness of aspirin cannot be accurately determined. Using a sensitivity analysis, the benefit of aspirin in reducing stroke would have to be greater than 58 per cent to be less costly and more effective than anticoagulation with warfarin. This is beyond even the optimistic 44 per cent reduction found in SPAF II. Therefore, anticoagulation with warfarin for the average patient with AF appears to be a very cost-effective strategy.

PAROXYSMAL AF

> Most studies of paroxysmal AF have found an incidence of stroke equal to that of chronic AF, although the data are sparse.

The pooled analysis of the randomized anticoagulation trials found that there was no difference in stroke occurrence compared to sustained AF in the 462 (12.5 per cent patients with paroxysmal AF at entry in the study. Furthermore, symptoms of AF are not always reliable. Page et al.[49] found asymptomatic episodes of AF 12 times more common in patients with paroxysmal AF than symptomatic episodes. It is unclear how prolonged the paroxysms need to be before anticoagulation is necessary. Patients in the Atrial Fibrillation Follow-Up Investigation of Rhythm Management (AFFIRM)[50] trial who had infrequent paroxysms of AF less than 1 hour in duration were not considered eligible for the trial because it was felt that anticoagulation was not clearly indicated. On the other hand, patients who have atrial fibrillation for less than 48 hours are considered appropriate for electrical cardioversion without prior anticoagulation.

Our practice is to consider anticoagulation seriously for patients with appropriate risk factors who are felt to have episodes of AF lasting 24 hours or more. Decisions regarding anticoagulation in these patients should be individualized.

PERI-CARDIOVERSION

Early studies found that patients undergoing cardioversion for AF without anticoagulation had a stroke risk of up to 7 per cent[51,52,53] over the hours to weeks after cardioversion. This led to the largely empiric strategy of anticoagulation with warfarin before and after cardioversion to promote clot dissolution and organization. This strategy proved effective, as retrospective studies have found that patients given 3 weeks of warfarin before cardioversion have the stroke risk reduced to approximately 0.8 per cent.[51] In addition, studies using transesophageal echocardiography have found that most atrial thrombi do resolve after 4 weeks of treatment with warfarin.[54]

Following cardioversion, there may be up to a 3-week delay before normal mechanical atrial contraction is restored, even though electrical sinus rhythm has been maintained.[55] This delay in return to normal atrial mechanical function following cardioversion has been termed 'stunning',[56,57] and appears to be independent of the method of cardioversion.[58] Although the mechanism of atrial 'stunning' after cardioversion remains unclear, the stroke risk does seem to persist for up to 3 weeks after cardioversion.

All patients with AF lasting over 48 hours should therefore undergo anticoagulation with warfarin to an INR of 2–3 for 3 weeks before, and 3–4 weeks after cardioversion.

Patients with known AF lasting less than 48 hours, by clear symptom history or documented telemetry, can undergo cardioversion without the preceding 3 weeks of warfarin.

The risk of stroke in patients cardioverted after less than 48 hours of AF is only 0.8 per cent.[59] There is evidence that patients with AF of less than 1 week's duration have a rapid return to normal atrial function and may be candidates for an abbreviated course of anticoagulation after cardioversion;[55,60] however this has not yet been studied in a prospective manner. Given the risk of early reversion to AF, and concerns about possible atrial mechanical dysfunction, even patients with AF <48 hours should be considered for anticoagulation with warfarin for at least 3 weeks after cardioversion.

The risk of stroke in patients with 'lone AF' undergoing cardioversion has not been studied. Although the risk of thromboembolism in these patients is low, most clinicians anticoagulate these patients because the perceived consequences of a stroke in a young patient are high. The currently published recommendations for anticoagulation with warfarin for 3 weeks before and 4 weeks after cardioversion in all patients do not require any thromboembolic risk factors.[61]

CARDIOVERSION GUIDED BY TRANSESOPHAGEAL ECHOCARDIOGRAPHY

The technology of transesophageal echocardiography has led to the development of a new strategy for early cardioversion. TEE allows direct visualization of the left atrial appendage, a structure that has been implicated in the formation of thrombus responsible for subsequent embolization. TEE has a much higher reported sensitivity (100 per cent) and specificity (99 per cent) for detecting atrial thrombus compared to traditional two-dimensional echocardiography.[62] Manning and colleagues demonstrated in a prospective study that, if there was no thrombus in the left atrial appendage as determined by TEE, the risk of thromboembolism with cardioversion was low (0 of 186 patients; 95 per cent confidence interval (CI) 0–1.6 per cent).[63] Shortly after this initial report, Black reported 13 patients who developed thromboembolism 2–7 days after TEE-guided cardioversion.[64] However, none of these patients were therapeutically anticoagulated at the time. In the Assessment of Cardioversion Using Transesophageal Echocardiography (ACUTE)[65] pilot study, there were no embolic events in 56 patients who underwent TEE-guided cardioversion followed by anticoagulation, versus one embolic event in 37 patients undergoing cardioversion after conventional anticoagulation. Continued anticoagulation after cardioversion is therefore an important part of the TEE-guided strategy. The ACUTE study, a large multicenter randomized prospective trial expected to recruit between 3000 and 5000 patients, is currently evaluating the safety of TEE-guided cardioversion. Nevertheless, TEE-guided cardioversion has already become a common clinical practice in many centers.

All patients undergoing TEE-guided cardioversion are anticoagulated with heparin for 24 hours before cardioversion, if possible. If the TEE demonstrates no evidence of left atrial appendage thrombus, immediate cardioversion is performed.

Although the two procedures can be performed separately, we generally perform electrical cardioversion immediately after the TEE, since the patient is already sedated. Patients should then be anticoagulated with warfarin for at least 4 weeks after cardioversion because of the risk of thromboembolism and recurrent AF, as outlined above.

The prevalence of atrial thrombi in patients undergoing TEE for AF is approximately 15 per cent, most of which are found in the left atrial appendage.[62] If an atrial

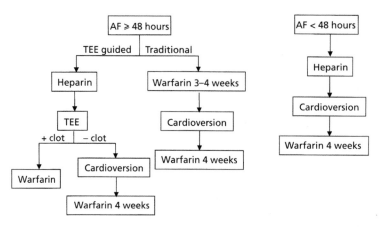

Figure 20.3 *A suggested algorithm for anticoagulation before and after cardioversion. Transesophageal echocardiography (TEE)-guided cardioversion should be reserved for patients intolerant of prolonged atrial fibrillation (AF) until this strategy is validated in a large prospective randomized trial. The treatment of patients with a left atrial appendage clot on TEE is still being refined (see text). The use of warfarin after cardioversion of AF lasting less than 48 hours depends on the underlying risk of thromboembolism.*

appendage clot is revealed during TEE, cardioversion should be delayed and anticoagulation continued for at least 4 weeks. The optimal strategy after an atrial appendage clot has been demonstrated is not clear. Manning has advocated repeat TEE at monthly intervals until the clot has resolved. A more empiric strategy is to give 3 months of anticoagulation followed by cardioversion. The ACUTE study may help clarify this controversial area.

The benefits of TEE-guided cardioversion include three fewer weeks of anticoagulation, immediate relief of patient symptoms, and the possibility of improving the likelihood of maintaining sinus rhythm. The risks include those of esophageal perforation (1/10 000), stroke, and conscious sedation, although since sedation will be required for cardioversion even without TEE, the overall risk is low. Until the safety of TEE-guided cardioversion is confirmed, it should in most cases be used in those patients who are hospitalized and intolerant of prolonged AF. A suggested algorithm for cardioversion is shown in Fig. 20.3. If proven safe, TEE-guided cardioversion promises the benefit of early return to sinus rhythm and shorter duration of anticoagulation. This could be important, as there is evidence that the longer a patient continues in AF, the less likely sinus rhythm will be maintained once restored.[66,67]

TEE also involves the added cost of hospital admission or observation, the echocardiographic charge, and the cardiologist's charge for performing the procedure. A cost-effectiveness analysis by Seto *et al.* found that the cost-effectiveness of TEE-guided cardioversion compared to a traditional approach (transthoracic echocardiogram followed by 4 weeks of warfarin) was dependent on the risk of thromboembolism after cardioversion.[68] If the risk of stroke after TEE-guided cardioversion was less than that of the traditional approach (relative risk < 0.95), then the TEE approach

was more cost effective. However, if the risk of stroke after TEE was slightly higher (relative risk 1.1), then the TEE-guided approach cost $50 000 per quality adjusted life-year gained. This analysis assumed that all patients were admitted to the hospital, and that patients undergoing the traditional route of anticoagulation all received a transthoracic echocardiogram. Since the true event rate after TEE-guided cardioversion will not be known until the ACUTE trial is completed, the cost-effectiveness of this method remains to be determined.

Cardioversion/maintenance of sinus rhythm

The decision of when to attempt cardioversion and aggressive maintenance of sinus rhythm versus acceptance of AF with anticoagulation and ventricular rate control is a difficult one.

> Most patients presenting with new-onset AF of relatively short duration (<1 year) should receive an initial attempt at cardioversion to sinus rhythm.

Since AF will recur in many patients, the addition of antiarrhythmic agents is often needed to help maintain sinus rhythm. However, even with antiarrhythmic treatment, the likelihood of maintaining sinus rhythm at 1 year is only 50–65 per cent.[69,70] In patients with left ventricular dysfunction or persistent symptoms of palpitations, fatigue, or exertional dyspnea, aggressive maintenance of sinus rhythm is certainly warranted. In the asymptomatic patient with prolonged AF and no contraindication to anticoagulation with warfarin, antiarrhythmic therapy has little benefit to offer and the potential for increasing morbidity and mortality. The Cardiac Arrhythmia Suppression Trial (CAST)[71] study highlighted the risk of antiarrhythmic drugs when it was discovered that patients with marked ventricular ectopy after myocardial infarction treated with type IC antiarrhythmic agents had an increase in mortality. A meta-analysis by Coplen[70] and a retrospective study of SPAF[72] further dampened enthusiasm for antiarrhythmic therapy by demonstrating an increase in mortality of patients in AF treated with class IA antiarrhythmic drugs.

There is currently no prospective data, however, demonstrating an increased mortality risk in patients with AF on antiarrhythmic therapy, and many patients do feel better in sinus rhythm. Many patients continue to have fatigue and palpitations in AF despite adequate heart rate control. Cardiac output and exercise tolerance are often reduced. Patients with an absolute contraindication to warfarin may have a lower stroke risk in sinus rhythm. Early restoration of sinus rhythm may promote long-term maintenance of sinus rhythm by preventing electrical remodeling of the atria.[65,66] A prospective randomized trial of anticoagulation and rate control of AF, versus aggressive attempts to maintain sinus rhythm, called AFFIRM, is currently under way and may help answer this question. Until the results of AFFIRM are available, the decision of whether to attempt maintenance of sinus rhythm should be individualized.

Many antiarrhythmic drugs are available for conversion and maintenance of sinus rhythm. They are the Vaughn Williams class IA, IC, and III antiarrhythmic drugs. A complete listing of drugs, dosages, and routes of administration is shown in Table 20.5.

DRUGS FOR CONVERSION/MAINTENANCE OF SINUS RHYTHM

Class IA

These drugs work by blocking fast sodium channels and potassium channels, thereby slowing conduction velocity and increasing refractoriness in the atrium. Quinidine,[69] disopyramide,[73] and procainamide[74] have all been demonstrated to improve the likelihood of maintaining sinus rhythm. Only quinidine is approved by the Food and Drug Administration for the treatment of AF. These drugs increase the QT interval on the ECG, creating the risk of a potentially fatal arrhythmia, *torsade de pointes*.[75] The incidence of *torsade* in patients receiving quinidine is estimated to be between 1.5 and 8 per cent per year.[76] Class IA drugs are also limited by their side effects. Quinidine often causes a dose-related nausea and diarrhea. A total of 20–30 per cent of patients on procainamide develop clinical symptoms of a lupus-like syndrome, with arthralgias, fever, pericarditis, and pleuritis.[77] Disopyramide has a significant anticholinergic effect, which can lead to urinary retention, dry mouth, constipation, and exacerbation of glaucoma.

Class IC

These drugs also block sodium channels, causing a marked slowing of conduction velocity. Flecainide and propafenone are both well tolerated and as effective as class IA agents in maintaining sinus rhythm. Propafenone has a weak β-blocker effect, and therefore it is often effective in controlling the ventricular response to AF. Because of the increased mortality found in the CAST study, flecainide should not be used in patients with significant structural heart disease. Since propafenone has a similar mechanism of action, it should also be used cautiously in patients with any structural heart disease. A small proportion of patients (2 per cent) may develop exacerbations of arrhythmias,[78] including atrial flutter with 1:1 atrioventricular conduction and a wide complex ventricular response mimicking ventricular tachycardia.[79] These events are most common in patients with underlying heart disease.[76] Some patients may experience gastrointestinal intolerance or a metallic taste in their mouth.

Class III

These drugs block potassium channels, causing marked increases in atrial refractoriness without slowing conduction velocity. Drugs in this class include sotalol, amiodarone, and ibutilide. Although sotalol and amiodarone have not been approved by the Food and Drug Administration for the treatment of AF, they have a favorable pharmacologic profile for this purpose and are used by many physicians experienced in arrhythmia management.

Sotalol is well tolerated and has potent β-blocking activity. It can also cause a dose-related increase in the QT interval and predispose to *torsade de pointes*. The incidence of *Torsade* is lower in men than women, and unlikely (<2 per cent) if the total dose is kept under 320 mg/day in patients with normal cardiac and renal function.[80]

Amiodarone has sodium-channel, calcium-channel, β-receptor and α-receptor blocking activity. Although the QT interval may be lengthened, amiodarone appears to have the lowest incidence of proarrhythmia of any antiarrhythmic drug. Significant side effects do exist, however, including pulmonary fibrosis, hepatotoxicity, hyperthyroidism and hypothyroidism, neuropathy, photosensitivity, optic neuritis, and corneal microdeposits.[81-84] Its beneficial effects must therefore be weighed carefully against potential side effects for each patient.

Ibutilide[85] is approved for acute cardioversion of AF to sinus rhythm. Efficacy at converting atrial flutter to sinus rhythm (63 per cent) is higher than for cardioverting atrial fibrillation (31 per cent). The major side effect is *torsades de pointes*, both non-sustained (6.7 per cent) and sustained (1.7 per cent). Patients given ibutilide need to be closely monitored during and for at least 4 hours after the initial dose, or until the QT interval returns to baseline. Contraindications to ibutilide administration include a corrected QT interval greater than 440 ms, hypokalemia, or previous *torsade*.

Table 20.5 *Drugs for conversion of atrial fibrillation to sinus rhythm. (Reproduced with permission from Gerstenfeld EP, Beaudette SP, Mittleman RS. Supraventricular tachycardias. In: Irwin RS, Cerra FB, Rippe JM, eds Intensive care medicine, 4th edn. Philadelphia: Lippincott–Raven, 1999)*

Drug	Most commonly used dosage	Half-life	Route of elimination	Major adverse effects	Comments
Quinidine	po: 300–600 mg q6hr (sulfate) po: 324–648 mg q8hr (gluconate)	6–8 hours	Hepatic	Gastrointestinal distress, diarrhea, thrombocytopenia, anemia, rash, *torsades de pointes*	Frequent early side effects
Procainamide	IV loading: 15 mg/kg at 20 mg/minute IV maintenance: 2–5 mg/minute po: 500–1000 mg q6hr	3–5 hours	Hepatic, renal	Lupus-like syndrome, nausea, diarrhea, rash, confusion, myalgias, *torsades de pointes*	60% develop antinuclear antibodies 20-30% developing clinical lupus-like syndrome NAPA (active metabolite) formed in the liver
Disopyramide	po: 100–200 mg q6hr po: 150–300 mg q12hr (sustained release)	6–7 hours	Renal	Anticholinergic effects: urinary retention, constipation, dry mouth; CHF; *torsades de pointes*	Greater negative inotropy than other class IA agents
Flecainide	po: 100–200 mg q12hr	20 hours	Hepatic	Dizziness, visual disturbances, bradycardia, sustained ventricular tachycardia	Increases mortality in patients with prior myocardial infarction
Propafenone	po: 150–300 mg q8hr	5–8 hours	Hepatic	Bradycardia, bronchospasm, CHF, sustained ventricular tachycardia	β-Blocker activity 1/40 that of propranolol
Amiodarone	po loading: 600–800 mg/day for 6 weeks, then 400 mg/day for 2 months, then 200 mg/day	50 days	Hepatic	Pulmonary fibrosis, hepatitis, hypothyroidism and hyperthyroidism, neuropathy, corneal deposits, photosensitivity	Use limited by dose-related toxicity. Increases digoxin level; lowers coumadin requirements
Sotolol	po: 80–160 mg q12hr	6–18 hours	Renal	Bronchospasm, CHF, AV block, bradycardia, hypotension, *torsades de pointes*	Potent β-blocker in addition to class III activity
Ibutilide	IV: 1 mg over 10 minute (0.01 mg/kg if weight < 60 kg) repeat initial dose in 10 minutes if no effect	6 hours	Hepatic	*Torsades de pointes* (6.7% non-sustained, 1.7% sustained)	QTc < 440 mseconds, correct hypokalemia Close monitoring for 4–6 hours after dose
Dofetilide	po: 250–500 µg twice daily	8 hours	Hepatic, renal	Torsade de pointes (2.9%)	Dose adjust for renal insufficiency

AV = atrioventricular; CHF = congestive heart failure; IV = intravenous; NAPA = N-acetyl procainamide; QTc = corrected Q-T interval; po = per os; SA = sinoatrial.

Dofetilide is a new class III agent approved for the treatment of atrial fibrillation. Two large studies by the Danish Investigators of Arrhythmia and Mortality in Dofetilide (DIAMOND) investigators demonstrated that dofetilide did not increase mortality compared to controls in patients with congestive heart failure (DIAMOND CHF[85a]). In DIAMOND CHF, patients who converted from AF to sinus rhythm were significantly more likely to remain in sinus rhythm at one year (80 per cent dofetilide *vs.* 40 per cent placebo). The major risk of defetilide was *torsade de pointes*, occurring in 2.9 per cent of patients. These findings led the FDA to mandate that physicians administering dofetilide need special certification, that dofetilide is only initiated in hospital, and that the dose is carefully adjusted for renal insufficiency.

ACUTE CARDIOVERSION

Acute conversion of AF to sinus rhythm can either be performed pharmacologically or electrically. Oral pharmacologic cardioversion has been performed with quinidine 600 mg (200 mg every 2 hours),[86] propafenone 600 mg,[87] or flecainide 200–300 mg[88] in patients without overt congestive heart failure or coronary artery disease. Intravenous cardioversion can be performed with procainamide or ibutilide, although a comparative study indicated that ibutilide is superior.[89] Electrical cardioversion is the most effective method (>85 per cent).[90] For resistant cases, intra-atrial cardioversion performed by experienced operators is safe and highly effective (91 per cent).[91]

Most outpatients still undergo electrical cardioversion because of time constraints. If chronic antiarrhythmic therapy is planned, this should be started before cardioversion to help maintain sinus rhythm.

A reasonable strategy for monitored in-patients or patients in the emergency department is to try single-dose pharmacologic therapy, and proceed to electrical cardioversion if unsuccessful. We reserve ibutilide for patients in the coronary or surgical intensive care units, because of the extensive monitoring required.

CHRONIC THERAPY

Patients with a first episode of AF and preserved left ventricular systolic function are often treated with cardioversion alone. Patients with recurrent, symptomatic AF, or reduced left ventricular function may require antiarrhythmic therapy to maintain sinus rhythm. Only quinidine, flecainide, and propafenone have been approved by the Food and Drug Administration for the treatment of AF. However, all the drugs mentioned above are in widespread clinical use.

The initial choice of drug depends on the patient's age, underlying heart disease, and risk of proarrhythmia. An assessment of coronary artery disease and left ventricular function should be performed in most patients before instituting therapy. For patients with structurally normal hearts and no manifest coronary artery disease, class IC agents are usually well tolerated[92] and relatively safe.[93] Patients with coronary artery disease or asymptomatic mild to moderate left ventricular dysfunction can be treated with either sotalol or amiodarone. For patients with symptomatic left ventricular dysfunction, amiodarone is the only drug that has a proven safety record.[94-96] Patients treated with amiodarone need to be monitored closely for signs of hepatic, pulmonary, or thyroid toxicity.[97] Class IA drugs have fallen out of favor because of their frequent side effects, however, there are cases where these drugs are useful. A decision analysis comparing the various antiarrhythmic strategies found that amiodarone was the most effective drug with the fewest side effects over a 5-year period.[98] Other studies have documented significant side effects and patient intolerance of amiodarone, even at low doses.[99] A suggested algorithm is shown in Fig. 20.4.

Complete suppression of AF is probably an unrealistic goal in many patients. Even with effective drug therapy, recurrence rates of AF are approximately 50 per cent at 1 year. Often, a more reasonable goal is a reduction in the *frequency* of AF recurrences. Therefore, each AF recurrence is not necessarily a 'failure' of therapy, and drug type or dosage need not be adjusted for infrequent recurrences.[100] The key to successful treatment of AF is tailoring therapy to the individual patient.

INITIATION OF THERAPY

It is not known whether the initiation of antiarrhythmic treatment for AF requires monitoring as an in-patient. Patients without structural heart disease can often be started on antiarrhythmic medications as an out-patient. It should be recognized that, even if a patient is admitted to the hospital to begin treatment, pro-arrhythmia could still occur after a week or more of treatment, by which time the patient has generally been discharged.

Our current practice is to admit patients routinely to initiate treatment with class IA drugs or sotalol, because of the concern about the early occurrence of *torsade de pointes*. We commonly initiate treatment with amiodarone, or class IC drugs in patients without structural heart disease, on an out-patient basis.[101] However, we monitor patients closely with weekly 12-lead electrocardiograms or transtelephonic event monitor recordings during loading to screen for bradycardia or proarrhythmia.

A cost-effectiveness analysis of in-patient initiation of antiarrhythmic therapy found that a 72-hour hospitalization for an average 60-year-old man cost $19 231 per year of life saved.[102] The added cost must therefore be weighed against the potential risks for each patient.

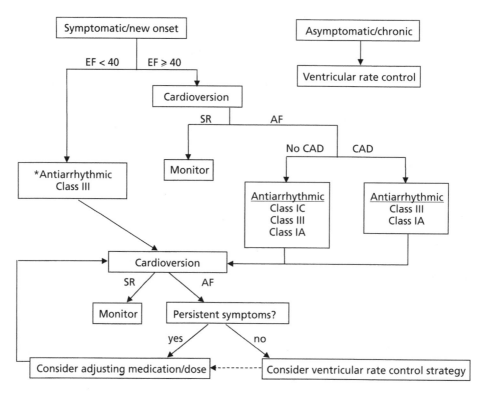

Figure 20.4 *A suggested algorithm for the management of patients with newly discovered atrial fibrillation (AF). Patients with chronic (>1 year) asymptomatic AF rarely benefit from cardioversion and antiarrhythmic drug use. Patients with symptoms, left ventricular dysfunction, or recent-onset AF are often cardioverted to sinus rhythm (SR). Patients with recurrences after antiarrhythmic treatment may undergo medication or dose adjustments, depending on the frequency of recurrence. The number of repeat cardioversions and antiarrhythmic drugs used before acceptance of AF is often determined by the frequency of recurrences and the patient's tolerance of chronic AF. Antiarrhythmic drug class is listed in order of preference. * Some physicians may elect to perform an initial cardioversion without antiarrhythmic therapy in these patients, although the likelihood of maintaining sinus rhythm is low. CAD = coronary artery disease; Class IA = quinidine, procainamide, disopyramide; Class IC =flecainide, propafenone; Class III = amiodarone, sotalol, dofetilide; EF = ejection fraction.*

CAN ANTICOAGULATION BE STOPPED AFTER RETURN TO SINUS RHYTHM?

Once a patient has been converted to sinus rhythm, the question of stopping anticoagulation always arises. There are currently no data to support the assertion that patients in sinus rhythm on antiarrhythmic treatment have a low risk of thromboembolism. Even patients with significant symptoms from AF can also have significant asymptomatic episodes. Therefore, the decision to use antiarrhythmic drugs should not necessarily be guided by the desire to withdraw anticoagulation with warfarin in the future. This is particularly important in patients at high risk of thromboembolism.

> Our clinical practice is to consider stopping warfarin in a reliable patient with a clear, abrupt onset of symptoms from AF who is at a low risk of stroke, provided that sinus rhythm has been maintained for a minimum of 1–3 months after cardioversion.

Patients are monitored closely and at least one Holter monitor recording is performed to exclude significant asymptomatic episodes of AF. Patients are also taught to monitor their own pulse on a regular basis. However, patients with a history of previous stroke or TIA, low ejection fraction, or rheumatic valvular disease are at high risk and should be strongly considered for lifelong anticoagulation regardless of antiarrhythmic therapy. We also continue anticoagulation in most patients who are asymptomatic, since these patients are often unable to recognize recurrences of AF.

NON-PHARMACOLOGIC THERAPY

Given the limitations of antiarrhythmic drug therapy, non-pharmacologic options for treatment of atrial fibrillation have been growing in popularity. These include the surgical MAZE procedure, atrioventricular node ablation and permanent pacemaker implantation, hybrid therapy, and ablation of atrial fibrillation triggers.

Cox and colleagues[103] developed the surgical MAZE procedure in the first effort to cure AF. Since maintenance of AF depends on a critical number of circulating wavelets, compartmentalizing the atrium surgically with linear incisions to prevent re-entrant circuits can eliminate AF. This procedure may be used as an adjunctive procedure in patients undergoing other forms of open heart surgery, particularly mitral valve replacement. However, the need for open heart surgery has limited the applicability of this technique in the general population.

The use of AV node ablation and permanent pacemaker implantation to control the ventricular response in patients with drug refractory AF has become increasingly popular.[30] This palliative procedure leaves the atria fibrillating, but allows the ventricular rate to be entirely controlled by a rate-responsive ventricular pacemaker. Although patients need to be maintained on chronic anticoagulation with warfarin, there is often a tremendous improvement in symptoms, exercise tolerance and even left ventricular function.

Some patients treated with class IC antiarrhythmic agents or amiodarone can organize from atrial fibrillation into typical atrial flutter. Combination therapy with an atrial flutter catheter ablation and continuation of antiarrhythmic therapy, so called 'hybrid' therapy, has been shown to provide excellent long-term maintenance of sinus rhythm (89 per cent maintained sinus rhythm at 14 months).[104] Patients with frequent atrial flutter and rare episodes of atrial fibrillation on drug therapy appear to be the best candidates for this procedure.

Several investigators attempted to mimic the surgical MAZE procedure using percutaneous intracardiac catheters in an attempt to develop a catheter-based cure of AF. Long linear burns were made between various anatomic landmarks in the right and left atrium in order to eliminate the substrate for re-entry.[105,106] Although these studies resulted in a 'proof of concept' by curing AF in some patients, long procedure time and complications including stroke, pulmonary vein stenosis, and recurrent atrial tachycardia have thus far prevented further development of this procedure. More recent data have revealed that some patients have focal 'triggers' of atrial fibrillation, most often originating in the pulmonary veins.[14a] In these patients, focal ablation at the site of the initiating trigger using standard percutaneous intracardiac catheters has been documented to eliminate or reduce recurrences of AF. In general, this technique has been limited to patients with paroxysmal AF and preserved left ventricular function who have multiple atrial premature beats of uniform morphology or runs of atrial tachycardia that initiate AF. However, as newer technology specifically designed for the treatment of atrial fibrillation evolves, these techniques may become applicable to a wider segment of patients with AF.

CLINICAL OVERVIEW

The current treatment of AF includes ventricular rate control, anticoagulation, and conversion/maintenance of sinus rhythm. It should be recognized that all patients have individual characteristics and no comprehensive treatment strategy can be developed which applies to all patients. Nevertheless, certain guidelines can be formulated. Rate control should initially be attempted with calcium-channel or β-receptor blockers, with digoxin added if a suboptimal result is achieved. Digoxin should be used as first-line therapy in patients with significant left ventricular dysfunction. In patients with persistent symptoms, adequate rate control should be confirmed objectively with exercise. A proposed algorithm is shown in Fig. 20.2.

All patients over age 75, or with at least one risk factor for stroke should be anticoagulated with warfarin to an INR of 2–3 if no contraindication to anticoagulation exists (Table 20.6). Patients with paroxysmal AF should, in general, be treated identically to patients with chronic AF. All patients should also be anticoagulated for at least 3 weeks before and 4 weeks after cardioversion, regardless of the method used.

Table 20.6 *Recommendations for anticoagulation*

Age	No risk factors	Risk factors[a]
< 65	Aspirin *vs* nothing	Warfarin
65–75	Warfarin[b]	Warfarin
> 75	Warfarin	Warfarin

[a]Risk factors include hypertension, diabetes mellitus, prior stroke, or transient ischemic attack.
[b]In patients with no history of angina or heart failure, aspirin therapy may be an option (see text).

The ACUTE trial is investigating whether TEE-guided cardioversion will safely reduce the length of anticoagulation before cardioversion. A proposed algorithm is shown in Fig. 20.3.

Patients with chronic, asymptomatic AF should be maintained on anticoagulation with ventricular rate control. Patients with symptomatic or recent-onset AF should undergo attempts at cardioversion and maintenance of sinus rhythm.

Antiarrhythmic drugs should be reserved for symptomatic patients who revert to AF after an initial cardioversion, or patients with symptoms from left ventricular dysfunction.

A proposed algorithm is shown in Fig. 20.4. Until the results of AFFIRM are available, the decision to maintain sinus rhythm will need to be individualized.

FUTURE DIRECTIONS

There are many advances in the management of AF on the horizon. Results of the AFFIRM trial will help guide medical management. New antiarrhythmic drugs are being developed. However, it is likely that continued breakthroughs in non-pharmacologic therapy will dominate the next decade.

Retrospective and prospective studies have demonstrated that patients receiving atrial-based pacing have less AF and fewer strokes than those receiving ventricular-based pacing.[107] Pacing strategies for the prevention of AF in the postoperative setting have shown promise.[108] Atrial-based pacing is currently being investigated as a primary therapy for the prevention of AF.[109] Implantable atrial defibrillators designed to cardiovert atrial fibrillation to sinus rhythm were limited in early studies by the need for device implantation and the pain associated with atrial shocks. Adding the capability of atrial defibrillation to pacing strategies may become available in the future.

Because of the long procedure time and complex techniques required for catheter ablation of AF triggers, these procedures are currently limited to select patients at a few tertiary care centers. Newer catheters are being designed specifically for electrically isolating the pulmonary veins, hopefully allowing safer and shorter procedures with lower AF recurrence rates after ablation. Expanding the indications for AF ablation to patients with persistent or even chronic AF could revolutionize our current treatment strategy.

Stroke remains the most feared complication of AF. Despite the strong evidence supporting the use of warfarin, many patients are not effectively anticoagulated because of poor medical care, noncompliance, or contraindications to anticoagulation. Since >90 per cent of emboli originate in the left atrial appendage, there are efforts underway to isolate the left atrial appendage through either surgical, thoroscopic, or even percutaneous catheter-based techniques in order to prevent stroke in high risk patients.

Risk stratification of patients with atrial fibrillation is clearly needed. Better methods to select patients for atrial pacing/defibrillation strategies, or particularly for the ablation of focal triggers are under investigation. In the future there may be a wide array of options open to patients with AF. However, the majority of AF patients have significant cardiac disease, co-morbid conditions, and chronic AF. While newer techniques will allow more effective therapy in some patients, drug therapy will likely remain the mainstay of our therapeutic regimen.

SUMMARY

- Control of the ventricular rate, anticoagulation, and consideration of cardioversion to sinus rhythm should be addressed in every patient with atrial fibrillation.
- β-Blockers or calcium-channel blockers are more effective at controlling ventricular rate during exertion than digoxin.
- All patients over the age of 75, or with at least one other risk factor for thromboembolism, should be anticoagulated with warfarin to an international normalized ratio (INR) of 2–3.
- The benefit of aspirin in preventing thromboembolism from atrial fibrillation is uncertain.
- Patients in atrial fibrillation for > 48 hours should be anticoagulated with warfarin for 3 weeks before, and 4 weeks after cardioversion to sinus rhythm.
- Transesophageal echocardiography-guided cardioversion may allow early cardioversion to sinus rhythm.
- Cardioversion to sinus rhythm should be attempted in most patients with recent onset atrial fibrillation, symptoms, or left ventricular dysfunction.
- Antiarrhythmic drug use should be individualized, after consideration of underlying heart disease, patient compliance, symptoms, and risk of proarrhythmia.

REFERENCES

♦1. Kannel WB, Abbott RD, Savage DD, et al. Epidemiologic features of chronic atrial fibrillation: the Framingham Study. N Engl J Med 1982; **306**: 1018.

2. Feinberg, WM, Blackshear JL, Laupicis A, Kronmal R, Hart RG. Prevalence, age distribution, and gender of patients with atrial fibrillation. Arch Intern Med 1995; **155**: 469–73.

♦3. Wolf PA, Dawber TR, Thomas HE, Kannel WB. Epidemiologic assessment of chronic atrial fibrillation and risk of stroke: the Framingham Study. Neurology 1978; **28**: 973.

4. Kuhn, DCG. Claudii Galeni opera omnia, Leipzig, Germany 1824; **8**, 294–6.

♦5. Withering W. An account of the foxglove and some of its medical uses: with practical remarks on dropsy, and other diseases. London: Paternoster-Row, 1785.

6. Kisch, B. The mechanics of flutter and fibrillation: a short review of a century of studies. Cardiologia 1950; **17**: 244–50.

7. Cushny AR. The action and uses of digitalis and its allies. London: Longmans Green and Co., 1925 (reprinted Birmingham, Alabama: Gryphon Editions, Inc., 1988, p 213).

8. Lewis T. Auricular fibrillation. In: The mechanism and graphic registration of the heartbeat. London: Shaw and Sons, 1920: 294–303.

9. Scherf D. Studies on auricular tachycardia caused by aconitine administration. Proc Soc Exp Biol Med 1947; **64**: 233–9.

10. Moe GK. On the multiple wavelet hypothesis of atrial fibrillation. *Arch Int Pharmacodyn Ther* 1962; **140**: 183.

11. Mayer AG. Rhythmical pulsation in Scyphomedusae. *Papers from the Tortugas Laboratory, Carnegie Institute, Washington DC* 1908; **1**: 115–31.

12. Mines GR. On dynamic equilibrium in the heart. *J Physiol* 1913; **46**: 350–83.

13. Garrey WE. The nature of fibrillatory contraction of the heart – its relation to tissue mass and form. *Am J Physiol* 1914; **33**: 397–414.

14. Allesie MA, Lammers WJEP, Bonke FIM, Hollen J. Experimental evaluation of Moe's multiple wavelet hypothesis of atrial fibrillation. In: Zipes DP, Jalife J, eds *Cardiac electrophysiology and arrhythmias*. Orlando, FL: Grune & Stratton, 1985: 265–75.

14a. Haissaguerre M, Jais P, Shah DC, *et al*. Spontaneous initiation of atrial fibrillation by ectopic beats originating in the pulmonary veins. *N Engl J Med* 1998; **339**: 659–66.

15. Benjamin EJ, Levy D, Vaziri SM *et al*. Independent risk factors for atrial fibrillation in a population-based cohort. The Framingham Heart Study. *JAMA* 1994; **271**: 840–4.

○16. Pritchett ELC. Management of atrial fibrillation. *N Engl J Med* 1992; **326**: 19.

17. Danias PG, Caulfield TA, Weigner MJ, Silverman DI, Manning WJ. Likelihood of spontaneous conversion of atrial fibrillation to sinus rhythm. *J Am Coll Cardiol* 1998; **31**: 588–92.

18. Kaplan MA, Gray RE, Iser LT, *et al*. Metabolic and hemodynamic responses to exercise during atrial fibrillation and sinus rhythm. *Am J Cardiol* 1968; **22**: 543–9.

19. Chai CY, Wang HH, Hoffman BF, *et al*. Mechanisms of bradycardia induced by digitalis substances. *Am J Physiol* 1967; **212**: 26.

20. Goldman S, Probst P, Selzer A, *et al*. Inefficacy of 'therapeutic' serum levels of digoxin in controlling the ventricular rate in atrial fibrillation. *Am J Cardiol* 1975; **35**: 651.

♦21. The Digitalis Investigation Group. The effect of digoxin on mortality and morbidity in patients with heart failure. *N Engl J Med* 1997; **336**: 525–33.

22. Atwood JE, Sullivan M, Forbes S, *et al*. Effect of beta-adrenergic blockade on exercise performance in patients with chronic atrial fibrillation. *J Am Coll Cardiol* 1987; **10**: 314–20.

23. Lang R, Klein H, Segni E, *et al*. Verapamil improves exercise capacity in chronic atrial fibrillation: double-blind crossover study. *Am Heart J* 1983; **105**: 820–4.

24. Platia EV, Michelson EL, Porterfield JK, Das G. Esmolol versus verapamil in the acute treatment of atrial fibrillation or atrial flutter. *Am J Cardiol* 1989; **63**: 925.

25. Salerno DM, Dias VC, Kleiger RE, *et al*. Efficacy and safety of intravenous diltiazem for treatment of atrial fibrillation and atrial flutter: The Diltiazem Atrial Fibrillation/Flutter Study Group. *Am J Cardiol* 1989; **63**: 1046.

26. Falk RH, Leavitt JI. Digoxin for atrial fibrillation: a drug whose time has gone? *Ann Intern Med* 1991; **114**: 573.

27. Waxman HL, Myerburg RJ, Appel R, *et al*. Verapamil for control of ventricular rate in paroxysmal supraventricular tachycardia and atrial fibrillation or flutter: A double-blind randomized cross-over study. *Ann Intern Med* 1981; **94**: 1.

28. Lewis RV, Laing E, Moreland TA, *et al*. A comparison of digoxin, diltiazem, and their combination in the treatment of atrial fibrillation. *Eur Heart J* 1988; **9**: 279.

29. David D, Di Segni E, Klein HO, *et al*. Inefficacy of digitalis in the control of heart rate in patients with chronic atrial fibrillation: beneficial effects of an added beta blocking agent. *Am J Cardiol* 1979; **44**: 1378.

30. Rodriguez LM, Smeets JLRM, Xie B, *et al*. Improvement in left ventricular function by ablation of atrioventricular nodal conduction in selected patients with lone atrial fibrillation. *Am J Cardiol* 1993; **72**: 1137–41.

♦31. Petersen P, Boysen G, Godtfredsen J, *et al*. Placebo-controlled randomized trial of warfarin and aspirin for prevention of thromboembolic complications in chronic atrial fibrillation: the Copenhagen AFASAK Study. *Lancet* 1989; **1**: 175–9.

♦32. The Boston Area Anticoagulation Trial for Atrial Fibrillation Investigators. The effect of low-dose warfarin on the risk of stroke in patients with nonrheumatic atrial fibrillation. *N Engl J Med* 1990; **323**: 1505.

33. Connolly SJ, Laupacis A, Gent M, *et al*., for the CAFA Study Coinvestigators: Canadian Atrial Fibrillation Anticoagulation (CAFA) Study. *J Am Coll Cardiol* 1991; **18**: 349.

♦34. The Stroke Prevention in Atrial Fibrillation Investigators. Stroke Prevention in Atrial Fibrillation Study: final results. *Circulation* 1991; **84**: 527–39.

35. The Stroke Prevention in Atrial Fibrillation Investigators. Warfarin versus aspirin for the prevention of thromboembolism in atrial fibrillation: Stroke Prevention in Atrial Fibrillation II Study. *Lancet* 1994; **343**: 687–91.

36. Ezekowitz M, Bridgers S, James K, *et al*., for the Veterans Affairs Stroke Prevention in Nonrheumatic Atrial Fibrillation Investigators: Warfarin in the prevention of stroke associated with nonrheumatic atrial fibrillation. *N Engl J Med* 1992; **327**: 1406.

♦37. Atrial Fibrillation Investigators. Risk factors for stroke and efficacy of antithrombotic therapy in atrial fibrillation: analysis of pooled data from five randomized trials. *Arch Intern Med* 1994; **154**: 1449.

38. The Stroke Prevention in Atrial Fibrillation Investigators. Predictors of thromboembolism in atrial fibrillation: II. Echocardiographic features of patients at risk. *Ann Intern Med* 1992; **116**: 6–12.

39. Kopecky SL, Gersh BJ, McGoon MD, *et al*. The natural history of lone atrial fibrillation. A population-based study over three decades. *N Engl J Med* 1987; **317**: 669–74.

40. The SPAF III Writing Committee for the Stroke Prevention in Atrial Fibrillation Investigators. Patients with nonvalvular atrial fibrillation at low risk of stroke during treatment with aspirin. *JAMA* 1998; **279**: 1273–7.

41. Fihn SD, Callahan CM, Martin DC, *et al*. The risk and severity of bleeding complications in elderly patients treated with warfarin. *Ann Intern Med* 1996; **124**: 970–9.

42. EAFT Study Group. Secondary prevention in nonrheumatic atrial fibrillation after transient ischemic attack or minor stroke. *Lancet* 1993; **342**: 1255–62.

♦43. The Stroke Prevention in Atrial Fibrillation Investigators. Adjusted-dose warfarin versus low-intensity fixed dose warfarin plus aspirin for high-risk patients with atrial fibrillation – Stroke Prevention in Atrial Fibrillation III randomized trial. *Lancet* 1996; **348**: 633–8.

♦44. Hylek EM, Skates SJ, Sheehan MA, Singer DE. An analysis of the lowest effective intensity of prophylactic anticoagulation for patients with nonrheumatic atrial fibrillation. *N Engl J Med* 1996; **335**: 540–6.

○45. Ansell, JE. Anticoagulation management as a risk factor for adverse events: grounds for improvement. *J Thromb Thrombol* 1998; **5**: S13–S18.

46. Eckman MH, Pauker SG. Decision analytic issues in the management of atrial fibrillation. In: Falk RH, Podrid PJ, eds *Atrial fibrilllation: mechanisms and management*, 2nd edn. New York. Lippincott-Raven, 1997.

47. Weinstein MC, Stason WB. Cost-effectiveness of interventions to prevent or treat coronary heart disease. *Ann Rev Public Health* 1985; **6**: 41–63.

48. Kelley MD. Hypercholesterolemia: the cost of treatment in perspective. *South Med J* 1990; **83**: 1421–5.

49. Page RL, Wilkinson WE, Clair WK, McCarthy ES, Pritchett EL. Asymptomatic arrhythmias in patients with symptomatic paroxysmal atrial fibrillation and paroxysmal supraventricular tachycardia. *Circulation* 1994; **89**: 224–7.

50. The Planning and Steering Committees of the AFFIRM Study for the NHLBI AFFIRM Investigators. Atrial fibrillation follow-up investigation of rhythm management – the AFFIRM study design. *Am J Cardiol* 1997; **79**: 1198–202.

51. Bjerkelund CJ, Orning OM. The efficacy of anticoagulant therapy in preventing embolism related to the D.C. cardioversion of atrial fibrillation. *Am J Cardiol* 1969; **23**: 208–16.

52. Weinberg DM, Mancini J. Anticoagulation for cardioversion of atrial fibrillation. *Am J Cardiol* 1989; **63**: 745–6.

53. Zeiler A, Mick MJ, Mazureck RP, Loop FD, Trohman RG. Role of prophylactic anticoagulation for direct current cardioversion in patients with atrial fibrillation or atrial flutter. *J Am Coll Cardiol* 1992; **19**: 851–5.

♦54. Collins LJ, Silverman DI, Douglas PS, Manning WJ. Cardioversion of non-rheumatic atrial fibrillation: reduced thromboembolic complications with 4 weeks of pre-cardioversion anticoagulation are related to atrial thrombus resolution. *Circulation* 1995; **92**: 160–3.

55. Manning WJ, Silverman DI, Katz SE, *et al*. Impaired left atrial mechanical function after cardioversion: relation to the duration of atrial fibrillation. *J Am Coll Cardiol* 1994; **23**: 1535–40.

56. Fatkin D, Kuchar DL, Thorburn CW, Feneley MP. Transesophageal echocardiography before and after direct current cardioversion of atrial fibrillation: evidence for 'atrial stunning' as a mechanism of thromboembolic complications. *J Am Coll Cardiol* 1994; **23**: 307–16.

57. Grimm RA, Stewart WJ, Maloney JD, *et al*. Impact of electrical cardioversion for atrial fibrillation on left atrial appendage function and spontaneous echo contrast: characterization by simultaneous transesophageal echocardiography. *J Am Coll Cardiol* 1993; **22**: 1359–66.

58. Grimm RA, Leung DY, Black IW, Stewart WJ, Thomas JD, Klein AL. Left atrial appendage 'stunning' after spontaneous conversion of atrial fibrillation demonstrated by transesophageal Doppler echocardiography. *Am Heart J* 1995; **130**: 174–6.

59. Weigner MJ, Caulfield TA, Danias PG. Risk for clinical thromboembolism associated with conversion to sinus rhythm in patients with atrial fibrillation lasting less than 48 hours. *Ann Intern Med* 1997; **126**: 615.

60. Shapiro EP, Effron MB, Lima S, Ouyang P, Siu CO, Bush D. Transient atrial dysfunction after cardioversion of chronic atrial fibrillation to sinus rhythm. *Am J Cardiol* 1988; **62**: 1202–7.

61. Laupacis A, Albers G, Dunn M, Feinberg W. Antithrombotic therapy in atrial fibrillation. *Chest* 1992; **102**: 426S.

62. Manning WJ, Weintraub RM, Waksmonski CA, *et al*. Accuracy of transesophageal echocardiography for identifying left atrial thrombi: a prospective intraoperative study. *Ann Intern Med* 1995; **123**: 817–22.

♦63. Manning WJ, Silverman DI, Keighley CS, Oettgen P, Douglas PS. Transesophageal echocardiographically facilitated early cardioversion from atrial fibrillation using short-term anticoagulation: final results of a prospective 4.5 year study. *J Am Coll Cardiol* 1995; **25**: 1354–61.

64. Black IW, Fatkin D, Sagar KB, *et al*. Exclusion of atrial thrombus by transesophageal echocardiography does not preclude embolism after cardioversion of atrial fibrillation: a multicenter study. *Circulation* 1994; **89**: 2509–13.

65. Klein AL, Grimm RA, Black IW, *et al*. Cardioversion guided by transesophageal echocardiography: the ACUTE pilot study: a randomized, controlled trial. *Ann Intern Med* 1997; **126**: 200.

66. Wijffels MCEF, Kirchhof CJHJ, Dorland R, *et al*. Atrial fibrillation begets atrial fibrillation. *Circulation* 1995; **92**: 1954–68.

67. Dittrich HC, Erickson JS, Schneiderman T, Blacky AR, Savides T, Nicod PH. Echocardiographic and clinical predictors for outcome of elective cardioversion of atrial fibrillation. *Am J Cardiol* 1989; **63**: 193–7.

68. Seto TB, Taira DA, Tsevat J, *et al*. Cost-effectiveness of transesophageal echocardiographic-guided cardioversion: a decision analytic model for patients admitted to the hospital with atrial fibrillation. *J Am Coll Cardiol* 1997; **29**: 122–30.

69. Gosselink, ATM, Crijns HJGM, Van Gelder IC, Hilige H, Wiesfeld ACP, Lie KI. Low-dose amiodarone for maintenance of sinus rhythm after carioversion of atrial fibrillation or fluttter. *JAMA* 1992; **267**: 3289–93.

70. Coplen SE, Antman EM, Berlin JA, *et al*. Efficacy and safety of quinidine therapy for maintenance of sinus rhythm after cardioversion: a meta-analysis of randomized control trials. *Circulation* 1990; **82**: 1106–16.

71. Echt DS, Liebson PR, Mitchell LB, *et al*. Mortality and morbidity in patients receiving encainide, flecainide, or placebo: the Cardiac Arrhythmia Suppression Trial. *N Engl J Med* 1991; **324**: 781.

72. Flaker GC, Blackshear JL, McBride R, Kronmal RA, Halperin JL, Hart RG, on behalf of the Stroke Prevention in Atrial Fibrillation Investigators. Antiarrhythmic drug therapy and cardiac mortality in fibrillation. *J Am Coll Cardiol* 1992; **20**: 527–32.

73. Karlson BW, Torstensson I, Abjorn C, Tansson GO, Peterson LE. Disopyramide in the maintenance of sinus rhythm after electrical cardioversion of atrial fibrillation – a placebo controlled one year follow up study. *Eur Heart J* 1988; **9**: 284–90.

74. Szekely P, Sideris DA, Batson GA. Maintenance of sinus rhythm after atrial defibrillation. *Br Heart J* 1970; **32**: 741–6.

75. Selzer A, Wray HW. Quinidine syncope: paroxysmal ventricular fibrillation occurring during treatment of chronic atrial arrhythmias. *Circulation* 1964; **30**: 17.

76. Grace AA, Camm AJ. Quinidine. *N Engl J Med* 1998; **338**: 35–44.

77. Adams LE, Baldkrishnan K, Roberts SM, *et al*. Genetic, immunologic and biotransformation studies of patients on procainamide. *Lupus* 1993; **2**: 89.

78. Podrid PJ, Anderson JL, for the Propafenone Multicenter Study Group. Safety and tolerability of long-term propafenone therapy for supraventricular tachyarrhythmias. *Am J Cardiol* 1996; **78**: 430–4.

79. Crijins HJ, van Gelder IC, Lie KI. Supraventricular tachycardia mimicking ventricular tachycardia during flecainide treatment. *Am J Cardiol* 1988; **62**: 1303–6.

80. Lehmann MH, Hardy S, Archibald D, *et al*. Sex differences in risk of Torsade de Pointes with d,l-Sotalol. *Circulation* 1996; **94**: 2534.

81. Greene HL, Graham EL, Werner JA, *et al*. Toxic and therapeutic effects of amiodarone in the treatment of cardiac arrhythmias. *J Am Coll Cardiol* 1983; **2**: 1114.

82. Raeder EA, Podrid PJ, Lown B. Side effects and complications of amiodarone therapy. *Am Heart J* 1983; **109**: 975.

83. Martin WJ, Rosenow EC. Amiodarone pulmonary toxicity: recognition and pathogenesis (part 1). *Chest* 1988; **93**: 1067.

84. Martin WJ, Rosenow EC. Amiodarone pulmonary toxicity: recognition and pathogenesis (part 2). *Chest* 1988; **93**: 1242.

85. Stambler BS, Wood MA, Ellenbogen KA, *et al*. Efficacy and safety of repeated doses of ibutilide for rapid conversion of atrial flutter or fibrillation. *Circulation* 1996; **94**: 1613.

85a. Torp-Pedersen C, Moller M, Bloch-Thomsen, *et al*. Dofetilide in patients with congestive heart failure and left ventricular dysfunction. *N Engl J Med* 1999; 341: 857–65.

86. Comparison of sotalol with digoxin-quinidine for conversion of acute atrial fibrillation to sinus rhythm (the sotalol-digoxin-quinidine trial). *Am J Cardiol* 1995; **76**: 495–8.

87. Boriani G, Biffi M, Capucci A, *et al*. Oral propafenone to convert recent-onset atrial fibrillation in patients with and without underlying heart disease: a randomized, controlled trial. *Ann Intern Med* 1997; **126**: 621.

88. Capucci A, Lenzi T, Boriani G, *et al*. Effectiveness of loading oral flecainide for converting recent-onset atrial fibrillation to sinus rhythm in patients without structural heart disease or with only systemic hypertension. *Am J Cardiol* 1992; 70: 69–72.

89. Volgman AS, Stambler BS, Kappagoda C, *et al*. Comparison of intravenous ibutilide versus procainamide for the rapid termination of atrial fibrillation or flutter. *PACE* 1996; **19**: 608 (abstract).

90. Lown B, Pelroth MG, Bey SK, *et al*. 'Cardioversion' of atrial fibrillation. A report on the treatment of 65 episodes in 50 patients. *N Engl J Med* 1963; **269**: 325.

91. Levy S, Lauribe P, Dolla E, *et al*. A randomized comparison of external and internal cardioversion of chronic atrial fibrillation. *Circulation* 1992; **86**: 1415–20.

92. Naccarelli GV, Dorian P, Hahnloser SH, Coumel P, for

the Flecainide Multicenter Atrial Fibrillation Study Group. Prospective comparison of flecainide versus quinidine for the treatment of paroxysmal atrial fibrillation/flutter. *Am J Cardiol* 1996; **77**: 53A–59A.

93. Chimienti M, Cullen MT, Casadei G, for the Flecainide and Propafenone Italian Study Investigators. Safety of long-term flecainide and propafenone in the management of patients with symptomatic paroxysmal atrial fibrillation. *Am J Cardiol* 1996; **77**: 60A–75A.

94. Doval HC, Nul DR, Grancelli HO, Perrone SV, Bortman GR, Curiel R, for the Grupo de Estudio de la Sobrevida en la Insuficiencia Cardiaca en Argentina (GESICA). Randomised trial of low-dose amiodarone in severe congestive heart failure. *Lancet* 1994; **344**: 493–8.

95. Singh SN, Fletcher RD, Fisher SG, *et al.*, for the Survival Trial of Antiarrhythmic Therapy in Congestive Heart Failure. Amiodarone in patients with congestive heart failure and asymptomatic ventricular arrhythmia. *N Engl J Med* 1995; **333**: 77–82.

96. Julian DG, Camm AJ, Grangin G, *et al.*, for the European Myocardial Infarct Amiodarone Trial Investigators. Randomized trial of the effect of amiodarone on mortality in patients with left-ventricular dysfunction after recent myocardial infarction: EMIAT. *Lancet* 1997; **349**: 667–74.

97. Singh BN. Amiodarone: the expanding role and how to follow a patient on chronic therapy. *Clin Cardiol* 1997; **20**: 608–18.

98. Disch DL, Greenberg ML, Holzberger PT, *et al.* Managing chronic atrial fibrillation: a Markov decision analysis comparing warfarin, quinidine, and low-dose amiodarone. *Ann Intern Med* 1994; **120**: 449–57.

99. Vorperian VR, Havighurst TC, Miller S, January CT. Adverse effects of low dose amiodarone: a meta analysis. *J Am Coll Cardiol* 1997; **30**: 791–8.

100. Waldo AL, Prystowski EN. Drug treatment of atrial fibrillation in the managed care era. *Am J Cardiol* 1998; **81**(5A): 23C–29C.

101. Gosselink ATM, Crijns HJGM, Van Gelder IC, Hillige H, Wiesfeld ACP, Lie KI. Low-dose amiodarone for maintenance of sinus rhythm after cardioversion of atrial fibrillation or flutter. *JAMA* 1992; **267**: 3289–93.

102. Simons GR, Eisenstein EL, Shaw LJ, Mark DB, Pritchett ELC. Cost effectiveness of inpatient initiation of antiarrhythmic therapy for supraventricular tachycardias. *Am J Cardiol* 1997; **80**: 1551–7.

103. Cox JL, Schuessler RB, D'Agostino HJ, *et al.* The surgical treatment of atrial fibrillation: development of a definitive surgical procedure. *J Thorac Cardiovasc Surg* 1991; **101**: 569.

104. Huang DT, Monahan KM, Zimetbaum P, *et al.* Hybrid pharmacologic and ablative therapy: a novel and effective approach for the management of atrial fibrillation. *J Cardiovasc Electrophysiol* 1998; **9**: 462–9.

105. Elvan A, Pride H, Eble J, *et al.* Radiofrequency catheter ablation reduces the inducibility and duration of atrial fibrillation in dogs. *Circulation* 1995; **91**: 2235.

106. Haissaguerre M, Gencel L, Fischer B, *et al.* Successful catheter ablation of atrial fibrillation. *J Cardiovasc Electrophysiol* 1994; **5**: 1045.

107. Andersen HR, Theusen L, Bagger JP, Vesterlund T, Thomsen PB. Prospective randomized trial of atrial versus ventricular pacing in sick-sinus syndrome. *Lancet* 1994; **344**: 1523–8.

108. Mittleman RS, Hill MRS, Mehra R, *et al.* Evaluation of the effectiveness of right atrial and biatrial pacing for the prevention of atrial fibrillation after coronary artery bypass surgery. *Circulation* 1996; **94**: I-68 (abstract).

109. Saksena S, Prakash A, Hill M, Krol RB, Munsif AN, Methew PP, Mehra R. Prevention of recurrent atrial fibrillation with chronic dual-site right atrial pacing. 1996; **28**: 687–94.

110. Murgatroyd FD, Slade AKB, Sopher SM, Rowland E, Ward DE, Camm AJ. Efficacy and tolerability of transvenous low energy cardioversion of paroxysmal atrial fibrillation in humans. *J Am Coll Cardiol* 1995; **25**: 1347–53.

21

Treatment of endocarditis and endovascular infections

ALAN J TAEGE AND SUSAN J REHM

Infective endocarditis continues to be a significant worldwide health problem. The demographics of the disease have evolved with patients being older and less rheumatic heart disease being seen. Subacute endocarditis is declining and more acute endocarditis is occurring. Prosthetic valves are being implanted more frequently for degenerative conditions, providing increased opportunities for prosthetic valve endocarditis. New criteria have been developed that include modern technological advances. Antibiotic prophylaxis for groups at risk continues to play a role in health care. The prophylactic regimens have been simplified and revised.

INTRODUCTION

Worldwide, infective endocarditis (IE) continues to be a significant source of morbidity and mortality. The pre-antibiotic era was able to offer only observation and comfort measures for this uniformly fatal disease.[1] The poignantly detailed self-observations of an afflicted medical student as submitted by Dr Weiss[2] etch a vivid description of this disease in our minds. The advent of antibiotics, along with improved microbiologic techniques, diagnostic abilities, and surgical intervention have vastly improved the prognosis and survival of these patients. Despite these advances, relapse and overall mortality may still run as high as 20 per cent.

Infective endocarditis implies a bacterial or fungal process on the endocardial surface of the heart. This includes not only the valves but the chordae, and any endocardial structure or device implanted therein. The early years of this disease were predominantly associated with rheumatic heart disease (RHD), which has declined in frequency. Improved health care and life expectancy have allowed degenerative and technology-associated infections to occur more commonly.

EPIDEMIOLOGY

The epidemiology and patient profile of IE has evolved. The pre-antibiotic era was notable for a predominance of young patients with rheumatic or congenital heart diseases.[3–6] Antibiotics markedly reduced the incidence of RHD and surgery has been able to correct many congenital defects. Patients are now more likely to have mitral valve prolapse, degenerative valvular disease, such as aortic sclerosis, congenital bicuspid aortic valves, prosthetic valves, permanent pacemakers or automatic

Table 21.1 *Native cardiac disease and risk of infective endocarditis (IE). (Adapted from Michel PL, Acar J. Native cardiac disease predisposing to infective endocarditis.* Eur Heart J 1995; **16**(suppl B): 2–6)

High	Moderate	Low or none
Cyanotic CHD	Mitral valve prolapse with regurgitation or leaf thickening	Isolated ASD
Previous IE	Mitral stenosis	Ischemic heart disease +/or previous cancer
Aortic valve disease	Tricuspid valve disease	Cancer
Mitral regurgitation	Pulmonary stenosis	Corrected left–right shunt without residual
Uncorrected left–right shunt (except ASD)	Hypertrophic cardiomyopathy	Calcified mitral annulus

The age groups involved have drifted upward, from the 2nd–4th decade,[4–6,8] with the majority in a recent review[9] coming from the 6th decade and beyond (Table 21.2).
ASD = atrial septal defect; CHD = congenital heart disease.

implantable cardiac defibrillators, (AICDs), or a history of intravenous drug use (Table 21.1).

The age groups involved have drifted upward, from the second to the fourth decade,[4–6,8] with the majority in a recent review[9] coming from the sixth decade and beyond (Table 21.2).

The annual number of cases in the USA is estimated to be 10 000–15 000[3] with an incidence of 3.8–6.2/100 000. There are roughly equal numbers of cases distributed between males and females.[9,10] A trend

Table 21.2 *Demographic features. (Adapted from Durack DT, Lukes AS, Bright DK. New criteria for diagnosis of infective endocarditis: utilization of specific endocardiographic findings.* Am J Med 1995; **96**: 200–9)

Age	
Median	43 years
Mean	47.8 years
Range	1 month to 92 years
Sex	
Female (%)	101 (50)
Male (%)	103 (50)
Race	
White (%)	108 (53)
Black (%)	90 (44)
Other (%)	9 (4)
Types of episode	
Acute (%)	102 (50)
Subacute (%)	93 (46)
Indeterminate (%)	9 (4)
Type of valve	
Native (%)	128 (63)
Prosthetic (%)	32 (16)
Primary treatment	
Antibiotics alone (%)	128 (63)
Antibiotics + surgery (%)	76 (37)
In-hospital mortality (%)	42 (21)

toward increasing aortic valve involvement and decreasing mitral valve involvement has been noted.[7,8]

IE occurs in 1–3 per cent of prosthetic valve replacements and accounts for approximately one-third of all cases of infective endocarditis.[5,11–14] Prosthetic valve endocarditis (PVE) has been arbitrarily divided into early onset (≤ 60 days postoperative) or late onset (≥ 60 days postoperative), although this classification has been debated.[15] Mechanical prostheses are more prone to infection in the early period and bioprostheses more likely to acquire infection in the late period.[12,13]

Intravenous drug use (IVDU) leads to a significant number of cases of IE.[3] Endocarditis in these patients typically involves the right side of the heart, although left-sided disease has been reported.[16] The overall prognosis of IE in IVDU is better than in non-IVDU patients.

Human immunodeficiency virus (HIV) patients comprise a subset of IE in IVDU. The endocarditis risk in HIV-infected patients is no different from that of HIV-negative individuals with the same risk factors[17] and the outcome is approximately the same except in advanced acquired immunodeficiency syndrome (AIDS), where mortality increases.[18]

MICROBIOLOGY

Virtually any microorganism can cause IE, but continuous bacteremia with certain typical microorganisms make the diagnosis of IE more likely and should alert the clinician to the possibility of this diagnosis. The microbiology of IE has evolved with time, technology, and lifestyles. Streptococci and staphylococci are the most common etiologic agents, comprising 70–80 per cent of all cases in Durack's 1995 series (Table 21.3).[9] Brandenburg's longitudinal study, however, demonstrated that the proportion of cases due to streptococci has declined, while the proportion due to staphylococci has increased (Table 20.4).[19] Most centers still report

Table 21.3 *Microbial etiologies of infective endocarditis. (Adapted from Durack DT, Lukes AS, Bright DK. New criteria for diagnosis of infective endocarditis: utilization of specific endocardiographic findings.* Am J Med *1995;* **96***: 200–9)*

Streptococci	88 (43)
Viridans	47 (23)
Enterococci	14 (7)
S. bovis	10 (5)
S. agalactiae	11 (5)
Other	6 (3)
Staphylococci	90 (44)
S. aureus	76 (37)
S. epidermidis	12 (6)
S. warneri	2 (1)
HACEK	7 (3)
Other species	9 (4)
Polymicrobic	3 (1)
Culture-negative	7 (3)

streptococci as being the most common etiologic agent of IE; however a large series from a community hospital demonstrated staphylococci as being the most common microorganism.[20] The apparent increase in staphylococcal cases may be based, at least in part, on the increased number of nosocomial cases, prosthetic valve cases, and cases associated with IVDU. After streptococcal and staphylococcal, enterococcal endocarditis is the third most common cause of native valve IE (NVE).

The streptococci responsible for IE may come from any group; however, viridans (including nutritional variants and *S. bovis*) and group B are most common. Group A, C, and G are infrequently associated with IE. Enterococci are considered separately from the rest of the streptococci.

Viridans streptococci cause approximately 50 per cent of NVE cases. These organisms are usually α- or γ-

hemolytic and reside in the oral cavity (hence the association with poor dentition and/or dental procedures) or the gastrointestinal (GI) tract. The most common species include *S. mitis, S. mutans, S. salivarius, S. sanguis, S. bovis*, the nutritional variants (*S. adjacens* and *S. defectivus*) and the *S. milleri* group (*S. anginosis, S. constellatus* and *S. intermedius*). The *S. milleri* group is associated with visceral abscess formation (brain, liver, kidney, or myocardium). *S. bovis* has been associated with intestinal polyps or malignancy, therefore an evaluation of this association should be undertaken in cases of *S. bovis* endocarditis.[21]

The nutritional variants have additional nutritional requirements for adequate growth (vitamin B_6 and thiol compounds). They have also been referred to as satelliting streptococci because of their ability to grow around colonies of *S. aureus* (which supply their nutritional supplements). This group of organisms is associated with higher rates of relapse, failure and mortality than other viridans streptococci.

There has been an increase of invasive Group B (*S. agalactiae*) streptococcal disease.[22] Normally found in the mouth, vagina, and urethra, it has usually been associated with puerpural sepsis, neonatal bacteremia, and meningitis. It is also a cause of endocarditis. Risk factors for acquisition are diabetes mellitus, liver disease, cancer, and neurologic disease. Mortality rates are high, secondary to its aggressive invasive nature.

Staphylococci are the second most common cause of IE, accounting for 40–50 per cent of cases of endocarditis depending upon the series. *S. aureus* of native left-sided heart valves and prosthetic valves is often an acute aggressive infectious process[23] with a fulminant course and high mortality. In contrast, right-sided IE with *S. aureus*, most commonly in IVDU, is less fulminant and aggressive[23] with a better treatment outcome. Studies have shown higher rates of colonization by *S. aureus* of IVDU;[24,25] a likely explanation for the frequency of this organism in IVDU-associated IE.

Coagulase-negative staphylococcus or *S. epidermidis* is

Table 21.4 *Etiologic trends in infective endocarditis. (Adapted from Brandenburg RO, et al. Infective endocarditis – a 25 year overview of diagnosis and therapy.* J Am Coll Cardiol *1983;* **1***: 281)*

	1951–1957		1970–1979	
	n	%	*n*	%
Viridans streptococci	91	53	149	39
Group D streptococci	28	16	79[a]	20
Staphylococcus aureus	24	14	72	18
S. epidermidis	4	2	16	4
Gram-negative bacilli	10	6	35	9
Other microorganisms	1	1	29	7
Negative blood cultures	14	8	13	3
Total	172	100	393	100

[a]Includes 26 *Streptococcus bovis* isolates.

most often associated with PVE, although they do cause NVE[26,27] with rheumatic or congenital abnormalities or mitral prolapse.[28] Coagulase-negative staphylococcus is ubiquitous on the skin and is the most common cause of contamination in blood cultures. This feature, as well as its typically indolent nature as an infective agent, may make diagnosis difficult.

Enterococci, typically inhabitants of the GI and genitourinary tracts, are the third most common cause of endocarditis.[29] They were previously classified as group D streptococci. They exhibit variable hemolysis. The three most common species are *Enterococcus faecalis, E. faecium* and *E. durans. E. faecalis* is the most common of the enterococci associated with endocarditis. They may infect normal, abnormal, or prosthetic valves.

Synergistic combinations of penicillin and gentamicin are necessary for bacterial killing as the enterococci are relatively resistant to either drug alone. Gentamicin resistance has emerged and needs to be evaluated in all isolates.[30] Furthermore, the emergence of vancomycin resistance poses another therapeutic dilemma.

A small but significant percentage of cases of native and prosthetic valve endocarditis are associated with a variety of less common pathogens.[31–39] The HACEK group[40] (*Haemophilis* sp., *Actinobacillus actinomycetemcomitans, Cardiobacterium hominis, Eikenella corrodens, Kingella kingae*) and *Pseudomonas aeruginosa* are the most common Gram-negative bacilli associated with endocarditis. HACEK organisms are most frequently associated with an oral origin but they do reside in the GI tract as well. *Pseudomonas* may be part of the normal human flora; it can also rapidly colonize hospitalized patients. IE from *Pseudomonas* in IVDU may be regional in origin and scope.[41] Infective endocarditis may occasionally be polymicrobic. The majority of documented cases are in IVDU.[42]

Q fever endocarditis is caused by the Gram-negative rickettsial organism *Coxiella burnetti*.[43] This zoonosis is uncommon in the USA, but more frequent in Europe, especially in handlers of farm animals. It is highly infectious and seldom cultured, therefore it is a difficult diagnosis to establish. Serology or the polymerase chain reaction (PCR) are most commonly employed in the diagnosis. Q fever is often a consideration in culture-negative IE.

Lactobacillus is an example of a modern-day opportunistic pathogen. This Gram-positive anaerobic or facultative anaerobic rod tends to cause disease in patients with underlying illness[44] and has been associated with endocarditis.[45]

Bartonella species are a group of rickettsial-like organisms that are emerging pathogens. A variable spectrum of clinical diseases from trench fever to peliosis hepatitis, bacillary angiomatosis, cat scratch disease, or endocarditis may be produced. A typical patient profile today is that of a homeless, alcoholic male. A recent series of cases of *Bartonella* endocarditis[46] points out the role of

this organism in many cases of what may have been previously classified as culture-negative endocarditis. Although the organism can be cultured, it is difficult to do so. Diagnosis is perhaps better established through serologic means or PCR.

Fungal infections and fungal endocarditis are largely a result of medical progress. Most cases are associated with prolonged use of antibiotics, intravenous catheters,[47–49] immunosuppression[50] and cardiac surgery.[51] IVDU is an additional known risk factor. The most common species are *Candida, Torulopsis*, and *Aspergillus*. Isolated cases of endocarditis due to other fungi, including some due to fungi of the order Mucorales, have been reported (Table 21.5).[47,52]

Table 21.5 *Fungal organisms associated with infectious endocarditis. (Adapted from Rubenstein E and Lang R. Fungal endocarditis.* Eur Heart J 1996; **16** (suppl B): 84)

Acremonium (Cephalosporium)	*Hansenula anomalia*
Arnium leporinum	*Histoplasma capsulatum*
Aspergillus sp.	*Lecycthophora* sp.
Blastomyces dermatitidis	*Paecilomyces* sp.
Blastoschizomyces capitatus	*Penicillum* sp.
Candida sp.	*Phycomyces*
Chrysosporium sp.	*Rhodotorula*
Coccidioides immitis	*Saccharomyces cerevisiae*
Coprinius sp.	*Scedosporium* sp.
Curvularia geniculata	*Torulopsis glabrata*
Cryptococcus neoformans	*Trichosporon beigelii*
Fusarium sp.	*Wangiella dematitidis*

Fungi are difficult to recover from blood cultures; this is particularly notable for *Aspergillus*, which is almost never isolated from blood. In fungal endocarditis, cultures of valve tissue and/or extracted emboli may be the best method for identifying the causative organism.

Five to ten per cent of all cases of endocarditis are culture-negative. The most common cause is felt to be prior antibiotic use (Table 21.6). As methods improve, it

Table 21.6 *Categories of apparent culture-negative infective endocarditis. (Adapted from van Scoy RE. Culture-negative endocarditis.* Mayo Clin Proc 1982; **57**: 150)

Prior antimicrobial treatment
'Fastidious' bacteria
Q-fever
Fungi
Acid-fast bacteria
Chlamydia
? L forms of bacteria
? Virus
Right-sided endocarditis

is likely that more of the suspected infectious causes will be elucidated. Non-infective conditions may be associated with symptoms mimicking IE (Table 21.7). They should be considered in the evaluation of patients with possible culture-negative IE.

Table 21.7 *Non-infective causes of endocardial disease. (Adapted from van Scoy RE. Culture-negative endocarditis.* Mayo Clin Proc *1982; **57**: 150)*

Myxoma
Rheumatic fever
Lupus non-bacterial verrucous endocarditis
Marantic endocarditis
Endocardial fibroelastosis
Fibroplastic endocarditis (Loeffler's)
Carcinoid

Table 21.8 *Symptoms of infective endocarditis. (Adapted from Von Reyn, et al. Infective endocarditis: an analysis based on strict case definitions.* Ann Intern Med *1981; **94**(1): 51)*

Symptom	n (%)
Fever	80 (86)
Malaise	62 (94)
Anorexia	47 (75)
Chills	35 (45)
Headache	29 (48)
Weight loss	28 (50)
Cough	28 (42)
Night sweats	28 (50)
Arthritis/arthralgia	24 (44)
Myalgia	21 (49)
Mental status change	20 (36)
Back pain	17 (37)
Rash	17 (31)
Dyspnea	16 (25)

CLINICAL PRESENTATION

Von Reyn's series[53] indicates that the signs and symptoms of IE continue to be non-specific (Tables 21.8 and 21.9). Concerns have been voiced over the possibility that referral bias (sicker patients being referred to academic centers) has skewed our views of the clinical aspects of IE.[54] Table 21.10 summarizes the characteristics of patients with IE presenting to a large community teaching hospital.[20]

The 'traditional' manifestations of Janeway lesions, Roth spots, splenomegaly, and subacute presentations have decreased, and are being replaced by more acute and fulminant disease with fewer extracardiac findings. This shift in presentation has been coincident with an emergence of more staphylococcal disease. Fever is the most consistent symptom and sign[55] but it may be absent

in as many as 30 per cent of cases of NVE. It is a more consistent finding in PVE (Table 21.11).

In uncomplicated IE, fever tends to dissipate rapidly.[56,57] Fifty per cent defervesce in 3 days and approximately 75 per cent by 1 week.[57] Prolonged fever is associated with *S. aureus, P. aeruginosa,* and culture-negative endocarditis. In addition, microvascular phenomena often are noted with prolonged fever. Tissue infarction may be the cause of the prolonged febrile episodes. Deep cardiac infections, ring and myocardial abscesses, are other factors to consider as is drug fever. On rare occasions metastatic visceral abscesses or antibiotic-resistant organisms may be responsible. Repeat blood cultures will assist in the diagnosis of these organisms or perhaps display persistent bacteremia leading one to search for deep abscesses. In the case of right-sided IE, septic pulmonary emboli and/or pulmonary infarction may be the etiology of prolonged fever.

Table 21.9 *Signs of endocarditis. (Adapted from Von Reyn, et al. Infective endocarditis: an analysis based on strict case definitions.* Ann Intern Med *1981; **94**(1): 51)*

Signs	On admission n (%)	After admission n	Total number n (%)
Fever	76 (73)	18	94 (90)
Rales	31 (30)	3	34 (33)
Splenomegaly	22 (21)	10	32 (31)
Mental status change	20 (19)	7	27 (26)
Conjunctival hemorrhage	17 (16)	3	20 (19)
Splinter hemorrhage	15 (14)	14	29 (28)
Petechiae	14 (13)	7	21 (20)
Hepatomegaly	13 (13)	1	14 (13)
Osler's node	10 (10)	7	17 (16)
Hemiparesis	9 (9)	3	12 (12)
Nuchal rigidity	7 (7)	3	10 (10)
Janeway lesion	3 (3)	2	5 (5)
Roth spot	2 (2)	6	8 (8)

Table 21.10 *Clinical features of infective endocarditis. (Adapted from Watanakunakorn C, Burkert T. Infective endocarditis at a large community teaching hospital, 1980–1990. A review of 210 episodes.* Medicine *1993; **72**: 95)*

	Host valves 148 episodes *n* (%)	Intravenous drug users 33 episodes *n* (%)	Prosthetic valves	
			Early 2 episodes *n*	Late 27 episodes *n* (%)
Prior surgical procedures	10 (6.7)	2 (6.1)	2	3 (11.1)
Infected intravascular devices	16 (10.8)			2 (7.4)
Symptoms				
Fever	98 (66.2)	29 (87.9)	1	21 (77.8)
Chills	63 (42.6)	25 (75.8)		12 (44.4)
Malaise	59 (39.9)	13 (39.4)		15 (55.6)
Arthralgias, myalgia	24 (16.2)	12 (36.4)		8 (29.6)
Mental confusion	33 (22.3)	2 (6.1)		2 (7.4)
Severe back pain	11 (33.3)	3 (9.1)		1 (3.7)
Pleuritic chest pain		12 (36.4)		
Temperature (°C)				
<37.8	35 (23.6)	8 (24.2)	1	8 (29.6)
37.8–38.9	62 (41.9)	11 (33.3)	1	10 (37.0)
>38.9	51 (34.5)	14 (9.5)		9 (33.3)
Cardiac murmur	120 (81.1)	31 (93.9)	2	27 (100)
Petechiae, embolic lesions	67 (45.3)	3 (9.1)		18 (66.6)
Osler's node, Janeway lesion, Roth spot	15 (10.1)	3 (9.1)		1 (3.7)
Congestive heart failure	77 (52.0)	7 (21.2)	2	10 (37.0)
Central nervous system manifestations	38 (25.7)	4 (12.1)		5 (18.1)
Renal insufficiency	45 (30.4)	5 (15.2)	1	8 (29.6)
Hemoglobin <10 g/dL	84 (56.8)	15 (45.5)	2	10 (37.0)
Hematuria	89 (60.1)	11 (33.3)	1	14 (51.9)
Two-dimensional echocardiogram (no. positive/no. done)	45/114 (39.4)	15/24 (69.5)	0/1	7/25 (28.0)

Table 21.11 *Clinical signs in prosthetic valve endocarditis (PVE). (Adapted from Chastre J, Tronillet JL. Early infective endocarditis on prosthetic valves.* Eur Heart J *1995; **16**(suppl B): 36)*

Finding	Early PVE (%)	Late PVE (%)
Fever	95–100	95–100
New/changing murmur	50–70	40–60
Congestive heart failure	30–100	30
Shock	33	0–10
Conduction abnormalities	15–20	5–10
Systemic emboli	5–30	10–40
Peripheral signs[a]	5	15

[a]Osler's nodes, Janeway lesions, Roth's spots.

Heart murmurs are not present in all cases. Murmurs tend to be more common in NVE with up to 85 per cent of patients manifesting a new or changing murmur.[14] Cases of PVE demonstrate murmurs in 50–70 per cent.[14]

Systemic embolic phenomena occur in less than half of patients with endocarditis and tend to be more common in NVE and late PVE. Patients infected with certain organisms – fungi, HACEK and *C. burnetti* – are more prone to embolic phenomena.

Neurologic manifestations may occur in 29–40 per cent of IE cases.[58–61] Symptoms may vary from headache and confusion to encephalopathy, seizure, or stroke (Table 21.12). Meningitis may result secondary to bacterial seeding, presumably from septic emboli. This complication occurs in approximately 6 per cent of cases.[58] Brain abscesses are uncommon but occur in 1–4 per cent of cases.[58–61] *Staphylococcus aureus* is most frequently responsible for meningitis and brain abscesses in IE.

As the average age of the IE patient has increased, it is important to recognize that the elderly report fewer symptoms than younger patients, making the clinical presentation even more non-specific.[55] Compared to patients <60 years of age, the elderly were less likely to complain of fever and chills. However, on admission, they are equally as likely to have an elevated temperature.

Table 21.12 *Neurologic complications[a] (Adapted from Pruitt AA, et al. Neurologic complications of bacterial endocarditis.* Medicine 1978; **57**: 332)

Complication	Frequency (%)
Cerebral infarction in territory of middle cerebral arteries	34(16)
Meningeal signs and symptoms	33(15)
Seizures	24(11)
Multiple microemboli	23(11)
Microscopic brain abscesses	8(4)
Visual disturbances[b]	6(3)
Cranial or peripheral neuropathy	5(2)
Cerebral infarction in territory of vertebrobasilar arteries	4(2)
Mycotic aneurysm	4(2)
Subarachnoid hemorrhage (without identifiable mycotic aneurysm)	5(2)
Cerebral infarcts in 'watershed areas' due to hypotension	3(1)
Intracerebral hemorrhage	4(2)
Subdural hemorrhage	2(1)
Macroscopic brain abscess	1(1)
Psychiatric disturbance	4(2)

[a]More than one complication was frequently observed in a single patient. Each complication is listed separately.
[b]Four patients developed retinal artery emboli, one a retinal artery hemorrhage, and one cortical blindness.

LABORATORY FINDINGS

The most important laboratory finding is sustained bacteremia. Two or three sets of blood cultures of 10 mL or more of blood prior to antibiotic initiation is sufficient.[62,63] Perhaps additional cultures may be necessary to capture the organism if prior antibiotics have been utilized. It is otherwise unnecessary to continue to obtain additional cultures beyond the initial two or three appropriately obtained specimens.

Anemia is common, particularly in subacute bacterial endocarditis (SBE), as is an elevated sedimentation rate.[55] The leukocyte count is unpredictable. It is more likely to be elevated in acute endocarditis, but it may be normal or depressed in SBE.

Immune-related phenomena such as the development of detectable rheumatoid factor (up to 50 per cent) and false-positive Venereal Disease Research Laboratories (VDRL) occur more commonly with SBE. Abnormal urinalyses may be found in approximately 50 per cent of cases. Abnormalities may vary from proteinuria to microscopic hematuria to red blood cell casts.

DIAGNOSIS

More than 100 years later, Osler's words, 'Few diseases present greater difficulties in the way of diagnosis than malignant endocarditis, difficulties which in many cases are practically insurmountable' still ring true.[64] IE is a systemic disease whose diagnosis is made on clinical grounds supported by laboratory and echocardiographic findings. As the clinical findings are numerous, it requires careful consideration and thought or it will easily be overlooked and missed.[65]

Osler's criteria of remittent fever, an old valvular lesion, embolic features, skin lesions, and progressive cardiac changes are largely true today. In general terms, our current criteria would include persistent bacteremia, echocardiographic features of vegetations and/or abscesses, and a typical clinical picture.

The Von Reyn criteria[53] for the diagnosis of IE were derived from strict case definitions. They were useful but were felt to be too restrictive and did not include echocardiographic data, nor did they include the risk of IVDU. They were supplanted by the more inclusive Duke criteria,[10] which in comparison are felt to be more helpful in diagnosis of current cases (Tables 21.13 and 21.14).[66] These criteria are used as a foundation from which to work in establishing a diagnosis of infective endocarditis. There are no perfect guidelines. The seasoned clinician will recognize that clinical judgement frequently is the final determinant.

Echocardiography has become an important tool to aid in the diagnosis of IE. Transthoracic echocardiography (TTE) is able to visualize vegetations in 30–80 per cent of cases.[67–69] Transesophageal echocardiogram (TEE) is more sensitive and specific,[70] and should be utilized if the findings of TTE are inconclusive. TEE is very useful in the diagnosis of valve ring and intracardiac abscesses, being superior to TTE for this purpose.[71] Likewise, TEE is the preferred mode of evaluation for prosthetic valve endocarditis because of its greater technical resolution.[72]

Table 21.13 *Proposed new criteria for diagnosis of infective endocarditis. (Adapted from Durack DT, Lukes AS, Bright DK. New criteria for diagnosis of infective endocarditis: utilization of specific echocardiographic findings. Am J Med 1995; **96**: 202)*

Definite infective endocarditis
Pathologic criteria
- Microorganisms: demonstrated by culture or histology in a vegetation, or in a vegetation that has embolized, or in an intracardiac abscess, *or*
- Pathologic lesion: vegetation or intracardiac abscess present, confirmed by histology showing active endocarditis
Clinical criteria, using specific definitions listed in Table 21.14
- 2 major criteria, *or*
- 1 major and 3 minor criteria, *or*
- 5 minor criteria

Possible infective endocarditis
Findings consistent with infective endocarditis that fall short of 'definite' but not 'rejected'

Rejected
Firm alternate diagnosis for manifestations of endocarditis, *or*
Resolution of manifestations of endocarditis, with antibiotic therapy for 4 days or less, *or*
No pathologic evidence of infective endocarditis at surgery or autopsy, after antibiotic therapy for 4 days or less

Table 21.14 *Definitions of terminology used in the proposed new criteria. (Adapted from Durack DT, Lukes AS, Bright DK. New criteria for diagnosis of infective endocarditis: utilization of specific echocardiographic findings. Am J Med 1995; **96**: 203)*

Major criteria
Positive blood culture for infective endocarditis
- Typical microorganism for infective endocarditis from two separate blood cultures
  Viridans streptococci,[a] *Streptococcus bovis*, HACEK group, *or*
  Community-acquired *Staphyloccus aureus* or enterococci, in the absence of a primary focus, *or*
- Persistently positive blood culture, defined as recovery of a microorganism consistent with infective endocarditis from:
  (i) Blood cultures drawn more than 12 hours apart, *or*
  (ii) All of three or a majority of four or more separate blood cultures, with first and last drawn at least 1 hour apart
Evidence of endocardial involvement
- Positive echocardiogram for infective endocarditis
  (i) Oscillating intracardiac mass, on valve or supporting structures, *or* in the path of regurgitant jets, *or* on implanted material, in the absence of an alternative anatomic explanation, *or*
  (ii) Abscess, *or*
  (iii) New partial dehiscence of prosthetic valve, *or*
- New valvular regurgitation (increase or change in pre-existing murmur not sufficient)

Minor criteria
- Predisposition: predisposing heart condition or intravenous drug use
- Fever: $\geq$38.0°C (100.4°F)
- Vascular phenomena: major arterial emboli, septic pulmonary infarcts, mycotic aneurysm, intracranial hemorrhage, conjunctival hemorrhages, Janeway lesions
- Immunologic phenomena: glomerulonephritis, Osler's nodes, Roth spots, rheumatoid factor
- Microbiologic evidence: positive blood culture but not meeting major criterion as noted previously[b] or serologic evidence of active infection with organism consistent with infective endocarditis
- Echocardiogram: consistent with infective endocarditis but not meeting major criterion as noted previously

HACEK = *Haemophilus* sp., *Actinobacillus actinomycetemcomitans, Cardiobacterium hominis, Eikenella* sp., and *Kingella kingae*.
[a]Including nutritional variant strains.
[b]Excluding single positive cultures for coagulase-negative staphylococci and organisms that do not commonly cause endocarditis.

BASIC PRINCIPLES OF TREATMENT

There are over 50 years of accumulated experience in the antimicrobial treatment of IE. The majority of the recommendations for treatment are the result of many small series of patients and the writings of several learned scholars.

Early diagnosis and initiation of treatment are the keys to successful therapy.[73] The longer the duration of infection the greater the potential for destruction of valvular structures, immunologic complications, and multisystem organ failure.

The practitioner must be alert to the possibility of IE in the appropriate setting despite its often non-specific presentation.

Appropriate therapy depends upon identification of the infecting organism. With proper microbiologic identification, the most effective antimicrobial agent can be utilized. Capable diagnostic microbiology and general laboratory facilities are necessary. The microbiology laboratory must have the ability to perform cultures and sensitivities on both routine and fastidious organisms (nutritionally deficient streptococci, fungi, HACEK organisms) and it should be capable of performing synergy testing. Drug levels are frequently necessary for monitoring therapy as well.

> The antimicrobial agent should be a cell-wall active bactericidal agent (β-lactam or glycopeptide) delivered in sufficient concentrations intravenously for the period of time necessary to sterilize the vegetation.[74,75] Synergistic combinations of antimicrobials (β-lactam or glycopeptide antibiotic and an aminoglycoside) may be necessary in the treatment of infections due to certain difficult organisms (enterococci and relatively resistant streptococci) and situations (PVE).

Empiric antimicrobial therapy is that which is initiated prior to the identification of the causative pathogen; it may become definitive therapy in culture-negative cases. The appropriate choice should be based on the patient, the presentation, and underlying conditions. For example, acute vs subacute, native vs prosthetic valve, community vs nosocomial or IVDU settings are associated with particular pathogens and treatment as previously discussed. There is no substitute for careful consideration of each individual patient situation.

MEDICAL TREATMENT

> Viridans streptococci are responsible for approximately 50 per cent of NVE cases.[76,77] Most will be penicillin sensitive minimum inhibitory concentration (MIC) ≤ 0.1 μg/mL) and can be treated using the recommendations of Table 21.15. A 4-week course of penicillin or ceftriaxone alone is generally adequate and acceptable.

Once-daily infusions of ceftriaxone are certainly more convenient for the patient and home therapy is facilitated by such regimens. A shorter 2-week course of synergistic combination therapy with penicillin and gentamicin is an option; however, this exposes the patient to the additional risk of aminglycoside nephrotoxicity – and ototoxicity, and the necessity to monitor drug levels and creatinine (with the added cost). Peak serum gentamicin levels of 3 μg/mL and trough levels of

<1 μg/mL are considered appropriate for synergism. Patients who have had symptoms of IE for >3 months may be more likely to relapse[78] and therefore should be considered for a longer course of therapy.

Many patients may report an allergy to penicillin. Frequently this is not a true hypersensitivity reaction; rather, the patient experienced an adverse event such as pain at an injection site, GI upset with oral dosing, etc. If a delayed hypersensitivity reaction occurred, cefazolin (first-generation cephalosporin) is an alternative. In the event of an immediate-type hypersensitivity reaction to penicillin, vancomycin can be utilized. Penicillin desensitization is an additional therapeutic option.

Some strains of streptococci may be relatively resistant to penicillin (MIC ⩾0.1 μg/mL but <0.5 μg/mL). Higher dose penicillin for 4 weeks with 2 weeks of synergistic gentamicin are recommended (Table 21.16). If a viridans streptococcus or S. bovis have a penicillin MIC ⩾ 0.5 μg/mL, they should be treated as an enterococcal endocarditis.

Enterococci are the third most common cause of endocarditis, accounting for 5 to 20 per cent of NVE cases.[77,79,80] They are uniformly more resistant to penicillin than streptococci and consequently more difficult to treat. A two-drug regimen combining a bactericidal cell wall-active agent and an aminoglycoside is necessary (Table 21.17). Cephalosporins are inappropriate for treatment of enterococcal endocarditis. Since enterococcal resistance is possible to virtually any of the currently available antibiotics, careful susceptibility testing for penicillin, ampicillin, vancomycin, and the aminoglycosides must be performed.

The duration of therapy (4–6 weeks) may be established, in part, by the duration of symptoms prior to diagnosis and therapy. Once again, symptom duration exceeding 3 months, especially with mitral valve involvement, is predictive of a higher likelihood of relapse and should be considered for 6 weeks of therapy.[79] Concomitant aminoglycoside therapy should be continued for the full course of therapy, if tolerated. Side effects may become a significant problem, with gentamicin causing more nephrotoxicity (reversible) and streptomycin more vestibular toxicity (usually not reversible). Despite enterococci being relatively more resistant to treatment, overall relapse rates are reported to be 0–14 per cent.[79,80] This rate of relapse is similar to the global rate for all types of IE.

Staphylococcal IE is a diverse and often aggressive infection requiring careful consideration during treatment. Separation of species, S. aureus vs coagulase-negative staphylococci, left- vs right-sided, native vs prosthetic valve, addict vs non-addict, and, finally, sensitivities to antibiotics are all necessary considerations for proper treatment.

When initiating therapy, it should be assumed that all staphylococci are penicillin resistant. A small minority may still be penicillin sensitive. If they are penicillin

Table 21.15 *Suggested regimens for therapy of native valve endocarditis due to penicillin-susceptible viridans streptococci and* Streptococcus bovis *(penicillin MIC ≤ 0.1 μg/mL). (Adapted from Wilson WR, Karchmer AW, Dajari AS, et al. Antibiotic treatment of adults with infective endocarditis due to streptococci, enterococci, staphylococci, and HACEK microorganisms. JAMA 1995; 274: 1707).*

Antibiotic	Dosage and route[a]	Duration, (weeks)	Comments
Aqueous crystalline penicillin G sodium	12–18 million U/24 hours iv either continuously or in 6 equally divided doses	4	Preferred in most patients older than 65 years and in those with impairment of the eighth nerve or renal function
or			
Ceftriaxone sodium	2 g once daily iv or im[b]	4	
Aqueous crystalline penicillin G sodium	12–18 million U/24 hours iv either continuously or in 6 equally divided doses	2	When obtained 1 hour after a 20–30 min iv infusion or im injection, serum concentration of gentamicin of approximately 3 μg/mL is desirable; trough concentration should be <1 μg/mL
With gentamicin sulfate[c]	1 mg/kg im or iv every 8 hours	2	
Vancomycin hydrochloride[d]	30 mg/kg per 24 h iv in 2 equally divided doses, not to exceed 2 g/24 hours unless serum levels are monitored	4	Vancomycin therapy is recommended for patients allergic to β-lactams; peak serum concentrations of vancomycin should be obtained 1 hour after completion of the infusion and should be in the range of 30–45 μg/mL for twice-daily dosing

[a]Dosages recommended are for patients with normal renal function. For nutritionally variant streptococci, *see* Table 21.17. iv = intravenous; im = intramuscular.
[b]Patients should be informed that im injection of ceftriaxone is painful.
[c]Dosing of gentamicin on a mg/kg basis will produce higher serum concentrations in obese patients than in lean patients. Therefore, in obese patients, dosing should be based on ideal body weight. (Ideal body weight for men is 50 kg + 2.3 kg per inch over 5 feet, and ideal body weight for women is 45.5 kg + 2.3 kg per inch over 5 feet). Relative contraindications to the use of gentamicin are age >65 years, renal impairment or impairment of the eighth nerve. Other potentially nephrotoxic agents (e.g. non-steroidal anti-inflammatory drugs) should be used cautiously in patients receiving gentamicin.
[d]Vancomycin dosage should be reduced in patients with impaired renal function. Vancomycin given 1 mg/kg basis will produce higher serum concentrations in obese patients than in lean patients. Therefore, in obese patients, dosing should be based on ideal body weight. Each dose of vancomycin should be infused over at least 1 hour to reduce the risk of the histamine-release 'red man' syndrome.

Table 21.16 *Therapy for native valve endocarditis due to strains of viridans streptococci and* Streptococcus bovis *relatively resistant to penicillin G (MIC >0.1 μg/mL and <0.5 μg/mL). (Adapted from Wilson WR, Karchmer AW, Dajari AS, et al. Antibiotic treatment of adults with infective endocarditis due to streptococci, enterococci, staphylococci, and HACEK microorganisms. JAMA 1995; 274: 1708).*

Antibiotic	Dosage and route[a]	Duration (weeks)	Comments
Aqueous crystalline penicillin G sodium	18 million U/24 hours iv either continuously or in six equally divided doses	4	Cefazolin or other first-generation cephalosporin may be substituted for penicillin in patients whose penicillin hypersensitivity is not of the immediate type
With gentamicin sulfate[b]	1 mg/kg im or iv every 8 hours	2	
Vancomycin hydrochloride[c]	30 mg/kg per 24 hours iv in two equally divided doses, not to exceed 2 g/24 hours unless serum levels are monitored	4	Vancomycin therapy is recommended for patients allergic to β-lactams

[a]Dosages recommended are for patients with normal renal function. iv = intravenous; im = intramuscular.
[b]For specific dosing adjustment and issues concerning gentamicin (obese patients, relative contraindications), *see* Table 21.15 footnotes.
[c]For specific dosing adjustment and issues concerning vancomycin (obese patients, length of infusion), *see* Table 21.15 footnotes.

Table 21.17 *Therapy for endocarditis due to enterococci. (Adapted from Wilson WR, Karchmer AW, Dajari AS, et al. Antibiotic treatment of adults with infective endocarditis due to streptococci, enterococci, staphylococci, and HACEK microorganisms. JAMA 1995; 274: 1709).*

Antibiotic	Dosage and route[a]	Duration (weeks)	Comments
Aqueous crystalline penicillin G sodium	18–30 million U/24 hours iv either continuously or in 6 equally divided doses	4–6	
With gentamicin sulfate[b]	1 mg/kg im or iv every 8 hours	4–6	4-week therapy recommended for patients with symptoms <3 months in duration; 6-week therapy recommended for patients with symptoms >3 months in duration
Ampicillin sodium	12 g/24 hours iv either continuously or in 6 equally divided doses	4–6	
With gentamicin sulfate[b]	1 mg/kg im or iv every 8 hours	4–6	
Vancomycin hydrochloride[c]	30 mg/kg per 24 hours iv in 2 equally divided doses; not to exceed 2 g/24 hours unless serum levels are monitored	4–6	Vancomycin therapy is recommended for patients allergic to β-lactams; cephalosporins are not acceptable alternatives for patients allergic to penicillin
With gentamicin sulfate[b]	1 mg/kg im or iv every 8 hours	4–6	

All enterococci causing endocarditis must be tested for antimicrobial susceptibility in order to select optimal therapy (see text). This table is for endocarditis due to gentamicin or vancomycin-susceptible enterococci, viridans streptococci with a minimum inhibitory concentration of >0.5 µg/mL, nutritionally variant viridans streptococci, or prosthetic valve endocarditis caused by viridans streptococci or *Streptococcus bovis*.
[a]Antibiotic dosages are for patients with normal renal function. iv = intravenous; im = intramuscular.
[b]For specific dosing adjustments and issues concerning gentamicin (obese patients, relative contraindications), *see* Table 21.15 footnotes.
[c]For specific dosing adjustment and issues concerning vancomycin (obese patients, length of infusion), *see* Table 21.15 footnotes.

sensitive, high doses of approximately 20 million units per day[81] should be utilized (Table 21.18). More likely, oxacillin or occasionally cefazolin may be appropriate. The addition of a short course of an aminoglycoside has been recommended for more rapid clearing of the bloodstream (therefore less valvular destruction and fewer peripheral complications would be anticipated).[82] Overall relapse rates and outcome, however, were not affected by this combination approach. A more recent study[83] suggests that the aminoglycoside may not be necessary.

Infections due to methicillin-resistant *Staphylococcus aureus* (MRSA) or methicillin-resistant *Staphylococcus epidermidis* (MRSE) require the use of vancomycin. Because there are no data to suggest an improved outcome, aminoglycosides are not routinely utilized in this setting of NVE. Furthermore, the use of vancomycin with aminoglycosides is associated with enhanced toxicity. Six weeks of parenteral antimicrobial therapy should be given to non-addicts with NVE. The duration of antimicrobial therapy will be influenced by the overall status of the patient and the presence of complications.

The HACEK organisms are a unique group of Gram-negative slow-growing fastidious bacteria of oral origin. They may be responsible for 5–10 per cent of the cases of IE.[76] If suspicious of these organisms, the laboratory should be requested to hold the cultures for 2 weeks to allow adequate time for growth.

Because of their fastidiousness, susceptibility testing may be difficult. Previous recommendations for the use of ampicillin should be supplanted by the use of ceftriaxone as the treatment of choice.[76,77] If sensitivity can be determined, specific therapy can be utilized. In NVE, duration of therapy is 3–4 weeks (Table 21.19).

Overall, fungal endocarditis is uncommon except in populations of drug addicts and patients with prosthetic cardiac valves. It is, unfortunately, very difficult to treat and cure. Combined medical and surgical therapy is the preferred approach to this difficult problem. Mortality ranges from 50 to 100 per cent depending upon the organisms and host.[47,84]

Amphotericin B is the preferred antimicrobial; however, duration of therapy is poorly defined. Doses totaling 2.5–3.0 g are considered appropriate in most circumstances. In situations of fluconazole susceptibility, long-term suppression may be appropriate for years. In spite of this, repeated relapses may occur.

Table 21.18 *Therapy for staphylococcal endocarditis in the absence of prosthetic material[a]. (Adapted from Wilson WR, Karchmer AW, Dajari AS, et al. Antibiotic treatment of adults with infective endocarditis due to streptococci, enterococci, staphylococci, and HACEK microorganisms. JAMA 1995; 274: 1710).*

Antibiotic	Dosage and route	Duration	Comments
A. Methicillin-susceptible staphylococci			
Regimens for non-β-lactam-allergic patients			
Nafcillin sodium or oxacillin sodium	2 g iv every 4 hours	4–6 weeks	
With optional addition of gentamicin sulfate[b]	1 mg/kg im or iv every 8 hours	3–5 days	Benefit of additional aminoglycoside therapy has not been established
Regimens for β-lactam-allergic patients			
Cefazolin (or other first-generation cephalosporins in equivalent dose	2 g iv every 8 hours	4–6 weeks	Cephalosporins should be avoided in patients with immediate-type hypersensitivity to penicillin
With optional addition of gentamicin[b] every 8 hours	1 mg/kg im or iv	3–5 days	
Vancomycin hydrochloride[c]	30 mg/kg per 24 hours in 2 equally divided doses, not to exceed 2 g/24 hours unless serum levels are monitored	4–6 weeks	Recommended for patients allergic to penicillin
B. Methicillin-resistant staphylococci			
Vancomycin hydrochloride[c]	30 mg/kg per 24 hours in 2 equally divided doses, not to exceed 2 g/24 hours unless serum levels are monitored	4–6 weeks	

[a]For treatment of endocarditis due to penicillin-susceptible staphylococci (minimum inhibitory concentration ≤0.1 µg/mL), aqueous crystalline penicillin G sodium (Table 21.15) can be used for 4–6 weeks instead of nafcillin or oxacillin. Shorter antibiotic courses have been effective in some drug addicts with right-sided endocarditis due to *Staphylococcus aureus*. iv = intravenous; im = intramuscular.
[b]For specific dosing adjustment and issues concerning gentamicin (obese patients, relative contraindications), *see* Table 21.15 footnotes.
[c]For specific dosing adjustment and issues concerning vancomycin (obese patients, length of infusion), *see* Table 21.15 footnotes.

Table 21.19 *Therapy for endocarditis due to HACEK microorganisms. (Adapted from Wilson WR, Karchmer AW, Dajari AS, et al. Antibiotic treatment of adults with infective endocarditis due to streptococci, enterococci, staphylococci, and HACEK microorganisms. JAMA 1995; 274: 1712).*

Antibiotic	Dosage and route[a]	Duration (weeks)	Comments
Ceftriaxone sodium[b]	2 g once daily iv or im[b]	4	Cefotaxime sodium or other third-generation cephalosporins may be substituted
Ampicillin sodium[c]	12 g/24 hours iv either continuously or in 6 equally divided doses	4	
with gentamicin sulfate[d]	1 mg/kg im or iv every 8 hours	4	

[a]Antibiotic dosages are for patients with normal renal function. iv = intravenous; im = intramuscular.
[b]Patients should be informed that im injection of ceftriaxone is painful.
[c]Ampicillin should not be used if laboratory tests show β-lactamase production.
[d]For specific dosing adjustment and issues concerning gentamicin (obese patients, relative contraindications), *see* Table 21.15 footnotes.

Culture-negative endocarditis

True culture-negative endocarditis is probably uncommon;[77] in many cases previous antibiotic use complicates attempts to isolate the causative microorganism.[43,85,86] Treatment is determined by careful consideration of the presenting case scenario; previous antibiotic use, subacute *vs* acute, native *vs* prosthetic valve, addict *vs* non-addict with additional consideration being given to the uncommon organisms such as *Coxiella*, *Legionella*, *Chlamydia*, or fungi. Endocarditis in IVDU constitutes a separate situation and should be treated according to the recommendations outlined below.

> Duration of treatment for culture-negative endocarditis will be dictated by the patient's response. If signs and symptoms remit in 1 week, the aminoglycoside should be used for a total of 2 weeks and the rest of the regimen continued for 6 weeks.[43]

If there is lack of response and no other explanation for continued fever and clinical failure, the regimen should be reconsidered.

> In the event of progression (enlarging vegetations, emboli, or perivalvular abscess formation), surgical intervention should be considered.

IVDU and IE

Treatment of IE in IVDU requires knowledge of the current microbiology of this infection in this population for a particular locale at that time. Specific organisms may be prevalent in certain locales.[41,87] Staphylococcal organisms predominate; however, Gram-negative and fungal organisms occur.

> Right-sided IE, especially tricuspid, is unique to this population and tends to respond very well to antibiotics.[43,88] A 2-week course of combined therapy with a semisynthetic penicillin (i.e. oxacillin 2 g iv 4-hourly) with a synergistic aminoglycoside (i.e. gentamicin 1 mg/kg 8-hourly) is the standard of therapy, resulting in success rates of 90 per cent for *Staphylococcus aureus*.[81,88,89]

A recent study demonstrated equal outcomes of single *vs* combination therapy (cloxacillin or cloxacillin and gentamicin) for 2 weeks in right-sided *S. aureus* endocarditis. If MRSA infection is present, vancomycin 1 g 12-hourly ± rifampin 600 mg/day for 4 weeks is recommended.[81]

Left-sided endocarditis in IVDU should be approached as recommended in non-addicts infected with the same microorganisms. Please refer to that section for guidelines.

Prosthetic valve endocarditis

Bloodstream infection in the postoperative period is a bad prognostic sign associated with significant mortality independent of the development of PVE.[90] The frequency of PVE in this group may range from 24 to 43 per cent.[91,92]

Treatment of PVE is often more difficult than that of NVE. Often a combined medical and surgical effort is necessary, especially in early-onset PVE (EO-PVE).[93–96] Specific indications for surgical intervention will be reviewed later. EO-PVE is more likely to be staphylococcal and late onset PVE (LO-PVE) is more likely to be streptococcal in origin. The microbiology of LO-PVE is more typical of community acquired organisms, whereas EO-PVE tends to reflect nosocomially acquired organisms.

> Antibiotic therapy is organism specific and given for 6 weeks. Penicillin combined with an aminoglycoside remains the cornerstone of treatment for streptococcal PVE.

The dosing recommendations follow that of NVE depending upon the sensitivity of the organism. Enterococci are almost always treated with at least 6 weeks of combination therapy.[97]

> All staphylococcal PVE (*S. aureus* or *epidermidis*) should be considered methicillin-resistant until proven otherwise, especially in EO-PVE as these infections tend to mirror nosocomial staphylococcal organisms.[15] Definitive treatment consists of 6 weeks of vancomycin or oxacillin with 2 weeks of an appropriate aminoglycoside combined with 6 weeks of oral rifampin.

Because of the tendency of resistance to develop easily to rifampin when used alone, it is suggested that two effective antistaphylococcal antibiotics be initiated prior to the use of rifampin (Table 21.20).

The overall duration of antibiotic therapy for bacterial PVE hinges on the clinical condition of the patient. If the initial response to antibiotic therapy was slow ($\geq$7 days persistent fever, 3–5 days to clear bacteremia) or the patient is severely debilitated and compromised by other medical conditions, i.e. diabetes mellitus, it is reasonable to extend the course of therapy an additional 1–2 weeks or more if the patient is tolerating the therapy. It is accepted practice to time the duration of therapy from the time of obtaining sterility of the blood cultures or replacement of the valve.

Fungal PVE can be even more challenging to treat than to diagnose. Fungi are responsible for 1.8 to 10 per cent of PVE.[98,99] Current opinion favors a combined medical and surgical approach.[47,100–103] There are, however, long-term survivors. The surgical intervention may

Table 21.20 *Treatment of staphylococcal endocarditis in the presence of a prosthetic valve or other prosthetic material[a]. (Adapted from Wilson WR, Karchmer AW, Dajari AS, et al. Antibiotic treatment of adults with infective endocarditis due to streptococci, enterococci, staphylococci, and HACEK microorganisms.* JAMA 1995; 274: 1711).

Antibiotic	Dosage and route	Duration (weeks)	Comments
A. Regimen for methicillin-susceptible staphylococci			
Nafcillin sodium or oxacillin sodium	2 g iv every 4 hours	≥6	First-generation cephalosporins or vancomycin should be used in patients allergic to β-lactams
With rifampin[b]	300 mg orally every 8 hours	≥6	Cephalosporins should be avoided in patients with immediate-type hypersensitivity to penicillin or with methicillin-resistant staphylococci
And with gentamicin sulfate[c]	1.0 mg/kg im or iv every 8 hours	2	
B. Regimen for methicillin-resistant staphylococci			
Vancomycin hydrochloride[d]	30 mg/kg per 24 hours iv in 2 or 4 divided doses, not to exceed 2 g/day unless serum levels monitored	≥6	
With rifampin	300 mg orally every 8 hours	≥6	Rifampin increases the amount of warfarin sodium required for antithrombotic therapy
And with gentamicin sulfate[c]	1.0 mg/kg im or iv every 8 hours	2	

[a] Dosages recommended are for patients with normal renal function. iv = intravenous; im = intramuscular.
[b] Rifampin plays a unique role in the eradication of staphylococcal infection involving prosthetic material; combination therapy is essential to prevent emergence of rifampin resistance.
[c] For specific dosing adjustment and issues concerning gentamicin (obese patients, relative contraindications), *see* Table 21.15 footnotes.
[d] For specific dosing adjustment and issues concerning vancomycin (obese patients, length of infusion), *see* Table 21.15 footnotes.

be deemed urgent and not emergent if the patient remains stable without signs of CHF, embolization or multisystem organ failure secondary to ongoing sepsis.[91]

Medical therapy with amphotericin B is the standard.[47,100,102] Flucytosine may be added to the regimen for synergism; however, the enhanced liver and bone marrow toxicities are deterrents to its use.[47] The total dose of amphotericin B is not uniformly agreed upon but ranges between 2–3 g total dose. If toxicity precludes continued use, a trial of lipid-based or liposomal amphotericin may be undertaken as these preparations may be associated with less nephrotoxicity than standard amphotericin B.[104] If tolerance to amphotericin B still remains poor, fluconazole at doses of at least 400 mg/day may be utilized.

Many feel that fungal PVE cannot be cured and that long-term (perhaps lifelong) suppressive therapy should be administered.[101,105–107] There are currently no long-term trials to validate this approach.[100] It is, however, being employed by many centers to cope with the problem of the high relapse rates of fungal PVE. Long-term suppressive therapy is particularly important for those patients who, for various reasons, are not surgical candidates for valve replacement.[101]

The timing of surgical intervention for valve replacement in fungal PVE is not uniform nor standardized. An approach toward earlier rather than later intervention seems accepted and warranted, with the intent of preventing embolization and other complications. Some have attempted to establish arbitrary preoperative total dose goals of amphotericin B,[108] while others hope to administer 'aggressive perioperative doses'.[100–102] A major determining factor will always be the status of the patient. If there is clinical deterioration in the setting of medical management, surgical intervention should not be delayed further.

There are many special cases and situations of bacterial and fungal endocarditis for which there exists no body of literature on which to base treatment.[32–38,109,110] An experienced infectious diseases physician should be consulted in these cases.

Pseudomonas endocarditis of the left heart is a special situation of note. This infection often occurs in the face of IVDU, but it sometimes occurs in other settings.[41] Accepted therapy involves high doses of an antipseudominal β-lactam antibiotic in combination with an effective aminoglycoside (gentamicin, tobramycin or amikacin depending on the sensitivity) for at least 6 weeks. Medical therapy is felt to be inadequate alone in most cases, therefore valve replacement is frequently undertaken. This may be an additional circumstance in which attempting long-term oral suppressive therapy is appropriate.

SURGICAL INTERVENTION

Surgical intervention plays an important role in the management of certain cases of infective endocarditis.[111,112] As already noted, it currently assumes a central role in cases of fungal, pseudomonal, and prosthetic valve endocarditis.

> Surgical intervention is utilized to correct valvular dysfunction, remove infected tissue (perivalvular abscess) and excise large vegetations.[112] The timing of the intervention requires a vigilant coordinated effort between the medical and surgical teams.

It has been shown that it is acceptable to perform surgery in the active period (prior to completion of the course of antibiotic therapy), if the patient is unstable or deteriorating, without an undue risk of relapse.[113] Mortality is, however, higher for the patient having valvular surgery in the active period. This most likely represents the severity of the illness that led to the operation. The aortic valve is involved in surgical intervention more often,[114] owing to its more hemodynamically significant function.[115] The tissue removed at the time of operation should always be cultured to be certain of the organism and its sensitivities to antibiotics. If the tissue is culture positive, a full course of antibiotics should be given from that point forward. Table 21.21 lists several indications for operation.

There is little doubt that valvular replacement or repair is indicated for a malfunctioning valve causing congestive heart failure. Previous congestive heart failure may be aggravated by the infectious process. If it cannot be controlled, surgical intervention may be necessary.

Investigation of persistently positive blood cultures will usually reveal a sequestered focus for which the antibiotics are ineffective. This generally indicates an abscess cavity – perivalvular, myocardial, aortic root, or a fistulous track. Occasionally a distant focus is the culprit (mycotic aneurysm). Surgical removal or obliteration is necessary. Development of a new conduction abnormality is often an indication of myocardial invasion by the infectious process; it should prompt a search for a myocardial abscess.

Failure of medical therapy is indicated by blood culture positivity with the same organism after an appropriate course of antimicrobial therapy. If the organism is a sensitive and easily treated one, most would repeat the

Table 21.21 *Indications for surgical intervention in infective endocarditis. (Adapted from references 15, 94, 111, 114–116)*

Congestive heart failure (CHF)
  New onset
  Inability to control previously controlled CHF
Valve dysfunction
  Obstruction
  Dehiscence-prosthetic
Uncontrolled infection
  Persistently positive blood cultures beyond 3 days of
    therapy
  Greater than 1 week of fever/sepsis syndrome
Perivalvular, myocardial, or aortic root abscess
New conduction abnormality
Recurrent systemic emboli
Failure of medical therapy
Fungal endocarditis
Other possible indications
  Large vegetations
  Pseudomonal endocarditis
  Early prosthetic valve endocarditis-staphylococcal
  Gram-negative infections

course of therapy provided no extracardiac focus (mycotic aneurysm, distant abscess) could be demonstrated and the patient was otherwise clinically stable. A second relapse or a relapse in the face of a prosthetic valve IE would be indications for operation. The indications for surgery of the tricuspid valve are similar except that recurrent embolization is manifest by either septic or bland pulmonary emboli.[117]

There may be rare situations (such as patients with repeated operations or extensive abscess cavities) when surgical repair cannot be performed. Cardiac transplantation may be the only hope of cure for these patients.

HOME PARENTERAL ANTIMICROBIAL THERAPY

Because of the prolonged course of treatment in endocarditis, there has been interest in identifying patients who can complete their therapy at home or in other settings other than the hospital, i.e. out-patient clinics, infusion centers, subacute care units, rehabilitation centers, or nursing homes. Like other patients receiving home therapy, the candidates must be medically stable, compliant, and tolerant of the anti-infective agent; the home situation must support the safe administration of the therapy.[118] Venous access is always secured prior to initiation of out-patient therapy. Careful ongoing clinical and laboratory monitoring is essential. In patients with penicillin-susceptible viridans streptococcal endocarditis, Stamboulian[119] and Francioli[120,121] have demonstrated that ceftriaxone therapy can be completed safely on an out-patient basis. In exceptional cases, patients received their entire course of therapy outside the hospital. The published experience with treatment of infective endocarditis due to organisms other than viridans streptococcus is anecdotal,[122] but it appears that many carefully evaluated patients may be candidates for completion of therapy in the out-patient clinic or community.[123]

Patients receiving two-drug therapy (often a β-lactam antibiotic or vancomycin along with gentamicin) present special challenges with regard to logistics and monitoring. The Infectious Disease Society of America's guidelines indicate that creatinine levels and other laboratory tests should be obtained at least twice weekly during therapy outside the hospital.[118] Patients should be examined by a physician on a regular basis; serial electrocardiograms and echocardiograms may be indicated.

> Endocarditis patients are different from the majority of patients receiving out-patient parenteral antibiotic therapy in that there is a chance of sudden significant or catastrophic events during the course of treatment. The risk of embolic events, arrhythmias, and cardiac decompensation does not disappear upon initiation of therapy. Thus, the challenge is to identify subsets of patients who may be at increased risk.[123]

Patients with surgical indications (Table 21.21) should probably remain in a hospital or another carefully supervised setting with immediate access to advanced cardiac and neurologic care. Ideally, they should undergo surgical intervention before being considered for therapy at another site. Patients with left-sided infective endocarditis due to organisms known to be associated with acute invasive disease (*Staphylococcus aureus*, *Enterococcus* sp., etc.) or embolic events (HACEK group, group B streptococci, *Candida* sp., nutritionally deficient streptococci) may be at increased risk for complications. Some clinicians would include individuals with very large vegetations in the high-risk group. At the very least, these patients should be well evaluated and stabilized in the hospital before they are considered for home therapy; a sizable proportion of patients in the risk group should remain hospitalized for the entire course of therapy.

PROPHYLAXIS

Antibiotic prophylaxis has long been an accepted therapy despite the lack of prospective clinical trials to validate the efficacy of its use.[124,125] The recommendations for prophylaxis are not uniformly agreed upon throughout the international medical community despite repeated reevaluations and discussions.[126] In addition, many cases of IE are not the result of invasive procedures.

Certain organisms have traditionally been responsible for the majority of cases of endocarditis (viridans streptococci, enterococci, and staphylococci). The ability of an organism to cause endocarditis appears to be a result of

Table 21.22 *Cardiac conditions associated with endocarditis. (Adapted from Dajani AS, Taubert KA, Wilson W, et al. Prevention of bacterial endocarditis. Recommendations by the American Heart Association.* JAMA 1997; **277**: 1795)

A. Endocarditis – prophylaxis recommended
High-risk category
    Prosthetic cardiac valves, including bioprosthetic and homograft valves
    Previous bacterial endocarditis
    Complex cyanotic congenital heart disease (e.g. single ventricle states, transposition of the great arteries, tetralogy of Fallot)
    Surgically constructed systemic pulmonary shunts or conduits
Moderate-risk category
    Most other congenital cardiac malformations (other than above and below)
    Acquired valvular dysfunction, e.g. rheumatic heart disease
    Hypertrophic cardiomyopathy
    Mitral valve prolapse with valvar regurgitation and/or thickened leaflets[a]

B. Endocarditis – prophylaxis not recommended
Negligible-risk category
    Isolated secundum atrial septal defect
    Surgical repair of atrial septal defect, ventricular septal defect, or patent ductus arteriosus (without residua beyond 6 months)
    Previous coronary artery bypass graft surgery
    Mitral valve prolapse without valvular regurgitation[a]
    Physiologic, functional, or innocent heart murmurs
    Previous Kawasaki disease without valvular dysfunction
    Previous rheumatic fever without valvular dysfunction
    Cardiac pacemakers (intravascular and epicardial) and implanted defibrillators

[a] See text for further details.

Table 21.23 *Dental procedures and endocarditis prophylaxis. (Adapted from Dajani AS, Taubert KA, Wilson W, et al. Prevention of bacterial endocarditis. Recommendations by the American Heart Association.* JAMA *1997;* **277**: *1797)*

A. Endocarditis – prophylaxis recommended[a]
Dental extractions

Periodontal procedures including surgery, scaling and root planing, probing, and recall maintenance

Dental implant placement and reimplantation of avulsed teeth

Endodontic (root canal) instrumentation or surgery only beyond the apex

Subgingival placement of antibiotic fibers or strips

Initial placement of orthodontic bands but not brackets

Intraligamentary local anesthetic injections

Prophylactic cleaning of teeth or implants where bleeding is anticipated

B. Endocarditis – prophylaxis not recommended
Restorative dentistry[b] (operative and prosthodontic) with or without retraction cord[c]

Local anesthetic injections (non-intraligamentary)

Intracanal endodontic treatment; post-placement and build-up

Placement of rubber dams

Postoperative suture removal

Placement of removable prosthodontic or orthodontic appliances

Taking of oral impressions

Fluoride treatments

Taking of oral radiographs

Orthodontic appliance adjustment

Shedding of primary teeth

[a]Prophylaxis is recommended for patients with high- and moderate-risk cardiac conditions.
[b]This includes restoration of decayed teeth (filling cavities) and replacement of missing teeth.
[c]Clinical judgement may indicate antibiotic use in selected circumstances that may create significant bleeding.

Table 21.24 *Other procedures and endocarditis prophylaxis. (Adapted from Dajani AS, Taubert KA, Wilson W, et al. Prevention of bacterial endocarditis. Recommendations by the American Heart Association.* JAMA *1997;* **277**: *1798)*

A. Endocarditis – prophylaxis recommended
Respiratory tract

    Tonsillectomy and/or adenoidectomy

    Surgical operations that involve respiratory mucosa

    Bronchoscopy with a rigid bronchoscope

Gastrointestinal tract[a]

    Sclerotherapy for esophageal varices

    Esophageal stricture dilation

    Endoscopic retrograde cholangiography with biliary obstruction

    Biliary tract surgery

    Surgical operations that involve intestinal mucosa

Genitourinary tract

    Prostatic surgery

    Cystoscopy

    Urethral dilation

B. Endocarditis – prophylaxis not recommended
Respiratory tract

    Endotracheal intubation

    Bronchoscopy with a flexible bronchoscope, with or without biopsy[b]

    Tympanostomy tube insertion

Gastrointestinal tract

    Transesophageal echocardiography[b]

    Endoscopy with or without gastrointestinal biopsy[b]

Genitourinary tract

    Vaginal hysterectomy[b]

    Vaginal delivery[b]

    Cesarean section

    In uninfected tissue:

        Urethral catheterization

        Uterine dilatation and curettage

        Therapeutic abortion

        Sterilization procedures

        Insertion or removal of intrauterine devices

Other

    Cardiac catheterization, including balloon angioplasty

    Implanted cardiac pacemakers, implanted defibrillators, and coronary stents

    Incision or biopsy of surgically scrubbed skin

    Circumcision

[a]Prophylaxis is recommended for high-risk patients; optional for medium-risk patients.
[b]Prophylaxis is optional for high-risk patients.

its adhesive properties to the platelet–fibrin matrix and, to some degree, an innoculum effect (experimental).[125] If we consider the usual anatomic residence of these organisms, in general, viridans streptococci should be covered during dental, oropharyngeal, and upper airway procedures, while entercocci are the major target of prophylaxis during gastrointestinal or urologic procedures.

The current American Heart Association (AHA) recommendations are the result of recent reconsiderations and revisions (Table 21.22). These recommendations are based on risk stratification and have been simplified from previously published regimens.

Mitral valve prolapse (MVP) is still a controversial topic. If the mitral prolapse is associated with regurgitation, prophylaxis is indicated; if it is associated only with a click (no murmur or regurgitation), prophylaxis need not be given. An exception may be a male >45 years of age with MVP in whom a consistent murmur cannot be

demonstrated. This age group appears to be at higher risk for IE and should be considered for prophylaxis.[124]

Tables 21.23 and 21.24 provide a history of procedures felt to result in significant bacteremia and therefore predispose the patient to IE.

In the latest AHA recommendations, dental, oral, respiratory tract, and esophageal procedure regimens have been simplified (Table 21.25). The oral dose of

Table 21.25 *Prophylactic regimens for dental, oral, respiratory tract, or esophageal procedures. (Adapted from Dajani AS, Taubert KA, Wilson W, et al. Prevention of bacterial endocarditis. Recommendations by the American Heart Association. JAMA 1997; 277: 1798)*

Situation	Agent	Regimen[a]
Standard general prophylaxis	Amoxicillin	Adults: 2.0 g; children: 50 mg/kg orally 1 hour before procedure
Unable to take oral medications	Ampicillin	Adults: 2.0 g intramuscularly (im) or intravenously (iv); children: 50 mg/kg im or iv within 30 minutes before procedure
Allergic to penicillin	Clindamycin or	Adults: 600 mg; children: 20 mg/kg orally 1 hour before procedure
	Cephalexin[b] or cefadroxil[b] or	Adults: 2.0 g; children: 15 mg/kg orally 1 hour before procedure
	Azithromycin or clarithromycin	Adults: 500 mg; children: 15 mg/kg orally 1 hour before procedure
Allergic to penicillin and unable to take oral medications	Clindamycin or	Adults: 600 mg; children: 20 mg/kg iv within 30 min before procedure
	Cefazolin[b]	Adults: 1.0 g; children: 25 mg/kg im or iv within 30 minutes before procedure

[a]Total children's dose should not exceed adult dose.
[b]Cephalosporins should not be used in individuals with immediate-type hypersensitivity reaction (urticaria, angiodema, or anaphylaxis) to penicillins.

amoxicillin has been reduced to 2 g for adults (50 mg/kg for children) and the post-procedure dose has been eliminated. Erythromycin is no longer recommended as a second-line agent and has been replaced by clindamycin or first-generation cephalosporins. Oral antibiotic doses should be given 1 hour prior to the procedure and intravenous (iv) doses 30 minutes beforehand.

The latest AHA-recommended regimens for GI and genitourinary procedures are found in Table 21.26. The backbone of prophylaxis remains ampicillin and gentamicin, with vancomycin being used in penicillin allergic patients. Parenteral doses should be used in patients classified as high risk and a follow-up dose given 6 hours later if ampicillin is used (repeat dose not necessary with vancomycin). A single oral dose of amoxicillin or ampicillin is adequate for moderate risk patients.

PACEMAKER/IMPLANTABLE CARDIAC DEFIBRILLATOR INFECTIONS

Device-related infections comprise a small and distinct subset of cardiac infections. However, with improving technology, the aging of the population and the increased frequency of implantation, the numbers of these infections will no doubt increase. Currently, the prevalence of pacemaker infections range from 0.13 to 12 per cent[127] probably averaging 3 per cent. It tends to be lower with initial implantations (1–7 per cent)[128] and increases with revision and repeated implantations.

Staphylococcal organisms are the predominant pathogen and are responsible for 75–89 per cent of cases.[127,129] Many other organisms have been cultured

from pacemaker infections, including Gram-negative bacteria, fungi, and anaerobes.[130]

Analogous to PVE, these infections can similarly be considered in categories of early and late infections. The early infections tend to be more acute and possibly more often associated with *S. aureus*, and the later infections are usually less acute and may be associated with *S. epidermidis* or other organisms of lower pathogenicity and aggressiveness.

Infections limited to the generator pocket present with local signs and symptoms. If the infection is related to the pacing lead, a tunnel-type infection and/or systemic symptoms are noted.

An interesting subset of pacemaker infections are those classified as pacemaker endocarditis, in which the atrial or ventricular lead becomes infected and the process spreads to the adjacent endocardial surface[129,131] Most are staphylococcal and behave as right-sided endocarditis with the typical manifestations of that entity.

Implantable cardiac defibrillators (ICDs) have similar rates of infection, occurring in approximately 2–6 per cent of cases.[132] The microbiology is similar with a preponderance of staphylococcal organisms.

Treatment consists of organism-specific antibiotics, usually antistaphylococcal, and total device removal.[132–135] Some advocate antibiotics, local pocket debridement, and antibiotic irrigation with subsequent salvage of the device in selected patients.[128]

There is a growing experience in the use of various left ventricular assist devices. Because of their size and externalized drive lines and power sources, they are prone to infection.[136–141] Antibiotic treatment is often prolonged, placing these already compromised patients at risk for multidrug-resistant bacterial superinfection and fungal

Table 21.26 *Prophylactic regimens for genitourinary and gastrointestinal (other than esophageal) procedures. (Adapted from Dajani AS, Taubert KA, Wilson W, et al. Prevention of bacterial endocarditis. Recommendations by the American Heart Association. JAMA 1997; 277: 1799)*

Situation	Agent[a]	Regimen[b]
High-risk patients	Ampicillin plus gentamicin	Adults: ampicillin 2.0 g intramuscularly (im) or intravenously (iv) plus gentamicin 1.5 mg/kg (not to exceed 120 mg) within 30 minutes of starting the procedure; 6 hours later, ampicillin 1 g im/iv or amoxicillin 1 g orally Children: ampicillin 50 mg/kg im or iv (not to exceed 2.0 g) plus gentamicin 1.5 mg/kg within 30 minutes of starting the procedure; 6 hours later, ampicillin 25 mg/kg im/iv or amoxicillin 25 mg/kg orally
High-risk patients allergic to ampicillin/amoxicillin	Vancomycin plus gentamicin	Adults: vancomycin 1.0 g iv over 1–2 hours plus gentamicin 1.5 mg/kg iv/im (not to exceed 120 mg); complete injection/infusion within 30 minutes of starting the procedure Children: vancomycin 20 mg/kg iv over 1–2 hours plus gentamicin 1.5 mg/kg iv/im; complete injection/infusion within 30 minutes of starting the procedure
Moderate-risk patients	Amoxicillin or ampicillin	Adults: amoxicillin 2.0 g orally 1 hour before procedure, or ampicillin 2.0 g im/iv within 30 minutes of starting the procedure Children: amoxicillin 50 mg/kg orally 1 hour before procedure, or ampicillin 50 mg/kg im/iv within 30 minutes of starting the procedure
Moderate-risk patients allergic to ampicillin/amoxicillin	Vancomycin	Adults: vancomycin 1.0 g iv over 1–2 hours; complete infusion within 30 minutes of starting the procedure Children: vancomycin 20 mg/kg iv over 1–2 hours; complete infusion within 30 minutes of starting the procedure

[a] Total children's dose should not exceed adult dose.
[b] No second dose of vancomycin or gentamicin is recommended.

invasion. Device-related bloodstream infection can usually be controlled with long-term antimicrobial drugs in these patients awaiting cardiac transplantation. Ultimately, only cardiac transplantation with attendant removal of the infected device results in cure.

CLINICAL OVERVIEW

Infective endocarditis continues to be a significant disease process. The introduction of antibiotics and the continual re-engineering of new agents have been the single most important advances in the treatment of IE. The refinement of microbiologic techniques have allowed the isolation, identification, and antimicrobial susceptibility testing of many of the microbes responsible for this illness. Technological advances in imaging techniques have provided improved diagnostic capabilities for IE and its systemic complications, while surgical advances have allowed interventions for many previously fatal complications. The relapse and mortality rate of approximately 20 per cent, however, attests to our incomplete conquest of this condition. The next significant change in the rates of disease and death related to endocarditis may be tied more to enhanced prevention

efforts than to the development of a 'breakthrough' drug or a new type of cardiac valve.

FUTURE DIRECTIONS

The persistence of relatively high rates of morbidity and mortality in patients with infective endocarditis will drive advances in prophylaxis, diagnostics, and therapeutics. Nonetheless, many practical aspects of endocarditis prevention and management can be improved, primarily through enhancement of physicians' awareness of currently available diagnostic and therapeutic measures.

Education of patients and their physicians is vital to the successful implementation of guidelines for antimicrobial prophylaxis of individuals at risk. Further investigation of surgical techniques that reduce the risk of perioperative contamination of prosthetic heart valves could lead to a reduction in the number of cases of early PVE.

Recognition of early or subtle manifestations of IE promotes early and accurate diagnosis. Further improvements in echocardiographic techniques will provide increasingly detailed images of cardiac valves and other endocardial structures, but clinical correlation will be more and more important in the interpretation of the images. Likewise, if it were possible to enhance blood culturing methodology and clinical algorithms to assist clinicians in distinguishing 'contaminants' from significant isolates in cases of possible PVE, patients would benefit through earlier diagnosis and, in some cases, avoidance of unnecessary courses of antimicrobial therapy.

When therapy is indicated, advances in antimicrobial therapy should make the treatment course safer and easier to administer. Development of antimicrobial agents with long half-lives and favorable safety profiles will also facilitate completion of therapy outside the hospital when it is indicated. Additional studies should help to delineate groups of patients at risk for serious complications from endocarditis and illuminate the decision-making process when surgical intervention or alternate sites of therapy are contemplated.

SUMMARY

- The epidemiology of infective endocarditis (IE) has evolved. In the past, younger patients with rheumatic heart disease were often affected; now older patients with degenerative valvular conditions or prosthetic valve/device-related infections are more typical. Intravenous drug abuse leads to a significant number of cases.
- A trend toward more cases of acute IE has been noted. Staphylococci are playing an increasing role, while streptococcal infection is declining.
- IE is a systemic disease whose diagnosis is made on clinical grounds supported by laboratory and echocardiographic findings. Fever, peripheral circulatory signs, sustained bacteremia, and valvular vegetations are the typical features.
- Treatment requires prolonged parenteral therapy with bactericidal agents, sometimes in synergistic combinations. Surgical intervention may be required in certain cases.
- Completion of parenteral antimicrobial therapy outside the hospital setting has been shown to be safe and effective in carefully selected and monitored patients.
- Despite a lack of prospective clinical trials, antibiotic prophylaxis of IE is endorsed.
- Approaches to treatment of patients with infected implantable cardiac devices are still evolving.
- Refinements in antibiotic prophylaxis, newer diagnostic techniques, and novel antibiotics and advances in antimicrobial therapy should lead to reductions in new cases of infective endocarditis, earlier diagnosis, and more effective management.

REFERENCES

1. Kelson SR, White PD. Notes on 250 cases of subacute bacterial (streptococcal) endocarditis studied and treated between 1927 and 1939. *Ann Intern Med* 1945; **22**: 40–60.
2. Weiss S. Self-observations and psychologic reactions of medical student A.S.R. to the onset and symptoms of subacute bacterial endocarditis. *J Mt Sinai Hosp* 1941; **9**: 1079–93.
3. Bayer AS. Infective endocarditis. *Clin Infect Dis* 1993; **17**: 313–22.
4. Gary IR. Infective endocarditis 1937–1987. *Br Heart J* 1987; **57**: 211–13.
5. Kaye D. Changing pattern of infective endocarditis. *Am J Med* 1985; **78**(suppl 6B): 157–62.
6. Hayward GW. Infective endocarditis: a changing disease. *Br Med J* 1973; **2**: 706–9, 764–6.
7. Michel PL, Acar J. Native cardiac disease predisposing to infective endocarditis. *Eur Heart J* 1995; **16**(suppl B): 2–6.
8. Hogevik H, Olaison L, Andersson R, et al. Epidemiologic aspects of infective endocarditis in an urban population. A 5-year prospective study. *Medicine* 1995; **74**: 324–39.
9. Durack DT, Lukes AS, Bright DK. New criteria for diagnosis of infective endocarditis: utilization of specific echocardiographic findings. *Am J Med* 1995; **96**: 200–9.
10. Griffin MR, Wilson WR, Edwards WD, et al. Infective endocarditis: Olmsted County, Minnesota, 1950 through 1981. *JAMA* 1985; **254**: 1199–202.
11. Zak O, Scheld WM, Sande MA. Rifampin in experimental endocarditis due to *Staphylococcus aureus* in rabbits. *Rev Infect Dis* 1983; **5**(suppl 3): S481–S490.
12. De Gevigney G, Pop C, Delahaye JP. The risk of infective endocarditis after cardiac surgical and interventional procedures. *Eur Heart J* 1996; **16**(suppl B): 7–14.
13. Chastre J, Trouillet JL. Early infective endocarditis on prosthetic valves. *Eur Heart J* 1995; **16**(suppl B): 32–8.
14. Lazenby D, Gold JP. Prevention and management of prosthetic valve endocarditis. *Infect Med* 1991; **8**: 15–16, 42–5.
15. Calderwood SB, Swinski LA, Waternaux CM, Karchmer AW, Buckley MJ. Risk factors for the development of prosthetic valve endocarditis. *Circulation* 1985; **72**: 31–7.
16. Graves MK, Soto L. Left-sided endocarditis in parenteral drug abusers: recent experience at a large community hospital. *South Med J* 1992; **85**: 378–80.
17. Currie PF, Sutherland GR, Jacob AJ, et al. A review of endocarditis in acquired immunodeficiency syndrome and human immunodeficiency virus infection. *Eur Heart J* 1995; **16**(suppl B): 15–18.
18. Nahass RG, Weinstein MP, Bartels J. Gocke DJ. Infective endocarditis in intravenous drug users: a comparison of human immunodeficiency virus type 1-negative and -positive patients. *J Infect Dis* 1990; **162**: 967–70.

19. Brandenburg RO, Giuliani ER, Wilson WR, Geraci JE. Infective endocarditis – a 25 year overview of diagnosis and therapy. *J Am Coll Cardiol* 1983; **1**: 280–91.

20. Watanakunakorn C, Burkert T. Infective endocarditis at a large community teaching hospital, 1980–1990. A review of 210 episodes. *Medicine* 1993; **72**: 90–102.

21. Beeching NJ, Christmas TI, Ellis-Pegler RB. *Streptococcus bovis* bacteraemia requires rigorous exclusion of colonic neoplasia and endocarditis. *Q J Med* 1985; **220**: 439–50.

22. Jackson LA, Hilsdon R, Farley MM, *et al*. Risk factors for group B streptococcal disease in adults. *Ann Intern Med* 1995; **123**: 415–20.

23. Chambers HF, Korzeniowski OM, Sande MA, *et al*. *Staphylococcus aureus* endocarditis: clinical manifestations in addicts and nonaddicts. *Medicine* 1983; **62**: 170–7.

24. Tuazon CU, Sheagren JN. Staphylococcal endocarditis in parenteral drug abusers: source of the organism. *Ann Intern Med* 1975; **82**: 788–90.

25. Tuazon CU, Sheagren JN. Increased rate of carriage of *Staphylococcus aureus* among narcotic addicts. *J Infect Dis* 1974; **129**: 725–7.

26. Caputo GM, Archer GL, Calderwood SB, *et al*. Native valve endocarditis due to coagulase-negative staphylococci. *Am J Med* 1987; **83**: 619–25.

27. Whitener C, Caputo GM, Weitekamp MR. Endocarditis due to coagulase-negative staphylococci. Microbiologic, epidemiologic, and clinical considerations. *Infect Dis Clin North Am* 1993; **7**: 81–96.

28. Baddour LM, Phillips TN, Bisno AL. Coagulase-negative staphylococcal endocarditis: occurrence in patients with mitral valve prolapse. *Arch Intern Med* 1986; **146**: 119–21.

29. Wilkowske CJ Jr. Enterococcal endocarditis. *Mayo Clin Proc* 1982; **57**: 101–5.

30. Lipman ML, Silva J Jr. Endocarditis due to *Streptococcus faecalis* with high-level resistance to gentamicin. *Rev Infect Dis* 1989; **11**: 325–8.

31. Geraci JE, Wilson WR. Symposium on infective endocarditis. III. Endocarditis due to gram-negative bacteria. Report of 56 cases. *Mayo Clin Proc* 1982; **57**: 145–8.

32. Shapiro DS, Kenney SC, Johnson M, *et al*. Brief report: *Chlamydia psittaci* endocarditis diagnosed by blood culture. *N Engl J Med* 1992; **326**: 1192–5.

33. Tunkel AR, Fisch MJ, Schlein A, *et al*. *Enterobacter* endocarditis. *Scand J Infect Dis* 1992; **24**: 233–40.

34. Choo PW, Gantz NM, Anderson C, *et al*. *Salmonella* prosthetic valve endocarditis. *Diag Microbiol Infect Dis* 1992; **15**: 273–6.

35. Fukushima N, Ishikawa N, Shimazaki Y, *et al*. *Salmonella* prosthetic valve endocarditis. *J Thorac Cardiovasc Surg* 1996; **112**: 840–2.

36. Thompson EC, Brantley D. Gonococcal endocarditis. *J Natl Med Assoc* 1996; **88**: 353–6.

37. Spach DH, Kaner AS, Daniels NA. *Bartonella (Rochalimaea)* species as a cause of apparent 'culture-negative' endocarditis. *Clin Infect Dis* 1995; **20**: 1044–7.

38. Binder D, Zibinden R, Widmer U, *et al*. Native and prosthetic valve endocarditis caused by *Rothia dentocariosa*: diagnostic and therapeutic considerations. *Infection* 1997; **25**: 22–6.

39. Gradon JD, Chapnick EK, Lutwick LI. Infective endocarditis of a native valve due to *Acinetobacter*: case report and review. *Clin Infect Dis* 1992; **14**: 1145–58.

40. Ellner JJ, Rosenthal MS, Lerner PI, *et al*. Infective endocarditis caused by slow-growing fastidious, gram-negative bacteria. *Medicine* 1979; **58**: 145–58.

41. Wieland M, Lederman MM, Kline-King C, *et al*. Left-sided endocarditis due to *Pseudomonas aeruginosa*: a report of 10 cases and review of the literature. *Medicine* 1986; **65**: 180–9.

42. Baddour LM, Meyer J, Henry B. Polymicrobial infective endocarditis in the 1980's. *Rev Infect Dis* 1991; **13**: 963–70.

43. Van Scoy RE. Culture-negative endocarditis. *Mayo Clin Proc* 1982; **57**: 149–54.

44. Husni RN, Gordon SM, Washington JA. *Lactobacillus* bacteremia and endocarditis: review of 45 cases. *Clin Infect Dis* 1997; **25**: 1048–55.

45. Sussman JI, Baron EJ, Goldberg SM, *et al*. Clinical manifestations and therapy of *Lactobacillus* endocarditis: report of a case and review of the literature. *Rev Infect Dis* 1986; **8**: 771–6.

46. Raoult D, Fournier PE, Drancourt M, *et al*. Diagnosis of 22 new cases of *Bartonella* endocarditis. *Ann Intern Med* 1996; **125**: 646–52.

47. Rubinstein E, Lang R. Fungal endocarditis. *Eur Heart J* 1996; **16**(suppl B): 84–9.

48. Rubinstein E, Noriega ER, Simberkoff MS, *et al*. Fungal endocarditis: analysis of 24 cases and review of the literature. *Medicine* 1975; **54**: 331–44.

49. Nasser RM, Melgar GR, Longworth DL, Gordon SM. Incidence and risk of developing fungal prosthetic valve endocarditis after nosocomial candidemia. *Am J Med* 1997; **103**: 25–32.

50. Woods GL, Wood RP, Shaw BW Jr. *Aspergillus* endocarditis in patients without prior cardiovascular surgery: report of a case in a liver transplant recipient and review. *Rev Infect Dis* 1989; **11**: 263–72.

51. Seelig MS, Speth CP, Kozinn PJ, *et al*. Patterns of *Candida* endocarditis following cardiac surgery: importance of early diagnosis and therapy (an analysis of 91 cases). *Prog Cardiovasc Dis* 1974; **17**: 125–60.

52. Erdos MS, Butt K, Weinstein L. Mucormycotic endocarditis of the pulmonary valve. *JAMA* 1972; **222**: 951–3.

53. Von Reyn CF, Levy BS, Arbeit RD, *et al*. Infective endocarditis: an analysis based on strict case definitions. *Ann Intern Med* 1981; **94**: 505–18.

54. Steckelberg JM, Melton LJ III, Ilstrup DM, *et al*. Influence of referral bias on the apparent clinical spectrum of infective endocarditis. *Am J Med* 1990; **88**: 582–8.

55. Terpenning MS, Buggy BP, Kauffman CA. Infective endocarditis: clinical features in young and elderly patients. *Am J Med* 1987; **83**: 626–34.

56. Douglas A, Moore-Gillon J, Eykyn S. Fever during treatment of infective endocarditis. *Lancet* 1986; **i** 1341–3.

57. Lederman MM, Sprague L, Wallis RS, Ellner JJ. Duration of fever during treatment of infective endocarditis. *Medicine* 1992; **71**: 52–7.

58. Jones HR Jr, Siekert RG. Neurological manifestations of infective endocarditis. *Brain* 1989; **112**: 1295–315.

59. Pruitt AA, Rubin RH, Karchmer AW, Duncan GW. Neurologic complications of bacterial endocarditis. *Medicine* 1978; **57**: 329–43.

60. Selky AK, Roos KL. Neurologic complications of infective endocarditis. *Semin Neurol* 1992; **12**: 225–33.

61. Bertorini TE, Gelfand M. Neurological complications of bacterial endocarditis. *Comp Ther* 1990; **16**: 47–55.

62. Washington JA. The microbiological diagnosis of infective endocarditis. *J Antimicrob Chemother* 1987; **20**(suppl A): 29–36.

63. Werner AS, Cobbs CG, Kaye D, Hook EW. Studies on the bacteremia of bacterial endocarditis. *JAMA* 1967; **202**: 127–31.

64. Osler W. Galstonian lectures on malignant endocarditis. *Lancet* 1885; **1**: 505–8.

65. Lerner PI, Weinstein L. Infective endocarditis in the antibiotic era. *N Engl J Med* 1966; **274**: 199–206, 259–66, 323–31, 388–93.

66. Bayer AS, Ward JI, Ginzton LE, Shapiro SM. Evaluation of new clinical criteria for the diagnosis of infective endocarditis. *Am J Med* 1994; **96**: 211–22.

67. Jaffe WM, Morgan DE, Pearlman AS, Otto CM. Infective endocarditis, 1983–1988: echocardiographic findings and factors influencing morbidity and mortality. *J Am Coll Cardiol* 1990; **15**: 1227–33.

68. Mugge A, Daniel WG, Frank G, Lichtlen PR. Echocardiography in infective endocarditis: reassessment of prognostic implications of vegetation size determined by the transthoracic and the transesophageal approach. *J Am Coll Cardiol* 1989; **14**: 631–8.

69. Shapiro SM, Bayer AS. Transesophageal and doppler echocardiography in the diagnosis and management of infective endocarditis. *Chest* 1991; **100**: 1125–30.

70. Shively BK, Gurule FT, Roldan CA, *et al.* Diagnostic value of transesophageal compared with transthoracic echocardiography in infective endocarditis. *J Am Coll Cardiol* 1991; **18**: 391–7.

71. Rohmann S, Erbel R, Mohr-Kahaly S, Meyer J. Use of transoesophageal echocardiography in the diagnosis of abscess in infective endocarditis. *Eur Heart J* 1995; **16**(suppl B): 54–62.

72. Vered Z, Mossinson D, Peleg E, *et al.* Echocardiographic assessment of prosthetic valve endocarditis. *Eur Heart J* 1995; **16**(suppl B): 63–7.

73. Fleming HA. General principles of the treatment of infective endocarditis. *J Antimicrob Chemother* 1987; **20**(suppl A): 143–5.

74. Carbon C, Cremieux A-C, Fantin B. Pharmacokinetic and pharmacodynamic aspects of therapy of experimental endocarditis. *Infect Dis Clin North Am* 1993; **7**: 37–51.

75. Besnier JM, Choutet P. Medical treatment of infective endocarditis: general principles. *Eur Heart J* 1995; **16**(suppl B): 72–4.

76. Wilson WR, Karchmer AW, Dajani AS, *et al.* Antibiotic treatment of adults with infective endocarditis due to streptococci, enterococci, staphylococci, and HACEK microorganisms. *JAMA* 1995; **274**: 1706–13.

77. Wilson WR. Recognition and treatment of infective endocarditis. *Heart Dis Stroke* 1992; **1**: 65–7.

78. Malacoff RF, Frank E, Andriole VT. Streptococcal endocarditis (nonenterococcal, non-group A): single vs combination therapy. *JAMA* 1979; **241**: 1807–10.

79. Wilson WR, Wilkowske CJ, Wright AJ, *et al.* Treatment of streptomycin-susceptible and streptomycin-resistant enterococcal endocarditis. *Ann Intern Med* 1984; **100**: 816–23.

80. Megran DW. Enterococcal endocarditis. *Clin Infect Dis* 1992; **15**: 63–71.

81. Bille J. Medical treatment of staphylococcal infective endocarditis. *Eur Heart J* 1995; **16** (suppl B): 80–3.

82. Korzeniowski O, Sande MA, National Collaborative Endocarditis Study Group. Combination antimicrobial therapy for *Staphylococcus aureus* endocarditis in patients addicted to parenteral drugs and in nonaddicts: a prospective study. *Ann Intern Med* 1982; **97**: 496–503.

83. Ribera E, Gomez-Jimenez J, Cortes E, *et al.* Effectiveness of cloxacillin with and without gentamicin in short-term therapy for right-sided *Staphylococcus aureus* endocarditis. A randomized, controlled trial. *Ann Intern Med* 1996; **125**: 969–74.

84. Fowler VG, Durack DT. Infective endocarditis. *Curr Opin Cardiol* 1994; **9**: 389–400.

85. Tunkel AR, Kaye D. Endocarditis with negative blood cultures (editorial). *N Engl J Med* 1992; **326**: 1215–17.

86. Oakley CM. The medical treatment of culture-negative infective endocarditis. *Eur Heart J* 1995; **16** (suppl B): 90–3.

87. Mathew J, Addai T, Anand A, *et al.* Clinical features, site of involvement, bacteriologic findings, and outcome of infective endocarditis in intravenous drug users. *Arch Intern Med* 1995; **155**: 1641–8.

88. Chambers HF. Short-course combination and oral therapies of *Staphylococcus aureus* endocarditis. *Infect Dis Clin North Am* 1993; **7**: 69–80.

89. Chambers HF, Miller TR, Newman MD. Right-sided *Staphylococcus aureus* endocarditis in intravenous drug abusers: two week combination therapy. *Ann Intern Med* 1988; **109**: 619–24.

90. Gordon SM, Keys TF. Bloodstream infections in patients with implanted prosthetic cardiac valves. *Semin Thorac Cardiovasc Surg* 1995; **7**: 2–6.

91. Fang G, Keys TF, Gentry LO, Harris AA, *et al.* Prosthetic

valve endocarditis resulting from nosocomial bacteremia: a prospective, multicenter study. *Ann Intern Med* 1993; **119**: 560–7.

92. Keys TF. Early-onset prosthetic valve endocarditis. *Cleve Clin J Med* 1993; **60**: 455–9.

93. Saffle JR, Garner P, Schoenbaum SC, *et al*. Prosthetic valve endocarditis: the case for prompt valve replacement. *J Thorac Cardiovasc Surg* 1977; **73**: 416–20.

94. Baumgartner WA, Miller DC, Reitz BA, *et al*. Surgical treatment of prosthetic valve endocarditis. *Ann Thorac Surg* 1983; **35**: 87–104.

95. Oakley CM. Treatment of prosthetic valve endocarditis. *J Antimicrob Chemother* 1987; **20** (suppl A): 181–6.

96. Lytle BW. Surgical treatment of prosthetic valve endocarditis. *Semin Thorac Cardiovasc Surg* 1995; **7**: 13–19.

97. Rice LB, Calderwood SB, Eliopoulos GM, *et al*. Enterococcal endocarditis: a comparison of prosthetic and native valve disease. *Rev Infect Dis* 1991; **13**: 1–7.

98. Ivert TSA, Dismukes WE, Cobbs CG, Blackstone EH, Kirklin JW, Bergdahl LAL. Prosthetic valve endocarditis. *Circulation* 1984; **69**: 223–32.

99. Arnett EN, Roberts WC. Prosthetic valve endocarditis: clinicopathologic analysis of 22 necropsy patients with comparison of observations in 74 necropsy patients with active infective endocarditis involving natural left-sided cardiac valves. *Am J Cardiol* 1976; **38**: 281–92.

100. Melgar GR, Nasser RM, Gordon SM, *et al*. Fungal prosthetic valve endocarditis in 16 patients. An 11-year experience in a tertiary care hospital. *Medicine* 1997; **76**: 94–103.

101. Gilbert HM, Peters ED, Lang SJ, *et al*. Successful treatment of fungal prosthetic valve endocarditis: case report and review. *Clin Infect Dis* 1996; **22**: 348–54.

102. Muehrcke DD. Fungal prosthetic valve endocarditis. *Semin Thorac Cardiovasc Surg* 1995; **7**: 20–4.

103. Nguyen MH, Nguyen ML, Yu VL. *Candida* prosthetic valve endocarditis: prospective study of six cases and review of the literature. *Clin Infect Dis* 1996; **22**: 262–7.

104. Hiemenz JW, Walsh TJ. Lipid formulations of amphotericin B: recent progress and future directions. *Clin Infect Dis* 1996; **22** (suppl 2): S133–44.

105. Johnston PG, Lee J, Domanski M. Late recurrent *Candida* endocarditis. *Chest* 1991; **99**: 1531–3.

106. Baddour LM. Long-term suppressive therapy for *Candida parapsilosis*-induced prosthetic valve endocarditis. *Mayo Clin Proc* 1995; **70**: 773–5.

107. Czwerwiec FS, Bilsker MS, Kamerman ML, *et al*. Long-term survival after fluconazole therapy of candidal prosthetic valve endocarditis. *Am J Med* 1993; **94**: 545–55.

108. Norenberg RG, Sethi GK, Scott SM, Takaro T. Opportunistic endocarditis following open-heart surgery. *Ann Thorac Surg* 1975; **19**: 592–604.

109. Lam S, Samraj J, Rahman S, *et al*. Primary actinomycotic endocarditis: case report and review. *Clin Infect Dis* 1993; **16**: 481–5.

110. Guerrero ML, Perea RT, Rodrigo JG, *et al*. Infectious endocarditis due to non-typhi *Salmonella* in patients infected with human immunodeficiency virus: report of two cases and review. *Clin Infect Dis* 1996; **22**: 853–5.

111. Dinubile MJ. Surgery in active endocarditis. *Ann Intern Med* 1982; **96**: 650–9.

112. Acar J, Michel PL, Varenne O, *et al*. Surgical treatment of infective endocarditis. *Eur Heart J* 1995; **16**(suppl B): 94–8.

113. Keys TF. Diagnosis and management of infective endocarditis. *Cleveland Clin J Med* 1990; **57**: 558–62.

114. Larbalestier RI, Kinchla NM, Aranki SF, *et al*. Acute bacterial endocarditis: optimizing surgical results. *Circulation* 1992; **86**(suppl II): 68–74.

115. Calderwood SB, Swinski LA, Karchmer AW, *et al*. Prosthetic valve endocarditis: analysis of factors affecting outcome of therapy. *J Thorac Cardiovasc Surg* 1986; **92**: 776–83.

116. Vlessis AA, Hovaguimian H, Jaggers J, *et al*. Infective endocarditis: ten-year review of medical and surgical therapy. *Ann Thorac Surg* 1996; **61**: 1217–22.

117. Chan P, Ogilby JD, Segal B. Tricuspid valve endocarditis. *Am Heart J* 1989; **117**: 1140–6.

118. Williams DN, Rehm SJ, Tice AD, *et al*. Practice guidelines for community-based parenteral anti-infective therapy. *Clin Infect Dis* 1997; **25**: 787–801.

119. Stamboulian D, Bonvehi P, Arevalo C, *et al*. Antibiotic management of outpatients with endocarditis due to penicillin-susceptible streptococci. *Rev Infect Dis* 1991; **13** (suppl 2): S160–S163.

120. Francioli P, Etienne J, Hoigne R, *et al*. Treatment of streptococcal endocarditis with a single daily dose of ceftriaxone sodium for four weeks: efficacy and outpatient treatment feasibility. *JAMA* 1992; **267**: 264–7.

121. Francioli PB. Ceftriaxone and outpatient treatment of infective endocarditis. *Infect Dis Clin North Am* 1993; **7**: 97–115.

122. Rehm SJ, Weinstein AJ. Home management. In: Magilligan DJ Jr, Quinn EL, eds *Endocarditis: medical and surgical management*. New York: Marcel Dekker, 1986: 117–27.

123. Rehm SJ. Outpatient parenteral antibiotic therapy for endocarditis. *Infect Dis Clin North Am* 1998; **12**: 879–901.

124. Dajani AS, Taubert KA, Wilson W, *et al*. Prevention of bacterial endocarditis. Recommendations by the American Heart Association. *JAMA* 1997; **277**: 1794–801.

125. Blatter M, Francioli P. Endocarditis prophylaxis: from experimental models to human recommendation. *Eur Heart J* 1995; **16**(suppl B): 107–9.

126. Leport C, Horstkotte D, Burckhardt D, *et al*. Antibiotic prophylaxis for infective endocarditis from an international group of experts towards a European consensus. *Eur Heart J* 1995; 16(suppl B): 126–31.

127. Bluhm G. Pacemaker infections. *Acta Med Scand (Suppl)* 1982; **699**: 1–62.

128. Lee JH, Geha AS, Rattehalli NM, *et al*. Salvage of infected ICDs: management without removal. *Pacing Clin Electrophysiol* 1996; **19**(pt 1): 437–22.

129. Arber N, Pras E, Copperman Y, *et al*. Pacemaker endocarditis. Report of 44 cases and review of the literature. *Medicine* 1994; **73**: 299–305.

130. Brook I, Frazier EH. Role of aerobic and anaerobic bacteria in pacemaker infections. *Clin Infect Dis* 1997; **24**: 1010–12.

131. Klug D, Lacroix D, Savoye C, *et al*. Systemic infection related to endocarditis on pacemaker leads. Clinical presentation and management. *Circulation* 1997; **95**: 2098–107.

132. Spratt KA, Blumberg EA, Wood CA, *et al*. Infections of implantable cardioverter defibrillators: approach to management. *Clin Infect Dis* 1993; **17**: 679–85.

133. Perez I, Nunain SO, Osswald S, *et al*. Management of patients with infected implantable cardioverter–defibrillator systems. *Pacing Clin Electrophysiol* 1994; **17**: 780.

134. Grimm W, Flores BF, Marchlinski FE. Complications of implantable cardioverter defibrillator therapy: follow-up of 241 patients. *Pacing Clin Electrophysiol* 1993; **16**(part II): 218–22.

135. Molina JE. Undertreatment and overtreatment of patients with infected antiarrhythmic implantable devices. *Ann Thorac Surg* 1997; **63**: 504–9.

136. McCarthy PM, Schmitt SK, Vargo RL, *et al*. Implantable LVAD infections: implications for permanent use of the device. *Ann Thorac Surg* 1996; **61**: 359–65.

137. Kormos RL, Murali S, Dew MA, *et al*. Chronic mechanical circulatory support: rehabilitation, low morbidity, and superior survival. *Ann Thorac Surg* 1994; **57**: 51–8.

138. McCarthy PM, Wang N, Vargo R. Preperitoneal insertion of the Heartmate 1000 IP implantable left ventricular assist device. *Ann Thorac Surg* 1994; **57**: 634–8.

139. Phillips WS, Burton NA, Marcmanus Q, *et al*. Surgical complications in bridging to transplantation: the Thermo Cardiosystems LVAD. *Ann Thorac Surg* 1992; **52**: 482–6.

140. Myers TJ, McGee MG, Zeluff BJ, *et al*. Frequency and significance of infections in patients receiving prolonged LVAD support. *Transactions* 1991; **37**: M283–M285.

141. McCarthy PM, Portner PM, Tobler HG, *et al*. Clinical experience with the Novacor ventricular assist system. *J Thorac Cardiovasc Surg* 1991; **102**: 578–87.

22

Clinical approach to preoperative risk stratification and management

KIM A EAGLE AND PETER HAGAN

Cardiovascular complications of surgery often result in significant morbidity, increase mortality and prolong patient length of stay. Cardiovascular disease is often occult prior to impending surgery. Several tools are available to aid the clinician in assessing perioperative risk. A stepwise approach, evaluating patient- and surgery-specific variables, is recommended. The role of invasive and pharmacologic therapy in perioperative risk adjustment needs further evaluation.

INTRODUCTION

Since the time of Hippocrates, the primary edict of medicine has been 'do no harm'. Surgical procedures may be complicated by cardiovascular disease, which is often clinically occult prior to surgery. Strategies for perioperative risk assessment are designed to estimate the risk and minimize complications in a rational fashion. With an increasing emphasis on evidence-based medicine and the increased interest in cost-effective care, perioperative risk assessment has evolved rapidly over the past 20 years. The scale of the problem is impressive. Approximately 10 per cent of the population of the USA undergoes surgery each year. About one-third of these have or are considered 'at risk' for cardiovascular disease with estimated in-hospital or long-term complications occurring in 1.5 million patients.[1,2] Variables pertaining to patient, procedure, physician, testing, and institution make the process of accurate risk assessment complex.

HISTORICAL LANDMARKS

Many variables have been assessed as markers of increased perioperative risk. However, review of the literature often reveals conflicting data. Many studies suffer from methodological deficiencies.[1] Also, the relevance of data gathered 10 or more years ago to modern practice is unclear. In an effort to stratify perioperative risk, many indices have been proposed. In 1963, the American Society of Anesthesiologists proposed a simple index based on the clinical status of the patient.[3] It is simple and correlates with outcome. The Goldman index developed a weighted score based on preoperative clinical markers.[4] The Detsky index was a simplified model which added angina and congestive heart failure to risk factors utilized in the Goldman model.[5] A five-variable Eagle index uses simple clinical markers to classify patients into low, intermediate, and high-risk groups.[6]

Assimilating much of the previously published data, a stepwise approach to preoperative coronary assessment was proposed by Paul and Eagle.[7] Subsequently, the American College of Cardiology/American Heart Association (ACC/AHA) published practice guidelines for perioperative cardiovascular evaluation for noncardiac surgery, outlining a similar stepwise approach.[8]

PREOPERATIVE CLINICAL EVALUATION

Perioperative myocardial infarction

The true incidence of perioperative myocardial infarction (MI) is difficult to estimate and varies with the surgical cohort and definition of infarction.[9] While older studies suggest the majority of events occurred within the first 3 days, a more recent study, in which there was a small number of events, documented all infarctions after day 3.[10] The proportion of events occurring intraoperatively may be less than 5 per cent.[11,12] Postoperative MIs are difficult to diagnose, as signs and symptoms are often subtle and diverse, such as fluctuations in blood pressure, arrhythmias, congestive heart failure, and confusion. Electrocardiographic monitoring frequently shows evidence of preceding prolonged ischemia.[1,11–14] Postmortem assessment of fatal MI after non-cardiac surgery shows the nearly uniform presence of severe fixed multivessel coronary artery disease (CAD) with predominantly regional myocardial damage, and evidence of acute coronary plaque disturbance in most cases. The pathophysiology of non-fatal MI may be different, perhaps more related to prolonged ischemia rather than acute plaque disruption.[15] Perioperative myocardial infarction is associated with a high perioperative mortality and reduced long-term survival.[11,16–18]

Preoperative risk assessment

HISTORY

A thorough history is the foundation of preoperative cardiovascular risk assessment.

The history should focus on patient- and surgery-specific variables that may affect perioperative risk.

The likelihood and significance of underlying cardiovascular disease as well as co-morbid illness, functional capacity, and type and urgency of surgery should be established. Time devoted to patient interaction develops rapport and an understanding of the individual's health and lifestyle, as well as their knowledge of cardiovascular disease, risk factors, and prevention.

History of prior or symptomatic CAD, congestive heart failure (CHF), or arrhythmia should be elicited. Coronary risk factors, such as cigarette smoking, hyperlipidemia, diabetes mellitus, family history of premature CAD, peripheral vascular occlusive disease (PVOD),

hypertension, and premature menopause should be evaluated. Specific attention should be given to prior cardiac diagnoses, assessments and treatments, congenital or valvular heart disease, or a past history of rheumatic fever. Co-morbid disorders that may affect perioperative risk and management include diabetes, pulmonary disease, renal failure, anemia, and malignancy. The social history should document substance abuse, especially alcohol and cocaine. Assessment of occupation and the domestic situation are important features of the general evaluation. Medications, dosages, adverse effects, and allergies should be evaluated.

Physical examination

General assessment includes evaluation for respiratory distress, pallor or cyanosis, cachexia or obesity, or markers of congenital or co-morbid disease. Pulse rate, rhythm, contour, and symmetry should be assessed and blood pressure in both arms, lying and supine, should be measured. The head and neck examination should assess for evidence of hyperlipidemia, carotid pulse and bruits, and jugular venous pressure and waveform. The precordial examination should assess apical impulse, heart sounds, murmurs, and added sounds. The remainder of the physical examination should include an assessment for pulmonary rales and wheezes, hepatomegaly or hepatic tenderness, aortic aneurysm, vascular bruits, peripheral pulses, and edema.

Clinical markers of perioperative risk

PRIOR MYOCARDIAL INFARCTION

Patients with known prior MI are at increased risk of perioperative MI, especially if the infarct is recent, although the risk may not be as high as previously thought.[8,15,16,19] Major changes in peri-infarct and long-term management, such as thrombolysis, primary and rescue percutaneous transluminal coronary angioplasty (PTCA), other medical therapy including angiotensin-converting enzyme (ACE) inhibitors, β-blockers and lipid-lowering agents, as well as postinfarct risk stratification, have probably reduced the overall impact of past myocardial infarction, although some elevation in risk remains. Factors that are likely to impact the patient with recent MI include the amount of residual ischemia, left ventricular compensation, and overall clinical status. For elective surgery, it is reasonable to wait 4–6 weeks after myocardial infarction to allow the coronary plaque and myocardium to heal. If a stress test shows no residual ischemia, the likelihood of perioperative reinfarction is low.[8]

UNSTABLE ANGINA

Unstable or severe angina pectoris (Canadian Cardiovascular Society class 3 or 4) is a major predictor for perioperative risk and warrants postponement of elective surgery and appropriate management.[8,20]

AGE AND GENDER

In Western populations, CAD risk increases almost linearly with age. Atherosclerotic plaques develop 10–20 years earlier in men than women.[21,22] Below age 55, CAD is approximately four times more common in men than women. CAD increases in postmenopausal women so that in older persons incidence rates are similar. The mortality of myocardial infarction associated with surgery increases with age.[4,23]

CONGESTIVE HEART FAILURE

Congestive heart failure is a marker of increased perioperative risk. Heart failure patients should be optimized prior to surgery, and special care given to salt and water balance. Patients with newly diagnosed heart failure should be investigated for the underlying etiology and treated accordingly.

VALVULAR HEART DISEASE

The three major considerations in patients with valvular heart disease are: hemodynamic effect, antibiotic prophylaxis, and anticoagulation. Severe symptomatic aortic stenosis is associated with a high risk of perioperative complications.[4] Except for emergent cases, surgery should be postponed until after valve replacement or valvuloplasty has been performed. Patients who must proceed to surgery with stenosis of the aortic valve are likely to be intolerant of major preload or afterload reduction or significant fluctuations in cardiac work, and may decompensate rapidly.

Mitral stenosis may be associated with postoperative tachyarrhythmias (particularly atrial fibrillation) and these are often poorly tolerated. Balloon valvuloplasty or surgery is often indicated in patients with symptomatic mitral stenosis that is discovered prior to elective surgery.[24]

Bradycardia may exacerbate the hemodynamic effects of a regurgitant aortic valve by prolonging diastolic filling time. Volume control and afterload reduction therapy are probably beneficial in reducing perioperative congestive heart failure in such patients.

Mitral regurgitation with prolapse or structural leaflet abnormality warrants perioperative antibiotic prophylaxis.[25] Again, volume control and afterload reduction are likely to be beneficial.

Perioperative management of anticoagulation and antibiotic prophylaxis in patients with prosthetic valves depends on the type of valve and procedure. In patients with valvular heart disease, anticoagulation and antibiotic prophylaxis should be administered according to published guidelines.[25,26]

ARRHYTHMIA AND CONDUCTION ABNORMALITIES

Arrhythmias and conduction abnormalities are important because they may reflect underlying cardiopulmonary pathology. They may progress during the perioperative period and cause hemodynamic compromise. In the absence of severe underlying pathology, such as advanced ischemia or left ventricular dysfunction, prognosis is favorable.[27,28] Conduction abnormalities should be approached as in the non-operative setting. Patients with bifasicular block appear to have less than 1 per cent risk of progressing to complete heart block during or following surgery.[28]

FUNCTIONAL CAPACITY

Assessment of functional capacity is a key element of the history. Many patients presenting for surgery may be asymptomatic but are functionally limited due to age, PVOD, or other factors. The stress of surgery may far exceed the patient's normal metabolic demands. Clearly, two asymptomatic patients, one who runs 10 miles and one who is wheelchair bound may have significantly different risk profiles for surgery. Functional status predicts future cardiac events.[29] One metabolic equivalent (MET) represents the oxygen consumption of a 40-year-old 70 kg male at rest. MET capacity during daily life or with treadmill stress testing correlates with perioperive events.[29] In an effort to quantify functional capacity by history, indices of activity have been developed.[30–32] Table 22.1 outlines metabolic demands of different activities. This provides subjective but semi-quantitative assessment of a patient's functional status.

Table 22.1 *Assessment of functional capacity from history*

Poor (< 4 METs)
Shower/ dress without stopping, make bed, light housework
Walk at 2.5 mph on level ground

Moderate (4–7 METs)
Walk 4 mph on level ground
Outdoor work gardening, raking
Golf, bowling, dancing

Excellent (> 7 METs)
Carry 24 lbs up 8 steps
Shovel snow, dig soil
Strenuous sports: swimming, singles tennis, skiing

METs = metabolic equivalents.

CORONARY REVASCULARIZATION WITHIN THE PAST 5 YEARS

Complete surgical revascularization or coronary angioplasty within 6 months to 5 years without a change in clinical status is associated with a low risk of perioperative cardiac events.[8] Also, if the patient has undergone adequate cardiac evaluation by means of stress testing or coronary angiography within the past 2 years without change in clinical status, then it is often acceptable to forego repeat testing.[7,8]

CO-MORBID DISEASE

Diabetes mellitus

Diabetes is a significant marker of increased risk of perioperative events. Diabetics frequently have advanced and clinically silent CAD. Diabetics, when compared with non-diabetics undergoing non-cardiac surgery with similar preoperative thallium stress test results, had double the perioperative event rate.[33] Perioperative ischemia and infarction are often silent in the diabetic population. Diabetics are at increased risk of perioperative cardiac events following vascular and coronary artery bypass surgery.[6,33-35] Poor longer term prognosis has also been reported in diabetics.[36,37] Diabetics frequently have other end organ damage, are at increased risk of poor wound healing and infection, and may have fluctuation in blood sugar levels that may complicate perioperative care.

Hypertension

Hypertension is often associated with CAD but moderate hypertension does not appear to be an independent risk factor for perioperative complications.[4-6,38,39] Hypertensive patients have greater variation in intraoperative blood pressure and electrocardiogram (ECG) evidence of ischemia is more common.[40,41] Diastolic pressure at or above 110 mm Hg warrants control prior to elective surgery.[8,38] β-Blockers are first-line therapy in the preoperative patient. Target organ damage should be assessed and secondary causes of hypertension considered. Antihypertensive medication should be continued during the perioperative period and discontinuation of drugs that may predispose to rebound phenomenon, such as clonidine, methyldopa, and β-blockers should be avoided. Volume status and electrolytes should be carefully monitored, especially in patients receiving diuretics.

Pulmonary disease

Since cigarette smoking is a common risk factor for premature coronary disease, it comes as no surprise that pulmonary disease and CAD frequently co-exist in smokers. Factors that frequently impact on perioperative care include hypoxia, hypercapnia, atalectasis, pneumonia, acidemia, and arrhythmias. β-Agonists and theophylline may cause tachycardia and other arrhythmias, and predispose to hypokalemia. β-Blockers may be contraindicated in patients with active bronchospasm.

Hematologic disorders

Anemia may significantly affect cardiac oxygen supply/demand balance. This may have an important role in the mechanism of perioperative ischemia.[42] Patients with platelet disorders may have abnormal coagulation, potentially predisposing to coronary thrombus formation or excessive blood loss.

Renal failure

Renal failure, hypertension, diabetes, and CAD are frequently associated. Renal insufficiency may interfere with fluid and electrolyte homeostasis and acid–base control. Drugs, especially ACE inhibitors and diuretics, may exacerbate renal dysfunction and electrolyte abnormalities.

SURGERY SPECIFIC VARIABLES

Perioperative risk varies depending upon the urgency and type of surgery as well as the individual surgeon and institution.[43,44] Emergent surgery may carry up to five times the risk of similar surgery performed on an elective basis.[1,4,5] Aortic abdominal and infrainguinal vascular surgery are associated with a high risk of perioperative complications.[5,45,46] On the other hand, opthalmologic, minor prostate, and day-case procedures carry a low risk of cardiac complications.[5,47-49] It is helpful to know the complication rates for particular procedures in your institution.

RISK STRATIFICATION

Stepwise approach (Figure 22.1)

Step 1: Urgency of surgery?

Step 2: Coronary revascularization within 5 years and asymptomatic?

Step 3: Coronary evaluation within 2 years with adequate assessment and asymptomatic? If the patient requires emergency surgery or has had recent revascularization (within 5 years) or cardiovascular evaluation (within 2 years) with no symptoms, then surgery should proceed without further work-up.

Step 4: Major predictor of risk? If the patient has a major clinical predictor of risk, then surgery should be postponed and the underlying condition fully evaluated and treated (Table 22.2).

Step 5: Intermediate predictor of risk? If the patient has intermediate predictors of risk, then functional capacity and surgery-specific risk should be evaluated in an attempt to determine which patients may benefit from further non-invasive testing (Table 22.3).

Step 6: Functional capacity and surgery-specific risk combined with intermediate predictors of risk. Patients with intermediate predictors of risk and moderate-to-excellent functional capacity can generally undergo intermediate risk surgery with a low risk of complications. Poor functional capacity or moderate functional capacity and higher risk surgery usually warrant non-invasive testing.

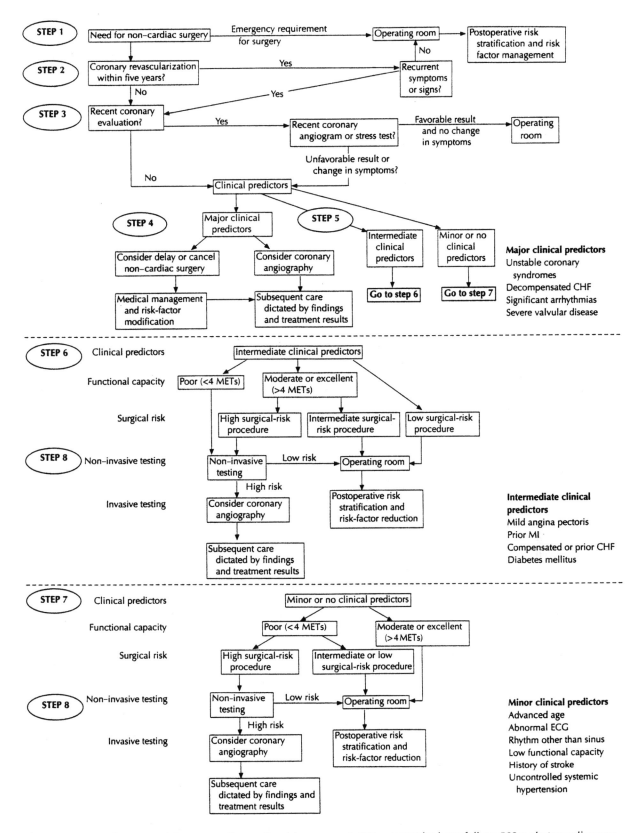

Figure 22.1 *Stepwise approach to preoperative cardiac risk assessment. CHF = congestive heart failure; ECG = electrocardiogram; MET = metabolic equivalent; MI = myocardial infarction.*

Table 22.2 *Clinical predictors of increased perioperative risk*

Major

Unstable coronary syndromes: myocardial infarction (MI) within 7–30 days with evidence of ischemia by history or non-invasive study; Canadian Class 3 or 4 angina

Decompensated heart failure

Significant arrhythmias

Severe valvular disease

Intermediate

Mild angina pectoris (Canadian Class 1 or 2)

Prior MI by history or pathological Q waves

Compensated or prior congestive heart failure

Diabetes mellitus

Minor

Advanced age

Abnormal electrocardiogram (left ventricular hypertrophy, left bundle branch block, ST-T abnormalities); rhythm other than sinus

Low functional capacity

Prior stroke

Uncontrolled systemic hypertension

Table 22.3 *Cardiac risk stratification for non-cardiac surgical procedures*

High

Emergent major surgery

Aortic and other major vascular

Peripheral vascular

Prolonged surgery associated with large fluid shifts

Intermediate

Carotid endarterectomy

Head and neck

Intraperitoneal and intrathoracic

Orthopedic

Prostate

Low

Endoscopic procedures

Cataract

Breast

Superficial procedure

Step 7:   Functional capacity and surgery-specific risk combined with low or no predictors of risk. In the absence of major or minor predictors of risk, and at least moderate functional capacity, proceeding with surgery is generally safe. In patients with several minor factors and poor functional capacity undergoing major surgery, further work-up may be warranted.

Step 8:   Non-invasive testing. Before proceeding with further testing, the effect the result will have on further patient care should be considered. Patients at low clinical risk generally do not need further risk stratification. Patients with major clinical markers are likely to have

significant underlying disease and may warrant an aggressive approach, perhaps including cardiac catheterization. Patients classified as intermediate risk may benefit most from further non-invasive testing.[6,49,50]

NON-INVASIVE TESTING

Exercise stress testing

If possible, exercise (as opposed to pharmacologic) stress testing is the method of choice to evaluate for coronary risk because of the added information provided by workload, maximum heart rate achieved, blood pressure response, onset of symptoms and ECG changes, and their duration into recovery. Patients unable to reach 75 per cent or 85 per cent of predicted maximum heart rate (PMHR) or >5 METs are at increased risk of perioperative events. If poor workload is associated with ECG evidence of ischemia, then the risk is greater.[1,51–53]

> The negative predictive value (NPV) of a normal, adequate, ECG stress test for perioperative MI or death is probably greater than 95 per cent.

The positive predictive value is much lower. However, many patients have baseline ECG abnormalities, which interfere with interpretation and up to 50 per cent of patients seen for preoperative assessment for major surgery are unable to perform adequate exercise testing.[6,54] Sensitivity may be improved by the addition of myocardial imaging for patients with baseline ECG abnormalities.[55]

Pharmacological stress testing

Dipyridamole is a coronary vasodilator that results in relatively greater flow to areas of normal perfusion. The major factor in determining the value of dipyridamole-thallium scintigraphy (DTS) in preoperative evaluation appears to be of patient selection, as the positive predictive value (PPV) is highly correlated to the underlying prevalence of disease and the pretest probability of an event.[6,56] In critical coronary stenosis, ischemia may occur as a result of a 'steal' phenomenon.[57] Dipyridamole may also cause bronchospasm and hypotension, and should be avoided in patients with bronchospasm and critical carotid stenosis. For various reasons, reported PPV rates are low and have fallen over time.[8] One study showed that thallium redistribution had a PPV of only 5 per cent for cardiac death or MI.[58]

> The negative predictive value of a normal scan, especially in vascular patients, is high, particularly in patients at intermediate risk by clinical markers.[6,59]

A fixed defect may be an independent predictor of risk and may better predict long-term events.[60] A fixed defect may represent an area of prior infarction or an area that demonstrates redistribution on late imaging that suggests severe restriction in baseline coronary flow to a viable region of myocardium.[61] Multiple defects on thallium scan correlates with greater perioperative risk as these patients are more likely to have multivessel CAD.[62] Ischemia on ECG associated with dipyridamole also correlates with an increased perioperative risk.[6] Left ventricular dilatation or increased lung uptake of tracer are worrisome features and may also indicate a high risk of periopertive complications.[63]

Adenosine, a coronary vasodilator, combined with thallium appears to yield similar results as those provided by dipyridamole thallium imaging.[57,64] Dobutamine is a β1 receptor agonist with positive inotropic and chronotropic effects. It may be substituted as the pharmacological stressor prior to perfusion imaging in patients at risk for bronchospasm, known serious arrhythmias, hypertension or hypotension, or patients who have ingested caffeine or theopylline. It is used less frequently, but predictive values appear comparable.[65,66]

Dobutamine stress echocardiography (DSE) is becoming a more commonly utilized method of preoperative stress testing, and predictive values appear to be similar to that of DTS.[67–69] Echocardiography provides additional information regarding cardiac structure and function, and is particularly useful in assessing valvular disease. DSE is safe and well tolerated, although arrhythmias and hypotension and hypertension may occur.[70,71] In patients with left bundle branch block, tachycardia induced during stress testing may result in abnormal septal wall motion. Therefore, vasodilator stress and myocardial perfusion studies are preferred modalities in these patients.[8] Patients with anticipated or proven poor-quality echo images should be referred for myocardial perfusion study.

Assessment of left ventricular function

> Routine assessment of resting left ventricular (LV) function is not indicated since its reliability in predicting perioperative complications is not clear.[8]

Assessment of LV function is appropriate in individual patients as part of a work-up of CHF, especially if CHF is recent or poorly controlled. Ambulatory ECG monitoring has been shown to predict perioperative ischemia. Interestingly, ischemia on Holter monitor in the early postoperative period is much more sensitive for perioperative complications than preoperative or intraoperative ischemia.[11] Some centers have used early postoperative ischemia monitoring to identify patients at

short- and long-term risk. However, the cost effectiveness of this approach over and above usual postoperative surveillance is not yet clear.

PREOPERATIVE THERAPY

Coronary artery bypass grafting

Patients who have undergone prior coronary artery bypass grafting (CABG) and remain asymptomatic are at low risk of perioperative complications.[36,37,71] Data from the Coronary Artery Surgery Study (CASS) registry shows 0.9 per cent perioperative cardiac mortality in prior CABG patients vs 0.5 per cent in the patients with no angiographic evidence of CAD, and 2.4 per cent event rate in those patients with angiographic evidence of 70 per cent or greater stenosis in one or more arteries who did not receive CABG.[71] CABG appears to improve long-term survival in certain subsets of patients with severe disease, whether or not they are identified in the preoperative setting.[36,72,73] However, performing CABG as a preoperative treatment to lower risk of non-cardiac surgery adds the 'up-front' risk of the bypass surgery, thus increasing the total short-term risk to the patient. The risk of CABG for many patients is low; higher rates of complications occur in elderly patients and/or those with PVOD. For such individuals, CABG itself confers such risk that it is rarely justified in order to simply lower perioperative risk of non-cardiac surgery.

> In general, indications for CABG prior to non-cardiac surgery are similar to those in the non-operative setting.

These include significant left main disease, three-vessel CAD with left ventricular dysfunction, or two-vessel disease with severe proximal left anterior descending artery stenosis when accompanied by uncontrolled symptoms or a positive stress test.[74]

Percutaneous coronary interventions

The value of PCI in reducing perioperative complications is unclear. There may be a role in certain symptomatic patients prior to high-risk surgery.[74–77] The same guidelines for the use of PCI in the non-operative setting apply.[78] The optimal timing of surgery in patients who have undergone PCI is not known. For recent coronary interventions it is reasonable to allow up to a month for endovascular stability to occur. However, prolonged delay (more than a few weeks) increases the risk of re-stenosis. After 6 months, re-stenosis is less likely to be a problem.

Medical therapy

Data on the use of medical therapy to reduce perioperative events are limited. β-Blockers appear to be associated with a reduction in perioperative events.[79]

> If possible, therapy should be started at least 48 hours prior to surgery and continued through the perioperative period.

Nitroglycerin may reduce the incidence of perioperative ischemia, but the effect on overall outcome remains unclear.[8,80,81] It is reasonable to use nitroglycerin intravenously in high-risk patients previously on nitrates who have active signs of myocardial ischemia without hypotension.[8] There are insufficient data to support the use of calcium-channel blockers. Aspirin frequently is discontinued prior to surgery in an effort to reduce perioperative bleeding. The role of aspirin in reducing perioperative events is not known, hence the overall risk–benefit effect of discontinuing this therapy in high-risk coronary patients is not defined.

Anesthesia

> The choice of anesthetic agent does not appear to affect the rate of perioperative cardiac complications.[81–86]

Indeed, it may not be the drug that matters as much as who gives it. Adequate pain control is especially important in the patient at increased risk of perioperative complications, since pain influences factors associated with myocardial ischemia including catecholamine levels.

Intraoperative monitoring

The role of pulmonary artery catheters is uncertain.[87,88] Pulmonary artery catheters are associated with important risks, and guidelines regarding their use were published in 1993.[89] They are helpful in managing the patient with significant ventricular dysfunction undergoing major surgery. Transesophageal echocardiography may be used to detect wall motion abnormalities during surgery, but sensitivity for identifying patient's risk is low. At present it is not recommended as a routine method of monitoring patients during non-cardiac surgery.[8]

Surveillance for postoperative infarction

The optimal protocol for detecting perioperative MI is not known. In patients without evidence of CAD, surveillance should be done only in those with signs of perioperative myocardial dysfunction.[8] In patients with known or suspected CAD undergoing high-risk surgery, serial ECG at baseline, in recovery room, and daily for 2 days is recommended. Measurement of cardiac enzymes should be limited to patients at high risk or those with evidence of ischemia. Creatine kinase (CK) assays vary between laboratories and non-cardiac sources may result in false-positive assays. The degree of elevation of CK appears to correlate to overall survival. Enzymes such as troponin T or I may be specific to the myocardium, but their role in defining perioperative ischemia or infarction is evolving.[8]

LONG-TERM RISK FACTOR ASSESSMENT AND MANAGEMENT

Perioperative risk stratification provides a special opportunity to reduce the risk of long-term cardiovascular disease. Since coronary heart disease remains the most common cause of death in the USA and the prevalence is increasing rapidly in some developing countries, every reasonable effort to identify and treat subclinical disease and its risk factors should be made. The Cleveland Clinic data shows that the 5-year mortality rate for patients undergoing vascular surgery was 40 per cent.

In the preoperative moment, many of these patients may be having a cardiovascular assessment for the first time. It is vital to identify coronary risk factors and focus on patient education. Perhaps, the single largest area for benefit is in the area of lipid control. There is substantial evidence to support the role of elevated cholesterol in the pathogenesis of CAD. Several clinical trials have demonstrated a significant reduction in CAD risk with cholesterol-lowering therapy.[90–94]

Patients should be encouraged to stop smoking and referred to a smoking cessation program. Emphasis should be placed on antihypertensive therapy and glycemic management to prevent long-term complications.

FUTURE CONSIDERATIONS

1 Clarify and modulate the neurohumoral and hemostatic factors that promote ischemia and plaque destabilization.
2 Clarify the role of PCI and stent treatment to lower perioperative risk.
3 Further study of pharmacologic agents, including new agents, such as angiotensin 2 receptor antagonists, in at risk patients.

CLINICAL OVERVIEW

Much change and progress in the area of perioperative care has occurred over recent years in an effort to simplify, rationalize, and improve patient care. The goal of perioperative cardiovascular assessment is to provide thorough risk-factor evaluation and modification as opposed to simply 'clearing' the patient for surgery. In general, the risk of perioperative events is low. Patients are categorized into low-, intermediate- or high-risk groups. Surgery-specific risk, prior cardiac evaluation, and/or revascularization and level of functional capacity are assessed to determine the need for further non-invasive or invasive testing. In general, indications for further testing are similar to those in the non-operative setting. The potential to modify long-term risk has been highlighted and should be part of every assessment. Special consideration should be given to diabetics, who represent a high-risk group. Long-term changes are best accomplished through effective communication with the patient, as well as within the health care team. Future advancements in perioperative risk stratification and treatment will undoubtedly improve perioperative patient care.

SUMMARY

- Perioperative cardiac risk varies with type and urgency of surgery. Aortic, peripheral vascular, and urgent surgery are high risk.
- Patients with a recent satisfactory cardiovascular assessment or revascularization procedure without subsequent symptoms usually do not require further evaluation.
- The history should focus on cardiovascular risk factors, co-morbidities and clinical markers of elevated risk, such as diabetes, congestive heart failure, arryhthmias, and valvular heart disease.
- Functional capacity correlates with perioperative risk; a higher functional capacity means lower perioperative risk.
- The approach to further cardiac assessment is similar to the non-operative setting.
- Exercise treadmill testing is the preferred form of stress testing but patient factors frequently preclude its use. Pharmacologic stress testing is a helpful alternative.
- Medications, especially antihypertensives, should be continued perioperatively, and β-blockers appear to reduce the incidence of perioperative ischemic events.
- The type of anesthesia does not appear to affect risk significantly.
- Diabetics represent a high-risk group.
- Long-term risk factor assessment and modification should be part of the perioperative assessment.

REFERENCES

♦1. Mangano DT. Perioperative cardiac morbidity. *Anesthesiology* 1990; **72**: 153–84.

2. National Center for Health Statistics. *Health United States 1988*. Public Health Service. Washington, DC; US Government Printing Office, 1989. DHSS publication (PHS) 89–1232: 10–17, 66, 67, 100, 101, 1989.

3. American Society of Anesthesiologists. New classification of physical status. *Anesthesiology* 1963; **24**: 111.

♦4. Goldman L, Caldera DL, Nussbaum SR, *et al*. Multifactorial index of cardiac risk in noncardiac surgical procedures. *N Engl J Med* 1977; **297**: 845–50.

5. Detsky AS, Abrams HB, Forbath N, Scott JG, Hilliard JR. Cardiac assessment for patients undergoing noncardiac surgery: a multifactorial clinical risk index. *Arch Intern Med* 1986; **146**: 2131–4.

♦6. Eagle KA, Coley CM, Newell JB, *et al*. Combining clinical and thallium data optimizes preoperative assessment of cardiac risk before major vascular surgery. *Ann Intern Med* 1989; **110**: 859–66.

7. Paul SD, Eagle KA. A stepwise strategy for coronary risk assessment for non cardiac surgery. *Med Clin North Am* 1995; **79**: 1241–62.

○8. Eagle KA, Brundage NH, Chaitman BR, *et al*. Guidelines for perioperative cardiovascular evaluation for noncardiac surgery. *Circulation* 1996; **93**: 1278–317.

9. Charlson ME, McKenzie CR, Ales KL, *et al*. The postoperative electrocardiogram and creatine kinase: implications for diagnosis of myocardial infarction after noncardiac surgery. *J Clin Epidemiol* 1989; **42**: 25–34.

♦10. Poldermans D, Fioretti PM, Forster T, *et al*. Dobutamine stress echocardiography for assessment of perioperative cardiac risk in patients undergoing major vascular surgery. *Circulation* 1993; **87**: 1507–12.

11. Mangano DT, Browner WS, Hollenberg M, London MJ, Tubau JF, Tateo IM. Association of perioperative myocardial ischemia with cardiac morbidity and mortality in men undergoing noncardiac surgery: the Study of Perioperative Ischemia Research Group. *N Engl J Med* 1990; **323**: 1781–8.

12. Mangano DT, Hollenberg M, Fegert G, *et al*. Perioperative myocardial ischemia in patients undergoing noncardiac surgery: incidence and severity during the 4 day perioperative period. *J Am Coll Cardiol* 1991; **17**: 843–50.

13. Landesberg G, Luria MH, Cotev S, *et al*. Importance of long-duration postoperative ST-segment depression in cardiac morbidity after vascular surgery. *Lancet* 1993; **341**: 715–19.

14. Raby KE, Barry J, Creager MA, Cook EF, Weisberg MC, Goldman L. Detection and significance of intraoperative and postoperative myocardial ischemia in peripheral vascular surgery. *JAMA* 1992; **268**: 222–7.

○15. Coley CM, Eagle KE. Pre-operative assessment and

management of cardiac ischemic risk in non-cardiac surgery. *Curr Probl Cardiol* 1996; **21**: 289–382.

16. Rao TL, Jacobs KH, El-Etr AA. Reinfarction following anesthesia in patients with myocardial infarction. *Anesthesiology* 1983; **59**: 499–505.

17. Mangano DT, Browner WS, Hollenberg M, Li J, Tateo IM. Long-term cardiac prognosis following noncardiac surgery: the Study of Perioperative Ischemia Research Group. *JAMA* 1992; **268**: 233–9.

18. Yeager RA, Moneta GL, Edwards JM, Taylor LM Jr, McConnell DB, Porter JM. Late survival after perioperative myocardial infarction complicating vascular surgery. *J Vasc Surg* 1994; **20**: 598–606.

19. Shah KB, Kleinman BS, Sami H, Patel J, Rao TLK. Reevaluation of perioperative myocardial infarction in patients with prior myocardial infarction undergoing noncardiac operations. *Anesth Analg* 1990; **71**: 231–5.

20. Unstable angina: diagnosis and management. Clinical practice guideline number 10. AHCPR publication #94-0602. 1995 GPO Washington DC.

21. Tejada C, Strong JP, Montenegro MR, Restrepo C, Solberg LA. Distribution of coronary and aortic atherosclerosis by geographic location, race, and sex. *Lab Invest* 1968; **18**: 509–26.

22. Castelli WP. Epidemiology of coronary heart disease: the Framingham study. *Am J Med* 1984; **76**: 4–12.

23. Detsky AS, Abrams HB, McLaughlin JR, *et al*. Predicting cardiac complications in patients undergoing non-cardiac surgery. *J Gen Intern Med* 1986; **1**: 211–19.

24. Reyes VP, Raju BS, Wynne J, *et al*. Percutaneous balloon valvuloplasty compared with open surgical commissurotomy for mitral stenosis. *N Engl J Med* 1994; **331**: 961–7.

25. Dajani AS, Bisno AL, Chung KJ, *et al*. Prevention of bacterial endocarditis: recommendations by the American Heart Association. *JAMA* 1990; **264**: 2919–22.

26. Stein PD, Alpert JS, Copeland J, Dalen JE, Goldman S, Turpie AGG. Antithrombotic therapy in patients with mechanical and biological prosthetic heart valves. *Chest* 1992; **102**(suppl): 445S–455S.

27. Kennedy HL, Whitlock JA, Sprague MK, Kennedy LJ, Buckingham TA, Goldberg RJ. Long-term follow-up of asymptomatic healthy subjects with frequent and complex ventricular ectopy. *N Engl J Med* 1985; **312**: 193–7.

28. Pastore JO, Yurchak PM, Janis KM, Murphy JD, Zir LM. The risk of advanced heart block in surgical patients with right bundle branch block and left axis deviation. *Circulation* 1978; **57**: 677–80.

29. Weiner DA, Ryan TJ, McCabe CH, *et al*. Prognostic importance of a clinical profile and exercise test in medically treated patients with coronary artery disease. *J Am Coll Cardiol* 1984; **3**: 772–9.

30. Hlatky MA, Boineau RE, Higginbotham MB, *et al*. A brief self-administered questionnaire to determine functional capacity (the Duke Activity Status Index). *Am J Cardiol* 1989; **64**: 651–4.

31. Nelson CL, Herndon JE, Mark DB, Pryor DB, Califf RM, Hlatky MA. Relation of clinical and angiographic factors to functional capacity as measured by the Duke Activity Status Index. *Am J Cardiol* 1991; **68**: 973–5.

32. Myers J, Do D, Herbert W, Ribisl P, Froelicher VF. A nomogram to predict exercise capacity from a specific activity questionnaire and clinical data. *Am J Cardiol* 1994; **73**: 591–6.

33. Brown KA, Rowan M. Extent of jeopardized viable myocardium determined by myocardial perfusion imaging best predicts perioperative cardiac events in patients undergoing non cardiac surgery. *J Am Coll Cardiol* 1993; **21**: 325–30.

34. Salomon NW, Page US, Okies JE, Stephens J, Krause AH, Bigelow C. Diabetes and coronary artery bypass: short term risks and long term prognosis. *J Thorac Cardiovasc Surg* 1983; **85**: 264–71.

35. Tischler MD, Lee TH, Hirsch AT, *et al*. Prediction of major events after peripheral vascular surgery using dipyridamole echocardiography. *Am J Cardiol* 1991; **68**: 593–7.

36. Hertzer NR, Young JR, Beven EG, O'Hara PJ, Graor RA, Ruschhaupt WF, Maljovec LC. Late results of coronary bypass in patients with peripheral vascular disease, I: five-year survival according to age and clinical cardiac status. *Cleveland Clin Q* 1986; **53**: 133–43.

37. Hertzer NR, Young JR, Beven EG, O'Hara PJ, Graor RA, Ruschhaupt WF, Maljovec LC. Late results of coronary bypass in patients with peripheral vascular disease, II: five-year survival according to sex, hypertension, and diabetes. *Cleveland Clin J Med* 1987; **54**: 15–23.

38. The fifth report of the Joint National Committee on Detection, Evaluation, and Treatment of High Blood Pressure (JNC V). *Arch Intern Med* 1993; **153**: 154–83.

39. Lette J, Waters D, Bernier H, *et al*. Preoperative and long-term cardiac risk assessment: predictive value of 23 clinical descriptors, 7 multivariate scoring systems, and quantitative dipyridamole imaging in 360 patients. *Ann Surg* 1992; **216**: 192–204.

40. Stone JG, Foex P, Sear JW, Johnson LL, Khambatta HJ, Triner L. Myocardial ischemia in untreated hypertensive patients: effect of a single small oral dose of alpha-adrenergic blocking agent. *Anesthesiology* 1988; **68**: 495–500.

41. Stone JG, Foex P, Sear JW, Johnson LL, Khambatta HJ, Triner L. Risk of myocardial ischaemia during anaesthesia in treated and untreated hypertensive patients. *Br J Anaesth* 1988; **61**: 675–9.

42. Juste RN, Lawson AD, Soni N. Minimising cardiac anaesthetic risk: the tortoise or the hare? *Anaesthesia* 1996; **51**: 255–62.

43. Hannan EL, Kilburn H Jr, O'Donnell JF, Bernard HR, Shields EP, Lindsey ML, Yazici A. A longitudinal analysis of the relationship between in-hospital mortality in New York State and the volume of abdominal aortic aneurysm surgeries performed. *Health Serv Res* 1992; **27**: 517–42.

♦44. Hannan EL, O'Donnell JF, Kilburn H Jr, Bernard HR, Yazici A. Investigation of the relationship between volume and mortality for surgical procedures performed in New York State hospitals. *JAMA* 1989; **262**: 503–10.

45. Ashton CM, Petersen NJ, Wray NP, Kiefe CI, Dunn JK, Wu L, Thomas JM. The incidence of perioperative myocardial infarction in men undergoing noncardiac surgery. *Ann Intern Med* 1993; **118**: 504–10.

46. Pedersen T, Eliasen K, Henriksen E. A prospective study of risk factors and cardiopulmonary complications associated with anaesthesia and surgery: risk indicators of cardiopulmonary morbidity. *Acta Anaesthesiol Scand* 1990; **34**: 144–55.

47. Backer CL, Tinker JH, Robertson DM, Vlietstra RE. Myocardial reinfarction following local anesthesia for ophthalmic surgery. *Anesth Analg* 1980; **59**: 257–62.

48. Warner MA, Shields SE, Chute CG. Major morbidity and mortality within 1 month of ambulatory surgery and anesthesia. *JAMA* 1993; **270**: 1437–41.

♦49. Wong T, Detsky AS. Preoperative cardiac risk assessment for patients having peripheral vascular surgery. *Ann Intern Med* 1992; 166 : 743–53.

50. L'Italien GJ, Cambria RP, Cutler BS, *et al.* Comparative early and late cardiac morbidity among patients requiring different vascular surgery procedures. *J Vasc Surg* 1995; **21**: 935–44.

51. Gerson MC, Hurst JM, Hertzberg VS, Baughman R, Rouan GW, Ellis K. Prediction of cardiac and pulmonary complications related to elective abdominal and noncardiac thoracic surgery in geriatric patients. *Am J Med* 1990; **88**: 101–7.

52. Cutler BS, Wheeler HB, Paraskos JA, Cardullo PA. Applicability and interpretation of electrocardiographic stress testing in patients with peripheral vascular disease. *Am J Surg* 1981; **141**: 501–6.

53. McPhail N, Calvin JE, Shariatmadar A, Barber GG, Scobie TK. The use of preoperative exercise testing to predict cardiac complications after arterial reconstruction. *J Vasc Surg* 1988; **7**: 60–8.

54. Browner WS, Li J, Mangano DT, for the Study of Perioperative Ischemia Group. In-hospital and long-term mortality in male veterans following noncardiac surgery. *JAMA* 1992; **268**: 228–32.

55. Botvinick EH. Stress imaging: current clinical options for the diagnosis, localization, and evaluation of coronary artery disease. *Med Clin North Am* 1995; **79**: 1025–61.

♦56. Baron JF, Mundler O, Bertrand M, *et al.* Dipyridamole–thallium scintigraphy and gated radionuclide angiography to assess cardiac risk before abdominal aortic surgery. *N Engl J Med* 1994; **330**: 663–9.

57. Marshall ES, Raichlen JS, Forman S, Heyrich GP, Keen WD, Weitz HH. Adenosine radionuclide perfusion imaging in the preoperative evaluation of patients undergoing peripheral vascular surgery. *Am J Cardiol* 1995; **76**: 817–21.

58. Mangano DT, London MJ, Tubau JF, *et al.* Dipyridamole thallium-201 scintigraphy as a preoperative screening test: a re-examination of its predictive potential. *Circulation* 1991; **84**: 493–502.

59. Marwick TH, Underwood DA. Dipyridamole–thallium imaging may not be a reliable screening test for coronary artery disease in patients undergoing vascular surgery. *Clin Cardiol* 1990; **13**: 14–18.

60. McEnroe CS, O'Donnell RF Jr, Yeager A, Konstam M, Mackey WC. Comparison of ejection fraction and Goldman risk factor analysis of dipyridamole–thallium 201 studies in the evaluation of cardiac morbidity after aortic aneurysm surgery. *J Vasc Surg* 1990; **11**: 497–504.

61. Dilsizian V, Rocco TP, Freedman NMT, Leon MB, Bonow RO. Enhanced detection of ischemic but viable myocardium by the reinjection of thallium after stress-redistribution imaging. *N Engl J Med* 1990; **323**: 141–6.

62. Josephson MA, Brown BG, Hecht HS, Hopkins J, Pierce CD, Petersen RB. Noninvasive detection of and localization of coronary stenosis in patients: comparison of resting dipyridamole and exercise thallium-201 myocardial perfusion imaging. *Am Heart J* 1982; **103**: 1008–18.

63. Lette J, Waters D, Cerino M, Picard M, Champagne P, Lapointe J. Preoperative coronary artery disease risk stratification based on dipyridamole imaging and a simple three-step, three-segment model for patients undergoing non-cardiac vascular surgery or major general surgery. *Am J Cardiol* 1992; **69**: 1553–8.

64. Shaw L, Miller D, Kong B, *et al.* Determination of perioperative cardiac risk by adenosine thallium-201 myocardial imaging. *Am Heart J* 1992; **124**: 861–9.

65. Elliott BM, Robison JG, Zellner JL, Hendrix GH. Dobutamine-201 thallium imaging: assessing cardiac risks associated with vascular surgery. *Circulation* 1991; **84**: III54–60.

66. Zellner JL, Elliott BM, Robison JG, Hendrix GH, Spicer KM. Preoperative evaluation of cardiac risk using dobutamine thallium imaging in vascular surgery. *Ann Vasc Surg* 1990; **4**: 238–43.

♦67. Lane RT, Sawada SG, Segar DS, *et al.* Dobutamine stress echocardiography for assessment of cardiac risk before noncardiac surgery. *Am J Cardiol* 1991; **68**: 976–7.

68. Lalka SG, Sawada SG, Dalsing MC, *et al.* Dobutamine stress echocardiography as a predictor of cardiac events associated with aortic surgery. *J Vasc Surg* 1992; **15**: 831–40.

69. Eichelberger JP, Schwarz KQ, Black ER, Green RM, Ouriel K. Predictive value of dobutamine echocardiography just before noncardiac vascular surgery. *Am J Cardiol* 1993; **72**: 602–7.

70. Prevateli M, Lanzarini L. Pharmacologic echocardiographic testing. *Coronary Artery Dis* 1992; **3**: 679–86.

71. Foster ED, Davis KB, Carpenter JA, Abele S, Fray D. Risk of noncardiac operation in patients with defined coronary disease: The Coronary Artery Surgery Study

(CASS) Registry Experience. *Ann Thorac Surg* 1986; **41**: 42–9.

72. European Coronary Surgery Study Group. Long-term results of prospective randomised study of coronary artery bypass surgery in stable angina pectoris. *Lancet* 1982; **2**: 1173–80.

73. Varnauskas E. Twelve-year survival in the randomized European Coronary Surgery Study. *N Engl J Med* 1988; **319**: 332–7.

74. Guidelines and indications for coronary artery bypass graft surgery: a report of the American College of Cardiology/American Heart Association Task Force on Assessment of Diagnostic and Therapeutic Cardiovascular Procedures (Subcommittee on Coronary Artery Bypass Graft Surgery). *J Am Coll Cardiol* 1991; **17**: 543–89.

75. Huber KC, Evans MA, Bresnahan JF, Gibbons RJ, Holmes DR Jr. Outcome of noncardiac operations in patients with severe coronary artery disease successfully treated preoperatively with coronary angioplasty. *Mayo Clin Proc* 1992; **67**: 15–21.

76. Elmore JR, Hallett JW Jr, Gibbons RJ, *et al*. Myocardial revascularization before abdominal aortic aneurysmorrhaphy: effect of coronary angioplasty. *Mayo Clin Proc* 1993; **68**: 637–41.

77. Allen JR, Helling TS, Hartzler GO. Operative procedures not involving the heart after percutaneous transluminal coronary angioplasty. *Surg Gynecol Obstet* 1991; **173**: 285–8.

78. Guidelines for percutaneous transluminal coronary angioplasty: a report of the American College of Cardiology/American Heart Association Task Force on Assessment of Diagnostic and Therapeutic Cardiovascular Procedures (Committee on Percutaneous Transluminal Coronary Angioplasty). *J Am Coll Cardiol* 1993; **22**: 2033–54.

♦79. Pasternack PF, Imparato AM, Baumann FG, *et al*. The hemodynamics of β-blockade in patients undergoing abdominal aortic aneurysm repair. *Circulation* 1987; **76**(suppl 3, pt 2): 1111–7.

80. Dodds TM, Stone JG, Coromilas J, Weinberger M, Levy DG. Prophylactic nitroglycerin infusion during noncardiac surgery does not reduce perioperative ischemia. *Anesth Analg* 1993; **76**: 705–13.

81. Godet G, Coriat P, Baron JF, Bertrand M, Diquet B, Sebag C, Viars P. Prevention of intraoperative myocardial ischemia during noncardiac surgery with intravenous diltiazem: a randomized trial versus placebo. *Anesthesiology* 1987; **66**: 241–5.

82. Cohen MM, Duncan PG, Tate RB. Does anesthesia contribute to operative mortality? *JAMA* 1988; **260**: 2859–63.

83. Leung JM, Goehner P, O'Kelly BF, Hollenberg M, Pineda N, Cason BA, Mangano DT. Isoflurane anesthesia and myocardial ischemia: comparative risk versus

sufentanil anesthesia in patients undergoing coronary artery bypass graft surgery. The SPI (Study of Perioperative Ischemia) Research Group. *Anesthesiology* 1991; **74**: 838–47.

84. Baron JF, Bertrand M, Barre E, Godet G, Mundler O, Coriat P, Viars P. Combined epidural and general anesthesia versus general anesthesia for abdominal aortic surgery. *Anesthesiology* 1991; **75**: 611–18.

85. Christopherson R, Beattie C, Frank SM, *et al*. Perioperative morbidity in patients randomized to epidural or general anesthesia for lower extremity vascular surgery: Perioperative Ischemia Randomized Anesthesia Trial Study Group. *Anesthesiology* 1993; **79**: 422–34.

86. Slogoff S, Keats AS. Randomized trial of primary anesthetic agents on outcome of coronary artery bypass operations. *Anesthesiology* 1989; **70**: 179–88.

87. Isaacson IJ, Lowdon JD, Berry AJ, Smith RB III, Knos GB, Weitz FI, Ryan K. The value of pulmonary artery and central venous monitoring in patients undergoing abdominal aortic reconstructive surgery: a comparative study of two selected, randomized groups. *J Vasc Surg* 1990; **12**: 754–60.

88. Joyce WP, Provan JL, Ameli FM, McEwan MM, Jelenich S, Jones DP. The role of central haemodynamic monitoring in abdominal aortic surgery: a prospective randomised study. *Eur J Vasc Surg* 1990; **4**: 633–6.

89. Practice guidelines for pulmonary artery catheterization: a report by the American Society of Anesthesiologists Task Force on Pulmonary Artery Catheterization. *Anesthesiology* 1993; **78**: 380–94.

90. Byington RP, Jukema JW, Salonen JT, *et al*. Reduction in cardiac events during pravastatin therapy: pooled analysis of clinical events of the Pravastatin Atherosclerosis Intervention Program. *Circulation* 1995; **92**: 2419–25.

91. Scandanavian Simvastatin Study Survival Group. Randomized trial of cholesterol lowering in 4444 patients with coronary heart disease: the Scandanavian Simvastatin Survival Study (4S). *Lancet* 1994; **334**: 1383–9.

92. Sacks FM, Pfeffer MA, Mote LA, *et al*., for the cholesterol and recurrent events trial Investigators. The effects of pravastatin in coronary events after myocardial infarction in patients with average cholesterol levels. *N Engl J Med* 1996; **335**: 1001–3.

93. Sheperd J, Cobbe SM, Ford I, *et al*., for the West of Scotland Coronary Prevention Study Group. Prevention of coronary heart disease with pravastatin in men with hypercholesterolemia. *N Engl J Med* 1995; **33**: 1301–7.

94. Summary of the second report of the National Cholesterol Education Program (NCEP) Expert Panel on Detection, Evaluation, and Treatment of High Blood Cholesterol in Adults (Adult Treatment Panel II). *JAMA* 1993; **269**: 3015–23.

23

Reducing hospital length of stay for cardiovascular disease states: cost-effective evaluation and treatment

DAVID N RUBIN AND ERIC J TOPOL

Achieving and maintaining high levels of patient care is the endeavor of all clinicians and health care providers. To this end, clinical pathways derived from consensus statements, randomized clinical trials and published guidelines represent a readily achievable means to standardize care within hospitals, ambulatory practices and multi-center clinical systems. The development and utilization of clinical pathways also provides a mechanism for tracking costs and patient outcomes, facilitating quality assurance efforts and change when needed.

INTRODUCTION

In this era of burgeoning health care costs, it has become critical to maximize efficiency in health care delivery in order to contain costs. The key to efficient health care delivery is a coordinated health care delivery system including the management of utilization. The hospital arena is ideal for studying the recent cost-efficiency changes affecting health care delivery in the USA. In this chapter, the hospital length of stay issues regarding various cardiac procedures are discussed. The focus will be on methods to reduce utilization as well as to enhance efficient use of resources.

UTILIZATION

A strong focus of cost containment in the health care industry is utilization management. By reducing the use

of inefficient and ineffective services, the total costs of health care are limited. Health management organizations have instituted some common methods to decrease utilization of medical services.

Many organizations will identify cases that are expected to involve large costs, and then prospectively review them. These concurrent reviews involve the tracking of specific cases for their length of stay, use of hospital resources, and discharge planning.

By having a utilization review team following the case and prompting efficient use of resources, costs can be minimized.

Concurrent reviews are tracked against previously determined criteria for utilization. These criteria are often published or are commercially available to facilitate concurrent reviews.[1-4] Many payers are now routinely using computer software to assist with concurrent reviews. The software generates maximum allowable length of stays, diagnostic and procedure codes, and review criteria. Information entered by the staff performing the review is used for tracking and statistics generation.

The most common review, however, is the precertification review. Prior to hospital admission for in-patient care or an out-patient procedure, the admitting physician, and often the hospital, will be required to notify the payer. The main purpose for precertification is not to act as a barrier to resource use, but to notify the payer concurrent review system that a case will be occurring.

> With precertification, the payer is made aware of a forthcoming case so that care can be better coordinated and discharge planning can be initiated.

Precertification also helps ensure that care takes place in the setting most advantageous to the payer. These settings include the out-patient department, centers with expertise in particular cases, or centers in alliance with the payer. Precertification also allows payers to assign guidelines for care and hospital length of stays at the time the admission is approved. Some payers have instituted maximum allowable length of stays for particular admission diagnoses. The payers will authorize payment for length of stays no longer than the preset maximum.

Once it is determined that hospital admission for an elective procedure is necessary, cost control can be implemented by performing routine preoperative tests as an out-patient. The patient is hospitalized on the day that the planned procedure is to be performed. Discharge planning is initiated as soon as admission plans are made. The patient's needs upon discharge are anticipated and follow-up is scheduled. Coordinated efforts from pre-admission to hospitalization to out-patient follow-up reduce utilization of resources and contain costs.

Payers will often perform retrospective reviews of specific cases. These reviews focus on patterns of utilization. The payers will identify patterns regarding length of stays, costs, and clinical outcomes for diagnoses and for health care providers. Once identified, sources of inefficient utilization can be addressed for improvement or abandonment, while sources of efficient utilization can be acknowledged for continued use.

CLINICAL PATHWAYS

Admission diagnoses that are common tend to carry a large cost burden, owing to the sheer volume of hospital days and other services accumulated for the population. Improving the efficiency of health care delivery for these common diagnoses and procedures would dramatically reduce health care costs. The health care industry has responded with the development of clinical pathways (also known as care maps, care plans, and care tracks).

> Clinical pathways are used to coordinate health care delivery. They are called clinical pathways because they identify all the activities that every patient with a particular diagnosis must accomplish.

Clinical pathways most often involve a flow chart of activities along with their expected duration. Activities that must precede others are usually identified. Clinical pathways vary in design. Highly detailed charts can be used to ensure that all aspects of patient care are addressed and that all health care providers and ancillary services are organized and understand the expected outcomes. Frequently, clinical pathway charts can be used as educational tools in discussions with patients and their families for ensuring realistic expectations during the hospital course.

Clinical pathways are obtained from either commercial sources or by designing them anew. Commercially available clinical pathways may require some customization for the particular institution planning to implement them. With the development of the electronic medical record, and computerization of hospitals, clinical pathways will likely become easier to implement. Diagnostic codes will be able to cue up clinical pathways as well as prompt hospital staff for necessary clinical pathway orders including medications, diet orders, monitoring orders, laboratory tests, and consultations with physical therapy and social services.

Two main benefits result from designing and implementing clinical pathways. The first is improved quality of care. Patient care is better planned, delivered, and communicated. The second benefit is more efficient use of resources with decreased hospitalization length of stays and costs. Uzark and associates reported the results from a trial of case management with clinical pathways for pediatric cardiology cases at the University of Michigan Medical Center.[5] Uzark compared the costs, readmission rates, and parental perceptions of discharge readiness for in-patient cases before and after the implementation of case management with clinical pathways. Of the 300 cases examined, 130 were prior to the implementation of case management. Case management with clinical pathways resulted in a 15 per cent increase of discharges within the expected length of stay (on-time discharges before case management = 66 per cent; with case management = 76 per cent; $\chi^2 = 3.89$, $P = 0.05$). Readmission rates were not significantly reduced with the implementation of case management. There was a 13.4 per cent increase in charges for surgical procedures over the years in which clinical pathways were in use. However, the data on costs did not reflect changes in hospital charges over the years of analysis.

CARDIAC CATHETERIZATION

Over the past decade, there has been a dramatic rise in the rate of cardiac catheterization utilization. More than one million diagnostic coronary angiograms are performed annually in the USA.[6] Being a common procedure with rising rates of use, the cardiac catheterization procedure has been targeted as a source where cost containment would yield great financial savings. Payers, health care providers, and national medical associations have developed guidelines for the use of cardiac catheterization.[7,8] These guidelines have addressed various issues including the appropriate use of diagnostic cardiac catheterization and standardization in the techniques, qualifications of operators, and need for surgical back-up for cardiac catheterizations.[9-11] In 1991, the American Heart Association and the American College of Cardiology jointly sponsored guidelines for cardiac catheterization that covered many of the above issues.[8] A controversial issue addressed in the guidelines was the use of ambulatory cardiac catheterizations and mobile laboratories. The balance among patient safety, accessibility, appropriateness, and cost containment were weighed. Because even low-risk cardiac catheterizations can result in hospitalization-requiring complications, the guidelines detailed precautions and protocols that should be implemented in the event complications during ambulatory cardiac catheterizations occurred. One such precaution is that all ambulatory catheterizations be performed in hospitals.

The 1992 Society for Cardiac Angiography and Interventions published guidelines similar to those of the 1991 American Heart Association and American College of Cardiology.[12] These more recent guidelines included more patients for whom ambulatory cardiac catheterization should be avoided. Table 23.1 describes patients for whom ambulatory cardiac catheterization should be avoided.

Ambulatory cardiac catheterization can be performed safely in a variety of patients with low risk of complications. These procedures can be performed safely from either the brachial or the femoral approach.[13-16]

At the Cleveland Clinic Foundation, nearly 5600 diagnostic cardiac catheterization procedures are performed annually. As a high-volume health care provider, the Cleveland Clinic Foundation developed several clinical pathways for patients undergoing diagnostic cardiac catheterization. These clinical pathways encompass the various diagnoses for which catheterizations are indicated, as well as patient hospitalization status. The clinical pathways detail the educational materials for the patients, the medication and pre-procedural tests, as well as postprocedural orders and care. In the cardiac catheterization laboratory, there are guidelines for the use of contrast agents, anticoagulants, and mechanical hemostasis devices. Checklists and pre-printed physician orders prompt the medical services to adhere to the clinical pathways.

CORONARY ANGIOPLASTY AND RELATED PROCEDURES

With over 400 000 percutaneous interventional procedures performed annually in the USA, coronary angioplasty is a frequently performed procedure requiring hospital admission.[6] It is currently recommended that all percutaneous interventional procedures be performed as an in-patient procedure. The costs associated with these interventional procedures are substantial and vary with the complexity of the procedure and patient characteristics.[17-25] Higher costs are associated with procedures performed on patients with multivessel disease, complex lesion morphology, diabetes mellitus, advanced age, and acute or recent myocardial infarction. Ellis and colleagues identified decision delay and weekend delay to be associated with marked increases in hospital costs of 86 per cent and 61 per cent, respectively.[18] With advances in medical technology, increased costs are also associated with the use of intra-aortic balloon counterpulsation pumps, rotational atherectomy, stents, perfusion balloons, directional coronary atherectomy, laser, and newer antiplatelet regimens.[18,19,26,27]

The Cleveland Clinic Foundation clinical pathway for coronary angioplasty and stents with or without the use of abciximab (Reopro®) is designed to coordinate patient care among the various allied health professionals. The goal is to provide high-quality and efficient care at an acceptable cost. The clinical pathway is applied to every patient undergoing the procedure, and is reviewed three times daily. The guideline length of stay of 1 day after the

Table 23.1 *Criteria for exclusion from ambulatory cardiac catheterization*

1. Unstable angina
2. Suspected left main coronary artery disease
3. Known left ventricular dysfunction or congestive heart failure
4. Significant ventricular dysrhythmias
5. Uncontrolled hypertension or severe pulmonary hypertension
6. Renal impairment (creatinine > 2 mg/dL)
7. Coagulation disorder
8. Age > 75 years
9. Percutaneous interventional procedure
10. Infancy
11. Presence of relative contraindication to cardiac catheterization (e.g. fever or active infection, severe anemia or electrolyte imbalance, digitalis excess, contrast media hypersensitivity)
12. Recent cerebrovascular event
13. Severe peripheral vascular disease
14. Severe insulin-dependent diabetes
15. Other data and testing suggestive of high risk for an adverse event
16. Severe obesity
17. Generalized debility or dementia

THE CLEVELAND CLINIC FOUNDATION
COORDINATED CARE TRACK (CCT)

Directions:
1. Review CCT approximately every 8°.
2. Appropriate and completed interventions need no additional documentation.
3. Cross through any interventions which are not applicable.
4. Circle any intervention *not* completed.
5. The plan of care--nursing interventions and outcome evaluation statements--may be added to the CCT as necessary.

DRG 112
LOS = 1night

Admit date: _____

Discharge date: _____

Procedure: _____

If Reopro given, refer to guidelines on next page

**PCI / Stent
with or without Reopro
(G90/91)**

Comorbid Conditions:
- ☐ ASHD
- ☐ IDDM/NIDDM
- ☐ Hypertension
- ☐ Renal Insufficiency
- ☐ COPD
- ☐ Peripheral Vascular Disease
- ☐ CVA
- ☐

Events leading to this admission:
_____
_____
_____
_____
_____

Imprint\Label

Medical complications during hospitalization:
- ☐ Vascular complication
- ☐ CHF
- ☐ Respiratory Failure
- ☐ CVA
- ☐ Cardiogenic Shock
- ☐ Dysrhythmia
- ☐ Renal Failure
- ☐ Infection/Sepsis
- ☐ GI Bleed
- ☐

Risk Factors:
- ☐ Smoking
- ☐ High Cholesterol
- ☐ Obesity
- ☐ Family Hx

Date	Problem List	Discharge Criteria	Date Initially Met	Met on Discharge	
				Yes	No
	1. Potential altered tissue perfusion (cardiopulmonary) 2. Knowledge deficit 3. Potential arterial access site bleeding	1. No cardiac ischemia since Interventional Procedure 2. Access site without active bleeding 3. Patient and/or family understand discharge medications, wound care, activity restrictions, and follow-up. Received written material on immediate discharge instructions and life-style changes. If pt. received Reopro or Stent, wallet cards received.			
		Explain any discharge criteria not met:			

REOPRO ADMINISTRATION GUIDELINES

Indications for Reopro Administration:
-Elective or urgent coronary revascularization
-Target artery diameter stenosis > 60%

Exclusion Criteria/ Contraindications:
-Active internal bleeding or history of hemorrhagic diathesis
-Major surgery/trauma in the last 6 weeks
-CVA within 2 years or CVA with residual deficit
-Puncture of a non-compressive vessel within 24 hours
-GI or GU bleeding within the last 6 weeks
-Uncontrolled hypertension
-INR > 1.2 times control
-Thrombocytopenia (Platelets < 100,000)
-CPR for > 5 minutes prior to procedure

Conditions which may increase bleeding:
-Weight less than 75 Kg. (unless weight dosed heparin given at 70u/Kg)
-Greater than 65 years old
-History of prior GI disease/bleeding
-Concurrent thrombolysis
-Advanced renal disease

Reopro (Abciximab) Administration:

PLANNED USE:

Bolus: 0.25 mg/kg over 1-2 min.

Infusion: 0.125 mcg/kg/min (max 10mcg/min- 12hrs)
Must have separate IV site & be delivered via pump with a low protein binding micron filter tubing set.

TARGET ACT: 200-300

Heparin administration: bolus 70 u/Kg (max 7000 u)
Then per nomogram post-procedure

UNPLANNED / BAILOUT USE:

Bolus: 0.25 mg/ kg over 1-2 min

Infusion: 0.125 mcg/kg/min (max 10 mcg/min - 12 hours)

Maintain ACT 300-350 until decision made to use REOPRO. If reopro used, **check ACT after REOPRO bolus--if > 400, consider reversal with protamine** (10-15 mg IV over 5 min, ACT in 10 min; repeat q.15 min until ACT < 300) ACT q. 30 minutes during procedure & 2-5 min after each bolus of heparin
Must have separate IV site & be delivered via pump with a low protein binding micron filter tubing set.

Heparin Administration: bolus should not exceed 100u/Kg (max 10,000u) in cath lab; then per nomogram post-procedure

THE CLEVELAND CLINIC FOUNDATION
DISCHARGE PLANNING RECORD

Plan	Team Members (INCLUDE BEEPER #)	Homegoing Equipment/Supplies	Has @ home	Ordered	Patient Education (Initiated in hospital)
Anticipated date of discharge:	Clinical Resource Manager: Physical Therapist:	Wheelchair	☐	☐	☐ Medications
		Bedside Commode	☐	☐	☐ Reopro Wallet Card
To: ☐ Home ☐ Home Care	Social Worker: Occupational Therapist:	Walker	☐	☐	☐ After Your Intervention
☐ Rehab ☐ SNF		Crutches	☐	☐	☐ CAD
☐ Intermediate care	Alternate Site Coordinator(s): Respiratory Therapist:	Hospital Bed	☐	☐	☐ LAF diet
☐ Hospital transfer		Dressing Supplies	☐	☐	☐ Treatment of angina
☐ Subacute Services		BP kit	☐	☐	☐ Access Site Care
☐ Other	Speech Therapist:	Pharmacy Supplies	☐	☐	☐ Activity
		Ventilator	☐	☐	☐ Return follow-up
APEX FORM COMPLETED AS APPROPRIATE:	Nutrition Service: Other:	Oxygen	☐	☐	☐ Discharge needs
					☐ Nutrition
_____ (date/initials of ASC)	Pastoral Care:	Other:	☐	☐	Diet _____
Person assisting with care at home _____					☐

NOTES:

Figure 23.1 Excerpts of clinical pathway outline for percutaneous revascularization. Shown here are lists for noting patient co-morbid conditions and complications as well as details for abciximab administration. This diagram is for illustration only and should not be used as a standard of care. © The Cleveland Clinic Foundation, 1997.

procedure is noted. The path outlines possible co-morbid conditions and medical complications during the hospitalization that may need to be addressed. Coronary artery disease risk factors are also displayed and are noted for each patient. A problem list with discharge criteria as well as when the criteria were met is charted. Any deviations from the discharge criteria are to be documented on the clinical pathway chart. Discharge plans and home-going equipment are all listed. Patient education on all aspects of health care are noted as they are completed. To facilitate patient management, important phone and pager numbers for the allied health care team members are listed on the clinical pathway. As with many of the Cleveland Clinic clinical pathways, the newer and more highly technical procedures are detailed on the clinical pathway (Figure 23.1). In the case of coronary interventions, guidelines for the administration of abciximab are provided. These guidelines include the indications, relative contraindications, higher risk patient profiles, and methods for administration and monitoring of abciximab. As for all clinical pathways, daily patient activities and expectations grouped by type of activity are detailed in chart format.

To assure implementing the clinical pathway, preprinted physician order forms with check boxes are used to assist physicians with complying with the clinical pathway guidelines. The order forms not only suggest procedures and activities to be performed or discontinued, but also their timing. The goal is to coordinate care for maximum efficiency and quality with the highest patient satisfaction while at a contained cost. At the Cleveland Clinic, the mean length of stay for percutaneous coronary revascularization patients has decreased steadily from 3.29 days in 1994 to 2.47 days in 1996. Over the same 3-year period, the proportion of patients discharged within the expected 2 days length of stay has increased from 55 per cent to 68 per cent. These data show that utilization of hospital resources is possibly declining. It is the efficient delivery of health care that make decreased utilization possible.

CARDIOTHORACIC SURGERY

Cardiovascular disease affects 57 million people and is responsible for nearly one million deaths annually at an annual cost of $259.1 billion in the USA.[28] With over 500 000 coronary artery bypass operations performed annually in the USA, a significant portion of this health care bill is attributed to surgical therapies.[6] Recently, Hlatky and colleagues reported long-term functional status and 5-year costs for angioplasty and surgery.[17] In that study, functional-status scores on the Duke Activity Status Index improved more over 3 years in patients assigned to surgery than in those assigned to angioplasty ($P<0.05$) for the 934 of the 1829 patients enrolled in the

randomized Bypass Angioplasty Revascularization Investigation. As expected, patients in the angioplasty group returned to work 5 weeks sooner than did patients in the surgery group ($P<0.001$). For the entire group after 5 years, the total medical cost of angioplasty was 95 per cent that of surgery ($P = 0.047$). The 5-year cost of surgery was lower than that of angioplasty among patients with three-vessel disease but not among patients with two-vessel disease.

Several recent studies have evaluated predictors that determine the cost of coronary artery bypass grafting (CABG).[22,23,29–37] In a study of 604 patients treated at Duke University Medical Center, it was found that individual patient predictors accounted for less than 25 per cent of the total variance in hospital costs for CABG.[31] However, those factors associated with higher costs were the presence of diabetes mellitus, extensive coronary artery disease, and impaired left ventricular systolic function. Older patients, female patients, and patients having had a prior bypass operation were also associated with higher costs for CABG. Interestingly, the attending surgeon was a major determinant of the cost, but not the outcome, of CABG.

In an Emory University study of 807 patients undergoing CABG, patient characteristics associated with higher cost included older age, higher angina class, previous MI, history of heart failure, and more extensive coronary artery disease.[30] There was only a trend towards higher costs for diabetic patients. Additionally, complications of CABG associated with significantly higher costs included septicemia, adult respiratory distress syndrome, pneumonia, neurological events, arrhythmias, and major bleeding events.

As technology changes, so do the costs associated with cardiothoracic surgery. Currently, there is a trend toward shorter length of stays for CABG and valvular surgery. The recently promoted minimally invasive surgeries for CABG and valvular operations may further reduce hospital length of stays, morbidity, and cost.[38]

The Cleveland Clinic performs over 3000 CABGs and over 1000 valvular operations annually. The hospital staff, both out-patient preoperative assessment teams and in-patient perioperative teams, are well versed in the details of the clinical pathways. The clinical pathways shown in Fig. 23.2 detail not only patient co-morbidities and complications, but also the team members and pager numbers, problem list, daily activities, discharge criteria, and home-going plans. Exact timing of laboratory tests and radiographs are also detailed. The plan is to accomplish high-quality perioperative care with high patient satisfaction at controlled costs. Ideally, patients receiving care based on the clinical pathways will be able to be transferred to regular patient wards on the first postoperative day, and ambulating in the halls by the third postoperative day. The clinical pathway aims for patient discharge to home on the fifth postoperative day. Out-patient follow-up is also detailed in the clinical

THE CLEVELAND CLINIC FOUNDATION
COORDINATED CARE TRACK (CCT)

Directions:
1. Review CCT approximately every 8'
2. Appropriate and completed interventions need no additional documentation.
3. Cross through any interventions which are not applicable.
4. Circle any intervention not completed.
5. The plan of care--nursing interventions and outcome evaluation statements--may be added to the CCT as necessary.

DRG 106/107   Expected LOS 5 days

Physician(s) _____

Admit
Date _____

Discharge
Date _____

Surgery/Procedure:
CABG with/without Cath

Date of Surgery/Procedure _____

Comorbid Conditions:
□ CHF
□ IDDM
□ Angina
□ ASHD
□ COPD
□ Hypertension
□ CHF
□

Imprint\Label

Complications during this admission:
□ Atrial fibrillation   □ CVA
□ Pleural effusion   □ GI Bleed
□ Pneumothorax   □ DVT
□ Hemodynamic instability/IABP

Risk Factors:
□ Obesity   □ ETOH/Substance Abuse   □ Smoking   □

Title: Coronary Artery Bypass Graft with/without Cath

Date	Problem List	Discharge Criteria	Date Initially Met	Met on Discharge	
				Yes	No
	1. Altered Cardiac Output	1. ADL's & activity are performed independently			
	2. Ineffective Airway Clearance	2. Medication & basic nutrition teaching and postop instructional objectives are met			
	3. Pain	3. Wound is pink, approximated, & has minimal or no drainage present			
	4. Knowledge Deficit	4. Pain is absent or controlled			
		5. Cardiac & respiratory status are stable			
	5. Anxiety	6. Anxiety levels are manageable			
		7. Home Health Care support is coordinated as needed			
		Explain any discharge criteria not met:			

CLEVELAND CLINIC FOUNDATION
COORDINATED CARE TRACK

Time Frame Location	Hospital Day POD - DOS Date ___ Unit ___	Hospital Day POD - 1 Date ___ Unit ___	Hospital Day POD - 2 Date ___ Unit ___	Hospital Day POD - 3 Date ___ Unit ___
Patient Satisfaction	"What can we do to enhance your stay with us?"	"What can we do to enhance your stay with us?"	"What can we do to enhance your stay with us?"	"What can we do to enhance your stay with us?"
Discharge Planning	Patient/family verbalize expected LOS & postop activities Primary Support person is identified	No dyspnea or cyanosis Consistent cardiac rhythm & rate Neurologically intact or at baseline Baseline renal status	Psychosocial needs are assessed Pt/family are able to restate expected LOS & postop activities	Social Work & Home Health Care needs are assessed
Patient Education	Family will wait in Surgical Waiting Room Patient is reoriented during emergence from anesthesia	Orient pt/family to new room Family may attend Family Resource Group at 0900 & Family Class at 1730 Daily activities are reviewed with pt/family	Family may attend Family Resource Group at 0900 (Monday-Friday)	Family may attend Family Resource Group at 0900 (Monday-Friday) Pt/family receive medication information Nutrition education/dietician
Tests/Procedures/ Consults	CXR; EKG; H&H; K+; SGOT; ABG; CT Anesthesia	CXR; SMA-16; EKG; H&H; CK-MB ABG; K+ at 1800; Anesthesia; CHIRP	KP-6; H&H; EKG; Anesthesia; CHIRP	K+; CHIRP; SW/HHC as needed
Allied Health Interventions	Wean ventilator within 4-6 hours Nutrition screen completed Nutrition education needs assessed	O₂ by nasal cannula Pulse oximetry/Anesthesia CHIRP evaluation RD assessment per protocol	Nutritional supplement initiated by RD per protocol	
Nursing/Medical Interventions	Turn side-to-side q2h Invasive monitoring/routine VS per nursing unit routine Autotransfusion D/C'd 12⁰ post-op Wean inotropic support as tolerated: Monitor I & O D/C NG tube after extubation NPO until extubated, then ice chips Incentive spirometry (IS) q1h after extubation Initiate rewarming per procedure Pain control per MD order	VS per floor routine → → Stand on stationary scale for weight Up in chair for all meals (20 minutes) Walk in room with assist (30 feet) before bedtime D/C Hemodynamic lines & CT per order Transfer to RNF via WC Cardiac liquid diet, adv as tol; I&O Telemetry - check q1h; IV @ KVO D/C foley at 2200 IS q1h while awake until D/C → Pain control per MD orders until D/C →	Up to chair for all meals Walk to bathroom for AM care w/assist Walk 2-4 minutes in room 2x w/assist Change IV to heparin lock Advance to preop diet; Monitor I&O D/C O₂ Daily weight at 0600 until D/C →	Up in chair for all meals Walk in hallway w/assist 2-4 minutes, 2-3 times Monitor I&O D/C pacemaker wires
			D/C telemetry	
Outcome Criteria	Patient/family satisfaction addressed Hemodynamically stable Extubated with adequate ABGs Dangled at bedside within one hour of extubation Nutrition criteria met with F/U per protocol	Patient/family satisfaction addressed Transferred to RNF Alert & oriented Stable hemodynamic, cardiac, neuro, renal and respiratory status Liquid diet is tolerated; reassess per standard Activity is tolerated	Patient/family satisfaction addressed Stable cardiac & respiratory status Ambulate in room 2x Comfort level maintained ADL's with assist Nutrition supplement tolerated to prevent protein/caloric malnutrition	Patient/family satisfaction addressed Stable cardiac & respiratory status Ambulate in hall Diet and supplement are tolerated

CLEVELAND CLINIC FOUNDATION
COORDINATED CARE TRACK

Time Frame Location	Hospital Day ___ POD - 4 Date ___ Unit ___	Hospital Day ___ POD - 5 Date ___ Unit ___	Hospital Day ___ POD ___ Date ___ Unit ___	Hospital Day ___ POD ___ Date ___ Unit ___
Patient Satisfaction	"What can we do to enhance your stay with us?"	"What can we do to enhance your stay with us?"	"What can we do to enhance your stay with us?"	"What can we do to enhance your stay with us?"
Discharge Planning	Home support plans are finalized	Patient signs Discharge Order Sheet		
Patient Education	**Family may attend Family Resource Group at 0900 (Monday-Friday)** Medication information reinforced Pt/family to view nutrition & CABG films, receive CHIRP booklets & video and "After your heart surgery" pamphlet Pt/family attends CHIRP discharge class Pt/family instructed on D/C procedure	**Family may attend Family Resource Group at 0900 (Monday-Friday)** Patient receives prescriptions & medication information handouts		
Tests/Procedures/ Consults	CBC; EKG; CXR; SMA-16 CHIRP → → → → → → →	CBC; EKG; CXR; SMA-16 CHIRP → → → → → → → D/C		
Allied Health Interventions	Basic nutrition information provided per protocol Nutrition supplement per protocol			
Nursing/Medical Interventions	Up in chair for all meals Walk in hallway 4-8 minutes, 3x w/stand-by assist Daily weight until D/C → → → → → → →	Ambulates independently → → → → → → → D/C		
Outcome Criteria	Patient/family satisfaction addressed Frequency of stools is normal for pt Shower with supervision Fluid balance adequate Basic diet goals can be stated Tolerating diet and supplements	Patient/family satisfaction addressed Discharge criteria are met Dietician appointment for 6 week followup Tolerates > 75% meals Labs show only mild/mod nutrition depletion		

Figure 23.2 *Clinical pathway outline for coronary artery bypass grafting surgery. This figure is for illustration only and should not be used as a standard of care. © The Cleveland Clinic Foundation, 1997.*

pathway and scheduled for the patient prior to discharge. The physician order forms are pre-printed with check boxes and fill-in blanks to assist the physicians with adhering to the clinical pathways. Overall, the Cleveland Clinic in 1996 achieved on-time discharges in 35 per cent of CABG operations. More than two-thirds of CABG patients were discharged by the seventh post-operative day.

TRANSPLANTATION

The number of Americans with heart failure has been growing over the past few decades.[28,39,40] Currently, nearly 5 million Americans have congestive heart failure, and approximately 400 000 new cases of heart failure will be diagnosed in 1997.[28] Congestive heart failure accounts for more hospitalizations in the elderly than any other primary diagnosis.[28] As heart failure becomes more prevalent, hospitalization and nursing home costs for heart failure will explode well beyond the current $13.5 billion annually.[28]

Hospitalization for heart failure cannot be completely eliminated. Episodic decompensation due to dietary indiscretions, medical non-compliance, complicating arrhythmias, and disease progression will occur. Certainly, there are two major determinants of hospitalization for heart failure: severity of the disease and patient age. The development of atrial fibrillation, increasing edema, and uncontrolled ischemia are the most common factors contributing to the need for hospitalization in this population.

With advances in pharmacological and non-pharmacological therapy, as well as in the initiation of case managers to follow out-patients closely, it may be possible to improve the course of the heart failure patient and to reduce the need for recurrent hospitalizations. Non-pharmacological therapies currently include cardiac transplantation, mechanical cardiac assist devices, high-risk coronary artery bypass grafting, myocardial volume reduction surgery, cardiomyoplasty, and transmyocardial laser revascularization. Of these, cardiac transplantation and high-risk coronary revascularization are the most widely accepted for improving the long-term prognosis.

The many aspects of cardiac transplantation are expensive and have been previously examined.[41–48] Prior to being accepted for cardiac transplantation, patients undergo rigorous testing, which may include coronary angiography, right heart catheterization, metabolic exercise stress testing, psychosocial testing, and often many other tests and procedures, including vascular ultrasonography and laboratory testing. The pre-transplant evaluation can cost between $10 000 and $20 000. Many more patients are evaluated for possible transplantation than are accepted for the listing. Of the few selected as candidates for transplantation, only a minority will ever undergo the surgical procedure. Owing to the donor shortage, only about 2200 cardiac transplantations take place annually in the USA. However, there are almost 3000 patients on the transplantation waiting list daily. The usual patient undergoing cardiac transplantation was listed for the transplant approximately 7 months. Not only is the pre-transplantation evaluation expensive, the intensive therapy required to care for advanced heart failure patients while awaiting cardiac transplantation can run as high as $100 000 or more. The operative procedure averages $123 000.[46,47,49] Therapy following cardiac transplantation is ongoing and costs approximately $15 000 annually.

The Cleveland Clinic Foundation performed 113 cardiac transplantations in 1998. Many of these patients are on chronic intravenous inotropic therapy or mechanical assist devices preoperatively. As can be expected, the care of these patients is highly technical. To coordinate this very complicated care, clinical pathways were devised that are themselves very detailed and extensive (Fig. 23.3). The patient's history, risk factors for complicated postoperative course, and co-morbidities are all outlined. Preoperative, intensive care unit, and postoperative activities are all detailed along a time line. Patients undergo intensive education throughout the pre-transplantation and post-transplantation periods. Allied health care professionals with particular expertise in cardiac transplantation are involved in each case from its initiation. The goal is to achieve hospital discharge on postoperative day 19 of a patient having experienced a high-quality and efficient hospital stay.

PACEMAKERS AND DEFIBRILLATORS

In 1958, the first cardiac pacemaker was implanted. There are currently over 500 000 patients with permanently implanted pacemakers in the USA. With the widespread use of permanent pacing, the American College of Cardiology and the American Heart Association devised guidelines for the implantation of cardiac pacemakers in 1984, and has since revised the guidelines in 1991.[50,51] The guidelines describe the indications for pacing and discuss the scientific evidence to support the indications. By devising and disseminating these guidelines, the use of permanent cardiac pacing may be standardized, and possibly limited. By devising and implementing clinical pathways, health care providers may be able to implant pacemakers efficiently and reduce hospital length of stays and costs.

Following in the wake of permanent cardiac pacing is the use of implantable cardioverter defibrillators (ICDs). The first device of this class was implanted in 1980. Since then, the use of these devices has grown to over 4000 implants in 1990, and is expected to be nearly 65 000

CLEVELAND CLINIC FOUNDATION
COORDINATED CARE TRACK -- Heart Transplant Surgery

Time Frame Location	Hospital Day #: _____ DOS Date Unit			
Patient Satisfaction	**What can we do to enhance your stay?**			
Discharge Planning	-Evaluate home-going resources and support systems -Identify pt.'s primary support person			
Patient Education	*-Preop:* Review Preop protocol including NPO status -Review Peri-op & post-op protocol -Family to wait in Surgical Waiting Room *-Postop:* Reorientation during emergence from anesthesia			
Tests/Procedures/ Consults	*-Preop:* APTT/PT/CBC/DIFF/SMA 17/T&C for 6 units Leukocyte depleted Packed Cells, 4 units FFP; CT Anesth. consult, CXR once line placed *-Postop:* ABG's/Ionized Ca/ CBC/ PT /APTT/SMA 17/ALT/PCXR, & EKG upon arrival to ICU. 2 red top tubes to tissue typing M&F. -Initiate standard immunosuppression protocol			

Figure 23.3 *Clinical pathway outline for cardiac transplantation. This figure is for illustration only and should not be used as a standard of care. © The Cleveland Clinic Foundation, 1997.*

implants in 2002. Recently, technological advances in pulse generators and leads have revolutionized ICD therapy. Major advances include transvenous single-lead positioning and reduced size, combined with prolonged longevity of the pulse generator. These advances have simplified implantation technique and provided for superior effectiveness and lower costs.[52] This suggests that a more favorable cost effectiveness is to be expected.

In 1992, O'Brien and colleagues reported an analysis of costs for the use of the defibrillator versus amiodarone in the UK.[53] At the time of their analysis, the defibrillators were implanted via left lateral thoracotomy, and were expected to reduce the 5-year overall mortality from 52.4 per cent to 35.8 per cent. The defibrillator was associated with an expected £15 400 per life-year gained. Transvenous, pre-pectorally implanted ICDs should be expected to provide even greater cost effectiveness.[52]

Hauer and associates have devised a cost-analysis model for the years 1996–2000 for ICD implants. For survivors of cardiac arrest due to malignant ventricular tachyarrhythmias, with a mean follow-up of 27 months, transvenous positioning of a pre-pectorally implanted ICD with 5-years longevity results in a cost of $44 537 ($51 per day alive) or a cost savings of $11 530 per patient when compared with intra-abdominally implanted transvenous ICDs.[54]

At the Cleveland Clinic, patients undergo cardioverter defibrillator implantation with an anticipated hospital stay of 2 days. All patients are assigned to a clinical pathway, and post-procedure physician orders are pre-printed to prompt coordinated care with the clinical pathway. In the out-patient clinic, patients are educated regarding their cardiac disease and the use of ICD therapy. Educational materials are provided for review at home. The hospital course is discussed with the patient and family. Assessment is made of the patient's ability to cope with the changes in lifestyle associated with the disease and the device. Pre-procedural laboratory and radiological tests are performed. The device leads and generator, as well as applicable research protocols are all planned during the out-patient visit. Following implantation of the device, laboratory tests and ICD checks are scheduled for the following day prior to hospital discharge. Patient and family education continues, and home-going needs are assessed. Out-patient follow-up is scheduled prior to patient discharge.

ELECTROPHYSIOLOGY TESTING

Over the past decade, the field of cardiac electrophysiology has come to encompass not only diagnostic, but also therapeutic techniques. Since the advent of endocardial catheter ablative techniques, the role of surgical techniques with thoracotomy has been markedly reduced. In 1995, a joint task force of the North American Society of Pacing and Electrophysiology, the American College of Cardiology, the American Heart Association, and the Working Groups on Arrhythmias and Cardiac Pacing of the European Society of Cardiology issued a report on radiofrequency catheter ablation.[55] The task force reported that radiofrequency ablation was superior to traditional cardiothoracic surgical procedures with respect to morbidity and mortality.

With the improved efficacy and techniques of electrophysiology testing and radiofrequency ablation comes the increased demand and utilization of these procedures. Electrophysiology testing and radiofrequency ablation will likely become increasingly popular for the nearly 4.5 million Americans with an arrhythmic disorder.[28]

The increased utilization of electrophysiology studies will lead to increased scrutiny by health care payers and providers for cost containment. Clinical pathways are useful to coordinate care among the many providers within the hospital arena. Hospital length of stays have been dramatically reduced over the years. As recently as 1994, length of stays of 4 days for supraventricular tachycardia ablative therapy was common practice. Today, many patients are released the day following the procedure. In many cases, diagnostic electrophysiology studies may be performed on an ambulatory basis. Although not a common practice, and not promoted by our group, some centers are performing ambulatory ablative procedures.[56] Efficient care for interventional procedures is promoted through the use of clinical pathways. Laboratory tests, patient education, and out-patient follow-up can all be addressed by clinical pathways.

SUMMARY

- Providing coordinated health care is the key to decreased utilization of resources and cost containment.
- Concurrent reviews track specific cases against previously determined criteria for utilization.
- With precertification of hospitalization cases, the concurrent review system can be activated to better coordinate care and discharge plans.
- Clinical pathways help coordinate health care delivery by identifying all the activities that most patients with a particular diagnosis must accomplish.
- Ambulatory cardiac catheterization can be performed safely in selected patients.
- Decision delay and weekend delay have been identified as the main determinants of higher costs in patients undergoing percutaneous revascularization procedures.

- Although many patient characteristics affect the overall cost of coronary artery bypass grafting, the attending surgeon is the most important determinant of cost.
- Recent advances in implantable cardioverter-defibrillator pulse generators and leads have reduced length of hospitalization and improved cost effectiveness of these devices.
- Advances in radiofrequency catheter ablation of arrhythmias has led to a decline in hospital length of stays.
- Clinical pathways are important tools to coordinate the health care delivery, to shorten hospital length of stays, and to contain health care costs.

REFERENCES

1. Doyle RL. *Healthcare management guidelines: inpatient and surgical care*. Seattle: Milliman & Robertson, 1990.
2. InterQual. *The ISD – a review system with adult criteria*. Chicago: InterQual, 1991.
3. InterQual. *Surgical indications monitoring SIM III*. Chicago: InterQual, 1991.
4. Utilization Management Associates. *Managed care appropriateness protocol (MCAP)*. Wellesley, MA: Utilization Management Associates, 1991.
5. Uzark K, LeRoy S, Callow L, Cameron J, Rosenthal A. The pediatric nurse practitioner as case manager in the delivery of services to children with heart disease. *J Pediat Health Care* 1994; **8**: 74–8.
6. American Heart Association. *Heart facts*. Dallas: American Heart Association, 1994.
7. Ross J Jr, Brandenburg RO, Dinsmore RE, *et al.* Guidelines for coronary angiography. A report of the American College of Cardiology/American Heart Association Task Force on Assessment of Diagnostic and Therapeutic Cardiovascular Procedures (Subcommittee on Coronary Angiography). *J Am Coll Cardiol* 1987; **10**: 935–50.
8. Pepine CJ, Allen HD, Bashore TM, *et al.* ACC/AHA guidelines for cardiac catheterization and cardiac catheterization laboratories. American College of Cardiology/American Heart Association Ad Hoc Task Force on Cardiac Catheterization. *Circulation* 1991; **84**: 2213–47.
9. Bernstein SJ, Hilborne LH, Leape LL, *et al.* The appropriateness of use of coronary angiography in New York State. *JAMA* 1993; **269**: 766–9.
10. Brook RH, Park RE, Chassin MR, Solomon DH, Keesey J, Kosecoff J. Predicting the appropriate use of carotid endarterectomy, upper gastrointestinal endocscopy, and coronary angiography. *N Engl J Med* 1990; **323**: 1173–7.
11. Bernstein SJ, Laouri M, Hilborne LH, *et al. Coronary angiography. A literature review and ratings of appropriateness and necessity*. Santa Monica, CA: RAND, 1992.
12. Clark DA, Moscovich MD, Vetrovec GW, Wexler L. Guidelines for the performance of outpatient catheterization and angiographic procedures. *Cathet Cardiovasc Diagnos* 1992; **27**: 5–7.
○13. Fierens E. Outpatient coronary arteriography. *Cathet Cardiovasc Diagnos* 1984; **10**: 27–32.
○14. Mahrer PR, Young C, Magnusson PT. Efficacy and safety of outpatient catheterization. *Cathet Cardiovasc Diagnos* 1987; **13**: 304–8.
15. Pink S, Fiutowski L, Gianelly RE. Outpatient cardiac catheterizations: analysis of patients requiring admission. *Clin Cardiol* 1989; **12**: 375–8.
♦16. Block PC, Ockene I, Goldberg RJ, *et al.* A prospective randomized trial of outpatient versus inpatient cardiac catheterization. *N Engl J Med* 1988; **319**: 1251–5.
17. Hlatky MA, Rogers WJ, Johnstone I, *et al.* Medical care costs and quality of life after randomization to coronary angioplasty or coronary bypass surgery. Bypass Angioplasty Revascularization Investigation (BARI) Investigators. *N Engl J Med* 1997; **336**: 92–9.
♦18. Ellis SG, Miller DP, Brown KJ, *et al.* In-hospital cost of percutaneous coronary revascularization. Critical determinants and implications. *Circulation* 1995; **92**: 741–7.
19. Cohen DJ, Breall JA, Ho KK, *et al.* Economics of elective coronary revascularization. Comparison of costs and charges for conventional angioplasty, directional atherectomy, stenting and bypass surgery. *J Am Coll Cardiol*. 1993; **22**: 1052–9.
20. Cohen DJ, Krumholz HM, Sukin CA, *et al.* In-hospital and one-year economic outcomes after coronary stenting or balloon angioplasty. Results from a randomized clinical trial. Stent Restenosis Study Investigators. *Circulation* 1995; **92**: 2480–7.
21. Cohen EA, Schwartz L. Coronary artery stenting: indications and cost implications. *Prog Cardiovasc Dis* 1996; **39**: 83–110.
♦22. Weintraub WS, Mauldin PD, Becker E, Kosinski AS, King SB III. A comparison of the costs of and quality of life after coronary angioplasty or coronary surgery for multivessel coronary artery disease. Results from the Emory Angioplasty Versus Surgery Trial (EAST). *Circulation* 1995; **92**: 2831–40.
23. Mushinski M. Average charges for coronary artery bypass grafts and percutaneous transluminal coronary angioplasties, 1995. *Statistical Bulletin – Metropolitan Insurance Companies* 1997; **78**: 20–8.
24. Mushinski M. Average hospital charges for percutaneous transluminal coronary angioplasty, 1993: geographic variations. *Statistical Bulletin – Metropolitan Insurance Companies* 1995; **76**: 10–17.
25. Vaitkus PT, Witmer WT, Brandenburg RG, Wells SK, Zehnacker JB. Economic impact of angioplasty salvage

techniques, with an emphasis on coronary stents: a method incorporating costs, revenues, clinical effectiveness and payer mix. *J Am Coll Cardiol* 1997; **30**: 894–900.

26. Goklaney AK, Murphy JD, Hillegass WB Jr. Abciximab therapy in percutaneous intervention: economic issues in the United States. *Am Heart J* 1998; **135**: S90–7.

27. Van Hout BA, van der Woude T, de Jaegere PP, *et al.* Cost effectiveness of stent implantation versus PTCA: the BENESTENT experience. *Semin Intervent Cardiol* 1996; **1**: 263–8.

28. American Heart Association. *1997 Heart and Stroke Statistical Update*. Dallas: American Heart Association, 1996.

29. Dudley RA, Harrell FE Jr, Smith LR, *et al.* Comparison of analytic models for estimating the effect of clinical factors on the cost of coronary artery bypass graft surgery. *J Clin Epidemiol* 1993; **46**: 261–71.

♦30. Mauldin PD, Weintraub WS, Becker ER. Predicting hospital costs for first-time coronary artery bypass grafting from preoperative and postoperative variables. *Am J Cardiol* 1994; **74**: 772–5.

31. Smith LR, Milano CA, Molter BS, Elbeery JR, Sabiston DC Jr, Smith PK. Preoperative determinants of postoperative costs associated with coronary artery bypass graft surgery. *Circulation* 1994; **90**: II124–8.

○32. Mark DB. Implications of cost in treatment selection for patients with coronary heart disease. *Ann Thorac Surg* 1996; **61**: S12–15.

33. Cowper PA, DeLong ER, Peterson ED, *et al.* Geographic variation in resource use for coronary artery bypass surgery. IHD Port Investigators. *Med Care* 1997; **35**: 320–33.

34. Cheng DC, Karski J, Peniston C, *et al.* Early tracheal extubation after coronary artery bypass graft surgery reduces costs and improves resource use. A prospective, randomized, controlled trial. *Anesthesiology* 1996; **85**: 1300–10.

35. Lee JH, Kim KH, van Heeckeren DW, *et al.* Cost analysis of early extubation after coronary bypass surgery. *Surgery* 1996; **120**: 611–17.

36. Kay GL, Sun GW, Aoki A, Prejean CA Jr. Influence of ejection fraction on hospital mortality, morbidity, and costs for CABG patients. *Ann Thorac Surg* 1995; **60**: 1640–50.

♦37. Longo KM, Cowen ME, Flaum MA, *et al.* Preoperative predictors of cost in Medicare-age patients undergoing coronary artery bypass grafting. *Ann Thorac Surg* 1998; **66**: 740–5; discussion 746.

38. King RC, Reece TB, Hurst JL, *et al.* Minimally invasive coronary artery bypass grafting decreases hospital stay and cost. *Ann Surg* 1997; **225**: 805–9; discussion 809–11.

39. Croft JB, Giles WH, Pollard RA, Casper ML, Anda RF, Livengood JR. National trends in the initial hospitalization for heart failure. *J Am Geriat Soc* 1997; **45**: 270–5.

40. Ho KK, Pinsky JL, Kannel WB, Levy D. The epidemiology of heart failure: the Framingham Study. *J Am Coll Cardiol* 1993; **22**: 6A–13A.

41. Mehta SM, Aufiero TX, Pae WE Jr, Miller CA, Pierce WS. Mechanical ventricular assistance: an economical and effective means of treating end-stage heart disease. *Ann Thorac Surg* 1995; **60**: 284–90.

♦42. Sharples LD, Briggs A, Caine N, McKenna M, Buxton M. A model for analyzing the cost of main clinical events after cardiac transplantation. *Transplantation* 1996; **62**: 615–21.

43. Loisance D, Sailly JC. Cost-effectiveness in patients awaiting transplantation receiving intravenous inotropic support. *Eur J Anaesthesiol Suppl* 1993; **8**: 9–13.

44. De Geest S, Kesteloot K, Degryse I, Vanhaecke J. Hospital costs of protective isolation procedures in heart transplant recipients. *J Heart Lung Transplant* 1995; **14**: 544–52.

45. Cloy MJ, Myers TJ, Stutts LA, Macris MP, Frazier OH. Hospital charges for conventional therapy versus left ventricular assist system therapy in heart transplant patients. *ASAIO J* 1995; **41**: M535–9.

46. Evans RW, Manninen DL, Dong FB. An economic analysis of heart–lung transplantation. Costs, insurance coverage, and reimbursement. *J Thorac Cardiovasc Surg* 1993; **105**: 972–8.

47. Evans RW, Manninen DL, Dong FB, Frist WH, Kirklin JK. The medical and surgical determinants of heart transplantation outcomes: the results of a consensus survey in the United States. *J Heart Lung Transplant* 1993; **12**: 42–5.

○48. Evans RW. Socioeconomic aspects of heart transplantation. *Curr Opin Cardiol* 1995; **10**: 169–79.

49. Evans RW. Organ transplantation and the inevitable debate as to what constitutes a basic health care benefit. *Clin Transplants* 1993: 359–91.

50. Frye RL, Collins JJ, DeSanctis RW, *et al.* Guidelines for permanent cardiac pacemaker implantation, May 1984. A report of the Joint American College of Cardiology/American Heart Association Task Force on Assessment of Cardiovascular Procedures (Subcommittee on Pacemaker Implantation). *Circulation* 1984; **70**: 331A–339A.

51. Dreifus LS, Fisch C, Griffin JC, Gillette PC, Mason JW, Parsonnet V. Guidelines for implantation of cardiac pacemakers and antiarrhythmia devices. A report of the American College of Cardiology/American Heart Association Task Force on Assessment of Diagnostic and Therapeutic Cardiovascular Procedures. (Committee on Pacemaker Implantation). *Circulation* 1991; **84**: 455–67.

♦52. Mushlin AI, Hall WJ, Zwanziger J, *et al.* The cost-effectiveness of automatic implantable cardiac defibrillators: results from MADIT. Multicenter Automatic Defibrillator Implantation Trial. *Circulation* 1998; **97**: 2129–35.

53. O'Brien BJ, Buxton MJ, Rushby JA. Cost effectiveness of the implantable cardioverter defibrillator: a preliminary analysis. *Br Heart J* 1992; **68**: 241–5.

54. Hauer RN, Derksen R, Wever EF. Can implantable cardioverter–defibrillator therapy reduce healthcare costs? *Am J Cardiol* 1996; **78**: 134–9.

55. Saksena S, Epstein AE, Lazzara R, *et al*. NASPE/ACC/ AHA/ESC medical/scientific statement special report – clinical investigation of antiarrhythmic devices: a statement for healthcare professionals from a Joint Task Force of the North American Society of Pacing and Electrophysiology, the American College of Cardiology, the American Heart Association, and the Working Groups on Arrhythmias and Cardiac Pacing of the European Society of Cardiology. *Pacing Clin Electrophysiol* 1995; **18**: 637–54.

56. Weerasooriya HR, Harris AH, Davis MJ. Cost effectiveness of day stay versus inpatient radiofrequency (RF) ablation for the treatment of supraventricular tachyarrhythmias. *Austral N Zealand J Med* 1996; **26**: 206–9.

24

Evaluation of cardiovascular diseases in competitive athletes

CHRISTOPHER A McGREW

Sudden cardiovascular death of a competitive athlete is a typically unexpected and certainly tragic occurrence. In attempting to prevent such tragedies, the prescribing physician must usually address one or both of the following issues. The first is screening of apparently healthy asymptomatic athletes during pre-participation examinations. The second is the evaluation of and decision making for athletes with known cardiovascular disease. These two areas are addressed in this chapter.

For the purposes of this chapter, the definition of competitive athlete will be 'one who participates in organized team or individual sport that requires regular competition against others as a central component, places a high premium on excellence and achievement, and requires some form of systematic training.[1]

EPIDEMIOLOGY

The number of competitive athletes involved at the high school, collegiate, and professional level in the USA is approximately five million. This does not include participants in youth, junior high, and masters athletic programs.

> The prevalence of cardiovascular disease in this athletic population is low. Although the precise risk of sudden cardiac death in athletes with underlying disease is unknown, it too is undoubtedly low.

The National Center for Catastrophic Injury Research reports approximately 12–15 sudden cardiac deaths in high school and college athletes each year.[2] It is not clear from these numbers as to what percentage of these individuals had pre-participation screening and/or known cardiovascular disease. A study reported by Maron *et al.* in 1996 discusses 158 sudden deaths in trained athletes from 1985 to 1995.[3] Of these 158 athletes, 134 died from cardiovascular causes. Thirty-six per cent had probable or definite evidence of hypertrophic cardiomyopathy. Another 10 per cent had possible hypertrophic cardiomyopathy. Nineteen per cent were seen to have coronary artery abnormalities. One hundred and thirty of the 134 had pre-participation evaluations. One hundred and fifteen had a standard screening with history and physical examination, of which one had a correct diagnosis (although this athlete was not disqualified). Fifteen of the athletes who underwent standard screening were sent on to further testing because of a positive family history, symptom, or other aspect of the screening examination. This further examination group had seven correct diagnoses made, of which two were officially disqualified from sports participation. Of the 130 athletes with some form of pre-participation medical evaluation, an appropriate cardiovascular diagnosis was ultimately achieved during life in only 6 per cent.

PRE-PARTICIPATION SCREENING

The American Heart Association (AHA) in 1996 published a scientific statement entitled 'cardiovascular preparticipation screening of competitive athletes'.[4] This section will rely heavily on information provided in this scientific statement. Reprints of this statement can be obtained by contacting the American Heart Association, 7272 Greenville Avenue, Dallas, Texas 75231-4596, USA.

> The first thing that must be remembered is that screening for cardiovascular disease in the competitive athlete is usually a part of a more general pre-participation physical examination.

This will include a history and physical examination, which cover a wide variety of areas, but primarily the musculoskeletal system along with the cardiovascular system. The most widely accepted guideline for this general pre-participation examination is the *Preparticipation physician evaluation* monograph,[5] which has been endorsed by two primary care and three sports medicine societies. The most recent revision was published in 1996. It has incorporated all the general guidelines promulgated in the AHA statement except for the frequency of the examination.

In conducting pre-participation evaluations of competitive athletes, it is important to take into account the normal variations resulting from the athlete's heart syndrome.[6] These differences from a general population's norm are related to the physiologic adaptations that occur as a result of training, especially for endurance. The higher vagal tone associated with training may lead to bradyarrhythmias, including marked sinus arrhythmia, atrial ventricular disassociation with junctional escape rhythm, intermittent types I and II atrioventricular (AV) blocks and, in rare cases, intermittent third-degree block. One should consider the higher forms of AV block to be normal variants, however, only if they are transient and disappear with exercise. On physical examination these arrhythmias can translate into cannon A waves owing to AV dissociation or hyperdynamic carotid pulses due to bradycardia and concomitantly increased stroke volume. Large stroke volumes can also produce a venous hum detectable on a neck examination or a systolic murmur related to turbulent flow through normal semilunar valves. The third and fourth heart sounds may also be a normal adaptation to training. The highly trained athlete can also exhibit a variety of alterations on the electrocardiogram (ECG), including changes in virtually every wave form, duration time, and interval. A full discussion of the variety of conduction defects and arrhythmias that are possible can be found in an article published by Zehender *et al.* in 1990.[7] In general, supraventricular ectopy, paroxysmal atrial tachycardia, and both simple and complex ventricular arrhythmias should be no more common – and no less alarming – in the well-trained athlete than his/her sedentary counterpart. A thorough search for underlying structural heart disease should be performed on any athlete with complex ventricular arrhythmias.[8]

It is generally accepted that a standardized screening program by history and physical examination alone will not guarantee detection of many critical cardiovascular abnormalities in large populations of young trained athletes. However, the AHA[4] recommends that some form of pre-participation cardiovascular screening for high school and college athletes is justifiable and compelling based on 'ethical, legal and medical grounds'.

> Non-invasive testing can enhance a diagnostic power of the standard history and physical examination; however, it is not prudent to recommend routine use of such tests as 12-lead electrocardiography, echocardiography, or graded exercise testing for detection of cardiovascular disease in large populations of athletes.

Given the large number of competitive athletes in the USA, the relatively low frequency with which the cardiovascular lesions responsible for these deaths occur, and the low rate of sudden cardiac death in the athletic community, there is concern that widespread use of non-invasive testing in athletic populations could result in many false-positive test results, creating unnecessary anxiety among substantial numbers of athletes and their families, as well as unjustified exclusion from life insurance coverage in athletic competition. Indeed, in such a circumstance with a low incidence of disease within the community, a great likelihood exists that the number of false-positive results would exceed that of true positive results.[4]

> The AHA recommends that athletic screening be performed by a health care worker with 'the requisite training, medical skills, and background to reliably obtain a detailed cardiovascular history and perform a physical examination and recognize heart disease' (*see* Table 24.1).

Specifically, athletic screening evaluations should include a complete medical history and physical examination, including brachial artery blood pressure measurement.

The cardiovascular history should include key questions designed to determine the following:

1 prior occurrence of exertional chest pain/discomfort or syncope/near syncope as well as excessive unexpected and unexplained shortness of breath or fatigue associated with exercise;
2 past detection of a heart murmur or increased systemic blood pressure; and

Table 24.1 *Pre-participation cardiovascular screening of competitive athletes: the American Heart Association scientific statement*

High school and college age athletes	Older athletes (over 35 years)
History and physical examination[a], performed prior to participation in organized high school or college sports	History and physical examination[a], including personal history of coronary risk factors and/or family history of premature ischemic heart disease
Screening repeated every 2 years	Selective exercise stress testing in men older than 40 (and women older than 50) who wish to engage in regular physical training and competitive sports, if physician suspects coronary artery disease on the basis of risk factors, either multiple (two or more other than age and gender) or single markedly abnormal risk
In intervening years (between screenings), an interim history should be obtained	Older athletes should also be warned specifically about prodromal cardiovascular symptoms (for example, exertional chest pain)

[a] The examination should be conducted in an environment conducive to optimal auscultation. It should be performed by a health care worker with requisite skills. The evaluation should emphasize elements critical to the detection of cardiovascular disease known to be associated with cardiac problems or sudden cardiac death in athletes.

3 family history of premature death (sudden or otherwise) or significant disability from cardiovascular disease in close relatives younger than 50 years old or specific knowledge of the occurrence of certain conditions, i.e. hypertrophic cardiomyopathy, dilated cardiomyopathy, long QT syndrome, Marfan's syndrome, or clinically important arrhythmias.

These questions obviously represent an ideal history; the accuracy of some of the responses elicited from athletes may be less than optimal. Parents/guardians should assist in completing the history forms with the athlete, if possible (*see* Table 24.2)

The cardiovascular physical examination should emphasize (but not necessarily be limited to):

1 precordial auscultation in both the supine and standing positions to identify any particular heart murmurs consistent with dynamic left ventricular outflow obstruction;
2 assessment of the femoral artery pulses to exclude coarctation of the aorta;
3 recognition of the physical stigmata of Marfan's syndrome; and
4 brachial blood pressure measurement in the sitting position (*see* table 24.2).

When cardiovascular abnormalities are identified or suspected by this screening examination, the athlete should be referred for further evaluation and/or confirmation. Skillful interpretation of high-quality echocardiography will play an important role in the resolution of many of these cases.

Table 24.2 *American Heart Association recommendations for cardiovascular screening of competitive athletes*

History
- Have you experienced chest pain, fainting or near-fainting with exertion?
- Have you experienced excessive, unexpected, or unexplained shortness of breath, or fatigue associated with exercise?
- Have you ever been found to have a heart murmur, or increased blood pressure?
- Have any of your close relatives developed significant disability from cardiovascular disease before age 50? Have any of your close relatives died from cardiovascular disease before age 50?
- Does anyone in your family have heart conditions, such as hypertrophic cardiomyopathy, dilated cardiomyopathy, long QT syndrome, Marfan's syndrome, or arrhythmias?

Physical examination
- Brachial blood pressure in the sitting position
- Precordial auscultation in both supine and standing position, specifically for heart murmurs consistent with dynamic left ventricular outflow obstruction
- Assessment of femoral artery pulses to exclude coarctation of aorta
- Recognition of physical stigmata of Marfan's syndrome

EVALUATION OF ATHLETES WITH KNOWN CARDIOVASCULAR DISEASE

Athletes with recognized cardiovascular abnormalities should be evaluated with respect to the 26th Bethesda Conference Guidelines.[9] In dealing with the athlete with

Table 24.3 *Classification of sports: based on peak dynamic and static components during competition. (Adapted with permission from* Medicine and Science in Sports and Exercise)

	Low dynamic	Moderate dynamic	High dynamic
Low static	Billiards Bowling Cricket Curling Golf Riflery	Baseball Softball Table tennis Tennis (doubles) Volleyball	Badminton Cross-country skiing (classic technique) Field hockey[a] Orienteering Race walking Racquetball Running (long-distance) Soccer[a] Squash Tennis (singles)
Moderate static	Archery Auto racing[a,b] Diving[a,b] Equestrian[a,b] Motorcycling[a,b]	Fencing Field events (jumping) Figure skating[a] Football (American) Rodeoing[a,b] Rugby[a] Running (sprint) Surfing[a,b] Synchronized swimming[b]	Basketball[a] Ice hockey[a] Cross-country skiing (skating technique) Football (Australian rules)[a] Lacrosse[a] Running (middle-distance) Swimming Team handball
High static	Bobsledding[a,b] Field events (throwing) Gymnastics[a,b] Karate/judo[a] Luge[a,b] Sailing Rock climbing[a,b] Water skiing[a,b] Weight lifting[a,b] Wind surfing[a,b]	Body building[a,b] Downhill skiing[a,b] Wrestling[a]	Boxing[a] Canoeing/kayaking Cycling[a,b] Decathlon Rowing Speed skating

[a] Danger of bodily collision.
[b] Increased risk if syncope occurs.

known cardiovascular disease, the clinician must have some idea of the demands of the chosen sport in determining, after appropriate evaluation, whether the athlete can return to that sport or will need to consider other options. (A classification of sports based on peak dynamic and static components during competition is shown in Table 24.3.) The 26th Bethesda Conference divided cardiovascular abnormalities into six basic areas. These included:

1 congenital heart disease;
2 acquired valvular heart disease;
3 hypertrophic cardiomyopathy, myocarditis and other myopericardial diseases and mitral valve prolapse;
4 systemic hypertension;
5 coronary artery disease; and
6 arrhythmias.

Only key areas under each of these topics will be touched upon in this chapter. For complete and compre-

hensive review of all of these areas, the reader is referred to the complete publication of the 26th Bethesda Conference.[9]

Congenital heart disease

There are relatively few congenital conditions that have been associated with sudden cardiovascular death during sports participation. The most common are hypertrophic cardiomyopathy, congenital coronary anomalies, Marfan's syndrome, aortic stenosis, and mitral valve prolapse.

HYPERTROPHIC CARDIOMYOPATHY

Hypertrophic cardiomyopathy[10] is of great importance because it is probably the most common cause of unexpected sudden cardiac death in young competitive athletes. The athlete with hypertrophic cardiomyopathy may be assessed by non-invasive testing using, in particular, clinical examination and history, echocardiography, 12-lead electrocardiogram (ECG), and ambulatory (Holter) ECG. Cardiac catheterization is usually not required for diagnostic purposes. The demonstration of unexplained left ventricular hypertrophy by two-dimensional echocardiography represents the key to clinical diagnosis. At present insufficient data are available that support particular invasive or non-invasive approaches for definitely stratifying risks for sudden death in individual patients with hypertrophic cardiomyopathy. This includes the use of electrophysiologic testing with programmed electrical stimulation because of its relatively low predictive accuracy. Programmed electrical stimulation does not, at present, permit definitive clinical decisions to be made in individuals with hypertrophic cardiomyopathy. Future investigative work in molecular genetics, electrophysiology, and evaluation of vascular responses will more accurately define parameters of hemodynamic and electrical instability, and may in the future permit more reliable identification of those athletes with this disease who are at particular risk for sudden cardiac death.

Recommendations for participation include the following.

1 Athletes with the unequivocal diagnosis of hypertrophic cardiomyopathy should not participate in most competitive sports with the possible exception of those with low intensity (class 1A). This recommendation includes those athletes with or without symptoms of left ventricular outflow obstruction.

2 In recognition of the observation that the risk for sudden cardiac death may be reduced in older individuals with hypertrophic cardiomyopathy, the Bethesda guidelines suggest that individual judgment in assessing eligibility may be utilized in selected older patients (i.e. greater than 30 years of age) for whom each of the following clinical features (judged or established to be unfavorable or potential risk factors for sudden death) are *absent*.

- Ventricular tachycardia (sustained or non-sustained) on the ambulatory ECG.
- Family history of sudden death due to hypertrophic cardiomyopathy, particularly, if occurring at less than 40 years of age.
- History of syncope or other clinically relevant episodes of impaired consciousness.
- Severe hemodynamic abnormalities, including a dynamic left ventricular outflow track gradient ($\geq$50 mm Hg).
- Exercise induced hypotension.
- Moderate to severe mitral regurgitation, enlarged left atrium ($\geq$50 mm), or paroxysmal atrial fibrillation.
- Evidence of abnormal myocardial perfusion.

CONGENITAL CORONARY ANOMALIES

Congenital coronary anomalies[11] are rarely identified because patients usually do not experience warning symptoms and non-invasive diagnosis is difficult. These abnormalities are rarely detected unless the athlete has significant chest pain (rare) or syncope on exertion. Sudden death may be the first manifestation of disease. These abnormalities should be considered in athletes with exertional syncope or near-fatal arrhythmias. Routine ECG is typically unremarkable as is an exercise stress test in the absence of ischemia. Detailed two-dimensional echocardiograms may give a clue to the diagnosis by indicating abnormal origins of the right and left coronary arteries. Other coronary abnormalities, such as hypoplastic vessels, may only be discoverable through angiography.

Recommendations include:

1 detection of these abnormalities should result in exclusion from all competitive sports participation;
2 sports participation $\geq$ 6 months after surgery would be permitted for an individual without ischemia during maximal exercise testing.

MARFAN'S SYNDROME

Marfan's syndrome[11] is typically characterized by arachnodactyly, tall stature, pectus excavatum, kyphoscoliosis, and monticular dislocation; there are, however, atypical presentations with no obvious physical stigmata. Cardiovascular manifestations are mitral valve prolapse and aortic dilatation. Aortic dissection is a known cause of sudden death in competitive athletes. Diagnosis is suspected by skeletal features and/or family history, and confirmed by eye examination (lens dislocation) and echocardiography.

Recommendations for participation are as follows.

1 Athletes without a family history of premature sudden death, and without evidence of aortic dilatation or mitral regurgitation can participate in moderate, low static, and low dynamic competitive sports (classes IA and IIA). Echocardiographic measurements of aortic dimension should be repeated every 6 months for continued sports participation.
2 Athletes with aortic dilatation can participate only in low intensity competitive sports (class IA).
3 Athletes with Marfan's syndrome should *not* participate in sports with the risk of bodily collision.

VALVULAR AORTIC STENOSIS[11]

Congenital aortic stenosis is usually identifiable by a constant apical ejection click and systolic ejection murmur heard maximally at the right upper sternal border. Differentiation between mild and moderate severe stenosis is readily accomplished with ECG and Doppler echocardiography as well as the physical examination. The distinction, however, between moderate and severe stenosis is more difficult and may require cardiac catheterization to clarify. Sudden death is more likely to occur in patients with severe disease, which is indicated by severe left ventricular hypertrophy, exertional syncope, chest pain or dyspnea, or left ventricular strain pattern on ECG. For purposes of sports recommendations, mild aortic stenosis is defined as having a resting peak instantaneous systolic pressure gradient (in the presence of normal cardiac output) of <20 mm Hg by catheterization or Doppler echocardiography. Moderate stenosis is defined between 21 and 49 mm Hg, and severe stenosis is defined as > 50 mm Hg. This classification is different from that used for making clinical decisions regarding balloon valvuloplasty or surgery and represents a conservative approach tailored to strenuous sports participation in this condition because of the known problems of sudden death with severe aortic stenosis and the difficulty in achieving an up to date appraisal of severity for a lesion that can progress with time.

Recommendations for participation are as follows.

1 Athletes with mild aortic stenosis can participate in all competitive sports if they have a normal ECG and exercise tolerance, and no history of exercise-related chest pain, syncope, or arrhythmia associated with symptoms.
2 Athletes with moderate aortic stenosis can participate in low static/low moderate dynamic and moderate static/low dynamic (classes IA and IB and IIA) competitive sports if the following conditions are met:
   • mild or no left ventricular hypertrophy by echocardiography and the absence of left ventricular strain on ECG;
   • normal exercise test with no evidence for ischemia or arrhythmia, normal exercise duration, and normal blood pressure response;
   • an absence of symptoms as defined above.
3 Athletes with severe aortic stenosis should *not* participate in competitive sports.

MITRAL VALVE PROLAPSE

Mitral valve prolapse,[10] a common abnormality that is benign in most persons, demands a comprehensive work-up when there is any of the following:

• history of syncope or near syncope;
• family history of sudden death; or
• complex ventricular activity.

This evaluation should include comprehensive echocardiography, exercise testing and long-term Holter monitoring while the athlete is performing his or her sport. Athletes with mitral valve prolapse *without* any of the following criteria can engage in all competitive sports:

• history of syncope documented to be arrhythmogenic in origin;
• a family history of sudden death associated with mitral valve prolapse;
• repetitive forms of sustained, non-sustained supraventricular arrhythmias or complex ventricular arrhythmias, particularly exaggerated by exercise;
• moderate to marked mitral regurgitation;
• a prior embolic event.

If athletes have any of the aforementioned criteria, they can participate in only low-intensity competitive sports (class IA).

ARRHYTHMOGENIC RIGHT VENTRICULAR DYSPLASIA[12]

This unusual primary disorder of the right ventricular myocardium has been cited as a leading cause of sudden death in athletes outside the USA. Athletes with arrhythmogenic right ventricular dysplasia can have normal ventricular performance, allowing them to attain high levels of physical performance. The most common clinical marker is ventricular arrhythmia with a left bundle branch block pattern; the mechanism of sudden death is the degeneration into ventricular fibrillation. Diagnosis is established with echocardiography and electrophysiology testing. The recommendation is that patients with arrhythmogenic left ventricular dysplasia should not be permitted to participate in competitive sports.

Other common problems

MYOCARDITIS

Myocarditis[10] is probably under-represented in statistics on sudden cardiovascular death in athletes. Myocarditis is suspected clinically by virtue of fatigue, exertional dyspnea, syncope, palpitations, arrhythmias, or acute congestive heart failure in the presence of left ventricular dilatation and associated with evidence of ventricular dysfunction (usual segmental wall motion abnormalities or ST-T changes on ECG).

Recommendations for participation are as follows.

1 Athletes judged probably to have myocarditis should be withdrawn from all competitive sports and should undergo a prudent convalescent period of about 6 months after the onset of clinical manifestations. Before the athlete may return to competitive athletic training, an evaluation of cardiac status should be undertaken, including assessment of ventricular function at rest and with exercise, preferably in conjunction with radionucleide angiography or echocardiography.
2 An athlete should be allowed to return to competition when ventricular function and also

cardiac dimensions have returned to normal and clinically relevant arrhythmias (repetitive forms of ventricular ectopic activity are sustained, supraventricular tachycardia) are absent on ambulatory monitoring.

3 Sufficient clinical data are not available to justify a strong recommendation to perform endomyocardial biopsy as a precondition to return to athletic competition after the proposed 6-month period of deconditioning. The role of invasive electrophysiologic testing in assessing the eligibility of athletes with myocarditis remains to be defined.

SYSTEMIC HYPERTENSION[13]

Athletes with any degree of persistent hypertension should have a thorough history and physical examination and limited laboratory testing in order to evaluate secondary causes and to target organ damage. Laboratory testing for most people observed to have mild to moderate hypertension[13] should be limited to a measurement of glucose, creatinine, electrolytes and cholesterol, hematocrit, urinalysis, and ECG. If these are abnormal or if features suggestive of secondary causes are noted by history or physical examination the subject should be referred for additional study and therapy. Echocardiography and exercise testing may be useful; however, there is an absence of data documenting that they provide either diagnostic or prognostic information about the eligibility for athletic computation in relation to hypertension and, therefore, they are not required for routine use.

Recommendations for participation are as follows.

1 Mild to moderate hypertension in the absence of target organ damage or concomitant heart disease should not limit the eligibility for any competitive sports. Once beginning a training program, the hypertensive athlete should have his or her blood pressure remeasured every 2–4 months.

2 Athletes with severe degrees of hypertension should be restricted, particularly from high static sports (classes IIIA , IIIB, and IIIC) until their hypertension is controlled by either lifestyle modification or drug therapy, and in the absence of evidence of target organ damage.

CORONARY ARTERY DISEASE[14]

The diagnosis of coronary artery disease is established if:

1 coronary angiography demonstrates coronary artery atherosclerotic luminal narrowing of at least one major coronary artery;

2 a history of myocardial infarction can be confirmed by conventional ECG or enzyme criteria; or

3 a history suggestive of angina pectoris is supported by objective data, such as ischemic ST segment or abnormal myocardial perfusion response to exercise.

There are no data directly relating the presence and severity of coronary artery disease to the risk of participating in competitive athletics. However, it is probable that the risk of cardiac events during competitive exercise increases with the presence of increasingly severe coronary artery disease, left ventricular dysfunction, and ventricular arrhythmias. Athletes with previously diagnosed coronary artery disease undergoing evaluation for competitive athletics, should have their left ventricular function assessed by two-dimensional echocardiography, radionucleide angiography, or left ventricular angiography. These athletes should also undergo maximal treadmill or bicycle exercise testing to assess their exercise capacity. When feasible, exercise testing should approximate closely the cardiovascular and metabolic demands of the planned competitive event and its training regimen. The presence or absence of provocable myocardial ischemia should also be determined by exercise ECG, radionucleide profusion imaging exercise, echocardiography or subjective evidence of ischemia.

Risk stratification is somewhat arbitrary but two levels have been defined on the basis of testing. These include 'mildly increased' risk and 'substantially increased' risk. 'Mildly increased' risk includes athletes that demonstrate each of the following:

1 normal or nearly normal resting left ventricular systolic function (i.e., ejection fraction >50 per cent);

2 normal exercise tolerance for age (see Table 24.5);

3 absence of exercise-induced ischemia by exercise testing;

4 absence of exercise-induced complex ventricular arrhythmias, including ventricular tachycardia;

5 absence of hemodynamically significant stenosis in all major coronary arteries (generally regarded as 50 per cent greater luminal diameter narrowing), if coronary angiography is performed; or successful myocardial revascularization by surgical or percutaneous techniques.

Table 24.5 *Normal exercise tolerance by age*

Age (years)	METs
<50	>10
50–59	>9
60–69	>8
>70	>7

METs = metabolic equivalents.

'Substantially increased risk' includes athletes that demonstrate any of the following:

1 impaired left ventricular systolic function at rest (ejection fraction < 50 per cent);

2 evidence of exercise-induced myocardial ischemia;

3 evidence of exercise-induced complex ventricular arrhythmias, including ventricular tachycardia;

4 hemodynamically significant stenosis of a major coronary artery (generally regarded as 50 per cent or greater luminal diameter narrowing) if coronary angiography was performed.

Recommendations for participation are as follows.

1 Athletes in the mildly increased risk group can participate in low and moderate static and low dynamic competitive sports (classes IA and IIA), and avoid intensely competitive situations. It is recognized that selected athletes with mildly increased risk may be permitted to compete in sports of higher levels of intensity when their overall clinical profile suggests very low risk. All athletes should understand that the risk of a cardiac event with exertion is increased once coronary artery disease is present. Athletes with mildly increased risk engaging in competitive sports should undergo re-evaluation of their risk stratification at least once a year.

2 Athletes in the substantially increased risk category should be generally restricted to low-intensity competitive sports (class IA). Those groups of patients judged to be at the highest risk because of severe abnormalities in left ventricular function, exercise intolerance, or exercise-induced cardiac arrhythmias should be prohibited even from low intensive competitive activity. Athletes allowed to participate in low-intensity activities should be re-evaluated at least every 6 months.

3 Athletes should be informed of the nature of ischemic symptoms and should be instructed to cease promptly their sports activity and to contact their physician if symptoms appear.

ARRHYTHMIAS[15]

Malignant arrhythmias are usually the final common pathway for the conditions that have been mentioned previously. On the other hand, there are primary abnormalities of the cardiac conduction system that can cause sudden death in athletes whose hearts may be structurally normal.

In general, all athletes with significant cardiac arrhythmias being considered for athletic activity should have a 12-lead ECG, echocardiogram, exercise test and long-term 24-hour ambulatory (Holter) monitoring, *if possible during the specific type of exercise being considered*. All athletes with an arrhythmia that are permitted to engage in athletics should be re-evaluated at intervals after they are trained to determine whether the condition process affected the arrhythmia. They also need to be evaluated frequently for adherence to their medicine regimens.

Special note should be made about unexplained syncope in the competitive athlete. This is a potentially important symptom that requires a thorough evalua-

tion. It may be due to a variety of causes, including cardiovascular disease. On the other hand, it may be completely unassociated with structural heart disease and due to such a common finding in highly trained athletes as vasovagal syncope. Caution, however, should be used in making the diagnosis of vasovagal syncope in highly trained athletes without first definitively excluding underlying structural heart disease. Tilt-table testing has been used to assess patients at risk for vaso-vagal syncope but the lack of specificity of this test (particularly in endurance-trained athletes) requires a particularly cautious interpretation of the result. Exercise testing is useful and optimally performed while recording the ECG during the sport activity in which the athlete participates. In certain athletes, when no other cause of the syncope has been identified with thorough evaluation, including ambulatory ECG, exercise testing and echocardiography, then invasive electrophysiologic testing should be considered.

FUTURE DIRECTIONS

Given the considerable lack of what could be considered solid, evidence-based medical documentation for various components of the pre-participation examination as well as some of the guidelines for patients with known cardiovascular disease, research must continue to look at these areas. In particular, in the area of the pre-participation examination, questions concerning the frequency of the examination, the optimal questionnaire, and the role of investigative technologies are areas that are ripe for continued investigation. Another area to look at is the cost effectiveness of the current protocol for pre-participation screening in this country. In the area of athletes with known cardiovascular disease, researchers continue to look at the problem of risk stratification within the group of athletes with hypertrophic cardiomyopathy in order to determine whether some of these athletes are indeed reasonably safe to participate in competitive sports. Additionally, it would be helpful for prospective studies to follow athletes that have been disqualified from organized competitive sports because of certain cardiovascular illnesses, such as hypertrophic cardiomyopathy, to follow their natural history of physical activity and participation in strenuous but not officially organized athletic activity.

FINAL CONSIDERATIONS

In general, providing athletic health care to competitive athletes is a very rewarding (and most of the time, fun) type of medical practice. As a group they tend to be healthy, enthusiastic, and very curious about finding out about their physiologic capabilities. It is important when dealing with them, whether it be in the pre-participation screening, or in the work-up of a known or potential cardiovascular disease, that good rapport be established.

> In particular, this rapport can be enhanced by understanding the demands of the sport that the athlete is involved in, knowing some of the 'jargon' (or be willing to listen and learn from the athlete), and being empathetic to the perceived value of the sport to each particular athlete.

Part of this empathy must include an understanding of the time urgency many athletes feel in their desire to return to active training and competition. This is not to say that any evaluation should be rushed or done in haste, but only to suggest that appropriate reflecting back to the athlete of your understanding of their concerns and your wishes to proceed as quickly and safely as possible should be conveyed. In addition, in working with athletes, one should be prepared to deal with questions and concerns that come from outside the 'typical family unit'. This may include coaches, school and sports team officials, and, in the case of professional athletes, agents. One should discuss thoroughly with the athlete with whom he or she would like information shared as the evaluation proceeds. Also, it should be admitted to the athlete in cases where little hard scientific data are available for that particular condition and that there are no guarantees as to the outcome, either good or bad, in all situations.

> Additionally, during the pre-participation examination, it must be clearly outlined that passing a standard evaluation prior to beginning competitive sports is no guarantee against sudden death.

Finally, the aforementioned recommendations, which have been derived primarily from the 26th Bethesda Conference, should be seen as guidelines that may be, in certain cases, individualized and modified, depending on the particular situation of the athletes.

SUMMARY

- Prevalence of cardiac disease is low in athletes.
- Sudden death in athletes is rare.
- Screening history and physical should be standardized.
- 26th Bethesda Guidelines are the standard for evaluation of athletes with known disease.
- Understanding athletes and their environment is important for effective evaluation and management.

REFERENCES

○1. Maron BJ, Mitchell JH. Revised eligibility of recommendations for competitive athletes with cardiovascular abnormalities. *Med Sci Sports Exercise* 1994; **26** (suppl 2): S223.

2. Mueller FO, Cantu RC, VanCamp SP. Catastrophic injuries in high school and college sports. *HK Sport Sci Monograph Ser* 1996; **8**: 23–39.

3. Maron BJ, Shirani J, Poliac L, *et al.* Sudden death in young competitive athletes. Clinical, demographic and pathological profiles. *JAMA* 1996; **276**: 199–204.

○4. American Heart Association. Cardiovascular preparticipation screening of competitive athletes: a statement for health professionals from the Sudden Death Committee (Clinical Cardiology) and Congenital Cardiac Defects Committee (Cardiovascular Disease in the Young). *Circulation* 1996; **94**: 850–6.

○5. American Academy of Family Physicians, *et al. Preparticipation physical evaluation*, 2nd edn. Minneapolis, MN: McGraw Hill Health Care, 1996.

6. Houston TP, Puffer JC, Rodney WM. The athletic heart syndrome. *N Engl J Med* 1985; **31**: 24–32.

○7. Zehender M, Minertz T, Keul J, *et al.* ECG variance and cardiac arrhythmias in athletes: clinical relevance and prognostic importance. *Am Heart J* 1990; **119**: 1378–91.

8. Rouzich RS. Cardiac evaluation for the athlete at risk. *Family Practice Recertification* 1994; **16**(8): 37–50.

9. Maron BJ, Mitchell JA, Raven PB, *et al.* 26th Bethesda Conference recommendations for determining eligibility for competition athletes with cardiovascular abnormalities. *Med Sci Sport Exercise* 1994; **26** (suppl 2): S223–83.

10. Maron BJ, Eisner JM, McKenna WJ. Task force 3. Hypertrophic cardiomyopathy, myocarditis and other myopericardial diseases in mitral valve prolapse. *Med Sci Sport Exercise* 1994; **26** (suppl 2): S261–7.

11. Graham TP, Bricker TJ, James FW, *et al.* Task force 1 – congenital heart disease. *Med Sci Sport Exercise* 1994; **26** (suppl 2): S246–53.

12. Furlanello R, Beitini R, Bertoldi A, *et al.* Arrhythmia patterns in athletes with arrhythmogenic right ventricular dysplasia. *Eur Heart J* 1989; **10** (suppl D): 16–19.

13. Caplan NM, Deveraux RV, Miller HS. Task force 4 – systemic hypertension. *Med Sci Sport Exercise* 1994; **26** (suppl 2): S268–70.

14. Thompson PD, Klocke FJ, Levine BD, VanCamp SP. Task force 5 – coronary artery disease. *Med Sci Sport Exercise* 1994; **26** (suppl 2): S271–5.

15. Zipes DP, Garson A. Task force 6 – arrhythmias. *Med Sci Sport Exercise* 1994; **26** (suppl 2): S276–83.

25

Out-patient management of thrombotic disorders

GRAHAM F PINEO AND RUSSELL D HULL

In recent years there has been an increasing trend to manage medical and surgical conditions in the out-patient setting. The advent of low-molecular-weight heparins has permitted the management of a number of thrombotic disorders in the out-patient setting. This chapter reviews the use of low-molecular-weight heparin in the management of venous thrombo-embolism, unstable angina and non-ST segment elevation myocardial infarction and intravenous unfractionated heparin by continuous infusion with particular reference to the out-patient setting.

INTRODUCTION

In recent years, there has been an increasing trend to manage medical and surgical conditions in the out-patient setting. This trend has been particularly prevalent in the management of thrombotic disorders where it has been shown to be both effective and safe when compared with in-hospital treatment; in addition, it is cost effective, and most patients prefer to have their treatment in their home environment wherever possible. Furthermore, the downsizing of hospitals in North America has made bed availability a constant problem, and this has encouraged the development of out-patient management programs to ensure that the limited number of hospital beds are properly utilized. The advent of the low-molecular-weight heparins has permitted the management of a number of thrombotic disorders in the out-patient setting. This chapter will review the use of low-molecular-weight heparin in the management of venous thromboembolism, unstable angina, and non-ST segment elevation myocardial

infarction, with particular reference to the out-patient setting. We also review the management of oral anticoagulants, with particular reference to the optimal duration of anticoagulation following an initial or recurrent episode of venous thromboembolism and the problems of interrupting oral anticoagulants for surgical procedures.

TREATMENT OF VENOUS THROMBOEMBOLISM

Anticoagulant properties of unfractionated heparin

Unfractionated heparin from either porcine or bovine sources has been available for clinical use for several decades. Although heparin has been studied extensively, much remains uncertain about its mode of action, and some of the complications have only recently been better understood.[1]

The anticoagulant activity of unfractionated heparin depends upon a unique pentasaccharide, which binds to antithrombin III (ATIII) and potentiates the inhibition of thrombin and activated Factor X (X_a) by ATIII.[2-4] About one-third of all heparin molecules contain the unique pentasaccharide sequence regardless of whether they are low or high in molecular-weight fractions. It is the pentasaccharide sequence that confers the high molecular affinity for ATIII.[3,5] The remaining two-thirds of heparin has minimal anticoagulant activity at the therapeutic concentrations that are used clinically. For the inhibition of thrombin, heparin must form a bridge between thrombin and ATIII, but for the inhibition of Factor X_a this bridging is not necessary.[4,5] It has been shown that molecules of heparin with fewer than 18 saccharide units are unable to bind thrombin and ATIII simultaneously and as a result cannot catalyse thrombin inhibition.[6] Heparin fragments with smaller numbers of saccharide units are capable of catalysing the inhibition of Factor X_a by ATIII, providing the high-affinity pentasaccharide sequence is present. Unfractionated heparin is unable to inhibit thrombin bound to fibrin, whereas the specific antithrombin agents do so.[7] Heparin does not inhibit Factor X_a bound to platelets.[8]

Heparin also catalyses the inactivation of thrombin by another plasma co-factor (co-factor II), which acts independently of ATIII.[9] Heparin has a number of other effects. Those related to the anticoagulant effects of heparin include the release of tissue factor pathway inhibitor,[10] binding to numerous plasma and platelet proteins, endothelial cells and leukocytes,[2,11] suppression of platelet function[8] and increase in vascular permeability.[12]

The anticoagulant response to a standard dose of heparin varies widely between patients. Heparin is poorly absorbed from the subcutaneous site, especially at lower doses.[13] The plasma clearance of heparin depends on a dose-related renal clearance and a non-dose-related saturable cellular mechanism.[14] The binding of heparin to plasma proteins, endothelial cells and platelets contributes to the unpredictable response.[10,11] Some patients develop relative heparin resistance and require a large dose of heparin to achieve a response in the activated partial thromboplastin time (aPTT).[15] Recent studies have documented a rebound thrombin generation when heparin is abruptly stopped.[16,17] It is therefore necessary to monitor the anticoagulant response of heparin frequently using either the aPTT or heparin levels, and to titrate the dose to the individual patient.

Unless a prescriptive heparin nomogram is used, many patients receive inadequate heparin in the initial 24–48 hours of treatment.[18-20] This inadequate therapy has been shown to increase the incidence of venous thromboembolism during follow-up.[21-23] Treatment is further complicated by the fact that there is a diurnal variation in the aPTT response in patients on a constant infusion of intravenous heparin.[24] A peak response is seen at 3 am and a reduction of heparin infusion in response to the high aPTT could result in subtherapeutic treatment later in the day.[24] There is a wide variation in the sensitivity of various thromboplastins used in performing the aPPT and even with the same thromboplastin, different coagulometers may yield different results.[25] It is necessary for each laboratory to define a therapeutic range with respect to aPTT in terms of heparin blood levels (therapeutic range 0.2–0.4 units/mL heparin).[25]

The use of heparin is associated with a number of complications, the most serious of which is bleeding. Bleeding is primarily related to underlying clinical risk factors but is also increased in females and individuals over the age of 65 years.[26] The relationship of bleeding to heparin dosage and aPTT levels is less clear-cut.

Heparin-induced thrombocytopenia is a well-recognized complication of heparin therapy, usually occurring within 5–10 days after heparin treatment has started.[27-30] Approximately 1–2 per cent of patients receiving unfractionated heparin will experience a fall in platelet count to less than the normal range, or a 50 per cent fall in the platelet count within the normal range. In the majority of cases, this mild to moderate thrombocytopenia appears to be a direct effect of heparin on platelets and is of no consequence. However, approximately 0.1–0.2 per cent of patients receiving heparin develop an immune thrombocytopenia mediated by immunoglobulin G (IgG) antibody directed against a complex of PF4 and heparin.[30]

The development of thrombocytopenia may be accompanied by arterial or venous thrombosis, which may lead to serious consequences such as death or limb amputation.[28-31] The diagnosis of heparin-induced thrombocytopenia, with or without thrombosis, must be made on clinical grounds, because the assays with the highest sensitivity and specificity are not readily available and have a slow turnaround time.[28-30]

> When the diagnosis of heparin-induced thrombocytopenia is made, heparin in all forms must be stopped immediately.[29]

In those patients requiring ongoing anticoagulation, several alternatives exist. The agents most extensively used currently include the heparinoid Danaparoid,[32] hirudin,[33] and, most recently, the specific antithrombin argatroban.[34-36] Danaparoid and hirudin are now available and argatroban has recently been approved by the Food and Drug Administration (FDA). Warfarin may be used but probably should not be started until one of the above agents has been used for 3 or 4 days to suppress thrombin generation. Insertion of an inferior vena cava filter may be indicated.

Other complications of heparin include osteoporosis (most frequently documented in pregnancy), elevated liver enzymes, hypoaldosteronism, hypersensitivity and allergic skin reactions, and heparin-induced skin necrosis.[1]

The hope that the low-molecular-weight heparins may overcome some of the problems related to heparin therapy and decrease some of the complications has stimulated a large number of trials comparing low-molecular-weight heparins with unfractionated heparin.

Antithrombotic properties of low-molecular-weight heparin

Over the past 15 years a number of low-molecular-weight heparin (LMWH) fractions of unfractionated heparin have become available for commercial use.[36] The LMWHs are manufactured from unfractionated heparin (usually of porcine origin) by controlled depolymerization using either chemical (nitrous oxide, alkaline hydrolysis, or peroxidative cleavage) or enzymatic (heparinase) techniques.[37] The low-molecular-weight fractions have a molecular weight between 4000 and 6000 with 60 per cent of the polysaccharide chains having a molecular weight between 2000–8000. The various LMWHs differ in terms of mean molecular weight, glycosoaminoglycans content and anticoagulant activity as measured by anti-Factor X_a and anti-Factor II_a activity.[37–44] The various fractions have different pharmacologic profiles in terms of bioavailability, plasma clearance, and release of tissue factor pathway inhibitor, and in experimental models they have demonstrated different antithrombotic and hemorrhagic properties.[37–44] The LMWHs that have been most thoroughly studied are shown in Table 25.1; the method of production, molecular weights and anti-Factor X_a to anti-Factor II_a ratio are shown as well. Because the LMWHs are different compounds with distinct pharmacological properties[37,42] and because different regimens have been used in clinical trials, it may be inappropriate to use meta-analyses for comparing the effects of LMWH with placebo, unfractionated heparin, dextran or warfarin.

Despite the various differences between the LMWHs, the clinical outcomes in clinical trials are very similar, particularly in prophylactic studies using lower doses. In the higher doses used in the treatment of thrombotic disorders, it is quite possible that differences in outcomes will become apparent.

There has been a hope that the LMWHs will have fewer serious complications, such as bleeding,[44–47] osteoporosis[48–51] and heparin-induced thrombocytopenia[52] when compared with unfractionated heparin. Evidence is accumulating that these complications are indeed less serious and less frequent with the use of LMWH.[1] Low-molecular-weight heparin has not been approved for the prevention or treatment of venous thromboembolism in pregnancy. These drugs do not cross the placenta[53,54] and small case series suggest that they are both effective and safe.[55–57] However, at the present time, the standard treatment for venous thromboembolism in pregnancy is twice-daily adjusted doses of subcutaneous unfractionated heparin.[58] The LMWHs all cross-react with unfractionated heparin and they can therefore not be used as alternative therapy in patients who develop heparin-induced thrombocytopenia. The heparinoid Danaparoid possesses a 10–20 per cent cross-reactivity with heparin and it can be safely used in patients who have no cross-reactivity.[32]

Advantages of LMWH over unfractionated heparin

The LMWHs differ from unfractionated heparin in numerous ways. Of particular importance are the following: increased bioavailability[40,41] (>90 per cent after subcutaneous injection); prolonged half-life[37,40] and predictable clearance enabling once or twice daily injection;[59] and predictable antithrombotic response based on body weight, permitting treatment without laboratory monitoring.[50] Patients or other caregivers in the home can be readily taught to inject LMWH, particularly from pre-filled syringes, and numerous clinical trials involving self-injection for three or four weeks or even longer, have

Table 25.1 *Some commercial low-molecular-weight heparins and some of their properties*

Trade name[a]	International non-proprietary name	Method of production	Mean molecular weight (Da)	Anti-Factor X_a/II_a ratio
Logiparin Innohep	Tinzaparin	HD	5866	1.9 : 1
Fragmin	Dalteparin	NAP	5819	2.1 : 1
Lovenox	Enoxaparin	AH	4371	2.7 : 1
Fraxiparin	Nadroparin	NAP	4855	3.2 : 1
Reviparin	Clivarin	NAP	4653	3.6–6.1[b]
Normoflo	Ardeparin	PC	6000	2.0 : 1

[a] Manufacturers: Logiparin – Novo Nordisk; Innohep – Dupont; Fragmin – Pharmacia-Upjohn; Lovenox – Aventis; Fraxiparin – Sonofi; Reviparin – Knoll AG; Normoflo – Wyeth-Ayerst.
[b] Range provided by Knoll AG.
Da = daltons; HD = heparinase digestion; NAP = nitrous acid depolymerization; AH = alkaline hydrolysis; PC = peroxidative cleavage.

documented that patient compliance is very high. Other possible advantages are their ability to inhibit platelet-bound Factor X_a,[60] resistance to inhibition by platelet factor 4,[8,11] and their decreased effect on platelet function[8] and vascular permeability[12] (possibly accounting for less hemorrhagic effects at comparable antithrombotic doses).[44–47]

LMWH IN THE TREATMENT OF VENOUS THROMBOEMBOLISM

In the treatment of established venous thromboembolism, LMWHs given by subcutaneous injection have a number of advantages over continuous intravenous unfractionated heparin: they can be given by once or twice daily subcutaneous injection, and the antithrombotic response to low-molecular-weight heparin is highly correlated with body weight, permitting administration of a fixed dose without laboratory monitoring.

In a number of early clinical trials (some of which were dose finding), LMWH given by subcutaneous or intravenous injection was compared with continuous intravenous unfractionated heparin with repeat venography at day 7–10 being the primary end point.[61–66] These studies demonstrated that LMWH was at least as effective as unfractionated heparin in preventing extension or increasing resolution of thrombi on repeat venography.[61–66] More recently the more relevant clinical end point of recurrent venous thromboembolism or death during follow-up have been used as end points.[67–71] These studies are not all comparable because different regimens of LMWHs were used, not all studies ensured that adequate intravenous heparin therapy was given or properly monitored, and some studies entered patients with distal as well as proximal deep vein thrombosis. Only one study was double blinded,[67] although others used blinded assessment of outcome measures for both efficacy and safety. In these studies, LMWH was given for 6–10 days with warfarin therapy starting either on day 2[67] or on day 7–10.[68–71] Warfarin was continued for 3 months with the target international normalized ratio (INR) range being 2.0–3.0. The outcomes in terms of recurrent venous thromboembolism, major bleeding and mortality for five clinical trials using clinical end points are summarized in Table 25.2. When the results of two clinical trials were pooled there was a striking decrease in mortality in the patients receiving LMWH, particularly for patients with cancer.[72] Most of the abrupt deaths could not be attributed to thromboembolic events, suggesting that the benefits of LMWH may not be entirely related to thrombotic events.

A recent study showed that once-daily LMWH was as effective as continuous intravenous unfractionated heparin in the initial treatment of patients presenting with pulmonary embolism.[73] In a previous study comparing the effectiveness and safety of LMWH versus intravenous heparin, all patients had ventilation/perfusion lung scans and chest x-ray within 24 hours of entering the study.[67] Of the 97 patients who had received LMWH, there were no new episodes of venous thromboembolism compared with seven of the 103 patients who had received intravenous heparin ($P = 0.01$).[74] The incidence of death and major bleeding did not differ. Results of this study therefore supported the results of the randomized clinical trial.[73]

In two recent meta-analyses, all randomized clinical trials comparing the use of LMWH and intravenous unfractionated heparin for the initial treatment of deep venous thrombosis were reviewed.[75,76] Both studies showed a significant decrease in mortality in patients receiving LMWH and a trend favouring LMWH for both recurrent venous thromboembolism and major bleeding.

Most of the early studies comparing subcutaneous

Table 25.2 *Randomized trials of low-molecular-weight heparin* vs *unfractionated heparin for the in-hospital treatment of proximal deep vein thrombosis: results of long-term follow-up*

Reference	Treatment	Recurrent venous thromboembolism (no.(%))	Major bleeding (no.(%))	Mortality (no.(%))
Hull *et al.*[67]	Tinzaparin	6/213 (2.8)	1/213 (0.5)[a]	10/213 (4.7)[a]
	Heparin	15/219 (6.8)	11/219 (5.0)	21/219 (9.6)
Prandoni *et al.*[68]	Fraxiparine	6/85 (7.1)	1/85 (1.2)	6/85 (7.1)
	Heparin	12/85 (14.1)	3/85 (3.8)	12/85 (14.1)
Lopaciuk *et al.*[69]	Fraxiparine	0/74 (0)	0/74	0/74
	Heparin	3/72 (4.2)	1/72 (1.4)	1/72 (1.4)
Simonneau *et al.*[70]	Enoxaparin	0/67	0/67	3/67 (4.5)
	Heparin	0/67	0/67	2/67 (3.0)
Lindmarker *et al.*[71]	Dalteparin	5/101 (5.0)	1/101(0.001)	2/101 (2.0)
	Heparin	3/103 (2.9)	0/103	3/103 (2.9)

[a] *P* <0.05 *vs* heparin.

LMWH with continuous intravenous, unfractionated heparin for the treatment of venous thrombosis used a twice-daily, subcutaneous injection of LMWH. This was based on the hypothesis that maintaining a more constant anti-Factor X_a level was important to suppress thrombus formation in the initial stages of treatment. In the study by Hull et al.,[67] a single injection of LMWH was given based on the hypothesis that achieving a therapeutic dose of LMWH would be as important as achieving therapeutic levels of heparin early on in the treatment of deep vein thrombosis to prevent recurrent thromboembolism. Recent studies with three different LMWHs have indicated that a once-daily subcutaneous injection is at least as effective and safe as twice-daily injections.[77–79] A recent meta-analysis[76] indicated that the use of once- or twice-daily LMWH was equally efficacious.

Therefore, once-daily administration of LMWH has become the preferred standard of care for the treatment of deep vein thrombosis.

COST EFFECTIVENESS OF LMWH IN THE TREATMENT OF PROXIMAL VENOUS THROMBOSIS

A cost-effectiveness analysis was conducted comparing the treatment of proximal venous thrombosis with subcutaneous LMWH vs intravenous heparin, based on a prospective clinical trial.[80] The cost data used in this study were based on actual costs at an urban hospital site in Alberta, and an urban hospital site in the mid-west USA. The cost data used were based on actual costs that were derived from patient care. Included in the costs were the cost of anticoagulant therapy (including drugs and laboratory tests), hotel costs of hospitalization (rooming, laundry, food), the cost of treating recurrent venous thromboembolism for 12 months, and the cost of major bleeding complications. In addition, multiple sensitivity analyses were performed. The following variables related to costs that were examined included: initial drug treatment with either LMWH or intravenous heparin; long-term anticoagulant therapy; pharmacy charges; laboratory monitoring; objective diagnosis and treatment of recurrent venous thromboembolism; management of hemorrhagic complications (major bleeding only); hotel costs of hospitalization; physician charges and number of hospital days attributable to recurrent venous thromboembolism. For each of these variables a range of 40–300 per cent was applied. These ranges were based on variations in regional unit costs observed among the centers in North America that participated in the clinical trial. The economic viewpoint of the analysis was that of a third-party payer, i.e. the Ministry of Health in Canada, or an insurance company in the USA.

The total cost and effects per 100 patients of the two alternative approaches to antithrombotic therapy of proximal venous thrombosis are shown in Table 25.3.[80] This cost analysis showed that LMWH, which was at least as effective and safe as continuous intravenous heparin, was less costly. The use of LMWH in this setting, therefore, was shown to both reduce cost and improve health care outcomes, a 'win–win situation'.

In the cost analysis, it was defined a priori that treatment could be given on an out-patient basis to patients without co-morbid conditions.[80] Thirty-seven per cent (79 of 213) of patients who were treated with low-molecular-weight heparin had uncomplicated proximal venous thrombosis, and could have been treated out of hospital. The impact of treating the 79 patients as out-patients with discharge from hospital on day 2 was examined. Also, the 95 per cent confidence limits for this proportion in the sensitivity analysis were used to evaluate the effects of varying the proportion treated as out-patients on the conclusions of the cost-effectiveness

Table 25.3 Total costs and effects per 100 patients of the alternative approaches for antithrombotic therapy for proximal vein thrombosis. (Reproduced with permission from Hull et al. Treatment of proximal vein thrombosis with subcutaneous low molecular weight heparin vs intravenous heparin. An economic perspective. Arch Intern Med 1997; **157**: 289–94)

Approach	Recurrent VTE[a]	Death[b]	Major bleeding complications	Cost ($ Cdn)	Cost ($ US)
IV heparin	7	10	5	414 655	375 836
LMWH	3	5	3	399 403	335 687
				(15 252)[c]	(40 149)

[a] Six (2.8%) of 213 patients who received LMWH and 15 (6.9%) of 210 patients who received iv heparin had recurrent VTE (P=0.07 by Fisher exact test; 95% confidence interval for the difference, 0.02– 8.1%).
[b] Ten patients (4.7%) who received LMWH died, compared with 21 patients (9.6%) who received iv heparin (P=0.06) by Fisher exact test; P=0.049 by the uncorrected χ^2 test; reduction in risk, 51%).
[c] Cost saving per 100 patients treated with LMWH.
VTE = venous thromboembolism; IV = intravenous; LMWH = low-molecular-weight heparin.

analysis. If 79 of the 213 patients (37 per cent) had been treated as out-patients, the total cost per 100 patients who received low-molecular-weight heparin would have been $318 919.00 (Cdn) or $284 504.00 (US).[46] The potential use of out-patient therapy with low-molecular-weight heparin in 37 per cent of patients increased the Canadian cost savings from $15 252.00 to $95 736.00 and the US cost savings from $40 149.00 to $91 332.00 in the treatment of 100 patients with proximal venous thrombosis.[80] Thus, it is clear that the out-patient management of acute proximal venous thrombosis with the use of LMWH will be more cost-effective than treatment using intravenous heparin in hospital.[81–83]

A cost analysis based on a recent meta-analysis indicated that the in-hospital use of LMWH was highly cost effective compared with unfractionated heparin and that treatment of even a small number of patients out-of-hospital with LMWH would be cost effective.[84]

OUT-PATIENT TREATMENT OF ACUTE DEEP VEIN THROMBOSIS USING LMWH

Three Level I clinical trials compared the use of LMWH given primarily in the out-patient setting with continuous, intravenous, unfractionated heparin given in-hospital in patients with proximal venous thrombosis.[85–87] The outcomes in terms of recurrent venous thromboembolism and major bleeding are shown in Table 25.4. All three studies showed that the treatment of selected patients with proximal venous thrombosis with LMWH predominantly in the out-patient setting was as effective and safe as treatment with continuous, intravenous unfractionated heparin in-hospital (Table 25.4). However, it is important to emphasize that these patients were carefully selected and not all eligible patients entered the study, so that the results may not be entirely generalizable. Also, there are many patients who will still require treatment of proximal

venous thrombosis in the hospital setting, with either intravenous heparin or LMWH.

In the study by Levine et al., patients were excluded if they had one or more previous episodes of deep vein thrombosis or pulmonary embolism, had concurrent symptomatic pulmonary embolism, had been on standard intravenous heparin for more than 48 hours, were at high risk of bleeding, or had the presence of a known inhibitor deficiency state.[85] They were also excluded if they were considered unable to be treated with low-molecular-weight heparin as an out-patient because of a co-existing condition, the likelihood of non-compliance, or if they were geographically inaccessible. Of the 2230 consecutive patients with proximal DVT who were screened, 1491 were excluded. Of the remaining 739 patients, 500 (68 per cent) gave informed consent, and 247 were randomized to receive low-molecular-weight heparin. One hundred and twenty of these patients were not hospitalized at all, 29 were admitted to hospital for treatment with LMWH, 76 were admitted to hospital at night or on weekends before randomization, and 22 had been hospitalized for other reasons. The 127 patients who were admitted spent an average of 2.2 days in hospital.

In the study by Koopman et al.,[86] the exclusion criteria were less stringent; the exclusion criteria included previous venous thromboembolism within 2 years, suspected pulmonary embolism at presentation, previous treatment with heparin for more than 24 hours, geographic inaccessibility, life expectancy of less than 6 months, overt post-thrombotic syndrome, age less than 18 years, and pregnancy. Of 692 eligible patients, 216 (31 per cent) were excluded. Of the 476 eligible patients, 76 (16 per cent) did not consent to participate, and 200 of the 400 patients were randomized to receive LMWH. Of these patients, 72 (36 per cent) were never admitted, 50 (25 per cent) were treated entirely in the hospital, 44 (22 per cent) were discharged in less than 48 hours, and 36 (18 per cent) were discharged after greater than 48 hours.

In the Columbus study[87] exclusion criteria included the use of heparin, LMWH and warfarin for more than

Table 25.4 Out-patient treatment of proximal deep vein thrombosis (DVT) with low-molecular-weight heparin vs in-patient treatment with intravenous heparin

Study	Treatment	Recurrent DVT	Major bleeding
Levine et al.[85]	Enoxaparin	13/247 (5.3%)	5/247 (2.0%)
	vs		
	heparin	17/253 (6.7%)	3/253 (1.2%)
Koopman et al.[86]	Fraxiparine	14/202 (6.9%)	1/202 (0.5%)
	vs		
	heparin	17/198 (8.6%)	4/198 (2.0%)
Columbus investigators[87]	Reviparin	27/510 (5.3%)	16/510 (3.1%)
	vs		
	heparin	24/511 (4.9%)	12/511 (2.3%)

24 hours, contraindication to anticoagulants, planned thrombolytic therapy, gastrointestinal bleeding within the previous 14 days, surgery requiring anaesthesia in the preceding 3 days, stroke within the previous 10 days, platelet count less than 100×10^9/L, pregnancy, age less than 18 years, and geographic inaccessibility. Of the 1745 consecutive patients screened, 424 (24 per cent) were excluded. Of the remaining 1321 eligible patients, 1021 (77 per cent) gave consent and 510 were randomized to LMWH. Of these patients, 27 per cent were not admitted to hospital and 15 per cent were discharged during the first 3 days.

> Recent observational studies demonstrate the feasibility of treating a large number of patients with deep vein thrombosis (DVT) and/or pulmonary embolism (PE) out of hospital.[88,89]

Certain exclusion criteria for the out-patient treatment of venous thromboembolism have been established. These include:

- proximal DVT with vascular compromise;
- PE with hemodynamic instability;
- patients at high risk of bleeding;
- patients with significant co-morbid conditions requiring hospitalization;
- geographic inaccessibility;
- non-compliant patients;
- previous heparin-induced thrombocytopenia.

The use of out-of-hospital LMWH, along with warfarin, has created a number of logistic problems, which so far defy easy solutions. This approach to treatment requires someone to either take responsibility for teaching the patients to self-inject or to ensure that the patients are given their daily injections of LMWH; it also requires that patients have daily measurement of their INR, and that somebody orders the appropriate dose of warfarin. Also, it is important that all of the members of the health care team are kept informed regarding the patient's progress. Payment for the LMWH, particularly for patients with no third-party insurance, is a further unresolved problem. The development of anticoagulation management clinics could provide solutions for some of these concerns.

ROLE OF LMWH IN THE MANAGEMENT OF UNSTABLE ANGINA AND NON-ST SEGMENT ELEVATION MYOCARDIAL INFARCTION

The short-term and long-term use of LMWH for the prevention of vascular events in patients with unstable angina is currently under active study. In a small, open study in patients with unstable angina, LMWH plus aspirin was compared with low-dose heparin plus aspirin or aspirin alone for a period of 5–7 days (or sooner if an end point occurred).[90] For the prevention of recurrent angina, myocardial infarction and revascularization procedures, LMWH plus aspirin was superior to the other two groups.

In six large multicenter studies, low molecular weight heparin has been compared with either placebo or intravenous unfractionated heparin for the prevention of recurrent angina, myocardial infarction, urgent revascularization or death in patients with unstable angina or non-Q wave myocardial infarction.[91–97] In the FRISC study (Fragmin® during instability in coronary artery disease), LMWH (dalteparin) was compared with an identical subcutaneous placebo given twice daily for the initial 5–8 days following a diagnosis of unstable angina or non-Q wave myocardial infarction (in-hospital phase).[91] Subsequently, dalteparin once-a-day or a corresponding placebo was continued for 35–45 days (out-of-hospital phase). All patients took aspirin and conventional anti-angina drugs throughout the study. During the in-hospital phase, the incidence of death and new myocardial infarction was significantly lower in the LMWH group, as was the need for intravenous heparin and the need for revascularization. During the 35–40 day long-term treatment (out-of-hospital phase), the incidence of death and new myocardial infarction, and the need for revascularization or heparin infusion remained lower with the LMWH group, although the difference was not significant. The addition of LMWH to aspirin did not increase the incidence of major bleeding.

In the FRIC study (Fragmin® in unstable coronary heart disease), twice-daily subcutaneous LMWH (dalteparin) was compared with intravenous heparin by continuous infusion for a period of 6 days, followed by long-term subcutaneous LMWH once a day, with an identical placebo for 40 days.[92] As with the FRISC study, the FRIC study was double-blind. During the in-hospital phase (6-day outcomes), the risk of death, myocardial infarction and recurrent angina, and the need for revascularization were similar. Also during the prolonged treatment phase (day 6–45) there was no difference in the composite end points of recurrent angina, myocardial infarction, death or revascularization. The incidence of major bleeding was similar in the two groups.

In the ESSENCE study (Efficacy and Safety of Subcutaneous Enoxaparin in non-Q-Wave Coronary Events),[93] LMWH (enoxaparin) given by twice-daily subcutaneous injection was compared with intravenous heparin by continuous infusion in patients with unstable angina and non-ST segment elevation myocardial infarction for an average of 3.5 days. All patients received aspirin. At 14 days, the incidence of recurrent angina, myocardial infarction and death were significantly lower in the LMWH group, compared with the intravenous heparin group. At 30 days, there was still a significant difference in the composite end points, favoring the LMWH group. There was no increase in the risk of major bleeding using LMWH.

In the FRISC II (Fragmin In Fast Revascularization during InStability in Coronary Artery Disease) study, invasive and non-invasive treatments were compared using a factorial design in patients with unstable angina or non-Q-wave myocardial infarction.[94,95] After open label treatment with dalteparin (120 IU/kg twice daily subcutaneously for 5 days) or intravenous unfractionated heparin in all patients, half the patients in each group were randomly assigned to long-term treatment with subcutaneous weight-adjusted dalteparin (7500 units bid subcutaneously) or placebo for 3 months. In the double-blind phase of the study, dalteparin treatment produced a non-significant reduction in the primary double end point of death or myocardial infarction at 90 days. However, death or myocardial infarction was significantly reduced early on at 30 and 45 days, as was the triple composite end point of death, myocardial infarction, or revascularization at 3 months. Long-term treatment with dalteparin was associated with an increased risk of major bleeding compared with placebo (3.3 vs 1.5 per cent) and minor bleeding (23.0 vs 8.4 per cent).

The Thrombosis in Myocardial Infarction (TIMI) 11B trial compared prolonged enoxaparin therapy with standard dose-adjusted unfractionated heparin in 3910 patients with unstable angina or non-Q-wave myocardial infarction.[96] During the acute in-hospital phase, patients received either enoxaparin 30 mg by intravenous bolus followed by 1 mg/kg subcutaneously every 12 hours, or unfractionated heparin administered in a bolus dose of 70 U/kg intravenously and an infusion rate of 15 U/kg per hour, adjusted to achieve an aPTT of 1.5–2.5 times control. The median duration of enoxaparin treatment was 4.6 days and for unfractionated heparin was 3 days. Analysis of the primary end point of death, myocardial infarction, and recurrent angina requiring urgent revascularization at day 14 revealed a significant reduction in the enoxaparin group (14.2 per cent vs 16.6 per cent; relative risk reduction 15.0 per cent, P<0.03) with the predominant effect evident in urgent revascularization. The largest risk reduction was evident at 48–72 hours. In the chronic phase, the benefits of enoxaparin were still evident at day 43 (17.3 per cent vs 19.6 per cent, relative risk reduction 12.0 per cent, P = 0.049). Out-patient enoxaparin treatment was associated with an excess of major hemorrhage (2.9 per cent vs 1.5 per cent, P<0.02).

In the FRAXIS Study (Fraxiparine in Ischemic Syndrome) patients were randomized to receive unfractionated heparin by intravenous infusion with a 5000-unit bolus followed by an activated partial thromboplastin time (aPTT) adjusted infusion of unfractionated heparin for 6 ± 2 days, or nadroparin 86 U/kg as an intravenous bolus followed by nadroparin 86 U/kg twice daily for either 6 ± 2 days or 14 days.[97] There was no significant difference among the three groups with respect to the primary outcome (cardiac death, myocardial infarction, refractory angina, or recurrent or unstable angina at day 14). There was an increased risk of major hemorrhage in the patients receiving nadroparin for 14 days compared with unfractionated heparin (3.5 per cent vs 1.6 per cent, P = 0.0035).

A recent meta-analysis analyzed the clinical trials comparing unfractionated heparin and LMWH in acute coronary syndromes without ST elevation.[98] In studies comparing either unfractionated heparin or LMWH with placebo or an untreated control, the summary odds ratio for myocardial infarction or death during short-term treatment (up to 7 days) was 0.53 (95 per cent confidence interval (CI), 0.38–0.73; P = 0.0001) in favor of LMWH or 29 events prevented per 1000 patients treated. In the clinical trials comparing short-term LMWH with short-term unfractionated heparin the odds ratio was 0.88 (95 per cent CI, 0.69–1.12; P = 0.34) in favor of LMWH. In the clinical trials comparing long-term LMWH (up to 3 months) with placebo or untreated control the odds ratio was 0.98 (95 per cent CI, 0.81–1.17; P = 0.80) in favor of LMWH. There was a significant increase in the risk of major bleeding with long-term LMWH compared with placebo (odds ratio 2.26, 95 per cent CI, 1.63–3.14; P<0.0001). This was equivalent to 12 major bleeding episodes per 1000 patients treated. In this meta-analysis assessing the firm end points of myocardial infarction or death, no difference was found between the various LMWHs and unfractionated heparin. When the less firm end points of unstable angina or requirement for revascularization were added to death or myocardial infarction, the studies with enoxaparin both showed a significant difference when compared with unfractionated heparin. It was concluded that in aspirin-treated patients with acute coronary syndromes without ST elevation, either short-term unfractionated heparin or LMWH significantly decreased the risk of myocardial infarction or death. There was no evidence to support the use of long-term LMWH beyond the first 7 days.

Also, in two recent reviews of the clinical trials comparing the use of LMWH versus unfractionated heparin in the acute coronary syndromes it was concluded that weight-adjusted LMWH was as effective and safe as intravenous unfractionated heparin in the management of these syndromes, with the added benefit of ease of administration without the need for laboratory monitoring.[99,100] It was concluded that the risk of major bleeding was equivalent with LMWH and unfractionated heparin, and this was in particular related to vascular instrumentation. Because of the long half-life of LMWH and the concern about blocking its activity, intravenous unfractionated heparin has remained the agent of choice in many centers. The differences in outcomes seen in the various studies, particularly with respect to the softer end points, probably relates to the populations being studied and to the study methodology rather than to differences in the intrinsic properties of the various LMWHs.

ORAL ANTICOAGULANTS IN THE MANAGEMENT OF THROMBOTIC DISORDERS – SPECIAL PROBLEMS

Oral anticoagulant therapy has been the mainstay of long-term treatment of both venous and arterial thrombotic disorders. The management of oral anticoagulants, particularly in the out-patient setting, is discussed in detail elsewhere in this book (see Chapter 32). This section will be devoted to two special problems: the optimal duration of oral anticoagulant treatment after an initial or recurrent episode of venous thromboembolism, and the problems related to the interruption of oral anticoagulants for surgical procedures.

Optimal duration of treatment

Patients with established venous thrombosis or pulmonary embolism require long-term anticoagulant therapy to prevent recurrent disease.[103] Warfarin therapy is highly effective and is preferred in most patients.[101] Adjusted-dose subcutaneous heparin is the treatment of choice where long-term oral anticoagulants are contraindicated, such as in pregnancy.[102] Adjusted-dose, subcutaneous heparin, or unmonitored low-molecular-weight heparin have been used for the long-term treatment of patients in whom oral anticoagulant therapy proves to be very difficult to control.

The use of a less intense warfarin regimen (INR 2–3), markedly reduces the risk of bleeding from 20 per cent to 4 per cent, without loss of effectiveness in comparison with more intense warfarin.[103] With the improved safety of oral anticoagulant therapy using a less intense warfarin regimen, there has been renewed interest in evaluating the long-term treatment of thrombotic disorders. In clinical trials in patients with atrial fibrillation, it has been shown that oral anticoagulant treatment can be given safely with a low risk of major bleeding complications (1–2 per cent per year).[104] In trials such as these, the safety of oral anticoagulant treatment depends heavily on the maintenance of a narrow therapeutic INR range. When the INR falls below the therapeutic range, the incidence of thrombotic stroke increases, whereas when the INR exceeds a level of 3.5–5.0, the incidence of major hemorrhage markedly increases. These and other studies have emphasized the importance of maintaining careful control of oral anticoagulant therapy, particularly with the use of anticoagulant management clinics if oral anticoagulants are going to be used for extended periods of time.

The high incidence of recurrent venous thromboembolism in clinical trials in patients with proximal deep vein thrombosis who are treated according to the current practice with intravenous heparin for several days, followed by oral anticoagulant treatment for 3–6 months, has been the reason for renewed interest in longer term treatment of venous thromboembolism.[101, 105–109] These studies indicate that patients with deep vein thrombosis who are treated according to current clinical practice face an unfavorable long-term prognosis. Three groups of patients who have a particularly poor prognosis have been identified: patients with idiopathic, recurrent venous thromboembolism; patients who are carriers of genetic mutations, which predispose to venous thromboembolism (such as the Factor V Leiden mutation or the patients with the antiphospholipid antibody syndromes); and patients with cancer.[110,111]

Prandoni et al. followed the long-term course of patients with a first episode of deep vein thrombosis who were treated in the classical fashion with initial heparin or LMWH, followed by oral anticoagulant therapy for 3 months.[105] The cumulative incidence of recurrent venous thromboembolism was 17.5 per cent after 2 years, 25 per cent after 5 years, and 30 per cent after 8 years. Their studies confirm that patients with an initial episode of symptomatic deep vein thrombosis have a high risk of recurrent thromboembolism, which can persist for many years. In an earlier study by Hull et al., it was shown that patients with recurrent venous thromboembolism, who are treated with heparin followed by warfarin for 3 months, had a 20 per cent incidence of documented recurrent venous thromboembolism and a 4.5 per cent incidence of fatal pulmonary embolism during the following year.[103]

Optimal duration after a first episode of deep vein thrombosis

It has been recommended that all patients with a first episode of venous thromboembolism receive warfarin therapy for 12 weeks.

Attempts to decrease the treatment to 4 weeks[112,113] or 6 weeks[108] resulted in higher rates of recurrent thromboembolism in comparison with either 12 or 26 weeks of treatment (11–18 per cent recurrent thromboembolism in the following 1–2 years). Most of the recurrent thromboembolic events occurred in the 6–8 weeks immediately after anticoagulant treatment was stopped, and the incidence was higher in patients with continuing risk factors, such as cancer and immobilization.[108,113] Treatment with oral anticoagulants for 6 months reduced the incidence of recurrent thromboembolic events, but there was a cumulative incidence of recurrent events at 2 years (11 per cent) and an ongoing risk of recurrent thromboembolism of approximately 5–6 per cent per year.[108] This continued risk of recurrent thromboembolism even with 6 months treatment after a first episode of deep vein thrombosis has encouraged the development of clinical trials evaluating the effectiveness of long-term anticoagulant treatment beyond 6 months.

In patients with a first episode of idiopathic venous thromboembolism (VTE) treated with intravenous heparin followed by warfarin for 3 months, continuation of warfarin for 24 months led to a significant reduction in the incidence of recurrent venous thromboembolism when compared with placebo (29 per cent per year *vs* 1 per cent per year; $P = 0.00003$).[114] Three patients on longer term warfarin had major bleeding compared with none on placebo. The authors conclude that more than 3 months of anticoagulation therapy is required after an initial episode of idiopathic venous thromboembolism.

> In the recent ACCP Consensus Conference on Antithrombotic Therapy, it was recommended that all patients with a first episode of idiopathic venous thromboembolism should receive treatment for at least 6 months.[115]

In view of the continued risk of recurrent disease in patients with a first episode of idiopathic venous thromboembolism, and the concern about the incidence of major bleeding with long-term anticoagulation, a number of clinical trials are underway to compare the efficacy and safety of long-term oral anticoagulant therapy with a targeted INR of 1.5–2.0 as compared with an INR of 2.0–3.0 or to a placebo control.[116] These trials will continue for a duration of 3–4 years and their outcomes are awaited with interest.

Optimal duration of treatment in patients with recurrent deep vein thrombosis

In a multicenter clinical trial, Schulman *et al.* randomized patients with a first recurrent episode of venous thromboembolism to receive either 6 months or indefinitely continued oral anticoagulants, with a targeted INR of 2.0–2.85.[109] Outcomes were assessed at 4 years. In the patients receiving anticoagulants for 6 months, recurrent thromboembolism occurred in 20.7 per cent, compared with 2.6 per cent of patients on the indefinite treatment ($P < 0.001$). However, the rates of major bleeding were 2.7 per cent in the 6 months group, compared with 8.6 per cent in the indefinite group. In the indefinite group, two of the major hemorrhages were fatal, whereas there were no fatal hemorrhages in the 6 months group. There were 16 deaths in the 6 months group (14.4 per cent) compared with 10 in the indefinite duration group (8.6 per cent) ($P = 0.21$). This study showed that extending the duration of oral anticoagulants for approximately 4 years resulted in a significant decrease in the incidence of recurrent venous thromboembolism, but with a higher

incidence of major bleeding. There were no fatal thromboembolic events in the 6-month duration group, whereas there were two fatal major bleeding events in the indefinite treatment group. There were fewer deaths in the indefinite duration group, although this did not achieve statistical significance. The relative risk of death with the 6-month treatment group was 1.7 (95 per cent CI 0.8–3.5). Without a significant mortality difference, the risk/benefit of extended warfarin treatment is uncertain, and will require further clinical trials large enough to have the power to reach firm conclusions, particularly relating to a mortality advantage.

Recommendations regarding long-term anticoagulation therapy

The committee on Antithrombotic Therapy for Venous Thromboembolic Disease for the 5th American College of Chest Physicians Consensus Conference on Antithrombotic Therapy,[115] made the following suggestions regarding long-term antithrombotic treatment of venous thromboembolism:

> 'patients with reversible or time limited risk factors should be treated for three to six months. Patients with a first episode of idiopathic venous thromboembolism should be treated for at least six months. Patients with recurrent venous thromboembolism or a continued risk factor such as cancer, inhibitor deficiency states or antiphospholipid antibody syndrome should be treated indefinitely. Patients with activated Protein C Resistance (Factor V Leiden) should probably receive indefinite treatment if they have recurrent disease, if they are homozygous for the gene or if they have multiple thrombophilic conditions.'

Management of patients who require surgical intervention

Physicians are commonly confronted with the problem of managing oral anticoagulants in individuals who require temporary interruption of treatment for surgery or other invasive procedures.[117–121] No randomized clinical trials comparing different approaches to the temporary cessation of anticoagulants in such circumstances have been performed, so that recommendations can only be made based on cohort studies, retrospective reviews, and expert opinions. Recommendations for temporary cessation of oral anticoagulants will depend on the underlying reason for long-term treatment, the most common indications being atrial fibrillation, mechanical or bioprosthetic heart valves and venous thromboembolism. In each of these settings, the risk of arterial or venous thromboembolism while anticoagulants have been discontinued must be weighed against the risks of bleeding if intravenous heparin therapy is applied before or after the surgical procedure. Many of the studies in patients with mechanical heart valves are from the 1960s and 1970s, when the likelihood of embolic complications was higher, but bleeding complications were higher as well because higher intensity warfarin therapy with respect to INR was being used.[116–119]

For patients with mechanical heart valves, it has been recommended that oral anticoagulants be discontinued for 3–5 days prior to operation, and recommenced following surgery.[122] A risk–benefit assessment must be made to assess the risk of arterial embolism vs the risk of bleeding with the use of heparin therapy. The possible choices based on the risk–benefit assessment include:

1 discontinuing warfarin for 3–5 days before the procedure, to allow the INR to return to normal, and then restarting therapy shortly after surgery;
2 lowering the warfarin dose to maintain an INR in the lower or subtherapeutic range during the surgical procedure; or
3 discontinuing warfarin and treating the patient in-hospital with intravenous heparin up to 2–4 hours before surgery and then reinstituting heparin therapy postoperatively when hemostasis has been secured.

In the latter approach, the patient is unprotected by anticoagulation for the shortest period of time, but hospitalization is required, and the cost-effectiveness of this practice has been questioned. This approach has been recommended for patients with the most thrombogenic prostheses, unless the heparin therapy can be given during the required hospitalization for the surgical procedure. In patients with mitral valve prostheses who are at the highest risk of arterial embolism and who are undergoing major surgery, placing them at risk of major bleeding, hospitalization with the use of intravenous heparin can be justified. For patients undergoing minimally invasive procedures such as dental extractions or superficial biopsies, the INR may be temporarily decreased to the low or subtherapeutic range for the procedure, and then oral anticoagulants started immediately after.[123] For all other patients, an individual approach may be required.

Low-molecular-weight heparin, which can be given by a once- or twice-daily subcutaneous injection in either prophylactic or therapeutic doses, offers a convenient alternative to intravenous unfractionated heparin. To date, no randomized clinical trials have compared the use of LMWH with unfractionated intravenous heparin for patients requiring temporary interruption of warfarin therapy for invasive procedures. In the largest cohort study reported to date, patients with mechanical heart valve, atrial fibrillation, or venous thromboembolism who required an interruption of anticoagulant therapy for various surgical procedures were placed on LMWH (dalteparin 100 U/kg subcutaneously twice daily) after their warfarin had been discontinued 4–5

days prior to the procedure.[124] LMWH was discontinued 12 hours before the procedure and recommenced within 8–12 hours following the surgery. With this protocol, patients were off warfarin therapy for an average of 5.4 days and they received LMWH for an average of 9.3 days. One patient experienced major bleeding. Continued use of this protocol indicates that it is both effective and safe (personal communication, Dr AGG Turpie). In two other small studies, LMWH either in therapeutic or prophylactic doses has also been shown to be effective and safe in patients on long-term oral anticoagulants for a variety of indications.[125,126] These studies therefore indicate that LMWH provides a convenient and less costly alternative to unfractionated heparin.

It should be noted that these recommendations are not based on Level 1 evidence. There are anecdotal reports of patients having embolic strokes when oral anticoagulants are temporarily discontinued. Therefore, until further randomized clinical trials are carried out in patients in whom anticoagulants must be temporarily discontinued, no firm recommendations can be made, but the above suggestions have proven to be useful in clinical practice.

SUMMARY

- Thrombotic disorders, including venous thromboembolism (deep vein thrombosis and pulmonary embolism), unstable angina and non-ST segment elevation myocardial infarction, are common disorders associated with significant morbidity and mortality.
- Traditionally these disorders have been treated initially with unfractionated heparin by continuous intravenous infusion.
- The introduction of the low-molecular-weight heparins, given by a once- or twice-daily subcutaneous injection without laboratory monitoring, has permitted the out-of-hospital treatment of these disorders.
- Clinical trials comparing the out-of-hospital use of low-molecular-weight heparin with in-hospital use of continuous intravenous unfractionated heparin for the treatment of proximal deep vein thrombosis has shown low-molecular-weight heparin to be both effective and safe.
- Several observational studies have demonstrated that out-of-hospital treatment of proximal deep vein thrombosis, upper extremity deep venous thrombosis, and pulmonary embolism is both feasible and safe in the majority of patients.
- Low-molecular-weight heparin by twice-daily subcutaneous injection has been compared with unfractionated heparin by continuous

intravenous infusion in the initial treatment of unstable angina or non-ST segment elevation myocardial infarction. Low-molecular-weight heparin is equally effective or more effective in the outcomes of myocardial infarctions, death, recurrent angina, or the requirement for urgent revascularization.

- The optimal duration of oral anticoagulant treatment after an initial episode of idiopathic deep vein thrombosis or in patients with recurrent disease is currently under intense investigation with most studies indicating that oral anticoagulation is required for longer periods than those recommended in the past.

REFERENCES

o1. Hirsh J, Raschke R, Warkentin TE. Heparin: mechanism of action, pharmacokinetics, dosing considerations, monitoring, efficacy, and safety. *Chest* 1998; **114**: 489S–510S.

2. Lane DA. Heparin binding and neutralizing protein. In: Lane DA, Lindahl U, eds *Heparin, chemical and biological properties, clinical applications*. London: Edward Arnold, 1989: 363–91.

♦3. Lindahl U, Backstrom G, Hook M. Structure of the antithrombin-binding site of heparin. *Proc Natl Acad Sci USA* 1979; **76**: 3198–302.

4. Lindahl U, Thunberg L, Backstrom G. Extension and structural variability of the antithrombin-binding sequence in heparin. *J Biol Chem* 1984; **259**: 12368–76.

♦5. Rosenberg RD, Lam L. Correlation between structure and function of heparin. *Proc Natl Acad Sci USA* 1979; **76**: 1218–22.

6. Casu B, Oreste P, Torri G, *et al.* The structure of heparin oligosaccharide fragments with high anti-(factor X$_a$) activity containing the minimal antithrombin III-binding sequence. *Biochem J* 1981; **197**: 599–609.

♦7. Weitz JI, Hudoba M, Massel D, *et al.* Clot-bound thrombin is protected from inhibition by heparin–antithrombin III but is susceptible to inactivation by antithrombin III-independent inhibitors. *J Clin Invest* 1990; **86**: 385–91.

8. Salzman EW, Rosenberg RD, Smith MH, *et al.* Effect of heparin and heparin fractions on platelet aggregation. *J Clin Invest* 1980; **65**: 64–73.

9. Tollefsen DM, Majerus DW, Blank MK. Heparin cofactor II. Purification and properties of a heparin-dependent inhibitor of thrombin in human plasma. *J Biol Chem* 1982; **257**: 2162–9.

10. Hoppensteadt D, Walenga JM, Fasanella A, *et al.* TFPI antigen levels in normal human volunteers after intravenous and subcutaneous administration of unfractionated heparin and low molecular weight heparin. *Thromb Res* 1995; **77**: 175–85.

11. Barzu T, Molho P, Tobelem G, *et al.* Binding of heparin and low molecular weight heparin fragments to human vascular endothelial cells in culture. *Nouv Rev Fr Haematol* 1984; **26**: 243–7.

12. Blajchman MA, Young E, Ofosu FA. Effects of unfractionated heparin, dermatan sulfate and low molecular weight heparin on vessel wall permeability in rabbits. *Ann New York Acad Sci* 1989; **556**: 245–54.

13. Bara L, Billaud E, Gramond G, *et al.* Comparative pharmacokinetics of low molecular weight heparin (PK 10169) and unfractionated heparin after intravenous and subcutaneous administration. *Thromb Res* 1985; **39**: 631–6.

14. Bjornsson T, Wolfram BS, Kitchell BB. Heparin kinetics determined by three assay methods. *Clin Pharmacol Ther* 1982; **31**: 104–13.

15. Levine M, Hirsh J, Gent M, *et al.* A randomised trial comparing activated thromboplastin time with heparin assay in patients with acute venous thromboembolism requiring large daily doses of heparin. *Arch Intern Med* 1994; **154**: 49–56.

♦16. Theroux P, Waters D, Lain J, *et al.* Reactivation of unstable angina after the discontinuation of heparin. *N Engl J Med* 1992; **327**: 141–5.

17. Granger CB, Miller JM, Bovill EG, *et al.* Rebound increase in thrombin generation and activity after cessation of intravenous heparin in patients with acute coronary syndromes. *Circulation* 1995; **91**: 1929–35.

18. Fennerty A, Thomas P, Backhouse G, *et al.* Audit of control of heparin treatment. *Br Med J* 1985; **290**: 27–8.

19. Wheeler AP, Jaquiss RD, Newman JH. Physician practices in the treatment of pulmonary embolism and deep-venous thrombosis. *Arch Intern Med* 1988; **148**: 1321–5.

20. Cruickshank MK, Levine MN, Hirsh J, *et al.* A standard nomogram for the management of heparin therapy. *Arch Intern Med* 1991; **151**: 333–7.

21. Hull RD, Raskob GE, Hirsh J, *et al.* Continuous intravenous heparin compared with intermittent subcutaneous heparin in the initial treatment of proximal-vein thrombosis. *N Engl J Med* 1986; **315**: 1109–14.

♦22. Raschke RA, Reilly BM, Guidry JR, *et al.* The weight-based heparin dosing nomogram compared with a 'standard care' nomogram. *Ann Intern Med* 1993; **119**: 874–81.

23. Brandjes DPM, Heijboer H, Buller HR, *et al.* Acenocoumarol and heparin compared with acenocoumarol alone in the initial treatment of proximal-vein thrombosis. *N Engl J Med* 1992; **327**: 1485–9.

24. Hull RD, Raskob GE, Rosenbloom DR, *et al.* Optimal

therapeutic level of heparin therapy in patients with venous thrombosis. *Arch Intern Med* 1992; **152**: 1589–95.

25. Brill-Edwards P, Ginsberg JS, Johnston M, *et al*. Establishing a therapeutic range for heparin therapy. *Ann Intern Med* 1993; **119**: 104–9.

26. Campbell NR, Hull RD, Brant GF, *et al*. Aging and heparin-related bleeding. *Arch Intern Med* 1996; **156**: 857–60.

27. Warkentin TE, Kelton JG. A 14 year study of heparin-induced thrombocytopenia. *Am J Med* 1996; **101**: 502–7.

♦28. Kelton JG, Sheridan D, Brian H, *et al*. Clinical usefulness of testing for a heparin-dependent platelet aggregation factor in patients with suspected heparin-associated thrombocytopenia. *J Lab Clin Med* 1984; **103**: 606–12.

♦29. Warkentin TE, Chong GH, Greinacher A. Heparin-induced thrombocytopenia: towards consensus. *Thromb Haemost* 1998; **79**: 1–7.

30. Arepally G, Reynolds C, Tomaski A, *et al*. Comparison of PF4/heparin ELISA assay with the $^{(14)}$C-serotonin release assay in the diagnosis of heparin-induced thrombocytopenia. *Am J Clin Path* 1995; **104**: 648–54.

○31. Warkentin TE. Heparin-induced thrombocytopenia: a clinicopathologic syndrome. *Thromb Haemost* 1999; **82**: 439–47.

32. Magnani HN. Heparin-induced thrombocytopenia (HIT): an overview of 230 patients treated with Orgaran (Org 10172). *Thromb Haemost* 1993; **70**: 554–61.

♦33. Greinacher A, Janssens U, Berg G, *et al*. Lepirudin (recombinant hirudin) for parenteral anticoagulation in patients with heparin-induced thrombocytopenia. Heparin-associated thrombocytopenia (HAT) investigators. *Circulation* 1999; **100**: 587–93.

34. Matsuo T, Kario K, Chikahira Y, *et al*. Treatment of heparin-induced thrombocytopenia by use of argatroban, a synthetic thrombin inhibitor. *Br J Haematol* 1992; **82**: 627–9.

35. Ahmad S, Iqbal O, Ahsan A, *et al*. Clinical laboratory monitoring of a synthetic antithrombin agent, argatroban, using high performance liquid chromatography and functional methods. *Int Angiol* 1999; **18**: 198–205.

36. Lewis BE, Cohen M, Leya F, *et al*. Argatroban use in patients with heparin-induced thrombocytopenia during percutaneous coronary intervention. *Chest* 2000; **118**: 261S.

○37. Hirsh J, Levine MN. Low molecular weight heparin. *Blood* 1992; **79**: 1–17.

38. Bara L, Samama MM. Pharmacokinetics of low molecular weight heparins. *Acta Chir Scand* 1988; **543**: 65–72.

39. Briant L, Caranobe C, Saivin SE, *et al*. Unfractionated heparin and CY216. Pharmacokinetics and bioavailabilities of the anti-Factor X_a and II_a. Effects of

intravenous and subcutaneous injection in rabbits. *Thromb Haemost* 1989; **61**: 348–53.

40. Anderson LO, Barrowcliffe TW, Holmer E, *et al*. Molecular weight dependency of the heparin potentiated inhibition of thrombin and activated factor X. Effect of heparin neutralization in plasma. *Thromb Res* 1979; **115**: 531–8.

41. Fareed J, Walenga JM, Racaneilli A, *et al*. Validity of the newly established low molecular weight heparin standard in cross referencing low molecular weight heparins. *Haemostasis* 1988; **3**(suppl): 33–47.

42. Barrowcliffe TW, Curtis AD, Johnson EA, *et al*. An international standard for low molecular weight heparin. *Thromb Haemost* 1988; **60**: 1–7.

43. Holmer E, Soderberg K, Bergqvist D, *et al*. Heparin and its low molecular weight derivatives: anticoagulant and antithrombotic properties. *Haemostasis* 1986; **16**(suppl 2): 1–7.

44. Carter CJ, Kelton JG, Hirsh J, *et al*. The relationship between the hemorrhagic and antithrombotic properties of low molecular weight heparins and heparin. *Blood* 1982; **59**: 1239–45.

45. Cade JF, Buchanan MR, Boneu B, *et al*. A comparison of the antithrombotic and hemorrhagic effects of low molecular weight heparin fractions: the influence of the method of preparation. *Thromb Res* 1984; **35**: 613–25.

46. Andriuoli G, Mastacchi R, Barnti M, *et al*. Comparison of the antithrombotic and hemorrhagic effects of heparin and a new low molecular weight heparin in the rat. *Haemostasis* 1985; **15**: 324–30.

47. Lensing AW, Prins MH, Davidson BL, *et al*. Treatment of deep venous thrombosis with low-molecular-weight heparins. *Arch Intern Med* 1989; **155**: 601–7.

48. Monreal M, Lafoz E, Salvador R, *et al*. Adverse effects of three different forms of heparin therapy: thrombocytopenia, increased transaminases, and hyperkalemia. *Eur J Clin Pharmacol* 1989; **37**: 415–18.

49. Monreal M, Vinas L, Monreal L, *et al*. Heparin-related osteoporosis in rats. A comparative study between unfractionated heparin and a low molecular weight heparin. *Haemostasis* 1990; **20**: 204–7.

50. Matzsch T, Bergqvist D, Hedner U, *et al*. Effects of low molecular weight heparin and unfragmented heparin on induction of osteoporosis in rats. *Thromb Haemost* 1990; **63**: 505–9.

51. Shaughnessy SG, Young E, Deschamps P, *et al*. The effects of low molecular weight and standard heparin on calcium loss from fetal rat calvaria. *Blood* 1995; **86**: 1368–73.

52. Warkentin TE, Levine MN, Hirsh J, *et al*. Heparin-induced thrombocytopenia in patients treated with low-molecular-weight heparin or unfractionated heparin. *N Engl J Med* 1995; **332**: 1330–5.

53. Forestier F, Daffos F, Capella-Pavlovsky M. Low molecular weight heparin (PH 10169) does not cross the placenta during the second trimester of

pregnancy: study by direct foetal blood sampling under ultrasound. *Thromb Res* 1984; **34**: 557–60.

54. Omri A, Delaloye FJ, Andersen H, *et al*. Low-molecular-weight heparin Novo (LHN-1) does not cross the placenta during the second trimester of pregnancy. *Thromb Haemost* 1989; **61**: 55–6.

55. Melissari E, Parker CJ, Wilson NV, *et al*. Use of low molecular weight heparin in pregnancy. T*hromb Haemost* 1992; **68**: 652–6.

56. Wahlberg TB, Kher A. Low molecular weight heparin as thromboprophylaxis in pregnancy. A retrospective analysis from 14 European clinics. *Haemostasis* 1994; **24**: 55–6.

57. Sanson BJ, Lensing AW, Prins MH, *et al*. Safety of low-molecular-weight heparin in pregnancy: a systematic review. *Thromb Haemost* 1999; **81**: 668–72.

58. Ginsberg JS, Hirsh J. Use of antithrombotic agents during pregnancy. *Chest* 1998; **114**: 524S–530S.

59. Boneu B, Caranobe C, Cadroy Y, *et al*. Pharmacokinetic studies of standard unfractionated heparin, and low molecular weight heparins in the rabbit. *Semin Thromb Hemost* 1988; **14**: 18–27.

60. Boneu B, Buchanan MR, Cade JF, *et al*. Effects of heparin, its low molecular weight fractions and other glycosaminoglycans on thrombus growth in vivo. *Thromb Res* 1985; **40**: 81–9.

61. Bratt G, Tornebohn E, Cranqvist S, *et al*. A comparison between low molecular weight heparin (KABI 2165) and standard heparin in the intravenous treatment of deep venous thrombosis. *Thromb Haemost* 1985; **54**: 813–17.

62. Holm HA, Ly B, Handeland GF, *et al*. Subcutaneous heparin treatment of deep venous thrombosis. A comparison of unfractionated and low molecular weight heparin. *Haemost* 1986; **16**: 30–7.

63. Albada J, Nieuwenhuis HK, Sixma JJ, *et al*. Treatment of acute venous thromboembolism with low molecular weight heparin (Fragmin): results of a double-blind randomized study. *Circulation* 1989; **80**: 935–40.

64. Bratt G, Aberg W, Johansson M, *et al*. Two daily subcutaneous injections of Fragmin as compared with intravenous standard heparin in the treatment of deep venous thrombosis (VDT). *Thromb Haemost* 1990; **64**: 506–10.

65. Harenberg J, Huck K, Bratsch H, *et al*. Therapeutic application of subcutaneous low molecular weight heparin in acute venous thrombosis. *Haemost* 1990; **20**(suppl 1): 205–19.

66. Siegbahan A, Y-Hassan S, Boberg J, *et al*. Subcutaneous treatment of deep venous thrombosis with low molecular weight heparin. A dose finding study with LMWH-Novo. *Thromb Res* 1989; **55**: 267–78.

67. Hull RD, Raskob GE, Pineo GF, *et al*. Subcutaneous low molecular weight heparin compared with continuous intravenous heparin in the treatment of proximal vein thrombosis. *N Engl J Med* 1992; **326**: 975–88.

68. Prandoni P, Lensing AW, Buller HR, *et al*. Comparison of subcutaneous low molecular weight heparin with intravenous standard heparin in proximal deep vein thrombosis. *Lancet* 1992; **339**: 441–5.

69. Lopaciuk S, Meissner AJ, Filipecki S, *et al*. Subcutaneous low molecular weight heparin vs. subcutaneous unfractionated heparin in the treatment of deep vein thrombosis: a Polish multicentre trial. *Thromb Haemost* 1992; **68**: 14–18.

70. Simonneau G, Charbonnier B, Decousus H, *et al*. Subcutaneous low-molecular-weight heparin compared with continuous intravenous unfractionated heparin in the treatment of proximal deep vein thrombosis. *Arch Intern Med* 1993; **153**: 1541–6.

71. Lindmarker P, Holmstrom M, Granqvist S, *et al*. Comparison of once-daily subcutaneous Fragmin with continuous intravenous unfractionated heparin in the treatment of deep venous thrombosis. *Thromb Haemost* 1994; **72**: 186–90.

72. Green D, Hull RD, Brant R, Pineo GF, *et al*. Lower mortality in cancer patients treated with low molecular weight versus standard heparin. *Lancet* 1992; **339**: 1476.

73. Simonneau G, Sors H, Charbonnier B, *et al*. Once daily low molecular weight heparin tinzaparin vs. unfractionated heparin in the treatment of acute pulmonary embolism. *Thromb Haemost* 1997; **3080**: 753.

74. Hull RD, Raskob GE, Brant RF, *et al*., for the American–Canadian Thrombosis Study Group. Low-molecular-weight heparin vs heparin in the treatment of patients with pulmonary embolism. *Arch Intern Med* 2000; **160**: 229–36.

75. Gould MK, Dembitzer AD, Doyle RL, *et al*. Low-molecular-weight heparins compared with unfractionated heparin for treatment of acute deep venous thrombosis: a meta-analysis of randomized, controlled trials. *Ann Intern Med* 1999; **130**: 800–9.

76. Dolovich LR, Ginsberg JS, Douketis JD, *et al*. A meta-analysis comparing low-molecular-weight heparins with unfractionated heparin in the treatment of venous thromboembolism. *Arch Intern Med* 2000; **160**: 181–8.

77. Fiessinger JN, *et al*. Once-daily subcutaneous Dalteparin, a low molecular weight heparin, for the initial treatment of acute deep vein thrombosis. *Thromb Haemost* 1996; **76**: 195–9.

78. Charbonnier BA, Fiessinger JN, Barqa JD, *et al*. Comparison of a once daily with a twice daily subcutaneous nadroparin calcium regiment in the treatment of deep vein thrombosis. The FRAXODI study. *Thromb Haemost* 1998; **79**(5): 897–901.

79. Spiro TE. Clinical use of low molecular weight heparins. *Thromb Haemost* 1997; **1527**: 373.

80. Hull RD, Raskob GE, Brant GF, *et al*. Treatment of proximal vein thrombosis with subcutaneous low

molecular weight heparin vs intravenous heparin. An economic perspective. *Arch Intern Med* 1997; **157**: 289–94.

81. van den Belt AGM, *et al.*, for the TASMAN Study Group. Replacing inpatient care by outpatient care in the treatment of deep venous thrombosis: an economic evaluation. *Thromb Haemost* 1998; **79**: 259–63.

82. O'Brien B, Levine M, Willan A, *et al.* Economic evaluation of outpatient treatment with low-molecular-weight heparin for proximal vein thrombosis. *Arch Intern Med* 1999; **159**: 2298–304.

83. Boccalon H, *et al.*, for the Vascular Midi-Pyrenees Network Group. Clinical outcome and cost of hospital vs home treatment of proximal deep vein thrombosis with a low-molecular-weight heparin – the vascular Midi-Pyrenees study. *Arch Intern Med* 2000; **160**: 1769–73.

84. Gould MK, Dembitzer AD, Sanders GD, Garber AM. Low-molecular-weight heparins compared with unfractionated heparin for treatment of acute deep venous thrombosis: a cost-effectiveness analysis. *Ann Intern Med* 1999; **130**: 789–99.

85. Levine M, Gent M, Hirsh J, *et al.* A comparison of low molecular weight heparin administered primarily at home with unfractionated heparin administered in the hospital for proximal deep vein thrombosis. *N Engl J Med* 1996; **334**: 677–81.

♦86. Koopman M, Prandoni P, Piovella F, *et al.* Treatment of venous thrombosis with intravenous unfractionated heparin administered in the hospital as compared with subcutaneous low-molecular-weight heparin administered at home. *N Engl J Med* 1996; **334**: 682–7.

♦87. The Columbus Investigators. Low molecular weight heparin is an effective and safe treatment of deep vein thrombosis and pulmonary embolism. *Blood* 1996; **88**: 626–24.

88. Harrison L, McGinnis J, Crowther M, *et al.* Assessment of outpatient treatment of deep vein thrombosis with low-molecular-weight heparin. *Arch Intern Med* 1998; **158**: 2001–3.

89. Wells P, Kovacs MH, Bormanis J, *et al.* Expanding eligibility for outpatient treatment of deep venous thrombosis and pulmonary embolism with low-molecular-weight heparin. *Arch Intern Med* 1998; **158**: 1809–12.

90. Gurfinkel EP, Santopinto J, Bozovich GE, *et al.* Low molecular weight heparin vs. regular heparin or aspirin in the treatment of unstable angina and silent ischemia. *J Am Coll Cardiol* 1995; **26**: 313–18.

91. Fragmin During Instability in Coronary Artery Disease (FRISC) Study Group. Low molecular weight heparin during instability in coronary artery disease. *Lancet* 1996; **347**: 561–8.

92. Klein W, Buchwald A, Hillis SE, *et al.*, for the FRIC Investigators. Comparison of low-molecular-weight heparin with unfractionated heparin acutely and with placebo for six weeks in the management of unstable coronary artery disease: Fragmin in Unstable Coronary Artery Disease Study (FRIC). *Circulation* 1997; **96**: 61–8.

♦93. Cohen M, Demers C, Gurfinkel EP, *et al.*, for the Efficacy and Safety of Subcutaneous Enoxaparin in Non-Q-Wave Coronary Events Study Group. A comparison of low-molecular-weight heparin with unfractionated heparin for unstable coronary artery disease. *N Engl J Med* 1997; **337**: 447–52.

♦94. FRagmin and Fast Revascularization during InStability in Coronary artery disease Investigators. Long-term low-molecular-weight heparin in unstable coronary-artery disease: FRISC II prospective randomised multicentre study. *Lancet* 1999; **354**: 701–7.

♦95. FRagmin and Fast Revascularization during InStability in Coronary artery disease Investigators. Invasive compared with non-invasive treatment in unstable coronary-artery disease: FRISC II prospective randomised multicentre study. *Lancet* 1999; **354**: 708–15.

♦96. Antman EM, McCabe CH, Gurfinkel EP, *et al.* Enoxaparin prevents death and cardiac ischemic events in unstable angina/non-Q-wave myocardial infarction: results of the Thrombolysis in Myocardial Infarction (TIMI) IIB trial. *Circulation* 1999; **2100**: 1593–601.

97. The FRAXIS Study Group. Comparison of two treatment durations (6 days and 14 days) of a low molecular weight heparin in the initial management of unstable angina or non-Q-wave myocardial infarction: FRAX.I.S. (FRAxiparin in Ischemic Syndrome). *Eur Heart J* 1999; **20**: 1553–62.

98. Eikelboom JW, Malmberg K, Weitz JI, *et al.* Unfractionated heparin and low-molecular-weight heparin in acute coronary syndrome without ST elevation: a meta-analysis. *Lancet* 2000; **355**: 1936–42.

99. Kaul S, Shah PK. Low molecular weight heparin in acute coronary syndrome: evidence for superior or equivalent efficacy compared with unfractionated heparin? *J Am Coll Cardiol* 2000; **35**: 1699–712.

100. Weitz JI, Bates SM. Beyond heparin and aspirin: new treatments for unstable angina and non-Q-wave myocardial infarction. *Arch Intern Med* 2000; **160**: 749–58.

101. Hull R, Hirsh J, Jay R, *et al.* Different intensities of oral anticoagulant therapy in treatment of proximal-vein thrombosis. *N Engl J Med* 1982; **307**: 1676–81.

102. Hull R, Delmore T, Carter C, *et al.* Adjusted subcutaneous heparin vs. warfarin sodium in the long-term treatment of venous thrombosis. *N Engl J Med* 1982; **306**: 189–94.

103. Hull RD, Delmore T, Genton E, *et al.* Warfarin sodium vs low-dose heparin in the long term treatment of venous thrombosis. *N Engl J Med* 1979; **301**: 855–68.

104. Laupacis A, Albers G, Dalen J, *et al.* Antithrombotic

therapy in atrial fibrillation. *Chest* 1995; **108**(suppl): 352S–359S.

105. Prandoni P, Lensing AWA, Cogo A, *et al*. The long-term clinical course of acute deep venous thrombosis. *Ann Intern Med* 1996; **125**: 1–7.

106. Beyth RJ, Cohen AM, Landefeld CS. Long-term outcomes of deep vein thrombosis. *Arch Intern Med* 1995; **155**: 1031–7.

107. Franzeck UK, Schaich I, Jager KA, *et al*. Prospective 12 year follow-up study of clinical and hemodynamic sequelae after deep vein thrombosis in low-risk patients (Zurich study). *Circulation* 1996; **93**: 74–9.

◆108. Schulman S, Rhedin AS, Lindmarker P, *et al*. A comparison of six week with six months of oral anticoagulation therapy after a first episode of venous thromboembolism. *N Engl J Med* 1995; **332**: 1661–5.

109. Schulman S, Granqvist S, Holmstrom M, *et al*. The duration of oral anticoagulant therapy after a second episode of venous thromboembolism. *N Engl M Med* 1997; **336**: 393–8.

110. Prandoni P, Lensing A, Buller H, *et al*. Deep vein thrombosis and the incidence of subsequent symptomatic cancer. *N Engl J Med* 1992; **327**: 1128–33.

111. Simioni P, Prandoni P, Lensing AWA, *et al*. The risk of recurrent venous thromboembolism in patients with an Arg[506]→Gin mutation in the gene for factor V (factor V Leiden). *N Engl J Med* 1997; **336**: 339–403.

112. Research Committee of the British Thoracic Society. Optimum duration of anticoagulation for deep vein thrombosis and pulmonary embolism. *Lancet* 1992; **340**: 873–6.

113. Levine MN, Hirsh J, Gent M, *et al*. Optimal duration of oral anticoagulant therapy: a randomized trial comparing four weeks with three months of warfarin in patients with proximal deep vein thrombosis. *Thromb Haemost* 1995; **74**: 606–11.

◆114. Kearon C, Gent M, Hirsh J, *et al*. A comparison of three months of anticoagulation with extended anticoagulation for a first episode of idiopathic venous thromboembolism. *N Engl J Med* 1999; **340**: 901–7.

115. Hyers T, Agnelli G, Hull R, *et al*. Antithrombotic therapy for venous thromboembolic disease. *Chest* 1998; **114**: 561S–578S.

116. Schulman S. Duration of anticoagulants in acute or recurrent venous thromboembolism. *Curr Opin Pulmon Med* 2000; **6**: 321–5.

117. McIntyre H. Management during dental surgery of patients on anticoagulants. *Lancet* 1966; **2**: 99–100.

118. Tinker JH, Tarhan S. Discontinuing anticoagulant therapy in surgical patients with cardiac valve prostheses. *JAMA* 1978; **239**: 738–9.

119. Katholi RE, Nolan SP, McGuire LB. The management of anticoagulation during noncardiac operations in patients with prosthetic heart valves. *Am Heart J* 1978; **96**: 163–5.

120. Bodnar AG, Hutter AM. Anticoagulation in valvular heart disease preoperatively and postoperatively. *Cardiovasc Clin* 1984; **14**: 247–64.

121. Eckman MH, Beshansky JR, Duranad-Zaleski I, *et al*. Anticoagulation for noncardiac procedures in patients with prosthetic heart valves. *JAMA* 1990; **263**: 1513–21.

122. Stein PD, Alpert JS, Copeland JG, *et al*. Antithrombotic therapy in patients with mechanical and biological prosthetic heart valves. *Chest* 1995; **108**: 371S–379S.

123. Wahl MJ. Dental surgery in anticoagulated patients. *Arch Intern Med* 1998; **158**: 1610–16.

124. Johnson J, Turpie AGG. Temporary discontinuation of oral anticoagulants: role of low molecular weight heparin. *Thromb Haemost* 1999; Suppl (Aug): 62–3.

125. Tinmouth A, Kovacs MJ, Cruikshank M, *et al*. Outpatient peri-operative and peri-procedure treatment with dalteparin for chronically anticoagulated patients at high risk for thromboembolic complications. *Thromb Haemost* 1999; Suppl (Aug): 662.

126. Spandorfer JM, Lynch S, Weitz HH, *et al*. Use of enoxaparin for the chronically anticoagulated patient before and after procedures. *Am J Cardiol* 1999; **84**: 478–80.

127. Ansell J, Hirsh J, Dalen J, *et al*. Managing oral anticoagulant therapy. *Chest* 2001; in press.

26

Clinical approach and diagnostic evaluation of the patient with hypertension

GLENN R KERSHAW

Although widespead treatment of hypertension has had a major impact on reductions in stroke and coronary mortality, the incidence of heart failure and end-stage renal disease climbs relentlessly. Underlying these trends is the disturbing observation that only one-half of treated hypertensive patients ever reach goal blood pressure. Optimal management involves the integration of home blood pressure measurements and, in special circumstances, 24-hour ambulatory BP data into reliable measurements of clinic BP. The hypertensive database addresses the potential for aggravating factors and secondary hypertension, an assessment of target organ status and identification of total cardiovascular risk. In most patients, a thorough history, physical examination and limited laboratory evaluation is sufficient to compile this database. The secondary hypertensive syndromes are suggested by specific clinical clues which prompt cost-effective screening tests. Increasingly complex renovascular patients with refractory hypertension, renal insufficiency and widespread atherosclerosis are now under consideration for renal revascularization. Interventional strategies among this group must be highly individualized.

INTRODUCTION

In 1995, more than 100 million Americans made office visits to their physician for management of hypertension; a diagnosis that ranks second to upper respiratory infections as an indication for physician visits.[1] Hypertension maintains its prominence among medical conditions because of the following two facts.

1 About 20–25 per cent of the US population has hypertension at any point in time, and most individuals will develop hypertension as they grow older.[2]
2 There is increased awareness by the public and a well-founded conviction by the medical community that hypertension is a major contributor to cardiovascular disease and that the progression of hypertension-induced disease can be slowed, if not halted, by its treatment. This perception is based partly on experimental and epidemiologic observations but primarily on the results of large-scale therapeutic trials.

Data from the National Health and Nutrition Examination Survey (NHANES) reveal that the percentage of Americans who are aware of their hypertension, who are being treated, and whose blood pressure (BP) is controlled, rose considerably from the 1970s to the 1990s. These changes contributed to dramatic reductions in the morbidity and mortality attributable to hypertension. Death rates from stroke declined by nearly 60 per cent and from coronary heart disease by 53 per cent. These trends are evident in men and women and in African Americans and whites. The benefit of reduction in stroke mortality is particularly striking in women beyond age 50: one-half of the benefit among white women and nearly two-thirds of the benefit among African American women is attributable to improved detection and treatment of hypertension.[3] Accompanying these improvements is a decline in disability among older Americans. These trends have

Table 26.1 *Trends in the awareness, treatment, and control of high blood pressure in adults: United States 1976–94.[a] (Reprinted from the Joint National Committee on Prevention, Detection, Evaluation, and Treatment of High Blood Pressure. The sixth report of the Joint National Committee on Prevention, Detection, Evaluation, and Treatment of High Blood Pressure (JNC VI). Arch Intern Med 1997; 157: 2413–46.)*

	NHANES II 1976–1980	NHANES III (Phase 1) 1988–1991	NHANES III (Phase 2) 1991–1994
Awareness	51%	73%	68.4%
Treatment	31%	55%	53.6%
Control[b]	10%	29%	27.4%

[a]Data are for adults age 18–74 years with systolic blood pressure (SBP) of 140 mm Hg or greater, diastolic blood pressure (DBP) of 90 mm Hg or greater, or taking antihypertensive medication.
[b]SBP below 140 mm Hg and DBP below 90 mm Hg.

important implications for reducing national health costs (Table 26.1).[4]

Over the past 5 years however, these dramatic improvements have slowed. The slope of the age-adjusted decline in coronary heart disease (CHD) is leveling off and the stroke rate has risen slightly.[5] Furthermore, the age-adjusted prevalence of heart failure is higher now than it was 10 years ago[6] and the incidence of end-stage renal disease climbs relentlessly.[7] These disturbing trends are paralleled by another: hypertension control rates have not continued to improve and, in fact, have slipped over the past 5 years. Only one-half of treated hypertensives are adequately controlled. Although the majority of inadequately treated hypertensives have only mild elevations in blood pressure, clinicians generally overlook the fact that, due to their sheer numbers, mildly (stage I) hypertensive patients contribute most to the cardiovascular mortality of the population at large.[8]

In the following two chapters, the current approach to the clinical management of hypertension is discussed. This section presents practical management strategies for the broad spectrum of hypertensive disorders encountered in clinical practice. My objective is to provide a resource for medical students, residents, and fellows in training as well as for nurse practitioners and primary care physicians already entrenched in practice. Many of the recommendations cited in these chapters derive from the Sixth Report of the Joint National Committee on Prevention, Detection, Evaluation, and Treatment of High Blood Pressure (JNC VI).[9] This set of national guidelines, developed by more than 100 expert contributors, is directed primarily at primary care clinicians. I encourage the reader to review this outstanding document. Standard texts on clinical hypertension should be consulted for a more in-depth discussion on selected topics.[10] We begin with a theme fundamental to hypertension management strategies, the measurement of blood pressure.

MEASUREMENT OF BLOOD PRESSURE

Office measurement using a sphygmomanometer

Hypertension detection and management begins with accurate determination of blood pressure. Blood pressure is most reliably measured by trained health professionals using a well-maintained mercury manometer. This indirect occluding cuff method has been used for over 100 years and remains the gold standard. Direct intra-arterial recordings are neither safe nor practical to employ in most clinical settings. Moreover, all epidemiologic data used to determine treatment guidelines were generated using indirect methodology. Although blood pressure measurement is one of the most frequently performed procedures by health professionals, it is often performed incorrectly. Errors in blood pressure measurement may lead to inappropriate or inadequate treatment.[11,12]

Guidelines for measurement of blood pressure

PATIENT FACTORS

- No caffeine or smoking 30 minutes before measurement.
- Routine *follow-up*: seated in chair for 5 minutes with back supported, arm bare, and supported at heart level.
- Establish concordance of BP (within 5 mm Hg) in both arms at *initial* visit; if disparity exists, use higher value.
- Postural BP at initial visit *and* at follow-up visits, particularly in the elderly, patients with diabetes and those on therapy.
5 minutes supine, immediately upon standing, and 2 minutes after standing.

EQUIPMENT

- Cuff bladder should encircle 80 per cent of the arm circumference, cover two-thirds of the arm length, and cover the brachial artery.
  Too large is preferred over too small.
- Mercury manometer is the most accurate; aneroid devices must be *calibrated* and electronic devices *validated*.

TECHNIQUE

- Approximate systolic pressure by rapid cuff inflation while palpating radial pulse, then deflate.
  Don't miss an auscultatory gap!
- Inflate cuff rapidly 30 mm Hg above systolic pressure.
- Place stethoscope diaphragm *gently* over brachial artery (ulnar side of anticubital fossa).
- Deflate bladder 3 mm Hg per second.
- Record first (appearance) and fifth (disappearance) Korotkoff sounds as systolic and diastolic pressure.
- Record pressure to nearest 2 mm Hg, position, arm, and cuff size.

FREQUENCY AND NUMBER

- Record 2–3 readings per session; separate readings by at least 2 minutes, longer if practical.
- For initial diagnosis, obtain three sets of readings at least 1 week apart.

The Joint National Committee's classification of hypertension is based on two or more clinic readings taken at each of two or more visits following the initial screen. (Table 26.2).

Self-monitoring of blood pressure

The measurement of blood pressure outside of the office setting provides information useful for the initial assessment of the patient with hypertension and for monitoring the response to treatment.[13,14] Several applications have been endorsed by JNC VI and are listed below.

1   Self-measurement distinguishes sustained hypertension from 'white coat hypertension', a condition characterized by consistent BP elevations in clinic but normal BP at other times. These patients are at a lower level of cardiovascular risk than those with sustained hypertension and are less suitable for antihypertensive drug treatment.[15,16]
2   Self-monitoring of blood pressure may prevent overtreatment or undertreatment of the patient with sustained hypertension. Patients on drug therapy often display a higher BP in clinic than at home. Conversely, clinic measurements may coincide with the peak effect of antihypertensive medication. Decidedly higher values may exist during morning and evening conditions.
3   Involvement of the patient in the monitoring process provides positive feedback and improves adherence to therapy.
4   Decreased reliance on multiple doctor/nurse clinic visits to record BP reduces cost.

An aneroid sphygmomanometer is the preferred device for self-monitoring. Mercury manometers are rarely available outside clinic settings. Digital electronic monitors are less reliable but are useful in patients unable to operate an aneroid device. Finger monitors are inaccurate. All automated devices should be validated against a mercury manometer in a clinic setting. Consumer publications rate the various automated monitors periodically.[17] Ideal home monitoring involves measurements in the morning and evening. Home pressures are generally 5–10 mm Hg lower than clinic pressures. Patients may under-report high BP levels or monitor only under relaxed conditions. Home pressures greater than 135/85 are considered elevated but no reli-

Table 26.2 *Classification of blood pressure for adults age 18 and older[a]. (Reprinted from the Joint National Committee on Prevention, Detection, Evaluation, and Treatment of High Blood Pressure. The sixth report of the Joint National Committee on Prevention, Detection, Evaluation, and Treatment of High Blood Pressure (JNC VI). Arch Intern Med 1997; **157**: 2413–46.)*

Category	Systolic (mm Hg)		Diastolic (mm Hg)
Optimal[b]	<120	and	<80
Normal	<130	and	<85
High-normal	130–139	or	85–89
Hypertension[c]			
Stage 1	140–159	or	90–99
Stage 2	160–179	or	100–109
Stage 3	≥180	or	≥110

[a]Not taking antihypertensive drugs and not acutely ill. When systolic and diastolic pressures fall into different categories, the higher category should be selected to classify the individual's blood pressure status.
[b]Optimal blood pressure with respect to cardiovascular risk is below 120/80 mm Hg. However, unusually low readings should be evaluated for clinical significance.
[c]Based on the average of two or more readings taken at each of two or more visits after an initial screening.

able outcome data exists for self-monitored BP values. In true normotensives, home pressures are usually similar to clinic pressures.

Ambulatory blood pressure monitoring

Commercially available monitors are widely available that record BP every 15–30 minutes throughout the day and night. Korotkoff sounds are accurately recorded by auscultation or oscillometry. Readings are downloaded on to a personal computer for analysis. A log of activities or symptoms may be included in the analysis. The ambulatory BP pattern is highly reproducible in normotensives and hypertensive subjects. Blood pressure is highest while awake and declines (*dipps*) during sleep only to rise again with early morning arousal.[13,14] Mean BP, average daytime BP or the BP load (percentage of readings >140 systolic or >90 diastolic) are common expressions of a single 24-hour ambulatory study. Ambulatory pressures correlate more closely with target organ damage (left ventricular hypertrophy (LVH), carotid wall thickness, and microalbuminuria) than do casual clinic values.[14,18,19] *Nondipping* is also associated with target organ damage and in some groups is an independent predictor of cardiovascular mortality.[20–22]

Ambulatory BP monitoring (ABPM) is a costly procedure ($150–400) and should not be used indiscrimi-

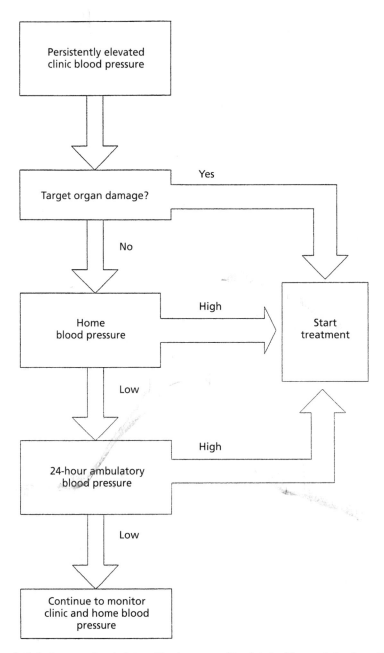

Figure 26.1 *Integration of clinic, home and ambulatory blood pressure. (Reprinted with permission from Pickering T. Hypertension handbook. New York: American Society of Hypertension, 1993.)*

nately. Medicare provides no reimbursement for ABPM and reimbursement by other insurers varies. A formal appeal to the Health Care Financing Administration was submitted in June 2000. In most patients, self-monitored BP readings can provide any supplementary data needed for clinical management decisions. A schema for using clinic, home and ambulatory monitoring in evaluating the patient with suspected hypertension is presented in Fig. 26.1.

Clinical situations in which ambulatory blood pressure monitoring may be helpful are:

- suspected white coat hypertension with no target organ damage;
- borderline hypertension with target organ damage;
- refractory hypertension;
- hypotensive symptoms while taking antihypertensive drugs;
- episodic hypertension;
- autonomic dysfunction with suspected nocturnal (supine) hypertension.

OFFICE EVALUATION OF THE HYPERTENSIVE PATIENT

Office evaluation of the patient with high blood pressure has three objectives:

1 to identify known causes of hypertension, specifically clinical features suggesting secondary forms of hypertension or factors aggravating primary hypertension;
2 to assess the status of target organs involved in the hypertensive process;
3 to identify other cardiovascular risk factors or concomitant disorders that may define prognosis and guide treatment.

The hypertension database is acquired through the medical history, a physical examination, and a focused laboratory evaluation.

Medical history

- Onset, duration, severity of hypertension; last recorded normal BP.
- Prior antihypertensive therapy: specific drugs, effectiveness, tolerance.
- Medications that may raise BP or blunt action of antihypertensive agents: oral contraceptives, non-steroidal anti-inflammatory drugs (NSAIDS), sympathomemetics, cyclosporine, steroids, erythropoietin.
- Dietary assessment: sodium, alcohol, saturated fat, caffeine.
- Family history of hypertension; premature coronary disease, stroke or sudden death; diabetes, renal disease.
- Symptoms suggesting secondary causes: spells of headache, sweats, palpitation; muscle weakness; flank pain or hematuria.
- Symptoms or history of target organ damage: angina, myocardial infarction, dyspnea; transient weakness, blindness or prior stroke; claudication.
- Additional cardiovascular risk factors: diabetes, hyperlipidemia, smoking, physical inactivity.
- Behavioral and psychosocial factors that may influence BP control: weight gain, employment status, educational level, family structure.

Physical examination

The initial physical examination includes a careful search for features suggesting secondary hypertension and an assessment of target organ damage. Important aspects of the examination are:

- blood pressure measurement: two or more readings separated by 2 minutes both supine or seated and after standing for at least 2 minutes according to guidelines described earlier;
- general appearance – weight and distribution of body fat;
- fundi – arteriolar narrowing, AV crossing changes, hemorrhage, exudate, disc edema;
- neck – carotid bruit, distended veins, thyromegaly;
- heart – rate, rhythm, size, abnormal sounds;
- lungs – rales, signs of bronchospasm;
- abdomen – enlarged kidneys, epigastric or femoral bruit;
- extremities – edema, distal pulses;
- neurological assessment.

Laboratory evaluation

A few routine laboratory tests are recommended on all hypertensive patients before initiating therapy.

A minimal laboratory evaluation includes urinalysis, complete blood count (CBC), blood chemistry (potassium, creatinine, glucose, total/high-density lipoprotein (HDL) cholesterol), and 12-lead electrocardiogram (ECG). These laboratory tests, coupled with the medical history and physical examination, are usually sufficient to exclude secondary forms of hypertension, estimate the extent of target organ involvement, and formulate a profile of cardiovascular risk.

Optional laboratory tests include creatinine clearance and 24-hour urinary protein excretion, microalbuminuria, triglycerides and low-density lipoprotein (LDL)

Table 26.3 *Renin profiling in hypertension. (Reprinted from Pickering T.* Hypertension handbook. *New York: American Society of Hypertension, 1993)*

	High renin	Normal renin	Low renin
Percentage of hypertensive patients	20	60	20
Common in	Malignant hypertension		African Americans, elderly
Secondary hypertension	Renovascular		Adrenocortical disorders, diabetes
Preferred drugs	β-blockers, ACE inhibitors		Diuretics, calcium channel blockers
Risk of CHD	Increased		

ACE = angiotensin–converting enzyme; CHD = Coronary heart disease.

cholesterol, glycosated hemoglobin, serum calcium and uric acid, thyroid-stimulating hormone and limited echocardiography.

Although *echocardiography* identifies LVH with greater sensitivity than does the ECG, cardiac 'echos' are not recommended as a routine procedure. Patients whose blood pressure remains above threshold values after several months of lifestyle modification warrant antihypertensive treatment irrespective of the presence of LVH. Blood pressure reduction with any of the first-line antihypertensive agents reverses LVH.[23,24] The cost of echocardiography is justified only if other specific indications exist. When the presence of LVH will serve as the deciding factor guiding institution of drug therapy, the limited (two-dimensional) echocardiogram provides useful prognostic information at half the cost of the comprehensive examination.[25]

The measurement of *plasma renin activity* (PRA) (Table 26.3) may be of value for three reasons:[26]

1 as a screening test for common secondary forms of hypertension;
2 to predict the BP response to specific anti-hypertensive agents;
3 to serve as an additional predictor of cardiovascular risk.[27]

Dietary sodium intake, posture and antihypertensive drugs influence PRA. A low-salt diet stimulates PRA, as does therapy with diuretics, angiotensin-converting enzyme (ACE) inhibitors and angiotensin antagonists. High dietary salt and β-blockers suppress PRA. The affects of calcium blockers vary. PRA is most meaningful when sampled on no antihypertensive agents and when indexed against 24-hour urinary sodium excretion, the renin–sodium profile. This patient preparation may be impractical in routine office settings. Extremes of PRA that override the stimulatory or suppressive effects of drug therapy may still provide valuable information, e.g. low PRA despite ACE inhibitor or high PRA despite β-blocker.

SECONDARY HYPERTENSION

Diagnostic screening for secondary hypertension is not recommended for most hypertensive subjects. The prevalence of these secondary syndromes is no more than 5 per cent and most forms of secondary hypertension are readily excluded with a high degree of confidence based on the history, physical findings, and laboratory features of the initial evaluation. Positive clinical clues gathered in the initial evaluation should prompt focused screening for specific secondary syndromes (Table 26.4).

Screening for secondary hypertension is also recommended in subjects who lack specific clinical clues but display 'inappropriate' hypertension. Features of 'inappropriate' hypertension include:

1 age of onset <20 or >55;
2 abrupt onset of hypertension;
3 escape from well-controlled hypertension;
4 BP >180/110;
5 hypertension refractory to three-drug regimen;
6 accelerated/malignant hypertension (with grade III or IV retinopathy).

Renovascular disease

Occlusive disease of the renal arteries (renovascular disease) may lead to two common clinical syndromes; elevations in arterial pressure (renovascular hypertension) and compromise of renal function (ischemic nephropathy). However, the relationships between renal artery stenosis (RAS), hypertension, and renal failure are complex. The impact of renal revascularization on blood pressure control and renal function are incompletely understood and often unpredictable. Many patients with renovascular hypertension never reach diagnostic consideration because blood pressure is well controlled on ACE inhibitors and potent dihydropyridine calcium

Table 26.4 *Guide for identifying secondary causes of hypertension*

Secondary condition	Clinical clue	Initial screen	Additional tests
Renovascular hypertension	Age of onset >60 years old Presence of carotid or ileofemoral disease Carotid, femoral, or abdominal bruit	Duplex – renal artery Captopril scan Captopril test	Arteriography
Renal parenchymal disease	Proteinuria, hematuria, azotemia		Renal ultrasound Renal biopsy
Primary aldosteronism	Hypokalemia: unprovoked or diuretic-induced	Plasma aldosterone, renin (aldo–renin ratio)	Saline suppression Adrenal CT Adrenal vein sampling Adrenal scintiscan
Cushing's syndrome	Truncal obesity Purple striae	Dexamethasone 1 mg hs followed by a.m. cortisol	24-hour urinary free cortisol Low-dose (2 mg) dexamethasone suppression
Pheochromocytoma	Paroxysmal headache, sweats, palpitation Paroxysmal hypertension	Spot urine for metanephrine, creatinine	Urinary catecholamines Clonidine suppression of plasma catechols Adrenal CT Adrenal scintiscan

aldo = aldosterone; CT = computed tomography.

channel blockers. Hence, patients who do reach diagnostic consideration for RAS are increasingly complex. More are now characterized by severe, resistant hypertension, declining renal function with widespread atherosclerosis and stenotic involvement of both renal arteries. New imaging techniques provide accurate, noninvasive screening tools to diagnose RAS.

However, the decision to revascularize patients with RAS is highly individualized and dependent upon clinical features including age, comorbid disease and life expectancy, renal function and BP control and the relative risks of intervention and nonintervention.

Comprehensive reviews of this highly controversial area have been published recently.[28–31] A diagnostic and management approach to the patient with suspected renovascular disease is provided in Fig. 26.2 a,b.

PATHOGENESIS AND NATURAL HISTORY

Renovascular hypertension (RVH) is the most common treatable form of secondary hypertension. The prevalence of RVH in the pre ACE-inhibitor era is cited as less than 1 per cent in a general office practice to as high as 15–30 per cent among a tertiary care referral population.[32] The pathophysiology of classic RVH involves renin–angiotensin activation induced by the ischemia of renal artery stenosis (RAS). Additional mechanisms include sodium retention, adrenergic activation and alterations in endothelial factors (nitric oxide, endothelin). Plasma renin activity often reverts to normal

with sustained hypertension thereby limiting the utility of renin assays in diagnosing RVH.

A variety of systemic conditions and lesions extrinsic to the renal artery can impair renal blood flow to initiate renovascular physiology. Most renovascular disease is caused by either fibromuscular dysplasia (FMD) or atherosclerotic renal artery stenosis, primary intrinsic diseases of the renal artery. Fibromuscular disease involves segmental medial thickening of the renal artery leading to a characteristic beaded appearance on angiography. FMD occurs most commonly in young women and involves the distal two-thirds of the renal artery and its branches. It is often bilateral but rarely does it progress to total occlusion. Atherosclerotic RAS accounts for 90 per cent of RAS. Atherosclerotic disease involves the proximal third of the renal artery, the ostium and the perirenal aorta. Progressive occlusive disease may lead to renal atrophy with irreversible loss of renal function. Over a 3–5 year observation period, atherosclerotic renal artery disease progresses in severity among 20–50 per cent of subjects and may progress to total occlusion (16–40 per cent) particularly in the setting of high grade (>75 per cent) stenosis.[33,34] Blood pressure control does little to arrest this process.

Ischemic nephropathy refers to renal functional compromise induced by global RAS, i.e. bilateral RAS or stenosis to a solitary functioning kidney. It is estimated that 10–15 per cent of the dialysis population is comprised of patients with ischemic nephropathy. Classic unilateral RAS is characterized by normal renal function. This is explained by autoregulatory adjustments of the stenotic kidney or offsetting increments in

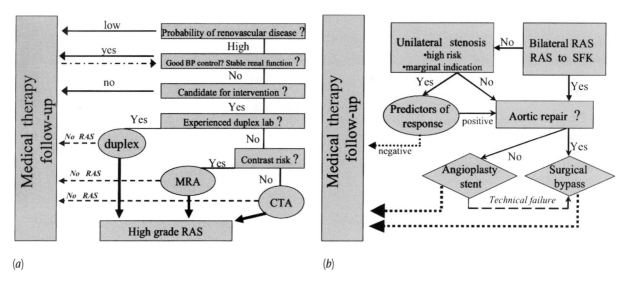

(a)   (b)

Figure 26.2 *Diagnostic and management approach in suspected renovascular disease. CTA = computed tomography angiography; MRA = magnetic resonance angiography; RAS = renal artery stenosis; SFK = solitary functioning kidney.*

filtration of the non-stenotic kidney. The large renal reserve of a kidney paired with a stenotic partner dictates that creatinine elevations in the setting of unilateral RAS imply intrinsic parenchymal disease (e.g. nephrosclerosis, diabetic nephropathy) of the non-stenotic kidney. Ischemic nephropathy does not encompass chronic renal failure in the setting of unilateral RAS.

CLINICAL DIAGNOSIS

Hypertensive subjects with RAS may be indistinguishable from those with essential hypertension. Clinical clues such as hypokalemia, negative family history, and even age of onset are more common among patients with renovascular disease but are insufficiently sensitive or specific to offer diagnostic direction. In addition to the features of 'inappropriate hypertension' cited earlier, certain clinical presentations increase the probability that a hypertensive patient may harbor RAS:

- abdominal, carotid, femoral bruits and/or widespread vascular disease;
- asymetry of renal size;
- flash pulmonary edema or unexplained episodes of congestive heart failure;
- ACE inhibitor-induced acute renal failure;
- progressive unexplained renal insufficiency.

SCREENING TESTS

Several non-invasive imaging studies are available that provide anatomic detail of the renal arteries at little or no morbidity.

Duplex ultrasonography permits direct, non-invasive interrogation of the renal arteries with little patient preparation. Stenotic lesions of the renal arteries are rarely directly visualized by duplex, but are identified by detecting high flow velocity across the stenosis. The velocity of the renal artery is compared to that of the aorta to generate a renal-aortic flow velocity ratio (RAR). A RAR of 3.5 or greater identifies significant (>60 per cent) stenosis with high sensitivity.[35] Duplex sonography can discern stenosed from occluded renal arteries but cannot grade the severity of stenosis. Therefore, duplex alone is not suitable to monitor the progression of pre-existing RAS. Kidney size can be readily measured during the duplex study and monitored during surveillance.[36,37] The duplex procedure also permits the recording of wave forms in smaller segmental arteries and the calculation of a renal resistance-index which may be predictive of the response to revascularization.[38] Duplex scanning requires little patient preparation, involves no radiation or contrast exposure and is relatively inexpensive. The technique identifies global RAS accurately and has no limitations posed by renal insufficiency. Bowel gas and obesity may preclude accurate localization of the renal arteries. Renal artery duplex evaluation is highly operator-dependent and may have limited screening value at inexperienced laboratories.[39]

Gadolinium-enhanced *magnetic resonance angiography* (MRA) permits visualization of main renal arteries with a precision that may approach conventional angiography.[40] Since gadolinium is not nephrotoxic, MRA can be used safely in patients with renal insufficiency. Visualization of distal intrarenal vessels and accessory renal arteries is poor.

Spiral *CT angiography* employs high dose (100mL) intravenous contrast to generate superb, three-dimensional images of main and accessory renal arteries which are superior to those generated by MRA.[41] The high-contrast load poses nephrotoxic risks in patients with underlying renal insufficiency. CT angiography and MRA are more costly than duplex ultrasonography.

Captopril renography employs radionuclides and a rapidly acting ACE inhibitor to unmask the action of angiotensin II on a stenotic kidney.[42–44] In RVH, the decline in renal perfusion pressure distal to a stenosis induces renin-angiotensin activation, constriction of efferent arterioles and maintenance of glomerular capillary pressure despite a decline in flow. Interruption of this angiotensin-mediated defense of GFR with captopril leads to acute glomerular capillary hypotension and a sharp decline in GFR. This response is easily detected by nuclear medicine techniques as delayed washout. Captopril renography is a functional study rather than an anatomic study. It does not detect RAS when systemic and renal renin are suppressed. Its sensitivity is limited in renal failure and it cannot discriminate between bilateral and unilateral disease.[45] Captopril-induced shifts in isotopic washout may be predictive of the interventional response to surgery or angioplasty.[43,46]

A captopril-stimulated rise in PRA may discriminate between essential hypertension and RVH whereas static measurements of PRA do not. Angiotensin II directly suppresses renin release. Captopril interrupts this negative feedback loop and stimulates renin release. Although a captopril-stimulated rise in PRA is seen in essential hypertensives this response is exaggerated in RVH and forms the basis for the *captopril test*. The study may be performed in an office setting or in conjunction with captopril renography.[47]

Formal renal angiography is generally reserved for patients with positive screening tests. Screening studies may be bypassed whenever the clinical probability of RAS is so great that a negative screen more likely reflects a false negative rather than a true negative finding.[48] Digital subtraction angiography (DSA) enhances a contrast image permitting renal artery visualization after a high-dose intravenous (IV-DSA) or low-dose intra-arterial (IA-DSA) bolus. With the emergence of MRA and high-resolution CT angiography, the utilization of digitally enhanced procedures as diagnostic studies is in decline. Invasive intra-arterial procedures are increasingly reserved as confirmatory studies performed in conjunction with renal angioplasty and stenting.

PREDICTORS OF INTERVENTIONAL RESPONSE

In *true RVH*, hypertension and RAS are linked by renal ischemia and renin–angiotensin activation. Hypertension improves with correction of stenosis. However, hypertension may merely coexist with RAS without a causal relationship, *incidental or nonfunctional RAS*. Incidental RAS and RVH are best distinguished retrospectively, but several diagnostic tests exist which may predict the blood pressure response to intervention.[49]

Renal vein renin determinations have been used to predict the response to subsequent intervention with some success.[50] Ipsilateral hypersecretion and contralateral suppression of renal renin is highly predictive (90 per cent) of a beneficial response to surgery. However, many RAS patients (>50 per cent) with non-lateralizing renins also improve with surgery or angioplasty.[51,52] This finding coupled with the invasiveness of the sampling and the lag-time involved in the renin assay conspire to make this impractical for modern use. A captopril-induced delay in isotopic washout identifies angiotensin dependency of GFR and predicts the BP response to revascularization.[43,46] Some studies refute this predictive potential of *captopril renography*.[53] The captopril scan has never been studied as a predictor of the GFR response to revascularization. *Doppler ultrasonography* may provide a simple yet powerful tool to predict the functional response to angioplasty. A recent study reports that a renal resistance index exceeding 80 reliably identifies patients with RAS in whom angioplasty or surgery will not improve BP or renal function.[38] This index is measured in segmental arteries beyond a stenosis and presumably reflects small vessel disease.

TREATMENT: MEDICAL THERAPY

The goals of therapy in managing RAS in the hypertensive subject are BP control and preservation of renal function. Therapeutic options are surgical revascularization, percutaneous transluminal angioplasty (PTRA) with or without endovascular stenting, and medical therapy. Medical therapy had been traditionally reserved for subjects who decline intervention or who carry an unacceptable risk for intervention.[54] However, more conservative management strategies have been fueled by recent randomized trials of medical therapy vs. angioplasty. In patients with unilateral RAS, these trials report a drug-sparing effect of angioplasty but comparable long term BP control.[55,56] A widely cited trial reports no difference in BP control or renal function 12 months following randomization.[57] However, this study has been criticized for its poor design and high crossover rate from medical therapy to angioplasty. Twenty-two of the 50 patients randomized to medical therapy underwent angioplasty at three months because of resistant hypertension or worsening renal function. The outcomes of these crossover patients were analyzed as if they had received medical therapy over the full 12 months.

Conservative medical management of patients with bilateral RAS or stenosis to a solitary functioning kidney involves considerable risk for progressive renal failure. Some series report a low (10–19 per cent) rate of renal deterioration with medical therapy;[58,59] others emphasize progression.[60] A retrospective analysis of 51 patients with severe bilateral RAS reports 38 per cent mortality and 12 per cent dialysis dependency over 5 years of medical management.[61] The impact of revascularization on these outcomes has never been tested systematically.

> Medical therapy is an appropriate management strategy in *unilateral* RAS with easily controlled hypertension and stable renal function.

ACE inhibitors effectively control BP in up to 85 per cent of patients with RAS[62] but carry a risk of autoregulatory failure and loss of filtration pressure beyond the stenosis. Such events may go undetected by creatinine monitoring alone. Significant creatinine increments in response to ACE inhibitors may signal global RAS.[63] Reductions in renal function in response to ACE inhibitors are usually reversible in RVH[64] occasionally after months of therapy. Calcium antagonists induce less renal dysfunction than do ACE inhibitors at equivalent degrees of BP reduction.[65] Any antihypertensive agent may compromise renal function if systemic pressure is reduced below a critical level needed to maintain post-stenotic pressure.[66] Medical management of unilateral RAS should include smoking cessation and lipid reduction. Ongoing surveillance of renal function, renal size and contralateral renal artery patency is imperative.

RENAL REVASCULARZATION

Renal revascularization is recommended for all patients with RAS due to fibromuscular dysplasia.[67] Older patients with unilateral atherosclerotic disease are candidates for revascularization when refractory to a three-drug regimen. The younger patients (<55 years old) with unilateral disease may be strong, low-risk candidates even when BP is well controlled. The BP response to conventional balloon angioplasty in atherosclerotic disease has been well established: 50 per cent improve and display reductions in BP, often on fewer agents; 15 per cent are cured and require no antihypertensive agents; and 35 per cent (failures) derive no BP benefit.[68,69] Predictors of interventional response may improve patient selection among marginal, higher risk candidates. Empiric revascularization is indicated for the refractory patient with severe hypertension.

Revascularization is also indicated to preserve or retrieve renal function, particularly in the setting of bilateral RAS or stenosis, to a solitary functioning kidney.[70-73] Functional outcomes are most favorable early in the course of renal failure.

> Renal function rarely improves when the serum creatinine exceeds 3 mg/dL at the time of angioplasty.[74] In global RAS, revascularizing a single kidney is often sufficient to stabilize renal function.

However, bilateral procedures are increasingly performed with high technical success and low morbidity. Revascularization rarely stablizes renal function in unilateral RAS. Revascularization of a kidney <7–8 cm rarely impacts favorably on BP control or renal function.

The advantages of PTRA over surgery are the ability to perform diagnostic and therapeutic maneuvers in the same session, reduced cost and reduced morbidity, particularly in high-risk patients. Technical response rates to conventional balloon angioplasty are 80 per cent. Stenosis recurs in 15–40 per cent over one year.[75,76] Complications of conventional balloon angioplasty include injury at access site (2.3 per cent), cholesterol emboli (1.1 per cent) and the need for renal surgery (2 per cent).[67]

The introduction of endovascular stents in renal revascularization has improved technical success (94–100 per cent) and reduced recurrent stenosis (10–20 per cent).[72,73,77,78] Stents oppose the elastic recoil of the aortic wall and prevent re-incursion of aortic atheromata into the ostial lumen. A recent series of renal artery stenting in patients with global RAS and renal failure (creatinine 1.5–4.0 mg/dL) reports uniform reversal or slowing of the decline in renal function.[79] Complications were few in this meticulously executed protocol and patient survival was 90 per cent over 20 months. Should a stented vessel require surgical intervention, anastomotic options are reduced. Stents cannot be removed.

Advances in surgical renal revascularization include improved preoperative screening for coronary and carotid disease and the development of microvascular techniques for branch artery lesions. The use of aortorenal bypass has declined considerably and has been replaced by the spleno–renal or hepato–renal bypass. This procedure avoids anastamoses to a friable, atherosclerotic aorta. Excellent outcomes (80–90 per cent BP response) at an operative mortality of 2 per cent are reported among carefully selected patients at highly experienced referral centers.[80] Long-term survival in this highly select group was excellent (80 per cent at 5 years).[81] A benefit in BP control was reported in 84 per cent of 631 patients who underwent surgical revascularization for atherosclerotic RAS.[82] Surgical mortality varies from 1.3–5.8 per cent; graft failure from 6–18 per cent at 5 years.[28] Azotemic subjects with RAS and widespread atherosclerosis may derive an impressive benefit from surgery; 80 per cent of 600 patients achieved improved or stable renal function 36 months following surgical revascularization.[75] Despite excellent surgical outcomes, most centers now regard renal angioplasty, with stenting, the intervention of choice for renal revascularization. Surgical revascularization of RAS is increasingly reserved for hypertensive/azotemic patients who:

1 require surgery for associated aortic disease (aortic aneurism, aortic occlusion);
2 develop recurrent stenosis in a stented renal artery;
3 require revascularization of an occluded renal artery.

Surgical revascularization of an occluded kidney is justified if the kidney is greater than 9 cm long *and* if one demonstrates *both* post-occlusive filling from collateral vessels on arteriography and viable glomeruli on biopsy.[83]

Primary aldosteronism

Primary aldosteronism accounts for less than 1 per cent of all cases of hypertension. The pathophysiology of this hypertensive syndrome involves autonomous secretion of aldosterone leading to sodium retention and volume expansion with suppression of PRA. Excess aldosterone coupled with enhanced distal sodium delivery accelerates potassium and proton secretion. Primary aldosteronism may be caused by a solitary adrenal adenoma (two-thirds of cases) or by bilateral adrenal hyperplasia (one-third of cases). Rare causes of primary aldosteronism include adrenal carcinomas, extra-adrenal adenomas and adrenocorticotrophic hormone (ACTH)-producing tumors.[84–87] Glucocorticoid-remediable aldosteronism (GRA) is a recently elucidated form of genetic hypertension in which the activity of the aldosterone synthase enzyme is ectopically expressed in the zona fasciculata.[88] Patients with GRA have mild hypertension that responds to glucocorticoids. Hypokalemia is notably absent. The prevalence and significance of GRA is not established.[89]

Primary aldosteronism presents as spontaneous hypokalemia (K <3.5 meq/L) or moderately severe diuretic-induced hypokalemia (K <3.0 meq/L). However, extensive screening has identified normokalemic forms with increasing frequency.[90,91] Hypernatremia and metabolic alkalosis are often present. Edema is absent but hypertension may be severe and refractory.

> The initial screen for primary aldosteronism involves measuring upright plasma aldosterone (PA) and plasma renin activity and then computing a PA: PRA ratio.[92] These measurements are best performed on no antihypertensive medication but the accuracy of the PA: PRA ratio in diagnosing primary aldosteronism is retained despite multidrug therapy.[93]

Most patients with 'primary aldosteronism' have a ratio greater than 25 and often greater than 50. A diagnostic PA:PRA ratio is usually followed by a spiral CT scan of the adrenals (3 mm cuts) with or without a saline suppression test.[94] Failure to suppress aldosterone (<10 ng/dL) following saline infusion confirms the autonomous secretion of the hormone. A diagnostic approach to the patient with suspected primary aldosteronism is presented in Fig. 26.3.

The CT finding of a large solitary adrenal mass and a normal contralateral gland is highly suggestive of adrenal adenoma and may be sufficient to proceed to adrenalectomy. However, the distinction between unilateral adrenal adenoma and bilateral hyperplasia by CT criteria alone is often unreliable.[95] A solitary adenoma may be concealed within normal-appearing, within bilaterally enlarged or bilaterally nodular adrenal glands. For this reason, confirmatory hormonal data are often integrated with CT findings: plasma aldosterone shows a paradoxical postural decline[96] and serum 18-hydroxy-corticosterone (18-OHB) concentrations are greater than 65ng/dL in adrenal adenomas.[97] If hormonal and imaging studies are concordant, appropriate therapeutic strategies are implemented; if discordant, adrenal venous sampling[98] or adrenal scintigraphy is performed.[99] The hormonal correlates of adrenal pathology have several pitfalls and adrenal scintigraphy requires experienced interpretation. Adrenal vein sampling, while invasive, is a low morbidity 'gold-standard' for distinguishing the two pathologies. Bilateral adrenal hyperplasia is managed with high dose spironolactone.[100] Adrenal adenomas are managed by laparoscopic adrenalectomy with a high expectation (80 per cent) that hypertension will be cured.[101] Long-term medical management of aldosterone-producing adrenal adenomas is a viable option for patients declining adrenalectomy.[102]

Pheochromocytoma

Pheochromocytoma is a tumor of chromaffin cells derived from the neural crest. The symptoms and signs of pheochromocytoma relate to excessive production and release of catecholamines. The most common findings are attacks of headache, sweating, and palpitation. In one study, this triad had a sensitivity and specificity of 90 per cent in the diagnosis of pheochromocytoma.[103] Pallor, nervousness, or nausea occur less commonly (20–40 per cent) as does weakness, dyspnea, chest, or abdominal pain. Flushing is so rarely a manifestation of pheochromocytoma that its presence casts doubt on the diagnosis. Paroxysms may be spontaneous or precipitated by a variety of physical or pharmacologic stimuli. Episodes vary in severity and frequency, but most patients experience at least one episode per week. In some (2–50 per cent) patients with pheochromocytoma, hypertension is intermittent and only accompanies attacks. The majority have sustained hypertension with superimposed surges of hypertension during attacks.[104,105]

Pheochromocytoma is diagnosed by identifying increased levels of catecholamines and/or metabolites in urine or plasma followed by an imaging procedure to localize the tumor.

The following screening tests are used.

- The simplest screening test for pheochromocytoma is measuring metanephrine and creatinine on a single-voided or overnight urine collection.[106] Normal values are similar whether expressed as mg/24 hours or as μg/mg creatinine. A normal value (metanephrine <1.3 μg/mg creatinine) excludes pheochromocytoma with 99 per cent confidence.
- Confirm an elevated spot metanephrine screen with 24-hour metanephrine and catecholamine.
- False-negative urinary metanephrines may be caused by propanolol or recent exposure to x-ray contrast.

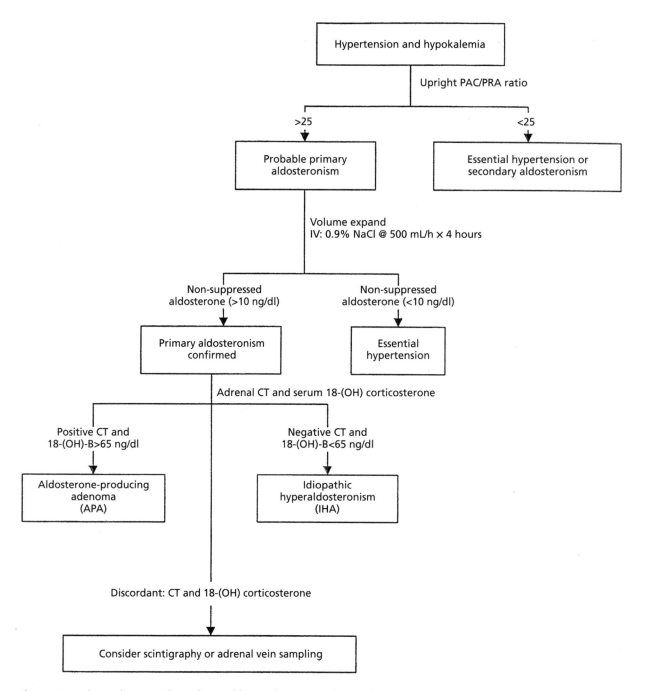

Figure 26.3 *Diagnostic approach to primary aldosteronism. PAC = plasma aldosterone concentration; PRA = plasma renin activity; CT = computed tomography; IV = intravenous. (Adapted from Kaplan N. Clinical hypertension. Baltimore: Williams & Wilkins, 1998.)*

Labetalol often causes false-positive elevations of urinary metanephrines and catecholamines.

- If metanephrine screen is negative and paroxysms persist, urinary catecholamines (epinephrine, norepinephrine) and creatinine should be measured in a specimen collected during and immediately after the episode. Patients with small active tumors may secrete predominantly free catecholamines.

- If urinary assays are equivocal, plasma catecholamines should be measured before and after oral clonidine 0.3 mg.[107]
- Measurement of plasma metanephrine is highly sensitive and specific in patients with suspected pheo. This assay is not yet commercially available.[108]
- Imaging studies are restricted to patients with biochemical confirmation of catecholamine excess.

- CT or magnetic resonance imaging (MRI) identifies pheochromocytoma with high sensitivity but MRI may be preferred.[109]
- MIBG scanning may localize pheochromocytoma in patients with hormonal evidence but negative CT or MRI examinations.[110] Up to 10 per cent of pheochromocytomas are bilateral, 10 per cent are extra-adrenal, and 10 per cent are metastatic.

Cushing's syndrome

Hypertension and the additional clinical features of Cushing's syndrome are due to hypercortisolism.[111] The syndrome may be suggested by truncal obesity, moon facies, plethora, muscle weakness, hirsuitism, emotional disturbance, and purple stria. Glucose intolerance, easy bruising, amenorrhea, decreased libido, and spontaneous fractures may be present. Rarely do patients exhibit all of these features but most exhibit some. Many more essential hypertensive patients are seen with cushingoid features than the few who prove to harbor the syndrome.[112]

Hypertensive patients with cushingoid features are screened by overnight suppression of plasma cortisol:[113]

- dexamethasone 1 mg at bedtime;
- plasma cortisol at 8.00 am;
- cortisol <5 µg/dL is normal suppression;
- few (<3 per cent) false-normals, 10–20 per cent false-positives.

Non-suppressible patients undergo low-dose dexamethasone suppression:

- dexamethasone 0.5 mg q 6 h for 2 days;
- 24-hour urinary free cortisol on day 2;
- normal cortisol suppression is <10 µg/day;
- unsuppressed patients proceed to high-dose dexamethasone suppression, ACTH, imaging studies.

Renal parenchymal disease

Renal parenchymal disease (RPD) refers to primary pathologic diseases of the kidney usually manifest as azotemia, proteinuria, or hematuria. Renal parenchymal disease does not refer to the various functional abnormalities of the kidney identified in essential hypertension nor does it include RVH or nephrosclerosis, a secondary parenchymal disease induced by the hypertensive process. Both RVH and nephrosclerosis, however, may manifest azotemia and low-grade (<2 gs/24 hours) proteinuria in advanced stages. The renal parenchymal diseases include glomerular, interstitial, cystic, and vascular diseases of the kidney other than RVH and nephrosclerosis.

The RPDs are usually associated with azotemia. Exceptions may include early polycystic kidney disease and reflux nephropathy with pyelonephritis. Historical data (family history, childhood urinary tract infections) and urinalysis (hematuria, pyuria) usually lead to appropriate diagnostic imaging studies (ultrasound) in these conditions. Glomerular disease is identified by proteinuria with or without hematuria. Quantification of proteinuria in a 24-hour collection will distinguish nephrotic from nephritic conditions. Glomerular sources of hematuria can be distinguished from urologic hematuria by the presence of proteinuria, red blood cell (RBC) casts or dysmorphic RBCs. Hematuric patients who lack supporting evidence of glomerular disease require urologic evaluation. Painful or gross hematuria almost always indicates urologic disease. The presence of proteinuria in a diabetic with retinopathy and neuropathy is sufficient to diagnose diabetic nephropathy. Historical clues and physical features may guide serologic diagnosis of glomerular disease in lupus, scleroderma, ANCA-positive GN and hepatitis C-associated MPGN.

SUMMARY

- Accurate measurement of arterial pressure in the clinic setting carries several pitfalls which must be avoided to plan adequate treatment.
- Self-monitoring of blood pressure and 24-hour ambulatory BP monitoring are valuable adjuncts to clinic BP in assuring appropriate management.
- The goals of the initial office evaluation are to identify features suggesting secondary hypertension, to assess the status of target organs, and to identify other factors contributing to total cardiovascular risk.
- Specific clinical clues suggest the presence of renovascular disease. Duplex ultrasonagraphy, magnetic resonance angiography and CT angiography are reliable screens for renal artery stenosis in hypertensive patients who are candidates for revascularization.
- Revascularization of patients with renal artery stenosis has the most favorable effect on long-term outcomes when applied to patients with severe/refractory hypertension or to patients with progressive renal insufficiency particularly when they feature stenosis of the total renal mass.
- When patients with spontaneous hypokalemia or inordinate diuretic-induced hypokalemia have an aldosterone: renin ratio exceeding 25, further diagnostic studies are indicated to discern adrenal adenoma from adrenal hyperplasia. A screening aldosterone: renin profile is appropriate for the drug-resistant patient, even in the presence of normal serum potassium.

REFERENCES

1. Woodell DA. *National ambulatory medical care survey: 1995 summary*. Advance data from Vital and Health Statistics; no. 286. Hyattsville, MD: National Center for Health Statistics, 1997.

2. Burt VL, Cutler JA, Higgins M, *et al*. Trends in the prevalence, awareness, treatment, and control of hypertension in the adult US population. Data from the Health Examination Surveys, 1960–91. *Hypertension* 1995; **26**: 60–9.

♦3. Data calculated by National Heart, Lung, and Blood Institute staff, J Culter, principal investigator, January 1997.

4. Manton KG, Corder L, Sallard E. Chronic disability trends in elderly United States populations: 1982–1994. *Proc Natl Acad Sci USA* 1997; **94**: 2593–8.

5. National Heart, Lung, and Blood Institute. *Fact book fiscal year 1996*. Bethesda, MD: US Department of Health and Human Services, National Institutes of Health, 1997.

♦6. Levy D, Larson MG, Vasan RS, Kannel WB, Ho KKL. The progression from hypertension to congestive heart failure. *JAMA* 1996; **275**: 1557–62.

♦7. US Renal Data System. *USRDS 1997 Annual Report*, Bethesda, MD: US Department of Health and Human Services, National Institute of Diabets and Digestive and Kidney Disease, 1997.

8. National High Blood Pressure Education Program Working Group. National High Blood Pressure Education Program Working Group report on primary prevention of hypertension. *Arch Intern Med* 1993; **153**: 186–208.

○9. Joint National Committee on Prevention, Detection, Evaluation, and Treatment of High Blood Pressure. The sixth report of the Joint National Committee on Prevention, Detection, Evaluation and Treatment of High Blood Pressure. (JNC VI). *Arch Intern Med* 1997; **157**: 2413–46.

10. Kaplan NM. *Clinical hypertension*. Baltimore, MD: Williams & Wilkins, 1998.

11. Perloff D, Grim C, Flack J, *et al.*, for the Writing Group. Human blood pressure determination by sphygmomanometry. *Circulation* 1993; **88**: 2460–7.

12. American Society of Hypertension. Recommendations for routine blood pressure measurement by indirect cuff sphygmomanometry. *Am J Hypertens* 1992; **5**: 207–9.

○13. Pickering T. For an American Society of Hypertension ad hoc panel. Recommendations for the use of home (self) and ambulatory blood pressure monitoring. *Am J Hypertens* 1995; **9**: 1–11.

♦14. Appel LJ, Stason WB. Ambulatory blood pressure monitoring and blood pressure self-measurement in the diagnosis and management of hypertension. *Ann Intern Med* 1993; **118**: 867–82.

15. Perloff D, Sokolow M, Cowan R. The prognostic value of ambulatory blood pressures. *JAMA* 1983; **249**: 2792–8.

16. Verdecchia P, Porcellati C, Schillaci G, *et al*. Ambulatory blood pressure: an independent predictor of prognosis in essential hypertension. *Hypertension* 1994; **24**: 793–801.

17. Consumer Reports. Blood-pressure monitors: convenience doesn't equal accuracy. *Consumer Rep* 1996; **61**: 50, 53–5.

18. Muiesan ML, Pasini GF, Salvetti M, *et al*. Cardiac and vascular structural changes. Prevalence and relation to ambulatory blood pressure in a middle-aged general population in northern Italy: The Vobarno Study. *Hypertension* 1996; **27**: 1046–52.

19. Hoegholm A, Bang LE, Kristensen KS, *et al*. Microalbuminuria in 411 untreated individuals with established hypertension, white coat hypertension, and normotension. *Hypertension* 1994; **24**: 101–5.

20. Kario K, Matsuo T, Kobayashi H, Imiya M, Matsuo M, Shimada K. Nocturnal fall of blood pressure and silent cerebrovascular damage in elderly hypertensive patients. Advanced silent cerebrovascular damage in extreme dippers. *Hypertension* 1996; **27**: 130–5.

♦21. Fagher B, Valind S, Thulin T. End-organ damage in treated severe hypertension: close relation to nocturnal blood pressure. *J Hum Hypertens* 1995; **9**: 605–10.

22. Ohkubo T, Imai Y, Tsuji I, *et al*. Relation between nocturnal decline in blood pressure and mortality. The Ohasama Study. *Am J Hypertens* 1997; **10**: 1201–7.

○23. Devereaux RB. Do antihypertensive drugs differ in their ability to regress left ventricular hypertrophy? *Circulation* 1997; **95**: 1983–5.

24. Gottdiener JS, Reda DJ, Massie BM, *et al*. VA Cooperative Study Group of Antihypertensive Agents. Effect of single-drug therapy on reduction of left ventricular mass in mild to moderate hypertension: comparison of six antihypertensive agents; the Department of Veterans Affairs Cooperative Study Group on Antihypertensive Agents. *Circulation* 1997; **95**: 2007–14.

25. Sheps SG, Frohlich ED. Limited echocardiography for hypertensive left ventricular hypertrophy. *Hypertension* 1997; **29**: 560–3.

26. Mueller FB, Laragh JH. Clinical evaluation and differential diagnosis of the individual hypertensive patient. *Clin Chem* 1991; **37**: 1868–79.

♦27. Alderman MH, Madhavan S, Ooi W, *et al*. Association of the renin-sodium profile with the risk of myocardial infarction in patients with hypertension. *N Engl J Med* 1991; **3**: 1098–104.

28. Safian R, Textor S. Renal-artery stenosis. *N Engl J Med* 2001; **344**: 431–42.

29. Eisenhauer A. Atherosclerotic renovascular disease: diagnosis and treatment. *Curr Op Nephrol Hypertens* 2000, **9**: 659–68.

30. Spitalewitz S, Reiser IW. Renovascular hypertension: diagnosis and treatment. In: Oparil S, Weber MA, eds *Hypertension: a companion to Brenner & Rector's the kidney*. Philadelphia: WB Saunders, 2000; 662–74.

31. Textor S. Revascularization in atherosclerotic renal artery disease. *Kidney Int* 1998; **53**: 799–811.

32. Nally JV. Medical management of renovascular disease. In: Izzo JL, Black HR, Taubert KA, eds *Hypertension primer*. Dallas, TX: American Heart Association, 1993; 360–2.

○33. Caps MT, Perissinotto C, Zierler RE, *et al*. Prospective study of atherosclerotic disease progression in the renal artery. *Circulation* 1998; **98**: 2866–72.

34. Pohl MA, Novick AC. Natural history of atherosclerotic and fibrous renal artery disease. Clinical implications. *Am J Kidney Dis*, 1985; **5**: 120–30.

♦35. Olin JW, Piedmonte MR, Young JR, *et al*. The utility of duplex ultrasound scanning of the renal arteries for diagnosing significant renal artery stenosis. *Ann Intern Med* 1995; **122**: 833–8.

36. Hoffmann U, Edwards JM, Carter S, *et al*. Role of duplex scanning for the detection of atherosclerotic renal artery disease. *Kidney Int* 1991; **39**: 1232–9.

37. Guzman RP, Zierler RE, Isaacson JA, *et al*. Renal atrophy and arterial stenosis. A prospective study with duplex ultrasound. *Hypertension* 1994; **23**: 346–50.

♦38. Radermacher J, Chavan A, Bleck J, *et al*. Use of doppler ultrasonography to predict the outcome of therapy for renal artery stenosis. *N Engl J Med* 2001; **344**: 410–17.

39. Postma CT, Bijlstra PJ, Rosenbusch G, Thien T. Pattern recognition of loss of early systolic peak by Doppler ultrasound has a low sensitivity for the detection of renal artery stenosis. *J Human Hypertens* 1996; **10**: 181–4.

♦40. Rieumont MJ, Kaufman JA, Geller SC, *et al*. Evaluation of renal artery stenosis with dynamic gadolinium-enhanced MR angiography. *Am J Roentgenol* 1997; **169**: 39–44.

♦41. Olbricht CJ, Pauk K, Prokop M, *et al*. Minimally invasive diagnosis of renal artery stenosis by spiral computed tomography angiography. *Kidney Int* 1995; **48**: 1332–7.

○42. Nally JV Jr, Black HR. State-of-the art review: captopril renography-pathophysiological considerations and clinical observations. *Semin Nucl Med* 1992; **22**: 85–97.

43. Fommei E, Ghione S, Hilson AJW, *et al*. Captopril radionuclide test in renovascular hypertension: a European multicentre study. *Eur J Nucl Med* 1993; **20**: 617–23.

44. Textor SC, Canzanello VJ. Radiographic evaluation of the renal vasculature. *Curr Opin Nephrol Hypertens* 1996; **5**: 541–51.

♦45. Mann SJ, Pickering TG, Sos TA, *et al*. Captopril renography in the diagnosis of renal artery stenosis: accuracy and limitations. *Am J Med* 1991; **90**: 30–40.

♦46. Setaro JF, Saddler MC, Chen CC, *et al*. Simplified captopril renography in diagnosis and treatment of renal artery stenosis. *Hypertension* 1991; **18**: 289–98.

♦47. Muller FB, Sealey JE, Case DB, *et al*. The captopril test for identifying renovascular disease in hypertensive patients. *Am J Med* 1986; **80**: 633–44.

48. Blaufox MD, Middleton ML, Bongiovanni J, Davis BR. Cost efficacy of the diagnosis and therapy of renovascular hypertension. *J Nucl Med* 1996; **37**: 171–7.

○49. Mann SJ, Pickering TG. Detection of renovascular hypertension. State of the art: 1992. *Ann Intern Med* 1992; **117**: 845–53.

50. Vaughan ED Jr. Renovascular hypertension. *Kidney Int* 1985; **27**: 811–27.

51. Rudnick MR, Maxwell MH. Limitations of renin assays. In: Narins RG, ed. *Controversies in nephrology and hypertension*. New York: Churchill Livingstone, 1984; 123–60.

52. Canzanello VJ, Textor SC. Noninvasive diagnosis renovascular disease. *Mayo Clin Proc* 1994; **64**: 1172–81.

○53. The diagnosis of renovascular hypertension: the role of captopril renal scintigraphy and related issues. *Eur J Nucl Med* 1993; **21**: 625–44.

54. Hollenberg NK. Medical therapy for renovascular hypertension. A review. *Am J Hypertens* 1988; **1**: 338S–43S.

55. Plouin PF, Chatellier BD, Raynaud A, for the ESSAI Multicentrique Medicaments vs. Angioplastie (EMMA) Study Group. Blood pressure outcome of angioplasty in atherosclerotic renal artery stenosis. A randomized trial. *Hypertension* 1998; **31**: 823–9.

56. Webster J, Marshall F, Abalalla M, *et al*. Randomized comparison of percutaneous angioplasty vs. continued medical therapy for hypertensive patients with atheromatous renal artery stenosis: Scottish and Newcastle Renal Artery Stenosis Collaborative Group. *J Hum Hypertens* 1998; **12**: 329–35.

♦57. Van Jaarsveld V, Krijnen P, Pieterman H, *et al*. The effect of balloon angioplasty on hypertension in atherosclerotic renal artery stenosis. *N Engl J Med* 2000; **342**: 1007–14.

♦58. Dean RH, Kieffer RW, Smith BM, *et al*. Renovascular hypertension: anatomic and renal function changes during therapy. *Arch Surg* 1981; **116**: 1408–15.

♦59. Chabova V, Schirger A, Stanson AW, *et al*. Outcomes of atherosclerotic renal artery stenosis managed without revascularization. *Mayo Clin Proc* 2000; **75**: 437–44.

♦60. Ying CY, Tifft CP, Garvas H, Chobanian AV. Renal revascularization in the azotemic hypertensive patient resistant to therapy. *N Engl J Med* 1984; **311**: 1070–5.

♦61. Baboolal K, Evans C, Moore RH. Incidence of end-stage renal disease in medically treated patients with severe bilateral atherosclerotic renovascular disease. *Am J Kidney Dis* 1998; **31**: 971–7.

62. Hollenberg NK. The treatment of renovascular hypertension: surgery, angioplasty and medical therapy with converting enzyme inhibitors. *Am J Kidney Dis* 1987; **10** (suppl I): 52–60.

♦63. Hricik DE, Browning PJ, Kopelman R, *et al*. Captopril-induced functional renal insufficiency in patients with bilateral renal-artery stenosis or renal-artery stenosis in a solitary kidney. *N Engl J Med* 1983; **308**: 373–6.

64. Kalra PA, Mamtora H, Holmes AM, Waldek S. Renovascular disease and renal complications of angiotensin-converting enzyme inhibitor therapy. *Q J Med* 1990; **77**: 1013–18.

65. Ribstein J, Mourad G, Mimram A. Contrasting acute effect captopril and nifedipine on renal function in renovascular hypertension. *Am J Hypertens* 1988; **1**: 239–44.

♦66. Textor SC, Novick AC, Tarazi RC, *et al*. Critical perfusion pressure for renal function in patients with bilateral atherosclerotic renal vascular disease. *Ann Intern Med* 1985; **102**: 308–14.

67. Kidney D, Deutsch LS. The indications and results of percutaneous transluminal angioplasty and stenting in renal artery stenosis. *Semin Vasc Surg* 1996; **9**: 188–97.

68. Aurell M, Jensen G. Treatment of renovascular hypertension. *Nephron* 1997; **75**: 373–83.

69. Ramsay LE, Waller PC. Blood pressure response to percutaneous transluminal angioplasty for renovascular hypertension: an overview of published series. *Br Med J* 1990; **300**: 569–72.

♦70. Bonelli FS, McKusick MA, Textor SC, *et al*. Renal artery angioplasty: technical results and clinical outcome in 320 patients. *Mayo Clin Proc* 1995; **70**: 1041–52.

♦71. Hansen KJ, Starr SM, Sands E, *et al*. Contemporary surgical management of renovascular disease. *J Vasc Surg* 1992; **16**: 319–31.

72. Rundback JH, Jacobs JM. Percutaneous renal artery stent placement for hypertension and azotemia: Pilot study. *Am J Kidney Dis* 1996; **28**: 214–19.

♦73. Harden PN, MacLeod MJ, Rodger RSC, *et al*. Effect of renal-artery stenting on progression of renovascular renal failure. *Lancet* 1997; **349**: 1133–6.

74. Sandy DT, Vidt DG. Serum creatinine prior to angioplasty: a predictor of clinical success in atherosclerotic renovascular disease. *J Am Soc Nephrol* 1995; **6**: 648.

75. Aurell M, Jensen G. Treatment of renovascular hypertension. *Nephron* 1997; **75**: 373–83.

76. Jenson G, Zachrisson B, Delin K, *et al*. Treatment of renovascular hypertension: one year results of renal angioplasty. *Kidney Int* 1995; **48**: 1936–45.

♦77. Van de Ven P, Kaatee R, Beutler J, *et al*. Arterial stenting and balloon angioplasty in ostial atherosclerotic renovascular disease: a randomised trial. *Lancet* 1999; **353**: 282–6.

♦78. Blum U, Krumme B, Flugel P, *et al*. Treatment of ostial renal artery stenoses with vascular endoprostheses after unsuccessful balloon angioplasty. *N Engl J Med* 1997; **336**: 459–65.

♦79. Watson P, Hadjipetrou P, Cox S, *et al*. Effect of Renal artery stenting on renal function and size in patients with atherosclerotic renovascular disease. *Circulation* 2000; **102**: 1671–7.

80. Novick AC. Surgical management of renovascular disease. In: Izzo JL, Black HR, Taubert KA, eds *Hypertension primer*. Dallas, TX: American Heart Association, 1993; 362–4.

81. Steinbach F, Novick AC, Campbell S, Dykstra D. Long-term survival after surgical revascularization for atherosclerotic renal artery disease. *J Urol* 1997; **158**: 38–41.

○82. Stanley JC. Surgical treatment of renovascular hypertension. *Am J Surg* 1997; **174**: 102–10.

♦83. Schefft P, Novick AC, Stewart BH. Renal revascularization in patients with total occlusion of the renal artery. *J Urol* 1980; **124**: 184–6.

○84. Blumenfeld JD, Sealey JE, Schlussel Y, *et al*. Diagnosis and treatment of primary hyperaldosteronism. *Ann Intern Med* 1994; **121**: 877–85.

○85. Bravo EL. Primary aldosteronism. Issues in diagnosis and management. *Endocrinol Metab Clin North Am* 1994; **23**: 271–83.

○86. Litchfield WR, Dluhy RG. Primary aldosteronism. *Endocrinol Metab Clin North Am* 1995; **24**: 593–612.

○87. Ganguly A. Primary aldosteronism. *New Engl J Med* 1998; **339** (25): 1828–34.

88. Lifton RP, Dluhy RG, Powers M, *et al*. Hereditary hypertension caused by chimaeric gene duplications and ectopic expression of aldosterone synthyase. *Nature Genet* 1992; **2**: 66–74.

89. Dluhy RG, Lifton RP, Glucocorticooid-remediable aldosteronism (GRA); diagnosis, variability of phenotype and regulation of potassium homeostasis. *Steroids* 1995; **60**: 48–51.

90. Rayner BL, Opie LH, Davidson JS. The aldosterone/renin ratio as a screening test for primary aldosteronism. *S Afr Med J* 2000; **90** (4): 394–400.

91. Fardella CE, Mosso L, Gomez-Sanchez C, *et al*. Primary hyperaldosteronism in essential hypertensives: prevalence, biochemical profile, and molecular biology. *J Clin Endocrinol Metab* 2000; **85** (5): 1863–7.

92. Weinberger MH, Fineberg NS. The diagnosis of primary aldosteronism and separation of two major subtypes. *Arch Intern Med* 1993; **153**: 2125–9.

93. Gallay BJ, Toivila B, Wasylenko M, Davidson RC. Insensitivity of the plasma aldosterone-renin ration to antihypertensive medication in screening for primary hyperaldosteronism [abstract]. *Am J Hypertens* 1997; 10(Part 2); 31A.

94. Holland O, Brown H, Kuhnert L, *et al*. Further evaluation of saline infusion for the diagnosis of primary aldosteronism. *Hypertension* 1984; **6**: 717–23.

○95. Doppmann J, Gill J, Miller D, *et al*. Distinction between hyperaldosteronism due to bilateral hyperplasia and unilateral aldosteronoma: reliability of CT[1]. *Radiology* 1992; **184**: 677–82.

96. Ganguly A, Dowdy AJ, Luetscher JA, Melada GA. Anamalous postural response of plasma aldosterone concentration in patients with aldosterone-producing adrenal adenoma. *J Clin Endocrinol Metab* 1973; **36**: 401–4.

97. Ulick S, Blumenfeld JD, Atlas SA, *et al*. The unique steroidogeneis of the aldosteronoma in the differential diagnosis of primary aldosteronism. *J Clin Endocrinol Metab* 1993; **76**: 873–8.

98. Doppman JL, Gill JR Jr. Hyperaldosteronism: sampling of adrenal veins. *Radiology* 1996; **198**: 309–12.

99. Shapiro B, Grekin R, Gross MD, Freitas JE. Interference by spironalactone on adrenocortical scintigraphy and other pitfalls in the location of adrenal abnormalities in primary aldosteronism. *Clin Nucl Med* 1994; **19**: 441–5.

100. Mantero F, Opocher G, Rocco S, *et al*. Long-term treatment of mineralocorticoid excess syndromes. *Steroids* 1995; **60**: 81–6.

101. Duh Q-Y, Siperstein AE, Clark OH, *et al*. Laparoscopic adrenalectomy. *Arch Surg* 1996; **131**: 870–6.

102. Ghose R, Hall P, Bravo E, *et al*. Medical management of aldosterone-producing adenomas. American College of Physicians-American Society of Internal Medicine. *Ann Intern Med* 1999; **131**: 105–8.

103. Bravo EL, Gifford RW Jr. Pheochromocytoma diagnosis, localization and management. *N Engl J Med* 1984; **311**: 1298–1303.

104. Ross EJ, Griffith DNW. The clinical presentation of phaeochromocytoma. *Q J Med* 1989; **266**: 485–96.

105. Werbel SS, Ober KP. Pheochromocytoma. Update on diagnosis, localization, and management. *Med Clin North Am* 1995; **79**: 131–53.

106. Kaplan NM, Kramer NJ, Holland OB, *et al*. Single-voided urine metanephrine assays in screening for pheochromocytoma. *Arch Intern Med* 1977; **137**: 190–3.

♦107. Bravo EL, Tarazi RC, Fouad FM, *et al*. Clonidine-suppression test. A useful aid in the diagnosis of pheochromocytoma. *N Engl J Med* 1981; **305**: 623–6.

108. Lenders J, Keiser H, Goldstein D, *et al*. Plasma metanephrines in the diagnosis of pheochromocytoma. *Ann Intern Med* 1995; **123**: 101–9.

109. Freitas JE. Adrenal cortical and medullary imaging. *Semin Nucl Med* 1995; **25**: 235–50.

110. Shapiro B, Fig LM. Management of pheochromo-cytoma. *Endocrinol Metab Clin North Am* 1989; **18**: 443–81.

111. Danese RD, Aron DC. Cushing's syndrome and hypertension. *Endocrinol Metab Clin North Am* 1994; **23**: 299–324.

112. Orth DN. Cushing's syndrome. *N Engl J Med* 1995; **332**: 791–803.

113. Kaye TB, Crapo L. The Cushing syndrome: an update on diagnostic tests. *Ann Intern Med* 1990; **112**: 434–44.

27

Comprehensive management of hypertension and its complications

GLENN R KERSHAW

The goal of antihypertensive therapy is to reduce cardiovascular complications by reducing arterial pressure and modifying total cardiovascular risk. Treatment strategies are based on a system of risk stratification which includes the status of target organs, traditional cardiovascular risk factors and the absolute level of blood pressure. The Joint National Committee (JNC VI) assigns preferred status to traditional antihypertensive agents (β-blockers, diuretics) based on outcome data from randomized controlled trials (RCTs). More recent RCTs suggest that newer antihypertensive agents (ACE-inhibitors, calcium channel blockers) are at the very least as protective and in some target organs, more protective than traditional agents. Patients with diabetes and the elderly carry a higher cardiovascular risk but derive a greater treatment benefit than does the general hypertensive population. In all hypertensive populations, the choice of agents and the goal BP is dictated by specific target organ involvement.

TREATMENT STRATEGIES

The objective of treating hypertension is to reduce cardiovascular risk and prolong life by the least intrusive means possible. Prospective randomized studies *have* demonstrated that antihypertensive treatment provides protection from stroke, coronary events, heart failure, and progression of renal disease.[1] However, the relationship between blood pressure (BP) and cardiovascular events is graded and continuous. Risk increases with increasing levels of blood pressure,[2] as does the benefit of treatment. The magnitude of cardiovascular risk, and the potential benefit of treatment, is also dependent upon the presence or absence of additional cardiovascular risk factors, the degree of target organ damage and clinical cardiovascular disease. These factors modify the risk for cardiovascular events independent of the level of blood pressure.

Risk stratification and initiation of therapy

The treatment of hypertension involves lifestyle modification and drug therapy. Lifestyle modification is a proven adjunct to drug therapy. It facilitates drug therapy and independently reduces cardiovascular risk. Lifestyle modification alone may be sufficient treatment in subjects with stage 1 hypertension (BP 140–159 mm Hg/90–99 mm Hg) who are otherwise at low risk. If blood pressure falls to target levels, as is often the case, the cost and risks of drug therapy are eliminated. In patients with stage 2 and 3 hypertension, drug therapy is indicated in conjunction with lifestyle modification once the diagnosis of hypertension is established.

Whenever an initial elevation in blood pressure is first detected, it should be verified with a minimum of three readings over at least 4 weeks before instituting drug therapy. This confirmation phase may be bypassed and drug therapy promptly instituted if target symptoms and/or severe hypertension (>180/110 mm Hg) are present.

Current guidelines (JNC IV) stratify patients according to absolute levels of blood pressure and the degree of cardiovascular risk. This matrix serves as a therapeutic guide in the newly diagnosed patient with hypertension (Tables 27.1 and 27.2).

Goals of therapy

The goal of therapy is to reduce and maintain systolic BP *below* 140 mm Hg and diastolic BP *below* 90 mm Hg, while controlling other modifiable risk factors for cardiovascular disease. Further BP reductions may be useful and well tolerated in many patients, and are recommended (<135/85 mm Hg; as low as 125/75 mm Hg) in proteinuric renal disease, diabetes, and heart failure.

A rationale for lower goal BP targets among the uncomplicated hypertensive population may emerge with the recent publication of the Hypertension Optimal Treatment (HOT) trial.[3] This large prospective trial randomized hypertensive subjects to one of three *target* diastolic blood pressures: below 90, below 85 or below 80 mm Hg. The *achieved* diastolic BP (DBP) fell short of target leading to overlap among groups. Final mean DBP was approximately 85, 83 and 81 mm Hg among the three groups respectively. The failure to clearly separate the three groups may account for the major disappointment of the HOT trial: no stastistically significant difference was noted in most cardiovascular events between the three randomized groups. However, major cardiovascular events did decline in relation to the randomized target BP and the lowest incidence of CV events was found at an achieved DBP of 82.6 mm Hg. Moreover, lower rates of cardiovascular events were found among HOT participants than among subjects in previous trials. This finding may be explained by the remarkable

Table 27.2 *Components of cardiovascular risk stratification in patients with hypertension. (Reprinted from the Joint National Committee on Prevention, Detection, Evaluation, and Treatment of High Blood Pressure. The sixth report of the Joint National Committee on Prevention, Detection, Evaluation, and Treatment of High Blood Pressure (JNC VI).* Arch Intern Med 1997; **157**: 2413–46)

Major risk factors
Smoking
Dyslipidemia
Diabetes mellitus
Age older than 60 years
Sex (men and postmenopausal women)
Family history of cardiovascular disease: women under age 65 or men under age 55

Target organ damage/clinical cardiovascular disease
Heart diseases
  Left ventricular hypertrophy
  Angina/prior myocardial infarction
  Prior coronary revascularization
  Heart failure
Stroke or transient ischemic attack
Nephropathy
Peripheral arterial disease
Retinopathy

achievement of the HOT trial: DBP was reduced and maintained below 90 mm Hg in 90 per cent of study subjects.

Concerns have been raised that aggressive reductions in diastolic blood pressure (DBP) may compromise coronary perfusion pressure and increase coronary events particularly in a susceptible elderly population.[4,5]

Table 27.1 *Risk stratification and treatment.[a] (Reprinted from the Joint National Committee on Prevention, Detection, Evaluation, and Treatment of High Blood Pressure. The sixth report of the Joint National Committee on Prevention, Detection, Evaluation, and Treatment of High Blood Pressure (JNC VI).* Arch Intern Med 1997; **157**: 2413–46)

Blood pressure stages (mm Hg)	Risk group A (no risk factors; no TOD/CCD)	Risk group B (at least one risk factor, not including diabetes; no TOD/CCD)	Risk Group C (TOD/CCD and/or diabetes, with or without other risk factors)
High-normal (130–139/85–89)	Lifestyle modification	Lifestyle modification	Drug therapy[b]
Stage 1 (140–159/90–99)	Lifestyle modification (up to 12 months)	Lifestyle modification[c] (up to 6 months)	Drug therapy
Stages 2 and 3 (≥160/≥100)	Drug therapy	Drug therapy	Drug therapy

For example, a patient with diabetes and a blood pressure of 142/94 mm Hg plus left ventricular hypertrophy should be classified as having stage 1 hypertension with target organ disease (left ventricular hypertrophy) and with another major risk factor (diabetes). This patient would be categorized as stage 1, risk group C, and recommended for immediate initiation of pharmacologic treatment.
[a]Lifestyle modification should be adjunctive therapy for all patients recommended for pharmacologic therapy.
[b]For those with heart failure, renal insufficiency, or diabetes.
[c]For patients with multiple risk factors, clinicians should consider drugs as initial therapy plus lifestyle modifications. TOD/CCD indicates target organ disease/clinical cardiovascular disease (*see* Table 27.2).

This *J-curve phenomenon* has been observed primarily with retrospective review of clinical studies. It is also described in hypertensive subjects on no therapy or on placebo.[6] Prospective trials in elderly hypertensives with isolated systolic hypertension have detected no increase in coronary events with further reductions in diastolic pressure.[7–9] The J-curve is probably a consequence of poor arterial compliance with associated coronary disease rather than a cause of coronary events.[10]

Many hypertensive patients, particularly those in low-risk strata, will derive no benefit from treatment. While it is true that treatment of stage I hypertension reduces relative cardiovascular risk by 30–60 per cent, the reduction in absolute risk is small. Nevertheless, despite the absence of symptoms, patients comply with recommended therapy to minimize cardiovascular risk. A therapy that may offer no benefit to an asymptomatic individual must aim to enhance, or at least maintain, quality of life (QOL).[11] This goal may or may not be attained. Perceived QOL may be compromised by the introduction of dietary restrictions, smoking cessation, and exercise programs leading to difficulties with adherence. On the other hand, these measures are safe, inexpensive, and may obviate the need for drug therapy.

When drug therapy is initiated, convenience, cost, and tolerability must be considered along with safety and efficacy. Once-daily formulations with 24-hour efficacy are preferred because of ease of administration, enhanced adherence and often lower cost. Long-acting preparations provide smooth and sustained BP control extending through the event-prone (sudden death, heart attack, stroke) period of early morning awakening when blood pressure rises. Although side effects may be induced by any antihypertensive agent, QOL is usually maintained and sometimes improved by any of the agents recommended for initial therapy. In the HOT study, only 2.2 per cent of subjects reported side effects at the end of the trial. There was improvement in the sense of 'well-being' compared to the baseline state and the magnitude of improvement was greatest in those randomized to the lowest target BP.

Choice of initial drug therapy

Drug therapy is indicated when hypertension is identified among high-risk patients with target organ damage or clinical cardiovascular disease. Drug therapy is also indicated when a trial of lifestyle modification fails to achieve goal BP in lower risk subjects. The choice of the initial agent is of great importance. Clinical trials have repeatedly demonstrated that about half of patients achieve BP control with the first agent regardless of which drug is chosen.[12,13] These patients are likely to continue on the 'first-choice agent' for many years over which time they accrue the costs and perhaps the side effects of the drug, while assuming optimal protection

from cardiovascular complications. The choice of this agent must be made with care.[14] Special considerations in the choice of the initial agent are:

- *demographics* – elderly and African American patients are more responsive to diuretics; young/middle-aged and white patients are more responsive to β-blockers, angiotensin-converting enzyme (ACE) inhibitors or angiotensin receptor blockers (ARBs);
- *quality of life* – awareness of side effects, including sexual dysfunction, sedation, and depression;
- *concomitant diseases and therapies* – either favorably or adversely affected by the agent;
- *physiologic/biochemical measurements*, e.g. body weight, heart rate, plasma renin activity;
- *cost/managed care* – the cost of diuretics < β-blocker < ACE inhibitor < Ca blocker, 'preferred' formulary drugs, generics < non-formulary, brand-name drugs.

> The sixth report of the Joint National Committee on Prevention, Detection, Evaluation and Treatment of Blood Pressure (JNC VI) recommends initiating antihypertensive drug treatment with either a diuretic or a β-blocker unless there are indications for another class of agent. These agents are recommended because they have been proven to decrease morbidity and mortality in randomized controlled trials (RCTs).[1,13]

At the publication of JNC VI, large scale studies with newer drug classes had not been completed. A large European RCT demonstrated that a dihydropyridine (DHP) calcium antagonist decreased stroke mortality in elderly patients with systolic hypertension.[7] A more recent Chinese trial among elderly hypertensives confirms the protective effects of DHPs.[15]

Many experts in the field of hypertension take issue with Joint National Committee's (JNC) guidelines and advocate first-line therapy with ACE inhibitors or calcium-channel blockers because of their favorable metabolic profiles, enhancement of insulin sensitivity, antihypertrophic and anti-atherosclerotic effects.[16,17] They argue that use of these 'modern' antihypertensive agents holds great promise to impact dramatically on coronary disease; RCTs of diuretics and β-blockers demonstrate only modest protection from coronary events.

Placebo controlled trials will never again be conducted in the United States and it is doubtful they will be conducted in Europe or Asia. Current and future clinical trials will compare the protective effects of different classes of antihypertensive agents. A RCT is now being conducted in which 42 000 hypertensive subjects were randomized to receive one of four agents: ACE inhibitor, calcium blocker, α-blocker (doxazocin) or diuretic. The doxazocin arm of the study has been terminated. When compared to the diuretic (chlorthalidone) arm, the patients treated with doxazocin had a 20 per cent higher risk of stroke and twice the risk of congestive heart failure.[18]

A large scale (11 000 subjects) post-JNC VI study (CAPP) that compared conventional therapy (β-blocker with/without diuretic) to captopril showed no difference in total cardiovascular end points.[19] Captopril-treated patients had a lower rate of myocardial infarction but a higher rate of stroke. The study is flawed by the fact that captopril-treated patients had higher initial and maintenance BP (2 mm Hg). Moreover, captopril was given only once a day to half the patients randomized to ACE-inhibitor. Nevertheless, the CAPP study is the first to demonstrate that an antihypertensive regimen based on ACE inhibitors is as effective as conventional treatment with diuretics and β-blockers in preventing cardiovascular events.

A second trial, conducted in the elderly (STOP Hypertension-2), pitted 'new' agents (enalapril/lisinopril or felodipine/isradipine) against older, conventional agents (β-blocker, thiazide).[20] Total cardiovascular mortality was identical in the two groups. Individually, calcium blocker and ACE-inhibitor were no better, and no worse, than conventional agents. Unlike CAPP study subjects, patients treated with these long-acting ACE-inhibitors showed no increased stroke rate. Moreover, they had fewer myocardial infarctions and a reduced frequency of CHF when compared to their counterparts taking calcium blockers. The interpretation of these studies in formulating JNC VII guidelines is speculative.

> Emerging evidence suggests that newer agents provide, at a minimum, equivalent cardiovascular protection and perhaps, in some organ systems or patient subsets, superior protection to that provided by conventional β-blocker/diuretic therapy. Additional RCTs are forthcoming.

The controversy over JNC guidelines applies exclusively to initial therapy of patients without concomitant medical conditions. In the setting of co-morbid disease, JNC VI supports a departure from first-line diuretic/β-blocker therapy whenever an alternative agent may prove beneficial. They recognize *compelling indications* to use specific agents in common clinical conditions based on outcome data from RCTs and they acknowledge other *indications* where specific agents are useful, even though outcome data are not yet available (Table 27.3).

> Therapy for most patients with uncomplicated stage 1 or 2 hypertension should begin with low doses of the initial agent. The primary goal is to introduce the agent without inducing troublesome side effects or an abrupt decline in blood pressure.

If BP remains above target values after 1–2 months, the dose is titrated upwards while lifestyle modifications are reinforced. It may take months to achieve target BP. It is useful to measure morning BP before taking antihypertensive agents, whether in office or home, to ensure control of the surge in BP that occurs with arising. Late afternoon values indicate adequacy of control throughout the day. Treatment goals based on out-of-office measurements should be lower than those based on office recordings.[21] Once BP is stabilized, follow-up at 3–6 month intervals is appropriate.

Monotherapy failure

Several strategies may be adopted if goal BP is not achieved with moderate doses of the initial agent. These are listed below and outlined in Fig. 27.1.

1 *Upward drug titration.* Titration beyond moderate dose ranges often leads to increased side effects and only modest further decrements in BP.[22] Counter-regulatory mechanisms (sodium retention, reflex vasoconstriction) often limit the response to escalating monotherapy. Titration to high (maximum)-dose monotherapy is reserved for patients whose goal systolic BP is within 5 mm Hg and who have no side effects on moderate dose monotherapy.

2 *Drug Combination.* If the patient is tolerating the first drug well, and has shown some response, add a second drug from a different class. If a diuretic is not the initial agent, it is often effective as a second agent since it potentiates the action of all antihypertensives. Low-dose diuretic is combined with β-blocker, ACE inhibitor, or angiotensin receptor blocker in a variety of fixed-dose preparations. Calcium-channel blockers (CCBs) complement the action of ACE inhibitors effectively,[23] while β-blockers do not. If target BP is achieved and sustained, consider withdrawing the first agent ('subtraction therapy').

3 *Drug substitution.* If the patient is tolerating the first drug poorly or shows no response, an agent from a different class should be substituted. If resistant to diuretic or CCBs, substitute β-blocker or ACE inhibitor. If resistant to β-blocker or ACE inhibitor, substitute diuretic or CCBs.

4 *Fixed-dose combination therapy* (Table 27.4). Low-dose combinations from different drug classes provide high efficacy while minimizing dose-related side effects. Fixed-dose combinations (FDCs) of antihypertensives are attractive because of their ease of administration and potential for improved compliance. In addition to the many useful FDCs that combine diuretic with the parent drug, several CCB/ACE inhibitor FDCs are now available, which may have a rationale in treating or preventing hypertensive cardiovascular disease. The cost of FDCs is often less than the cost of the constituent agents prescribed separately. The use of FDCs is

Table 27.3 *Considerations for individualizing antihypertensive drug therapy.[a] (Reprinted from the Joint National Committee on Prevention, Detection, Evaluation, and Treatment of High Blood Pressure. The sixth report of the Joint National Committee on Prevention, Detection, Evaluation, and Treatment of High Blood Pressure (JNC VI). Arch Intern Med 1997;* **157**: *2413–46)*

Indication	Drug therapy
Compelling indications unless contraindicated	
Diabetes mellitus (type 1) with proteinuria	ACE-I
Heart failure	ACE-I, diuretics
Isolated systolic hypertension (older patients)	Diuretics (preferred), CA (long-acting DHP)
Myocardial infarction	β-Blockers (non-ISA), ACE I (with systolic dysfunction)
May have favorable effects on co-morbid conditions[b]	
Angina	β-Blockers, CA
Atrial tachycardia and fibrillation	β-Blockers, CA (non-DHP)
Cyclosporine-induced hypertension (caution with the dose of cyclosporine)	CA
Diabetes mellitus (types 1 and 2) with proteinuria	ACE-I (preferred), CA
Diabetes mellitus (type 2)	Low-dose diuretics
Dyslipidemia	α-Blockers
Essential tremor	β-Blockers (non-CS)
Heart failure	Carvedilol, losartan potassium
Hyperthyroidism	β-Blockers
Migraine	β-Blockers (non-CS), CA (non-DHP)
Myocardial infarction	Diltiazem hydrochloride, verapamil hydrochloride
Osteoporosis	Thiazides
Pre-operative hypertension	β-Blockers
Prostatism (BPH)	β-Blockers
Renal insufficiency (caution in renovascular hypertension and creatinine ≥265.2 mmol/L (3 mg/dL)	ACE-I
May have unfavorable effects on co-morbid conditions[b,c]	
Bronchospastic disease	β-Blockers[d]
Depression	β-Blockers, central α-agonists, reserpine[d]
Diabetes mellitus (types 1 and 2)	β-Blockers, high-dose diuretics
Dyslipidemia	β-Blockers (non-ISA), diuretics (high-dose)
Gout	Diuretics
2° or 3° heart block	β-Blockers,[d] CA (non-DPH)[d]
Heart failure	β-Blockers (except carvedilol), CA (except amlodipine besylate, felodipine)
Liver disease	Labetalol hydrochloride, methyldopa[d]
Peripheral vascular disease	β-Blockers
Pregnancy	ACE I, angiotensin II receptor blockers[d]
Renal insufficiency	Potassium-sparing agents
Renovascular disease	ACE I, angiotensin II receptor blockers

[a]For initial drug therapy recommendations, *see* Fig. 27.1.
[b]Conditions and drugs are listed in alphabetical order.
[c]These drugs may be used with special monitoring unless contraindicated.
[d]Contraindicated.
ACE-I = angiotensin-converting enzyme inhibitors; BPH = benign prostatic hyperplasia; CA = calcium antagonists; DHP = dihydropyridine; ISA = intrinsic sympathomimetic activity; non-CS = non-cardioselective.

endorsed by leaders in the field of clinical hypertension[24] and by JNC VI. The use of these preparations is often restricted by closed formularies and managed care.

Two-drug failure

When adding a third agent to an antihypertensive regimen, a drug with a mechanism of action lacking in the existing regimen should be chosen. A diuretic should be one component of any three-drug regimen. The potential for secondary hypertension should be assessed once more and one should be wary of non-adherence to therapy.

Adherence to antihypertensive drug therapy may be no more than 50 per cent.[25,26] Methods for assessing adherence in clinical practice (patient self-reporting, clinician opinion) are often unreliable. Information

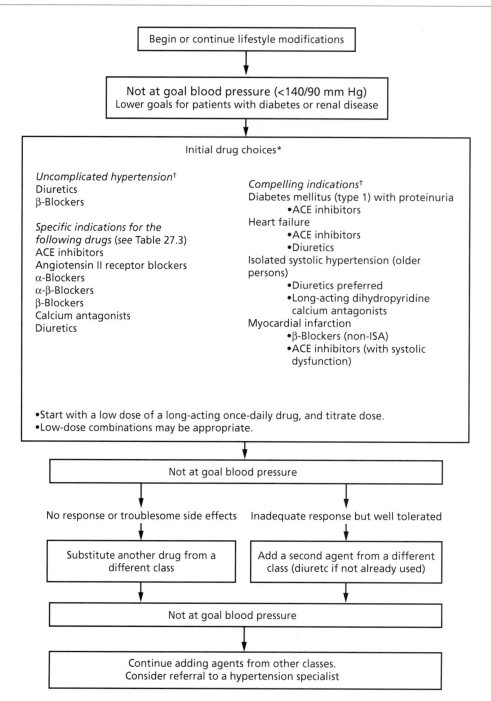

Figure 27.1 *Algorithm for the treatment of hypertension. *Unless contraindicated. †Based on randomized controlled trials. ACE = angiotensin-converting enzyme; ISA = intrinsic sympathomimetic activity. (Reprinted from the Joint National Committee on Prevention, Detection, Evaluation, and Treatment of High Blood Pressure. The sixth report of the Joint National Committee on Prevention, Detection, Evaluation, and Treatment of High Blood Pressure (JNC VI). Arch Intern Med 1997:* **157***: 2413–46)*

from spouses may be helpful, as are reports from pharmacists on the frequency of prescription refills. Some characteristics identify the patient at greatest risk for non-adherence:

- young;
- elderly;
- complicated regimen;

- missed appointments;
- failure to refill prescriptions;
- adverse effects;
- financial problems;
- history of alcoholism or substance abuse.

Recommendations to enhance adherence have been made by the Joint National Committee (Table 27.5).

Table 27.4 *Combination drugs for hypertension. (Reprinted from the Joint National Committee on Prevention, Detection, Evaluation, and Treatment of High Blood Pressure. The sixth report of the Joint National Committee on Prevention, Detection, Evaluation, and Treatment of High Blood Pressure (JNC VI).* Arch Intern Med 1997; 157: 2413–46)

Drug	Trade name
Adrenergic blockers and diuretics	
Atenolol, 50 or 100 mg/chlorthalidone, 25 mg	Tenoretic
Bisoprolol fumarate, 2.5, 5, or 10 mg/hydrochlorothiazide, 6.25 mg	Ziac[a]
Metoprolol tartrate, 50 or 100 mg/hydrochlorothiazide, 25 or 50 mg	Lopressor HCT
Nadolol, 40 or 80 mg/bendroflumethiazide, 5 mg	Corzide
Propranolol hydrochloride, 40 or 80 mg/hydrochlorothiazide, 25 mg	Inderide
Propranolol hydrochloride (extended release), 80, 120, or 160 mg/hydrochlorothiazide, 50 mg	Inderide LA
Timolol maleate, 10 mg/hydrochlorothiazide, 25 mg	Timolide
ACE inhibitors and diuretics	
Benazepril hydrochloride, 5, 10, or 20 mg/hydrochlorothiazide, 6.25, 12.5, or 25 mg	Lotensin HCT
Captopril, 25 or 50 mg/hydrochlorothiazide, 15 or 25 mg	Capozide*
Enalapril maleate, 5 or 10 mg/hydrochlorothiazide, 12.5 or 25 mg	Vaseretic
Lisinopril, 10 or 20 mg/hydrochlorothiazide, 12.5 or 25 mg	Prinzide, Zestoretic
Angiotensin II receptor antagonists and diuretics	
Losartan potassium, 50 mg/hydrochlorothiazide, 12.5 mg	Hyzaar
Calcium antagonists and ACE inhibitors	
Amlodipine besylate, 2.5 or 5 mg/benazepril hydrochloride, 10 or 20 mg	Lotrel
Diltiazem hydrochloride, 180 mg/enalapril maleate, 5 mg	Teczem
Verapamil hydrochloride (extended release), 180 or 240 mg/trandolapril, 1, 2, or 4 mg	Tarka
Felodipine, 5 mg/enalapril maleate, 5 mg	Lexxel
Other combinations	
Triamterene, 37.5, 50, or 75 mg/hydrochlorothiazide, 25 or 50 mg	Dyazide, Maxide
Spironolactone, 25 or 50 mg/hydrochlorothiazide, 25 or 50 mg	Aldactazide
Amiloride hydrochloride, 5 mg/hydrochlorothiazide, 50 mg	Moduretic
Guanethidine monosulfate, 10 mg/hydrochlorothiazide, 25 mg	Esimil
Hydralazine hydrochloride, 25, 50, or 100 mg/hydrochlorothiazide, 25 or 50 mg	Apresazide
Methyldopa, 250 or 500 mg/hydrochlorothiazide, 15, 25, 30, or 50 mg	Aldoril
Reserpine, 0.125 mg/hydrochlorothiazide, 25 or 50 mg	Hydropres
Reserpine, 0.10 mg/hydralazine hydrochloride, 25 mg/hydrochlorothiazide, 15 mg	Ser-Ap-Es
Clonidine hydrochloride, 0.1, 0.2, or 0.3 mg/chlorthalidone, 15 mg	Combipres
Methyldopa, 250 mg/chlorothiazide, 150 or 250 mg	Aldochlor
Reserpine, 0.125 or 0.25 mg/chlorthalidone, 25 or 50 mg	Demi-Regroton
Reserpine, 0.125 or 0.25 mg/chlorthiazide, 250 or 500 mg	Diupres
Prazosin hydrochloride, 1, 2, or 5 mg/polythiazide, 0.5 mg	Minizide

[a]Approved for initial therapy.
ACE = angiotensin-converting enzyme.

Non-drug therapy

Modifications in lifestyle should be strongly encouraged in all hypertensive subjects. These measures offer the potential of preventing hypertension in 'high normal' subjects[25,27] or normalizing blood pressure in patients with stage 1 hypertension without resorting to drug therapy. Lifestyle modifications have value in the drug-treated patient; they often permit reduced dosing of antihypertensive medication.[28–30] and several modifications reduce cardiovascular risk independent of blood pressure reduction (Table 27.6).[12] Several interventions potentiate each other. Although the protective effect of these interventions against cardiovascular disease has never been demonstrated, their efficacy in reducing BP is well established. In the Trial of Mild Hypertension Study (TOMHS), lifestyle modification reduced average BP from 141/91 to 130/83 mm Hg for 234 participants after 1 year.[12]

Successful implementation requires explicit education, ongoing support and close follow-up. A systematic, team approach involving nurses, dieticians, and community professionals is preferred. When lifestyle modifications are prescribed, the patient must understand that drug therapy will be initiated if target BP is not achieved within a given trial period. Promises of non-adherent

Table 27.5 *General guidelines to improve patient adherence to antihypertensive therapy. (Reprinted from the Joint National Committee on Prevention, Detection, Evaluation, and Treatment of High Blood Pressure. The sixth report of the Joint National Committee on Prevention, Detection, Evaluation, and Treatment of High Blood Pressure (JNC VI). Arch Intern Med 1997; **157**: 2413–46)*

- Be aware of signs of patient non-adherence to antihypertensive therapy
- Establish the goal of therapy: to reduce blood pressure to non-hypertensive levels with minimal or no adverse effects
- Educate patients about disease, and involve them and their families in its treatment. Have them measure blood pressure at home
- Maintain contact with patients; consider telecommunication
- Keep care inexpensive and simple
- Encourage lifestyle modifications
- Integrate pill-taking into routine activities of daily living
- Prescribe medications according to pharmacologic principles, favoring long-acting formulations
- Be willing to stop unsuccessful therapy and try a different approach
- Anticipate adverse effects, and adjust therapy to prevent, minimize, or ameliorate side effects
- Continue to add effective and tolerated drugs, stepwise in sufficient doses to achieve the goal of therapy
- Encourage a positive attitude about achieving therapeutic goals
- Consider using nurse case management

Table 27.6 *Lifestyle modifications advocated for managing hypertension, either as definitive or adjunctive treatment. (Reprinted from AHA. Hypertension primer. Izzo JL, Black HR, Taubert KA, eds. From the Council on High Blood Pressure Research, American Heart Association, 1993)*

Effective in reducing BP (in approximate order of effectiveness):
1. Weight reduction by at least 10 lb (preferably more) for patients >10% above ideal body weight
2. Limitation of alcohol intake to ≤1 oz of ethanol daily (equivalent to 2 oz of whiskey, 8 oz of wine, or 24 oz of beer)
3. Limitation of dietary sodium to <2.3 g daily (equivalent to 5 g sodium chloride)
4. Aerobic exercise (brisk walking for 30–45 minutes 3–5 times a week has been shown to be beneficial in reducing BP modestly)

Not demonstrated to be effective in reducing BP:
1. Supplements of calcium,[a] potassium,[a] magnesium,[a] fish oil
2. Stress management
3. Macronutrients
4. Garlic and onion

Effective for reducing cardiovascular risk but not for reducing BP:
1. Tobacco avoidance
2. Reduction of dietary saturated fat and cholesterol

[a]While dietary supplements of calcium, potassium, and magnesium have not been shown to reduce BP for hypertensive patients, deficiency of these minerals might result in elevated BP, so minimal daily requirements are recommended.
BP = blood pressure.

patients to do better in the future should not postpone drug therapy. A step-down from drug therapy may be implemented at a future date. Among patients with more severe hypertension or target organ damage, trials that advocate lifestyle modifications may carry risk and thus must be delayed while immediate antihypertensive therapy is instituted.

Weight reduction of as little as 10 lb reduces blood pressure in a large percentage of overweight hypertensive subjects.[27,31,32] A monitored program which combines caloric restriction and increased physical exercise is most effective. In order to achieve a weight loss of 1 lb per week, most patients require a daily intake reduction of 500 calories or a daily reduction of 300 calories coupled with a 200 calorie increase in daily expenditure (exercise program).[33] Anorectic agents should be used only with great caution; they may raise blood pressure, induce valvular heart disease or pulmonary hypertension. Recidivism may be discouraged by the feedback reward of reducing cardiovascular risk and step-down from antihypertensive therapy.

Excessive *alcohol intake* (>2 drinks/day) is a risk factor for hypertension,[25] stroke[34] and may cause resistance to

therapy.[35] Moderate alcohol (up to 2 drinks/day) reduces coronary risk compared to abstinence.[36] Hypertension may accompany alcohol withdrawal but resolves in several days.

Although multiple epidemiologic studies demonstrate a relationship between *sodium intake* and the level of blood pressure,[37] 'salt sensitivity' varies widely among hypertensive subjects.[38] The blood pressure of African Americans, elderly and diabetics is particularly sensitive to manipulations of dietary sodium.[38] In addition to a direct antihypertensive action, sodium restriction may enhance the action of antihypertensive agents, reduce diuretic-induced potassium losses,[39] and reverse left ventricular hypertrophy.[40] Extremes of sodium restriction are not practical and may carry risk. Moderate sodium restriction is feasible and beneficial.[41,42] Salt (sodium chloride) is 40 per cent sodium.

Daily dietary sodium should be restricted to 110 mmol or 2400 mg (6 g salt). Processed foods account for 75 per cent of dietary sodium intake in the American diet.[43]

Salt substitute (potassium chloride) is advocated by some as an alternative to table salt but most 'liberal salters' quickly lose their taste for salt soon after it is withdrawn. Compliance with a dietary sodium prescription can be monitored by measuring 24-hour urinary sodium. This monitoring tool retains its validity on chronic diuretic therapy.

Regular aerobic *physical activity* enhances weight loss and reduces cardiovascular risk.[44-46] The risk of developing hypertension decreases with increased physical activity[47] and established stage 1 hypertension may be reversed by a regular regimen of moderate exercise.[48] Regular exercise may lower BP in hypertensives from 5 to 15 mm Hg systolic and 5 to 10 mm Hg in diastolic pressure.[46,49,50] The effect in lean hypertensive subjects may be less than that seen in the sedentary, overweight patient with hypertension. The most effective forms of exercise are aerobic, dynamic activities in which large muscle groups are used repeatedly to maintain heart rate at target intensity for a sustained period. Brisk walking for 30–45 minutes, 4–5 times per week satisfies these criteria. Jogging, swimming, and cycling are also effective. High-intensity, vigorous exercise provides no additional antihypertensive or cardioprotective benefit. Intensive weightlifting raises blood pressure acutely.[51] More moderate strength and weight training is safe but induces only a modest decline in BP or none at all. Most patients can safely increase their level of activity without extensive medical evaluation. Formal cardiac stress testing and/or referral to a medically supervised exercise program is recommended for those with known coronary disease or a profile of high coronary risk. Regular exercise improves the lipid profile, decreases platelet aggregability and enhances insulin sensitivity.[52]

Deficiencies of *calcium, magnesium, and potassium* are associated with elevations in blood pressure.[53-55] Meta-analyses of RCTs employing calcium supplements or potassium supplements in hypertensive subjects show only small reductions in systolic (2–4 mm Hg) and diastolic (0–2 mm Hg) pressure.[56,57] An adequate intake of potassium (50–90 mmol/day) in the form of fruits and vegetables is recommended, but supplements are justified only in cases of potassium deficiency. Adequate calcium intake in the form of low-fat dairy products is important in general health maintenance, but there is no rationale for recommending calcium supplements to prevent or treat hypertension. A similar rationale applies to magnesium supplementation. The effects of mineral supplements on hypertension could be additive. The recently published Dietary Approaches to Stop Hypertension (DASH) trial reported that a diet rich in fruits, vegetables, and low-fat dairy foods reduced the systolic (−11.5 mm Hg) and diastolic (−5.5 mm Hg) pressure of patients with stage 1 hypertension substantially more than an equicaloric control diet of equal sodium content.[58]

Emotional stress can raise blood pressure acutely and job strain may be involved in the development of hypertension. The role of stress management in treating hypertension remains unproven. *Relaxation and biofeedback techniques* may lower blood pressure transiently,[59,60] but these techniques are impractical for most patients. More importantly, relaxation therapy provides no sustained reduction in blood pressure.[61-63] If available and acceptable to a motivated patient, relaxation techniques may be tried. There is no basis for using these therapies as definitive treatment for hypertension. There is no evidence that tranquilizers or sedatives lower blood pressure.

Cigarette smoking raises blood pressure acutely[64] and is a powerful risk factor for cardiovascular disease.

> Continued tobacco use may offset the beneficial effect of antihypertensive therapy.[65] Patients must be told repeatedly and unambiguously to stop smoking and they should be given some assistance in doing so.

Nicotine patches do not raise blood pressure and are a useful adjunct to counseling.[66] Patients often need help curbing the weight gain that follows. The cardiovascular benefit of quitting cigarette smoking is realized within 1 year.[67,68] While a diet low in saturated fat and cholesterol may reduce overall cardiovascular risk, it has little effect on BP.[69]

DRUG THERAPY

A list of oral hypertensive drugs is presented in Table 27.7.

Diuretics

Diuretics have been used to treat hypertension since the mid-1950s. Thiazides were the first well-tolerated highly effective agent available and they formed the cornerstone of regimens throughout the step-care era of the 1960s and 1970s. Thiazide use dropped during the 1980s when the decline in coronary artery disease fell short of that projected by epidemiologic estimates. It was suggested that the adverse metabolic effects of thiazides (hypokalemia, hypomagnesemia, and a tendency toward increased serum lipids) offset the beneficial effects achieved by blood pressure reduction.[70,71] Thiazides have enjoyed resurgence recently with the publication of studies refuting this hypothesis[72-74] and with the endorsement of these agents by JNC V and JNC VI as first-line drugs with proven efficacy in reducing stroke and coronary events.[75] Diuretics are the least expensive antihypertensive drugs.

All diuretics induce natriuresis by blocking sodium reabsorbtion at a discrete nephron site. The antihypertensive action of diuretics involves contraction of the extracellular fluid (ECF) volume and a decline in cardiac output at early stages (weeks), but a decline in vascular

Table 27.7 *Oral antihypertensive drugs[a]. (Reprinted from the Joint National Committee on Prevention, Detection, Evaluation, and Treatment of High Blood Pressure. The sixth report of the Joint National Committee on Prevention, Detection, Evaluation, and Treatment of High Blood Pressure (JNC VI).* Arch Intern Med *1997; **157**: 2413–46)

Drug	Trade name	Usual dose range, total mg/day[a] (frequency per day)	Selected side effects and comments
Diuretics (partial list)			*Short-term*: increase cholesterol and glucose levels. *Biochemical abnormalities*: decrease potassium, sodium, and magnesium levels, increase uric acid and calcium levels. *Rare*: blood dyscrasias, photosensitivity, pancreatitis, hyponatremia
Chlorthalidone (G)[b]	Hygroton	12.5–50 (1)	
Hydrochlorothiazide (G)	Hydrodiuril, Microzide, Esidrix	12.5–50 (1)	
Idapamide	Lozol	1.25–5 (1)	(Less or no hypercholesterolemia)
Metolazone	Mykrox	0.5–1.0 (1)	
	Zaroxolyn	2.5–10 (1)	
Loop diuretics			
Bumetanide (G)	Bumex	0.5–4 (2–3)	(Short duration of action, no hypercalcemia)
Ethacrynic acid	Edecrin	25–100 (2–3)	(Only nonsulfonamide diuretic, ototoxicity)
Furosemide (G)	Lasix	40–240 (2–3)	(Short duration of action, no hypercalcemia)
Torsemide	Demadex	5–100 (1–2)	
Potassium-sparing agents			Hyperkalemia
Amiloride hydrochloride (G)	Midamor	5–10 (1)	
Spironolactone (G)	Aldactone	25–100 (1)	(Gynecomastia)
Triamterene (G)	Dyrenium	25–100 (1)	
Adrenergic inhibitors			
Peripheral agents			
Guanadrel	Hylorel	10–75 (2)	(Postural hypotension, diarrhea)
Guanethidine monosulfate	Ismelin	10–150 (1)	(Postural hypotension, diarrhea)
Reserpine (G)[c]	Serpasil	0.05–0.25 (1)	(Nasal congestion, sedation, depression, activation of peptic ulcer)
Central α-agonists			Sedation, dry mouth, bradycardia, withdrawal hypertension
Clonidine hydrochloride (G)	Catapres	0.2–1.2 (2–3)	(More withdrawal)
Guanabenz acetate (G)	Wytensin	8–32 (2)	
Guanfacine hydrochloride (G)	Tenex	1–3 (1)	(Less withdrawal)
Methyldopa (G)	Aldomet	500–3000 (2)	(Hepatic and 'autoimmune' disorders) Postural hypotension
α-Blockers			
Doxazosin mesylate	Cardura	1–16 (1)	
Prazosin hydrochloride (G)	Minipress	2–30 (2–3)	
Terazosin hydrochloride	Hytrin	1–20 (1)	
β-Blockers			Bronchospasm, bradycardia, heart failure, may mask insulin-induced hypoglycemia. Less serious: impaired peripheral circulation, insomnia, fatigue, decreased exercise tolerance, hypertriglyceridemia (except agents with intrinsic sympathomimetic activity)
Acebutolol[d,e]	Sectral	200–800 (1)	
Atenolol (G)[d]	Tenormin	25–100 (1–2)	
Betaxolol[d]	Kerlone	5–20 (1)	
Bisoprolol fumarate[d]	Zebeta	2.5–10 (1)	
Carteolol hydrochloride[e]	Cartrol	2.5–10 (1)	
Metoprolol tartrate (G)[d]	Lopressor	50–300 (2)	
Metoprolol succinate[d]	Toprol-XL	50–300 (2)	
Nadolol (G)	Corgard	40–320 (1)	
Penbutolol sulfate[e]	Levatol	10–20 (1)	

Drug	Trade name	Usual dose range, total mg/day[a] (Frequency per day)	Selected side effects and comments
Pindolol (G)[e]	Visken	10–60 (2)	
Propranolol hydrochloride (G)	Inderal	40–480 (2)	
	Inderal LA	40–480 (1)	
Timolol maleate (G)	Blocadren	20–60 (2)	
Combined α- and β-blockers			Postural hypotension, bronchospasm
Carvedilol	Coreg	12.5–50 (2)	
Labetalol hydrochloride (G)	Normodyne, Trandate	200–1200 (2)	
Direct vasodilators			Headaches
Hydralazine hydrochloride (G)	Apresoline	50–300 (2)	(Lupus syndrome)
Minoxidil (G)	Loniten	5–100 (1)	(Hirsutism)
Calcium antagonists			
Non-dihydropyridines			Conduction defects, worsening of systolic dysfunction, gingival hyperplasia
Diltiazem hydrochloride	Cardizem SR	120–360 (2)	(Nausea, headache)
	Cardizem CD, Dilacor XR, Tiazac	120–360 (1)	
Mibefradil dihydrochloride (T-channel calcium antagonist)	Posicor	50–100 (1)	(No worsening of systolic dysfunction; contraindicated with terfenadine (Seldane), astemizole (Hismanal), and cisapride (Propulsid)
Verapamil hydrochloride	Isoptin SR, Calan SR	90–480 (2)	(Constipation)
	Verelan, Covera HS	120–480 (1)	
Dihydropyridines			Edema of the ankle, flushing, headache, gingival hypertrophy
Amlopidine besylate	Norvasc	2.5–10 (1)	
Felodopine	Plendil	2.5–20 (1)	
Isradipine	DynaCirc CR	5–20 (2)	
	DynaCirc	5–20 (1)	
Nicardipine	Cardene SR	60–90 (2)	
Nifedipine	Procardia XL	30–120 (1)	
	Adalat CC		
Nisoldipine	Sular	20–60 (1)	
ACE inhibitors			Common: cough; rare: angioedema, hyperkalemia, rash, loss of taste, leukopenia
Benazepril hydrochloride	Lotensin	5–40 (1–2)	
Captopril (G)	Capoten	25–150 (2–3)	
Enalapril maleate	Vasotec	5–40 (1–2)	
Fosinopril sodium	Monopril	10–40 (1–2)	
Lisinopril	Prinivil, Zestril	5–40 (1)	
Moexipril	Univasc	7.5–15 (2)	
Quinapril hydrochloride	Accupril	5–80 (1–2)	
Ramipril	Altace	1.25–20 (1–2)	
Trandolapril	Mavik	1–4 (1)	
Angiotensin II receptor blockers			Angioedema (very rare), hyperkalemia
Losartan potassium	Cozaar	25–100 (1–2)	
Valsartan	Diovan	80–320 (1)	
Irbesartan	Avapro	150–300 (1)	

[a]These dosages may vary from those listed in the *Physicians' desk reference* (51st edition), which may be consulted for additional information. The listing of side effects is not all-inclusive, and side effects are for the class of drugs except where noted for individual drugs (in parenthesis); clinicians are urged to refer to the package insert for a more detail listing.
[b](G) indicates generic availability.
[c]Also acts centrally.
[d]Cardioselective.
[e]Has intrinsic sympathomimetic activity.

resistance accompanied by restoration of volume and cardiac output with chronic administration (months and beyond).[76]

> Diuretics may be particularly effective, even critical to blood pressure control, in African Americans, the elderly, and the obese. These agents potentiate the action of all other antihypertensive agents.

They are also indicated in patients with edema. The effectiveness of diuretics in treating hypertension may be over-ridden by excess dietary sodium.

Diuretics can be classified into the following four groups:

- *Thiazide or thiazide-like diuretics*: these block the distal nephron, are preferred antihypertensive diuretics owing to their long duration of action (12–18 hours HCTZ, 24–72 hours chlorthalidone), and are used in most clinical trials.
- *Indoline derivatives*: indapamide rarely elevates lipids at a 1.25-mg dose, and has a 24-hour effect.
- *Loop diuretics*: these act at Henle's ascending loop, are potent natriuretics but are short acting (4–6 hours furosemide, bumetinide) with rebound sodium retention, and are preferred with chronic renal failure (creatinine >2.5); use twice daily as an antihypertensive; ethycrynic acid is the only alternative for patients with sulfur allergy.
- *Potassium-sparing diuretics*: these act at the cortical collecting duct, and are weak diuretics used primarily with thiazides as fixed combination agents to prevent or correct potassium depletion; there is a hyperkalemic risk with ACE inhibitors or renal insufficiency.

Diuretics are usually well tolerated. Sexual dysfunction, noted among 5–10 per cent of patients using diuretics, is often responsive to reduced or alternate-day dosing.[77] Most of the antihypertensive effect of HCTZ is achieved with a small (12.5 mg) or moderate (25 mg) dose. Higher dosing aggravates the metabolic side effects of diuretics while adding little to its antihypertensive action. A dose of HCTZ as small as 6.25 mg may be sufficient to potentiate the action of an ACE inhibitor as in a fixed combination agent.

The metabolic side effects of diuretics are dose related and are minimized by low-dose therapy. Except for hypokalemia, none of the metabolic alterations have been proven to carry increased morbidity and some experts believe these negative effects have been over-stated.

HYPOKALEMIA

Diuretic-induced renal losses are a consequence of enhanced sodium delivery to the aldosterone-sensitive, distal exchange site. Following HCTZ 25 mg, serum potassium falls from 0.2 to 0.7 mmol/L.[79] Hypokalemic

symptoms include muscle weakness, polyuria, and a tendency toward arrhythmias. Patients with left ventricular hypertrophy (LVH) and those taking digitalis are more prone to hypokalemia-induced arrhythmias.[79] The association between diuretic-induced hypokalemia and ventricular arrhythmias remains somewhat controversial but most of the evidence suggests a dose-dependent increase in sudden death among patients taking high-dose, non-potassium-sparing (naked) diuretics. Two case-control (retrospective) studies report that the risk of sudden death among patients on high doses of naked diuretics was twice that of patients on combinations of potassium-sparing agents plus thiazide.[80,81] A more recent retrospective analysis reports similar findings in patients with left ventricular dysfunction (ejection fraction <36 per cent). The use of naked diuretics increased the risk of arrhythmic death (RR, 1.33) compared to patients who did not take diuretics. Interestingly, potassium supplementation did not modify this risk. Combinations of K-sparring agents with thiazides and K-sparring agents alone carried no risk in this population.[82]

Diuretic-induced hypokalemia involves several management strategies:

- the prevention of K+ losses by reducing dietary sodium and supplement dietary K+ with citrus juices (1 meq /oz) and/or bananas (1 meq / inch);
- the prevention of K+ losses by using potassium-sparing diuretic combinations (e.g. aldactazide, dyazide) or thiazide/ACE inhibitor combinations as initial therapy;
- assessing serum potassium 2–4 weeks following initiation of diuretic therapy – *never initiate diuretics without pre-diuretic K+*;
- replete with KCl (20–40 meq/day) if prevention fails; microencapsulated forms are more acceptable than liquids, consider potassium-containing salt substitutes;
- the use of K+ supplements with caution in patients taking ACE inhibitors, angiotensin receptor blockers, and in patients with renal failure and/or diabetes.

EFFECTS ON LIPIDS

Small elevations (5–7 per cent) of serum cholesterol may be seen within 3–12 months of initiating high-dose thiazide (HCTZ 50 mg) therapy.[83] Levels often decline over time even if the thiazide is continued.[77,84] The effects on HDL cholesterol are negligible. All elevations involve LDL and total cholesterol as well as triglycerides.[85] Lower dose thiazide (HCTZ 25 mg) usually induces no change. There is no evidence that diuretic-induced lipid effects are harmful and thiazides are not contraindicated in the hypertensive patient with hyperlipidemia.[86] Lipid levels should be monitored in all hypertensive subjects whether or not thiazides are prescribed. Significant elevations may be managed by a low-fat diet, lipid-lowering agents, and/or discontinuing diuretic therapy.

INSULIN RESISTANCE AND GLUCOSE INTOLERANCE

Thiazides have been reported to increase levels of plasma insulin and impair glucose disposal (insulin resistance).[87] Worsening diabetic control and precipitation of frank diabetes are well described.[88,89] The impact of diuretic-induced insulin resistance and impaired glucose tolerance is uncertain. Elderly Type II diabetics treated with diuretics (low-dose chlorthalidone) experienced the same 34 per cent reduction in coronary events as did non-diabetics (SHEP trial).[90] In a large case-control study, diabetes developed no more frequently in diuretic-treated patients than in patients treated with ACE inhibitors, β-blockers or calcium-channel blockers.[91] A recent prospective study of 12 550 nondiabetics over 6 years is also reassuring: the risk of developing diabetes was no greater among thiazide users than among patients taking no antihypertensive agents.[92] Some investigators, however, report increased morbid events among diabetics treated with thiazide diuretics, generally in high doses.[93]

HYPERURICEMIA

Hyperuricemia is found among 30 per cent of untreated hypertensive subjects.[94] Diuretics compete with uric acid transport into the tubular lumen and raise serum uric acid by about 1 mg/dL. Susceptible individuals may experience higher elevations. Frank gout is precipitated among 5 per cent of diuretic-treated patients whose uric acid level exceeds 9 mg/dL.[95] Treatment of the gouty patient with allopurinol or probenecid may permit ongoing use of diuretics. Asymptomatic hyperuricemia poses no threat to renal function or survival and requires no therapy. Hyperuricemia is now under scrutiny as an independent cardiovascular risk factor.[96]

HYPONATREMIA

Thiazide diuretics compromise the cortical diluting site and stimulate release of antidiuretic hormone sometimes leading to modest, asymptomatic declines in serum sodium.[97] Rarely, severe, abrupt symptomatic hyponatremia develops with the institution of thiazide therapy.[98,99] This side effect has been observed almost exclusively in elderly women. Unlike thiazides, loop diuretics enhance free water excretion and may be used safely in patients with problematic hyponatremia.

β-Blockers

β-blockers are traditional first-line antihypertensive agents. Although they are no more effective than other agents in reducing BP, they are endorsed as 'preferred' first-line therapy by JNC VI because of their proven effect in reducing cardiovascular mortality in RCTs.

Although β-blockers provide convincing secondary cardioprotection following myocardial infarction,[100] the evidence that they provide any unique primary cardioprotection is less compelling.

In two large trials, β-blockers were no more protective than were diuretics.[101,102] In another major trial among the elderly, β-blockers were less effective than diuretics in preventing coronary events.[103] A recent review of β-blocker trials among uncomplicated, elderly hypertensives reports poor BP control. As monotherapy, β-blockers controlled less than one-third of elderly subjects and they were ineffective in preventing coronary heart disease and cardiovascular mortality.[104]

β-Blockers reduce blood pressure by suppressing renin release and by reducing cardiac output. Depression of central and peripheral adrenergic outflow may be additional mechanisms. Although all β-blockers act by this mechanism, several pharmacological differences exist among β-blocking agents that influence their duration of action and pattern of side effects (Table 27.8).[105]

CARDIOSELECTIVITY

β-1 receptors are distributed primarily in the heart and kidney while β-2 receptors are distributed in the bronchial tree and peripheral vasculature. β-1 stimulation increases heart rate and contractility and stimulates renin release while β-2 stimulation mediates bronchodilation and vasodilation. All β-blockers antagonize β-1 receptors but some have lower affinity for the β-2 site. When compared to non-selective β-blockers, the cardio-(β-1)-selective agents may preserve pulmonary and vascular dilatory responses and offer advantages to hypertensive patients with chronic pulmonary disease or peripheral vascular disease. However, no β-blocker is entirely cardioselective and no tissue contains exclusively one type of β-receptor. All β-blockers are best avoided in the setting of asthma. The benefits of low dose selective β-blockers probably exceed risks among patients with claudication who almost always have coexisting cororary disease. When compared to non-selective β-blockers, β-1 selective agents induce fewer disturbances of carbohydrate and lipid metabolism[106] and provide better secondary protection following myocardial infarction.[107]

LIPID SOLUBILITY

Highly lipophilic agents are readily extracted by the liver and have a short duration of action. Highly lipid-soluble agents may also enter the brain more readily and induce central nervous system (CNS) side effects more commonly.[108] β-Blockers with low lipid solubility are excreted by the kidney and have a prolonged half-life. The cardioprotective effect of β-blockers may be restricted to the lipid-soluble agents.[107]

Table 27.8 *Pharmacologic properties of some β-blockers. (Reprinted from Kaplan N. Clinical hypertension, 7th edn. Baltimore: Williams & Wilkins, 1998)*

Drug	US trade name	β$_1$-Selectivity	Intrinsic sympathomimetic activity	α-Blockage	Lipid solubility	Usual daily dosage (frequency)
Acebutolol	Sectral	+	+	−	++	200–800 mg (1)
Atenolol	Tenormin	++	−	−	−	25–100 mg (2)
Betaxolol	Kerlone	++	0	−	−	5–20 mg (1)
Bisoprolol	Zebeta	++	0	−	++	2.5–10 mg (1)
Carteolol	Cartrol	−	+	−	−	2.5–10 mg (1)
Carvedilol	Coreg	−	0	+	++	12.5–50 mg (2)
Celiprolol	Selectol	++	+	−	−	200–400 mg (1)
Esmolol	Brevibloc	++	0	−	−	25–300 µg/kg per minute iv
Labetalol	Normodyne, Trandate	−	+	+	+++	200–1200 mg (2)
Metoprolol	Lopressor, Toprol XL	++	−	−	+++	50–200 mg (2, 1)
Nadolol	Corgard	−	−	−	−	40–320 mg (1)
Penbutolol	Levatol	−	+	−	+++	10–20 mg (1)
Pindolol	Visken	−	+++	−	++	10–60 mg (2)
Propranolol	Inderal, LA	−	−	−	+++	40–480 mg (2, 1)
Timolol	Blocadren	−	−	−	+++	20–60 mg (2)

+ = increase; — = decrease; 0 = no effect; iv = intravenous.

INTRINSIC SYMPATHOMEMETIC ACTIVITY (ISA)

Agents with ISA stimulate β-receptors when background sympathetic activity is low but block β-receptors when activity is high. β-Blockers with partial agonist activity may induce less bradycardia, less bronchospasm and less peripheral vasoconstriction than do agents which act as pure antagonists.

α-BLOCKADE

Labetalol and carvedilol combine α-blockade with non-selective β-blocking effects. These agents lower blood pressure by reducing vascular resistance but have little effect on cardiac output. Both drugs require twice-daily dosing. Labetalol has been widely used both orally and intravenously to treat hypertensive emergencies.[109] Carvedilol has antioxidant and antiproliferative properties, which probably underlie its proven cardioprotective effect in patients with heart failure.[110] Unlike most pure β-blockers, the combined α–β-blockers commonly induce postural hypotension, particularly at high doses and when initiating therapy.

The antianginal and antiarrhythmic actions of β-blockers make them particularly useful in hypertensive patients with coexisting coronary disease. Following myocardial infarction, the greatest degree of secondary protection from reinfarction is provided by cardio-selective, lipid-soluble, non-ISA agents (metoprolol).[107] β-Blockers are also useful in hypertensive patients with hypertrophic cardiomyopathy, marked stress and anxiety, migraine, and variceal bleeding.

SIDE EFFECTS

The side effects of β-blockers reflect blockade of β-1 and β-2 receptors. Cardioselective, water-soluble agents are better tolerated.

CNS effects

Insomnia, nightmares, and depressed mood occur in some patients. The capacity of β-blockers for inducing clinical depression has been overstated.[111]

Cardiac effects

β-Blockers are contraindicated in high degrees of heart block. Despite negative inotropic actions in the laboratory, β-blockers are *not* contraindicated in CHF. A recent large scale trial has shown convincingly that a long-acting preparation of metoprolol improves survival in patients with CHF.[112] β-Blockers may compromise exercise capacity by inducing fatigue and by interfering with the metabolic and circulatory responses to exercise.[113]

Pulmonary effects

Patients with chronic obstructive pulmonary disease (COPD) usually have little difficulty with β-blockers. Cardioselective, ISA or combined α–β agents are preferred. All β-blockers are best avoided in asthma.[114]

Carbohydrate metabolism

β-Blockers mask the adrenergic symptoms (tachycardia, tremor) that develop in response to hypoglycemia. Sweating may be the only reactive symptom retained and this may even be enhanced by β-blocking agents.[115] β-Blockers also delay the recovery from hypoglycemia. These agents may depress insulin release and raise blood sugar in subjects on oral hypoglycemics.[116] The use of β-blockers in nondiabetics increases the risk of developing diabetes (28 per cent).[92] Despite these difficulties, β-blockers should not be withheld from diabetic patients with firm indications (post-myocardial infarction).

Lipid metabolism

β-Blockers without ISA raise triglycerides and lower high-density lipoprotein (HDL) cholesterol. There is little effect on total or low-density lipoprotein (LDL) cholesterol.

Discontinuation syndromes

Abrupt withdrawal of β-blockers often leads to nervousness, anxiety or palpitation – indicators of heightened adrenergic activity. These symptoms abate with resetting of β-receptor number and affinity. The most serious discontinuation syndrome appears among patients with coronary artery disease in whom angina, infarction, or sudden death may follow abrupt discontinuation.[117] Since hypertensives may harbor occult coronary disease, slow tapering regimens (cutting the dose in half every 3 days) are recommended when discontinuing β-blockers.

Calcium-channel blockers

Calcium-channel blockers are vasodilators. They lower blood pressure by inhibiting the entry of calcium into vascular smooth muscle cells. Several classes of CCBs are available for clinical use. They vary in their cardiovascular effects.[118,119] CCBs block the slow, voltage-operated, L-type calcium channels, which are distributed in vascular smooth muscle and the heart. *Verapamil* and *diltiazem* are non-selective and may depress cardiac contractility and slow AV conduction in addition to dilating vascular smooth muscle. The *dihydropyridines*, nifedipine, and particularly amlodipine, are vascular-selective CCBs and have no cardiac effects. *Mibefradil*, a recently released CCB, which inhibits T-type as well as L-type channels, has been recalled by the Food and Drug Administration (FDA) due to a high incidence of adverse events and multiple drug interactions. Most CCBs undergo extensive first-pass metabolism in the liver thus limiting the bioavailability of a single dose. Many agents have been reformulated into sustained-release preparations to permit once-daily administration. Amlodipine escapes first-pass metabolism and is an intrinsically long-acting agent.

The available CCBs are of comparable antihypertensive potency.[120] In hypertensives with a fast heart rate or atrial fibrillation, non-dihydropyridines (nonDHP) are preferred. Subjects with bradycardia, whether intrinsic or β-blocker induced, or with conduction defects do better on dihydropyridines (DHPs).[121] Amlodipine, a DHP, is the preferred CCB in hypertensives with impaired systolic function (ejection fraction <30 per cent).[122] Agents from either class are useful for reversing diastolic dysfunction. The combination of nonDHP and a β-blocker may induce heart block or systolic dysfunction and should be avoided.[123] Up to 40 per cent of stage 1 and 2 hypertensives are controlled with CCB monotherapy. African Americans, the elderly, and liberal salt users may show preferential responses. Response rates rise to 75 per cent with the addition of a diuretic.[124] CCBs also have additive antihypertensive effects when combined with ACE inhibitors. Several fixed-dose, CCB/ACE inhibitor preparations are available.

The most common side effects of the nonDHPs are constipation and nausea. Disturbances in cardiac conduction and contractility with use of nonDHPs are infrequent. Gastrointestinal and conduction problems are less frequent with cardizem than verapamil. The major side effects of the DHPs are vasodilatory (headache, tachycardia, flushing, ankle edema) but are less common with the advent of slow-release, long-acting preparations. Dependent edema develops in as many as 15 per cent of patients on DHPs, particularly in women, and is often refractory to diuretics. The mechanism of DHP-induced edema involves local vasodilation of pre-capillary arterioles. This process exposes the capillary bed to systemic pressure and drives fluid into the interstitium.[125] The concomitant use of ACE inhibitors may prevent DHP-induced edema by dilating postcapillary sphincters and normalizing capillary hydrostatic pressure.[126] CCBs have no effect on glucose or lipid metabolism.

The protective effects of CCBs on coronary events have been repeatedly challenged over the past 5 years. A well publicized case-controlled study reported an increased risk (65 per cent) of myocardial infarction among patients taking *short-acting* CCBs.[127] This association was confirmed in a second population-based, case-control analysis in which the risk of coronary events among users of short-acting CCBs was four times that of patients using β-blockers.[128] Neither study indicted long-acting or extended-release CCBs. Long-acting CCBs were not in use during the first study and carried a lower coronary risk (0.76) than did β-blockers in the second study.

Subsequent prospective trials have shown that, when compared to placebo, CCBs reduce the incidence of coronary events and heart failure and provide impressive protection from stroke.[10,20,23,129,130] However, CCBs may provide less coronary protection than do other agents.

Two recent meta-analyses of prospective trials compare cardiovascular end points of patients treated with CCBs to that of patients treated with other antihypertensive drugs.[131,132] In one analysis of nine trials involving 27 743 participants, patients receiving CCBs as first-line therapy had a 25 per cent greater risk of myocardial infarction and heart failure. No differences existed in systolic or diastolic blood pressure. The stroke risk was lower among CCB-treated patients and all-cause mortality was similar. A second meta-analysis reports that among placebo-controlled trials, the risk reductions of CCB treatment for heart failure (28 per cent), coronary heart disease (21 per cent) and total mortality (13 per cent) were similar to those achieved with β-blockers or diuretics. Head-to-head trials of CCBs vs conventional therapy report a significant (14 per cent) reduction in stroke risk with CCBs, but a non-significant (12 per cent) increase in the risk of coronary disease and heart failure (15 per cent). Additional RCTs of these widely prescribed agents as first-line therapy are ongoing. Until these trials are completed, caution should be exercised in prescribing CCBs as initial therapy among patients at high coronary risk. By contrast, CCBs may be the initial agent of choice in patients at high risk for stroke (Asian populations). No data suggest an increased coronary or heart failure risk when CCBs are used as add-on therapy to achieve goal BP.

Angiotensin-converting enzyme inhibitors

ACE inhibitors are widely used, well-tolerated, and highly effective antihypertensive agents. ACE not only circulates in plasma, but is also bound to vascular endothelium and widely distributed in kidney, heart, brain, and a host of other tissues.[133,134] The enzyme has a dual effect: (1) ACE cleaves two amino acids from the inactive peptide, angiotensin I, to yield angiotensin II (AII), a potent vasoconstrictor and stimulator of aldosterone; (2) ACE, or kininase II, cleaves fragments from bradykinin (BK), a dilator and permeability promoter, to yield inactivated peptides. Inhibition of ACE (kininase II) leads to decreased generation of AII and increased accumulation of BK (Fig. 27.2).[135]

ACE inhibitors lower blood pressure by reducing angiotensin II-mediated constriction. Bradykinin contributes to the hemodynamic response both directly as a dilator substance and indirectly as a stimulator of prostaglandin production. Variable sensitivity of vascular beds to AII and BK favors preferential vasodilation during ACE inhibition and increased regional blood flow to vital organs (heart, kidneys, and brain).[136] ACE inhibitors dilate both venous and arterial beds leading to decreases in preload as well as afterload. These agents also blunt sympathetic outflow in response to vasodilation. The sympatho-inhibitory and venodilating effects of ACE inhibition explain the absence of reflex tachycardia characteristic of direct vasodilators. Little change in cardiac output is seen in hypertensive subjects with

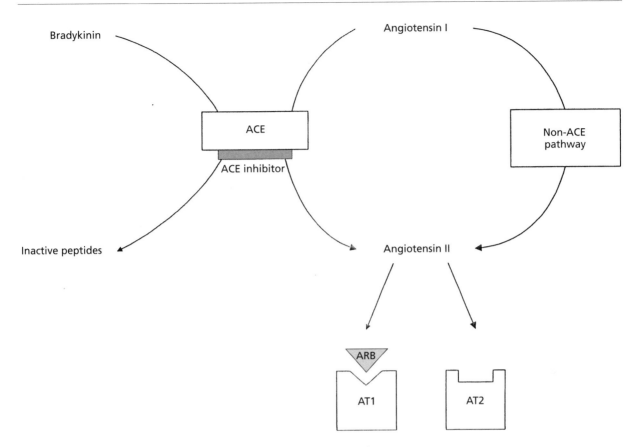

Figure 27.2 *Pharmacology of ACE inhibitors and angiotensin receptor blockers.*

normal left ventricular (LV) function.[133] ACE inhibitors depress aldosterone secretion and induce a mild diuresis.[137]

The beneficial effects of ACE inhibitors in reducing cardiovascular disease probably go far beyond blood pressure control. ACE inhibitors reverse left ventricular hypertrophy[138] and curb cardiac remodeling following myocardial infarction.[139–141] They slow the progression of proteinuric renal disease[142,143] and they prevent athero-sclerosis in animal models.[144]

In a recent landmark trial, treatment with an ACE inhibitor reduced the incidence of stroke, myocardial infarction or death from cardiovascular events across a broad range of high-risk patients with normal ejection fraction and no clinical CHF.[145] The benefit could not be ascribed to the small reduction in blood pressure (3/2 mm Hg) and is best explained by suppression of the tissue renin-angiotensin system at the level of the vasculature, heart and kidneys.

Non-hemodynamic actions by which ACE-inhibitors may provide cardiovasular protection include:

- stimulation of nitric oxide and reversal of endothelial dysfunction;[146–148]
- enhancing glucose disposal and sensitivity to insulin;[149]
- antiproliferative effects on vascular smooth muscle and cardiac myocytes;
- inhibition of monocyte adherence to and migration through endothelium;[150]
- favorable shifts in fibrinolytic balance via depression of plaminogen activator inhibitor (PAI-1) and stimulation of tPA;[151]
- inhibition of collagen deposition;[152]
- stabilization of atherosclerotic plaque.[153]

ACE inhibitors differ in the chemical structure of the active site which binds to ACE.[135] The majority of ACE inhibitors contain a carboxyl group at the active site. Captopril contains a sulfhydryl group, which may confer unique free-radical scavenging and prostaglandin stimulating actions, while fosinopril contains a phosphoryl group that enhances hepatic excretion. The remaining ACE inhibitors are cleared by the renal route and may require dosage adjustment in patients with renal insufficiency. Most ACE inhibitors are pro-drugs and have a delayed onset and prolonged (24-hour) duration of action since they require hepatic de-esterification to generate active drug. Captopril is an active drug and has a rapid onset (30–60 minutes) and shorter duration of action (6–12 hours) than other ACE inhibitors. Differences in tissue binding exist among ACE inhibitors but the clinical significance of these differences is not established. Cost, familiarity, and ease of administration (once-daily dosing) should guide the selection of a specific agent.

When employed as monotherapy, ACE inhibitors effectively control up to 60 per cent of patients with mild to moderate hypertension. Response rates are lower in African Americans. The elderly respond as well as do younger patients. The addition of a diuretic increases response rates to 85 per cent.[136] Several ACE inhibitor/diuretic fixed combinations are available. Calcium-channel blockers complement the action of ACE inhibitors nicely. Several fixed combinations have been introduced. ACE inhibitors have a proven benefit beyond their blood pressure lowering effect in patients with diabetic proteinuria, heart failure, and in the post-myocardial infarction setting with systolic dysfunction.[143,154,155] Whenever these 'compelling indications' coexist with hypertension, the medical regimen should include an ACE inhibitor.

ACE inhibitors are usually well tolerated. The most troublesome side effects are listed below.

- *Cough:* This occurs in 15–20 per cent of patients and women more than men; the onset is usually with initiation of therapy, is *not* dose-related, and resolves within a few weeks of drug withdrawal. It recurs when rechallenged with any ACE inhibitor, and is mediated by BK or substance P, which lower the threshold of tracheobronchial irritability. Treat by substituting the angiotensin receptor antagonist.[156,157]
- *Azotemia:* This may be new onset or aggravation of pre-existing azotemia. It is more common with concomitant diuretics, exaggerated hypotensive response, bilateral renal artery stenosis; mediated by decline in glomerular capillary pressure; generally reversible.
- *Hyperkalemia:* This occurs primarily with underlying renal insufficiency and in diabetics, owing to depression of AII-mediated aldosterone secretion; treat by adding diuretic.
- *Angioedema:* This is rare but potentially life-threatening swelling of the face, lips, tongue, or airway; kinin-mediated.
- *Allergic/toxic reactions:* These are rash, taste disturbance, and leukopenia.

Angiotensin receptor blockers

Angiotensin receptor blockers (ARBs) lower blood pressure by blocking the constrictor effect of AII on vascular smooth muscle. The clinical efficacy and side effects of these agents are similar to ACE inhibitors but they induce no cough. When used as monotherapy, up to 60 per cent of patients respond and their effect is amplified by salt restriction or diuretics.[158–160] Animal studies and several clinical trials report ancillary actions in congestive heart failure, ventricular hypertrophy, and protein-

uric renal disease, which are comparable to those of ACE inhibitors.[161–163] Many studies are now under way which test the efficacy of ARBs in clinical settings where ACE inhibitors have proven benefit. Additional studies are comparing the efficacy of combination ARB/ACE inhibitor therapy with ACE inhibitor alone in heart failure and in other cardiovascular diseases.

ACE inhibitors and ARBs have distinctive pharmacologic differences that may hold clinical significance (see Fig. 27.2).[159]

BRADYKININ METABOLISM

Unlike ACE inhibitors, ARBs do not inhibit kinninase II (ACE), do not raise plasma BK and do not induce cough. However, enhanced BK activity may mediate some of the protective effects of ACE inhibitors in cardiovascular disease (stimulating fibriolysis, enhanced endothelial function). These effects may not be realized with ARB monotherapy.

INCOMPLETE ANGIOTENSIN BLOCKADE

The blockade of the renin-angiotensin system following ACE inhibitors may be incomplete.[164] Significant concentrations of AII persist in plasma and tissue during chronic ACE inhibitor therapy. This persistence may be due to non-sustained suppression of ACE, increased angiotensin I (AI) generation, and/or ongoing AII generation via alternate (ACE-independent) pathways.[165] Blockade of the renin-angiotensin system with ARBs may be more complete. ARBs specifically block the angiotensin receptor and the blockade is independent of the pathways for AII synthesis.

DIFFERENTIAL EFFECT ON AT1 AND AT2 RECEPTOR

AT1 and AT2 are receptor subtypes, both of which bind angiotensin II (AII). Angiotensin receptor blockers (ARBs) competitively displace AII from binding to the AT1 receptor but leave the AT2 receptor vacant. The AT1 receptor mediates most of the known effects of AII, including vasoconstriction, cell proliferation, and stimulation of aldosterone secretion. Activation of the AT1 receptor also *suppresses* renin release. Angiotensin receptor blockade removes this suppressive effect, stimulates renin release, and leads to the generation of AII, which, in the setting of AT1 blockade, is diverted to the AT2 receptor. Although the role of the AT2 receptor is not fully elucidated, evidence is emerging that AT2 stimulation mediates vasodilatory and antiproliferative actions.[166–168] The hypotensive effect of losartan in salt-depleted animals is blunted by AT2 blockade.[169] This observation supports the concept that the blood-pressure-lowering effects of ARBs involve a dual action: inhibition of a pressor receptor (AT1) and stimulation of a depressor receptor (AT2).

Several ARBs are now FDA approved. Losartan has been the most widely studied. Some data suggest twice-daily dosing may be optimal. Valsartan and irbesartan have sustained 24-hour antihypertensive efficacy, as do candesartan and telmisartan. The effects of tasosartan may last 48 hours. In patients with renal insufficiency, ARBs may induce less hyperkalemia and less functional deterioration than do ACE inhibitors.[170] In patients with normal renal and adrenal function, ARBs have no adverse laboratory effects. ARBs have the lowest incidence of side effects of all classes of antihypertensive agents. Side-effect profiles are no different than placebo.

Direct vasodilators

Direct vasodilators enter vascular smooth muscle cells where they act to mediate vasodilation. This mechanism differs from that of agents which vasodilate by alternative mechanisms, such as blocking production of a constrictor hormone, antagonizing a pressor receptor or by inhibiting calcium entry into vascular smooth muscle. Two vasodilators, hydralazine and minoxidil, have been available to treat hypertension for many years. Both agents elicit a baroreceptor-mediated sympathetic response to increase heart rate, stroke volume, and cardiac output. Sympathetic stimulation and sharp declines in blood pressure lead to reactive sodium retention. These compensatory responses induce troublesome side effects and they restrain the antihypertensive effect. For this reason, direct vasodilators are almost always used as part of a triple-drug regimen that includes an antiadrenergic agent to counter the sympathetic discharge and a diuretic to restore sodium balance.[171]

Hydralazine was widely used during the 1950s and 1960s in combination with reserpine and diuretic. By the early 1970s, hydralazine was the most commonly used third-step agent added to a β-blocker/diuretic regimen. With the arrival of newer agents, hydralazine is infrequently prescribed. When ACE-inhibitor-induced azotemia complicates the management of heart failure, hydralazine is sometimes employed as an alternative afterload reducing agent.[172] Unlike ACE inhibitors, hydralazine has no significant effect on intrarenal hemodynamics. In these settings, the agent is most effective when given three or even four times daily. Hydralazine inactivation is by hepatic acetylation; the activity of this enzyme is genetically determined.[173] A lupus-like syndrome with induction of antinuclear antibodies (ANAs) is an intriguing and fully reversible side effect.[174,175] Positive ANAs are more often identified in the absence of the syndrome. Both are dose related.

Minoxidil, a far more potent dilator than hydralazine, should always be used with an anti-adrenergic agent, preferably a β-blocker, and a diuretic. Loop diuretics are often required. Minoxidil was introduced in the early 1970s as an alternative to nephrectomy in managing the most severe forms of hypertension (malignant hypertension and sclerdermal renal crisis). Despite the subsequent introduction of ACE inhibitors and calcium-channel blockers, minoxidil has maintained its distinction as the mainstay of therapy (the 'big gun') in patients with severe hypertension often associated with renal insufficiency.[176] Minoxidil controls more than 75 per cent of patients resistant to mutidrug regimens and, unlike hydralazine, it can be given as a single daily dose.[177] The potent dilatory action of minoxidil induces hirsuitism in most (80 per cent) patients. This side effect precludes any long-term use in women.

α-Blockers

The selective α-1 blockers act at the synapse between the terminal sympathetic neuron and the vascular smooth muscle cell. These agents block catecholamine-induced vasoconstriction by blocking the α-1 adrenergic receptor on vascular smooth muscle but, unlike non-selective α-blockers (phentolamine, phenoxybenzamine), the presynaptic α-2 receptor remains unblocked. The overflow of norepinephrine (NE) from the synaptic cleff stimulates the unblocked presynaptic receptors, which mediate a negative feedback effect on ongoing NE release. Escape and tachyphalaxis is not a feature of selective α-1 blockade. These agents improve outlet obstruction in the setting of benign prostatic hypertrophy.

Despite proven efficacy and a favorable metabolic profile (decreased lipids, improved insulin resistance),[83,178] the α-blockers have a relatively small share of the antihypertensive market. Their use will probably decline further. In the ALLHAT trial, patients randomized to α-blockers (doxazocin) as step-one therapy had twice the risk of CHF than did patients randomized to diuretics.[18] No biologic mechanism exists whereby α-blockade would depress myocardial function. The increased heart failure risk is best explained by withdrawl from ACE-inhibitors as specified in the ALLHAT protocol.

Three α-blockers are available: *prazocin, terazocin, and doxazocin*. Doxazocin is the most widely used because it induces the fewest side effects and is a proven once-daily agent. As monotherapy, α-blockers are as effective as any of the four leading classes of drugs though their utilization is primarily as add-on therapy to two-drug regimens. The initial dose (1 mg) should be given at bedtime to safeguard against a first-dose phenomena of syncope.[179] The drug may be titrated by doubling the dose to achieve the target response. The dose of doxazocin may be titrated to 16–20 mg or more.

Central adrenergic agents

Central α-agents stimulate inhibitory neurons and decrease sympathetic outflow from the CNS. The marked decline in sympathetic activity induces both the antihypertensive effects and the common side effects (dry mouth, sedation, and drowsiness). In clinical trials, central agents effectively reduce BP in a high percentage of subjects, particularly when combined with a diuretic, but side effects lead to poor quality-of-life and high rates of dropout.[180]

Methyldopa was the most popular agent added to a diuretic throughout the 1960s and early 1970s. Its use rapidly declined with the introduction of β-blockers. A wide range of side effects occur commonly. Sedation, headache, depression, postural hypotension, and impotence are most prevalent. Autoimmune phenomena (fever, hepatitis, and positive Coombs' test) are peculiar to methyldopa. The only clinical niche reserved for this agent is in the management of hypertension during pregnancy.

Clonidine use had been curtailed because of concern over rebound and overshoot hypertension, if there is non-adherence to therapy. Its availability as a transdermal preparation eased concern (or diverted attention) over withdrawal syndromes and led to resurgence in its use. The clonidine patch delivers drug continuously over a 7-day interval and seems to induce milder side effects.[181] This preparation is employed commonly in nursing-home and institutionalized settings. Some clinicians use the clonidine patch as add-on therapy to avert the introduction of 'another pill'.

The oral preparation has its onset within 30 minutes and has been used in repeated, hourly doses to gradually reduce BP in hypertensive urgencies.[182] Clonidine prevents reflex sympathetic overreactivity and is useful as an alternative to β-blockers in asthmatic patients on direct vasodilator therapy.[180] Clonidine is dosed twice daily. It also serves a diagnostic role in screening patients with suspected pheochromocytoma.[183] *Guanabenz and guanfacine* are clonidine-like drugs. Guanfacine enters the brain more slowly and has a more sustained antihypertensive effect. This translates into fewer side effects, once daily dosing and less withdrawal symptoms.[184] All central adrenergic agents can be used safely in diabetics.

Peripheral adrenergic agents

Reserpine and guanethidine are infrequently used antihypertensive agents primarily of historical significance. They reduce sympathetic outflow by blocking the release of norepinephrine from the adrenergic nerve ending. The antihypertensive action of reserpine was first reported in 1942. It was introduced into the USA in the early 1950s and widely used throughout the 1960s. Reserpine was a key agent in the first randomized trial to prove cardiovascular benefit from BP reduction.[185,186] When combined with a diuretic, the average BP reduction was 14/11 mm Hg.[187] It was formulated into a fixed-dose combination with thiazide and hydralazine, which was quite popular in the community practice of the

1960s. Ser-Ap-Es, which is still available, retains the distinction as the only triple-drug combination to gain FDA approval.

Side effects associated with reserpine use (nasal stuffiness, sedation, and occasionally depression) are common with high doses. When used in low doses (0.05–0.1 mg/day) it is usually well tolerated. Despite its efficacy and tolerability, reserpine use in the USA and Europe has all but disappeared. With the introduction of each new generation of antihypertensive drug, reserpine became increasingly outdated. A cancer scare, since refuted,[188] sealed its demise. Because of reserpine's very low cost, once-daily dosing, and general efficacy in combination with diuretics, it is still widely used in some countries, such as Germany, Switzerland, and South Africa.

Guanethidine was once widely used as a step-three agent to treat moderate and severe hypertension. Guanethedine has a steep dose–response curve, which permitted stepwise titration of drug to achieve goal BP. Its use was limited by side effects of diarrhea, failure of ejaculation, and postural hypotension, which was often quite severe. In-patient management of malignant hypertension sometimes employed tilting a patient's bed to potentiate the action of high-dose guanethidine. *Guanadrel* is closely related to guanethedine but has a shorter duration of action, which makes it more tolerable.

SPECIAL POPULATIONS

African Americans

African Americans have the highest prevalence of hypertension in the USA and one of the highest of any population in the world. Compared with whites, hypertension develops at an earlier age and is more severe at any age.[189,190] This burden of hypertension among the African American population is associated with an 80 per cent higher stroke mortality, a 50 per cent higher cardiac mortality, and a 320 per cent greater rate of end-stage renal disease than the general population.[191,192]

The African American Study of Kidney Disease and Hypertension (AASK) is testing the role of specific antihypertensive agents and the intensity of BP control in preventing progressive renal disease among hypertensive African Americans with early renal impairment (GFR 20–65 mL/min). The NIH has stopped the calcium-channel blocker (amlodipine) arm of the AASK trial.

When compared to patients treated with ACE inhibitor or β-blocker, proteinuric patients treated with amlodipine displayed an increased risk of progressive renal failure.[193]

The AASK trial will conclude in 2002.

Environmental and genetic factors contribute to the high

prevalence of hypertension in African Americans.[194]

- *Socioeconomic:* more poverty, lower levels of education, decreased access to care.
- *Nutritional:* increased salt sensitivity, reduced dietary potassium and calcium. Greater age-related increases in obesity among women.
- *Neurohumoral:* tendency to low-renin state/sodium retention, enhanced constrictor response to stress.
- *Hemodynamic:* propensity to left ventricular hypertrophy, lesser decline in nocturnal BP.

African Americans receiving adequate treatment achieve blood pressure control equivalent to that of whites and gain protection from cardiovascular complications.[195,196] Lifestyle modification must be the cornerstone of therapy in African Americans given the high prevalence of obesity, type II diabetes, and cigarette smoking. Sodium restriction and potassium supplementation are likely to have a greater blood pressure lowering effect in African Americans than in whites.[197] When drug therapy is employed, diuretics are the initial agent of choice. Calcium-channel blockers and α-blockers are also effective.[198] Monotherapy with β-blockers and ACE inhibitors are less effective in African Americans; diuretics markedly augment the response. When special indications for the use ACE inhibitors and/or β-blockers exist, these agents should not be withheld for lack of an antihypertensive effect.

Women

Hypertension is less common in women than men up to age 65 in whites, and age 45 for African Americans. In the older age groups, prevalence rates are slightly higher for women, reflecting the longer life span of women.

> Women and men share many of the same risk factors for hypertension, but obesity and salt intake are stronger risk factors in women.[199] Even modest adult weight gain (2–5 kg) increases the risk for hypertension in women and risk increases with the magnitude of the weight gain.

Weight loss reduces the risk for hypertension.[200] Even though women were excluded from several earlier large hypertension trials, many trials, including trials in the elderly, have included women in sufficient number and have demonstrated no important gender differences in blood pressure response or in outcomes.[201,202] Prevalence rates for hypertension are higher among African American women than white women at all age groups. African American women consistently demonstrate greater reductions in cardiovascular complications with treatment than do white women. Women are more likely than men to have hypertension diagnosed, to be receiving antihypertensive medication, and to have BP adequately controlled.[199,203]

ORAL CONTRACEPTIVES

A small increase in systolic and diastolic blood pressure is seen in most women after initiating oral contraceptives (OCs), but blood pressure usually remains within the normotensive range. Some, particularly obese and older women, experience greater BP elevations, often to hypertensive levels.[204] Guidelines for the use of OCs have been issued by experts:

- dispense *no more than* a 6-month supply of the lowest effective dose of estrogen and progesterone;
- monitor BP every 6 months;
- if BP rises to hypertensive ranges, discontinue OCs and provide alternative form of contraception;
- if BP does not normalize after 3 months, investigate and treat hypertension;
- if no alternative to OCs, prescribe antihypertensives with OCs;
- cigarette smokers >35 years old must quit; if they do not, continued use of OCs is strongly discouraged.

HORMONE REPLACEMENT THERAPY

Observational studies have found lower rates of coronary heart disease (CHD) in post-menopausal women who take estrogen than in women who do not. The apparent protective effect of estrogens is particularly strong among women with pre-existing CHD. However, two recent prospective trials in women with known CHD weaken the case for hormone replacement therapy (HRT) in secondary prevention.[205,206] When compared to placebo treatment, HRT did not reduce the rate of coronary events over a 4.1 year follow-up nor did it alter the severity of coronary stenoses.

> The role of HRT in primary prevention of CHD and a role for earlier and more extended use of HRT in secondary prevention are unknown.

A 10-year study of estrogen use will address these issues with the completion of the Women's Health Initiative in 2005. The low doses of estrogen employed in HRT rarely elevate and often lower blood pressure.[207–209]

HYPERTENSION IN PREGNANCY

Hypertension may exist prior to pregnancy (chronic hypertension) or may be induced by pregnancy (pre-eclampsia). Normotensive and chronic hypertensive women both experience a decline in blood pressure during the first trimester. Diastolic pressure is often 7–10 mm Hg below baseline at 6 weeks. Several comprehensive reviews on the management of hypertension in pregnancy have been published. The goals of therapy are minimizing short-term maternal risk without fetal compromise.[210–213]

Chronic hypertension

- BP >140/90 mm Hg prior to pregnancy or *before* the 20th week of pregnancy;
- diuretics and most other agents may be continued if taken prior to pregnancy;
- ACE inhibitors and ARBs may induce renal failure/fetal death, and should be avoided;
- methyldopa and hydralazine have the longest history of safety; drugs of choice when initiating therapy;
- β-blockers are safe in later pregnancy but may retard fetal growth in early pregnancy.

Pre-eclampsia

- Pregnancy-specific hypertensive condition associated with proteinuria and edema;
- increase in systolic BP by 30 mm Hg or diastolic BP 15 mm Hg *vs* baseline or BP >140/90 mm Hg after 20 weeks;
- occurs primarily during first pregnancy with onset *after* 20th week;
- abnormalities in coagulation, liver function, renal function may signal progression to convulsive phase (eclampsia);
- low-dose aspirin or supplemental calcium does *not* prevent pre-eclampsia;
- home BP monitoring; restricting activity lowers BP and promotes diuresis;
- drug therapy (similar to chronic hypertension) for diastolic BP >100 mm Hg; diuretics usually avoided.

Elderly

Hypertension is common in the elderly and carries high cardiovascular risk. Blood pressure elevations are found in 60 per cent of white Americans and 70 per cent of African Americans age 60 and over.[190] Systolic BP (SBP) is a powerful predictor of stroke, coronary disease, heart failure, end-stage renal disease, and all-cause mortality in all age groups, but more so in the elderly.[202] Pulse pressure (SBP–DBP) is the strongest predictor of cardiovascular risk.[214,215] The risks and treatment of isolated systolic hypertension (SBP >160 mm Hg + DBP <90 mm Hg) are no different than those of combined systolic and diastolic hypertension. Several large prospective randomized trials have shown that older patients benefit from antihypertensive therapy as much if not more than younger individuals.[7,216–218] The value of treating elderly patients beyond age 80 who have a SBP greater than 160 mm Hg has recently been demonstrated but the value of treating stage 1 hypertension (SBP 140–159 mm Hg) is still unproven.[219,220]

Care must be taken in the measurement of blood pressure. Osler's maneuver may identify the excessive vascular stiffness which falsely elevates systolic pressure (pseudohypertension).[221]

High variability in SBP and 'white-coat hypertension' are more prevalent in the elderly, especially among women.[222] Out of office BP measurements are almost essential in this age group and ambulatory BP monitoring may be quite cost-effective, particularly in the absence of target organ damage.

Most elderly hypertensives have primary hypertension which has carried over from middle age but many have secondary hypertension. Atherosclerotic renovascular disease is particularly common and should be suspected in patients with onset of hypertension after age 60 or escape from long-standing control. Target organ damage is common in the elderly and should be thoroughly assessed. Standing BPs are imperative at initial and follow-up visits.[223]

Weight loss and sodium restriction have proven useful in lowering the BP of elderly hypertensives and reducing the need for drug therapy.[31] The elderly are excellent candidates for sodium restriction. Sodium intake is often excessive because of lessened taste sensitivity or because of their dependency on processed foods. In addition, the response of BP to changes in salt intake is greater in the elderly than in younger hypertensive patients.[224]

Several factors may complicate antihypertensive drug therapy in the elderly.[202] Diminished baroreceptor activity and a tendency toward volume contraction predispose to orthostatic hypotension often unmasked by antihypertensive agents. Depression and confusion may be compounded by BP medication. Cerebral autoregulatory problems may precipitate excessive drowsiness with only modest reductions in blood pressure. Hypokalemia may carry greater arrhythmogenic risk in the elderly given their high prevalence of LVH and widespread use of digitalis. Polypharmacy is common, as is the potential for drug interactions. Reductions in renal function and alterations in hepatic blood flow are common. These factors support a strategy of '*be in the know, start low and go slow*' when prescribing antihypertensive drugs to the elderly.

Recommendations for drug treatment in the elderly hypertensive patient.[225]

- treat patients up to age 80 with SBP >160 mm Hg;
- goal BP <140/90 mm Hg if tolerated; interim goal of SBP <160 acceptable with marked systolic hypertension (>200 mm Hg);
- individualize initial therapy according to co-morbid conditions/end-organ compromise;
- if no co-morbid conditions, *low-dose (thiazide plus K-sparing) diuretics or long-acting calcium-channel blockers preferred* as both classes have proven protective value in randomized trials of the elderly;[7,216]
- newer drugs (ACE inhibitors, calcium blockers) provide cardiovascular protection in the elderly equivalent to that of conventional drugs (β-blockers, diuretics);[20]

- β-blockers are useful in patients with angina or prior myocardial infarction;
- in absence of angina/prior myocardial infarction, β-blockers are no more effective than placebo in preventing coronary disease and less effective than diuretics;[101,104]
- avoid sedating central adrenergic agents;
- judicious use of α-blockers, high-dose diuretics because of orthostatic effects;
- initiate all agents as half-dose;
- be aware of cost issues in this fixed-income population.

Diabetics

Hypertension occurs 2–3 times more frequently in diabetic patients than in non-diabetics. Most type I diabetics who develop nephropathy (40 per cent) have hypertension but, in those with no nephropathy, the prevalence is similar to the general population.[226] Most hypertensive diabetics have type II or non-insulin-dependent diabetes (NIDDM), which is almost always obesity-induced. Patients with NIDDM, many of whom are insulin-requiring, comprise 80 per cent of the diabetic population. The incidence of cardiovascular events among diabetics is 2–3 times that of non-diabetics and hypertension accelerates complications.[227,228]

The glucose intolerance of the obese patient with NIDDM is due to insulin resistance and is identified by high circulating levels of plasma insulin. Lipid abnormalities are common. Insulin resistance may be the common factor that links hypertension, hyperlipidemia, and obesity.[229,230] Several lines of evidence support this premise:

- insulin levels in obese hypertensives are increased several-fold over normal levels of obese normotensives;
- insulin resistance is often seen among lean hypertensives with no overt diabetes;
- agents that sensitize tissues to the action of insulin (troglitazone) also lower BP.

When hypertension is detected in a diabetic, management should involve lifestyle modification and immediate drug therapy. Weight loss and exercise enhance insulin sensitivity and lower insulin levels, improve lipid profiles and reduce blood pressure.[231,232] Discontinuation of cigarette smoking is crucial and excessive alcohol should be curbed. Despite the importance of non-drug therapy in diabetic hypertension, concomitant drug therapy is recommended at the time of diagnosis before observing the response to lifestyle modification. JNC VI recommends initiating drug therapy even when blood pressure is at the high-normal range (130–139/85–89 mm Hg). Goal BP is <130/85 mm Hg.

> Intensive hypertension management is imperative in the diabetic patient. Diabetics treated with antihypertensive agents derive a cardioprotective effect that equals or even exceeds that of patients without diabetes.[233–235]

Aggressive antihypertensive therapy reduces macrovascular and microvascular complications more effectively than does aggressive glycemic control.[235] Type II diabetics who participated in the Hypertension Optimal Treatment (HOT) Study derived the greatest reduction in cardiovascular risk at the greatest reduction of diastolic pressure. In fact, the risk of having diabetes was virtually abolished among patients randomized to the lowest stratum of BP control (diastolic BP <80 mm Hg).[3] JNC VI, which preceded the HOT trial, recommends goal BP <130/85 mm Hg. Further reductions in goal BP (<125/80 mm Hg) among diabetics are justified and achievable with multidrug regimens.

ACE inhibitors, α-blockers, calcium channel blockers and low-dose diuretics are the preferred agents in diabetic hypertension because they have no adverse effects on glucose metabolism or lipid profiles.[83,87] *ACE inhibitors* enhance insulin sensitivity (captopril) and offer renoprotection particularly in the presence of microalbuminuria.[237] These agents may offer protection from proliferative retinopathy[238] and ischemic heart disease as well.[239,240] Two recent large prospective trials report major reductions in a wide range of cardiovascular events among diabetics randomized to ACE inhibitor.[19,241] ACE inhibitors are lipid neutral. Unless contraindicated (bilateral renal artery stenosis, hyperkalemia), ACE inhibitors are best suited for initial therapy. The protective effects of angiotensin receptor blockers in diabetic cardiovascular complications have not yet been reported in large clinical trials. Nevertheless, these agents are a good first-line alternative for patients intolerant of ACE inhibitors.

Calcium-channel blockers are lipid neutral and have no effect on insulin resistance. Renoprotective effects are reported but dihydropyridine CCBs may aggravate proteinuria in NIDDM.[242,243] Two recent small randomized trials among hypertensive patients with NIDDM report fewer cardiovascular events among ACE-inhibitor-treated patients than in patients treated with dihydropyridine CCBs.[239,240] Many experts interpret these findings as an anti-ischemic action of ACE inhibitor rather than a pro-ischemic action of dihydropyridine. Remarkably, the lowest rate of cardiovascular complictions in one of these trials was in patients treated with the *combination* of ACE inhibitor and calcium blocker.[244] Several larger-scale trials are in progress that test agent-specific outcomes. *Alpha-blockers* lower cholesterol and triglycerides, and consistently enhance insulin sensitivity. Orthostatic side effects may limit their application in diabetic patients with autonomic insufficiency. Alpha-

Table 27.9 *95th percentile of blood pressure by selected ages in girls and boys, by the 50th and 75th height percentiles.[a] (Reprinted from the Joint National Committee on Prevention, Detection, Evaluation, and Treatment of High Blood Pressure. The sixth report of the Joint National Committee on Prevention, Detection, Evaluation, and Treatment of High Blood Pressure (JNC VI). Arch Intern Med 1997; **157**: 2413–46)*

| Age (years) | Girls' SBP/DBP | | Boys' SBP/DBP | |
	50th percentile for height	75th percentile for height	50th percentile for height	75th percentile for height
1	104/58	105/59	102/57	104/58
6	111/73	112/73	114/74	115/75
12	123/80	124/81	123/81	125/82
17	129/84	130/85	136/87	138/88

[a]From the report by the NHBPEP Working Group on Hypertension Control in Children and Adolescents.
SBP = systolic blood pressure; DBP = diastolic blood pressure.

blocker monotherapy does not protect against the development of heart failure.[18]

Diuretic therapy must be used with discretion. High-dose thiazide therapy often worsens the lipid profile and heightens insulin resistance. *Low-dose thiazide* (12.5–25 mg) induces fewer metabolic effects, many of which are offset by concomitant use of ACE inhibitors. Elderly diabetics receive the same cardioprotection as do non-diabetics when (low-dose) thiazide-based regimens are used to control hypertension.[90] Loop diuretics may be needed as antihypertensive therapy (twice daily) with advanced renal disease and/or gross edema. *β-Blockers* consistently aggravate insulin resistance, raise triglycerides and lower HDL.[87] Hypoglycemic symptoms are masked by these agents and recovery from hypoglycemia is delayed.[116] β-Blockers should be reserved for diabetics in the post-myocardial infarction setting, in congestive heart failure or for angina pectoris.

Children and adolescents

Hypertension in children and adolescents is defined as *sustained* blood pressure readings at or beyond the 95th percentile according to height, age, and sex (Table 27.9). Children who have a single casual BP elevation should have readings repeated, preferably in out-of-office settings. Subsequent readings are likely to be normal in non-obese children with no hypertensive parent.[244a,245] The fifth Korotkoff sound is used to define diastolic BP for all ages.

Office evaluation is similar to that of the hypertensive adult but with a more astute eye towards renal disease. Increasingly, more children and adolescents are identified with essential hypertension. A comprehensive history, physical examination, and limited laboratory evaluation will identify the common secondary syndromes if present. The likelihood of identifying secondary forms of hypertension in children relates

directly to level of blood pressure and inversely to age. Severe elevations warrant aggressive evaluations (renal arteriography, endocrine tests). Mild elevations of BP, slightly above 95th percentile, are rarely due to secondary conditions.[246] Evaluation is uncomplicated and aims mainly to identify renal disease (Table 27.10)

Table 27.10 *Evaluation of asymptomatic children and adolescents with persistently elevated blood pressure levels. (Adapted from Kaplan N. Clinical hypertension, 7th edn. Baltimore: Williams & Wilkins, 1998)*

History
Family
    Primary hypertension and/or its complications
    Familial obesity, hyperlipidemia
    Genetic disorders associated with hypertension
    Blood pressure (BP) elevations in siblings
Patient
    Past or present history of events that influence BP (e.g. radiation to kidney, recurrent urinary tract infection, drugs with pressor properties)
    Dietary intake; calories, sodium

Physical examination
Vital signs: pulse, height, weight
BP in the right upper arm (by convention) and one leg
Clues to secondary causes: coarctation, Cushing's syndrome, abdominal mass, or bruits
Target organ damage: funduscopic, cardiac

Laboratory studies (limited)
Urinalysis
Hematocrit
BUN/creatinine; electrolytes
Lipid levels
Echocardiography
Renal ultrasound; isotope scan

BUN = blood urea nitrogen

Lifestyle intervention is recommended in the absence of reversible hypertension. Drug therapy is indicated for higher levels of blood pressure. Dosing must be adjusted with care. Detailed recommendations for treating hypertension in children and adolescents have been recently published.[247]

Table 27.11 *Causes of inadequate responsiveness to therapy. (Reprinted from the Joint National Committee on Prevention, Detection, Evaluation, and Treatment of High Blood Pressure. The sixth report of the Joint National Committee on Prevention, Detection, Evaluation, and Treatment of High Blood Pressure (JNC VI). Arch Intern Med 1997; 157: 2413–46)*

Pseudoresistance
'White-coat' hypertension or office elevations
Pseudohypertension in older patients
Use of regular cuff on very obese arm

Non-adherence to therapy (*see* Table 27.5)

Volume overload
Excess salt intake
Progressive renal damage (nephrosclerosis)
Fluid retention from reduction of blood pressure
Inadequate diuretic therapy

Drug-related causes
Doses too low
Wrong type of diuretic
Inappropriate combinations
Rapid inactivation, e.g. hydralazine
Drug actions and interactions:
   Sympathomimetics
   Nasal decongestants
   Appetite suppressants
   Cocaine and other illicit drugs
   Caffeine
   Oral contraceptives
   Adrenal steroids
   Licorice (as may be found in chewing tobacco)
   Cyclosporine, tacrolimus
   Erythropoietin
   Antidepressants
   Non-steroidal anti-inflammatory drugs

Associated conditions
Smoking
Increasing obesity
Sleep apnea
Insulin resistance/hyperinsulinemia
Ethanol intake of more than 1 oz (30 mL) per day
Anxiety-induced hyperventilation or panic attacks
Chronic pain
Intense vasoconstriction (arteritis)
Organic brain syndrome, e.g. memory deficit

Secondary causes of hypertension

SPECIAL SITUATIONS

Resistant hypertension

Resistant hypertension is defined as BP >140/90 mm Hg (>160 in isolated systolic hypertension) while taking three antihypertensive agents.[248]

> According to JNC VI, resistance exists only when the patient is adherent to an adequate and appropriate triple-drug regimen that includes a diuretic, with all three drugs prescribed in near-maximal doses.[249]

Various causes of inadequate response to therapy are listed in Table 27.11.

In a large series of patients resistant to three drugs, the most common mechanisms were inadequate or omitted diuretic (43 per cent), non-compliance (10 per cent), or intolerance to medication (22 per cent). Secondary hypertension was identified in 11 per cent of resistant patients.[250] Alcohol-related problems and non-compliance are common among resistant patients in an inner-city population.[251] Ambulatory BP monitoring has demonstrated that many 'resistant' patients are indeed well controlled in an out-of-office setting.[252] Patients who remain uncontrolled on maximum doses of an ACE inhibitor, CCB, diuretic regimen may be effectively managed with a minoxidil-based regimen.[253] Patients who fail to achieve goal blood pressure may still derive some cardiovascular protection. Resistant patients may benefit from referral to a hypertension specialist.

Hypertensive emergencies and urgencies

Hypertensive emergencies are situations that require immediate reduction of blood pressure, usually with parenteral agents, to prevent or limit acute target organ damage.[254,255] Examples include hypertensive encephalopathy, intracranial hemorrhage, acute myocardial infarction or unstable angina, acute pulmonary edema, dissecting aneurysm or eclampsia. A variety of parenteral antihypertensive agents are available and are listed in Table 27.12.

Dosing is titrated against the target BP by adjusting constant infusions (nitroprusside, nicardipine) or by repeating boluses (labetalol) at brief intervals (10–15 minutes).

> Immediate normalization of blood pressure is not the goal of therapy. Following abrupt declines in BP to normotensive (or even to lower but still hypertensive) levels, autoregulatory adjustments may fail to support vital organ perfusion.[256]

Older literature is replete with reports of stroke induced by overzealous treatment of a hypertensive emergency.[257] To avert such complications, JNC VI recommends a

Table 27.12 Parenteral drugs for treatment of hypertensive emergencies.[a] (Reprinted from the Joint National Committee on Prevention, Detection, Evaluation, and Treatment of High Blood Pressure. The sixth report of the Joint National Committee on Prevention, Detection, Evaluation, and Treatment of High Blood Pressure (JNC VI). Arch Intern Med 1997; **157**: 2413–46)

Drug	Dose[b]	Onset of action	Duration of action	Adverse effects[c]	Special indications
Vasodilators					
Sodium nitroprusside	0.25–10 μg/kg per minute as iv infusion[d] (maximal dose for 10 minutes only)	Immediate	1–2 minutes	Nausea, vomiting, muscle twitching, sweating, thiocyanate and cyanide intoxication	Most hypertensive emergencies; caution with high intracranial pressure or azotemia
Nicardipine hydrochloride	5–15 mg/hour iv	5–10 minutes	1–4 hours	Tachycardia, headache, flushing, local phlebitis	Most hypertensive emergencies except acute heart failure; caution with coronary ischemia
Fenoldopam mesylate	0.1–0.3 μg/kg per minute iv infusion	<5 minutes	30 minutes	Tachycardia, headache, nausea, flushing	Most hypertensive emergencies; caution with glaucoma
Nitroglycerin	5–100 μg/minute as iv infusion[d]	2–5 minutes	3–5 minutes	Headache, vomiting, methemoglobinemia, tolerance with prolonged use	Coronary ischemia
Enalaprilat	1.25–5 mg every 6 hours iv	15–30 minutes	6 hours	Precipitous fall in pressure in high-renin states; response variable	Acute left ventricular failure; avoid in acute myocardial infarction
Hydralazine hydrochloride	10–20 mg iv / 10–50 mg im	10–20 minutes / 20–30 minutes	3–8 hours	Tachycardia, flushing, headache, vomiting, aggravation of angina	Eclampsia
Diazoxide	50–100 mg iv bolus repeated, or 15–30 mg/minute infusion	2–4 minutes	6–12 hours	Nausea, flushing, tachycardia, chest pain	Now obsolete; when no intensive monitoring available
Adrenergic inhibitors					
Labetalol hydrochloride	20–80 mg iv bolus every 10 minutes / 0.5–2.0 mg/minute iv infusion	5–10 minutes	3–6 hours	Vomiting, scalp tingling, burning in throat, dizziness, nausea, heart block, orthostatic hypotension	Most hypertensive emergencies except acute heart failure
Esmolol hydrochloride	250–500 μg/kg per minute for 1 minute, then 50–100 μg/kg per minute for 4 minute; may repeat sequence	1–2 minutes	10–20 minutes	Hypotension, nausea	Aortic dissection, perioperative
Phentolamine	5–15 mg iv	1–2 minutes	3–10 minutes	Tachycardia, flushing, headache	Catecholamine excess

[a]These doses may vary from those in the Physicians' Desk reference (51st edition).
[b]iv = intravenous; im = intramuscular.
[c]Hypotension may occur with all agents.
[d]Require special delivery system.

Table 27.13 *Hypertensive emergencies and treatment. (Adapted from Kitiyakara C, Guzman N. Malignant hypertension and hypertensive emergencies.* J Am Soc Nephrol *1998;* **9***: 133–42)*

Type of emergency	Drugs of choice	Alternative or second-line drug	Relative contraindications	Comments and goals
Hypertensive encephalopathy	Nitroprusside	Labetalol	Trimethophan, clonidine	Promptly lower MAP 25% / BP 160/100 mm Hg at 2 hours / Encephalopathy resolves over 24–48 hours
Intracranial hemorrhage	Labetalol	Nitroprusside	Vasodilators[a]	BP 140/90 mm Hg in subarachnoid hemorrhage / Nimodipine reduces cerebral vasospasm
Left ventricular failure and pulmonary edema	Nitroprusside ± loop diuretics ± ACEI	Nitroglycerine	Labetalol, β-blockers, verapamil	Relieve hypoxia, dyspnea / Systolic BP 140 mm Hg usually well tolerated
Acute myocardial infarction, unstable angina	Nitroglycerin ± β-blockers	Nitroprusside, labetalol	Vasodilators[a]	Render pain free / Target BP 140/90 mm Hg
Adrenergic crisis	Nitroprusside ± β-blockers, phentolamine	Labetalol	Monotherapy with β-blockers	Pheochromocytoma, cocaine or amphetamine overdose / Resume clonidine in clonidine withdrawal
Dissecting aortic aneurysm	β-Blockers + nitroprusside trimethophan	Labetalol, verapamil	Vasodilators[a]	Render pain free / Target systolic BP 100–120 mm Hg
Eclampsia	Hydralazine, labetalol	Nifedipine[b]	ACEI, nitroprusside[c]	Occurs at moderate BP elevation / Target systolic BP 90–110 mm Hg before delivery

ACEI = angiotensin-converting enzyme inhibitors; BP = blood pressure.

[a]Vasodilators with reflex sympathetic stimulation, e.g. hydralazine, minoxidil, diazoxide, and short-acting nifedipine.

[b]Hypotensive effects of magnesium may be potentiated by nifedipine.

[c]Nitroprusside may be considered if BP cannot be controlled by other means.

prompt 25 per cent reduction of mean arterial pressure (MAP) followed by reductions to 160/100 mm Hg within 2 hours.[249] While this guideline is appropriate for hypertensive encephalopathy, malignant hypertension, and other conditions, more aggressive BP reductions are indicated in aortic dissection and eclampsia (systolic BP 110–120 mm Hg). In cardiac hypertensive emergencies, therapy is aimed at relief of symptoms. Whatever the clinical setting, the management of all hypertensive emergencies includes monitoring indicators of vital organ perfusion (neurologic status, angina, urine flow) and adjusting drug infusion rates to optimize blood pressure. The choice of specific parenteral agents is determined by the presenting condition (Table 27.13).[254,255]

Hypertensive urgencies are situations where the absence of symptoms or the lower acuity of target organ damage permits the use of oral agents to reduce blood pressure over several hours. The distinction between an emergency and urgency depends upon the immediate threat to end organs and not the severity of hypertension. Examples include uncomplicated accelerated-malignant hypertension, high levels of stage III hypertension, sclerodermal renal crisis, and severe perioperative or rebound hypertension. Considerable overlap exists between emergencies and urgencies. The route of drug therapy is often dictated by clinical judgement and available resources. Many oral agents are available which effectively lower BP in 1–2 hours (Table 27.14).

Patients are often encountered with uncontrolled severe hypertension who are asymptomatic and in no immediate danger. This condition does not constitute a hypertensive emergency or urgency.[258] If a patient with very high BP is a known hypertensive and has discontinued a well-tolerated, effective regimen, it should be resumed; if ineffective or poorly tolerated, the regimen should be revised. If a newly diagnosed hypertensive, therapy may be initiated and the patient referred for follow-up in 24–48 hours. Pain, anxiety, and other precipitants should be addressed. Some physicians choose to verify the response to an oral agent and observe the patient for a few hours following an office or ER dose.

> Sublingual nifedipine capsules have been prescribed for routine use postoperatively or in nursing home patients whenever BP reaches a threshold value.[259] This practice represents mere blood pressure cosmetics and should be avoided.

The inability to control the rate and magnitude of hypotension makes this agent unacceptable for use in these 'pseudoemergencies' as well as in true emergency/urgency settings.[260] Precipitous drops in blood pressure are of no proven benefit and serious adverse effects have been reported. Short-acting nifedepine carries no FDA approval for use in hypertension.

Anesthesia and surgery

The hypertensive patient without coronary disease has no greater anesthesia risk provided BP is controlled entering surgery.[261] Blood pressure elevations of 180/110 mm Hg or greater are associated with a high risk of perioperative ischemic events. When possible, surgery should be postponed until BP is better controlled.[262] Surgical patients with less severe hypertension, many of whom harbor occult coronary disease, derive a cardioprotective effect from β-blockers administered 2 hours prior to induction.[263] These agents may provide unique perioperative protection to this population by blocking the 'adrenergic arousal' so commonly seen before, during, and after surgery.[264] β-Blockers are probably the agent of choice in managing the untreated or poorly controlled hypertensive surgical patient.

Treated hypertensive patients should be maintained on their regular regimen until the time of surgery. The regimen should be resumed as soon as possible after surgery barring hypotensive/hypovolemic complications. If oral intake is interrupted, most classes of antihypertensive agents can be administered parenterally (diuretics, β-blockers, ACE inhibitors) and clonidine as a transdermal patch. Surgery and anesthesia may induce a non-specific blood pressure lowering effect requiring adjustment of the regimen in the postoperative, convalescent period.[265] In most cases, the admission regimen should be resumed upon discharge.

Table 27.14 *Oral agents for hypertensive urgencies*

Drug	Class	Dose	Onset	Duration
Captopril	Angiotensin-converting enzyme inhibitor	6.5–50 mg	15 minutes	4–6 hours
Clonidine	Central α-agonist	0.2 mg initial then 0.1 mg/hour, up to 0.8 mg total	½–2 hours	6–8 hours
Labetalol	α–β-blocker	200–400 mg	½–2 hours	8–12 hours
Minoxidil	Vasodilator	5–10 mg	½–1 hours	12–16 hours

PATIENTS WITH TARGET ORGAN DAMAGE

Cerebrovascular disease

Epidemiologic observations show a strong direct relationship between systolic and diastolic pressure and the risk of stroke.[266] Moreover, randomized trials of primary prevention in patients with hypertension demonstrate that BP lowering reduces the stroke risk after only a few years of treatment.[267] Trials of antihypertensive therapy for secondary prevention of stroke are substantially fewer and less conclusive.[268] All experts agree nevertheless that clinically evident cerebrovascular disease is a compelling indication for antihypertensive therapy. A major, large-scale, randomized trial of ACE-inhibitor-based therapy in hypertensive and normotensive patients with a history of stroke or transient ischemic attack (TIA) is now under way.[269]

There are no randomized trials of antihypertensive therapy during the acute phase of ischemic stroke. Blood pressure is frequently elevated at presentation but usually falls spontaneously over the first 24–48 hours, although not always to normotensive levels.[270] Rapid, drug-induced reductions of blood pressure during the early stages of ischemic stroke is often associated with neurologic deterioration as BP falls below the lower limits of cerebral autoregulation.[271]

Parenteral drugs may be indicated if acute stroke is accompanied by another indication for rapid BP control (aortic dissection, myocardial infarction). In the absence of these conditions, antihypertensive drugs are withheld unless systolic BP exceeds 220 mm Hg or MAP exceeds 130 mm Hg.[272,273]

In such instances, labetalol or enalaprilat are the preferred parenteral agents since they can be easily titrated and have a minimal effect on cerebral blood flow. Most patients can be treated with oral agents. The aim of treatment is to reduce MAP by 25 per cent over 24 hours. Oral or sublingual nifedipine should be avoided. In the presense of intracranial hemorrhage, more aggressive approaches to BP control are usually intiated but outcome is influenced largely by surgical issues.[272,274]

Coronary artery disease

Patients with coronary artery disease (CAD) and hypertension are at high cardiovascular risk. The benefits and safety of blood pressure reduction in preventing coronary events is well established even though the protective effect is less impressive than that for stroke.[275] Concerns over the 'J'-shaped curve, which suggested increased coronary events when diastolic BP is reduced below a critical threshold has been dispelled.[7–10] Randomized trials have shown no such relationship. Diuretic-based trials have proven that coronary events are reduced by antihypertensive therapy. Small trials suggest that ACE inhibitors may prevent coronary events in type II diabetics.[239,240] Among patients with pre-existing coronary disease participating in the HOPE trial, the ACE inhibitor ramapril reduced the incidence of worsening angina or myocardial infarction.[145] The benefit was observed whether or not patients were taking aspirin or β-blockers. Trials of ACE inhibitor therapy in the primary prevention of ischemic heart disease among non-diabetics are now being conducted.

In hypertensives with CAD, BP should be lowered below 140/90 mm Hg and even lower if angina persists. Agents which induce reflex cardioacceleration and sympathetic stimulation (naked dilators or naked nifedipine) increase cardiac demand and should be avoided.[276] β-Blockers and calcium-channel blockers are quite useful in patients with angina but short-acting CCBs should not be used.[127,128] In the post-myocardial infarction setting, non-ISA β-blockers reduce sudden death and recurrent myocardial infarction, while ACE inhibitors limit cardiac remodeling and curb the progression of asymptomatic systolic dysfunction to gross congestive heart failure.[155] If β-blockers are ineffective or contraindicated, verapamil or diltiazem may be used as each has improved survival modestly following non-Q myocardial infarction with preserved LV function.[277–279] Lifestyle modifications and aggressive lipid management are key adjunctive measures in managing total cardiovascular risk.

Aspirin and 'statin' therapy both have proven efficacy in reducing reinfarction rates among myocardial infarction survivors.[280–282]

Left ventricular hypertrophy

Left ventricular hypertrophy is a major independent risk factor for sudden cardiac death, myocardial infarction, stroke and other cardiovascular events.[283,284] Hypertensive patients with LVH have a higher prevalence of ventricular irritability (PVCs) than do normotensive patients or hypertensives with no LVH.[285] This finding probably reflects supply–demand mismatching of the coronary microcirculation as the hypertrophied ventricle outstrips its nutrient flow. Angina without coronary disease, seen in some hypertensives with severe LVH, reflects the same mismatch phenomenon.[249]

The evidence that PVCs predict sudden death in LVH is inconclusive in men and negative in women. Reversal of LVH reduces LVH-associated arrhythmias but no data links LVH regression to decreased incidence of sudden death.[286] Observational data indicate that regression of electrocardiographic LVH is associated with reduced cardiovascular events but no controlled study suggests that LVH reversal offers a benefit beyond that derived from blood pressure reduction alone.[287,288] Most antihypertensive agents (except hydralazine and minoxidil) reverse LVH but their potency varies: ACE inhibitors are most effective followed by CCBs > diuretics > β-blockers.[138] Reversal of LVH has recently been reported in response to valsartan.[163] Echocardiography is more sensitive than electrocardiography in identifying LVH but is too expensive for routine use.

Congestive heart failure

Hypertension is the major cause of left ventricular failure in the USA.[289] High BP triples the risk of developing congestive heart failure (CHF) and is present in 90 per cent of patients who develop the condition.[290] Epidemiologic data suggest that antihypertensive therapy postpones the development of CHF by several decades.[277,291] The pathogenesis of hypertensive CHF involves an interaction of LVH and ischemic heart disease which leads to alterations in ventricular structure and function (Fig. 27.3).[292]

CHF may be due to systolic dysfunction or diastolic dysfunction. This classification has therapeutic and prognostic significance. *Systolic dysfunction* is marked by ventricular dilation and identified by an ejection fraction (EF) less than 40 per cent. Following myocardial infarction, ACE inhibitors prevent the development of clinical CHF among asymptomatic survivors with modestly reduced EF.[139–141] In patients with symptomatic CHF, ACE inhibitors reduce morbidity and mortality when used alone or in conjunction with digoxin or diuretics.[141] Patients intolerant of ACE inhibitors may be treated with an angiotensin receptor blocker. In a small randomized

trial, losartan was superior to captopril in reducing mortality among elderly patients.[293] A larger study could not confirm this survival advantage.[294] Among heart failure patients maintained on ACE inhibitors, the addition of valsartan leads to further declines in systolic pressure and in pulmonary capillary wedge pressure.[295] These favorable hemodynamic changes persist at four weeks. The combination of hydralazine and nitrates is an alternative regimen for patients intolerant of renin–angiotensin blockade.[296] The rate-slowing CCBs (verapamil, diltiazem) may worsen LV function and should be avoided. Amlodipine and felodipine are safe in treating angina and hypertension in patients with advanced LV dysfunction.[122,297] β-Blockers had been traditionally contraindicated in CHF. However, randomized trials with carvedilol, metoprolol, and bisropolol all demonstrated improved survival in patients with CHF.[112,298–300] The addition of spironalactone to standard (digoxin, diuretic, ACE inhibitor) therapy reduces morbidity and mortality among patients with an ejection fraction below 35 per cent.[301] The management of heart failure with the vasopeptidase inhibitor, omapatrilat, offers great promise.[302]

Forty per cent of hypertensives with CHF have *diastolic dysfunction* marked by normal or high EF. Filling pressures are elevated because the ventricle is thickened and fails to relax during diastole. In the most advanced form of diastolic dysfunction, severe concentric hypertrophy obliterates the ventricular cavity. In such cases, ACE inhibitors and diuretics may induce hypotension. β-Blockers and CCBs induce diastolic relaxation and are the cornerstone of treatment. Digoxin has no role in the management of CHF due to diastolic dysfunction.

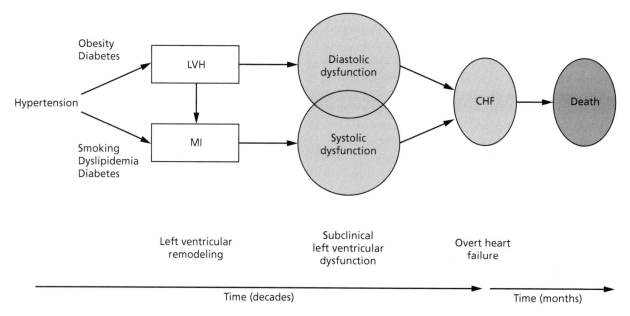

Figure 27.3 *Pathogenesis of hypertensive congestive heart failure (CHF). LVH = left ventricular hypertrophy; MI = myocardial infarction. (Reprinted from Kaplan N. Clinical hypertension, 7th edn. Baltimore: Williams & Wilkins, 1998.)*

Diastolic dysfunction carries a better prognosis than systolic dysfunction.[303] The evaluation and management of patients with CHF is discussed in detail elsewhere in the text.

Renal disease and proteinuria

Hypertension may cause renal disease or may exist as a consequence of renal disease. Hypertensive nephrosclerosis is second only to diabetes as a cause of end-stage renal disease (ESRD) and accounts for 25–30 per cent of the dialysis population.[304] Chronic renal disease is usually associated with hypertension and accounts for half of all secondary hypertension.[305] In both primary renal disease and in hypertensive nephrosclerosis, persistent hypertension leads to glomerular capillary hypertension, which plays a pivotal role in accelerating renal damage.[306–308]

Early detection of renal disease is essential. A small increment in serum creatinine (0.2 mg/dL) reflects significant loss of glomerular filtration rate (GFR) and should trigger an assessment of the adequacy of therapy and potential for reversibility.[309] Renal artery stenosis, obstruction and regular non-steroidal anti-inflammatory drug (NSAID) use may be identified and corrected. Ultrasound findings of small, 'echogenic' kidneys with a thin cortical rim speaks for advanced nephrosclerosis. Identification of polycystic kidney disease or asymmetry of renal size prompt additional management strategies. Urine analysis and quantification of proteinuria (24-hour urine *or* spot urine protein/creatinine) are fundamental.

ANTIHYPERTENSIVE THERAPY

Chronic renal failure is an independent risk factor for cardiovascular events. Data from the Framingham Study and from the Hypertension Detection and Follow-up Program document the high prevalence of cardiovascular disease among patients with mild chronic renal insufficiency.[310,311] A recent subgroup analysis of HOT Study participants reports an increased risk of cardiovascular events (RR 2.05) and cardiovascular mortality (RR 3.24) among those with entry creatinine values exceeding 1.5 mg/dL.[312] Risk was adjusted for the intensity of blood pressure control, for pre-existing cardiovascular disease and for traditional cardiovascular risk factors. These findings alone make a compelling case for comprehensive cardiovascular risk management, including aggressive antihypertensive therapy in this population.

A second rationale for aggressive antihypertensive management is to curb the progression of renal insufficiency. Chronic renal failure usually progresses relentlessly even after inciting causes have been arrested. Data documenting a renoprotective effect of antihypertensive therapy in non-diabetic renal disease are surprisingly limited.[313] This may relate to inadequate control of BP. In proteinuric patients with chronic renal disease, aggressive BP control (MAP 92 = 125/75 mm Hg) proved more renoprotective than did usual BP control (MAP 107 = 140/90 mm Hg).[314,315] This finding forms the basis for the JNC VI-recommended target BP for slowing progressive damage in patients with hypertension and chronic renal failure:

> Blood pressure should be controlled to 130/85 mm Hg – or lower (125/75) in patients with proteinuria in excess of 1 g/24 hours – with whatever antihypertensive therapy is necessary.[316,317]

Proteinuria is both a marker and a mediator of renal injury. Tubular reabsorbtion of protein activates a host of cytokines which have direct pathogenic actions on the kidney.[318] The magnitude of proteinuria is an important predictor of the rate of progression of renal disease.[319,320] The reduction in proteinuria in response to treatment predicts the efficacy of renoprotection.[321,322] Therefore, the treatment of renal disease should not only be aimed at blood pressure control but at reducing proteinuria as well. Goal proteinuria should be less than 1 g/24 hours. Multidrug regimens will usually be required.

ACE inhibitors exhibit unique intrarenal (efferent arteriolar vasodilatory) effects to lower glomerular capillary pressure which may provide renoprotection beyond a systemic antihypertensive effect.[142,323] Moreover, these agents exert unique antiproliferative, antithrombotic and antifibrotic actions which may curb the progression of renal injury. In clinical trials among diabetics and among non-diabetics with subnephrotic proteinuria (1–3 g/24 hours), ACE inhibitors reduce proteinuria and slow progression of renal failure more effectively than does conventional therapy.[143,324–326] Some smaller clinical trials report no renoprotective superiority of ACE inhibitors over conventional therapy.[327,328] In nonproteinuric states (interstitial nephritis, polycystic kidney disease, nephrosclerosis) ACE inhibitors may offer no unique renal benefit but may still provide a general cardiovascular benefit. More important than the choice of agent is the adequacy of BP control. Any intrarenal, renal sparing effect of ACE inhibition is squandered by persistently elevated systemic pressure.

Hyperkalemia often limits the use of ACE inhibitors in advanced renal insufficiency. Dietary potassium restriction (2 g) and concomitant use of diuretics often permit ongoing ACE inhibitor therapy. Modest elevations of serum potassium (5.5–5.8 mmol) generally incur little risk and do not require discontinuing therapy. Angiotensin receptor blockers may induce less hyperkalemia than do ACE inhibitors and provide the same renoprotection.[170] Long-term trials with these agents are in progress.

Calcium-channel blockers exhibit intrarenal (afferent arteriolar vasodilatory) effects, which could raise glomerular capillary pressure and aggravate progressive renal damage.[329] This hemodynamic action is restricted to the dihydropyridine (DHP) class of CCBs. Indeed, among proteinuric African Americans, amlodipine, a DHP agent, increased proteinuria and accelerated loss of renal function.[193] However, in a large European randomized trial of patients with chronic renal failure, most of whom were proteinuric, the DHP nifedipine was as renoprotective as captopril.[330] In experimental renal disease, CCBs reduce glomerular size, lower glomerular tension and exhibit cytoprotective effects.[331] The combination of ACE inhibitor and CCB may be more renoprotective than either agent alone.[332] Failure to reach goal reductions in proteinuria may prompt substitution of non-DHP for DHP among the antihypertensive regimen. The potent, non-CCB dilator, *minoxidil* is useful in managing refractory hypertension.

Diuretics counter the major defect of renal parenchymal hypertension (sodium retention) and are often the key component in achieving goal BP. Thiazides are the preferred diuretic in early renal disease but are rarely effective when serum creatinine exceeds 2.0 mg/dL. Beyond this range, single doses of loop diuretics (furosemide, bumetinide) are sequentially doubled until a ceiling dose is reached identified by diuresis and weight loss.[333] The ceiling dose is then used once or preferably twice daily. Thiazides occasionally have an additive effect to loop diuretics. Metolazone, a potent thiazide-like agent with 24-hour efficacy, often maintains excellent diuresis where standard thiazides, and sometimes loop agents, have failed. Effects of metolazone and loop diuretics are also additive. Potassium supplements are often not needed given the potassium-retaining effects of renal insufficiency and ACE inhibitor therapy. Potassium-retaining diuretics are employed with strict caution. Asymptomatic hyperuricemia is of no threat to renal function and need not be treated in the absence of gout or a kidney stone. Care should be taken to avoid prerenal exacerbations of chronic renal failure induced by overdiuresis.

Increments in the serum creatinine may occur during the first few months of aggressive antihypertensive therapy.[334] Bilateral renal artery stenosis (BRAS) should be suspected if the creatinine rise exceeds 1 mg/dL in an euvolemic patient.[335] Among such patients, ACE inhibitors or angiotensin receptor blockers should be discontinued, since these agents have unique intrarenal actions to lower filtration pressure in BRAS. Lesser increments in creatinine should prompt no adjustment in therapy unless there is volume contraction (postural hypotension) or suspected drug toxicity (rash, eosinophilia, and fever). Creatinine 'bumps' with sustained BP reductions may be transient, but more often persist with ongoing therapy. Immediate reductions of glomerular capillary pressure induce short-term declines in GFR, an acceptable trade-off for long-term preservation of renal function. Declining proteinuria – in the absence of sharp increments in creatinine – often predict a stay in the progressive course toward ESRD.

ADDITIONAL THERAPY

Sodium restriction in the range of 1–2 g (44–88 meq) per day is both feasible and often necessary to achieve goal BP in patients with chronic renal disease. Reduced dietary sodium intake exerts antiproteinuric effects independent of its potentiating effect on antihypertensive agents.[315,336] High dietary salt may over-ride the antiproteinuric effects of ACE inhibitors or CCBs.[337,338] A 24-hour urinary sodium (and creatinine) collection is a reliable index of sodium intake and may be used to monitor dietary adherence. This monitoring tool retains its validity on diuretic therapy as long as steady-state conditions exist.

Chronic *metabolic acidosis* suppresses hepatic albumin synthesis and accelerates progressive tubular injury. Sodium bicarbonate therapy (baking soda, 1 teaspoon = 50 meq) is employed when serum bicarbonate falls below 18 mmol. Bicarbonate therapy often requires further reduction of dietary sodium and/or increasing diuretic therapy.

Dietary protein restriction induces afferent arteriolar constriction, reduces glomerular capillary pressure and confers renoprotection in experimental renal disease.[339] A meta-analysis of several clinical trials in progressive (diabetic and non-diabetic) renal disease suggest improved renal and patient survival with moderate (0.7 g/kg) dietary protein restriction.[340,341] However, a single large, multicenter trial, sponsored by the National Institute of Health, showed no compelling benefit.[342] One report of an additive antiproteinuric effect of dietary protein restriction and ACE inhibition exists but skepticism is prevalent among the nephrology community.[343,344] Quality-of-life and adherence concerns also exist. Whenever protein restriction is prescribed, as in a highly motivated proteinuric subject, malnutrition must be avoided by assuring adequate energy (caloric) intake.

Hyperphosphatemia and secondary hyperparathyroidism should be managed with dietary phosphate restriction and phosphate binders (calcium carbonate) with meals. Intact parathyroid hormone (iPTH) should be assayed in plasma when serum creatinine exceeds 2.5 mg/dL. Therapy with oral 1,25-dihydroxy vitamin D is instituted when iPTH is 2–3 times normal.

DIABETIC NEPHROPATHY

Diabetic nephropathy is the leading cause of ESRD. Patients with diabetes account for 35 per cent of the dialysis population. Type I and type II patients are equally represented. Approximately 40 per cent of both type I and type II patients develop diabetic nephropathy, but many type II patients die of cardiovascular complications before reaching dialysis dependency.[345] The mortality from coronary and renal disease among

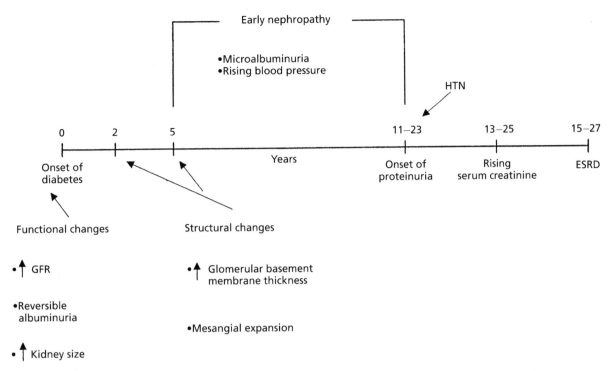

Figure 27.4 *Natural history of diabetic nephrology. ESRD = end-stage renal disease; GFR = glomerular filtration rate; HTN = hypertension (Reprinted from Greenberg A, ed.* Primer on kidney diseases, 2nd edn. *National Kidney Foundation, 1998)*

patients with diabetic nephropathy is 37 times that of the general population.[346] The risk of developing diabetic nephropathy is greater in some minority populations (African Americans, Mexican Americans, and American Indians) and their progression to ESRD is more rapid.[347] The hypertension that almost invariably accompanies diabetic nephropathy, accelerates the multiple macrovascular complications as well as the renal disease. Aggressive antihypertensive therapy (goal BP <130/85 mm Hg or lower) slows the progression of renal disease and reduces cardiovascular events. The management of hypertension in the diabetic and in the setting of target organ damage is discussed in earlier sections of this chapter.

The pathogenesis of diabetic nephropathy involves both metabolic and renal hemodynamic mechanisms.[348,349] The chemical interaction of glucose with tissue proteins leads to the accumulation of advanced glycosylation end products (AGEs), which may be responsible for end organ damage. In experimental diabetes, high renal plasma flows and activation of the intrarenal renin–angiotensin system lead to glomerular capillary hypertension, hyperfiltration, and glomerular sclerosis.[350] Animals develop proteinuria, progressive renal insufficiency, and die a uremic death. Normalization of glomerular pressure by decreasing angiotensin-mediated efferent arteriolar constriction (with enalapril) prevents proteinuria and preserves glomerular structure. Evidence exists for identical renal hemodynamic abnormalities during the evolution of clinical diabetic

nephropathy.[351,352] The natural history of diabetic nephropathy may extend over 30 years from the onset of disease (Fig. 27.4).

Microalbuminuria is the first sign of morphologic renal abnormalities.[353,354] Persistent microalbuminuria (30–300 mg/24 hours) must be distinguished from the transient albuminuria seen in early diabetes, which reverses with blood sugar control. The appearance of persistent microalbuminuria predicts the development of overt proteinuria and subsequent progressive renal insufficiency over the next 10–15 years. Microalbuminuric diabetics are also at increased risk for the development of cardiovascular complications, neuropathy, and retinopathy. Microalbuminuria can be detected by a complete 24-hour urine collection or on a spot morning urine with measurement of the albumin:creatinine ratio. Hypertension may not be present but more often precedes and may predict the development of microalbuminuria, as does poor glycemic control. Screening recommendations for microalbuminuria are listed in Table 27.15.

Aggressive blood pressure reduction with ACE inhibitors and strict glycemic control reduces microalbuminuria and prevents the development of overt proteinuria. ACE inhibitors also reduce microalbuminuria in normotensive subjects. A management plan is suggested below in Fig. 27.5.[237]

The management of overt diabetic nephropathy is similar to that of non-diabetic renal disease. *ACE inhibitors* lower BP, reduce proteinuria and slow the

Table 27.15 *Measurement of microalbuminuria. (Reprinted from Greenberg, A, ed.* Primer on kidney diseases, *2nd edn, National Kidney Foundation, 1998)*

- Test IDDM patients of greater than 5 years duration every year
- Test NIDDM patients at the time of diagnosis and every year
- Rule out causes of transient microalbuminuria: hyperglycemia, UTI, PE, essential HTN, CHF, water loading
- If the albumin excretion rate is elevated, repeat three times over 3–6 months to define persistent microalbuminuria
- Normal albumin excretion: <30 mg/24 hours; microalbuminuria: 30–300 mg/24 hours; proteinuria: >300 mg/24 hours

IDDM = insulin-dependent diabetes mellitus; NIDDM = non-insulin-dependent diabetes mellitus; UTI = urinary tract infection; PE = physical exercise; HTN = hypertension; CHF = congestive heart failure.

progression of renal insufficiency in type I and probably in type II disease. A large, placebo-controlled trial in type I diabetics with established nephropathy (>500 mg proteinuria/24 hours, creatinine 2.5 mg/dL) reported a renoprotective advantage of captopril over conventional antihypertensive agents. The patients receiving captopril had a 50 per cent reduction in the risk of doubling serum creatinine and a similar reduction in the risk of death or ESRD. The renoprotective effect was independent of its effect on systemic blood pressure.[143] Normotensive subjects received an identical benefit.

The findings of several smaller studies are compiled into a meta-analysis, which suggests a greater antiproteinuric effect of ACE inhibitor over conventional therapy at equivalent degrees of blood pressure reduction.[242] However, long-term (9 years) stabilization of proteinuria and GFR is well documented among patients with diabetic nephropathy treated with aggressive *non-ACE inhibitor regimens*.[355] Nondihydropyridine CCBs and amlodipine have antiproteinuric effects, which may be additive to those of ACE inhibitors.[243,256–358] Nifedipine increases proteinuria in diabetic nephropathy and is best avoided.[242]

Angiotensin receptor blockers are suitable alternatives for patients intolerant of ACE inhibitors. In Type I diabetics with macroalbuminuria, the ARB losartan had an antiproteinuric effect equivalent to that of enalapril.[359] In a Type II population with microalbuminuria, dual blockade with ARB and ACE inhibitor was more effective in reducing blood pressure and microalbuminuria than either drug alone.[360] Clinical trials assessing the effect of ARBs and dual renin-angiotensin blockade on progressive diabetic nephropathy are in progress.

Among 1440 type I diabetics in the Diabetes Control and Complication Trial (DCCT), those randomized to *intensive gycemic control* (Hgb A1C of 7 per cent) had a reduced risk of developing microalbuminuria and a reduced risk of microalbuminuria progressing to overt nephropathy than did conventionally treated diabetics (Hgb A1C of 9 per cent).[361] Several small studies report a beneficial effect of a *low-protein diet* in slowing the progression of diabetic renal disease.[340] An additive renoprotective effect of low-protein diet to that of ACE inhibitors has never been established. An additive antiproteinuric effect could be tested on an individual basis.

FUTURE DIRECTIONS

In the 1940s and 1950s, an elevation of arterial pressure was considered 'essential' to normal organ perfusion and was viewed as a harmless physical finding. The term 'benign hypertension', to be distinguished from the more fulminant malignant form, persists in our medical vocabulary as a remnant of that era of ignorance. In 1967, the Veterans Administration were the first to demonstrate in a randomized trial that lowering BP reduces cardiovascular events.[187] The next 30 years were marked by an explosion of knowledge about hypertension and the development of more effective and better tolerated antihypertensive agents. Additional trials advanced the benefits of treating hypertension and elevated it to its current prominence as the most common condition for which adults attend a physician's office.

The dramatic decline in stroke and coronary heart disease over the past 30 years is often viewed as the payoff of modern antihypertensive management, but disturbing trends are appearing. Stroke mortality rates have leveled off – and may be climbing – and the total number of deaths from cardiovascular disease actually increased in both men and women in 1993 and 1995, the first increase since 1972.[362] The incidence of end-stage renal disease continues to rise steeply[304] and we have an epidemic of heart failure (JNC VI). Have we hit bottom in antihypertensive therapy? Can we improve upon antihypertensive management and bring about further reductions in target organ disease? If so, where will the advances be made?

History tells us that great strides will be made in understanding the pathogenesis of hypertension and the mechanisms of target organ damage. A major theme now unfolding is the ever-broadening role of angiotensin in cardiovascular disease.[363] Only 20 years ago, the renin–angiotensin system was viewed exclusively as a circulating endocrine system that served pressor functions and body fluid homeostasis. It is now established that the renin–angiotensin operates at a tissue level where it mediates vascular hypertrophy and cardiac remodeling by regulating cellular proliferation and programmed cell death (aptosis). Angiotensin has

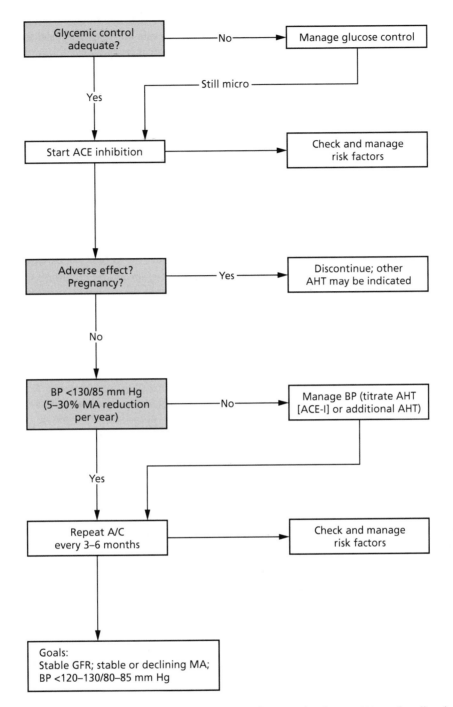

Figure 27.5 *Management of microalbuminuria in diabetes. AHT = antihypertensive therapy; MA = microalbuminuria; A/C = urinary albumin and creatinine. (Reprinted from Kaplan N.* Clinical hypertension, *7th edn. Baltimore: Williams & Wilkins, 1998)*

atherogenic and pro-ischemic actions; it stimulates monocytes to adhere to endothelium and to migrate into the subintima where they become lipid-laden macrophages. Angiotensin also tips fibrinolytic balance in favor of thrombosis. These insights carry particular therapeutic significance as the unique class of potent angiotensin receptor blockers penetrate our pharmaceutical market. These agents have a potential to reduce cardiovascular events by mechanisms that extend far beyond a

simple blood-pressure-lowering effect. A host of clinical trials are now assessing the role of ARBs in the prevention and treatment of heart failure, ischemic heart disease, stroke, peripheral vascular disease, and progressive renal damage.

We will continue to refine our understanding of the role of the endothelium in hypertension and cardiovascular disease.[364] This tissue is no longer viewed as a passive, porous interface between plasma and vessel. We now appreciate the endothelium as a target for mechanical and paracrine stimuli, and the source of potent vasoactive substances (endothelin, nitric oxide). A final major pathogenetic theme is the concept of insulin resistance and its relationship to hypertension, abnormal lipid, and glucose metabolism and the pathogenesis of atherosclerosis.[229] This conundrum will ultimately be solved and with it specific approaches for managing total cardiovascular risk.

Advances in therapeutics will keep pace with progress in pathophysiology. Increasingly potent and specific ARBs will lead the way over the next 5 years. A whole family of angiotensin receptor subtypes are now being described. Specific antagonists will be engineered for each. Endothelin antagonists are now in human clinical trials.[365] These agents confer dramatic renoprotection in hypertensive laboratory models and hold great promise, particularly for the African American population, so ravaged by hypertensive end-stage renal disease.[366] Several systems are now in development that potentiate the activity of nitric oxide and protect endothelium. Vasopepidase inhibitors, which simultaneously potentiate dilator/natriuretic peptides while blocking ACE, have proven to be potent and highly protective agents in the laboratory.[367] Promising stage III trials with these agents are ongoing in patients with heart failure and in uncomplicated hypertension.[302,368] Renin inhibitors, dopamine agonists, and potassium-channel openers are other exciting antihypertensive agents of the future.

Genetic advances will impact on diagnosis and treatment. Specific hypertensive genes have been cloned, which, when identified, confirm a specific monogenic hypertensive diagnosis (glucocorticoid remediable hypertension).[369] Mutations in the minerlocorticoid receptor (MR)[370] and in the epithelial sodium channel (ENaC) are now described which influence the renal handling of salt and water. These mutations have been demonstrated to both raise and lower BP in humans.[371] Gene polymorphism (variation) within components of the renin–angiotensin system have been linked to variations in the incidence of cardiovascular events and target organ damage.[372] Gene polymorphism will be integrated into systems of risk stratification. Genetic techniques will also be used to individualize therapy. Up to 30 per cent of the population are homozygous for a deletion within the gene encoding for ACE (DD genotype). Hypertensive patients with the DD-ACE genotype have higher circulating and tissue ACE activity. Patients with diabetic nephropathy and immunoglobulin A (IgA) nephropathy who carry the DD genotype exhibit a preferential renoprotective response to ACE inhibition and would be the best candidates for therapy.[373,374]

We need not wait for the arrival of genetic, pharmacologic and pathophysiologic advances to halt the resurgence in cardiovascular disease. Cardiovascular risk can be reduced now by intensifying our use of currently available antihypertensive agents. The findings of clinical trials will delineate future standards of practice. The Antihypertensive and Lipid-Lowering Heart Attack Prevention Trial (ALLHAT) is the largest (40 000 patients) of several trials to address agent-specific end-organ protection.[375] Hypertensive patients with additional cardiovascular risk factors have been randomized to one of four agents: amlodipine, lisinopril, doxazosin, or diuretic. Additional open-label agents are used to achieve target BP control in all four arms of the study. Aspirin and 'statins' are incorporated into the study design. ALLHAT, and other smaller trials, will advance one drug class over another for cardioprotection or for renoprotection. Agents will surface from the ALLHAT trial which carry 'preferred use status' in special populations (women, elderly, diabetics, African Americans).

Revised guidelines for treating hypertension will reduce cardiovascular disease only if embraced and implemented by the medical community at large. Guidelines for BP management exist today (goal BP <140/90 mm Hg), as they have for 30 years, yet adherence is poor. The most recent National Health and Nutrition Evaluation Survey (NHANES III),[376] conducted in 1991–1994, indicates that of the 50 million hypertensive Americans, 75 per cent are identified, 50 per cent are treated, and 27 per cent are controlled (BP <140/90 mm Hg). While the percentage with controlled hypertension is higher than surveys done in the 1970s and 1980s, it is lower than the 29 per cent control rate found in an identical survey in 1989–1991 (see Table 26.1). Adequacy of BP control continues to be poor by more recent surveys.[377]

It is estimated that over 35 million Americans are at risk for otherwise preventable cardiovascular events due to uncontrolled hypertension. Our future direction must be one of improved strategies for detecting hypertension and the creation of a multidisciplinary referral network for risk assessment and treatment. Public health initiatives must focus on the pre-hypertensive state in adolescents and young adults and on controlling the epidemic of obesity. Access to care must improve among disadvantaged minorities and managed care must be an advocate for aggressive preventative health maintenance in cardiovascular disease. Most critical to the future direction of hypertension is a renewed commitment by physicians to effective blood pressure control. A recent survey of over 11 000 hypertensive patients in Europe revealed that two-thirds were over target BP levels. More disturbing is the fact that in 82 per cent of cases, no alteration in the regimen was made to achieve better BP control.[378] Ambitious health-delivery programs, evidence-based guidelines, and scientific breakthroughs will be squandered if today's complacency is adopted by the next generation of practitioners.

SUMMARY

- In hypertensive disease, the urgency and threshold for drug therapy is based upon a system of patient risk stratification which includes a composite of traditional cardiovascular risk factors, the presence of target organ disease and the absolute level of blood pressure.
- On the basis of randomized clinical trials (RCTs), The Joint National Committee (JNC VI) recommends initiating antihypertensive therapy with diuretics or β-blockers unless there exist co-morbid conditions, compelling indications or other specific indications for alternative agents.
- Several RCTs completed since the formulation of JNC VI guidelines suggest that calcium-channel blockers and particularly ACE inhibitors offer equivalent if not superior cardiovascular protection to that provided by conventional diuretic/β-blocker therapy.
- Thiazide diuretics, when used in low doses and in combination with other agents, induce no significant adverse metabolic effect to compromise their proven role in reducing cardiovascular events.
- While ACE inhibitors are widely effective antihypertensive agents, their protective effect in cardiovascular disease also involves antiatherogenic, antiproliferative, antifibrotic and other non-hemodynamic effects exerted at several tissue sites.
- Elderly patients with hypertension are at greater risk for cardiovascular events and derive a greater benefit from antihypertensive therapy than do younger patients with hypertension.
- Systolic pressure and particularly pulse pressure are powerful predictors of stroke, coronary disease, heart failure and end stage renal disease.
- The rationale for aggressive management of hypertension in the patient with diabetes is based upon the threefold increase in cardiovascular risk compared to that of non-diabetics and proven incremental reductions in cardiovascular risk with increasing intensity of BP control.
- Severe elevations in blood pressure that acutely threaten target organ function are managed to goal BP by parenteral agents specific for the individual presenting condition. Severe but asymptomatic elevations of BP carry no acute target organ risk and are best managed with oral agents.
- Left ventricular hypertrophy (LVH) is a major independent risk factor for sudden cardiac death, myocardial infarction, stroke and other cardiovascular events. BP control with most antihypertensive agents reverses LVH but ACE inhibitors are most effective.
- Hypertension is present in 90 per cent of patients who develop congestive heart failure (CHF); chronic antihypertensive therapy delays the development of CHF by several decades.
- Treatment goals in the proteinuric patient with hypertension are reduction of BP to values less than 125/75 mm Hg *and* reduction of proteinuria to <1 g/24 hours. Targets are achieved with multidrug regimens which incorporate ACE-inhibitors, diuretics and additional agents.

REFERENCES

♦1. Psaty BM, Smith NL, Siscovick DS, *et al*. Health outcomes associated with antihypertensive therapies used as first-line agents: a systematic review and meta-analysis. *JAMA* 1997; **277**: 739–45.

2. MacMahon S, Peto R, Cutler J, *et al*. Blood pressure, stroke, and coronary heart disease. Part 1, Prolonged differences in blood pressure: prospective observational studies corrected for the regression dilution bias. *Lancet* 1990; **335**: 765–74.

♦3. Hansson L, Zanchetti A, Carruthers SG, *et al*. for the HOT Study Group. Effects of intensive blood pressure lowering and low-dose aspirin in patients with hypertension. Principal results of the Hypertension Optimal Treatment (HOT) randomised trial. *Lancet* 1998; **351**: 1755–62.

4. Farnett L, Mulrow CD, Linn WD, Lucey CR, Tuley MR. The J-curve phenomenon and the treatment of hypertension: is there a point beyond which pressure reduction is dangerous? *JAMA* 1991; **265**: 489–96.

5. Coope J, Warrander TS. Randomised trial of treatment of hypertension in elderly patients in primary care. *Br Med J* 1986; **293**: 1145–51.

♦6. Staessen J, Bulpitt C, Clement D, *et al*. Relation between mortality and treated blood pressure in elderly patients with hypertension: report of the European Working Party on High Blood Pressure in the elderly. *Br Med J* 1989; **298**: 1552–6.

♦7. Staessen JA, Fagard R, Thijs L, *et al*., for the Systolic Hypertension–Europe (Syst-Eur) trial investigators. Morbidity and mortality in the placebo-controlled European trial on isolated systolic hypertension in the elderly. *Lancet* 1997; **350**: 757–64.

8. Collins R, MacMahon S. Blood pressure, antihypertensive drug treatment and the risks of stroke and of coronary heart disease. *Br Med Bull* 1994; **50**: 272–98.

♦9. Systolic Hypertension in the Elderly Program Cooperative Research Group. Implications of the Systolic Hypertension in the Elderly Program. *Hypertension* 1993; **21**: 335–43.

10. Fletcher AE, Bulpitt CJ. How far should blood pressure be lowered? *N Engl J Med* 1992; **326**: 251–4.

11. Gifford RW Jr. Approach to treatment of hypertension. In: Izzo JL, Black HR, Taubert KA, eds *Hypertension primer*. Dallas, TX: American Heart Association, 1993.

12. Neaton JD, Grimm RH, Prineas RJ, *et al.* Treatment of Mild Hypertension Study: final results. *JAMA* 1993; **270**: 713–24.

13. MacMahon S, Rodgers A. The effects of blood pressure reduction in older patients: an overview of five randomized controlled trials in elderly hypertensives. *Clin Exp Hypertens* 1993; **15**: 967–78.

○14. Kaplan NM, Gifford RW. Choice of initial therapy for hypertension. *JAMA* 1996; **275**: 1577–80.

15. Wang JG, Staessen JA, Gong L, *et al.* Chinese trial on isolated systolic hypertension in the elderly. Systolic Hypertension in China (Syst-China) Collaborative Group. *Arch Intern Med* 2000; **160** (2): 211–20.

16. Tobian L, Brunner HR, Cohn JN, *et al.* Modern strategies to prevent coronary sequelae and stroke in hypertensive patients differ from the JNC V consensus guidelines. *Am J Hypertens* 1994; **7**: 859–72.

17. Current recommendations for initial therapy in hypertension: are they still valid? *Am J Hypertens* 1992; **11**(6), part 2.

♦18. The ALLHAT Officers. Major cardiovascular events in hypertensive patients randomized to Doxazosin vs Chlorthalidone: *JAMA* 2000; **283**: 1967–75.

♦19. Hansson L, Lindholm L, Niskanen L, *et al.* Effect of angiotensin-converting-enzyme inhibition compared with conventional therapy on cardiovascular morbidity and mortality in hypertension: the Captopril Prevention Project (CAPP) randomised trial. *Lancet* 1999; **353**: 611–16.

♦20. Hansson L, Lindholm L, Ekborn T, *et al.* Randomised trial of old and new antihypertensive drugs in elderly patients: cardiovascular mortality and morbidity the Swedish Trial in Old Patients with Hypertension –2 study. *Lancet* 1999; **354**: 1751–6.

21. Pickering T. For an American Society of Hypertension ad hoc panel. Recommendations for the use of home (self) and ambulatory blood pressure monitoring. *Am J Hypertens* 1995; **9**: 1–11.

22. Johnston GD. Dose-response relationships with antihypertensive drugs. *Pharmacol Ther* 1992; **55**: 53–9.

23. Gradman AH, Cutler NR, Davis PJ, *et al.* Combined enalapril and felodipine extended release (ER) for systemic hypertension. *Am J Cardiol* 1997; **79**: 431–5.

○24. Epstein M, Bakris G. Newer approaches to antihypertensive therapy: use of fixed-dose combination therapy. *Arch Intern Med* 1996; **156**: 1969–78.

♦25. Stamler R, Stamler J, Gosch FC, *et al.* Primary prevention of hypertension by nutritional-hygienic means: final report of a randomized, controlled trial. *JAMA* 1989; **262**: 1801–7.

26. Monane M, Bohn RJ, Gurwitz JH, *et al.* The effects of initial drug choice and co-morbidity on antihypertensive therapy compliance: results from a population-based study in the elderly. *Am J Hypertens* 1997; **10**: 697–704.

27. Trials of Hypertension Prevention Collaborative Research Group. Effects on weight loss and sodium reduction intervention on blood pressure and hypertension incidence in overweight people with high-normal blood pressure: the Trials of Hypertension Prevention, phase II. *Arch Intern Med* 1997; **157**: 657–67.

28. Singer DRJ, Markandu ND, Cappuccio FP, *et al.* Reduction of salt intake during converting enzyme inhibitor treatment compared with addition of thiazide. *Hypertension* 1995; **25**: 1042–4.

29. Wassertheil-Smoller S, Blaufox MD, Oberman AS, *et al.* Antihypertensive Interventions and Management (TAIM) Study: adequate weight loss, alone and combined with drug therapy in the treatment of mild hypertension. *Arch Intern Med* 1992; **152**: 131–6.

30. Darne B, Nivarong M, Tugaye A, *et al.* Hypocaloric diet and antihypertensive drug treatment. A randomized controlled clinical trial. *Blood Pressure* 1993; **2**: 130–5.

♦31. Whelton PK, Apple LJ, Espeland MA, *et al.* Sodium reduction and weight loss in the treatment of hypertension in older persons. *JAMA* 1998; **279**: 11.

♦32. Schotte DE, Stunkard AJ. The effects of weight reduction on blood pressure in 301 obese patients. *Arch Intern Med* 1990; **150**: 1701–4.

33. Moser M. Lifestyle modifications. In: *Clinical management of hypertension*, 2nd edn. Professional Communications Inc., 1997.

34. Gill JS, Shipley MJ, Tsementzis SA, *et al.* Alcohol consumption – a risk factor for hemorrhagic and nonhemorrhagic stroke. *Am J Med* 1991; **90**: 489–97.

35. Puddey IB, Parker M, Bellen LJ, Vandongen R, Masarei JRL. Effects of alcohol and caloric restrictions on blood pressure and serum lipids in overweight men. *Hypertension* 1992; **20**: 533–41.

36. Camargo CA Jr, Stampfer MJ, Glynn RJ, *et al.* Moderate alcohol consumption and risk for angina pectoris or myocardial infarction in U.S. male physicians. *Ann Intern Med* 1997; **126**: 372–5.

♦37. Elliott P, Stamler J, Nichols R, *et al.*, for the Intersalt Cooperative Research Group. Intersalt revisited: further analyses of 24 hour sodium excretion and blood pressure within and across populations. *Br Med J* 1996; **312**: 1249–53.

○38. Weinberger MH. Salt sensitivity of blood pressure in humans. *Hypertension* 1996; **27**(2): 481–90.

39. Ram CVS, Garrett BN, Kaplan NM. Moderate sodium restriction and various diuretics in the treatment of hypertension: effects of potassium wastage and blood pressure control. *Arch Intern Med* 1981; **141**: 1015–19.

40. Liebson PR, Grandits GA, Dianzumba S, *et al.*, for the

Treatment of Hypertension Study Research Group. Comparison of five antihypertensive monotherapies and placebo for change in left ventricular mass in patients receiving nutritional hygienic therapy in the Treatment of Mild Hypertension Study (TOMHS). *Circulation* 1995; **91**: 698–706.

∘41. Cutler JA, Follmann D, Allender PS. Randomized trials of sodium reduction: an overview. *Am J Clin Nutr* 1997; **65**(suppl): 643S–51S.

♦42. Midgley JP, Matthew AG, Greenwood CMT, Logan AG. Effect of reduced dietary sodium on blood pressure: a meta-analysis of randomized controlled trials. *JAMA* 1996; **275**: 1590–7.

43. US Department of Agriculture and US Department of Health and Human Services. *Nutrition and your health: dietary guidelines for Americans*, 4th edn. Home and Garden Bulletin No. 232. Washington, DC: US Department of Agriculture, 1995.

44. Paffenbarger RS Jr, Hyde RT, Wing AL, *et al*. The association of changes in physical-activity level and other lifestyle characteristics with mortality among men. *N Engl J Med* 1993; **328**: 538–45.

♦45. Kokkinos PF, Narayan P, Colleran JA, *et al*. Effects of regular exercise on blood pressure and left ventricular hypertrophy in African-American men with severe hypertension. *N Engl J Med* 1995; **333**: 1462–7.

∘46. Papademetriou V, Kokkinos PF. The role of exercise in the control of hypertension and cardiovascular risk. *Curr Opin Nephrol Hypertens* 1996; **5**: 459–62.

47. Blair SN, Goodyear NN, Gibbons LW, Cooper KH. Physical fitness and incidence of hypertension in healthy normotensive men and women. *JAMA* 1984; **252**: 487–90.

48. US Department of Health and Human Services. *Physical activity and health: A report of the Surgeon General*. Atlanta, GA: Centers for Disease Control and Prevention, National Center for Chronic Disease Prevention and Health Promotion, 1996.

49. Nelson L, Jennings GL, Esler MD, Korner PI. Effect of changing levels of physical activity on blood pressure and haemodynamics in essential hypertension. *Lancet* 1986; **2**: 473–6.

50. Martin J, Dubbert PM, Cushman WC. Controlled trial of aerobic exercise in hypertension. *Circulation* 1990; **81**: 1560–7.

51. MacDougall JD, McKelvie RS, Moroz DE, *et al*. Factors affecting blood pressure during heavy weight lifting and static contractions. *J Appl Physiol* 1992; **73**(4): 1590–992.

52. Cushman WC. Physical activity, fitness, and blood pressure. In: Izzo JL, Black HR, Taubert KA, eds *Hypertension primer*. Dallas, TX: American Heart Association, 1993.

53. Stamler J, Caggiula AW, Grandits GA. Relation of body mass and alcohol, nutrient, fiber, and caffeine intakes to blood pressure in the special intervention and usual care groups in the multiple risk factor intervention trial. *Am J Clin Nutr* 1997; **65**(suppl): 338S–65S.

54. Ascherio A, Hennekens C, Willett C, *et al*. Prospective study of nutritional factors, blood pressure, and hypertension among US women. *Hypertension* 1996; **27**: 1065–72.

55. Cappuccio FP, Elliott P, Allender PS, *et al*. Epidemiologic association between dietary calcium intake and blood pressure: a meta-analysis of published data. *Am J Epidemiol* 1995; **142**: 935–45.

♦56. Whelton PK, He J, Cutler JA, *et al*. Effects of oral potassium on blood pressure: meta-analysis of randomized controlled clinical trials. *JAMA* 1997; **277**: 1624–32.

♦57. Allender PS, Cutler JA, Follmann D, *et al*. Dietary calcium and blood pressure: a meta-analysis of randomized clinical trials. *Ann Intern Med* 1996; **124**: 825–31.

♦58. Appel LJ, Moore TJ, Obarzanek E, *et al.*, for the DASH Collaborative Research Group. A clinical trial of the effects of dietary patterns on blood pressure. *N Engl J Med* 1997; **336**: 1117–24.

59. van Montfrans GA, Karemaker JM, Wieling W, Dunning AJ. Relaxation therapy and continuous ambulatory blood pressure in mild hypertension: a controlled study. *Br Med J* 1990; **300**: 1368–72.

60. Alexander CN, Schneider RH, Staggers F, *et al*. Trial of stress reduction for hypertension in older African Americans. II. Sex and risk subgroup analysis. *Hypertension* 1996; **28**: 228–37.

61. Hunyor SN, Henderson RJ, Lal SKL, *et al*. Placebo-controlled biofeedback blood pressure effect in hypertensive humans. *Hypertension* 1997; **29**: 1225–31.

62. Johnston DW, Gold A, Kentish J, *et al*. Effect of stress management on blood pressure in mild primary hypertension. *Br Med J* 1993; **306**: 963–6.

63. Eisenberg DM, Delbanco TL, Berkey CS, *et al*. Cognitive behavioral techniques for hypertension: are they effective? *Ann Intern Med* 1993; **118**: 964–72.

64. Mikkelsen KL, Wiinberg N, Hoegholm A, *et al*. Smoking related to 24-h ambulatory blood pressure and heart rate. *Am J Hypertens* 1997; **10**: 483–94.

65. Greenberg G, Thompson SG, Brennan PJ. The relationship between smoking and the response to antihypertensive treatment in mild hypertensive in the Medical Research Council's trial of treatment. *Int J Epidemiol* 1987; **16**: 25–30.

66. Khoury Z, Comans P, Keren A, *et al*. Effects of transdermal nicotine patches on ambulatory ECG monitoring findings: a double-blind study in healthy smokers. *Cardiovasc Drugs Ther* 1996; **10**: 179–84.

67. US Department of Health and Human Services. *The health benefits of smoking cessation: a report of the Surgeon General*. Rockville, MD: Centers for Disease Control, Center for Chronic Disease Prevention and Health Promotion, Office on Smoking and Health, DHHS publication no. (CDC), 1990: 90–8416.

♦68. Kawachi J, Colditz GA, Stampfer MJ, et al. Smoking cessation and time course of decreased risks of coronary heart disease in middle-aged women. Arch Intern Med 1994; **154**: 169–75.

69. Sacks FM. Macronutrients, fiber and blood pressure. In: Izzo JL Jr, Black HR, Taubert KA, eds Hypertension primer. Dallas, TX: American Heart Association, 1993, 176–7.

70. Holland OB, Nixon JV, Kuhnert L. Diuretic-induced ventricular ectopic activity. Am J Med 1981; **70**: 762–8.

71. Duke M. Thiazide-induced hypokalemia: association with acute myocardial infarction and ventricular fibrillation. JAMA 1978; **239**: 43–5.

♦72. Madias JE, Madias NE, Gavras HP. Nonarrhythmogenicity of diuretic-induced hypokalemia: its evidence in patients with uncomplicated hypertension. Arch Intern Med 1984; **144**: 2171–6.

♦73. Papademetriou V, Price M, Notargiacomo A, et al. Effect of diuretic therapy on ventricular arrhythmias in hypertensive patients with or without left ventricular hypertrophy. Am Heart J 1985; **110**: 595–9.

○74. Freis ED. Critique of the clinical importance of diuretic-induced hypokalemia and elevated cholesterol level. Arch Intern Med 1989; **149**: 2640–8.

75. The Fifth Report of the Joint National Committee on Detection, Evaluation and Treatment of High Blood Pressure. Arch Intern Med 1993; **153**: 154–83.

76. Frohlich ED. Long-term thiazide therapy in essential hypertension. Circulation 1970; **41**: 709.

77. Moser M. Diuretics. In: Clinical management of hypertension, 2nd edn. Professional Communications Inc, 1997.

○78. Weir MR, Flack JM, Applegate WB. Tolerability, safety, and quality of life and hypertensive therapy: the case for low-dose diuretics. Am J Med 1996; **101**: 83S–92S.

79. James MA, Jones JV. An interaction between LVH and potassium in hypertension? J Hum Hypertens 1991; **5**: 474–8.

80. Hoes AW, Grobbee DE, Lubsen J, et al. Diuretics, β-blockers, and the risk for sudden cardiac death in hypertensive patients. Ann Intern Med 1995; **123**: 481–7.

♦81. Siscovick DS, Raghunathan TE, Wicklund KG, et al. Diuretic therapy for hypertension and the risk of primary cardiac arrest. N Engl J Med 1994; **330**: 1852–7.

♦82. Cooper HA, Dries DL, Davis CE, Shen YL, Domanski MJ. Diuretics and risk of arrhythmic death in patients with left ventricular dysfunction. Circulation 1999; **100**: 1311–15.

♦83. Kasiske BL, Ma JZ, Kalil RSN, Louis TA. Effects of antihypertensive therapy on serum lipids. Ann Intern Med 1995; **122**: 133–41.

♦84. Grimm RH Jr, Flack JM, Grandits GA, et al. Long-term effects on plasma lipids of diet and drugs to treat hypertension. JAMA 1996; **275**: 1549–56.

85. Weidmann P, Uehlinger DE, Gerber A. Antihypertensive treatment and serum lipoproteins. J Hypertens 1985; **3**: 297–306.

86. Manttari M, Tenkanen L, Manninen V, et al. Antihypertensive therapy in dyslipidemic men. Effects on coronary heart disease incidence and total mortality. Hypertension 1995; **25**: 47–52.

87. Lithell HOL. Effect of antihypertensive drugs on insulin, glucose, and lipid metabolism. Diabetes Care 1991; **14**: 203–9.

88. Samuelsson O, Hedner T, Berglund D, et al. Diabetes mellitus in treated hypertension: incidence, predictive factors and the impact of non-selective β-blockers and thiazide diuretics during 15 years treatment of middle-aged hypertensive men in the primary prevention trial Goteborg, Sweden. J Hum Hypertens 1994; **8**: 257–63.

89. Goldner MG, Zarowitx H, Akgun S. Hyperglycemia and glycosuria due to thiazide derivatives administered in diabetes mellitus. Med Intel 1960; **262**: 403–5.

♦90. Curb JD, Pressel SL, Cutler JA, et al. Effect of diuretic-based antihypertensive treatment on cardiovascular disease risk in older diabetic patients with isolated systolic hypertension. JAMA 1996; **276**: 1886–92.

91. Gurwitz JH, Bohn RL, Glynn RJ, et al. Antihypertensive drug therapy and the initiation of treatment of diabetes mellitus. Ann Intern Med 1992; **118**: 273–8.

♦92. Gress T, Nieto F, Shahar E, et al. Hypertension and antihypertensive therapy as risk factors for type 2 diabetes mellitus. New Engl J Med 2000; **342**: 905–12.

93. Warren JH, Laffel LMB, Valsania P, et al. Excess mortality associated with diuretic therapy in diabetes mellitus. Arch Intern Med 1991; **151**: 1350–6.

94. Langford HG, Blaufox MD, Borhani NO, et al. Is thiazide-produced uric acid elevation harmful? Analysis of data from the hypertension detection and follow-up program. Arch Intern Med 1987; **147**: 644–9.

95. Campion EW, Glynn RJ, DeLabry LO. Asymptomatic hyperuricemia. Risks and consequences in the normative aging study. Am J Med 1987; **82**: 421–6.

96. Culleton B, Larson M, Kannel W, et al. Serum uric acid and risk for cardiovascular disease and death: the Framingham Heart Study. Ann Intern Med 1999; **131**: 7–14.

○97. Nader PC, Thompson JR, Alpern RJ. Complications of diuretic use. Semin Nephrol 1988; **8**: 364–87.

98. Clark BA, Shannon RP, Rosa RM, et al. Increased susceptibility to thiazide-induced hyponatremia in the elderly. J Am Soc Nephrol 1994; **5**: 1106–11.

♦99. Ashraf N, Locksley R, Arieff A. Thiazide-induced hyponatremia associated with death or neurologic damage in outpatients. Am J Med 1981; **70**: 1163–8.

100. Frishman WH, Furberg CD, Friedewald WT. β-

Adrenergic blockade for survivors of acute myocardial infarction. *N Engl J Med* 1984; **310**: 830–7.

♦101. Medical Research Council Working Party. MRC trial of treatment of mild hypertension: principal results. *Br Med J* 1985; **291**: 97–104.

102. Wilhelmsen L, Berglund G, Elmfeldt D, *et al*. β-Blockers versus diuretics in hypertensive men: main results from the HAPPHY trial. *J Hypertens* 1987; **5**: 561–72.

♦103. Medical Research Council Working Party. Medical Research Council trial of treatment of hypertension in older adults: principal results. *Br Med J* 1992; **304**: 404–12.

♦104. Messerli F, Grossman E, Goldbourt U. Are β-blockers efficacious as first-line therapy for hypertension in the elderly. *JAMA* 1998; **279**: 1903–7.

○105. Frishman WH. β-Adrenergic blockers. *Med Clinics North Am* 1988; **72**: 37–81.

106. Dujovne CA, Eff J, Ferraro L, *et al*. Comparative effects of atenolol versus Celiprolol on serum lipids and blood pressure in hyperlipidemic and hypertensive subjects. *Am J Cardiol* 1993; **72**: 1131–6.

107. Soriano JB, Hoes AW, Meems L, Grobbee DE. Increased survival with β-blockers; importance of ancillary properties. *Prog Cardiovasc Dis* 1997; **39**: 445–6.

108. McDevitt DG, Nicholson AN, Wright NA, Zetlein MB. Central effects of repeated administration of atenolol and captopril in health volunteers. *Eur J Clin Pharmacol* 1994; **46**: 23–8.

109. Lebel M, Langlois S, Belleau LJ, Grose JH. Lebetalol infusion in hypertensive emergencies. *Clin Pharmacol Ther* 1985; **37**: 614–18.

♦110. Packer M, Bristow MR, Cohn JN, *et al*. The effect of carvedilol on morbidity and mortality in patients with chronic heart failure. *N Engl J Med* 1996; **334**: 1349–55.

111. Gerstman BB, Jolson HM, Bauer M, *et al*. the incidence of depression in new users of β-blockers and selected antihypertensives. *J Clin Epidemiol* 1996; **49**: 809–15.

112. MERIT-HF Study Group. Effect of metoprolol CR/XL in chronic heart failure: Metoprolol CR/XL Randomised Intervention Trial in congestive heart failure (MERIT – HF). *Lancet* 1999; **353**: 2001–7.

113. Gullestad L, Birkeland K, Nordby G, *et al*. Effects of selective β$_2$-adrenoceptor blockade on serum potassium and exercise performance in normal men. *Br J Clin Pharmacol* 1991; **32**: 201–7.

114. Lammers JWJ, Folgering HTM, van Herwaarden CLA. Ventilatory effects of long-term treatment with pindolol and metoprolol in hypertensive patients with chronic obstructive lung disease. *Br J Clin Pharmacol*, 1985; **20**: 204–10.

115. Molnar GW, Read RC, Wright FE. Propranolol enhancement of hypoglycemic sweating. *Clin Pharmacol Ther* 1974; **15**: 490–6.

116. Donhorst A, Powell SH, Pensky J. Aggravation by propranolol of hyperglyceaemic effect of hydrochlorothiazide in type II diabetics without alteration of insulin secretion. *Lancet* 1985; **1**: 123–6.

117. Psaty BM, Koepsell TD, Wagner EH, *et al*. The relative risk of incident coronary heart disease associated with recently stopping the use of β-blockers. *JAMA* 1990; **263**: 1653–7.

118. Triggle DJ. Pharmacologic and therapeutic differences among calcium channel antagonists: profile of mibefradil, a new calcium antagonist. *Am J Cardiol* 1996; **78**: 7–12.

119. Epstein M. Calcium antagonists in the management of hypertension. In: Epstein M, ed. *Calcium antagonists in clinical medicine*. Philadelphia: Hanley & Belfus, Inc, 1992: 213–30.

○120. Cummings DM, Amadio P Jr, Nelson L, Fitzgerald JM. The role of calcium channel blockers in the treatment of essential hypertension. *Arch Intern Med* 1991; **151**: 250–9.

121. Weir M. Calcium entry blockers. In: Izzo JL, Black HR, Taubert KA, eds, *Hypertension primer*. Dallas, TX: American Heart Association, 1993.

♦122. Packer M, O'Connor CM, Ghali JK, *et al*. Effect of amlodipine on morbidity and mortality in severe chronic heart failure. *N Engl J Med* 1996; **335**: 1107–14.

123. Carruthers SG, Freeman DJ, Bailey DG. Synergistic adverse hemodynamic interaction between oral verapamil and propranolol. *Clin Pharmacol Ther* 1989; **46**: 469–77.

124. Moser M. Calcium channel blockers. In: *Clinical management of hypertension*. Professional Communications Inc., 1997.

125. Iabichella ML, Dell'Omo G, Melillo, Pedrinelli R. Calcium channel blockers blunt postural cutaneous vasoconstriction in hypertensive patients. *Hypertension* 1997; **29**: 751–6.

126. Gradman AH, Cutler NR, Davis PJ, *et al*. Combined enalapril and felodipine extended release (ER) for systemic hypertension. *Am J Cardiol* 1997; **79**: 431–5.

♦127. Psaty BM, Heckbert SR, Koepsell TD, *et al*. The risk of myocardial infarction associated with anti-hypertensive drug therapies. *JAMA* 1995; **274**: 620–5.

♦128. Aldeman MH, Cohen H, Roque R, Madhavan S. Effect of long-acting and short-acting calcium antagonists on cardiovascular outcomes in hypertensive patients. *Lancet* 1997; **349**: 594–8.

129. Messerli F. Case-control study, meta-analysis, and bouillabaisse: putting the calcium antagonist scare into context. *Ann Intern Med* 1995; **123**: 880–9.

130. Hansson L, Hedner T, Lund-Johansen P, *et al*. Randomised trial of effects of calcium antagonists compared with diuretics and beta blockers on cardiovascular morbidity and mortality in hypertension: the Nordic Diltiazem (NORDIL) study. *Lancet* 2000; **356**: 359–65.

♦131. Pahor M, Psaty B, Alderman M, *et al*. Health outcomes associated with calcium antagonists compared with other first-line antihypertensive therapies: a meta-analysis of randomised controlled trials. *Lancet* 2000; **356**: 1949–54.

♦132. Blood Pressure Lowering Treatment Trialists Collaboration. Effects of ACE inhibitors, calcium antagonists, and other blood-pressure-lowering drugs: results of prospectively designed overviews overviews of randomised trials. *Lancet* 2000; **356**: 1955–64.

○133. Dzau VJ, Re R. Tissue angiotensin system in cardiovascular medicine. A paradigm shift? *Circulation* 1994; **89**: 493–8.

134. Paul M, Bachmann J, Ganten D. The tissue renin-angiotensin systems in cardiovascular disease. *Trends Cardiovasc Med* 1992; **2**: 94–9.

○135. Brown NJ, Vaughan DE. Angiotensin-converting enzyme inhibitors. *Circulation* 1998; **97**: 1411–20.

136. Gavras H. Angiotensin-converting enzyme inhibitors. In: Izzo JL, Black HR, Taubert KA, eds *Hypertension primer*. Dallas, TX: American Heart Association, 1993.

137. Gavras H, Gavras I, Textor S, *et al.* Effect of angiotensin converting enzyme inhibition on blood pressure, plasma renin activity and plasma aldosterone in essential hypertension. *J Clin Endocrinol Metab* 1977; **46**: 220–6.

138. Schmieder RE, Martus P, Klingbeil A. Reversal of left ventricular hypertrophy in essential hypertension. A meta-analysis of randomized double-blind studies. *JAMA* 1996; **275**: 1507–13.

139. Vaughan DE, Pfeffer MA. Post-myocardial infarction ventricular remodeling: animal and human studies. *Cardiovasc Drugs Ther* 1991; **8**: 453–60.

♦140. Pfeffer MA, Braunwald E, Moye LA, *et al.* Effect of captopril on mortality and morbidity in patients with left ventricular dysfunction after myocardial infarction. *N Engl J Med* 1992; **327**: 669–77.

141. Garg R, Yusuf S. Overview of randomized trials of angiotensin-converting enzyme inhibitors on mortality and morbidity in patients with heart failure. *JAMA* 1995; **273**: 1450–6.

♦142. Anderson S, Rennke HG, Brenner BM. Therapeutic advantage of converting enzyme inhibitors in arresting progressive renal disease associated with systemic hypertension in the rat. *J Clin Invest* 1986; **77**: 1993–2000.

♦143. Lewis EJ, Hunsicker LG, Bain RP, Rohde RD. The effect of angiotensin-converting-enzyme inhibition on diabetic nephropathy. *N Engl J Med* 1993; **329**: 1456–62.

144. Chobamiam AV, Haudenschild CC, Nickerson C, Drago R. Antiatherogenic effect of captopril in the Watanabe heritable hyperlipidemic rabbit. *Hypertension* 1990; **15**: 327–31.

♦145. The Heart Outcomes Prevention Evaluation Study Investigators. Effects of an angiotensin-converting-enzyme inhibitor, ramipril, on cardiovascular events in high-risk patients. *New Engl J Med* 2000; **342**: 145–54.

146. Gibbons GH. Endothelial function as a determinant of vascular function and structures: a new therapeutic target. *Am J Cardiol* 1997; **79**(5A): 3–8.

147. Pepine CJ. Improved endothelial function with angiotensin-converting enzyme inhibitors. *Am J Cardiol* 1997; **79**(5A): 29–32.

♦148. Mancini GBJ, Henry GC, Macaya C, *et al.* Angiotensin-converting enzyme inhibition with quinapril improves endothelial vasomotor dysfunction in patients with coronary artery disease. *Circulation* 1996; **94**: 258–65.

149. Pollare T, Lithell H, Berne C. A comparison of the effects of hydrochlorothiazide and captopril on glucose and lipid metabolism in patients with hypertension. *N Engl J Med* 1989; **321**: 868–73.

150. Hahn AW, Jonas U, Buhler FR, Resink TJ. Activation of human peripheral monocytes by angiotensin II. *Fed Eur Biochem Soc* 1994; **347**: 178–80.

151. Vaughan DE. The renin-angiotensin system and fibrinolysis. *Am J Cardiol* 1997; **79**(5A): 12–16.

152. Intengan HD, Thibault G, Li JS, *et al.* Resistance artery mechanics, structure, and extra-cellular components in spontaneously hypertensive rates: effects of angiotensin receptor antagonism and converting enzyme inhibition. *Circulation* 1999; **100**: 2267–75.

153. Rabbani R, Topol EJ. Strategies to achieve coronary arterial plaque stabilization. *Cardiovasc Res* 1999; **41**: 402–17.

♦154. Pfeffer MA, Braunwald E, Moye LA, *et al.*, for the SAVE investigators. Effect of captopril on mortality and morbidity in patients with left ventricular dysfunction after myocardial infarction: results of the survival and ventricular enlargement trials. *N Engl J Med* 1992; **327**: 669–77.

○155. Hennekens CH, Albert CM, Godfried SL, *et al.* Adjunctive drug therapy of acute myocardial infarction – evidence from clinical trials. *N Engl J Med* 1996; **335**: 1660–7.

156. Wood R. Bronchospasm and cough as adverse reactions to the ACE inhibitors captopril, enalapril, and lisinopril. A controlled retrospective cohort study. *Br J Clin Pharmacol* 1995; **39**: 264–70.

157. Israili ZH, Hall WD. Cough and angioneurotic edema associated with angiotensin-converting enzyme inhibitor therapy. *Ann Intern Med* 1992; **117**: 234–42.

○158. Messerli FH, Weder MA, Bruner HR. Angiotensin II receptor inhibition. *Arch Intern Med* 1996; **156**: 1957–65.

○159. Goodfriend TL, Elliott ME, Catt KJ. Angiotensin receptors and their antagonists. *N Engl J Med* 1996; **334**: 1649–54.

160. Bauer JH, Reams GP. The angiotensin II type I receptor antagonists. A new class of anti-hypertensive drugs. *Arch Intern Med* 1995; **155**: 1361–8.

♦161. Pitt B, Segal R, Martinez FA, *et al.* Randomized trial of losartan vs. captopril in patients over 65 with heart failure (evaluation of losartan in the elderly study, ELITE). *Lancet* 1997; **349**: 747–52.

162. Villa E, Rabano A, Cazes M, *et al*. Effects of UP269–6, a new angiotensin II receptor antagonist, and captopril on the progression of rat diabetic nephropathy. *Am J Hypertens* 1997; **10**: 274–81.

163. Thurmann PA. Angiotensin receptor blockers and left ventricular hypertrophy. *Am J Hypertens* 1998; **11**(4) part 2: 252a.

164. Husain A. The chymase-angiotensin system in humans. *J Hypertens* 1993; **11**: 1155–9.

165. Cohn JN. Effects of ARB-ACEI combination therapy on morbidity and mortality in heart failure. *Am J Hypertens* 1998; **11**(4): 257a.

166. Stoll M, Steckelings UM, Paul M, Bottari SP, Metzger R, Unger T. The angiotensin AT$_2$-receptor mediates inhibition of cell proliferation in coronary endothelial cells. *J Clin Invest* 1995; **95**: 651–7.

167. Siragy HM. Functional significance of angiotensin receptors. *Am J Hypertens* 1998; **11**(4): 251a.

168. Siragy HM, Carey RM. The subtype 2 (AT$_2$) angiotensin receptor mediates renal production of nitric oxide in conscious rats. *J Clin Invest* 1997; 264–9.

169. Gigante B, Natale A, Piras O, Volpe M. Selective blockade of AT$_2$ receptors offsets the blood pressure lowering effect of losartan in salt-restricted rats. *Am J Hypertens*, 1998; **11**: 18a.

170. Weir, M. Personal communication. *American Society of Hypertension*, New York City, 1998.

◆171. Zacest R, Gilmore E, Koch-Weser J. Treatment of essential hypertension with combined vasodilation and β-adrenergic blockade. *N Engl J Med* 1972; **286**: 617–22.

172. Cohn JN, Archibald DG, Ziesche S, *et al*. Effect of vasodilator therapy on mortality in chronic congestive heart failure. Results of a Veterans Administration Cooperative Study. *N Engl J Med* 1986; **314**: 1547–52.

173. Ramsay LE, Silas JH, Ollerenshaw JD, *et al*. Should the acetylator phenotype be determined when prescribing hydralazine for hypertension? *Eur J Clin Pharmacol* 1984; **26**: 39–42.

174. Cameron HA, Ramsay LE. The lupus syndrome induced by hydralazine: a common complication with low dose treatment. *Br Med J* 1984; **289**: 410–12.

175. Mansilla-Tinoco R, Harland SJ, Ryan PJ, *et al*. Hydralazine, antinuclear antibodies, and the lupus syndrome. *Br Med J* 1982; **284**: 936–9.

176. MacKay A, Isles C, Henderson I, *et al*. Minoxidil in the management of intractable hypertension. *Q J Med* 1981; **50**: 174–90.

177. Johnson BF, Errichetti A, Urbach D, *et al*. The effect of once/daily minoxidil on blood pressure and plasma lipids. *J Clin Pharmacol* 1986; **26**: 534–8.

○178. Lithell HO. Hyperinsulinemia, insulin resistance, and the treatment of hypertension. *Am J Hypertens* 1996; **9**: 150S–4S.

179. Stokes GS, Graham RM, Gain JM, Davis PR. Influence of dosage and dietary sodium on the first-dose effects of prazocin. *Br Med J* 1977; **1**: 1507–8.

180. Moser M. Central agonists. In: *Clinical management of hypertension* 2nd edn. Professional Communications Inc, 1997.

181. Weber MA. Transdermal antihypertensive therapy: Clinical and metabolic considerations. *Am Heart J* 1986; **112**: 906–12.

182. Houston MC. Treatment of hypertensive emergencies and urgencies with oral clonidine loading and titration. *Arch Intern Med* 1986; **146**: 586–9.

183. Bravo EL, Tarazi RC, Fouad FM, *et al*. Clonidine-suppression test. A useful aid in the diagnosis of pheochromocytoma. *N Engl J Med* 1981; **305**: 623–6.

184. Lewin A, Alderman MH, Mathur P. Antihypertensive efficacy of guanfacine and prazocin in patients with mild to moderate essential hypertension. *J Clin Pharmacol* 1990; **30**: 1081–7.

◆185. Veteran's Administration Cooperative Study Group on Antihypertensive Agents. Effects of treatment on morbidity in hypertension. Results in patients with diastolic BPs averaging 115 through 129 mm Hg. *JAMA* 1967; **202**: 116–22.

◆186. Veteran's Administration Cooperative Study Group on Antihypertensive Agents. Effects of treatment on morbidity in hypertension. Results in patients with diastolic BPs averaging 90 through 114 mm Hg. *JAMA* 1970; **213**: 1143–52.

187. Veteran's Administration Cooperative Study on Antihypertensive Agents. *Double blind control study of antihypertensive agents, II; further report on the comparative effectiveness of reserpine, reserpine and hydralazine, and three ganglion blocking agents, chlorisondamine, mecamylamine, and pentolinium tartrate. Arch Intern Med* 1962; **110**: 222–9.

188. Horwitz RI, Feinstein AR. Exclusion bias and the false relationship of reserpine and breast cancer. *Arch Intern Med* 1985; **145**: 1873–5.

189. Hall WD, Ferrario CM, Moore MA, *et al*. Hypertension-related morbidity and mortality in the southeastern United States. *Am J Med Sci* 1997; **313**: 195–206.

◆190. Burt VL, Wheaton P, Roccella EJ, *et al*. Prevalence of hypertension in the US adult population; results from the third National Health and Nutrition Examination Survey 1988–1991. *Hypertension* 1995; **25**: 303–13.

191. Singh GK, Kochanek KD, MacDorman MF. Advance report of final morbidity statistics, 1994. *Mon Vital Stat Rep* 1996; **45** (3, suppl): 1–76.

◆192. Klag MJ, Wheaton PK, Randall BL, Neaton JD, Brancati FL, Stamier J. End-stage renal disease in African-American and white men: 16-year MRFIT findings. *JAMA* 1997; **277**: 1293–8.

193. Mediview Express Report—From data presented at The American Society of Nephrology (ASN) 33rd annual meeting, October 13–16, 2000, Toronto, Canada.

194. Kaplan N. Primary hypertension: natural history, special populations, and evaluation. In: *Clinical hypertension* 7th edn. Baltimore: Williams & Wilkins, 1998.

195. Hypertension Detection and Follow-up Program Cooperative Group. Five-year findings of the Hypertension Detection and Follow-up Program: mortality by race-sex and blood pressure level: a further analysis. *J Commun Health* 1984; **9**: 314–27.

♦196. Ooi WL, Budner NS, Cohen H, Madavan S, Alderman MH. Impact of race on treatment response and cardiovascular disease among hypertensives. *Hypertension* 1989; **14**: 227–34.

197. Reed JW. Treatment of hypertensive patients in minorities. In: Izzo JL, Black HR, Taubert KA, eds *Hypertension primer*. Dallas, TX: American Heart Association, 1993.

♦198. Materson BJ, Reda DJ, Cushman WC, *et al.*, for the Department of Veterans Affairs Cooperative Study Group on AntiHypertensive Agents. Single-drug therapy for hypertension in men: a comparison of six antihypertensive agents with placebo. *N Engl J Med* 1993; **328**: 914–21.

199. LaCroix AZ. Gender effects and hypertension in women. In: Izzo JL, Black HR, Taubert KA, eds *Hypertension primer*. Dallas, TX: American Heart Association, 1993.

200. Huang Z, Willett W, Manson J, *et al.* Body weight, weight change, and risk for hypertension in women. *Ann Intern Med* 1998; **128**: 81–8.

201. Gueyffier F, Boutitie F, Boissel JP, *et al.*, for the INDANA Investigators. Effect on antihypertensive drug treatment on cadiovascular outcomes in women and men: a meta-analysis of individual patient data from randomized, controlled trials. Ann Intern Med 1997; 126: 761–7.

○202. National High Blood Pressure Education Program Working Group. National High Blood Pressure Education Program working group report on hypertension in the elderly. *Hypertension* 1994; **23**: 275–85.

203. Anastos K, Charney P, Charon RA, *et al.* Hypertension in women: what is really known? The Woman's Caucus Working Group on Woman's Health of the Society of General Internal Medicine. *Ann Intern Med* 1991; **115**: 287–93.

○204. Woods JW. Oral contraceptives and hypertension. *Hypertension* 1988; **11** (suppl II): II-11–II-15.

♦205. Hulley S, Grady D, Bush T, *et al.* Randomized trial of estrogen plus progestin for secondary prevention of coronary heart disease in postmenopausal women. *JAMA* 1998; **280**: 605–13.

♦206. Herrington DM, Reboussin DM, Brosnihan KB, *et al.* Effects of estrogen replacement on the progression of coronary artery atherosclerosis. *N Engl J Med* 2000; **343**: 522–9.

207. Nabulsi AA, Folsom AR, White A, *et al.* Association of hormone-replacement therapy with various cardiovascular risk factors in postmenopausal women. *N Engl J Med* 1993; **328**: 1069–75.

208. Akkad A, Halligan A, Abrams K, Al-Azzawi F. Differing responses in blood pressure over 24 hours in normotensive women receiving oral or transdermal estrogen replacement therapy. *Obstet Gynecol* 1997; **89**: 97–103.

209. Writing Group for the PEPI Trial. Effects of estrogen or estrogen/progestin regimens on heart disease risk factors in postmenopausal women: the Postmenopausal Estrogen/Progestin Interventions (PEPI) Trial. *JAMA* 1995; **273**: 199–208.

○210. Sibai BM. Treatment of hypertension in pregnant women. *N Engl J Med* 1996; **335**: 257–65.

211. National High Blood Pressure Evaluation Program. *Working Group Report on high blood pressure in pregnancy*. Washington, DC: US Department Health and Human Service (NIH Publication) 1990; 90–3029.

212. Lindheimer MD. Hypertension in pregnancy. *Hypertension* 1993; **22**: 127–37.

○213. Lindheimer MD. Pre-eclampsia-eclampsia 1996: Preventable? Have disputes on its treatment been resolved? *Curr Opin Nephrol Hypertens* 1996; **5**: 452–8.

214. Madhavan S, Ooi WL, Cohen H, Alderman MH. Relation of pulse pressure and blood pressure reduction to the incidence of myocardial infarction. *Hypertension* 1994; **23**: 395–401.

♦215. Franklin S, Khan S, Wong N, *et al.* Is pulse pressure useful in predicting risk for coronary heart disease? The Framingham Heart Study. *Circulation* 1999; **100**: 354–60.

♦216. SHEP Cooperative Research Group. Prevention of stroke by antihypertensive drug treatment in older persons with isolated systolic hypertension: final results of the Systolic Hypertension in the Elderly Program (SHEP). *JAMA* 1991; **265**: 3255–64.

♦217. Dahlof B, Lindholm LH, Hansson L, Schersten B, Ekbom T, Wester PO. Morbidity and mortality in the Swedish trial in Old Patients with Hypertension (STOP-Hypertension). *Lancet* 1991; **338**: 1281–5.

♦218. Kostis JB, Davis BR, Cutler J, *et al.* Prevention of heart failure by antihypertensive drug treatment in older persons with isolated systolic hypertension. *JAMA* 1997; **278**: 212–16.

219. Sagie A, Larson MG, Levy D. The natural history of borderline isolated systolic hypertension. *N Engl J Med* 1993; **329**: 1912–17.

220. Gueyffier F, Bulpitt C, Boissel J, *et al.* Antihypertensive drugs in very old people: a subgroup meta-analysis of randomised controlled trials. *Lancet* 1999; **353**: 793–6.

221. Messerli FH. Osler's maneuver, pseudohypertension and true hypertension in the elderly. *Am J Med* 1986; **80**: 906–10.

222. Wiinberg N, Hoegholm A, Christensen HR, *et al.* 24-h ambulatory blood pressure in 352 normal Danish subjects, related to age and gender. *Am J Hypertens* 1995; **8**: 978–86.

223. Ooi WL, Barret S, Hossain M, Kelley-Gagnon M, Lipsitz LA. Patterns of orthostatic blood pressure change and

their clinical correlates in a frail, elderly population. *JAMA* 1997; **277**: 1299–304.

224. Geleijnse JM, Witteman JCM, Bak AAA, *et al*. Reduction in blood pressure with a low sodium, high potassium, high magnesium salt in older subjects with mild to moderate hypertension. *Br Med J* 1994; **309**: 436–40.

○225. Beard K, Bulpitt C, Mascie-Taylor H, *et al*. Management of elderly patients with sustained hypertension. *Br Med J* 1992; **304**: 412–16.

226. Norgaard K, Rasmussen E, Jensen T, *et al*. Nature of elevated blood pressure in normoalbuminuric type I diabetic patients. Essential Hypertension? *Am J Hypertens* 1993; **6**: 830–6.

227. Kannel WB, D'Agostino RB, Wilson PWF, Belanger AJ. Diabetes, fibrinogen, and risk of cardiovascular disease: the Framingham experience. *Am Heart J* 1990; **120**: 672–6.

○228. Sowers JR, Epstein M. Diabetes mellitus and associated hypertension, vascular disease, and nephropathy. *Hypertension* 1995; **26** (Part I): 869–79.

○229. Reaven GM, Lithell H, Landsberg L. Hypertension and associated metabolic abnormalities – the role of insulin resistance and the sympathoadrenal system. *N Engl J Med* 1996; **334**: 374–81.

○230. National High Blood Pressure Education Program Working Group. National High Blood Pressure Education Program working group report on hypertension and diabetes. *Hypertension* 1994; **23**: 145–58.

231. Perseghin G, Price TB, Petersen KF, *et al*. Increased glucose transport-phosphorylation and muscle glycogen synthesis after exercise training in insulin-resistant subjects. *N Engl J Med* 1996; **335**: 1357–62.

232. Ikeda T, Gomi T, Hirawa N, *et al*. Improvement of insulin sensitivity contributes to blood pressure reduction after weight loss in hypertensive subjects with obesity. *Hypertension* 1996; **27**: 1180–6.

♦233. Curb JD, Pressel SL, Cutler JA, *et al*. Effect of diuretic-based antihypertensive treatment on cardiovascular disease risk in older diabetic patients with isolated systolic hypertension. *JAMA* 1996; **276**: 1886–92.

234. Shorr RI, Ray WA, Daugherty JR, Griffin MR. Antihypertensives and the risk of serious hypoglycemia in older persons using insulin or sulfonylures. *JAMA* 1997; **278**: 40–3.

♦235. Tuomilehto J, Rastenyte D, Birkenhager W, *et al*. Effects of calcium-channel blockade in older patients with diabetes and systolic hypertension. *N Engl J Med* 1999; **340**: 677–84.

♦236. Adler AI, Stratton IM, Neil HA, *et al*. Association of systolic blood pressure with macrovascular and microvascular complications of type 2 diabetes (UKPDS 36): Prospective observational study. *Br Med J* 2000; **321**: 412–9.

237. Mogensen CE, Keane WF, Bennett PF, *et al*. Prevention of diabetic renal disease with special reference to microalbuminuria. *Lancet* 1995; **346**: 1080–4.

238. Skinner S, Kelley D, Moravski C, Cooper M, Wilkinson-Berka J. Retinal renin and proliferative retinopathy. *Am J Hypertens* 1998; **11**(4), part 2: 236a.

♦239. Estacio RO, Jeffers BW, Hiatt WR, Biggerstaff SL, Gifford N, Schrier RW. The effect of nisoldipine as compared with enalapril on cardiovascular outcomes in patients with non-insulin-dependent diabetes and hypertension. *N Engl J Med* 1998; **338**: 645–52.

240. Tatti P, Pahor M, Byington R, DiMauro P, Guarisco R, Strollo G, Strollo F. Outcome results of the fosinopril versus amlodipine cardiovascular events randomized trial (FACET) in patients with hypertension and NIDDM. *Diabetes Care* 1998; **21**(4): 597.

♦241. Heart Outcomes Prevention Evaluation (HOPE) Study Investigators. Effects of ramipril on cardiovascular and microvascular outcomes in people with diabetes mellitus. Results of the HOPE study and MICRO-HOPE substudy. *Lancet* 2000; **355**: 253–9.

242. Weidmann P, Schneider M, Bohlen L. Therapeutic efficacy of different antihypertensive drugs in human diabetic nephropathy: an updated meta-analysis. *Nephrol Dial Transplant* 1995; **10**(suppl 9): 39–45.

♦243. Bakris GL, Copley JB, Vicknair N, Sadler R, Leurgans S. Calcium channel blockers versus other antihypertensive therapies on progression of NIDDM associated nephropathy. *Kidney Int* 1996; **50**: 1641–50.

♦244. Sowers J. Comorbidity of hypertension and diabetes: The Fosinopril versus Amlodipine Cardiovascular Events Trial (FACET). *Am J Cardiol* 1998; **82**: 15R–19R.

244a.Fixler DE, Laird WP, Ptizgerald V, *et al*. Hypertension screening in schools: results of the Dallas study. *Pediatrics* 1979; **63**: 32–6.

245. Rames LK, Clarke WR, Connor WE, *et al*. Normal blood pressures and the evaluation of sustained blood pressure elevation in childhood: the Muscatine study. *Pediatrics* 1978; **61**: 245–51.

○246. Sinaiko AR. Hypertension in children. *N Engl J Med* 1996; **335**: 1968–73.

○247. National High Blood Pressure Education Program Working Group on Hypertension Control in Children and Adolescents. Update on the 1987 task force report on high blood pressure in children and adolescents: a working group report from the National High Blood Pressure Education Program. *Pediatrics* 1996; **98**: 649–58.

○248. Setaro JF, Black HR. Refractory hypertension. *N Engl J Med* 1992; **327**: 543–7.

249. Joint National Committee on Prevention, Detection, Evaluation, and Treatment of High Blood Pressure. The sixth report of the Joint National Committee on Prevention, Detection, Evaluation and Treatment of High Blood Pressure. (JNC VI). *Arch Intern Med* 1997; **157**: 2413–46.

♦250. Yakovlevitch M, Black HR. Resistant hypertension in a tertiary care clinic. *Arch Intern Med* 1991; **151**: 1786–92.

251. Shea S, Misra D, Ehrlich MH, *et al*. Predisposing factors for severe, uncontrolled hypertension in an inner-city minority population. *N Engl J Med* 1992; **327**: 776–81.

252. Redon J, Campo C, Lozano JV, *et al*. Prognostic value of ambulatory blood pressure monitoring in refractory hypertension. *Am J Hypertens* 1997; **10**(2): 6A (abstract).

253. Pontremoli R, Robaudo C, Gaiter A, *et al*. Long-term minoxidil treatment in refractory hypertension and renal failure. *Clin Nephrol* 1991; **35**: 39–43.

○254. Kitiyakara C, Guzman NJ. Malignant hypertension and hypertensive emergencies. *J Am Soc Nephrol* 1998; **9**: 133–42.

○255. Calhoun DA, Oparil S. Treatment of hypertensive crisis. *N Engl J Med* 1990; **323**: 1177–83.

256. Strandgaard S, Olesen J, Skinhfj, Lassen NA. Autoregulation of brain circulation in severe aterial hypertension. *Br Med J* 1973; **1**: 507–10.

257. Ledingham JGG, Rajagopalan B. Cerebral complications in the treatment of accelerated hypertension. *Q J Med N S* XLVIII 1979; **189**: 25–41.

258. Fagan TC. Acute reduction of blood pressure in asymptomatic patients with severe hypertension: an idea whose time has come and gone. *Arch Intern Med* 1989; **149**: 2169–70.

259. Rehman F, Mansoor GA, White WB. 'Inappropriate' physician habits in prescribing oral nifedipine capsules in hospitalized patients. *Am J Hypertens* 1996; **9**: 1035–9.

260. Grossman E, Messerli FH, Grodzicki T, Kowey P. Should a moratorium be placed on sublingual nifedipine capsules given for hypertensive emergencies and pseudoemergencies? *JAMA* 1996; **276**: 1328–31.

○261. Estafanous FG. Hypertension in the surgical patient: management of blood pressure and anesthesia. *Clev Clin J Med* 1989; **56**: 384–93.

○262. Eagle KA, Brundage BH, Chaitman BR, *et al*. Guidelines for perioperative cardiovascular evaluation for noncardiac surgery: report of the American College of Cardiology/American Heart Association Task Force on Practice Guidelines (Committee on Perioperative Cardiovascular Evaluation for Noncardiac Surgery). *J Am Coll Cardiol* 1996; **27**: 910–48.

♦263. Mangano DT, Layug EL, Wallace A, Tateo I, for the Multicenter Study of Perioperative Ischemia Research Group. Effect of antenlol on mortality and cardiovascular morbidity after noncardiac surgery. *N Engl J Med* 1996; **335**: 1713–20.

264. Riles TS, Fisher FS, Schaefer S, Pasternack PF, Baumann FG. Plasma catecholamine concentrations during abdominal aortic aneurysm surgery: the link to perioperative myocardial ischemia. *Ann Vasc Surg* 1993; **7**: 213–19.

265. Volini IF, Flaxman N. The effect of nonspecific operations on essential hypertension. *JAMA* 1993; **12**: 2126–8.

266. MacMahon S, Peto R, Cutler J, *et al*. Blood pressure, stroke and coronary heart disease. Part I: Effects on prolonged differences in blood pressure. Evidence from nine prospective observational studies corrected for the regression dilution bias. *Lancet* 1990; **335**: 765–74.

♦267. Collins R, Peto R, MacMahon S, *et al*. Blood pressure, stroke, and coronary artery disease, part II: Effects on short-term reductions in blood pressure. An overview of the unconfounded randomized drug trials in an epidemiologic context. *Lancet* 1990; **335**: 827–38.

♦268. MacMahon S, Rodgers A, Neal B, Chalmers J. Blood pressure lowering for the secondary prevention of myocardial infarction and stroke. *Hypertension* 1997; **29**: 537–8.

♦269. PROGRESS Management Committee. Blood pressure lowering for the secondary prevention of stroke: design and rationale for PROGRESS. *J Hypertens* 1996; **14**(suppl 2): 41–6.

270. Britton M, Carlsson A, de Faire U. Blood pressure course in patients with acute stroke and matched controls. *Stroke* 1986; **17**: 861–4.

271. Lavin P. Management of hypertension in patients with acute stroke. *Arch Intern Med* 1986; **146**: 66–8.

○272. Gifford Jr, RW. Management of hypertensive crises. *JAMA* 1991; **266**(6): 829–35.

○273. Adams HP, Brott TG, Crowell RM, *et al*. *Guidelines for the management of patients with acute ischemic stroke*. American Heart Association Special Report, Dallas: American Heart Association, 1994.

274. Phillips SJ, Whisnant JP. Treatment of hypertensive patients with cerebrovascular disease. In: Izzo JL, Black HR, Taubert KA, eds *Hypertension primer*. Dallas, TX: American Heart Association, 1993.

275. MacMahon S, Rodgers A, Neal B, Chalmers J. Blood pressure lowering for the secondary prevention of myocardial infarction and stroke. *Hypertension* 1997; **29**: 537–8.

276. Sullivan JM. Treatment of hypertensive patients with ischemic heart disease. In: Izzo JL, Black HR, Taubert KA, eds *Hypertension primer*. Dallas, TX: American Heart Association, 1993.

♦277. Moser M, Hebert PR. Prevention of disease progression, left ventricular hypertrophy and congestive heart failure in hypertension treatment trials. *J Am Coll Cardiol* 1996; **27**: 1214–18.

278. Gibson RS, Boden WE. Calcium channel antagonists: friend or foe in postinfarction patients? *Am J Hypertens* 1996; **9**: 172S–6S.

279. Ryan TJ, Anderson JL, Antman EM, *et al*. ACC/AHA guidelines for the management of patients with acute myocardial infarction: a report of the American College of Cardiology/American Heart Association Task Force on Practice Guidelines (Committee in Management of Acute Myocardial Infarction). *J Am Coll Cardiol* 1996; **28**: 1328–428.

♦280. Sacks FM, Pfeffer MA, Moye LA, *et al*., for the Cholesterol and Recurrent Events Trial Investigators.

The effect of pravastatin on coronary events after myocardial infarction in patients with average cholesterol levels. *N Engl J Med* 1996; **335**: 1001–9.

♦281. Shepherd J, Cobbe SM, Ford I, *et al.*, for the West of Scotland Coronary Prevention Study Group. Prevention of coronary heart disease with pravastatin in men with hypercholesterolemia. *N Engl J Med* 1995; **333**: 1301–7.

282. Nyman I, Larsson H, Wallentin L. Prevention of serious cardiac event by low-dose aspirin in patients with silent myocardial ischemia. *Lancet* 1992; **340**: 497–501.

♦283. Koren MJ, Devereaux RB, Casale PN, Savage DD, Laragh JH. Relation of left ventricular mass and geometry to morbidity and mortality in uncomplicated essential hypertension. *Ann Intern Med* 1991; **114**: 345–52.

♦284. Liao Y, Cooper RS, McGee DL, Mensah GA, Ghali JK. The relative effects of the left ventricular hypertrophy coronary artery disease, and ventricular dysfunction on survival among black adults. *JAMA* 1995; **273**: 1592–7.

285. Messerli FH, Ventura HO, Elizardi DJ, *et al.* Hypertension and sudden death. Increased ventricular ectopic activity in left ventricular hypertrophy. *Am J Med* 1984; **77**: 18–22.

286. Messerli FH. Hypertension, cardiac arrhythmias, and sudden death. *Am J Hypertens* 1998; **11**(4), part 2: 250a.

287. Muiesan ML, Salvetti M, Rizzoni D, *et al.* Association of change in left ventricular mass with prognosis during long-term antihypertensive treatment. *J Hypertens* 1995; **13**: 1091–5.

288. Devereaux RB, Agabiti-Rosei E, Dahlof B, *et al.* Regression of left ventricular hypertrophy as a surrogate end-point for morbid events in hypertension treatment trials. *J Hypertens* 1996; **14**: S94–S102.

289. Vasan RS, Levy D. The role of hypertension in the pathogenesis of heart failure: a clinical mechanistic overview. *Arch Intern Med* 1996; **156**: 1789–96.

♦290. Levy D, Larson MG, Vasan RS, *et al.* The progression from hypertension to congestive heart failure. *JAMA* 1996; **275**: 1557–62.

○291. Kannel WB, Ho K, Thom T. Changing epidemiological features of cardiac failure. *Br Heart J* 1994; **72**(suppl): S3–S9.

○292. Vasan RS, Levy D. The role of hypertension in the pathogenesis of heart failure. *Arch Intern Med* 1996; **156**: 1789–96.

♦293. Pitt B, Segal R, Martinez FA, *et al.*, for the ELITE Study Investigators. Randomized trial of losartan versus captopril in patients over 65 with heart failure (Evaluation of Losartan in the Elderly Study, ELITE). *Lancet* 1997; **349**: 747–52.

♦294. Pitt B, Poole-Wilson PA, Segal R, *et al.* Effect of losartan compared with captopril on mortality in patients with symptomatic heart failure: randomised

trial—the Losartan Heart Failure Survival Study ELITE II. *Lancet* 2000; **355**: 1582–7.

♦295. Baruch L, Anand I, Cohen IS, *et al.* Augmented short and long-term hemodynamic and hormonal effects of an angiotensin receptor blocker added to angiotensin converting enzyme inhibitor therapy in patients with heart failure. Vasodilator Heart Failure Trial (V-HeFT) Study Group. *Circulation* 1999; **99**: 2658–64.

♦296. Cohn JN, Archibald DG, Ziesche S, *et al.* Effect on vasodilator therapy on mortality in chronic congestive heart failure. Results of a Veterans Administration Cooperative Study. *N Engl J Med* 1986; **314**: 1547–52.

297. Cohn JN, Ziesche S, Smith R, *et al.*, for the Vasodilator-Heart Failure Trial. Effect of the calcium antagonist felodipine as supplementary vasodilator therapy in patients with chronic heart failure treated with enalapril: V-HeFT III. *Circulation* 1997; **96**: 856–63.

♦298. Packer M, Bristow MR, Cohn JN, *et al.*, for the US Carvedilol Heart Failure Study Group. The effect of carvedilol on morbidity and mortality in patients with chronic heart failure. *N Engl J Med* 1996; **334**: 1349–55.

299. Australia/New Zealand Heart Failure Research Collaborative Group. Randomized, placebo-controlled trial of carvedilol in patients with congestive heart failure due to ischaemic heart disease. *Lancet* 1997; **349**: 375–80.

300. Anonymous. The Cardiac Insufficiency Bisoprolol Study II (CIBIS-II): a randomised trial. *Lancet* 1999; **353**: 9–13.

♦301. Pitt B, Zannad F, Remme W, *et al.* The effect of spironolactone on morbidity and mortality in patients with severe heart failure. *N Engl J Med* 1999; **341**: 709–17.

♦302. Rouleau J, Pfeffer M, Stewart D, *et al.* Comparison of vasopeptidase inhibitor, omapatrilat and lisinopril on exercise tolerance and morbidity in patients with heart failure: IMPRESS randomised trial. *Lancet* 2000: **356**: 615–20.

♦303. Gaasch WH. Diagnosis and treatment of heart failure based on left ventricular systolic or diastolic dysfunction. *JAMA* 1994; **271**: 1276–80.

304. US Renal Data System. *USRDS 1997 Annual Data Report*. Bethesda, MD: National Institutes of Health, National Institute of Diabetes and Digestive and Kidney Diseases, April 1997.

305. Buckalew VM Jr, Berg RL, Wang S-R, *et al.* Prevalence of hypertension in 1,795 subjects with chronic renal disease: the modification of diet in renal disease study baseline cohort. *Am J Kidney Dis* 1996; **28**: 811–21.

○306. Preston RA, Singer I, Epstein M. Renal parenchymal hypertension: current concepts of pathogenesis and management. *Arch Intern Med* 1996; **156**: 602–11.

307. Perry HM Jr, Miller JP, Fornoff JR, *et al.* Early predictors of 15-year end-stage renal disease in hypertensive patients. *Hypertension* 1995; **25**: 587–94.

◆308. Klag MJ, Whelton PK, Randall BL, *et al*. Blood pressure and end-stage renal disease in men. *N Engl J Med* 1996; **334**: 13–18.

○309. National High Blood Pressure Education Program Working Group. 1995 update of the working group reports on chronic renal failure and renovascular hypertension. *Arch Intern Med* 1996; **156**: 1938–47.

310. Culleton BF, Larson MG, Wilson PWF, Evans JC, Parfrey PS, Levy D. Cardiovascular disease and mortality in a community-based cohort with mild renal insufficiency. *Kidney Int* 1999; **56**: 2214–19.

311. Shulman NB, Ford CE, Hall WD, Blaufox MD, Simon D, Langford HG, Schneider KA. Prognostic value of serum creatinine and effect of treatment of hypertension on renal function. Results from the Hypertension Detection and Follow-up Program. The Hypertension Detection and Follow-up Program Cooperative Group. *Hypertension* 1989; **13**(Suppl 5): 1180–93.

312. Ruilope L, Salvetti A, Jamerson K, *et al*. Renal function and intensive lowering of blood pressure in hypertensive participants of the Hypertension Optimal Treatment (HOT) Study. *J Am Soc Nephrol* 2001; **12**: 218–25.

313. Toto RD, Mitchell HC, Smith RD, *et al*. 'Strict' blood pressure control and progression of renal disease in hypertensive nephrosclerosis. *Kidney Int* 1995; **48**: 851–9.

◆314. Peterson JC, Adler S, Burkart JM, *et al*. Blood pressure control, proteinuria, and the progression of renal disease. The modification of diet in renal disease study. *Ann Intern Med* 1995; **123**: 754–62.

○315. Weir M, Dworkin L. Antihypertensive drugs, dietary salt, and renal protection: How low should you go and with which therapy? *Am J Kidney Dis* 1998; **32**(1): 1–22.

316. Lazarus JM, Bourgoignie JJ, Buckalew VM, *et al*., for the Modification of Diet in Renal Disease Study Group. Achievement and safety of a low blood pressure goal in chronic renal disease: the Modification of Diet in Renal Disease Study Group. *Hypertension* 1997; **29**: 641–50.

◆317. Klag MJ, Whelton PK, Randall BL, Neaton JD, Brancati FL, Stamler J. End-stage renal disease in African-American and white men: 16-year MRFIT findings. *JAMA* 1997; **277**: 1293–8.

◆318. Klahr S. Mechanisms of progression of chronic renal damage. *J Nephrol* 1999; **12** (Suppl 2): S53–62.

319. The GISEN Group. Randomised placebo-controlled trial of effect of ramipril on decline in glomerular filtration rate of terminal renal failure in proteinuric, non-diabetic nephropathy. *Lancet* 1997; **349**: 1857–63.

320. Peterson JC, Alder S, Burkart JM, *et al*. Blood pressure control, proteinuria and the progression of renal disease. *Ann Intern Med* 1995; **123**: 752–62.

321. El Nahas AM, Masters-Thomas A, Brady SA, *et al*. Selective effects of low protein diets in chronic renal diseases. *Br Med J* 1984; **289**: 1337–41.

322. Apperloo AJ, de Zeeuw D, de Jong PE. Short-term antiproteinuric response to antihypertensive therapy predicts long-term GFR decline in patients with non-diabetic renal disease. *Kidney Int* 1994; **45** (suppl 45): 174–8.

323. Kakinuma Y, Kawamura T, Bills T, *et al*. Blood pressure-independent effect of angiotensin inhibition on vascular lesions of chronic renal failure. *Kidney Int* 1992; **42**: 46–55.

◆324. Giatras I, Lau J, Levey AS. For the angiotensin-converting enzyme inhibition and progressive renal disease study group. Effect of angiotensin-converting enzyme inhibitors on the progression of nondiabetic renal disease: a meta-analysis of randomized trials. *Ann Intern Med* 1997; **127**: 337–45.

◆325. Maschio G, Alberti D, Janin G, *et al*. Effect of the angiotensin-converting enzyme inhibitor benazepril on the progression of chronic renal insufficiency. *N Engl J Med* 1996; **334**: 939–45.

326. Ruggenenti P, Perna A, Gherardi G. Renoprotective properties of ACE-inhibition in non-diabetic nephropathies with non-nephrotic proteinuria. *Lancet* 1999; **354**: 359–64.

327. Van Essen GG, Apperloo AJ, Sluiter WJ, *et al*. Is ACE inhibition superior to conventional antihypertensive therapy in retarding progression in non-diabetic renal disease. *J Am Soc Nephrol* 1996; **7**: 1400 (abstract).

328. Hannedouche T, Landais P, Goldfarb, *et al*. Randomised controlled trial of enalapril and β-blockers in non-diabetic chronic renal failure. *Br Med J* 1994; **309**: 833–7.

329. Tolins JP, Raij L. Antihypertensive therapy and the progression of chronic renal disease. Are there reno-protective drugs? *Semin Nephrol* 1991; **11**: 538–48.

◆330. Zucchelli P, Zuccala A, Borghi M, *et al*. Long-term comparison between captopril and nifedipine in the progression of renal insufficiency. *Kidney Int* 1992; **42**: 452–8.

331. Epstein M. Calcium antagonists in the management of hypertension. In: Epstein M, ed. *Calcium antagonists in clinical medicine*. Philadelphia: Hanley & Beltus, 1992: 213–30.

332. Epstein M. The benefits of ACE inhibitors and calcium antagonists in slowing progressive renal failure: focus on fixed-dose combination antihypertensive therapy. *Renal Failure* 1996; **18**: 813–32.

○333. Brater DC. Use of diuretics in chronic renal insufficiency and nephrotic syndrome. *Semin Nephrol* 1988; **8**: 333–41.

◆334. Klahr S, Levey AS, Beck GL, *et al*., for the Modification of Diet in Renal Disease Study Group. The effects of dietary protein restriction and blood-pressure control on the progression of chronic renal disease. *N Engl J Med* 1994; **330**: 877–84.

335. Textor SC. Renal failure related to angiotensin-converting enzyme inhibitor. *Semin Nephrol* 1997; **17**: 67–76.

336. Mallamaci F, Leonardis D, Bellizzi V, Zoccali C. Does high salt intake cause hyperfiltration in patients with essential hypertension? *J Human Hypertens* 1996; **10**: 157–61.

♦337. Heeg JE, deJong PE, van der Hem GK, deZeeuw D. Efficacy and variability of the antiproteinuric effect of ACE inhibition by lisinopril. *Kindey Int* 1989; **36**: 272–9.

338. Bakris GL, Smith A. Effects of sodium intake on albumin excretion in patients with diabetic nephropathy treated with long-acting calcium antagonists. *Ann Intern Med* 1996; **125**: 201–4.

○339. Hostetter TA, Meyer TW, Rennke HG, Brenner BM. Chronic effects of dietary protein on renal structure and function in the rat with intact and reduced renal mass. *Kindey Int* 1986; **30**: 509.

340. Pedrini MT, Levey AS, Lau J, *et al.* The effect of dietary protein restriction on the progression of diabetic and nondiabetic renal diseases: a meta-analysis. *Ann Intern Med* 1996; **124**: 627–32.

341. Fouque D, Wang P, Laville M, Boissel JP. Low protein diets delay end-stage renal disease in non-diabetic adults with chronic renal failure. European Renal Association-European Dialysis and Transplant Association. *Nephrol Dial Transplant* 2000; **15**: 1986–92.

○342. Klahr S, Levey AS, Beck GJ, Caggiula AW, Hunsicker L, Kusek JW, Striker G. The effects of dietary protein restriction and blood pressure control on the progression of chronic renal disease. *N Engl J Med* 1994; **330**: 877–84.

343. Kasiske BK, Lakatua JD, Ma JZ, Louis TA. A meta-analysis of the effects of dietary protein restriction on the rate of decline in renal function. *Am J Kidney Dis* 1998; **31**(6): 954–61.

344. Gansevoort RT, de Zeeuw D, de Jong PE. Additive antiproteinuric effect of ACE inhibition and a low protein diet in human renal disease. *Nephrol Dial Transpl* 1995; **10**: 497–504.

345. Perneger TV, Brancati FL, Whelton PK, Klag MJ. End-stage renal disease attributable to diabetes mellitus. *Ann Intern Med* 1994; **121**: 912–18.

346. Borch-Johnsen K, Kreiner S. Proteinuria: value as predictor of cardiovascular mortality in insulin dependent diabetes mellitus. *Br Med J* 1987; **294**: 1651–4.

347. Breyer J. Diabetic nephropathy. In: Greenberg, ed. *Primer on kidney diseases*. National Kidney Foundation, 1998; 215.

348. DeFronzo RA. Diabetic nephropathy: etiologic and therapeutic considerations. *Diabetes Rev* 1995; **3**: 510–64.

○349. Hostetter TH. Mechanisms of diabetic nephropathy. *Am J Kidney Dis* 1994; **23**: 188–92.

♦350. Zatz R, Dunn RB, Meyer TW, Anderson S, Rennke HG, Brenner BM. Prevention of diabetic glomerulopathy by pharmacological amelioration of glomeruler capillary hypertension. *J Clin Invest* 1986; **77**: 1925–30.

♦351. Mogensen CE, Christensen CK. Predicting diabetic nephropathy in insulin-dependent patients. *N Engl J Med* 1984; **311**: 89–93.

352. Nelson RG, Bennett PH, Beck GJ, *et al.* Development and progression of renal disease in Pima Indians with non-insulin-dependent diabetes mellitus. *N Engl J Med* 1996; **335**: 1636–42.

○353. Breyer JA. Medical management of nephropathy in type I diabetes mellitus: current recommendations. *J Am Soc Nephrol* 1995; **6**: 1523–9.

○354. Ritz E, Stefanski A. Diabetic nephropathy in type II diabetes. *Am J Kidney Dis* 1996; **27**: 167–94.

♦355. Parving H-H. Impact of blood pressure and antihypertensive treatment on incipient and overt nephropathy, retinopathy, and endothelial permeability in diabetes mellitus. *Diabetes Care* 1991; **14**: 260–9.

356. Velussi M, Brocco E, Frigato F, *et al.* Effects of cilazapril and amlodipine on kidney function in hypertensive NIDDM patients. *Diabetes* 1996; **45**: 216–22.

♦357. Bakris GL, Weir M, deQuattro V, *et al.* Renal hemodynamic and antiproteinuric response to ACE inhibitor, trandolapril (T) or calcium antagonists, verapamil (V) alone or in fixed-dose combination in patients with diabetic nephropathy: a randomized multi-center study. *J Am Soc Nephrol* 1996; **7**: 1546.

♦358. Bakris GL, Weir MR, DeQuattro V, McMahon FG. Effects of an ACE inhibitor/calcium antagonist combination on proteinuria in diabetic nephropathy. *Kidney Int* 1998; **54**: 1283–9.

♦359. Andersen S, Tarnow L, Rossing P, Hansen BV, Parving HH. Renoprotective effects of angiotensin II receptor blockade in type I diabetic patients with diabetic nephropathy. *Kidney Int* 2000; **57**: 601–6.

360. Mogensen C, Neldam S, Tikkanen I, *et al.* Randomised controlled trial of dual blockade of renin–angiotensin system in patients with hypertension, microalbuminuria, and non-insulin dependent diabetes; the candesartan and lisinopril microalbuminuria (CALM) study. *Br Med J* 2000; **321**: 1440–4.

♦361. Diabetes Control and Complications Trial Research Group. The effect of intensive treatment of diabetes on the development and progression of long-term complications in insulin-dependent diabetes mellitus. *N Engl J Med* 1993; **329**: 977–86.

362. *Heart & stroke facts – statistical supplement for 1998.* Dallas, TX: American Heart Association, 1998.

363. Lonn EM, Yusuf S, Jha P, *et al.* Emerging role of angiotensin-converting enzyme inhibitors in cardiac and vascular protection. *Circulation* 1994; **90**: 2056–69.

364. Inagami T, Naruse M, Hoover R, *et al.* Endothelium as an edocrine organ. *Ann Rev Physiol* 1995; **57**: 171–89.

365. Krum H, Viskoper RJ, Lacourciere Y, Budde M, Charlon V. The effect of an endothelin-receptor antagonist, bosentan, on blood pressure in patients with essential hypertension. *N Engl J Med* 1998; **338**: 784–90.

366. Orth SR, Esslinger JP, Amann K, Schwarz U, Raschack M, Ritz E. Nephroprotection of an ET_A-receptor blocker (LU 135252) in salt-loaded uninephrectomized stroke-prone spontaneously hypertensive rats. *Hypertension* 1998; **31**: 995–1001.

367. Burnett JC. Vasopeptidase inhibition: a new concept in blood pressure management. *J Hypertens* 1999; **17** (suppl 1): S37–S43.

368. Weber M. Emerging treatments for hypertension: potential role for vasopeptidase inhibition. *Am J Hypertension* 1999; **12**: 139S–47S.

369. Lifton RP, Dluhy RG, Powers M. *et al*. Hereditary hypertension caused by chimaeric gene duplications and ectopic expression of aldosterone synthase. *Nature Genet* 1992; **2**: 66–74.

♦370. Geller D, Farhi A, Pinkerton N, *et al*. Activating mineralocorticoid receptor mutation in hypertension exacerbated by pregnancy. *Science* 2000; **289**: 119–23.

371. Lifton R. Molecular genetics of human blood pressure variation. *Science* 1996; **272**: 676–80.

♦372. Cambien F, Poirier O, Lecerf L, *et al*. Deletion polymorphism in the gene for angiotensin-coverting enzyme is a potent risk factor for myocardial infarction. *Nature* 1992; **359**: 641–4.

♦373. Marre M, Jeunemaitre X, Gallois Y, *et al*. Contribution of genetic polymorphism in the renin–angiotensin system to the development of renal complications in insulin-dependent diabetes. *J Clin Invest* 1997; **99**: 1585–95.

374. Harden PN, Geddes C, Rowe PA, *et al*. Polymorphisms in the angiotensin-converting enzyme gene and progression of IgA nephropathy. *Lancet* 1995; **345**: 1540–2.

375. Davis BR, Cutler JA, Gordon DJ, *et al*. Rationale and design for the antihypertensive and lipid lowering treatment to prevent heart attack trial (ALLHAT). *Am J Hypertens* 1996; **9**: 342–60.

376. Burt VL, Cutler JA, Higgins M, *et al*. Trends in the prevalence, awareness, treatment, and control of hypertension in the adult US population: data from the health examination surveys, 1960–1991. *Hypertension* 1995; **26**: 60–9.

♦377. Berlowitz D, Ash A, Hickey E, *et al*. Inadequate management of blood pressure in a hypertensive population. *N Engl J Med* 1998; **339**: 1957–63.

378. Sever PS. Blood pressure control for the hypertensive patient. *Am J Hypertens* 1997; **10**: 128S–30S.

PART 4

Advanced practice nursing

28

Advanced practice nursing: establishing a program and expanding roles in the current health care environment

MARIE BOSAK, THERESA MAZZARELLI AND JEANNE CORRAO

The design and implementation of patient care delivery models are driven in part by fiscal environments and available care providers. As health care reform alters the configuration of tertiary care facilities, the acute care nurse practitioner (ACNP) emerges as a valuable mid-level practitioner. Educated at graduate level, the ACNP conducts comprehensive health assessments, and demonstrates expertise in formulating clinical decisions required to manage acute and chronic illness. The University of Massachusetts Memorial Hospital has successfully integrated the ACNP into a patient care delivery model responsible for patients admitted for cardiac catheterization and percutaneous coronary intervention. The responsibilities of this practitioner and an overview of collaborative relationships in the model are presented.

THE ADVANCED PRACTICE NURSE: HISTORICAL OVERVIEW

Clinical expertise and specialization in nursing are long-standing. Historically, the nursing literature identifies four specialist roles: the nurse practitioner (NP), clinical nurse specialist (CNS), certified nurse midwife (CNM), and certified registered nurse anesthetist (CRNA). Each role has evolved along specialty areas of practice and is associated with a high degree of proficiency and autonomy.

The NP and CNS share a relatively short 30-year history (Table 28.1). The origins of each role stem from a need by both the recipients and providers of health care for nurses with clinical expertise to manage select populations in the ambulatory and acute care settings. Traditionally, the major distinction between these practitioners has been the practice setting.

Nurse practitioners are recognized as valuable providers of primary care in ambulatory settings.[1] The role emerged in the 1960s when a lack of primary care physicians resulted in medically undeserved populations. Nurse practitioners provide comprehensive, collaborative, and specialty care for individuals, families, and communities. The role affords independence and autonomy in activities of health screening, health promotion, and the management of patients during wellness and illness.

The clinical nurse specialist role originated in the 1950s for the purpose of improving nursing care provided to acutely ill hospitalized patients.[2] The role evolved along the lines of specialty areas of practice as new technologies altered and defined the configuration of acute care facilities. The CNS is responsible for the management of specific groups of patients presenting with complex problems. Additional activities specific to

Table 28.1 *Historical landmarks in the development of the advance practice nurse role*

1954	Rutger's University offers the first clinical nurse specialist (CNS) graduate program. Program specialty area of practice: psychiatric nursing
1965	University of Colorado establishes first nurse practitioner (NP) program for academic credit. Program specialty are of practice: pediatrics
1970s	CNS role identified as clinical expert in acute care facilities. Practice setting: critical care units, pediatrics, psychiatry
	NP role identified as valuable providers of primary care. Practice setting: ambulatory care
1986	American Nurses Association (ANA) Council of Clinical Nurse Specialists and Council of Primary Health Care Nurse Practitioners editorial suggests CNS and NP role responsibilities are similar prompting formal inquiry
1990	ANA Council of Clinical Nurse Specialists and Primary Health Care Nurse Practitioners merge, establishing the Council of Nurses in Advanced Practice
1992	ANA and American Nurses Credentialing Center (ANCC) require a Master's degree for NP preparation and certification
	ANA Congress of Nursing Practice approve the definition of advanced clinical practice
	Establishment of Acute Care Nurse Practitioner programs at Case Western Reserve University, University of Pittsburgh, and the University of Connecticut
1994	Nurse leaders and educators at the national level vote to support the merger of NP/CNS role in graduate education curricula
1997	Medicare approves third-party reimbursement of advanced practice nurse (APN) services

consultation, education, and research serve to effect the nursing care provided within an institution. The mission of an individual organization continues to delineate CNS role implementation specific to the institution.

In the 1980s, critical appraisal of NP and CNS practice responsibilities produced data supporting the fact that more similarities than differences existed between these roles.[3,4] Results revealed that the actual practice setting was the major determinant of role definition for nurses practising in a specialized role. The ensuing decade witnessed the movement of NP and CNS practices across formerly well-delineated boundaries. Nurse practitioners moved into acute care, while some CNSs obtained specific NP skills, including advanced physical assessment and prescriptive privileges.[5] Despite these changes, each role has become well established in a variety of health care delivery models.[6–10]

In 1992, responding to data confirming the similarities in the responsibilities of nurses in specialist practice (i.e. NP, CNS, CRNA, CNM), the American Nurses

Association (ANA) concluded that one broad title should encompass the four specialist titles. One intent of single titling was to clarify to health care providers and consumers the academic preparation and scope of practice of these specialists (Table 28.2). The title advanced practice nurse (APN) was selected and the following definition generated:

> Nurses in advanced clinical practice have a graduate degree in nursing. They conduct comprehensive health assessments, demonstrate a high level of autonomy, possess expert skills in the diagnosis and treatment of complex responses of individuals, families, and communities to actual or potential health problems. They formulate clinical decisions to manage acute and chronic illness and promote wellness. Nurses in advanced practice integrate education, research, management, leadership and consultation into their clinical role and function in collegial relationships with nursing peers, physicians, professionals and others who influence the health environment.[11]

Table 28.2 *Academic preparation and scope of practice of advanced practice nurses*

- Graduate degree in nursing
- Conduct comprehensive health assessments
- Demonstrate a high level of autonomy and expert skill in the diagnosis and treatment of complex responses of individuals, families, and communities to actual or potential health problems
- Formulate clinical decisions to manage acute and chronic illness, and promote wellness
- Integrate education, research, management, leadership, and consultation into the clinical role
- Function in collegial relationships with nursing peers, physicians, and those who influence the health environment

In addition to defining the title APN, qualifications and core competencies of APN practice were delineated (Table 28.3). Shortly thereafter, nurse leaders and educators at the national level moved to support the merging of NP/CNS roles in graduate education curricula. This reflected a growing sentiment among the profession that this combined APN role would bridge gaps between in-patient and out-patient settings, and between medicine and nursing to provide holistic and continuous care to specific patient groups.[12,13] In addition to preparing graduates to provide expert direct patient care, professional responsibilities associated with education, administration, consultation, and research were integrated into graduate education. One expected outcome is an advanced practice nursing role that is technically and clinically competent, flexible in collaborating across disciplines, and is highly marketable[12] (Table 28.4).

Table 28.3 *Criteria and competencies of advanced nursing practice. (Adapted from Hamric AB, Spross JA, Hanson CM. Advanced nursing practice: an integrative approach. Philadelphia: WB Saunders, 1996: 48–51)*

Primary criteria

- Earned graduate degree with a concentration in an advanced practice nurse (APN) category
- Professional certification of practice at an advanced level within a specialty
- Participates in a practice having a clinical focus

Core competencies

- Expert clinician
- Provides consultation and collaboration
- Demonstrates ethical decision-making skills
- Utilizes, conducts, and evaluates research consistent with graduate level of education preparation
- Performs activities as a change agent
- Demonstrates clinical and professional leadership

Table 28.4 *Common goals of advance practice nurse (APN) practice*

- Improve access to care
- Increase interdisciplinary collaboration within the health care system and between providers
- Expand the knowledge base for clinical decision making
- Provision of services in new arenas
- Increase professional autonomy and eligibility for reimbursement

ONE APN ROLE IN ACUTE CARE: THE ACUTE CARE NURSE PRACTITIONER

The role of the acute care nurse practitioner (ACNP) is to provide advanced nursing care across the continuum of acute care services to patients who are acutely or critically ill. The focus of ACNP care is restorative and provided within a collaborative model of practice (Table 28.5).[14] In 1995, the ANA produced the document 'Standards of Clinical Practice and Scope of Practice for the Acute Care Nurse Practitioner'. It delineates the scope, functions, and role of the ACNP in clinical practice, validating the practice of ACNP as a new role of advanced practice nursing.

> The ACNP assesses complex, acutely ill patients through history-taking, physical and mental status examination, and risk appraisal for complications. Diagnostic reasoning and advanced therapeutic interventions, consultation, and referral to other nurses, physicians and providers are intrinsic components of this role. ACNPs incorporate and apply appropriate theories to guide their practice. Care is provided using a collaborative model involving patients, families, significant others, nurses, and other health care providers.[14]

Table 28.5 *Role responsibilities and scope of practice of the acute care nurse practitioner (ACNP). (Adapted from ANA/AACN. Standards of clinical practice and scope of practice for the acute care nurse practitioner. Washington DC: American Nurses Publishing, 1995: 11–12)*

- To provide advanced nursing care in collaboration with patient, family, and members of the health care team to patients acutely or critically ill
- ACNP care is continuous and comprehensive, and provided across the continuum of acute care services
- ACNP assessment includes the health history and risk appraisal; physical and mental status examination
- Intrinsic components of the role include: diagnostic reasoning, advanced therapeutic interventions, consultation and referral to other direct care providers
- The short-term goal of ACNP care is stabilization of the patient, minimizing complications, and providing physical and psychological care measures
- The long-term goals of ACNP care is to restore maximal health potential while evaluating risk factors in achieving this outcome

The ACNP role has been described as a hybrid of the traditional CNS and NP roles. The advanced assessment and diagnostic skills traditionally emphasized in NP education combined with specialty practice, and clinical teaching skills traditionally emphasized in CNS education, have become requisites for the ACNP to be effective on an interdisciplinary health care team in the complex and diverse hospital setting.[15] Responsibilities of the ACNP vary by specialty and institution setting. The scope of ACNP practice is determined by many variables, most importantly, individual state Nurse Practice Acts (Table 28.6).

Health delivery models using advance practice nurses to provide care to acutely ill patients are not new. Recognition of APNs as valuable and viable mid-level practitioners is gaining momentum as health care reform alters the environment of tertiary care facilities. One of the most striking recent changes is the decline in the number of resident and fellowship positions in medical specialities. This is intended to accommodate changes in medical education programs committed to preparing physicians in primary care. Within existing residency programs there is increased emphasis on out-

Table 28.6 *Variables directing the scope of practice for the acute care nurse practitioner*

- Patient population
- Practice setting
- State legislation
- State Nurse Practice Acts
- Professional standards of practice set forth by specific specialty organizations

patient educational experiences.[16–18] The ramifications of this for institutions with academic affiliations is the maintenance of in-patient care services with a decreasing number of direct care providers. This one factor has contributed to the unprecedented growth of APN practice models in the acute care setting.

In response to anticipated shortages of primary health care providers, the American College of Physicians Task Force on Physician Supply examined the roles of NPs and physicians assistants as mid-level providers.[19] Both are viewed favorably as participants in models of collaborative practice. The College supports expanded roles for NPs and physician's assistants working in hospital and ambulatory settings as substitutes for physician house staff. Recommendations to explore the development of joint continuing education programs with these practitioners is valued by the American College of Physicians and intended to foster collaborative practice models.

There are various organizational models incorporating the ACNP in acute care. Three models predominate: the physician practice model, the nursing model, and the joint practice model.[20] While the scope of clinical practice may be similar, the models vary in reporting and fiscal responsibilities.

In a physician practice model, the ACNP is hired by a physician or group practice. Reporting responsibilities are to the practice members. ACNP responsibilities may encompass patient assessment during hospitalization to follow-up care post-discharge. In the nursing model, the ACNP reports to nursing leadership within the institution. The ACNP may be placed in a particular clinical area requiring the expertise of advanced practice nursing. In addition to direct care responsibilities, the ACNP may be expected to participate in organizational planning activities, such as quality improvement projects. Finally, the joint-practice model is a model of collaborative practice. The ACNP and physician have shared responsibilities in assessing and managing patient care. In this model, the ACNP has dual reporting responsibilities. Clinical issues are collaboratively addressed with the physician director, while issues relative to professional practice are directed to nursing leadership.

A MODEL OF COLLABORATIVE PRACTICE: THE CARDIOLOGY ACNP AT UMMC

Background

The university campus affiliated with the UMass Memorial Medical Center is a 384-bed tertiary care facility. In 1992, the Division of Cardiology was confronted by increasing numbers of patients admitted for diagnostic and intervention procedures. The increased volume of cardiac patients proved logistically burdensome for the medical house staff and potentially compromised objectives of the institutions' medical residency training program. The dilemma faced by UMass Memorial Medical Center (UMMC) was how to best care for a procedure-based population, and continue to accommodate graduate medical education and the growing physician referral base from surrounding communities.

Several collaborative practice models were evaluated and served to guide the development of the Cardiology ACNP service at UMMC.[21,22] The Cardiac Medicine Interventional Model at Boston's Beth Israel Hospital had been established in 1988. It utilizes APNs to manage patients admitted for interventional cardiac procedures. The model is effective in moving patients through in-patient and out-patient systems, while providing comprehensive and continuous care.

More recently, a collaborative practice model at the University Hospitals of Cleveland was established. The Collaborative Clinical Service provides in-patient medical care without medical residents. The APN is responsible for performing history and physical examinations, establishing a plan of care in collaboration with the patient's attending physician, reviewing the plan with the unit's medical director, and facilitating the plan to discharge. Protocols are in place to guide clinical practice. Consultations are obtained if a change in clinical status warrants additional management strategies.

Responding to the need to change the way UMMC provided care to their procedure-based cardiac population, its Division of Cardiology identified a subset of patients to be managed in a collaborative model, independent of medical residents and interns. The goal of this collaborative practice model was, and continues to be, to ensure expert, continuous, humanistic, and holistic care within a fiscally responsible framework.

Patients presenting for elective cardiac catheterization and/or coronary angioplasty are admitted to an area of an existing telemetry unit designated the 'short stay unit'. The cardiology fellow, cardiology ACNP, and nursing staff, together with the attending physician, coordinate and provide care before and after the procedure, inclusive of facilitating discharge plans (Fig. 28.1). The management responsibilities of the unit are shared by a medical director and nurse manager.

The initial success of this collaborative practice service was validated by measurement of patient satisfaction. As part of a system-wide quality improvement project, UMMC used a modified Picker-Commonwealth Patient Satisfaction Survey to monitor the experiences of those having non-emergent coronary angioplasty. With a 53 per cent return rate, patients responded favorably to the caliber of nursing services provided before and after coronary angioplasty. Anecdotal information cited the positive impact the ACNP had on the patient's hospital experience or issues specific to health status. Cardiology attending and referring physicians, nursing staff, and hospital administrators consistently expressed satisfac-

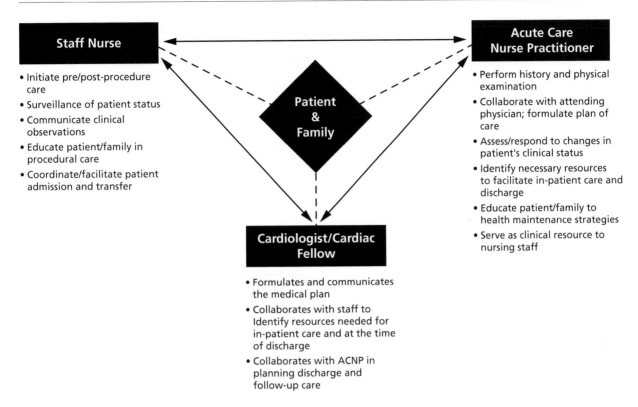

Staff Nurse

- Initiate pre/post-procedure care
- Surveillance of patient status
- Communicate clinical observations
- Educate patient/family in procedural care
- Coordinate/facilitate patient admission and transfer

Patient & Family

Acute Care Nurse Practitioner

- Perform history and physical examination
- Collaborate with attending physician; formulate plan of care
- Assess/respond to changes in patient's clinical status
- Identify necessary resources to facilitate in-patient care and discharge
- Educate patient/family to health maintenance strategies
- Serve as clinical resource to nursing staff

Cardiologist/Cardiac Fellow

- Formulates and communicates the medical plan
- Collaborates with staff to Identify resources needed for in-patient care and at the time of discharge
- Collaborates with ACNP in planning discharge and follow-up care

Figure 28.1 *Cardiac short stay unit – staff responsibilities.*

tion with the care provided by the ACNPs and their use of system resources.

The cardiology ACNP service proved effective in enhancing nursing care while appreciating a positive fiscal impact. Prior to the opening of the short stay unit, patients requiring arterial and venous sheaths were transferred to the coronary care unit (CCU), which augmented CCU costs. Once sheaths were removed, patients then transferred to the telemetry unit. The logistics of bed flow became increasingly difficult as the cardiac catheterization laboratory began to experience a 25–30 per cent yearly increase in interventional procedures. This placed a strain on CCU staffing and bed utilization. While the majority of patients undergoing interventional procedures did not require this level of critical care monitoring, they did require clinical expertise in prompt assessment in the management of complications after the procedure. The ACNPs worked with the short stay unit staff nurses providing education and standards of care for the management of arterial and venous lines, assessment and management of postprocedure chest pain and vasovagal episodes, electrocardiogram (ECG) interpretation, and arrhythmia monitoring. The outcome was an enhanced level of nursing care at the bedside, improved bed utilization, and improved utilization of staffing resources. Despite the fact that the majority of these patients no longer transferred to the CCU, this did not adversely impact the CCU census. After calculating expenses related to 'boarding' costs and

staffing patterns, a fiscal benefit of decreasing prior annual CCU costs by \$110 000 was appreciated.

This collaborative practice model at UMMC was developed with the advanced practice nurse at the forefront; however, the APNs utilized in the model have differed since the model's inception. This in part reflects the issues specific to APN role evolution discussed earlier and the needs of our particular organization. Initially, a clinical nurse specialist and primary health care nurse practitioner contributed to the model's development. It evolved into a model amenable to specialist practice and clinical nurse specialists were the APNs utilized. More recently, these CNSs achieved ACNP credentialing. The merit of this was viewed by the CNSs as being twofold. First, this credentialing was necessary to maintain autonomy as mid-level practitioners as defined by the state of Massachusetts. Secondly, UMMC's commitment to utilize ACNPs in other acute care settings warranted credentialing consistent with the institution's bylaws.

The UMMC Cardiology ACNP collaborative practice model evolved over time. Its development and implementation warranted numerous considerations (Table 28.7). Conquering the logistic barriers inherent in program development is only one part of the total process. The success of our collaborative practice model reflects the professional growth of the ACNP role, the strength of collaborative relationships established by the ACNP (Fig. 28.2) and a commitment by the Division of Cardiology and UMMC to the advanced practice nurse.

Table 28.7 *Issues for consideration in establishing a collaborative practice model utilizing the advanced practice nurse (APN) role*

- Assess the organization's mission and goals:
  What are the needs of both the patient population and the organization?
- Examine State Nurse Practice Act:
  Are there specific regulations/restrictions of APN scope of practice?
  Does the NP and CNS have limitations in their prescriptive authority?
- Examine State Board of Medicine regulations:
  What are the responsibilities of the supervising physician for mid-level practitioners?
- Review institution bylaws:
  Is the language specific to mid-level practitioners current?
- Determine funding sources
- Select a clinical practice model:
  Does it delineate medical and nursing leadership responsibilities?
  Where is the APN placed in the organization?
  What is the reporting structure for the APN?
- Delineate staffing patterns:
  What is anticipated level of acuity?
  Who provides off hour coverage?
- Generate and approve guidelines for clinical practice:
  How will emergencies, triaging, and changes in patient acuity be managed?
  Are conditions which require consultation identified?
- Introduce and market the APN collaborative practice model to both within the institution and to referring physicians and agencies

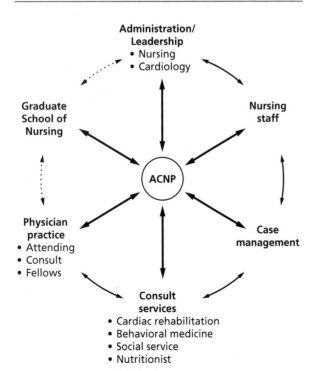

Figure 28.2 *UMass Medical Center cardiology acute care nurse practitioner service collaborative practice relationships.*

UMMC Cardiology ACNP Service

ADMINISTRATIVE CONSIDERATIONS

The Cardiology ACNP Service provides coverage 7 days a week, from 7.30 am to 7.30 pm. The ACNPs 'sign-out' their patient caseload to a physician who is responsible for off-hour coverage. The service is staffed with five full-time equivalent (FTEs) positions. Fiscal responsibility for ACNP salaries are assumed by the Division of Nursing. Staffing patterns typically comprise two to three ACNPs scheduled Monday through Friday. One ACNP provides weekend coverage. On average, daily census ranges from 14 to 22 patients.

Within the organizational structure, the ACNPs report directly to the medical director of the short stay unit. Regularly scheduled meetings afford time to discuss clinical and administrative issues. ACNP performance reviews are the responsibility of the medical director. There is a component of peer review among the ACNPs within the group. The ACNPs maintain less formal reporting lines to the director of the Division of Cardiology and to the director of Cardiovascular Medicine Patient Care Services, the latter having responsibilities of nurse manager for the short stay unit.

Clinical considerations

PATIENT SELECTION

In recognition of the high level of clinical expertise and initial success of the earliest model, the cardiology attending physicians and ACNPs have expanded upon the acuity of cardiac patients admitted to the service. Patients are admitted to the Cardiology ACNP Service from varied points in the system and with varied diagnoses (Table 28.8).

The majority of patients are admitted electively or transferred from an outside facility for a diagnostic or interventional procedure. Those presenting to the emergency department or cardiovascular clinic with unstable angina, congestive heart failure, or dysrhythmias without hemodynamic compromise may be admitted to the service. Another significant population are the patients leaving the CCU after a myocardial infarction. Upon transfer, ACNP care is focused on refinement of medication regime, patient education, and management of physical and psychosocial sequela of the cardiac event.

Triage decisions are made jointly by the cardiology attending physician and the ACNP. Considerations for admitting a patient to a resident house staff team include hemodynamic instability, clinical situations requiring frequent orders or assessment (particularly if needed during off-hour ACNP coverage) or when clinical presentation is deemed an interesting case with much learning potential for the resident team. Collaborative assessment of patient census and level of acuity by the

Table 28.8 *Overview of the cardiology acute care nurse practitioner service*

Point of admission	Admission diagnoses	Related procedures/interventions
Elective 'same day' admission Transfer from outlying hospital Intra-hospital areas: • Emergency department • Coronary care unit • Ambulatory clinics	Unstable angina R/O myocardial infarction Post-myocardial infarction: • Requires cardiac rehabilitation • Requires coronary revascularization Cardiac dysrhythmias Congestive heart failure	Cardiac catheterization Coronary revascularization Interventional procedures: • Angioplasty • Stent placement • Atherectomy Cardiac surgery: • Bypass grafting • Valve replacement Electrophysiology studies/procedures: • Radiofreqency catheter ablation • Pacemaker insertion/revision • ICD placement/revision • Cardioversion: chemical or electrical

R/O = rule out; ICD = implantable cardioverter defibrillator.

attending physician and ACNP is given consideration when admitting to either the resident or ACNP Service.

UMMC cardiology ACNP practice responsibilities

DIRECT CARE/PATIENT MANAGEMENT

Patient management is the core of the ACNP role. The ACNP collaborates with the attending cardiologist in performing the history and physical examination, communicating the findings, determining goals for hospitalization, developing a therapeutic plan, and ordering appropriate diagnostic tests. Additional technical skills associated with ACNP practice includes performing procedures inclusive of but not limited to arterial blood gases, phlebotomy, and insertion of nasogastric tubes.

ACNP practice is directed to a large extent by practice guidelines. These are systematically developed statements based on available scientific evidence and expert opinion. Practice guidelines contain specific recommendations for care to be provided in various clinical situations or for individuals or groups of patient populations. Sources of professional standards of practice utilized include Agency for Health Care Policy and Reform (AHCPR) and American Association of Critical Care Nurses (AACN) guidelines, Advanced Cardiac Life Support (ACLS) protocols, and American Heart Association/American College of Cardiology (AHA/ACC) standards of practice. These serve to support the development of patient care guidelines specific to the cardiology ACNP patient population.

Health care team members are apprised of the plan of care via documentation in the patient's medical record and daily attending rounds. The ACNP, in collaboration with the attending physician, initiates consultations and referrals with other services contingent upon changes in

a patient's clinical status. Coordination of care is also facilitated by a case manager who is responsible for discharge planning, referrals to other facilities, utilization review, and making appointments for follow-up physician and/or clinic visits. Patients' readiness for discharge is assessed collaboratively but is contingent upon the attending physician's approval. The discharge process is expedited by the cooperative effort of the ACNP and the case manager, who share the responsibility of completing the required paperwork and arranging appropriate referrals. The ACNP writes necessary prescriptions, completes appropriate discharge summary paperwork, dictations, and patient care referral forms required at the time of discharge.

TEACHING/MENTORING

The ACNP is responsible not only for educating colleagues and consumers, but for mentoring students and health care professionals. All ACNPs have clinical faculty appointments at the University of Massachusetts Medical Center Graduate School of Nursing. Responsibilities include precepting graduate ACNP students in the clinical setting as well as classroom instruction.

Actively involved in staff development, the ACNPs provide in-service education, both in the classroom and at the bedside, for the nursing and ancillary staff. Instruction in topics such as hemodynamic monitoring, 12-lead electrocardiogram (ECG) interpretation, and cardiovascular assessment, has broadened the nurses' knowledge base while enhancing the quality of nursing care. The ACNPs have been instrumental in increasing the competency of the nursing staff of the short stay unit, thereby enabling them to care for acutely ill patients.

Education of patients and families is a priority of ACNP practice. All patients are assessed for individual learning needs and appropriate teaching is instituted.

Patient and family education needs are individualized by the ACNP. Education focuses upon understanding the pathophysiology producing a change in health status (unstable angina, congestive heart failure, dysrhythmias), instructions specific to health maintenance strategies and symptom management, and assisting with referrals to community services.

Individual ACNP continuing education needs are met by attending interdisciplinary conferences. This is made possible by a philosophical and fiscal commitment from UMMC leadership. Additionally, the ACNPs attend daily attending rounds and grand rounds. These forums promote a high level of information sharing between the ACNPs and house staff. This socialization combined with the mutual exchange of knowledge serves to increase house staff awareness of ACNP expertise and foster interdisciplinary collaboration.

LEADERSHIP

The leadership provided by the ACNP at UMMC is primarily through clinical education and role modeling interdisciplinary collaboration. Although ACNPs are not involved in management or evaluation of staff, they are aware of nursing issues and either formally or informally participate in problem-solving in conjunction with the Director of Cardiovascular Services, nurse managers, and CNSs. There is a strong collegial relationship between the ACNPs and the unit-based CNS, which is characterized by active collaboration on professional nursing practice issues, quality improvement, risk management, and clinical education.

ACNP participation in committee activities and meetings is balanced with patient care responsibilities. Knowledge of systems management and change theory position the ACNP as an active and effective contributor to hospital-wide committee and redesign teams. For example, participation in the cardiac catheterization laboratory redesign team allowed the process of patient transfers from outlying facilities to be streamlined. Presently, a multidisciplinary documentation tool is being developed to minimize repetitive data collection while meeting all Joint Commission on Accreditation of Hospitals and Health Care Organizations (JCAHO) documentation requirements.

All ACNPs maintain membership in a variety of professional organizations, such as the AHA, the American Association of Critical Care Nurses, and the ANA. There is participation in the APN group at UMMC, which meets on a monthly basis and offers not only professional support but also continuing education programs.

Research

Presently, the majority of ACNP activities specific to research are at a collaborative level working with primary investigators conducting clinical trials. ACNP activities include identifying appropriate study candidates, limited data collection, and system management intended to ensure protocol compliance.

Despite initial limited experiences with independent nursing research, the ACNPs recognize their responsibility to identify clinical situations amenable to nursing research. One example is a study the ACNPs conducted to examine the risk of hematoma formation or bleeding relative to patient position after elective cardiac catheterization. This randomized clinical study, designed by the cardiology ACNPs and approved by the institution's investigational review board, revealed that patients could safely self-select a position of comfort in the immediate post-catheterization period without increasing the risk of bleeding or hematoma formation. The data supported favorable changes made in the nursing care provided after cardiac catheterization.

The ACNPs value participation in both nursing and interdisciplinary studies. The degree of participation is contingent upon individual interest, but nonetheless supported by all ACNPs on the service. It is projected that future studies will be generated from relationships with a doctorally prepared nursing faculty, physicians conducting clinical trials, and non-clinical staff involved in systems analysis. Areas of inquiry will include measurement of patient outcomes, clinical and fiscal efficacy of the ACNP collaborative practice model, and validation of therapeutic nursing interventions.

Evaluation

Individual ACNP performance is evaluated using a performance criteria tool generated by the cardiology ACNPs based on the ANA Statement of Professional Standards of Practice (Table 28.9). ACNP skills specific to direct patient care (assessment, diagnosis, outcome identification, planning, implementation, and evaluation) are accomplished through chart review and discussion. ACNP performance review is the responsibility of the medical director of the short-stay unit. There is a component of peer review, although it is less structured. ACNP activities associated with indirect patient care responsibilities (participation in quality improvement projects, systems management, education, consultation, collaboration, and research) are also evaluated.

Inherent in the inception of any new nursing role or care delivery program is the need to evaluate its impact on the health care system. This requires technical support to establish and maintain the infrastructure that will be used to gather and analyze selected data. Variables relative to clinical and system outcomes amenable to evaluation are identified in Table 28.10.

Table 28.9 *Cardiology acute care nurse practitioner (CACNP) performance criteria*

I. Standard: direct care

The cardiology acute care nurse practitioner (CACNP) provides advanced nursing care across the continuum of acute care services to cardiology patients who are acutely ill. Continuous, comprehensive, direct care is provided using a collaborative model involving patients, families, physicians, case manager, and other health care providers.

A. Assessment
1. Collects pertinent data using appropriate assessment techniques and supporting diagnostic information
2. Obtains data sensitive to cultural diversity, ethnicity, gender, and lifestyle choices obtained from the patient, significant others, health care providers, and the medical record
3. Performs ongoing data collection, acknowledging the dynamic nature of acute illness
4. Synthesizes, prioritizes, and documents the database in a retrievable form

B. Diagnosis
1. Derives diagnoses that encompass nursing and medical problems from the assessment data
2. Discusses, validates, and prioritizes diagnoses with the patient, family, and health care providers
3. Re-evaluates new or additional data as it becomes available

C. Outcome identification
1. Identifies outcomes consistent with current scientific knowledge and clinical cardiology practice guidelines
2. Formulates outcomes in accordance with the patient's present and potential capabilities
3. Communicates mutually formulated outcomes with patient, family, and health care team

D. Planning
1. Develops patient-specific care plans
2. Articulates diagnostic strategies and therapeutic interventions to the patient, family, and health care providers
3. Anticipates and addresses the continuing needs of the patient
4. Documents the plan of care in a retrievable format

E. Implementation
1. Prescribes interventions consistent with practice guidelines/protocols, institutional bylaws, and American Nurses Association/American Association of Critical Care Nurses (ANA/AACN) Standards of Clinical Practice and Scope of Practice for the ACNP
2. Performs interventions in accordance with advanced nursing level of education and practice
3. Documents patient's response to interventions

F. Evaluation
1. Provides ongoing evaluation of the patient's condition and responses to therapeutic interventions
2. Documents results and communicates findings to health care team
3. Utilizes quality indicators to assess the patient's progress toward expected outcomes

II. Standard: indirect care

The CACNP provides indirect care services to support patient care within the cardiology service line by participating in activities related to quality assessment and improvement, education, collaboration, consultation, and research.

A. Quality improvement (QI)
1. Participates in QI activities through interdisciplinary data analysis of clinical practice based on institutional standards/ guidelines
2. Recommends changes in clinical practice considering cost containment/effectiveness, length of stay, and patient satisfaction

B. Systems management
1. Identifies organizational barriers impacting on patient care
2. Participates in strategic planning within the cardiology division to provide structures and processes to optimize patient care
3. Participates in the development, implementation, and evaluation of practice guidelines
4. Facilitates the resolution of ethical dilemmas through individual or systems approach

C. Education
1. Applies teaching/learning theory to patient, family, and members of the health care team in order to influence patient outcomes
2. Acquires and maintains current knowledge in field of specialization (cardiology) and in advanced practice nursing
3. Disseminates nursing knowledge through presentations, in-services, and publications
4. Serves as mentors/preceptors for undergraduate or graduate nursing students, staff nurses, and others

D. Consultation
1. Serves as resource to nursing and medical colleagues in the area of specialization
2. Participates in appropriate interdisciplinary redesign committees

E. Collaboration
1. Collaborates with other disciplines and makes referrals to ensure continuity of care

F. Research
1. Evaluates current research findings and determines applicability to clinical cardiology practice
2. Participates in nursing and medical research activities

Table 28.9 *(continued)*

III. Standard: professional growth/role development

The CACNP engages in professional role activities appropriate to education, position, and practice setting, and maintains required credentialling

A. Maintains current knowledge in area of specialty (cardiology) through attendance at advanced nursing and medical conferences, continuing education offerings, journal readings, attending and grand rounds
B. Maintains educational standards required for advanced nursing/nurse practitioner licensure
C. Maintains requisite documentation for prescriptive authority as dictated by institutional bylaws and state regulations
D. Participates in professional organizations
E. Develops and implements plan for professional growth/role development
F. Maintains JCAHO-required competencies
G. Maintains certifications as ACLS and BLS providers

JCAHO = Joint Commission on Accreditation of Hospital and Health Care Organizations; ACLS = advanced cardiac life support; BLS = basic life support.

Table 28.10 *Measures of clinical and system outcomes*

Clinical outcomes
- Mortality
- Morbidity
- Complications
- Functional health status
- Symptom severity
- Patient satisfaction
- Patient knowledge level before and after discharge
- Patient and family psychosocial well-being
- Patient and family compliance with follow-up care

System outcomes
- Physician satisfaction with collaborative process
- Length of stay
- Recidivism rates
- Cost of care
- Hospital resource use
- Consultation requests
- Revenue generation
- Number of procedures

ISSUES IN THE EVOLUTION OF THE ACNP ROLE

Although the ACNP role is widely valued in the clinical arena, a plethora of issues must be addressed in order to promote further evolution of the role. Some of the critical issues include ACNP role confusion, organizational fit of the ACNP, prescriptive authority, cost containment and reimbursement issues, and practice settings.

Some members of the medical profession perceive ACNPs as 'physician extenders', who are attempting to assume more aspects of medical management. Clearly, many physicians are not familiar with the qualifications, academic preparation, and capabilities of the nurse practitioner.[23] They may confuse ACNPs with other mid-level practitioners, such as physician's assistants, who are legally bound to work under the supervision of physicians.

Much of the confusion and reticence on the part of the medical community can be explained by the multiplicity of titles inherent in advanced practice nursing. With all of the varying levels of advanced practice and diverse nomenclature, it is no wonder that physicians are reluctant to accept shared levels of care. Uncertainty of ACNPs' clinical abilities and lack of recognition or understanding of APN titles threaten the collaborative process, particularly in the acute care setting.[23]

Another consequence of role confusion is the lack of recognition of varying responsibilities between ACNPs, house staff, and physician's assistants. Overlaps in patient care management activities, such as taking histories and performing physical examinations, and prescription of diagnostic studies, treatments, and medications can foster a sense of competition. Resistance at the attending physician level may translate into non-support of the ACNP role with relationships being supervisory rather than collaborative. Ostensibly, the most effective method of education occurs when patients are admitted to the ACNP service, and referring, attending and house physicians experience the role first hand.

Placement of the ACNP within an organization warrants consideration. If ACNPs are hired and salaried by physicians, they may be discouraged from participating in nursing activities, thereby estranging them from pertinent clinical nursing issues and creating a loss of credibility among nursing staff.[20] In a model where ACNPs report to a nursing director, ties are strengthened within the nursing network. However, this relationship may be disadvantageous when nursing administrators are faced with budgetary constraints and downsizing, necessitating discontinuation of ACNP positions.[24] Most authors[20,24,25] recommend a reporting relationship to nursing administration with a matrixed line to physician colleagues, thereby allowing for coordination of care as well as evaluation of clinical performance.

Prescriptive authority varies widely from state to state and constitutes a potential burden to the implementation of the ACNP role. In some states, clinical nurse specialists are granted prescriptive authority upon completion of a requisite number of classroom hours of pharmacology, whereas, in other states, nurse practitioners have limitations on the drugs that they may prescribe.

Currently, there is no direct reimbursement mechanism for ACNPs. Although Medicaid and Medicare provide reimbursement of all health care providers, individual states control which providers are eligible, and many do not reimburse for services not provided directly by physicians.[26] Unlike nurse anesthetists and nurse midwives, ACNPs cannot bill patients or payers a professional fee for care they provide as part of a hospital admission. Hence, existing hospital in-patient reimbursement systems must cover ACNP services. This may be perceived as a barrier to the growth of ACNP practice in a tertiary care system that views the ACNP as another expense against a fixed revenue stream.[27]

Reduction of other expenses associated with hospitalization is the key to cost-effective delivery of health care. To the extent that the ACNP is able to demonstrate not only revenue-generating potential by allowing physician partners to expand their caseloads, but also cost containment by ordering fewer tests and interventions, and by decreasing length of stay, the added ACNP salary is justifiable. Relative to salary structure negotiations, nursing experts emphasize the importance of monitoring productivity by differentiating ACNP hospital care components from provider fee components that are reimbursed. Delineating contributions made by each provider through separate reimbursement would permit more accurate monitoring of actual costs.[23]

When viewed as physician extenders, ACNPs may be perceived as being more costly than house staff who work longer hours for lower salaries. Whereas the use of residents may be a less costly short-term option, the spiraling costs of health care are ultimately driven upward due to the oversupply of specialists produced by an overgrowth of residency training programs.[27]

Barriers to the scope of practice across various settings have created artificial boundaries and discontinuity of care. However, economic, insurer, and consumer demands are challenging advanced practice nurses to create new paradigms by expanding the spectrum of care beyond the traditional acute care system. The potential exists for the provision of a system of seamless services across the continuum of care. By virtue of educational preparation, advanced nursing practice experience, and specialization, the ACNP is a highly capable manager of the sequela of episodic illness. When placed strategically within the health care system, the ACNP can optimize patient outcomes across settings and boundaries.

Conclusion

Implementation of the ACNP role in cardiology specialty practice at UMMC has been a professionally and personally rewarding experience. Advanced knowledge coupled with pioneering innovation have gained the ACNPs prestige, recognition, and credibility from physicians, nurses, and administrators. As a result of this acceptance and support, the ACNPs have been allowed to remain autonomous in clinical decision-making while complementing the collaborative relationships with all health care professionals.

In marketing APN roles and present and potential contributions to administrators, insurers, and consumers, strong partnerships with APN colleagues must be maintained. Political proactivity in the legislative arena as well as familiarity with state regulations regarding prescriptive authority and reimbursement will benefit present and future advanced practitioners. This underscores the importance of educating health care recipients in the value of the advanced nurse practitioner in the acute care setting.

Removing legal, financial, and practice barriers to the APN role is key to actualizing its full potential. The advanced nurse practitioner's ability to develop innovative strategies in a strained, yet evolving health care environment, while supporting patient-focused initiatives, will ensure continued growth of the role.

SUMMARY

- Nurses in advanced practice are educated at the graduate level and are specialists in population-based care.
- Advanced practice nursing roles include the nurse practitioner, clinical nurse specialist, nurse midwife, and certified registered nurse anesthetist.
- Role responsibilities of advanced practice nurses include direct patient care, consultation, education, research, and leadership.
- The acute care nurse practitioner is one advanced practice role that has recently emerged in response to changes in acute care brought about by health care reform.
- The acute care nurse practitioner provides advanced nursing care across the continuum of acute care services.
- The UMass-Memorial Medical Center has successfully developed a patient care delivery model incorporating acute care nurse practitioners within the Division of Cardiology.
- Issues relative to prescriptive authority, reimbursement, and regulation of practice continue to be potential barriers to practice for advanced practice nurses.

REFERENCES

○1. Romaine-Davis A. *Advanced practice nurses: education, roles, trends*. Sudbury, MA: Jones and Bartlett Publishers, 1997.

○2. Hamric AB. History and overview of the CNS role. In: Hamric AB, Spross JA, eds *The clinical nurse specialist in theory and practice*, 2nd edn. Philadelphia, PA: WB Saunders, 1989: 3–18.

3. Elder RG, Bullough B. Nurse practitioners and clinical nurse specialists: are the roles merging? *Clin Nurse Specialist* 1990; **4**: 78–84.

4. Forbes KE, Radson J, Spross JA, Kozlowski D. Clinical nurse specialist and nurse practitioner core curricula survey results. *Nurse Practitioner* 1990; **15**: 46–8.

5. Mastrangelo R. Merging the NP and CNS roles. *Advance Nurse Practitioners* 1993; 23–4.

6. Thompson MW. Clinical nurse specialist: making the shift from critical care to home care. *Dimen Crit Care Nursing* 1996; **15**: 40–7.

○7. Giacolone MB, Mullaney D, DeJoseph D, Cosma M. Development of a nurse managed unit and the advanced practice role. *Crit Care Clin North Am* 1995; **7**: 35–41.

8. Gates S. Continuity of care: the orthopedic nurse practitioner in tertiary care. *Orthop Nursing* 1993; **12**: 48.

9. Shultz J, Liptak G, Fioravanti J. Nurse practitioners' effectiveness in the NICU. *Nursing Management* 1994; **25**: 50–3.

10. Kegal L. Advanced practice nurses can refine the management of heart failure. *Clin Nurse Management* 1995; **9**: 76–81.

11. American Nurses Association. ANA definition of advanced practice registered nurses. In: *Capitol notes*. Kansas City: American Nurses Association, 1993.

12. Busen N, Engleman S. The CNS with practitioner preparation: an emerging role in advanced practice nursing. *Clin Nurse Specialist* 1996; **10**: 145–50.

13. American Association of Colleges of Nursing. *Nursing education agenda for the 21st century (position paper)*. Washington DC: AACN, 1993.

14. American Nurses Association, and American Association of Critical-Care Nurses. *Standards of clinical practice and scope of practice for the acute care nurse practitioner*. Washington DC: American Nurses Publishing, 1995: 12.

15. Daly B, Genet C. Influence of the health care environment. In: Daly B, ed. *The acute care nurse practitioner*. New York: Springer Publishing, 1997: 29–56.

16. Schwartz A, Ginsberg PB, Leroy LB. Reforming graduate medical education: summary report of the physician payment review commission. *JAMA* 1993; **270**: 1079–82.

17. Groeger JS, Strosberg MS, Halpern NA, *et al.* Descriptive analysis of critical care units in the United States. *Crit Care Med* 1992; **20**: 856–63.

18. Kindig D, Cultice J, Mullan F. The elusive generalist physician: can we reach a 50% goal? *JAMA* 1993; **270**: 1069–73.

○19. American College of Physicians. Physicians assistants and nurse practitioners. *Ann Intern Med* 1994; **121**: 714–16.

20. Parrinello KM. Advanced practice nursing: an administrative perspective. *Crit Care Nursing Clin North Am* 1995; **7**: 9–16.

21. Clark L, *et al.* On the scene at Beth Israle Hospital, Boston. *Nurs Admin Q* 1994; **18**: 10–37.

22. Genet C, Brennan PF, Ibbotson-Wolf S, Phelps C, *et al.* Nurse practitioners in a teaching hospital. *Nurse Practitioner* 1995; **20**: 47–54.

○23. Gedwill A, Mack S, Mlaker D, Vanek R. Actualization of the ACNP role: the experience of University Hospitals of Cleveland. In: Daly BJ, ed. *The acute care nurse practitioner*. New York: Springer Publishing, 1997: 141–70.

24. Lott JW, Polak JD, Kenyon TB, Kerner CA. Acute care nurse practitioner. In: Hamric AB, Spross JA, Hanson CM, eds *Advanced nursing practice: an integrative approach*. Philadelphia, PA: WB Saunders, 1996: 363–5.

25. Richmond T, Keane A. Acute care nuse practitioners. In: Hickey JV, Ouimette RM, Venegoni SL, eds *Advanced practice nursing: changing roles and clinical applications*. Philadelphia, PA: Lippincott, 1996: 325.

26. Lott JW, Polak JD, Kenyon TB, Kerner CA. Acute care nurse practitioner. In: Hamric AB, Spross JA, Hanson CM, eds *Advanced nursing practice: an integrative approach*. Philadelphia, PA: WB Saunders, 1996: 370.

27. Parrinello KM. An administrative perspective on the acute care nurse practitioner role. In: Daly BJ, ed. *The acute care nurse practitioner*. New York: Springer Publishing, 1997: 111–39.

29

Integrating managerial and clinical leadership: a successful nursing management model

JAY CYR AND TAMMY B RETALIC

The importance of the communication, employee relations and resource utilization role has been discussed both generically and more specifically in the cardiovascular service line of the UMass-Memorial Medical Center. Each of these role components is critical for the success of the director and the service line. Emphasizing one and neglecting another can lead to disruption of an effective program. The successful director must recognize the pivotal role they play in implementing a service line. Key to their success is providing both clinical leadership and managerial leadership and blending the critical elements of both areas of expertise into seamless leadership structure.

Managerial

CARDIOVASCULAR SERVICE LINE: A JOINT EFFORT

Introduction

Successful operation of a patient care service line in today's complex health care system requires input from both clinical and managerial nursing leaders (Fig. 29.1). With these two complementary professionals, a balance is maintained focusing on the best care with the most efficient use of resources.

Historically, in-patient acute care and intensive care units elevated the most clinically competent and willing nurse to the Head Nurse or Nurse Manager position. This practice was quite effective for many years during an era when the key requirement of mid-level nursing leadership involved helping to make patient care-related decisions at the bedside.

As health care has become more complex the ability to maintain both a clinical and managerial focus has become more difficult. Downsizing has led to the elimination of many nursing managerial positions, most notably positions at the Assistant Director of Nursing (ADON) level between the Nurse Manager and Director of Nursing. Work previously performed by ADONs has been pushed down to the nurse manager level in many nursing departments.

From a more clinical perspective, reductions in nursing departments have also led to a decrease in size if not complete elimination of nursing education departments. Here again, work formally performed by this group has been shifted to the unit or service-based clinical nursing leaders. Both of these changes have forced many nursing leadership professionals to focus on either the clinical or managerial leadership role.

This chapter has been structured to provide the reader

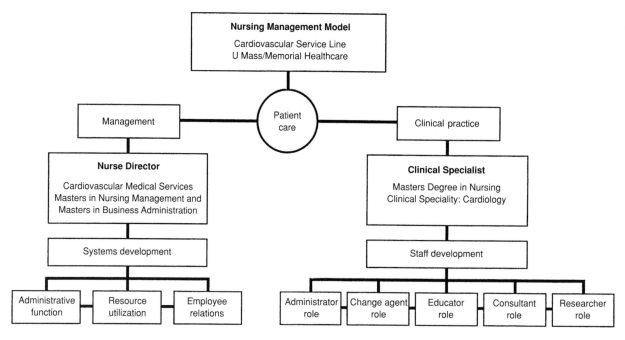

Figure 29.1 *Clinical and managerial operational structure for cardiac medical services. Success of this model requires two nursing professionals, one with formal nursing management training and education, the other formal clinical and teaching training and education.*

with an understanding of what is needed to operationalize the clinical and managerial aspects of professional nursing weaving together the principles, knowledge, and experience from both areas into an effective leadership team.

Evolution of the nursing managerial leadership role

Prior to the downsizing and merger activity that permeates health care today, most hospitals maintained a one unit–one nurse manager model for their critical care and acute care units. This philosophy stemmed from a practice that utilized the role as a liaison between daily nursing operations and medical practice. Forced to re-examine the nursing management structure as cost concerns became critical, many acute care hospitals began to investigate the possibility of a nurse manager overseeing more than one nursing unit.

Most often this process occurred through attrition. As a nurse manager resigned the position vacated was electively not filled. Instead, an existing nurse manager took on the oversight of the additional unit. As this process continued, it became evident that managers would be unable to oversee multiple units and maintain similar job functions as their predecessors or other managers with single-unit responsibility. Coinciding with this change was a need for nurse managers to become more involved in resource utilization. Both of these changes forced the nurse manager to give up many of their

bedside clinical duties and focus on more traditional management responsibilities, such as budgeting, staffing, scheduling, and cost accounting.

Interestingly, around the same time, many thought that the traditional nursing management role was an '*endangered species*'.[1] Initially, many nurse managers may have been offended by this concept and the above article. However, on closer inspection it has become clear that the prior nursing management role was outdated.

UMass/Memorial Healthcare experience

At the UMass/Memorial Healthcare (HC), the nursing management structure has been extensively reorganized. Originally the organizational structure consisted of a director of nursing, two associate vice-chairs, and 25 nurse managers. Administrative oversight of the in-patient units were divided between the two nursing vice presidents (VPs) with each nurse manager responsible for one unit.

Through a combination of attrition and position re-allocation, this structure was flattened to the present chief nursing officer and 11 directors of nursing services. Each of the directors report to either the chief nursing officer or one of two associate hospital administrators. This reorganization has effectively expanded the role of the former nurse manager and provided an avenue for direct communication with the associate hospital administrator level.

This change in organizational structure is exactly what

the aforementioned article alluded to, not an elimination of the nurse manager role but an evolution to a higher level of operation.

Cardiovascular medical services

Cardiovascular medical services at UMass/Memorial HC led the way in developing and operationalizing this innovative organizational structure. Through attrition and reorganization a director of cardiovascular medical services position was developed, who maintains direct-line supervisory responsibility for the 14-bed cardiac intensive care unit, a 52-bed cardiac telemetry step-down unit, a 12-bed cardiac diagnostic and interventional unit, a 14-bed critical care unit, a 25-bed acute care unit, the non-invasive cardiology laboratories, and the cardiology out-patient clinics. Additionally, the director of cardiovascular medical services acts as the nursing liaison for the electrophysiology and cardiac catheterization laboratories.

On initial glance, this reporting structure may look overwhelming; however, each section has a clinical leader who works directly with the managerial leader using a team approach to oversee the operations of each patient care area.

Regardless of the structure, effective nursing management requires a focus on resource utilization, employee relations, and communication. These three areas will be discussed at a general level and then the application to the cardiovascular service line will be addressed.

COMMUNICATOR ROLE: INTERDEPARTMENTAL COMMUNICATION

Nursing department communication

Transferring information throughout an organization is a difficult task but one essential for success. At the hospital department level, effective communication is critical but the number of employees, the complexity of shift work as well as staff working in multiple locations adds to an already difficult communication task.

Interdepartmental communication in the past was often left to the assistant director of nursing level and managerial counterparts from other hospital departments. Nursing leaders at this level attended department meetings where hospital-wide issues were discussed and often potential solutions examined. Unfortunately, much of the decision-making process was delayed as many of the personnel directly involved were outside the immediate communication loop.

Redesigning the nursing organizational structure has brought many of the key players into the communication loop, allowing for more streamline and effective communication and subsequent decision-making

regarding hospital-wide and nursing department issues. For example, at UMass/Memorial HC weekly nursing management council meetings are held. Two meetings per month are dedicated to nursing practice issues. These meetings are attended by the directors of nursing services, clinical nurse specialists, the clinical leaders in their service line and the chief nursing officer. These two meetings focus on the discussion of issues directly related to patient care and making informed decisions in a timely manner.

Once per month the meeting is opened up to other department heads (pharmacy, infection control, dietary, multidisciplinary service, etc.). Issues that require input from this group of hospital leaders are discussed and decisions made without undue delay. The final meeting is held with just the Directors of the Nursing Service Lines to discuss issues and make decisions related to service line operations.

Another aspect of the communicator role is maintaining effective links between the staff nurses and the director. As the role has evolved, it has become clear that the amount of time spent on any given unit is reduced. Any attempt to maintain the same physical presence allowed for in the former nurse manager role will be unsuccessful. Instead the new director of a service line must learn to communicate more effectively and more efficiently. Communication by walking around is an important part of the director's approach, as well as using electronic mail and even utilizing something as simple as a message or communication board. Additionally, the director must carry a beeper for in-house communication as well as a cellular phone, which is helpful in keeping the lines of communication open.

All of these communication tools assist the director in maintaining effective links with the staff in multiple units; however, if all communication is left to these mechanisms, the director may find themselves frequently out of the communication loop. Face to face formal communication forums are essential and must continue on a regular basis.

The Director of a Nursing Service cannot spend endless hours in staff meetings repeating the same information over and over. Efforts to streamline this mode of communication are critical for success. For example, prior to the implementation of the new model in the cardiovascular medical area (director of cardiovascular medical services (CMS)), the cardiology floor (coronary care unit) (CCU), acute care telemetry floor, acute care medical floor and cardiac interventional unit) had three nurse managers. In the past, the nurse managers held separate monthly staff meetings with their respective staffs to communicate information and discuss practice issues. Most of the information being communicated and the issues being discussed were similar among all three units. Regardless, the organizational structure at the time promoted multiple meetings each month on each of these units. At the time this process seemed to be an efficient and effective communication process.

Examining this process on the service line level instead of the unit level provides a perspective on the opportunities afforded through economies of scale. Now two staff meetings are held each month, the cardiac intensive care unit continues to have a separate meeting, and the acute care and interventional units hold a joint meeting. Both sets of meetings attract a large number of staff, providing a forum to discuss issues impacting the entire service line. Having a larger group focused on the care of the medical cardiology patient provides an arena for discussion of staffing concerns, quality improvement projects and their results, interdepartmental and intradepartmental relations, new policies, and other pertinent information.

In addition to the economies of scale this new organizational structure affords the cardiovascular service line, it also provides an environment that promotes input from staff with a range of experience, knowledge, and care perspectives. This meeting format has been very effective in assisting staff to better understand and accept the often difficult decisions in health care regarding resource utilization. However, this group also provides a strong patient advocacy voice when patient satisfaction or patient care issues surface.

Communication to other non-nursing departments in the cardiovascular service line has also been enhanced by this new managerial leadership model. Although all areas in the department focus on providing quality services to the cardiac patient, in the past these services and the employees worked in isolation to a degree, either through physical barriers or managerial barriers. Reorganizing this service and having one administrative person for the entire service has helped to break down the managerial barriers and recognize the limitations of physical barriers. For example, during Joint Commission on Accreditation of Healthcare Organizations (JCAHO) reviews, all employees in all cardiac areas were provided with the same information, regardless of service, in preparation for the site visit. Cardiac technicians, nurses, secretaries, nursing assistants, and other support personnel all understood the general patient and employee safety and documentation guidelines that were applicable throughout the service as well as knowing the specific issues related only to their area.

This communication approach was time efficient and ensured that the correct message was delivered during staff meetings and other discussions related to the JCHAO review. Results from this review indicated that clear and concise communication was the standard, and this practice yields positive patient care outcomes.

Another example of the importance of effective intra-departmental communication results from the never-ending changes in reimbursement. When these changes occur, action is required quickly in all effected departments to prevent substantial loss of income. Here again, having one unified administrative voice helps to keep individual departments abreast of new information and provides a change agent who can communicate any alterations in practice that must occur.

The director of CMS plays a pivotal role in both intradepartmental and interdepartmental communication. A key aspect of the role is functioning as a central conduit for communication among units in the service line and between hospital departments. Uniform and accurate information communicated to all staff in a concise and timely manner assists in the goal of improving patient care outcomes to all cardiovascular medical patients.

RESOURCE UTILIZATION ROLE

During the past decade, resources in health care have become exceedingly scarce. This is not a function of nursing personnel shortages, similar to the situation in the late 1980s and early 1990s, nor has this been a function of the unavailability of health care products. Unfortunately, the scarcity of resources in health care is due to a shortage of reimbursement for services. Since health care reimbursement issues are very complex and beyond the scope of this chapter, the following discussion will focus on the effect of lowered reimbursement not the cause.

Successful health care providers are able to provide high-quality care satisfying patients and families, while keeping the cost of this care reasonable, which satisfies payers. Deployment of resources efficiently and effectively has become the focus of virtually all health care organizations expecting to survive this era of rapid change.

One way that other industries have navigated the rough waters of change is by utilizing principles of economies of scale. Many industry leaders have implemented cost reductions and continued to provide a quality product by consolidating fixed resources and spreading their associated costs across a large manufacturing or service base.

In the health care industry these same principles began to surface soon after reimbursements began to decline. Initial efforts aimed at purchased goods engaged hospitals in re-evaluating their purchase practices, attempting to eliminate expensive individual unit-based buying and focusing on better controls, with the purchasing department orchestrating all buying.

These efforts were effective but the results failed to yield the savings needed to offset rapidly shrinking reimbursement. Enter a new era in the concept of economies of scale – providers joining together with the possibilities of real savings looming brightly ahead. As in many other industries, a service industry's fixed costs are negatively affected if patient volume is not maintained. Decreasing volumes were being seen across the country as the

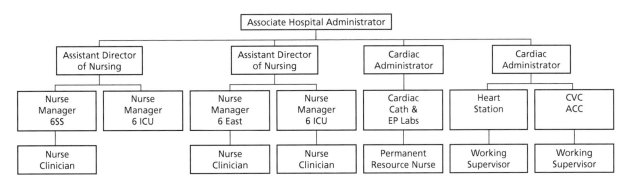

Figure 29.2 *Previous organizational chart for the cardiovascular service line. ACC = anticoagulation clinic; Cath = catheterization; CVC = cardiovascular clinic; EP = electrophysiology; ICU = intensive care unit; SS = short stay.*

average hospital length of stay was dramatically reduced and many services began to be shifted to the out-patient setting.

If efforts to reduce fixed costs could not be implemented, they would begin to consume an inordinate portion of the reimbursement dollar. With that understanding, it became imperative that consolidation or merger plans began immediately. Although large-scale merger operations have been the topic of much discussion, the focus of this chapter is taking the same principles of organizational merger and applying them to a service line, such as cardiovascular medicine.

Opportunities to reduce fixed costs and utilize variable costs more efficiently have never been more important. In the past, most patient care areas, in-patient or out-patient, functioned independently and to some degree in isolation. This type of operation utilized higher levels of fixed personnel resources than necessary. Although the development of the cardiovascular service line model was discussed above, the detail of its operations was not addressed completely.

Prior to the development of this model, the cardiac in-patient floor at our institution consisted of three separate patient care areas and required a nurse manager and nurse clinician in each unit (Fig. 29.2). Although this group worked well together, there was substantial

overlap in their job duties. Applying the same consolidation of resource concepts regularly applied in other industries, the leadership structure was reorganized resulting in one director of nursing services and three clinical leaders (Fig. 29.3). Concurrently, a fourth patient care area was added, which was folded into the leadership structure. This reorganization has reduced the clinical/managerial and support full-time equivalents (FTEs) from 8.2 in 1995 to the present 5.0 (Table 29.1) for the cardiac in-patient and interventional services. This decrease in total FTEs amounts to $214 452 in annual salary and benefit savings (Tables 29.2–29.4). However, this is only part of the total savings that result

Table 29.1 *Payroll cost reductions: change in clinical leadership*

	Clinical FTEs			
	6E	6W	6I	Total
Prior structure: FY98	1.0	1.0	1.2	3.2
Present structure: FY20	1.0	1.0	1.0	3.0
Cost savings	FTEs: 0.02			
Salary/benefits	$13 727			

FTEs = full-time equivalents; 6 E = 6 East; 6 W = 6 West; 6 I = 6 Intensive care unit; FY = financial year.

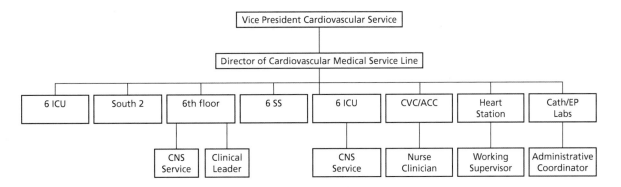

Figure 29.3 *Present organizational chart for the cardiovascular service line. ACC = anticoagulation clinic; CNS = clinical nurse specialist; CVC = cardiovascular clinic; EP = electrophysiology; ICU = intensive care unit; SS = short stay.*

Table 29.2 *Payroll cost reductions: change in managerial leadership*

	Management FTEs			
	6E	6W	6I	Total
Prior structure: FY98	1.0	1.0	1.0	3.0
Present structure: FY20	—	—	—	1.0
Cost savings	FTEs: 2.0			
Salary/benefits	$168 350			

For explanation of abbreviations, *see* Table 29.1.

Table 29.3 *Payroll cost reductions: change in clerical support*

	Clerical FTEs			
	6E	6W	6I	Total
Prior structure: FY98	1.0	0.5	0.5	2.0
Present structure: FY20	—	—	—	1.0
Cost savings	FTEs: 1.0			
Salary/benefits	$32 375			

For explanation of abbreviations, *see* Table 29.1.

Table 29.4 *Payroll cost reductions: total change*

	Clinical FTEs			
	NM	NC	Sec	Total
Prior structure: FY98	3.0	3.2	2.0	8.2
Present structure: FY20	1.0	3.0	1.0	5.0
Cost savings	FTEs: 3.2			
Salary/benefits	$214 452			

FTEs = full-time equivalents; NM = nurse manager; NC = nurse clinician; Sec = secretary; FY = financial year.

from re-organizing several patient care areas into a service line.

The savings from this reorganization come from both a one-time reduction in managerial/clinical leadership and support staff salary reductions, and the ongoing staffing economies of scale.

In addition to the salary savings, there is also a substantial reduction in staffing problems on the entire floor resulting from the ability to shift patient care resources where they are needed. Although the census remains high on the cardiac patient care areas, there are occasions when the census in one unit may be lower than normal. When this occurs, staffing resources are shifted to another unit if needed, and overtime or per diem can be eliminated or a staffing shortage can be averted.

Beyond the ability to reassign staff resources for an entire shift, the opportunity to shift resources at short notice and for brief periods of time is present. Frequently, patient care needs peak for an hour or two

during a shift. Utilizing overtime would be excessively costly, if available on short notice. However, without the use of overtime, patient care needs would not be met, leading to both staff and patient dissatisfaction. With the present managerial leadership structure resources can be reassigned without having to negotiate with several nurse managers from different units. The ability to react to staffing needs quickly (when resources are available) provides an economy of scales framework previously not employed in patient care services.

For example, a staffing shortage occurred in the cardiac intensive care unit. Help from the critical care float pool was unavailable but there was help available in the acute care float pool. This scenario is not uncommon at our institution, as the percentage of critical care beds to total beds is rather high, leading to frequent needs for critical-care float-pool support. To address this staffing situation, a nurse was sent from the acute care float pool to the telemetry floor. Next, a nurse from the telemetry floor was sent to the interventional unit and, finally, a nurse from the interventional unit was sent to the cardiac intensive care unit. At first glance, this floating scenario may seem complex and inefficient. However, on closer examination it becomes evident that effective cross-training enables nurses to care for patients competently at two and sometimes three levels of the acuity continuum, critical care (CCU), intermediate care (cardiac interventional unit), and acute care (telemetry floor).

Cross-training these nurses is an involved process but the results are worthwhile. Initially, some of the telemetry nurses volunteered to cross-train to work in the interventional unit. During cross-training, the acute care nurses were taught hemodynamic monitoring skills, enabling them to care for postangioplasty patients who have femoral sheaths in for several hours while awaiting their coagulation stabilization. Nurses in this area are also trained to monitor patients on several vasoactive intravenous medications. This first phase provided a pool of nurses who were competent to care for patients on both the telemetry floor and the cardiac interventional unit. This step was necessary as the cardiac interventional unit is only twelve beds, six beds utilized for out-patient cardiac catheterization patients and six beds used for same-day admit angioplasties or in-patient diagnostic catheterizations. Maintaining a full independent staff for this unit, which opens from 0600 to 2400, 5 days per week, would have been expensive and the fluctuating census would result in cost inefficiencies. Presently, there are 5.8 registered nurse (RN) FTEs permanently assigned to the unit and the additional needs are met by utilizing the pool of cross-trained telemetry nurses.

In the next phase of cross-training, several of the nurses who consistently work in the cardiac interventional unit were selected to be cross-trained to the cardiac intensive care unit. This was done for two reasons.

Cross-training staff provides an expanded pool of competent nurses capable of providing care to patients in the cardiac intensive care unit (ICU). This group of nurses is utilized when there is a need to fill an entire shift or if the need is to support higher acuity for a portion of a shift. In either circumstance patient care and staff satisfaction is maintained and the costs are minimized. In addition to the economical benefits and the benefits to the cardiac ICU, the nurses in the cardiac interventional unit have been fully trained to function independently as critical care nurses, this cross-training has helped them become better cardiac short-stay nurses, improving the overall quality of care in both areas.

Another method of reducing payroll costs comes in the form of an effective hire practice. As a regional tertiary care medical center, UMass/Memorial HC lures nurses who desire to practice in a fast-paced, innovative, professional nursing environment. Patients in need of the most advanced cardiovascular diagnostic and interventional treatments are referred to UMass/Memorial HC. Having the opportunity to provide cutting-edge cardiovascular nursing is a major factor in attracting top-level nurses from throughout the region.

As with many nursing departments, per diem staff are often utilized to augment permanent staff. Our practice of hiring only experienced critical care and acute care nurses with excellent clinical skills as per diem workers has been effective in supporting the staffing needs of the unit, while maintaining staffing and scheduling flexibility.

Per diem nurses are brought along depending on their ability to adapt to the medical center environment. Initially, they are assigned to stable patients on the unit. As the per diem nurse becomes more familiar with the flow of the unit and the permanent staff become more comfortable with his or her level of expertise, the nurse is assigned more complex and demanding patients. Eventually (usually after 6–12 months), the successful per diem staff nurse is allowed to care for more complex and challenging patients depending on the needs of the unit.

Additionally, an unexpected positive outcome of this practice has been the development of an excellent professional nursing pool to draw from when hiring permanent staff into the units. As permanent positions become available, per diem staff are encouraged to apply. Their clinical skills and work habits are well known to the staff, which provides a seamless transition from per diem to permanent staff status. Not only does this reduce orientation costs, which can range from $6000–15 000, it also greatly increases the probability of a successful hire. During the past 5 years, over $100 000 have been saved on orientation costs and 95 per cent (one nurse left due to husband's job transfer) of the nurses who make the transition from per diem to permanent status remain as staff nurses in the cardiovascular service line.

Maintaining an effective per diem pool and providing cross-training to permanent staff assists the cardiovascular service line managerial and clinical leaders in providing excellent clinical care to the patient in a variety of patient care settings. In addition to the human resource management issues that surface continuously, there are also non-payroll or non-staff related issues that, if addressed, can reduce waste of both time and money. Inefficiencies in general stores supply, capital equipment, utilization of clinical laboratory, radiology, non-invasive cardiology, and pharmacy resources lead to increased overall costs and dissatisfied patients, families, providers, and payers. A few examples warrant discussion.

Pharmacological intervention plays a major role in cardiac care. This is especially true in the critical care environment where patient acuity requires frequent and often expensive drug therapy. One area in which critical care nurses play a major role is the treatment of patients who are confused, disoriented, agitated, or withdrawing from alcohol or drug abuse. This patient population requires close monitoring and aggressive drug therapy to help minimize the impact of mental status changes, regardless of the cause, from complicating the treatment of the underlying disease process.

Providing accurate information regarding which drug regimens are effective from both a cost and clinical perspective can make a substantial difference in the overall utilization of payroll (additional RNs, constant observation staff) and non-payroll (cost of sedatives) resources. For example, providing information to staff nurses and physicians regarding the most effective methods of safely sedating critically ill patients can have positive financial and clinical outcomes. Unknowingly, many patients in need of extended sedation remain on continuous intravenous infusions of costly sedatives. However, both empirical data and literature reviews support the use of oral agents when sedation requirements extend beyond the initial critical time frame. A continuous intravenous infusion of lorazepam can cost upwards of $1500/day, while using oral lorazepam would only be a few dollars per day.

Implementing this change required the expertise of both the clinical and managerial nursing leadership. Obtaining information regarding the clinical effects and educating staff on this issue is clearly a clinical leadership role, while obtaining financial information and administratively initiating the change is more of a managerial leadership role. This is another excellent example of how both leaders can work together to improve patient care and reduce clinically unnecessary expenses.

EMPLOYEE RELATIONS

A final area that both the managerial and clinical nursing leader must be cognizant of is employee relations.

Probably the most important step a manager can take to maintain positive employee–management relations is simply being there. An absent manager will have a difficult time understanding staff concerns as well as trying to communicate management concerns to staff.

However, in a time when nursing leaders oversee multiple units, the ability to maintain visibility is difficult. For example, the director of CMS at the UMass/Memorial HC, as previously mentioned, is responsible for three cardiac clinics, six in-patient units, and is the nurse liaison for the cardiac catheterization and electrophysiology laboratories. These patient care areas are located on four different floors in two separate buildings. Maintaining visibility in these areas, some with 2–3 different shifts of staff per day is a strenuous task in itself. In order to maintain open lines of communication and visibility, the nurse leader must come in on off-shifts and weekends. This measure will help the director meet with staff on a regular basis to discuss hospital-wide and unit-specific issues, gain staff input in these areas, and maintain an open communication pathway. Meetings can be in the form of simple one on one discussions or more formal staff meetings held during off-shift hours.

In addition to attending staff meetings during off-shifts and weekends and coming in to meet one on one with staff, managers can also use other creative measures to maintain open lines of communication with staff. For example, recently the Coronary Care Unit Practice Council, comprised of staff nurses from all shifts, planned a meeting to discuss some nursing practice and employee relation concerns. Unfortunately, the director of CMS, who usually attends these meetings, was unable to be at the hospital at the time of the meeting (19:30), but was actually available at that time. In order to maintain the open line of communication, a speaker phone was brought into the nurses' conference room and the director was hooked up by telephone. Although this may seem unconventional, it allowed the director to hear staff concerns and partake in some important discussions. Without this creative approach, the above meeting would have had to have been followed by another meeting with Council members to be apprised of staff concerns without the director having the opportunity to hear first hand the discussions that ensued during the original meeting. This approach does not take the place of the traditional staff meeting but it goes a long way in maintaining positive employee relations through a show of commitment via creative steps.

Regardless of the mechanism, a high degree of visibility is a critical step in preventing staff and management becoming distant (resulting in miscommunication), misinformation (which can easily lead to resource – payroll and non-payroll – misuse and waste), employee dissatisfaction and, most troubling, customer dissatisfaction.

In addition to visibility, credibility is important in maintaining positive employee–management relations. If staff nurses and other health care providers see management as not listening and having poor follow through, then their credibility with these employees will suffer, leading to poor employee relations. Two major changes that occurred in the cardiac service line provides a good example of the importance of visibility, communication, and credibility.

An important issue developed and then redeveloped on the cardiac telemetry unit; at both times this required extensive and detailed communication with the staff. Approximately 3½ years ago, the cardiac telemetry unit underwent a staffing mix change. This change was due to fiscal constraints and a need to provide more personnel on the floor at all times. Originally, the telemetry unit was staffed with five RNs and two nursing assistants (NAs). This provided seven patient care personnel on the floor. A plan was developed to change the mix to four RNs and four NAs. This new staffing pattern provided more coverage on the floor, but would cost slightly less. Over the course of 4 months, this issue was discussed with the entire staff on the patient care unit. Meetings were held at all hours, including the night shift and weekends. Considering the controversial nature of this issue, it was important to ensure that each staff member had ample opportunity to discuss their concerns regarding this substantial change.

In June of 1995, the staffing mix change was made. Managerial and clinical leaders maintained a strong physical presence on the floor to answer questions and provide support. This staffing pattern was successfully implemented, in large part due to maintaining strong employee relations during a difficult change.

Although this staffing mix change was successfully implemented and operated for 2 years, several important changes throughout the institution over the past 2–3 years led to a need to re-examine the staffing pattern. Two factors that forced staffing on the telemetry floor to be looked at were the number of admissions and the consolidation of acute care floors. Owing to proactive steps taken by UMass/Memorial leaders, the number of admissions and patient days have increased over the past 2–3 years. This is quite remarkable at a time when many hospitals are closing and others, including university teaching institutions, are seeing dramatic decreases in admissions and patient days. In an effort to improve efficiencies, nursing units have been consolidated to capitalize on economies of scale. With this consolidation has come a higher volume of admissions per remaining floor as well as an increasing level of acuity. Both of these hospital-wide factors have affected the patient care requirements on the telemetry floor. Additionally, a decision to allow patients with continuous intravenous infusions of vasoactive medications on the floor has increased the overall nursing workload. These changes have led to the need to re-examine the staffing pattern on the telemetry unit.

Positive employee–management relations helped move this change along quickly. In addition to the pure number issues, other factors played important roles in this change. Comments from patients and family to staff and on patient-satisfaction surveys indicated that many thought the nurses were often too busy to address simple patient and family requests. Staff concurred with this customer observation, and were most concerned with their feeling of being unable to spend enough time with patients. Although satisfaction surveys indicated patients were pleased with the clinical care they received, it was clear that patients perceived staff to be rushed and unable to address some non-clinical yet very important customer satisfaction issues.

These insights have led to another change in staffing mix, this time to a five RN and three NA ratio. Although there are times when the four RN and four NA mix is used, the frequency is decreasing as new staff are brought on board. Without high visibility, credibility and communication, this issue may have resulted in untoward patient occurrences and loss of valuable staff members. Positive employee relations have led to an important change that will improve patient and staff satisfaction.

Clinical practice

INTRODUCTION

The nursing management model has a management and clinical component. The clinical practice component (Fig. 29.1) focuses primarily on the clinical practice and achievement of quality patient outcomes through the development of clinical expertise of nursing staff. Patient outcomes are the focal point of decision making. Each clinical and management decision should always consider the question 'how would this affect patient care?' Patient outcomes should not only be determined by the health care organization but through feedback from patients and families. By integrating both clinical and management roles effectively, achievement of patient-focused outcomes are possible. The clinical practice model emphasizes staff development as the main focus of the Clinical Nurse Specialists (CNS) role, not the direct patient care role, which was the primary focus in past models. This approach to staff development provides empowerment and increases the level of expertise that ultimately enhances quality care. We will explore the implementation of the CNS role components as it relates to staff and system development, and the achievement of patient-focused outcomes.

CNS ROLE COMPONENTS

So how do these role components guide the clinical nurse specialist in staff development? We need to discuss the concepts present in the clinical practice model and answer the question 'how can the CNS affect patient outcomes through development of staff and systems?'

Administrative role

The administrative role is a leadership role. This role helps shape and improve existing systems and deter-mines and initiates new ones. Within the nursing management system model, this role complements the director's role. Successful integration of management and clinical roles are necessary when implementing the nursing management system model. There are two components to an administrator role: management and leadership.

These two roles should complement one another: 'good management controls complexity; effective leadership produces useful change'.[2] Within this framework of management and clinical dimensions, there must exist a complementary situation. When management and leadership complement one another, productivity, value, and quality are attained. This type of relationship diversifies talents and fosters communication about the mission and vision of the organization. People can exhibit elements of both characteristics, although one dimension is more likely to be dominant. An overlap of the director and CNS roles most often occurs within this administrative function.

Communication and division of responsibilities must be established and updated by the director and the CNS to avoid duplication and provide efficiency within the management structure. An example of this delineation of responsibilities includes the following roles that the CNS oversees (rather than the director) from an administrative perspective: (1) adherence to Joint Commission Standards; (2) completion of performance reviews; and (3) acting as a liaison for management and staff goals (Table 29.5).

Table 29.5 *Administrative functions of the clinical nurse specialist*

Joint commission standards
Performance reviews
Management and staff agendas

JOINT COMMISSION STANDARDS

The CNS meets with quality managers and coordinators to determine and understand the current Joint Commission standards. Awareness of these standards enable the CNS to direct staff towards the desired outcomes and assist them to apply these standards into practice. Participation on hospital-wide and department-wide committees and work groups is a necessary step of the process. It is critical that the CNS stays updated on new standards, and is able to articulate these standards to staff, and adapt systems and processes as needed.

PERFORMANCE REVIEWS

Within this management model, performance reviews are delegated to the CNS rather than the director. The CNS is very visible on the unit and acutely aware of practice and clinical abilities. Day-to-day interactions with staff are routine. A crucial aspect of staff development is providing specific feedback regarding clinical practice, and assisting with the development of educational and professional goals – all congruent with a performance review format. Performance reviews offer an opportunity for staff to articulate strengths and weaknesses, and determine an action plan for the upcoming year. Achievement of the goals is facilitated by the CNS.

MANAGEMENT AND STAFF AGENDAS

Empowerment of staff is best achieved by allowing their areas of interest and concerns to be represented. The goal is actively to listen, meet concerns when feasible and appropriate, and collaborate to incorporate management and staff goals. It is very important that staff hear about the hospitals' visions and missions and the strategic plans of the institution. In order to be effective, the CNS should be active in hospital-wide committees/teams, and gain knowledge and access to future plans and initiatives. Frequent communication with the director of the service line is essential in establishing a unit-based plan that is congruent with hospital-wide goals. In addition, CNS/advanced practice nurses should meet together to form a common philosophy and educational plan. Agendas should have similar themes and ultimately have patient care at the center.

Change agent role

Change is inevitable. Ongoing modifications of systems, alteration of clinical practice/standards, and newly acquired missions and philosophy require constant adjustment. The CNS must be able to apply the change theory to ensure that change is systemic and purposeful so as to alleviate chaos. Using a change theory model provides reassurance when resistance is high and can create the impetus from which to continue. Welch discusses Lippitt's stages of change, which provide a comprehensive and detailed framework from which to plan effective change.[3] According to Welch, 'Lippitt emphasized problem-solving as well as the interpersonal aspects of the change process' (p. 313).[3] Lippitt's change theory is sequential and the structure meaningful when altering systems or processes in the health care setting. The CNS must develop networks across all settings (Fig. 29.4).

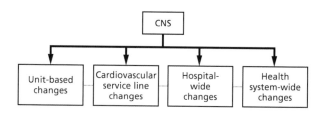

Figure 29.4 *The change agent role across the continuum.*

INTRAVENOUS PUSH POLICY

Networking is essential when creating hospital-wide practice changes. Upon review of the hospital medication policy, discussion occurred surrounding the difficulty of maintaining accurate lists of medications approved for unit use. Each specialty floor had its own list of accepted medications that could be pushed or infused on their units. Standardization across settings was difficult. Implementing an area hospital's medication decision flow chart policy that was already working greatly improved consistency of standards, enhanced patients outcomes, stressed collaboration with physicians, and improved critical thinking skills of the nursing staff (*see* Fig. 29.5). An intravenous (iv) reference book was selected as the standard for medication administration throughout the hospital. This selected reference provided the clinical information necessary for staff to make appropriate decisions regarding safe administration of a medication. Initially, this change created fear and concern among both pharmacy and nursing personnel. Education and discussion about the unique nature of this policy ensued. After a year of preparing and overcoming barriers, the final implementation of the medication policy prevailed. At this time, the policy has been well received. Patients are no longer transferred to areas for medications that could be given safely on all units. Pharmacy no longer has to update medication lists, and standardization is evident.

INITIATION OF INTRAVENOUS INFUSIONS

Once the main iv policy allowed for flexibility a year later, the decision by the director of the service line and the CNS was made to initiate iv infusions (nitroglycerin, renal dose dopamine, dobutamine, diltiazem, and lidocaine) on the acute care telemetry unit. This change

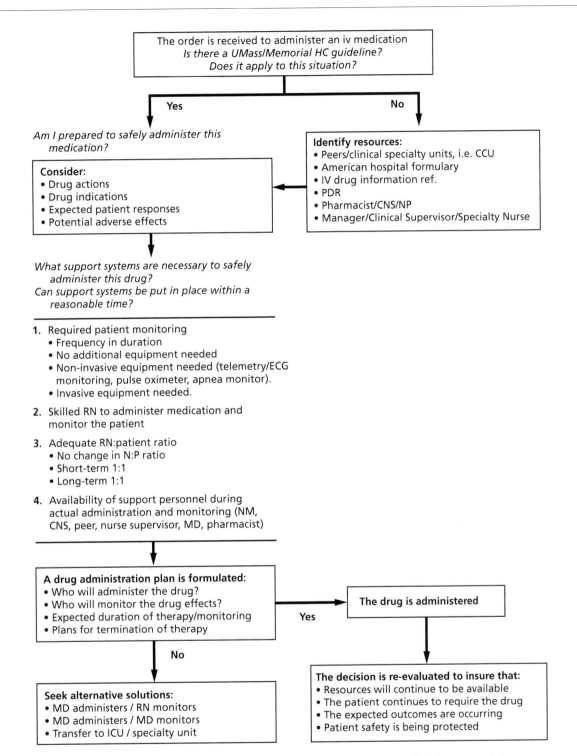

Figure 29.5 *Intravenous medication decision flow chart. CCU = coronary care unit; CNS = clinical nurse specialist; ECG = electrocardiogram; ICU = intensive care unit; IV = intravenous; MD = doctor of medicine; N = nurse; NM = nurse manager; NP = nurse practitioner; P = patient; PDR = physician desk reference; RN = registered nurse.*

(initially considered as a unit-based change) impacted patient care and patient flow hospital-wide. Prior to this change, all patients on iv nitroglycerin were admitted to the intensive care unit. A large percentage of the telemetry patients were diagnosed with unstable angina and were awaiting coronary bypass graft. It was not uncommon for this population to have repeated episodes of chest pain requiring increased nursing demand as their pain was managed with sublingual nitroglycerin. If these patients continued to experience pain, iv nitroglycerin was initiated and warranted transfer to the intensive care unit. Admitting these patients to an intensive care unit setting places increased stress on both the patient and his or her family, a situation that is not ideal prior to open heart surgery.

The CNS, being aware of these issues, was able to develop specific guidelines for selected medications used to treat stable cardiac conditions. The goals of this change were to:

1 allow patients who are hemodynamically stable (systolic blood pressure >90 mm Hg, no electrocardiographic changes) to remain on the telemetry unit;
2 reduce stress and anxiety for the patients and their families;
3 decrease the workload of nursing staff by reducing the frequency of chest pain events.

Intensive care beds that had been utilized for these patients were now open and able to take more critically ill patients. The intensive care unit could now transfer patients stable on these selected medications out to the acute care floor to make room for new admissions.

NURSING DOCUMENTATION

A system-wide change project was initiated and facilitated by the CNS in the area of documentation. The previous documentation system did not clearly highlight the patient's progress or response to specific treatment. There were several forms making it difficult to determine the current condition of patients. The CNS, as a change agent, was able to identify the issues and determine an action plan. Applying change theory was essential to reducing resistance and creating successful change. Getting staff 'buy-in' was achieved by inviting nursing staff to a documentation retreat day. The purpose of the retreat was to pull together all existing forms and attempt to develop one comprehensive form that would meet all required documentation standards. The staff was successful in developing this form (Fig. 29.6). Monitoring compliance of this form, now in practice, resulted in high compliance with documentation standards. Staff report much improved written communication from shift to shift as well as clarity regarding the patients' response and progress to medical and nursing interventions.

Educator role

The educator role comprises the largest proportion of the CNS' time. Education and enhancement of the knowledge base of the staff has a direct link to increased expertise. According to Benners' research on clinical practice, there are five stages of clinical development that range from novice to expert.[4] A nurse takes experiences, incorporates the information into their own internal database for storage. Clinical encounters trigger a retrieval of information that enables a nurse to anticipate, organize, and respond. The degree and the pace to which this is accomplished is correlated with their stage of clinical development. The role of the CNS is to facilitate critical thinking and increase an individual's knowledge base, which can artificially increase their 'experiences'. An increased knowledge base hastens the process of clinical development by enlarging the internal database. More staff can move from the 'competent stage' to 'proficient' and 'expert' stages, thereby improving the quality of care provided on the unit.

The CNS must be able to utilize both formal and informal mechanisms when educating staff (Table 29.6). Increased patient acuity, reduced lengths of stays, and limited financial resources create a challenging environment for education. The CNS must consider these elements and use innovative techniques and ideas in order to overcome these obstacles.

Table 29.6 *Educator role of the clinical nurse specialist*

Informal educational opportunities
Hallway discussions
Policy and procedure updates

Formal education programs
1-hour educational offerings
Day-long workshops
Basic and advanced life support classes

INFORMAL EDUCATION OPPORTUNITIES

Informal education to staff (hallway, conference room discussions) are the primary educational mechanism during the work day. The education occurs quickly, is usually one on one, and meets an immediate need. The CNS must be able to utilize this time to teach staff critical thinking. This is often done by asking staff, 'what do you think?' or 'where might we find this information?'. They then help the staff nurse determine the appropriate intervention. This process helps increase the internal database so, if a future situation occurs, the nurse can retrieve the information and respond without assistance. Their response will be much quicker than the initial experience and will help move them to the next stage of clinical development.

Educating staff about new policy and procedures is another example of informal education to staff. Copies of the new policies are displayed in the nurses conference rooms and changes are highlighted for quick association. Discussion about the changes are articulated during staff meetings and attached to the minutes. Hallway reminders are provided on a daily basis when the policy is being observed.

FORMAL EDUCATIONAL PROGRAMS

Formal educational classes are the more traditional method of education. Prior to developing programs, a learning needs survey should be completed. Classes should be developed according to the assessed needs of staff. Timing of the classes must be considered. An hour before or after a shift can significantly improve attendance. When designing educational classes, time must be dedicated to case study and application of information. The staff need to be able to walk away from the class with an 'experience'. Information without clinical application may not be 'stored'. Without internal storage, critical thinking and improved organization can not occur, stagnating clinical development.

Coordinating day-long workshops is another method of formal education. Co-sponsoring of programs with other institutions is economical. Access to area clinical experts enhances the overall quality of the program. Selecting a specific month annually and standardizing the goals of the program can increase dissemination of education to staff. Each year an intensive care forum presents the newest trends in critical care. This type of programming provides consistent and accurate information to health care providers in the regional area.

Annual certification of nursing staff, particularly in basic and advance life support education, is another important role of the CNS. The CNS should be certified as an instructor in this area. As an instructor, the hospital or unit does not need to fund an education department to provide this requirement. The CNS has the flexibility to coordinate these programs based on staff needs and the ability of staff to attend. This aspect of the educator role as well as coordination of formal programs can be economical and time appropriate for a hospital.

Consultation role

The consultation role develops by building trust with staff, demonstrating clinical expertise, and being readily available to respond to questions. Initially, boundaries must be established regarding this role so that staff do not utilize the CNS to 'play catch up' during busy times. Helping the staff learn to use the CNS as a consultant takes time. Communication is critical, particularly in the early phases of the role. The staff need to feel that they are the primary caregivers and that the interaction with the CNS adds to their ability to provide care without threatening their clinical competency. Gurka discusses the Lippitt and Lippitt's consultant model as a way to conceptualize the role of consultant.[5] Consults can be formal (round system) or informal (verbal request). On one level this role appears straightforward; however, personal experience suggests that successful implemen-

Table 29.7 *Consultation role of the clinical nurse specialist: key concepts*

Establish credibility and trust of staff
Empower staff by increasing clinical decision-making skills

tation is dependent on two key concepts: credibility and trust; and empowerment of nursing staff (Table 29.7).

CREDIBILITY AND TRUST

Establishing credibility as a clinical expert is crucial in the success of this role. Both clinical and judgment skills must be perceived at an expert level. Educating staff about your clinical expertise must be done delicately. In the early phases of this role, the CNS should offer assistance to the nurses whenever practical. Assisting with transferring of patients on and off stretchers and aiding during emergency situations. During these opportunities, the CNS can quickly assess patients' clinical and emotional conditions. Asking staff questions about how they are managing the patient respects their clinical competence and encourages dialogue. Strategies for improving care can be offered and, if staff perceive these suggestions as helpful to *their* plan of care, then credibility and trust is established. Once staff view the CNS in a positive manner, the consultant relationship between the CNS and staff can greatly improve the quality of care provided in a patient care area.

EMPOWERMENT OF STAFF

An effective consultant does not dictate practice. Telling staff how to care for patients will not foster a professional work environment. Staff need to feel in charge of their practice. Asking staff for feedback and ideas regarding the care of their patients leads to discussion and sharing of ideas. Often, while discussing a patient with a nurse, the CNS will ask another staff member to join in the discussion. This promotes joint problem-solving and encourages staff to utilize each other's clinical strengths. This type of interaction with staff is collegial and empowers the staff.

A list of all the clinical specialists, with their specialty and beeper numbers, was developed and distributed to nursing staff. This type of resource utilization fits the philosophy of the CNS: develop all staff to an expert level so they are self-sufficient, resourceful, and efficient and clinical experts.

Researcher role

The final role of the CNS in the clinical practice branch of the nursing management model is the researcher role. The ability to utilize research findings in practice is an important aspect of the advanced practice role. Actually conducting research on a unit is a goal, but difficult to complete with the limited resources available in the current health care climate. A strong commitment to research leads to innovation in the way that this role is operationalized. Altering practice standards with support of research findings will continue to improve patient care outcomes. The CNS plays a valuable role in developing a research-based practice for nurses.

DATE: _____

DIAGNOSIS: _____

PRECAUTIONS: _____

DATE:

NAME:

ADDRESS: SEX:

BIRTHDATE/AGE:

UNIT NUMBER:

ASSESSMENT/REASSESSMENT/CRITICAL PATH REVIEWED			
0700-1900		1900-0700	
0700-1500	1500-2300		2300-0700
PATIENT OUTCOME		1500-1900	1900-2300	

	PATIENT OUTCOME	0700-1500	1500-1900	1900-2300	2300-0700
N E U R O L O G I C A L	Alert and oriented x 3 behavior appropriate to situation, PERRL. Active ROM all extremities with symmetry. No c/o pain or weakness. Verbalization clear and understandable. Gag and cough reflex present. **Treatment/Action Plan**	☐ Meets outcome	☐ Meets outcome	☐ Meets outcome	☐ Meets outcome
P U L M O N A R Y	Respiratory rate 10-20/min, regular, non-labored. Breath sounds present all lobes. No adventitious sounds. Pt. will have adequate oxygenation. **Treatment/Action Plan**	☐ Meets outcome	☐ Meets outcome	☐ Meets outcome	☐ Meets outcome
C A R D I O V A S C U L A R	Apical pulse regular, 60-90 beats per minute. Rhythm regular. BP WNL. Peripheral (radial, pedal) pulses palpable and equal. No edema. Extremities warm. Capillary refill 1-3 sec. **Treatment/Action Plan**	☐ Meets outcome	☐ Meets outcome	☐ Meets outcome	☐ Meets outcome
G E N I T O U R I N A R Y	Voiding without pain or discomfort. Urine is clear or amber in color. No penile, urethral, or vaginal discharge. **Treatment/Action Plan**	☐ Meets outcome	☐ Meets outcome	☐ Meets outcome	☐ Meets outcome

		ASSESSMENT/REASSESSMENT/CRITICAL PATH REVIEWED			
G A S T R O I N T E S T I N A L	Pt. without nausea, vomiting. Abdomen soft, non-tender, bowel sounds present x 4 quadrants. Perirectal area non-tender and intact. Stools heme test negative. Oral mucosa moist and intact. Treatment/Action Plan	☐ Meets outcome	☐ Meets outcome	☐ Meets outcome	☐ Meets outcome
P S Y C H O S O C I A L	Appropriate affect, addresses needs and emotions in an effective manner. Support systems/significant other available to patient Treatment/Action Plan	☐ Meets outcome	☐ Meets outcome	☐ Meets outcome	☐ Meets outcome
S K I N / H Y G I E N E	Skin warm, dry, intact, color w/in pt's norm. No risk present. Treatment/Action Plan	☐ Meets outcome Braden Score:_____ ☐ Independent ☐ Assist ☐ Total	☐ Meets outcome Braden Score:_____ ☐ Independent ☐ Assist ☐ Total	☐ Meets outcome Braden Score:_____ ☐ Independent ☐ Assist ☐ Total	☐ Meets outcome Braden Score:_____ ☐ Independent ☐ Assist ☐ Total
S A F E T Y	Pt. will be provided a safe environment *RESTRAINT: ☐ None ☐ Type: _____ (Specify) **Treatment/Action Plan** Patient/Family/S.O. under-stands and accepts need for restraints. ☐ Yes ☐ Not available ☐ Dr. order obtained	Fall Risk Assessment: ☐ No/low risk ☐ High Risk due to:_____ RESTRAINT: Type: _____ Continue due to: ☐ Agitation ☐ Behavioral management ☐ Other _____ Psychological Response: Tolerated well: ☐ Yes ☐ No ☐ Calm ☐ Agitated☐ Restless	Fall Risk Assessment: ☐ No/low risk ☐ High Risk due to:_____ RESTRAINT: Type: _____ Continue due to: ☐ Agitation ☐ Behavioral management ☐ Other _____ Psychological Response: Tolerated well: ☐ Yes ☐ No ☐ Calm ☐ Agitated☐ Restless	Fall Risk Assessment: ☐ No/low risk ☐ High Risk due to:_____ RESTRAINT: Type: _____ Continue due to: ☐ Agitation ☐ Behavioral management ☐ Other _____ Psychological Response: Tolerated well: ☐ Yes ☐ No ☐ Calm ☐ Agitated☐ Restless	Fall Risk Assessment: ☐ No/low risk ☐ High Risk due to:_____ RESTRAINT: Type: _____ Continue due to: ☐ Agitation ☐ Behavioral management ☐ Other _____ Psychological Response: Tolerated well: ☐ Yes ☐ No ☐ Calm ☐ Agitated☐ Restless
		Safety check q_____Hr	Safety check q Hr	Safety check q Hr	Safety check q Hr
		Side rails up x _____	Side rails up x	Side rails up x	Side rails up x
		Other interventions:	Other interventions:	Other interventions:	Other interventions:
O T H E R	Treatment/Action Plan				

Figure 29.6 *Nursing clinical assessment and outcomes pathway within normal limits. PERRL = pupils equal, round and reactive to light; ROM = range of motion; c/o = complaints; Pt = patient; BP WNL = blood pressure within normal limits; SO = significant other.*

APPLICATION OF RESEARCH FINDINGS

Staying updated about clinical practice through periodic literature reviews is necessary. Advances in practice should be articulated to staff by changing policy and procedures to match the research recommendations. Revising standards of practice based on research findings is a CNS responsibility. The interventional unit at the UMass-Memorial Medical Center changed their practice of transducing all arterial sheaths post-cardiac catherterization. The literature stated favorable outcomes when flushing sheaths with heparinized saline and not transducing the lines. This practice change decreased cost (transducing equipment was no longer needed) and reduced the nursing staff workload.

QUALITY IMPROVEMENT

On a concrete level, the CNS implements the researcher role component through a quality improvement program. The role of the CNS in this context is to identify standards that require monitoring (documentation), provide structure (develop data collection tools), and assist staff with data analysis and identification of solution. Involving staff in the quality improvement monitoring is a primary level of research. Assisting with literature reviews and interpreting research findings for possible application to practice is very important when devising policies and procedures. Currently, all staff participate in data collection and their feedback elicited when formulating solutions. Identified interventions are monitored to ensure expected outcomes.

OVERVIEW AND FUTURE PLANS

Overall, this nursing management model applied to the Cardiovascular Service Line at UMass-Memorial Medical Center has been extremely successful in reducing costs, increasing efficiencies, and improving patient outcomes. Integrating clinical and management priorities, and outlining clear delineation of roles reduces duplication and enhances creativity. Goals for future projects can be delineated into management and clinical practice components. Future plans for the CNS are summarized in Table 29.8. Utilizing the CNS role components as the theoretical model for staff development will continue. Expanding the role to meet the needs throughout the health system is the newest challenge.

SUMMARY

- The UMass-Memorial Medical Center and Healthcare systems utilize a nursing management model that integrates key managerial and clinical concepts for their cardiovascular medicine service line.
- The management model utilizes a nurse with a degree in business administration and nursing management to develop systems by coordinating administrative functions, resource utilization, and employee relations.
- Clinical practice models utilize a 'master-prepared' nurse to coordinate the following clinical specialist role components: administrative, change agent, educator, consultant, and researcher roles.
- Division of responsibilities within the nursing management model is essential to reduce duplication of efforts and maximize strengths of the leadership roles.
- Developing systems and flexible resource utilization are critical to successful financial management.
- Developing clinical and critical thinking skills with nursing staff elevates the nurses level of practice and impacts patient care.

Table 29.8 *Future plans for the clinical nurse specialist role*

Administrative role
Revise current performance review
Format to enhance professional development

Change agent role
Coordinate and implement multidisciplinary patient assessment and standardization of patient care·

Educator role
Coordinate educational offerings throughout the health system

Consultant role
Provide clinical consultation services to other institutions in the health system

REFERENCES

1. Anonymous. Nurse managers: a blessing, a bother? an endangered species? *Intensive Care Nursing* 1986; **1**: 117–18.
2. Kotter JP. What leaders really do. *Harvard Business Rev* 1990; May–June: 103.
3. Welch LB. Planned change in nursing: the theory. *Nursing Clinics North Am* 1979; **14**: 307–21.
4. Benner P. *From novice to expert.* Menlo Park, CA: Addison-Welsey, 1984.
5. Gurka AM. Process and outcome components of clinical nurse specialist consultation. *Dimensions Crit Care Nursing* 1991; **10**: 169–75.

PART 5

Post-hospital management strategies

30

Cardiovascular rehabilitation

ANN WARD, JEAN EINERSON AND PATRICK MCBRIDE

Patients with cardiovascular diseases can benefit from an individualized comprehensive secondary prevention program that involves medical evaluation, prescribed exercise, nutritional counseling, risk factor management (lipids, hypertension, weight, diabetes, and smoking), psychosocial management, and physical activity counseling. Candidates for secondary services include patients with stable angina, myocardial infarction, stable heart failure, coronary artery bypass grafting, percutaneous transluminal coronary angioplasty, heart transplant, heart-valve surgery, peripheral vascular disease and congenital heart disease. Patients participating in secondary prevention/rehabilitation programs today tend to be older and sicker and have more co-morbidities, thus requiring risk stratification and individualized treatment plans. Benefits include improved exercise tolerance, risk factors, and sense of well-being and reduced mortality.

WHAT IS CARDIAC REHABILITATION?

Cardiac rehabilitation is a combination of interventions that help patients with cardiovascular disease to improve their functional abilities (particularly their tolerance for physical activity), to decrease their symptoms, and to achieve and maintain optimal health. Cardiac rehabilitation is characterized by comprehensive long-term programs involving medical evaluation, prescribed exercise, cardiac risk factor modification, education, counseling, and behavior modification. The main aims of cardiac rehabilitation are 'to limit the physiologic and psychological effects of cardiac illness, reduce the risk of sudden death or reinfarction, control cardiac symptoms, stabilize or reverse the atherosclerotic process and enhance the psychosocial and vocational status of selected patients'.[1] Cardiac rehabilitation services are physician directed and implemented by a variety of health care professionals, such as nurses, exercise physiologists, dietitians, physical therapists, occupational therapists, psychologists, and behavioral medicine specialists.

Candidates for cardiac rehabilitation[2] include patients with:

- stable angina (7 million);
- myocardial infarction (1 million survivors/year);
- stable heart failure (4.7 million);
- coronary artery bypass grafting (309 000 in 1993);
- percutaneous transluminal coronary angioplasty (362 000 in 1993);
- heart transplant (2000/year);
- heart-valve surgery;
- peripheral vascular disease;
- congenital heart disease.

Unfortunately, cardiac rehabilitation services are underutilized. Only 11–38 per cent of eligible patients participate in cardiac rehabilitation programs.[2] Barriers to participation include lack of physician referral, the patient's lack of interest, problems of reimbursement, and lack of access to appropriate services.[3]

Authoritative organizations such as the American Association of Cardiovascular and Pulmonary Rehabilitation (AACVPR), American College of Cardiology (ACC), American Heart Association (AHA), and the American College of Sports Medicine (ACSM) have produced detailed publications addressing the structure and organization of cardiac rehabilitation and secondary prevention programs.[4-7a] The purpose of this chapter is not to duplicate these publications, but to provide an overview of cardiac rehabilitation services, some key issues in delivery of the services, and principal outcomes.

HISTORICAL DEVELOPMENT OF CARDIAC REHABILITATION

Only a few decades ago, treatment for a heart attack consisted of weeks of bed rest. The prolonged bed rest led to deconditioning and weakness and increased morbidity and mortality. Cardiac care was revolutionized in the 1950s when Dr Paul Dudley White encouraged President Eisenhower, after he suffered a serious heart attack, to continue as president and to stay physically active.

Cardiac rehabilitation was formally introduced in the 1960s on an in-patient basis when it was discovered that patients improved and complications were reduced when they were ambulating rather than lying in bed for extended periods. The early out-patient cardiac rehabilitation programs involved primarily exercise and only limited risk factor modification. Most patients enrolled in exercise training programs were those who had recovered from uncomplicated myocardial infarction. In subsequent years, patients with complications of myocardial infarction were considered for more limited and gradual exercise rehabilitation. Gradually, cardiac rehabilitation expanded to include patients with coronary artery bypass grafting (CABG), percutaneous transluminal coronary angioplasty (PTCA), heart failure, heart transplantation, and other cardiovascular conditions. In recent years, risk stratification procedures have been developed. Patients at low risk are able to exercise safely with less supervision. A greater emphasis has been placed on education, counseling, and risk factor modification in the last two decades. Consequently, cardiac rehabilitation services provide an excellent model for secondary prevention and disease management.

The ACSM has led the profession in establishing guidelines and a certification program for professionals working in fitness and cardiopulmonary rehabilitation programs. In 1975, the first edition of *ACSM's Guidelines for Exercise Testing and Prescription*[8] for developing exercise programs for apparently healthy individuals and cardiac patients was published. The sixth edition of the *Guidelines* was published in 2000.[7] In 1986, the AACVPR was formed and represented the first professional organization dedicated exclusively to the practice of cardiovascular and pulmonary rehabilitation. Since 1990 this organization has published three editions of *Guidelines for Cardiac Rehabilitation and Secondary Prevention Programs*.[4,9,10] Recently, AACVPR implemented a certification program for cardiac and pulmonary rehabilita-

tion programs based on an essential standard of care. The goal of program certification is to ensure programs are following a standard of care and to enhance the practice of cardiac rehabilitation around the country. Programs can submit documentation to AACVPR demonstrating that they meet the standard of care guidelines. The guidelines and application may be obtained by contacting AACVPR.

In 1995, the Clinical Practice Guideline *Cardiac Rehabilitation*[2] was published by the Agency for Health Care Policy and Research. This landmark document represents the first comprehensive, objective examination of the outcomes of delivery of the two components of cardiac rehabilitation services: exercise training, and education, counseling, and behavioral interventions. The Guideline provides broad recommendations for cardiac rehabilitation based on the evaluation of the scientific evidence. The expert panel that reviewed the evidence and prepared the guideline concluded that cardiac rehabilitation is an essential component of the management of patients with heart disease.

CARDIAC REHABILITATION SERVICES AND SECONDARY PREVENTION

Components of cardiac rehabilitation

The AHA and AACVPR have recommended specific core components to assist cardiac rehabilitation staff in the design and development of their programs.[7a] These components are: (1) baseline patient assessment; (2) nutritional correcting; (3) risk factor management (lipids, hypertension, weight, diabetes, and smoking); (4) psychosocial management; (5) physical activity counseling; and (6) exercise training. These components can be tailored to the needs and preferences of the individual patient. Therefore, patients who are at greatest risk, or the most deconditioned, are excellent candidates for supervised cardiac rehabilitation. The exercise component is individually prescribed and is designed to improve the patient's exercise tolerance and ability to perform activities of daily living. The exercise can be supervised or unsupervised, and involves a variety of modes of activity. The educational, counseling, and behavioral interventions are designed to help patients stop smoking, lower their blood pressure, change their eating habits, lose weight, improve their cholesterol levels, and improve their psychosocial well-being.

A multifactorial program of cardiac rehabilitation services that includes all the core components is more effective than any of the components as a sole intervention.[2] The goal is to tailor the delivery of services individually to the specific needs of the patient.

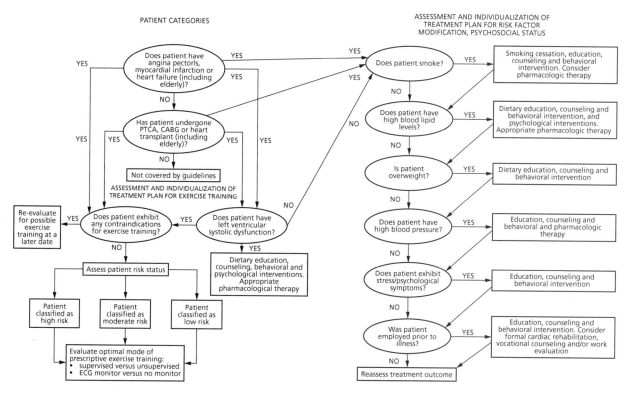

Figure 30.1 *Decision tree for cardiac rehabilitation services. Ovals represent yes–no decision points; rectangles represent intervention strategies or other clinical decision-making by the provider of cardiac rehabilitation services: PTCA = percutaneous transluminal coronary angioplasty; CABG = coronary artery bypass grafting; ECG = electrocardiogram. (Reprinted from Wenger NK, Froelicher ES, Smith LK, et al. Cardiac rehabilitation. Clinical Practice Guideline Number 17. Rockville, MD: US Department of Health and Human Services, Public Health Service, Agency for Health Care Policy and Research and the National Heart, Lung, and Blood Institute. AHCPR Publication No. 96-0672, 1995.)*

The AHCPR Clinical Practice Guideline developed a decision tree for cardiac rehabilitation services (Fig. 30.1), which provides an individualized approach to assessing patient status and implementing intervention strategies.[1] The figure describes patient categories as well as the patient assessment and treatment strategies involved in the delivery of cardiac rehabilitation services.

Risk stratification

Stratifying patients based on the level of risk can be useful in determining the appropriateness of exercise training, deciding level of supervision and monitoring needed during exercise training, and determining types of activities the patient can participate in safely. Several systems have been developed for determining a patient's risk of future cardiac events.[4–6] Generally, risk levels are designated as low, moderate or intermediate, and high. Patients should be stratified not only for risk of an event during exercise, but also for risk of disease progression. The risk stratification adopted by the University of Wisconsin Preventive Cardiology Program incorporates psychosocial assessments (Table 30.1).

Over half of cardiac patients fall in the low-risk category. Low-risk patients can perform reasonable levels of physical activity without adverse consequences and are good candidates for home-based programs.

High-risk patients often have a low peak exercise capacity, early onset of myocardial ischemia, serious arrhythmias, ventricular dysfunction, or combinations of these problems with exercise and thus need a higher level of surveillance and assistance with recovery and reducing risk.

Phases of cardiac rehabilitation

Cardiac rehabilitation provides a continuum of care between in-patient and out-patient settings and beyond, and has traditionally been thought of as three to four phases:[4]

1 in-patient hospital period generally lasting 4–14 days (longer for some transplant patients);
2 medically supervised out-patient programming in a cardiac rehabilitation center of generally 3 or more months in duration;

Table 30.1 *University of Wisconsin Preventive Cardiology Program risk stratification*

Low risk stratification (Presence of ALL factors)
- Uncomplicated MI, CABG, PCI. Absence of CHF or signs/symptoms indicating post-event ischemia
- No significant left ventricular dysfunction (EF >40%)
- No resting or exercise-induced complex dysrhythmias
- Normal hemodynamics responses with exercise and in recovery
- Absence of clinical depression measured by standardized psychological testing tool

Moderate risk stratification (Assumed for patients who do not meet the classification of either high or low risk)
- Moderately impaired left ventricular function (EF 30–40%)
- Signs/symptoms including angina or anginal equivalents at an exercise intensity above an appropriate prescribed training level, or in recovery
- Evidence of moderate clinical depression measured by standardized psychological testing tool

Highest risk stratification (Presence of any one factor)
- Exercise-induced ischemia as indicated by one or more of the following: anginal pain; 2 mm or more of ST segment depression on electrocardiogram; reversible filling defect(s) on radionuclear scan; ischemic wall motion abnormalities on stress echocardiogram, or medically-managed ischemia and no immediate intervention planned
- Severely depressed left ventricular function (EF >30%)
- Complex ventricular arrhythmias appearing or increasing with exercise; medically managed
- Abnormal hemodynamic responses with exercise (flat or decreasing systolic blood pressure or chronotropic incompetence with increasing workload)
- Survivor of cardiac arrest or sudden death
- Recent (<30 days) myocardial infarction complicated by arrhythmias or CHF
- Presence of one or more psychosocial risk factors including clinically significant levels of: (1) emotional distress; (2) depression; (3) pervasive hostility; (4) social isolation as determined by professional assessment and/or standardized psychological testing tools
- Compensated and medically-managed CHF

EF = ejection fraction; MI = myocardial infarction; CABG = coronary artery bypass grafting; CHF = congestive heart failure; METs = metabolic equivalents; PCI = percutaneous coronary intervention.

3 variable length program of intermittent or no electrocardiographic monitoring under supervision;
4 unsupervised maintenance (lifelong–community facility or at home).

> More recently, the addition of risk stratification has led to a format where the program is more individualized in terms of duration, degree of electrocardiogram (ECG) monitoring and level of clinical supervision.

The new format includes the addition of transition zones: (1) transition care between in-patient and out-patient settings (subacute facility, home care, and pre-training at home lasting up to 6 weeks); and (2) transition from supervised to unsupervised exercise with an emphasis on self-monitoring and management skills. Also, cardiac rehabilitation programs are beginning to include periodic follow-up visits to enhance long-term compliance and update the exercise prescription. Figure 30.2 shows the progression through the cardiac rehabilitation phases. Each phase has its own set of goals for exercise, and education, counseling, and behavioral interventions.

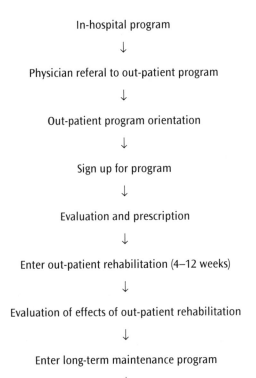

In-hospital program
↓
Physician referal to out-patient program
↓
Out-patient program orientation
↓
Sign up for program
↓
Evaluation and prescription
↓
Enter out-patient rehabilitation (4–12 weeks)
↓
Evaluation of effects of out-patient rehabilitation
↓
Enter long-term maintenance program
↓
Regular follow-up and updated prescription/treatment plan

Figure 30.2 *Progression through cardiac rehabilitation.*

In-patient and transitional settings

The in-patient phase is characterized by decreasing length of hospital stays. Rehabilitation begins as soon as the patient is stable, usually within 24–48 hours after an infarct or bypass surgery. The objectives of the in-patient program have focused on avoiding problems associated with extended bed rest, assessing functional tolerance to activities of daily living, counseling patients on activity, facilitating self-care, educating the patient about the components and benefits of a healthy lifestyle, and planning discharge from the hospital.

> Early physical activity reduces the risk of thrombi, maintains muscle tone and joint mobility, and reduces orthostatic hypotension.[11]

In many in-patient programs, cardiac rehabilitation services are initiated by standing orders. The rehabilitation staff reviews the patient's chart, assesses the patient and determines if he/she has any contraindications to activity. According to AACVPR guidelines,[4] patients are considered stable and ready to begin rehabilitation if they meet the following criteria:

- no new/recurrent chest pain for 8 hours;
- no new signs of uncompensated failure (dyspnea at rest with bibasilar rales);
- no new significant, abnormal rhythm or ECG changes in the past 8 hours.

> The therapy is closely supervised and monitored. Initial therapy in the first several days consists of low-intensity exercise (intermittent sitting or standing and walking) and a range of motion activities of approximately 2–3 METs (metabolic equivalents; 1 MET is equivalent to the resting metabolic rate and is approximately 3.5 mL/kg per minute).

Initial functional capacity should be assumed to be low, at approximately 3–5 METs, because functional capacity is generally unknown at this stage. Although patients at this stage require considerable individualization in program design, general guidelines recommended by ACSM[7] are:

Intensity
- Rating of perceived exertion (RPE) <13 (6–20 scale)
- Post-myocardial infarction (MI): heart rate (HR) <120 beats/minute or resting heart rate (HR_{rest}) + 20 beats/minute
- Post-surgery: HR_{rest} + 20 beats/minute or +12 if on a β-blocker

Duration
- intermittent bouts lasting 3–5 minutes for a total duration up to 20 minutes with rest periods lasting 1–2 minutes

Frequency
- 2–4 sessions per day.

Patients should gradually progress to longer duration sessions and increased intensity. Progression may vary from a more rapid increase in activity in the low-risk CABG or uncomplicated MI to a slower progression in a higher risk more debilitated patient (*see* Tables 30.2–30.4 for sample progressions for CABG, MI, and cardiac transplant patients). Compared to controls, patients who participated in in-hospital rehabilitation programs made substantial improvements in self-confidence and in performance of daily activities.[12]

> Education and counseling are integral components of the in-patient cardiac rehabilitation program.

With the trend toward early discharge, patients and their families need further explanations about how best to live with heart disease and how to develop lifestyle-change strategies. Assessments should include the patient's cardiovascular risk factors to determine those that will require management to reduce the risk of future events. Staff should also assess the patient's understanding of the disease, determine symptom pattern, and identify patient goals for rehabilitation. To implement risk changes, information about the various risk factors and practical techniques to alter behavior are provided.

Such education can occur in formal sessions with group support or on a one-to-one basis. To be effective, the educational program must be carefully structured, taking into account the patient's needs, the issues included in the treatment and techniques for lifestyle change. The short hospital stay often makes teaching difficult. A variety of techniques including audiovisual aids, booklets and video/audio tapes should be used. Patients can take written materials home to refer to after discharge.

DISCHARGE PLANNING

If available, an organized out-patient program should be recommended, particularly for moderate to high-risk patients.

> The discharge plan should include strategies for risk factor modification, dietary guidelines, education on medications, and an exercise prescription for use at home or until enrollment in an out-patient program.

Patients should receive specific exercise guidelines including recommendations for stair climbing and other activities of daily living, and instruction in measurement of HR.

Table 30.2 *University of Wisconsin Hospital and Clinics Preventive Cardiology Program activity and exercise guidelines for post-myocardial infarction patients*

Level	Supervised activity	MICU/Ward activities	Comments
1 (1 MET)	• Send consult to Preventive Cardiology • Assess functional status, risk factor profile and discharge needs	• Complete bed rest • Assisted care or partial self-care • Bedside commode • Dangle at bedside	Level 1 may continue for complicated MI. Usually unnecessary for uncomplicated MI after 24 hours
2 (2.0–2.5 METs)	• Orthostatic challenge (2 minutes standing with BP and HR at 30 seconds and 2 minutes) • Rehabilitation staff: monitored ambulation 2–5 minutes • HR = RHR +20/minutes (+10 on β-blocker) • SBP >90 mm Hg or well tolerated if <100 mm Hg • Nursing staff: supervised ambulation on telemetry 2–5 minutes BID–TID.	**Uncomplicated MI** • Full self-care/bathing • Up in room/chair 20–30 minutes TID–QID **Complicated MI** • Continue assisted bathing	Orthostatic responses: SBP >90 mm Hg; HR <110 beats/minute usual values for uncomplicated MI **Complicated MI** • Up in chair BID–TID as tolerated, ambulate 2–3 minutes BID–TID • HR = RHR +15–20/minute (+5–10 minutes on β-blocker)
3 (2.0–4.0 METS)	• Rehabilitation staff: monitored ambulation to 5 minutes • HR = RHR +20/minute (+10 on β-blocker) • SBP >90 mm Hg • Risk factor education • Nursing staff: supervised ambulation 5 minutes TID, then up *ad lib*.	**Uncomplicated MI** • Full self-care and shower • Up *ad lib*. **Complicated MI** • Assisted shower and self-care • Advance as tolerated	**Complicated MI** • Progress walk +1 minute/day as tolerated
4 Pre-discharge (2.0–5.0 METs)	• Low-level ETT/thallium in ECG laboratory **Discharge activity/guidelines** • Progressive walking program • Referral to local cardiac rehabilitation and/or lipid clinic	Maintain above protocol	**Complicated MI** • Thallium ETT • May be given exercise or ADL guidelines • Referal to local cardiac rehabilitation and/or lipid clinic

MICU = medical intensive care unit; MET = metabolic equivalent; MI = myocardial infarction; BP = blood pressure; HR = heart rate; RHR = resting heart rate; SBP = systolic blood pressure; BID = twice a day; TID = three times a day; QID = four times a day; ETT = exercise tolerance test; ECG = electrocardiogram; ADL = activities of daily living.

Out-patient rehabilitation and long-term maintenance

The out-patient program is a continuation of the in-patient program with the goals of independence in activities of daily living, resumption of occupational and recreational activities, and initiation of positive lifestyle modifications for secondary prevention. The out-patient exercise program is based on the patient's functional capacity. Contraindications to exercise training are listed below:[4]

• unstable ischemia;
• heart failure that is not compensated;
• uncontrolled arrhythmias;
• uncontrolled diabetes;
• severe and symptomatic aortic stenosis;
• hypertrophic obstructive cardiomyopathy;

• severe pulmonary hypertension;
• third-degree heart block without pacemaker therapy;
• other conditions that could be aggravated by exercise, e.g. resting systolic blood pressure ≥200 mm Hg or resting diastolic blood pressure ≥110 mm Hg, active or suspected myocarditis or pericarditis, suspected or known dissecting aneurysm, thrombophlebitis, and recent systemic or pulmonary embolus;
• orthopedic or arthritic problems that would prohibit significant exercise;
• acute systemic illness or fever.

EXERCISE PRESCRIPTION

A low-level exercise test at discharge provides useful information for prescribing exercise. Often, a low-level test is not performed at discharge.

Table 30.3 *University of Wisconsin Hospital and Clinics Preventive Cardiology Program exercise guidelines for post-CABG/valve surgery patients*

Level	Fast track recovery	Slow to recover[a]	Comments
Preoperative	Send Consult to Preventive Cardiology Up *ad lib.* Preoperative teaching by nursing and rehabilitation staff Assess functional status, risk factor profile and discharge needs		
1 I ICU/ward 1.5–2.0 METs POD 1–2	Assess postoperative clinical status Send consult if not sent preoperatively • Assisted self-care bathing • Up in chair as tolerated • Nursing ICU activity protocol	• Bed rest/intubation may continue • ICU activity protocol	
2 2.0–2.5 METs POD 2–3	Orthostatic BP/HR • One monitored ambulation 2–5 minutes; Nursing: continue BID, TID as tolerated • One to two (5–10) minute exercise sessions on TM or bike RPE 11–13 • Increase MET level as tolerated	 • Chair as tolerated • ICU activity protocol	**Orthostatic response** Desirable values: HR<120 beats/minute, SBP>90 mm Hg **Ambulation/exercise** • HR (+20–25/minute) • SBP >90 mm Hg • Patients with chest tubes and no air leak can be put to H_2O seal for ambulation
3 3.5 Mets POD 4	• Monitored ambulation 5 minutes TID (nursing) • Full self-care/bathing • Two exercise sessions on TM or bike, increase by 1–2 minutes/session as tolerated • Risk factor education • Stair climbing protocol • Monitored arm exercises	• Monitored ambulation with rehabilitation 2–3 minutes; Nursing: continue BID, TID as tolerated • Begin rehabilitation exercise sessions on TM or bike 5–10 minutes as tolerated • Assisted self-care/bathing	• Defer stair climbing until chest tubes are disconnected • Some pts may not tolerate TM or bike exercise; these pts will be monitored during hall ambulation
4 3.0–4.0 METs POD 5	• Up *ad lib.* • Two (15–20) minute exercise sessions on TM or bike • Monitored arm exercises • Home exercise instructions • Follow-up: refer to hometown rehabilitation facility; clinic visit at UWH 3–4 months post-operatively if no local rehabilitation program	• Monitored ambulation TID 2–5 minutes with nursing • Two exercise sessions on TM or bike; increase by 1–2 minutes/session as tolerated • Monitored arm exercises • Full self-care/bathing	• Some pts may not tolerate monitored hall ambulation (poor balance); these pts will be monitored with the restorator bike.
4 (cont.) POD 6		• Ambulate 5 minutes TID with minimal or no assistance • Two exercise sessions on TM or bike, 10–15 minutes BID as tolerated • Risk factor education • Stair climbing protocol	• Physical therapy will monitor stair climbing for patients with assist devices or severe functional impairments

Table 30.3 (*Continued*)

Level	Fast track recovery	Slow to recover[a]	Comments
5 POD 7		• Two exercise sessions on TM or bike, 15–20 minutes BID as tolerated • Monitored arm exercises • Home exercise instructions • Follow-up: refer to hometown rehabilitation facility; clinic visit at UWH 3–4 months post-operatively if no local rehabilitation program	

[a]Slow to recover patients may have the following: perioperative MI; CHF/low ejection fraction (EF <40%); uncontrolled diabetes or renal disease; infection; surgical complication, e.g. bleeding; lung disease; age >75 years; assistance device preop; second CABG; dysrhythmia.
CABG = coronary artery bypass grafting; METs = metabolic equivalents; POD = postoperative day; ICU = intensive care unit; HR = heart rate; SBP = systolic blood pressure; RPE = rating of perceived exertion; TM = treadmill; BID = twice a day; TID = three times a day; pts = patients; UWH = University of Wisconsin Hospital.

Table 30.4 *University of Wisconsin Hospital and Clinics Preventive Cardiology Program activity and exercise guidelines for post-cardiac transplant patients*

Level	Supervised activity	Ward activities	Comments
1 (Ward) 1.0–2.0 METs	• Send Consult to Preventive Cardiology • Orthostatic BP challenge (2 minutes standing with BP and HR at 30 seconds and 2 minutes) • Assess functional status, risk factor profile and discharge needs	• Assisted self-care/bathing • Up in room/chair as tolerated BID–TID	
2 (Ward) 2.0–3.0 METs	• Supervised ambulation on telemetry 3–5 minutes, BID–TID • HR +30/minute • SBP > 90 mm Hg or well tolerated if <90 mm Hg • Begin daily bicycle exercise 5–10 minutes as tolerated	As above	Patients with a positive biopsy (rejection grade 1–4) or who have elevated WBC may continue with exercise if they are medically stable (receiving treatment)
3 (Ward) 2.0–3.0 METs	• Increase biking by 1–2 minutes every day • RPE of 13 • HR +30 beats above standing rest • BP <160/100 mm Hg at rest (with appropriate increase with exercise) • Begin resistance training per protocol	Full self-care/bathing	• Patients that cannot tolerate the treadmill or exercycle will be monitored during hall ambulation • Appropriate SBP is 8–12 mm Hg/MET
4 (Rehabilitation room) Pre-discharge 3.0–5.0 METs	• Pre-discharge monitored session on a treadmill or bike to 3–5 METs • RPE 13–15 • HR +30 beats above standing rest, resting BP <160/100 mm Hg • Exercise prescription based on submaximal test	As above	
5 Out-patient rehabilitation	• Monitored exercise on a treadmill or exercise bike (MES) 3 times per week • Increase exercise intensity when 20 minutes duration is reached Workload: > 150 kpm on bike > 3 METs on treadmill • RPE, HR, and BP as above • Risk factor education • Continue resistance training	None	• Refer to local area cardiac rehabilitation program • Three-month follow-up VO$_2$ arranged by transplant office

METs = metabolic equivalents; BP = blood pressure; HR = heart rate; BID = twice a day; TID = three times a day; SBP = systolic blood pressure; RPE = rating of perceived exertion; WBC = white blood count; kpm = kilopond meters per minute.

A submaximal exercise evaluation can be performed at one of the initial out-patients visits to establish an exercise prescription.

McConnell et al.[13] compared patients with and without an exercise test prior to entry into out-patient cardiac rehabilitation and reported that the patients without an exercise test could be progressed safely and had outcomes similar to the patients with an entry exercise test. Exercise sessions are generally three times per week for approximately 1 hour.

Length of stay in the out-patient program is determined by disease severity, risk stratification, goal attainment, and evidence that the participant is clinically stable.

General guidelines recommended by ACSM for exercise prescription are listed below:[7]

Intensity
- 55–90 per cent of maximum HR or
- 40–85 per cent of maximum oxygen consumption or HR reserve
- if an exercise tolerance test (ETT) is not available, +20–25 beats/minute above standing rest or +10–12 beats/minute above standing rest if on a β-blocker
- RPE 11–15 (6–20 scale).

Duration
- 20–60 minutes of continuous aerobic activity
- multiple sessions of short duration (~10 minutes) for severely deconditioned individuals.

Frequency
- patients with functional capacity <3 METs – 2–3 short (5–10 minutes) exercise bouts daily
- patients with functional capacity 3–5 METs – daily
- patients with functional capacity >5 METs – 3–5 sessions per week.

Progression
- based on initial physical condition, medical condition, functional goals for daily activities, recreation or vocation and weight loss goal. Patients are progressed for 2–5 minutes per session over 2–3 weeks to a goal of 30 minutes at their target intensity. Intensity is increased when participants demonstrate a training effect and stable blood pressure responses.

The upper limit for exercise intensity should be based on when myocardial ischemia occurs during exercise. Generally, a peak exercise HR of 10 beats/minute below the ischemic threshold is appropriate. Lower intensity exercise (40–70 per cent) provides greater safety during unsupervised exercise as well as potentially promoting improved adherence to exercise training.

TO MONITOR OR NOT TO MONITOR

Continuous ECG monitoring was in wide use in the 1970s and 1980s. However, controversy exists as to whether continuous ECG monitoring is necessary.

Current data suggest that continuous monitoring does not provide added safety during supervised exercise for low-risk cardiac patients.[14,15]

Decisions regarding the extent of ECG monitoring and supervision can be facilitated using the risk stratification process and information found in Table 30.1. The shift from continuous ECG monitoring to intermittent or periodic monitoring should be individualized. No specific guidelines have been developed regarding the duration of continuous monitoring. Characteristics of patients most likely to benefit from continuous ECG monitoring during cardiac rehabilitation based on experience in the UW Preventive Cardiology Program and the literature[4-6] are listed in Table 30.5.[5]

Table 30.5 *Criteria for electrocardiographic monitoring*

Severely depressed left ventricular function (ejection fraction below 30%)
Resting complex ventricular arrhythmia
Ventricular arrhythmias appearing or increasing with exercise
Decrease in systolic blood pressure with exercise
Survivors of sudden cardiac death
Survivors of myocardial infarction complicated by congestive heart failure, cardiogenic shock, serious ventricular arrhythmias, or some combination of the three
Patients with severe coronary artery disease and marked exercise-induced ischemia (ST segment depression ≥ 2 mm)
Inability to self-monitor heart rate because of physical or intellectual impairment
Recurrence of cardiac symptoms

RESISTANCE TRAINING

Strength training was traditionally considered contraindicated for cardiac patients.

However, recent studies have documented that mild to moderate resistance exercise is beneficial for selected patients.[16]

Improvements in strength could benefit patients' performance of activities of daily living, tasks in the workplace, and leisure activities. Most studies have been limited to low-risk male patients aged 70 or younger with normal left ventricular function. The training ranged from 25 to 80 per cent of the one-rep maximum (1 RM; the maximal effort an individual can perform during a resistance exercise in one full range of motion), 2–3 days per week for 6–26 weeks. Adverse outcomes have not been observed in low-risk patients during supervised resistance training. The safety of resistance training in high-risk patients has not been evaluated. Resistance training is indicated for all patients except for those with the contraindications listed in Table 30.6.

Table 30.6 *Contraindications to resistance training*

Absolute contraindications
Severe hypertensive responses to low-level dynamic exercise (blood pressure > 200 mm Hg)
Untreated heart failure
Active retinopathy
Joint abnormalities, which preclude stress-bearing or safe range of motion
Anterior wall myocardial infarction within two months

Relative contraindications
Decreased left ventricular function (rest ejection fraction < 30%)
Decreased joint mobility or impaired musculoskeletal function
Recent (<3 weeks) abdominal or thoracic surgery
Borderline hypertensive responses to dynamic exercise

Most patients begin their resistance training program following hospital discharge with one set of 10–15 reps using 2–5 lb free weights or elastic resistance bands. Caution is used with patients with healing sternal incisions from CABG surgery. Patients may progress to heavier weights (30–60 per cent 1 RM) using either free weights or weight machines, 1–3 sets of 10–15 reps, 2–3 days per week. After 6 months, intensity can be increased to 60–80 per cent of 1 RM in selected patients. The rate pressure product should not exceed that during endurance exercise.

HOME-BASED PROGRAMS

Many patients are not enrolled in supervised out-patient programs due to travel distance or convenience. Home-based programs serve as a good alternative.

> In clinically stable, low- to moderate-risk patients, medically directed home-based programs are safe, inexpensive and effective.[17,18]

Advantages of home-based programs include improved accessibility, improved flexibility of time, lower cost, and greater independence in exercising. Drawbacks include the limited opportunity for patient education and counseling and the lack of medical surveillance, emergency care, and peer support. Periodic visits to the out-patient cardiac rehabilitation clinic or regular telephone contact between patients and rehabilitation staff can be used to overcome some of these limitations.

MAINTENANCE PROGRAMS

Patients are moved into the exercise maintenance stage when cardiovascular and physiological responses to exercise therapy have been obtained or no additional progress is evident. Patients who should remain in a clinically supervised program include those at high risk for cardiovascular complications and those unable to self-monitor. Most patients participate in a clinically supervised program for 12 weeks to facilitate exercise and lifestyle management changes. After 12 weeks, patients may go to a non-clinically supervised facility or home program. Development of self-management skills is important for a successful maintenance program. Regular follow-up visits can be used to assess the maintenance of outcome goals and adherence to lifestyle management changes. Patients may be transferred up and down through the various phases of rehabilitation as the disease progresses, regresses, or appears unchanged.

Case management and assessment of outcomes

The cardiac rehabilitation staff are ideally positioned to coordinate secondary prevention among the primary care physician, cardiologist, and other health care professionals because they have regular and continued contact with the patient.

> Many programs use a case-management approach to individualize patient care.

Each patient is assigned to a cardiac rehabilitation professional who is responsible for assessing the patient's needs and developing a treatment plan. The case manager is responsible and accountable for providing and/or coordinating the patient's care throughout the rehabilitation process. DeBusk et al.[19] found that a physician-directed, nurse-managed case-management system was a successful and cost-effective approach to reducing risk factors. A medical director who establishes policies and is involved in the day-to-day operations is important to the success of the program. A second important factor is the cardiac rehabilitation staff maintaining consistent contact with patients through formal education and exercise sessions, telephone calls, written correspondence, and follow-up visits, and then keeping the referring physicians appraised of their patients' progress through regular reports and telephone contacts.

Case management consists of three steps:[20]

- an initial assessment of the patient's status: medical, nutritional, psychosocial, educational, and vocational (including the impact of existing cardiac or other diseases);
- a specific treatment plan based on the initial assessment and an outcome-based long-term assessment; and

- an effective follow-up for compliance and reinforcement of behavior changes.

Each patient will require an individualized evaluation.

The evaluation should include a medical and family history (may be available from the medical chart), assessments of symptoms, risk factors, nutritional status and stress level, and measurements of resting blood pressure, body weight, and height. Laboratory studies should include at least one fasting lipid profile with total cholesterol, high-density lipoprotein (HDL) cholesterol, triglycerides, calculated low-density lipoprotein (LDL) cholesterol, and blood glucose values. We also recommend measurement of lipoprotein a (Lp (a)) and homocysteine to quantify risk and guide the aggressiveness of therapy and family evaluation. In some patients, functional stress testing is useful to define physical work capacity, blood pressure responses and evidence of ischemia. Information from the initial evaluation can be used to risk stratify the patient and develop an individualized treatment plan.

The treatment plan should include both short-term and long-term goals.

Guidelines from the AHA for comprehensive risk reduction[21] can be used as long-term goals. Goals established by the University of Wisconsin (UW) Preventive Cardiology Program are listed in Table 30.7. The goals for smoking, blood lipids, physical activity, blood pressure and diet are consistent with national guidelines.[22-24] The National Heart, Lung and Blood Institute (NHLBI) has established a body mass index (BMI) of <25 as desirable.[25] This goal is not attainable for most patients by the time of discharge from the out-patient program and for some patients may never be attainable. The UW Preventive Cardiology Program establishes realistic short-term and long-term goals for weight loss in consultation with the patient. The key is to develop goals for body weight that are realistic and achievable. Once the goal has been met, a new goal can be established if desired.

Implementation of the treatment plan involves education, counseling, and behavior modification strategies.

Some of the education needs may be met individually or through group classes. For some risk factor interventions, the cardiac rehabilitation professional may refer the patient to other professionals such as dietitians for follow-up. Routine referral to a dietitian for dietary evaluation and counseling is recommended. Due to the common problems of significant anxiety and depression in CAD patients during recovery, scales to evaluate these problems are recommended and referral made to a therapist for high-risk patients. The cardiac rehabilitation professional will also need to work with the referring physician to order diagnostic tests and prescribe medications to manage risk factors.

Documentation of outcomes using reliable and valid measurement tools is essential.

Objectively measured outcomes not only assess the progress of the individual patient, but help evaluate the effectiveness of the rehabilitation program as a whole. The AACVPR Outcomes Committee has identified three outcome domains: health, which includes morbidity, mortality and quality of life; clinical, which includes physical, psychological, and social functions; and behavioral, which includes those behaviors patients attempt to change to reduce risk such as diet and smoking.[26]

The committee recommends that rehabilitation programs measure at least one parameter in each domain, e.g. a quality of life measure, one functional activity or exercise-related measure, and one behavioral measure and has developed a synopsis of the tools available for measuring outcomes in the different domains.[26,27]

Table 30.7 *Goals for secondary prevention at the University of Wisconsin Preventive Cardiology Program*

Risk factor	Goal	
Smoking	Complete cessation	
Lipids	Primary:	LDL<100 mg/dL
	Secondary:	HDL>35 mg/dL for men, >45 for women
		TG<150 mg/dL
Physical activity	30 minutes, 3–4 days per week	
Weight management	Mutually acceptable short-term (Phase II discharge) and long-term goals	
Blood pressure	<140/90 mm Hg	
Diet	AHA Step II diet:	total fat < 30%
	or as specified	saturated fat < 7%
	by the dietitian	

LDL = low-density lipoprotein; HDL = high-density lipoprotein; TG = triglycerides; AHA = American Heart Association.

Other important outcome measures include patient's report of recurrent cardiac events and hospitalizations.

Many of the goals will not be attained during the formal cardiac rehabilitation program, but will require long-term follow-up.

> A computerized tracking system is a key component to an effective system for documentation of outcomes and long-term follow-up.

Tracking systems are available commercially (Quinton, Merck, Heartwatchers, Scott Care) or individuals can develop their own. Figure 30.3 shows the UW Hospital and Clinics Preventive Cardiology tracking system.

> Typically, the supervised out-patient program lasts 3 months followed by periodic follow-up sessions.

Table 30.8 shows the progression through the UW Preventive Cardiology Outpatient Program. The orientation and first 3–5 exercise sessions are one-on-one visits with the case manager. The orientation lasts approximately 1 hour and includes reviewing the patient's medical history, describing the program services, fees, and schedule, stratifying the patient based on his/her risk (see Table 30.1) and scheduling the first exercise session. In the first session, the Medical Outcomes Trust Short Form-36 Health Survey (SF-36)[28] is administered to assess quality of life and physical, emotional, and social function. The Symptom Check List (SCL-90)[29,30] is administered to assess the patient's psychological profile including anxiety and depression. Following completion of the questionnaires the patient undergoes ECG-monitored exercise.

The Eating Pattern Assessment Tool (EPAT)[31] and Modified Cardiac Self Efficacy Tools (SET)[32] are administered during the second session. The EPAT is a food frequency questionnaire that provides an estimate of the intake total fat and saturated fat, and a percentage of total calories. The SET was refined from the work of Sullivan et al.[32] and is appropriate to use with out-patient and long-term follow-up of cardiac patients. The SET consists of two scales: Self-Efficacy/Controlling Symptoms and Self-Efficacy/Maintaining Behaviors. Positive changes in the two scales denote greater self-efficacy and better health outcomes.

In the third session, the patient is scheduled for a stress management consultation and dietitian consultation if needed. During the fourth and fifth sessions, the case manager works with the patient to develop personal short-term and long-term goals. The goals are documented in the database (Fig. 30.3) and a printed copy is given to the patient. After the sixth session, patients are either mainstreamed into the supervised group program or start a home-based program. The case manager sends letters to the primary physician and cardiologist describing the patient's goals and progress. At 6 weeks,

patients in the group exercise and home-based programs undergo an ECG-monitored session, and the case manager reviews the patient's treatment plan and personal goals. The plan is updated and a letter is sent to the primary physician if needed. At discharge, usually at 12 weeks, another ECG-monitored session is scheduled and the SF-36, SCL-90, EPAT, and SET are readministered to assess outcomes. The treatment plan is updated, the first post-discharge follow-up visit (3 months) is scheduled, and letters are sent to the primary physician and cardiologist. The case manager calls the patient at 1 month post-discharge to check on exercise compliance and assess coronary artery disease (CAD) symptoms. Follow-up visits consist of ECG-monitored exercise, administration of the EPAT, SCL-90, and SET, and updating of the treatment plan. A letter is sent to the physician following each follow-up visit summarizing the patient's status and progress toward personal treatment goals.

What are the benefits of cardiac rehabilitation and secondary prevention?

The AHCPR Practice Guideline *Cardiac Rehabilitation*[2] conducted a comprehensive and objective review of the scientific literature examining the specific outcomes of cardiac rehabilitation. The findings from that review are presented in Table 30.9. Reports reviewed included randomized controlled trials, non-randomized controlled studies, and observational studies. Most of the studies involved primarily men and outcomes were not analyzed by gender. For most outcomes limited data are available for patients over age 65.

> In general, multifactorial programs of cardiac rehabilitation, including exercise training and education, counseling and risk factor modification, are more effective than any of the components as sole interventions.

The beneficial effects of a comprehensive rehabilitation program include an improvement in exercise tolerance, fewer symptoms, improved lipid levels, reduction in cigarette smoking, improvement in psychosocial well-being, and reduction in rates of death from cardiovascular disease.[2] Cardiac rehabilitation and efforts targeted at exercise, lipid management, hypertension control, and smoking cessation can reduce cardiovascular mortality,[31,32] improve functional capacity, attenuate myocardial ischemia, retard the progression, and foster the reversal of coronary atherosclerosis, and reduce the risk of further coronary events.[6] Randomized trials of cardiac rehabilitation after myocardial infarction show consistent trends toward a survival benefit among patients enrolled in rehabilitation programs. Data from two meta-analyses of the randomized trials have demon-

Area	Date:	Results of assessment						Next assessment		INIT	Comments
Smoking		0	1	2	3	4	Asked?	6w	3m		
Measure:	Ask	–	–	–	–	–		–	–		
Goal:	Cessation	–	–	–	–	–		–	–		
Interventions:	Ask	–	–	–	–	–		–	–		
	Advise										
	Arrange										
Lipids		0	1	2	3	4	Panel?				
Measure:	Lipid panel	–	–	–	–	–		–	–		
Goals:	1° = LDL < 100	–	–	–	–	–		–	–		
	TG < 150	–	–	–	–	–		–	–		
Interventions:	Diet consult										
Diet		0	1	2	3	4	Consult?				
Measure:	EPAT	–	–	–	–	–		–	–		
Goal:	Pt 1 ≤ 15	–	–	–	–	–		–	–		
Interventions:	Diet consult										
Weight		0	1	2	3	4	WT				
Measure:	Weight	–	–	–	–	–		–	–	Goal:
Goal:	± 5lbs of goal	–	–	–	–	–		–	–		
Interventions:	Exercise Rx										
	Diet consult										
BP		0	1	2	3	4	RBP				
Measure:	Avg. BP	–	–	–	–	–		–	–		
Goal:	1° = < 140/90	–	–	–	–	–		–	–		
		–	–	–	–	–		–	–		
Interventions:	1° MD referral										
	Lifestyle chgs										
Physical		0	1	2	3	4					
Measure:	Assess	–	–	–	–	–		–	–		
Goal:	↑ FC, ADLs	–	–	–	–	–	–	–	–		
	↓ angina freq.	–	–	–	–	–	–	–	–		
Interventions:	1° MD referral										
	(if warranted)										
Psychosocial		0	1	2	3	4	Consult?				
Measure:	SF-36	–	–	–	–	–	–	–	–		
Goal:	Complete tool	–	–	–	–	–		–	–		
Interventions:	SR consult										
Activity		0	1	2	3	4					
Measure:	Assess	–	–	–	–	–		–	–		
Goal:	30', 3d/wk min	–	–	–	–	–		–	–		
Interventions:	Exercise Rx	–	–	–	–	–		–	–		

Assessment results codes: 0 = Not at goal, 1 = At goal, 2 = Not applicable, 3 = Not measured, 4 = Tool not completed.

Figure 30.3 *University of Wisconsin Hospital and Clinics Preventive Cardiology secondary prevention and goals outcomes. INIT = Clinician's initials; 6w = 6 weeks; 3m = 3 months; LDL = low-density lipoprotein; TG = triglycerides; EPAT = Eating pattern assessment tool; Pt = patient; WT = weight; Rx = prescription; BP = blood pressure; RBP = resting blood pressure; MD = Doctor of Medicine; FC = Functional capacity; ADLs = activities of daily living; SF-36 = Medical Outcomes Trust Short Form-36 Health Survey; 30', 3d/wk min = 30 minutes, 3 days/week minimum.*

Table 30.8 *University of Wisconsin Hospital and Clinics Preventive Cardiology Cardiac Rehabilitation Protocol*

Sessions	
Orientation	Review medical history
	Give program information (services, fees, schedule)
	Risk stratify
	Schedule one-on-one visits if appropriate
First	Give SF-36/SCL-90 tools prior to exercise
	ECG/hemodymanic monitoring with exercise
	Assess secondary prevention areas
	Document on patient assessment form
Second	Continue monitoring from first session
	Exercise
	Give EPAT/SET
Third	Continue monitoring from second session
	Exercise
	Sign patient up for stress management class/consultation
	Schedule diet consultation as needed
Fourth	Continue monitoring if clinically indicated
	Exercise
	Review program/goals with patient
Fifth	Review assessment results
	Document in database
	Develop and document treatment plan
	Document personal goals/print out for patient
Sixth	Start supervised group or home program
	Schedule 6-week follow-up session
	Letters to primary physician and cardiologist
Week 6	ECG monitor
	Review patient plan/personal goals
	Update plan and document
	Letters to primary physician and cardiologist (optional)
Discharge	ECG monitored exercise
	Review patient plan/personal goals
	Repeat SF-36, EPAT, SCL-90, SET
	Update plan and document outcomes
	Schedule post-discharge (DC) follow-up
	Letters to primary physician and cardiologist
1 month post-DC	Phone follow-up on exercise, CAD symptoms
	Enter in database
3 months post-DC	ECG-monitored exercise
	EPAT, SCL-90, SET
	Review outcomes, laboratories, appointments
	Enter in database
9 months post-DC	ECG-monitored exercise
	EPAT, SCL-90, SET
	Review outcomes, laboratories, appointments
	Enter in database
Subsequent follow-up visits	ECG-monitored exercise (if indicated)
	EPAT, SCL-90, SET
	Review medical history, laboratories, appointments, tests, outcomes
	Enter in database

SF-36 = Medical Outcomes Trust Short Form-36 Health Survey; SCL-90 = Symptom check list; ECG = electrocardiogram; EPAT = Eating pattern assessment tool; SET = Modified cardiac self-efficacy tools; CAD = coronary artery disease.

strated a significant 20–25 per cent reduction in cardiovascular death, but no change in the occurrence of nonfatal reinfarction in patients assigned to medically supervised and prescribed exercise programs.[33,34]

Safety of cardiac rehabilitation

The data on the safety of exercise training for coronary patients are based on two large surveys using pooled data

Table 30.9 *Benefits of cardiac rehabilitation*

Benefit	Comment
Increased exercise tolerance	Cardiac rehabilitation exercise training consistently improves objective measures of exercise tolerance without significant cardiovascular complications or other adverse outcomes
Improved strength	Strength training improves skeletal muscle strength and endurance in clinically stable coronary patients
Decreased symptoms	Exercise rehabilitation decreases angina pectoris in patients with coronary disease and decreases symptoms of heart failure in patients with left ventricular dysfunction
Smoking cessation	Exercise training alone has little effect on smoking cessation. However, the combination of cardiac rehabilitation education, counseling, and behavioral interventions leads to smoking cessation and relapse prevention in up to 25% of patients who smoke
Improved lipid levels	Exercise training alone is not recommended for lipid modification. Education, counseling, and behavioral interventions about nutrition improve dietary fat and cholesterol intake and, with and without pharmacologic lipid-lowering therapy, result in significant improvement in blood lipid levels. Benefits have been demonstrated in patients of all ages, but no study reported lipid outcomes by gender
Weight loss	Nutritional education, counseling and behavioral interventions in combination with exercise training can help patients lose weight
Blood pressure control	Expert opinion on the control of hypertension supports a strategy incorporating education and behavioral intervention with pharmacologic therapy and exercise training. Neither exercise training nor education counseling and behavioral interventions as sole modalities can control elevated blood pressure levels
Improved psychological well-being and social adjustment	Exercise training, with and without other cardiac rehabilitation services, generally results in improvements in psychological status and functioning. Multifactorial cardiac rehabilitation including education, counseling, and/or psychosocial interventions result in improved psychological well-being and social adjustment and functioning
Return to work	Cardiac rehabilitation exercise training exerts less influence on the rate of return to work than do many non-exercise factors (e.g. employer attitudes, prior employment status, economic incentives), nor have education, counseling, and behavioral interventions been shown to improve rates of return to work
Mortality	Meta-analyses of randomized controlled trials indicate that cardiac rehabilitation is associated with a 20–25% reduction in mortality. A greater reduction in mortality has been demonstrated with multifactorial cardiac rehabilitation

from multiple centers.[35,36] Overall, the rates of cardiovascular complications occurring during cardiac rehabilitation exercise training are very low. The initial survey involved 30 cardiac rehabilitation programs in the USA and Canada during a period from 1960 to 1977.[35] One non-fatal and one fatal event occurred every 34 673, and 116 402 person-hours, respectively. In a larger survey of 142 supervised exercise rehabilitation programs (1980–1984), Van Camp and Peterson estimated the risk of cardiac arrests during exercise to be 1 per 111 966 person-hours, myocardial infarction rate of 1 per 293 990 person-hours and the risk of death at 1 per 783 972 person-hours of exercise.[36] These surveys antedate the current use of risk stratification procedures.

Also, contemporary patients are generally older with more co-existing illnesses. More recently, Vongavanich *et al.*[37] reported on a small single center study over a 9-year period (1986–1995). In that study, 268 503 patient exercise hours were recorded for 4752 patients (73 per cent men). Three arrests and one myocardial infarction occurred, all events non-fatal. The results of these studies are summarized in Table 30.10.

Economics

Cost–benefit data are limited. However, comprehensive cardiac rehabilitation programs have been shown to

Table 30.10 *Safety of cardiac rehabilitation exercise training*

Study (year)	Patient exercise hours	Cardiac arrest	Fatal events
Haskell (1960–1977)	1 629 634	1/32 593	1/116 402
Van Camp (1980–1984)	2 351 916	1/111 996	1/783 972
Vongavanich (1986–1995)	268 503	1/89 501	0/268 503

reduce rehospitalization rates and lessen the need for cardiac medications.[2] Oldridge *et al.*[38] assessed the incremental cost (subtracting the cost of usual care) of services in a randomized trial of an 8-week comprehensive cardiac rehabilitation program at $480 per patient. Ades *et al.*[39] estimated that cardiac rehabilitation saved $739 in reduced hospital admissions after 21 months. Comparing the estimated $480 per patient cost with the savings estimate of $739 in reduced hospital admissions, the net savings would be $259 per patient.

CLINICAL OVERVIEW

Patients with cardiovascular disease can benefit from a comprehensive cardiac rehabilitation program. Benefits include improved exercise tolerance, improved symptoms, improved blood lipid levels, smoking cessation, an improved sense of well-being, and reduced mortality. The population considered eligible for cardiac rehabilitation has expanded from the patients with uncomplicated myocardial infarction to include the elderly (>65 years old) and patients with CABG, PTCA, stable angina, heart valve surgery, heart failure, peripheral vascular disease, and congenital heart disease and post-cardiac transplant patients.

> The delivery of cardiac rehabilitation services is changing from an exercised-based and group-oriented format to one that is multifactorial, individualized, and outcome driven.

The transition is a result of varying lengths of hospital and out-patient stay, alternate sites of services, and an increased emphasis on cost effectiveness. Patient demographics have also changed. Patients tend to be older, sicker, and have more co-morbidities. In this new framework, patients are stratified in relation to risk factors and ability to exercise, and the program is individualized based on the risk stratification.

Many programs use a case-management approach to assess the patient, individualize the program and follow-up. Each cardiac rehabilitation professional follows a defined group of patients from rehabilitation entry to discharge. The case manager is responsible and accountable for providing and/or coordinating his/her patients' care. The process involves a comprehensive initial assessment, development of a specific treatment plan based on the patient's individualized problem list, documentation of intervention and assessment of outcomes. Frequently, not all outcomes are met during the formal supervised cardiac rehabilitation program. Consequently, long-term follow-up is being built into many programs. Home programs offer an alternative to supervised out-patient programs in select low-risk patients.

FUTURE DIRECTIONS

Cardiac rehabilitation has made tremendous strides in the last 50 years. The expert panel that prepared the Clinical Practice Guideline *Cardiac Rehabilitation* concluded that cardiac rehabilitation is an essential component of the management of patients with cardiovascular diseases. However, as we move into the twenty-first century, we need to address several issues, which are listed below.

- Less than one-third of the eligible patients participate in cardiac rehabilitation. We need to increase referrals of all eligible patients and reduce the barriers to participating in cardiac rehabilitation.
- Demographics are changing: the population is aging. Over one-half of eligible patients are over age 65 years and the proportion of older patients will continue to increase. More women are beginning to participate. The patients tend to be sicker and have more co-morbidities. For many patients, the goals of cardiac rehabilitation have shifted from return to work to maintaining function in independent living. Cardiac rehabilitation will need to develop programing to meet the needs of this population.
- We need to assess the outcomes and cost-effectiveness resulting from different methods of delivering cardiac rehabilitation services: home-based approaches will need to be expanded. Newer technologies should be integrated to deliver education and counseling components of cardiac rehabilitation for those following home programs.
- The degree of medical supervision and ECG monitoring is controversial. We need objective evidence to develop appropriate guidelines for which patients need continuous ECG monitoring and for how long.
- Most of the research on safety and efficacy of cardiac rehabilitation included primarily men. We have very limited information on the elderly, women of all ages, and ethnic minorities. We also need more research on the safety and efficacy of rehabilitation in patients with heart failure and impaired ventricular function.
- We need to evaluate the safety and efficacy of resistance training in higher risk patients.
- Strategies for maintaining long-term compliance should be devised: patients make significant changes in lifestyle behavior during the supervised rehabilitation program. However, after discharge from the program, patients begin to return to their old behaviors. Smith[40] reported that almost half of all patients receiving risk reduction therapy discontinue their intervention within a year. We found that up to 35 per cent of patients who were meeting treatment goals for smoking cessation, lipid levels, blood pressure, and exercise at discharge from the cardiac

rehabilitation program were no longer meeting the goals 6 months after discharge.[41] We need to obtain data on what constitutes effective follow-up and develop strategies for helping patients make and maintain behavior changes even after they have been discharged from the program.[41]

SUMMARY

- Cardiac rehabilitation is an essential component in the management of patients with cardiovascular disease. A combination of interventions is designed to help patients improve their functional abilities, decrease their symptoms, and achieve and maintain optimal health.
- Cardiac rehabilitation is underutilized. Only 11–38 per cent of eligible patients participate in cardiac rehabilitation programs.
- Comprehensive cardiac rehabilitation involves medical evaluation, prescribed exercise, risk factor modification, education and counseling. Patients can be stratified based on level of risk.
- Cardiac rehabilitation services should be individualized based on the patient's level of risk, goals, and needs.
- The use of continuous electrocardiogram (ECG) monitoring for all cardiac patients is controversial. Continuous ECG monitoring may be useful in high-risk cardiac patients, but does not provide added safety during supervised exercise for low-risk patients.
- Strength or resistance training can safely be included in the exercise-based rehabilitation of clinically stable coronary patients with appropriate instruction and surveillance.
- Documentation of outcomes using reliable and valid measurement tools is essential.
- Patients who undergo exercise training show consistent improvements in measures of exercise tolerance with no significant cardiovascular complications.
- Comprehensive cardiac rehabilitation reduces mortality.
- Cardiac rehabilitation is cost effective.

REFERENCES

○1. Feigenbaum E, Carter E. *Cardiac rehabilitation services*. Health technology assessment report, 1987, no. 6. Rockville, MD: US Department of Health and Human Services, Public Health Service, National Center for Health Services Research and Health Care Technology Assessment. DHHS publication no. PHS 88-3427, August 1988.

○2. Wenger NK, Froelicher ES, Smith LK, *et al*. *Cardiac rehabilitation*. Clinical Practice Guideline no. 17. Rockville, MD: US Department of Health and Human Services, Public Health Service, Agency for Health Care Policy and Research and the National Heart, Lung, and Blood Institute. AHCPR Publication No. 96-0672, 1995.

3. Filip JE, Han RE, McGillen, C *et al*. Barriers to participation in cardiac rehabilitation: do they differ by gender? *Circulation* 1998; **97**: 821.

○4. American Association of Cardiovascular and Pulmonary Rehabilitation. *Guidelines for cardiac rehabilitation and secondary prevention programs*, 3rd edn. Champaign, IL: Human Kinetics, 1999.

○5. American College of Cardiology. Position report on cardiac rehabilitation. *J Am Coll Cardiol* 1986; **7**: 451–3.

○6. American Heart Association. Cardiac rehabilitation programs: a statement for health care professionals from the American Heart Association (position statement). *Circulation* 1994; **90**: 1602–10.

○7. American College of Sports Medicine. *ACSM's guidelines for exercise testing and prescription*, 6th edn. Baltimore: Williams & Wilkins, 2000.

7a. Balady GJ, Ades PA, Cosmos, P, *et al*. Core components of cardiac rehabilitation/secondary prevention programs: a statement for healthcare professionals from the American Heart Association and the American Association of Cardiovascular and Pulmonary Rehabilitation. *Circulation* 2000; **102**: 1069–73.

8. American College of Sports Medicine. *ACSM's guidelines for graded exercise testing and exercise prescription*. Philadelphia: Lea & Febiger, 1975.

9. American Association of Cardiovascular and Pulmonary Rehabilitation. *Guidelines for cardiac rehabilitation programs*. Champaign, IL: Human Kinetics, 1991.

10. American Association of Cardiovascular and Pulmonary Rehabilitation. *Guidelines for cardiac rehabilitation programs*, 2nd edn. Champaign, IL: Human Kinetics, 1994.

○11. ACSM Position Stand. Exercise for patients with coronary artery disease. *Med Sci Sports Exercise* 1994; **26**: i–v.

12. Knapp D, Gutmann M, Regis S, *et al*. Follow-up activity level among coronary artery bypass surgery (CABS) patients. *Med Sci Sports Exercise* 1982; **14**: 178.

13. McConnell TR, Klinger TA, Gardner JK, Laubach CA Jr, Herman CE, Hauck CA. Cardiac rehabilitation without exercise tests for post-myocardial infarction and post-bypass surgery patients. *J Cardiopulm Rehabil* 1998; **18**: 458–63.

14. Fagan ET, Wayne VS, McConachy DL. Serious ventricular arrhythmias in a cardiac rehabilitation programme. *Med J Aust* 1984; **141**: 421–4.

♦15. Van Camp SP, Peterson RA. Cardiovascular complications of outpatient cardiac rehabilitation programs. *JAMA* 1986; **256**: 1160–3.

○16. Franklin BA, Bonzheim K, Gordon S, Timmis GC. Resistance training in cardiac rehabilitation. *J Cardiopulm Rehabil* 1991; **11**: 99–107.

♦17. DeBusk RF, Haskell WL, Miller NH, *et al.* Medically directed at home rehabilitation soon after clinically uncomplicated acute myocardial infarction: A new model for patient care. *Am J Cardiol* 1985; **55**: 251–7.

♦18. DeBusk RF, Blomqvist CG, Kouchoukos NT, *et al.* Identification and treatment of low-risk patients after acute myocardial infarction and coronary artery bypass surgery. *N Engl J Med* 1986; **313**: 161–6.

♦19. DeBusk RF, Miller NH, Superko HR, *et al.* A case management system for coronary risk factor modification following acute myocardial infarction. *Ann Intern Med* 1994; **120**: 721–9.

○20. Swan HJC, Gersh BJ, Graboys TB, Ullyot DJ. Task Force 7. Evaluation and management of risk factors for the individual patient (case management). *J Am Coll Cardiol* 1996; **27**: 1030–9.

21. Smith SC, Blair SN, Criqui MH, *et al.* Preventing heart attack and death in patients with coronary disease. *Circulation* 1995; **92**: 2–4.

22. Summary of the Second Report of the National Cholesterol Education Program (NCEP) Expert Panel on Detection, Evaluation and Treatment of High Blood Cholesterol in Adults (Adult Treatment Panel II). *JAMA* 1993; **269**: 3015–23.

23. The Fifth Report of the Joint National Committee on Detection, Evaluation, and Treatment of High Blood Pressure (JNCV). *Arch Intern Med* 1993; **153**: 154–83.

24. Jonas MA, Oates JA, Ockene JK, Hennekens CH. Statement on smoking and cardiovascular disease for health care professionals. American Heart Association. *Circulation* 1992; **86**: 1664–9.

25. National Institutes of Health, National Heart, Lung, and Blood Institute. *Clinical guidelines on the identification, evaluation, and treatment of overweight and obesity in adults: the evidence report.* Rockville, MD: National Institutes of Health National Heart, Lung, and Blood Institute, 1998.

○26. Pashkow P, Ades PA, Emery CF, *et al.* Outcomes measurement in cardiac and pulmonary rehabilitation. *J Cardiopulm Rehabil* 1995; **15**: 394–405.

○27. Pashkow P, Emery CF, Frid DJ, *et al. AACVPR outcomes tools resource guide.* Middleton, WI: American Association of Cardiovascular and Pulmonary Rehabilitation, 1996.

28. Ware JE, Sherbourne CO. The MOS36-item short-form health survey (SF-36): I. Conceptual framework and item selection. *Med Care* 1992; **30**: 473–83.

29. Derogatis LR. *SCL-90: administration, scoring and procedure manual.* Baltimore: Clinical Psychometrics Research, 1983.

○30. Allison TG, Williams DE, Miller TD, Patten CA, Bailey KR, Squires RW, Gau GT. Medical and economic costs of psychologic distress in patients with coronary artery disease. *Mayo Clin Proc* 1995; **70**: 734–42.

31. Peters JR, Quiter ES, Brekke ML. The eating pattern assessment tool: a simplified instrument for assessing dietary fat and cholesterol intake. *Am J Diet Assoc* 1994; **94**: 1008–13.

32. Sullivan MD, LaCroix AZ, Russo J, Katon WJ. Self-efficacy and self-reported functional status in coronary heart disease: a six-month prospective study. *Psychosom Med* 1998; **60**: 473–8.

♦33. Oldrigde NB, Guyatt GH, Fischer ME, Rimm AA. Cardiac rehabilitation after myocardial infarction: combined experience of randomized clinical trails. *JAMA.* 1988; **260**: 945–50.

♦34. O'Connor GT, Buring JE, Yusuf S, Goldhaber SZ, Olmstead EM, Paffenbarger RS Jr, Hennekens CH. An overview of randomized trials of rehabilitation with exercise after myocardial infarction. *Circulation* 1989; **80**: 234–44.

♦35. Haskell WL. Cardiovascular complications during exercise training of cardiac patients. *Circulation* 1978; **57**: 920–5.

♦36. Van Camp SP, Peterson RA. cardiovascular complication of outpatient cardiac rehabilitation programs. *JAMA* 1986; **256**: 1160–3.

37. Vongavanich P, Paul-Labrador MJ, Bairey Merz NC. Safety of medically supervised exercise in a cardiac rehabilitation center. *Am J Cardiol* 1996; **77**: 1383–5.

♦38. Oldridge N, Rurlong W, Feeny D, Torrance G, Guyatt G, Crowe J, Jones N. Economic evaluation of cardiac rehabilitation soon after acute myocardial infarction. *Am J Cardiol* 1993; **72**: 154–61.

39. Ades PA, Huang D, Weaver SO. Cardiac rehabilitation participation predicts lower rehospitalization costs. *Am Heart J* 1992; **123**: 916–21.

40. Smith SC Jr. Risk-reduction therapy: the challenge to change. Presented at the 68th Scientific Sessions of the American Heart Association November 13, 1995, Anaheim (AHA President's Address). *Circulation* 1996; **93**: 2205–11.

41. Einerson J, Vitcenda M, Ward A, McBride P. Secondary prevention outcomes in cardiac patients at discharge and follow-up. *J Cardiopulm Rehabil* 1999; **19**: 5.

31

Visiting nurse programs, subacute care, and home health care: the expanding paradigm

MINDY FAIN

The demand for out of hospital care of cardiovascular disease is growing rapidly, fueled by health care financing and enabled by medical technology, information systems, and patient preferences. Traditional Medicare home health agencies, newer comprehensive home care programs, and subacute care services represent options for management. Physicians are responsible for medical authorization and overseeing care. Patients with many cardiovascular disorders, including congestive heart failure and venous thromboembolic disease, can be managed in these alternative sites, achieving cost-effective, high quality outcomes.

INTRODUCTION

The potential role of home care programs and subacute care in the overall management of the patient with cardiac disease is currently being defined. The combination of advances in medical techniques and equipment, sophisticated information systems, patient preferences for comfort and control, and health care financing that promotes alternative sites of care has opened the door to a new paradigm for care. Physicians, although reluctant in the past to become actively involved in nursing home and home care activities, have always been and continue to be responsible for medical authorization and overseeing these activities. Greater physician understanding and involvement in the design and provision of these new programs is needed. Physicians, now and in the future, will be responsible for the care of patients in nontraditional, alternative sites.

Increased economic pressures over the past 15 years initially changed the role of nursing homes and home care services in the delivery of care to patients. Since Medicare's Prospective Payment System (PPS) was implemented in 1983, patients have been discharged from the hospital 'sicker and quicker', prompting an increase in the number and use of skilled nursing facilities (SNFs) and home health agencies (HHAs). Hospitals rushed into the home care business. As the acuity of the case mix increased, SNFs and HHAs responded to meet the increased clinical care demands. Subacute care units were developed within nursing homes and hospitals to expand the type and intensity of care and services available in the postacute hospital setting. Visiting nurse agencies (VNAs), seen as a means to reduce the length of hospital stay and ease the transition from hospital to home, responded with 'high-tech' treatment and monitoring capabilities. Lastly, home health care (HHC) teams with a highly integrated physician role emerged to provide comprehensive home care for emergent/urgent problems and chronic disease management.

OVERVIEW

The demand for organized health care delivery systems and alternative sites for care continues to grow. Visiting nurse agencies, home health care, and subacute care units are the sites and programs involved in this new paradigm of care. These programs have the potential to facilitate early hospital discharge, reduce hospital admissions, and provide quality, cost-effective care.

Visiting nurse programs – the Medicare Home Health Model

HISTORICAL PERSPECTIVE

From the late eighteenth century, home nursing visits to support indigent families were funded by religious orders and secular groups. One of the first home nursing services was established in Boston in 1796. At that time, much of the care at home was linked to public health problems and preventative care issues. By the end of the nineteenth century, visiting nurse associations, funded by philanthropy, were delivering most of the home care services in the USA. Home visits by physicians comprised a central role in general patient care. The modern hospital era began in the late nineteenth and early twentieth century, but most sick people still preferred to remain at home with the support of their families, privately paid visiting nurses, and physician house calls.[1]

By the 1940s and 1950s physician home visits were on the decline for a number of reasons. Facility-based care was encouraged after World War II because of federal funding legislation. In addition, the combination of improved public transportation and advanced medical technology promoted centralized patient care sites in offices and hospitals. Malpractice litigation at the time favored the newer, high-technological treatments, and made 'low-tech' home care even more unappealing to the physician. The hospital became the standard place for the treatment of serious ailments, and represented the gold standard of care. There was a brief renewal of home care during the polio epidemics in the 1950s and 1960s, when patients were sent home with life-support machines, and some physicians became skilled in high-technology home care. Ultimately, though, provisions for comprehensive home care services in the original Medicare and Medicaid legislation in the 1960s emphasized only nursing, rehabilitation, and other ancillary services. Although physician supervision was required, reimbursement was not commensurate with other physician activities. This ultimately solidified the physician's declining presence in home care.[2] The hospital represents the current paradigm for acute medical care.

Home care, 'the provision of care and services in a patient's home rather than an institutional setting or a provider's office', continues to be defined by public policies. For example, the 1965 Medicare legislation required home health agencies to provide nursing service plus one additional service, such as physical therapy, occupational therapy, speech therapy, medical social service' or home health aide.[3] Thus, the term 'visiting nurse' is a misnomer, as a variety of health care professionals and paraprofessionals are typically members of the care team (Table 31.1).

Medicare legislation and resulting funding priorities were originally conceived as a way to discharge patients from the hospital earlier and to reduce nursing home utilization. Before 1980, eligibility through Medicare was limited to those beneficiaries who had previously been hospitalized for at least 3 days. In 1980, this requirement was eliminated, and in 1988–1989 home health care eligibility was again liberalized and standardized.[4] This legislation resulted in an explosion of home health agencies, nurse-directed teams serving the patient's medical, nursing, rehabilitative, social, nutritional, and other needs.

Table 31.1 *Typical members of the visiting nurse agency team*

Registered nurses[a]
Occupational therapists[a]
Speech pathologists[a]
Physical therapists[a]
Medical social services[a]
Dietitians[a]
Home health aides[a]
Respiratory therapists
Clinical psychologists
Licensed practical nurses
Homemaker
Companions
Respiratory therapists

[a] Seven services covered under the Medicare home health benefit.

The 1990s have also shown substantial increases in physicians' direct involvement in home care. Market reform and integrated systems of care have made it more economically feasible for the physician to participate in home care management. Since 1998 there are nine current procedural terminology (CPT) codes for physician home visits of new and established patients, and a home care plan overseeing code[5] (Table 31.2). Although increased, physician payment is still low, and most physi-

Table 31.2 *Current procedural terminology (CPT) codes for home visits and oversight*

Home visit, new patient	99341 Focused
	99342 Expanded
	99343 Detailed
	99344 Comprehensive 1
	99345 Comprehensive 2
Home visit, established patient	99347 Focused
	99348 Expanded
	99349 Detailed
	99350 Comprehensive
Care plan oversight	G0181 30 minutes/month/ patient

Table 31.3 *Barriers to physician involvement in home health care*

Communication with agency inefficient and disruptive
Lack of physician understanding about home care
Inadequate physician reimbursement for services provided
Complex regulatory and legal issues

cians, though responsible for authorization and overseeing, tend merely to ratify the plans of others. There are multiple barriers to physician involvement in home care, outlined in Table 31.3.[6]

REGULATORY AND LEGAL ISSUES

Current regulations complicate the ability of the physician to provide coordinated care in the home. At the time of the original Medicare regulations, medical fraud and physician financial involvement in home health agencies was of great concern. Limitations were set on financial interest in home health agencies to less than 5 per cent of total assets, stock or profit, or less than $25 000 in salary or other benefits; above that, the physician could not refer patients to the home health agency. This often prevented a medical director of a home health agency from providing care, case management, or house calls for agency patients.

The original Medicare Act 'Anti Kickback' laws and the recent Stark II self-referral legislative provisions further complicate the situation, especially when health care providers employ physicians and provide home health services.[7] These providers include hospitals, home health agencies, and other health clinics. Under these circumstances, (1) if a home health agency is owned by a hospital, and (2) the hospital-employed physician (who may provide direct patient care at various hospital clinics and out-patient settings) is compensated in excess of $25 000, then (3) that physician may not refer patients to that home health agency. In addition, that physician may not establish or review the plan of treatment, or certify/re-certify the need for home health care. (If the home health agency is separately incorporated, then this would not limit hospital-employed physicians). Collaborative practices, however, such as physicians employing and working closely with physician assistants or nurse practitioners (as is seen in nursing homes and hospitals), are also affected by these laws when delivering home care services.

The passage of the Health Insurance Portability and Accountability Act is also relevant to home care. This legislation expanded the fraud and abuse provisions.[8] Physicians who knowingly approve care that does not meet Medicare guidelines are made subject to heavy fines. This would apply to physicians who falsely certify (with deliberate ignorance and reckless disregard) that a patient meets all of Medicare's requirements for home care. However, many physicians are distanced from the day-to-day activities of home health agencies and often poorly educated about home care in general, limiting their ability to effectively provide for certification/re-certification and care plan overseeing. In addition, there are no requirements for a home health agency to have a medical director (unlike nursing homes or hospices), thus further limiting physicians' involvement in the process of care. To begin to remedy this, in 1995 a Care Plan Oversight payment code was introduced to encourage physician home care case management.[9] In 1996, the American Medical Association recommended that all home care agencies hire a medical director.

Although this was meant to limit fraud and abuse, and avoid overutilization of home health services, the unintended consequences of these regulations are disruption of coordinated care across the continuum, making effective on-site care in the home by the physician more difficult. These regulations need to be considered when developing a home care program that includes highly integrated physician services. Depending upon the arrangement, home health agencies and hospital-based agencies are at risk. There is a call for some of these physician certification regulations to be revised. Questions or requests for clarification should be submitted to the Health Care Financing Administration (HCFA).

Lastly, laboratory regulatory requirements under the Clinical Laboratory Improvement Amendments (CLIA) limit the number of tests that can be performed in the home and remain cost effective.[10] It is argued that the CLIA regulations were based on high-volume, independent laboratories, where wet control calibrations of traditional equipment every 8 hours is possible. Currently only a few tests can be done in the home with electronically calibrated equipment, such as portable blood analyzers (blood urea nitrogen (BUN), glucose, hemoglobin, electrolytes, calcium, and arterial blood gases). However, the HCFA reviewed the CLIA regulations in 1996 and continues to support these restrictions in order to maintain and improve quality.

PRESENT STATUS

Approximately six million people receive home care services nationally each year, and the care and services available to the homebound population, along with costs, continue to grow. Home health reimbursements currently account for more than 8 per cent of the total Medicare budget. As the fastest growing portion of Medicare expenses, costs were projected to reach $20 billion by 1998.[11]

Certain criteria must be met for Medicare-sponsored patients to receive home care services, and third-party payers often follow these same Medicare guidelines to determine eligibility[2] (Table 31.4). There is a wide variety of care and services available in the home, including

Table 31.4 *Medicare criteria for home care reimbursement*

Patient is homebound
- Requires considerable, taxing effort to leave the home
- Patient may have absences from the home for medical care or spiritual services
- Patient may reside in a board-and-care home, but not a nursing home

Services must be intermittent
Services must be reasonable
Services must be medically necessary
Services must be ordered by a physician
Services must be provided by a certified home health agency

Table 31.6 *Indications for physician home visits (adapted from AMA guidelines[12])*

Sick patients responding poorly to medical therapy
Discrepancies in the patient's reported functioning
Acute declines in health or function
Unexplained failure to thrive
Unexplained failure of the care plan
Patients with multiple chronic illnesses and interacting psychosocial problems
Terminally ill patients who wish to die at home
Suspected cases of patient abuse or high caregiver stress
Need for patient/family meeting to make an important decision
Request by another team member or family/patient
Assessment of an acute illness to determine management options

comprehensive home assessment, skilled nursing assessment, education, and counseling, physical therapy, occupational therapy and speech therapy, diet assessment and education. In addition, there are newly available procedures and treatments. Advances in technology that led medical care away from home and into hospitals now makes aggressive care possible in the home (Table 31.5). The AMA Guidelines for the Medical Management of the Home Care Patient[12] and the Council on Scientific Affairs Report[13] identified several indications for a physician home visit (Table 31.6), recognizing that it is often difficult to determine when a physician needs to be on site, or whether the assessment from home health nurses and therapists is sufficient for management of the homebound patient. The frequency of continuing assessments should assure that the physician knows the current status of the patient, and be comparable to the visit frequency required to manage the condition in other settings.

Although rooted in transitional care of the patient from hospital to home, and able to provide a more intensive, high-tech category of home care, visiting nurse programs are now primarily used to provide long-term management of chronic disease, with a majority of

patient visits no longer predominantly linked to acute care needs. The overwhelming majority of home visits are made by nurses (40 per cent) and home health aides (50 per cent). This care provides much needed support for the elderly and infirm at home, and can optimize the quality of life and enhance the function of the frail and dependent patient. It often substitutes for care previously provided by family or friends, and intuitively appears to be a cost-effective means of assistance if only minimal services are required to avoid costly hospitalizations or institutionalization.[4]

COST EFFECTIVENESS

Despite these observations, clinical studies have not shown that visiting nurse programs save money. There are many reasons why it is difficult to measure and demonstrate the cost effectiveness of home care, including the heterogeneity of the population served, the complex health service interventions, problems of client selection and recruitment, logistics of follow-up, dropouts, and the consent and cooperation of the controls.[14] Indeed, in many studies survival has not improved, functional impairment has not slowed, and total costs of care may have been higher. A recent analysis failed to demonstrate that these conventional, chronic care services replaced hospital services or nursing home services, and additionally, raised questions about how successful Medicare's home health care program is in reducing expenditures for other services.[4]

Observers question whether it is possible for visiting nurse programs to be cost effective for several reasons. First, the home health agency under the fee-for-service system served as both the provider and the manager of care, a financial incentive that leads to a 'more is better' approach. However, since October 2000, Medicare home health agencies are being paid under the new Prospective Payment System (PPS), reversing these incentives. Second, there is a limited ability for home care agencies

Table 31.5 *Newer care and services available in the home*

Intravenous therapy, including antibiotics, hydration, TPN, diuretics, inotropics, blood products, chemotherapy, narcotics
Enteral feeding (gastrostomy or nasogastric tube)
Comprehensive wound management
Bladder catheterization and training
Cardiac rehabilitation and advanced cardiac care assessment and monitoring (post-MI, post-CABG, endocarditis, pre-transplant)
Pulse oximetry and spirometry
Ventilator management
Maintenance of percutaneous indwelling cathether lines, Groshong and Hickman catheters
On-site laboratory, electrocardiogram, radiology services

CABG = coronary artery bypass grafting; MI = myocardial infarction; TPN = total parenteral nutrition.

to manage cases across the continuum of care. Also the physician is often not in the position within the home care agency to manage sites of care and services, and its attendant costs optimally, especially if the patient begins to fail at home. Many times, a trip to the emergency room or urgent care is the solution. Third, hospitals traditionally viewed home care as a way to offset costs and increase revenue. In the traditional fee-for-service world, as length of hospital stays shortened, and hospital revenues declined, a home care service was a source for profit building for the hospital. It was an opportunity to generate revenue, shift overhead, and create margins. Very little focus had been placed on reducing the number of hospital admissions.

With the introduction of managed care, the role of the home health agency is shifted from a revenue generator to a cost center. These programs will be evaluated as to their ability to reduce total patient costs – shortening the length of stay, and delaying patient admission to both hospitals and nursing homes. The model of visiting nurse programs will likely be most cost effective when utilized to reduce hospital length of stay for patients with specific care needs, such as continuation of wound care, and delivery of intravenous antibiotics. Further studies are needed to determine the role of traditional visiting nurse programs as part of a cost-effective, comprehensive, coordinated system of care.

Additionally, home care is not for everyone. It can be physically and emotionally draining for the family. Lack of health insurance or limits on coverage create financial strains. Lost income of caregivers, especially daughters, who serve as unpaid caregivers instead of receiving outside wages, can be especially difficult. For some families providing high-tech care, the stress of a bedroom turned into an intensive care unit can be overwhelming. The caregiver may also not be capable of delivering the care that is required. Physicians must recognize when home care is not an appropriate alternative for a family, but rather a solution forced upon them by reimbursement policies. In these instances, advocacy by the physician for consideration of acute hospitalization, subacute care, or skilled nursing home care would be more appropriate.

There is growing concern about fraud in the home health care industry. Home care patients are often vulnerable, underserved, and isolated. They include the frail elderly with complex medical, psychological, and social problems, and are among the highest users of medical services. Fraud and abuse on the part of home health agencies, durable medical equipment vendors, and physicians, is a real problem. Home care is provided by private agencies (both for-profit and not-for-profit), hospitals, public health departments, and the Veterans Affairs. Over half the recipients of home care in the five highest-use states are served by for-profit agencies, which is approximately twice the national average. For-profit agencies provide many more visits per client than

other agencies.[4] The combination of explosive growth, reduced review of Medicare claims because of budget cuts, relaxation of eligibility criteria, and lack of physician surveillance fuels the concern about fraud. As noted previously, multiple statutory and regulatory restraints are in place to reduce fraud and abuse, but these restrictions have been shown also to hinder the implementation of new diagnostic and treatment modalities in the home. A balance needs to be found to provide quality, cost-effective care.

Home health care

HISTORICAL PERSPECTIVE

For the purposes of this discussion, an emerging form of team care at home will be termed 'home health care'. The distinguishing characteristic of HHC is the active involvement of the physician in the planning and implementation of care by the team in the home, including the house call. It has been well recognized that, without physician house calls, the care of the seriously and chronically ill elderly and terminal patients has been relegated to urgent care facilities, emergency rooms, crisis hospitalizations, and long-term care facilities. This has occurred despite the chronic support by traditional visiting nurse programs. The growing population of homebound patients has been seriously deprived of access to physicians in their homes, and hospitalization is a major risk for older persons. Iatrogenic complications, and the interaction of aging, hospitalization, and its associated bed rest, often leads to an irreversible decline[15] (Table 31.7). The introduction of the physician as an integral part of the team expands the team's capabilities to optimize a treatment regimen, and to include on-site assessment and management of many acute illnesses, including emergency room diversion techniques and home health care treatment intervention termed 'home hospitalization' (HH) (Table 31.8). In this model, the critical components of hospital care – physician, nursing, medicines and technology – are brought to

Table 31.7 *Hazards of hospitalization and bed rest for the elderly*

Decreased muscle strength and mass
Diminished aerobic capacity
Loss of plasma volume
Orthostatic hypotension
Reduced arterial oxygen tension (PO_2)
Accelerated bone loss
Urinary incontinence, functional
Pressure sores
Reduced sensory input leading to confusion
Malnutrition and dehydration
Delirium

Table 31.8 *Examples of the expanded range of care and services with physician home visit*

Medical care of complex patients (heart failure, ischemic heart disease, chronic obstructive pulmonary disease (COPD), diabetes, Parkinson's disease)

Pain and other symptom management in complex, terminally ill patients (seizures, vomiting, bowel obstruction)

Diagnostic/therapeutic paracentesis or thoracentesis

Treatment of pressure sores, including debridement

Drainage of superficial abscesses

Diagnosis and treatment on-site of certain acute illnesses:
- Exacerbation of COPD and heart failure
- Angina pectoris
- Community-acquired pneumonia
- Cellulitis
- Urinary tract infections

the home, avoiding acute hospitalization. Cost containment and managed care pressures have led to increased demand for this type of care.

PRESENT STATUS

In 1947, Montefiore Hospital in New York City established the first hospital-based home care program, uniting two systems of home care – physician's house calls and visiting nurses' care. This program, however, entered the health care arena simultaneously with the explosion of hospital-based, high-tech care, and thus was not timed historically for success. Similar models of home care have been developed over the years, focused on the chronically ill, elderly population.[14]

One of the longest standing models of home health care is the Veteran's Affairs (VA) Medical Center Home Based Primary Care Programs (HBPC, formerly HBHC). This program was created in response to a demographic imperative noted by the VA – the large number of aging World War II veterans.[16]

First developed in the 1970s, the HBPC program consists of a multidisciplinary team directed by a physician and based on a nurse case-manager model. The program provides primary health care to medically complex, functionally disabled patients in their own homes. Services provided include medical, nursing, social work, rehabilitative, pharmacy, psychological, and dietetic care. A nurse case manager coordinates care for a changing panel of selected veterans.

The model of HBPC differs from traditional (e.g. Medicare reimbursed) visiting nurse agencies. The HBPC physician is an active participant, working closely with the home care team, making home visits, developing the plan of care during weekly team meetings, and making timely management decisions. Home hospitalization services are provided, and key clinical interventions, at times, may be highly intense and time-consuming. The nursing care and services are not subject to Medicare restrictions, requiring home services to be

'part-time' and 'intermittent' for reimbursement. This provides the flexibility to meet fluctuating patient care needs, common in chronic diseases.

Studies have demonstrated that the HBPC model improves patient and caregiver satisfaction and is cost effective, reducing hospital costs and ambulatory care use.[16]

Recently, a model of care specifically for patients with congestive heart failure (CHF) was developed by Rich *et al.*[17] Patients with CHF are a high-cost group with complex care needs. A prospective, randomized trial of 282 patients was conducted to assess the effect of this nurse-directed, multidisciplinary intervention. The treatment regimen provided intensive education, individualized medications regimens and dietary instruction, and close follow-up including active medical management. This model was shown to improve quality of life and reduce hospital use and medical costs for elderly patients with CHF. Unlike other conventional home care approaches, this strategy included substantial medical management, with success likely due in part to more effective responses to the early signs of cardiac failure.

Physician on-site home care has also been found to be cost effective for selected patients on managed care contracts.[13] A 1995 study by Kaiser Permanente in San Diego evaluated the use of a physician-staffed mobile emergency van unit to provide care on-site at home when Kaiser facilities were overloaded. FHP Health Plan in California instituted a program of physician home visits for homebound patients with subacute illness. Both studies, though small, indicated cost savings.

A larger, recent study from Israel of a 'home hospital' program[18] demonstrated that, for selected elderly patients, substitution of home care instead of traditional hospitalization saved hospital days and nursing home days, and provided a favorable cost–benefit ratio. Central to the success of this program was the prompt medical intervention, with capabilities for on-site diagnosis and treatment. The HH program staff consisted of a treating physician and additional paramedical support required for home care, including a nurse, social worker, and therapist. The most common medical diagnoses for this group of patients was heart failure, ischemic heart disease, and obstructive pulmonary disease. Early detection and treatment of life-threatening complications such as intercurrent infection and exacerbation of heart failure enabled patients to remain in their homes. There are limitations, however, to the applicability of this particular model to the USA and its health care system. This study was not randomized, and the controls were not optimal. Analysis did not take into consideration the shift of costs to family caregivers.

These home care strategies include substantial medical management, with nurses, nurse practitioners, and clinical nurse specialists delivering much of the care. New technologies continue to be introduced, rapidly expanding diagnostic and treatment capabilities available during a home visit. Portable blood analyzers, 12-lead electrocardiogram machines, x-ray machines, including on-site processing, ultrasound machines, and miniaturized and simplified devices for parenteral drug delivery allow physicians to complete a diagnostic evaluation and begin treatment in one encounter, at home.

Mobile units with interactive communication and biotelemetry (transmission of data, video, voice, and imaging) further expands diagnostic considerations and therapeutics. There continues to be new opportunities for innovative HHC programs for those patients who are at high risk and for whom multidisciplinary intervention is appropriate.

COST EFFECTIVENESS

In recent years, the models of HHC and HH have been increasingly accepted as cost-effective alternatives. Physicians in predominantly fee-for-service markets have viewed HHC and HH as a management option that increases paperwork, telephone calls, and workload, without meaningful reimbursement. However, a substantial part of health care is now managed care, and for managed care groups accepting full capitation, these alternate-site options offer cost savings. Indeed, the concern is that economic considerations alone may force its use without proper validation. Physician involvement is critical in developing practice guidelines, including patient selection criteria, clinical assessment and monitoring, and outcomes measurements.

There are inherent difficulties in the design of studies to evaluate the cost effectiveness of HH. Patients selected for HH should be sick enough to have required hospital care, but not so sick that the level of surveillance is insufficient at home. This selection is further complicated by the current lack of accepted criteria for hospital admission for many diseases. General guidelines for hospital admission are currently being developed for some acute illnesses (e.g. community-acquired pneumonia), and exacerbations of chronic illnesses (chronic obstructive pulmonary disease). Randomizing patients may be difficult because many patients believe that hospital care is the best care. Also, most of the studies have not taken into consideration the cost of shifting the burden of care to the family or other caregiver, both financially and emotionally. Therefore, although HHC and HH systems are a feasible model for caring for ill older persons, further evaluation is needed.

DEVELOPING A HOME HEALTH CARE PROGRAM

The development of a home health care program does not necessarily incur major start-up costs. As an outreach of an office-based or hospital-based clinical practice, a nurse case-manager together with a physician constitute the basic team requirements. Liaisons between physician groups and established visiting nurse programs, especially with the guidance of an involved medical director of the home health agency, can provide effective, comprehensive home care. Expanding committed team coverage to 24 hours/day and ensuring clear lines of communication between the patient, case manager, and primary care physician, are the major hurdles. Home visits and telephone calls are, for the most part, handled by the nurse. The physician, in addition to case management and overseeing, makes home visits when indicated.

An expanded multidisciplinary team or home hospitalization team requires more commitment of time and resources. Various program options include a designated home care team providing care within a managed care group or integrated health care system, or a hospital-based home care team providing home hospitalization options.

The ultimate structure will depend upon multiple variables, including population needs, regulatory and legal restrictions, reimbursement options, and the acuity of on-site assessment and treatment to be provided (Table 31.9).

Table 31.9 *Developing a home care program*

Identify mission, vision, and values

Develop organizational structure

Identify the care and services (considerations: patient needs/ special populations, reimbursement, legal and regulatory issues)

Identify program staffing requirements

Determine patient selection criteria/clinical characteristics (considerations: availability of caregiver, geographic restrictions, high risk criteria)

Develop referral process and linkage with community resources

Establish clinical pathways (education, assessment, counseling, monitoring, treatment)

Identify equipment required for care of patients on-site (e.g. portable electrocardiography, oximeter, intravenous pumps, portable imaging)

Develop system integrated communication and medical information systems

Devise measurement strategies to evaluate the program's effectiveness (cost and quality)

Subacute care facilities

HISTORICAL PERSPECTIVE

Nursing homes in the early 1900s were highly unregulated facilities delivering inferior care to the poor and mentally ill. Initial changes came in 1935 with the passage of the Social Security Act, providing funds for the elderly, which could be used for long-term institutional care. However, nursing homes were still largely unregulated until 1965 when Title 18 and 19 of the Social Security Act was passed (Medicare/Medicaid) and the Federal Government assumed a major role in quality management. Throughout the next two decades, however, care in nursing homes was still considered poor, and attempts to improve the quality of care ultimately resulted in the passage of the Nursing Home Reform Amendments of the Omnibus Budget Reconciliation Act (OBRA) of 1987. Currently more than one and a half million people reside in nursing homes at a cost of $53 billion dollars in 1990.[19] The quality of care has greatly improved over the last decade, despite taking care of a sicker population under more regulations and with decreased funding. A major barrier, however, is the unavailability of sufficient trained professional staff on site. In many nursing homes there are still not enough capable health care providers, especially registered nurses and involved physicians, to assure quality on-site care.

PRESENT STATUS

In response to the Medicare Prospective Payment System and other financing systems, service utilization patterns have changed, and acute care hospitals, rehabilitation hospitals, and nursing homes have responded with 'intermediate care facilities' (ICFs) or 'subacute care' units (SCUs).[20] These units, compared to typical nursing home beds, provide more acute nursing and medical care for both diagnosis and therapy, along with laboratory and imaging services, and the capacity for intravenous therapies. The clinical care team represents a variety of backgrounds, including clinical nurse practitioners, respiratory, physical, occupational and speech therapists, and other health professionals. The goal of these units is to provide less costly sites of care for hospitalized patients, or avoid acute hospitalization entirely. Approximately 80 per cent of patients are hospital transfers and 20 per cent are direct admissions. Medicare reimbursement requires a 3-day hospital stay prior to transfer to a SCU.[21]

Subacute care, as defined by the Joint Commission on Accreditation of Healthcare Organizations (JCAHO), requires an interdisciplinary team, and is 'goal-oriented, comprehensive, in-patient care designed for an individual who has had an acute illness, injury, or exacerbation of a disease process' but does not require acute hospital care. Treatment should be directed towards one or more specific, active, complex medical conditions, or to administer one or more technically complex treatments, but the patient's care should not depend heavily on high-tech monitoring or complex diagnostic procedures. Patients in these units require frequent assess-

ments and treatments for a limited time (daily to weekly) until the condition has stabilized, or the course of care completed. A registered nurse is on site at all times to assess the patients. The American Medical Association recommended that a medical director be assigned to subacute units, and developed guidelines for physicians providing care to patients in subacute care units[20] (Table 31.10). These guidelines differ from JCAHO requirements.

Table 31.10 *Guidelines for physician responsibilities in subacute care*

Physicians are responsible to their patients 24 hours a day, 7 days a week

Physicians are responsible for the supervision and coordination of care

Physicians should complete an initial assessment within 24 hours of admission that identifies the medical services needed (*JCAHO – 48 hours)

Physicians should make an on-site visit within 72 hours to review the interdisciplinary plan of care

Physicians should determine the number of medically necessary follow-up visits; these may occur daily, but never less than weekly (*JCAHO – every 2 weeks)

Physician activity should be documented

JCAHO = Joint Commission on Accreditation of Healthcare Organizations.

Technically there is no designated 'subacute' care coverage category under Medicare. There are also no specific billing codes for 'subacute patients' other than one of standard nursing facility visit codes, but there are approved prolonged visit codes for extended visits to patients in nursing facilities, along with no limitation on billing for medically necessary visits (Table 31.11). Accreditation standards for subacute care have recently been developed by the JCAHO, and surveying began in 1995. In 1994, the Commission on Accreditation of Rehabilitation Facilities released in-patient rehabilitation standards for ICFs and SCUs.

Common admission diagnoses include orthopedic problems, post-stroke, pressure sores, post-surgical patients with deconditioning or wound issues, cancer, and decompensated heart and lung disease. The range of services considered 'subacute' is very broad, and includes infusion therapy, respiratory and cardiac care and monitoring, wound care, rehabilitation services, postoperative recovery programs for large joint replacements, cancer treatments and acquired immunodeficiency syndrome (AIDS) care[21] (Table 31.12). Typically, patients spend 1–3 weeks, and ultimately are discharged home.

Many hospitals and nursing homes are eager to develop SCUs, a fast-growing field that currently has revenues of $3 billion. Health care providers are viewing subacute care as an opportunity to market to managed

Table 31.11 *CPT coding for physician services to sub-acute patients*

Comprehensive assessment, new or established patient	99301	Low complexity	30 minutes
Comprehensive assessment, new or established patient	99302	Moderate	40 minutes
Comprehensive assessment, new or established patient	99303	High complexity	50 minutes
New or established patient, not comprehensive	99311	Low complexity	15 minutes
New or established patient, not comprehensive	99312	Moderate	25 minutes
New or established patient, not comprehensive	99313	High complexity	35 minutes
Prolonged visit codes for extended visits to patients in nursing facilities	99356, 99357		> 65 minutes

- Prior billing for same patient that day
- Time counted includes only direct care
- Medical record documents the content
- Typical time of visit code has been exceeded by 30 minutes

Table 31.12 *Examples of subacute care and services*

Intravenous antibiotics
Skilled nurse observations for heart failure, liver failure, renal failure
Physical therapy 5 days/week
Occupational therapy 5 days/week
Weaning from oxygen therapy with arterial blood gases (ABGs) 3 times/week
Tracheal suction 2 times/shift
Respiratory therapy 3 times/day
Blood glucose check 2 times/day with insulin therapy
Wound care daily
Bladder training

care businesses, claiming quality post-acute care hospital services for less cost than traditional hospital care. Some SCUs market special programs of care – ventilator weaning, burn care, or cancer chemotherapy, for example. Enthusiasm is tamed, however, by the complex regulations and reimbursement rules governing this newly developing field, leading to operational, financial, and policy hurdles.[22]

COST EFFECTIVENESS

Subacute care provides services in a less costly environment for patients who are appropriate candidates. Many of the patients now being cared for in SCUs would have been cared for in a traditional rehabilitation hospital or acute medical facility, with higher daily costs. Growth has been dramatic. Medicare outlays for post-acute care jumped from $3.3 billion dollars in 1985 to $12.2 billion dollars in 1991. Of these alternative sites, nursing homes claim to offer subacute services at a cost 30–60 per cent less than units operated by acute hospitals or rehabilitation facilities ($300–$550 per day *vs* $700–$1000 per day).[23]

Since selection criteria for subacute care is still being developed, some patients are referred to SCUs at a higher level of care, with attendant higher costs, rather than receiving care in a skilled nursing facility. A recent study[24]

compared the difference in outcomes of Medicare patients with strokes and hip fractures discharged from hospital to two types of nursing homes (rehabilitative and regular), and to rehabilitative facilities. (The rehabilitative nursing home is a type of subacute care program.) In this study, patients managed in nursing homes, subacute care units, or rehabilitation hospitals all had similar outcomes. Although this raises important questions, the study was not a randomized controlled trial. More work is needed to establish what sort of patients are most likely to benefit from a higher level of subacute care.

The cost effectiveness of SCUs is difficult to assess for a number of reasons. First, the clinical data do not yet exist that would guide specific patients to the type of post-hospital care that would produce the best results. Second, there are varied service sites – acute hospital designated units, nursing home units, and within rehabilitation hospitals – all with different overheads, equipment and other costs. Third, Medicare's payment policy for subacute care exempted new providers for 3 years from the cost limits used by the Federal Government to determine reimbursement levels. This results in certain costs, while integrated delivery systems capable of negotiating sophisticated managed care contracts will be allocated different costs. Lastly, measurement of quality of care and outcomes for this diverse population is in its most early stages. For instance, patients admitted to SCUs have a relatively high rate of re-admissions to the acute hospital.[21] This negatively impacts total costs, quality of care, and outcome measurements. Cost is not the only criterion on which to judge subacute care.

MANAGEMENT OF COMMON CARDIOVASCULAR PROBLEMS WITHIN THE NEW PARADIGM

Overview

Cardiovascular disease management is a major contributor to the national home care and nursing home bills.

Traditionally, management of advanced heart failure, ischemic heart disease, and postoperative cardiac care have always included a prominent nursing component. Co-morbid illness, functional impairments and available social support systems dictated the site of care: home care with visiting nurse services, or nursing home placement. Over the past decade, as alternative approaches to the delivery of care have evolved, the management of many costly cardiovascular conditions is on the cusp of change, and a new standard of care is being evaluated.

Advances in cardiac rehabilitation have resulted in increased numbers of patients receiving cardiac rehabilitation in their homes, decreasing costs while preserving safety and efficacy for selected patients.[25] DeBusk[26] described a home-based case-management system for coronary risk factor modification after acute myocardial infarction, instituted in a large health maintenance organization. This physician-directed, nurse-managed program addressed smoking cessation, home-based exercise training, and diet-drug therapy for hyperlipidemia. It was considerably more effective than usual medical care and cost less than traditional cardiac rehabilitation programs, the primary focus of which is often limited to exercise training. Other advances in electrocardiographic (ECG) technology, such as portable heart rate monitors and transtelephonic ECG monitoring (TEM), can extend the surveillance of patients by rehabilitation professionals into home exercise training locations. These alternate approaches to the delivery of cardiac rehabilitation services still have to be assessed in more diverse populations of patients with stable coronary heart disease, especially elderly patients and those with higher risk status. Limited data suggest that comprehensive cardiac rehabilitation is a cost-effective use of medical services. Home-based cardiac rehabilitation programs have the potential to increase availability widely while decreasing costs.[25]

The American Heart Association's recently published recommendations for treating infective endocarditis contain substantial changes allowing for easier treatment of certain strains of streptococci highly susceptible to penicillin in the home setting. Previously used parenteral regimens required two or three daily injections. The newer regimen consists of 2 g ceftriaxone administered intravenously or intramuscularly once daily for 4 weeks, and is reserved for hemodynamically stable patients who have no complications of endocarditis. Nonetheless, it is a major advance in terms of cost and convenience.[27]

Fast track recovery from coronary artery bypass surgery emphasizing early mobilization and home management is increasingly accepted as a standard of care for selected patients.[28]

In the following section, selected cardiovascular conditions are matched to new paradigms of care to illustrate management strategies, which are capable of improving quality of care and reducing total costs.

Venous thromboembolic disease

The management of patients with venous thromboembolic disease (VTE) is changing because of the development and clinical acceptance of low-molecular-weight heparins. Visiting nurse programs, home health care and sub-acute care units provide appropriate sites and services of care for many of these patients.

HISTORICAL PERSPECTIVE

It is current practice to treat patients with acute proximal deep vein thrombosis (DVT) with standard (unfractionated) heparin followed by long-term oral anticoagulant therapy. Hospitalization is required for continuous intravenous infusion of heparin, or frequent injections, and individual adjustment of the dosage of heparin to keep the activated partial thromboplastin time within the desired therapeutic range. In the hospital, patients are monitored for recurrent thromboembolic events such as pulmonary embolus, and bleeding complications of the heparin therapy.[29] In the 1980s patients were usually hospitalized for 7–14 days. It has been shown that total hospital days could be safely reduced to five if oral anticoagulation was begun at the same time as intravenous heparin.[30] In the USA, over a quarter of a million patients are hospitalized yearly for treatment of venous thromboembolic disease.

Low-molecular-weight heparins (LMWH), prepared by the depolymerization of heparin, have been developed in the last decade for clinical use. Compared with standard heparin, LMWH preparations have distinct advantages: better bioavailability, a longer plasma half-life, more predictable anticoagulant activity, and possibly more effective anticoagulant activity. This combination of properties allow for LMWHs to be given once or twice daily, subcutaneously, and without the requirement for laboratory monitoring.[31] This has opened the door to a different approach to the prevention and treatment of VTE disease.

OUTCOMES, COSTS, AND QUALITY OF LIFE ISSUES

Initial studies focused on the efficacy and safety of LMWHs in the prevention of venous thromboembolism in high-risk patients.[31] More recently, attention has been directed towards the use of LMWHs as the initial treatment for acute deep venous thrombosis (DVT). Based upon favorable comparative studies between LMWH and standard heparin, and the unique properties of LMWH, primary out-patient management of acute proximal DVT is a clinical option.[32] Two initial multi-institutional randomized trials demonstrated the efficacy and safety of LMWH administered at home to selected patients as the primary treatment for acute DVT in selected patients.[33,34] In particular, recurrent thromboembolic events and bleeding complications were no different in either treatment group, and recurrent life-threatening pulmonary embolism was extremely rare. LMWHs may be more effective than unfractionated heparin in preventing recurrence and cause less major bleeding.[29] More than 50 clinical trials have been published, along with seven meta-analyses of clinical trials.[35] The use of LMWHs as out-patient therapy for VTE has dramatically increased over the next few years. However, the move from in-hospital to home care raises questions in addition to demonstrated efficacy and safety: is the therapy cost effective? how is the patient's quality of life affected? how difficult will it be to disseminate this care into routine practice? And, lastly, if home care is elected, what are the specific management protocols?

> The simplicity of LMWH administration – subcutaneous injections in a dose determined by the patient's weight, in the patient's home, without laboratory monitoring – intuitively suggests that this would be much more cost-effective than current standard therapy.

In one study, patients with acute proximal DVT were randomly assigned to receive either intravenous standard heparin in the hospital, or LMWH primarily at home.[33] Half of the patients in the LMWH group did not need to be hospitalized at all, and of those who did, the mean length of stay in the hospital was approximately 1 day. A similar study also found markedly reduced hospital utilization in a randomly assigned LMWH group.[34] This group averaged two out-patient visits and two telephone calls per patient. A later study was designed to perform an economic evaluation of standard heparin therapy *vs* LMWH therapy in a randomized trial of over 400 patients. The use of LMWH was associated with cost savings of $40 000–90 000 per 100 patients.[36] Multiple cost analysis studies have been completed since, and demonstrate that LMWH treatment in the out-patient setting is cost-effective.[37]

Quality of life issues are more difficult to assess. For the most part, improvement of physical activity at home, maintenance of social functioning, and remaining in control of one's environment are seen as desirable by patients. However, patients with co-morbid illness, marked functional impairment, or limited social support may find it difficult to stay at home. Treatment at home shifts much of the burden of care – financial, physical, cognitive, and emotional – to the patient and/or caregiver who may or may not be capable of assuming the burden. In addition, some patients may become more apprehensive when treated for an acute illness outside of the walls of the hospital.

Lastly, how applicable is this treatment to the general population? Approximately 50 per cent of patients with acute proximal DVT were excluded from the randomized studies for a number of reasons, such as coexisting conditions (renal dysfunction), recurrent DVT or

pulmonary embolus, concurrent symptomatic pulmonary embolus, current active bleeding, concerns about compliance, and geographic inaccessibility.[33,34] In addition, for patients with other risk factors for hemorrhage (severe liver disease, thrombocytopenia) or patients with a high risk for falls, supervised treatment with heparin in the acute hospital setting may be more appropriate (Table 31.13). Therefore, a flexible approach to the management of acute DVT is required, matching the patient's needs to available resources. Home treatment with LMWH remains a safe and effective therapy for selected patients.

Table 31.13 *Typical exclusion criteria for out-patient treatment of deep vein thrombosis*

1. Two or more previous episodes of DVT or pulmonary embolus
2. Current or recent active bleeding, or peptic ulcer disease
3. Major surgery within 2 weeks
4. Evidence of concurrent pulmonary embolus at presentation
5. Coexisting condition that requires hospitalization
6. Severe renal or liver disease
7. Pregnancy
8. Geographic inaccessibility
9. No phone accessibility
10. Strong likelihood for non-compliance
11. Patient/family refuses home treatment
12. Acute functional impairments without adequate home support
13. Home safety issues

CLINICAL MANAGEMENT OF DVT: THE NEW PARADIGM

Within the next few years, management of most patients with acute proximal DVT will be home-based, except for those patients whose coexisting conditions, potential non-compliance, and geographic difficulties make them ineligible. These patients should be considered for treatment in a SCU. In addition, patients residing in a nursing home will likely not require transfer to an acute hospital for treatment of an intercurrent DVT, but rather be treated on site.

General guidelines for the out-patient management of acute proximal DVT are as follows.

1 *Establish the diagnosis.* Nearly three-quarters of patients in whom DVT or pulmonary embolus is suspected do not have these conditions on objective testing. Establishing the diagnosis is necessary, whether the patient is to be treated in the hospital, in the home, or in the nursing home.
2 *Review eligibility criteria* (Table 31.13). Randomized trials utilized highly selective eligibility criteria, and it is likely that certain restrictions will ease with the coming years of clinical experience. Eligibility includes patient consent for care at home.

3 *Initiate dosing regimen.* There are many low-molecular-weight heparins available, and they differ in cost and effectiveness. A typical dosing protocol is outlined in Table 31.14.

Table 31.14 *Dosing protocol for low-molecular-weight heparin (LMWH) (Enoxaparin)*

1. Determine patient's weight (kg). If weight >30% ideal body weight, use an adjusted weight for dosing
2. Begin subcutaneous fixed-dose LMWH. Example: enoxaparin 1 mg/kg per dose subcutaneously twice daily, or 1.5 mg/kg per dose once daily[37a]
3. Begin coumadin on first or second day of therapy
4. Daily laboratory monitoring and coumadin-dose adjustment to achieve international normalized ratio (INR) between 2.0 and 3.0 (target INR 2.5)
5. Discontinue LMWH when:
   - heparin has been given for at least 5 days; and
   - the INR has been > 2.0 for 2 consecutive days

4 *Contact the appropriate home health program:*
   - Visiting nurse programs. Visiting nurse services are the model program to facilitate early hospital discharge, or avoid hospitalization for the patient with acute DVT. The visiting nurse provides patient and family education, teaches and supervises subcutaneous injections and oral medications, monitors the patient's clinical condition, performs blood draws and obtains laboratory test results, and communicates and coordinates care with the patient's primary care physician. The agency chosen should have services available 24 hours a day, 7 days a week. Patients should be contacted daily by the agency, and reinforced to call the nurse or report to the clinic on an emergency basis with signs and/or symptoms of bleeding or recurrent venous thromboembolism.
   - Home health care teams. It is likely that, with continued experience, patients with more complex clinical conditions and co-morbid illnesses would be eligible to receive out-patient treatment. In these cases, HHC teams, with on-site evaluation and treatment capabilities by the nurse, physician, social worker, and other professionals, are better equipped to provide safe and effective comprehensive home management. Some patients, especially those at risk for bleeding, will require initiation of treatment in the hospital for 1 or 2 days, with early discharge to home. While at home, daily nursing visits and more frequent laboratory monitoring may be necessary. More patients in this group may require professional assistance with subcutaneous injections, clinical monitoring, and personal care

needs. The home health care physician may be called upon to make a home visit for assessment and on-site management. Once the acute management phase has been completed, the patient can be transferred back to the referring primary care physician for long-term management.
   - Subacute care units. Patients who are not candidates for home treatment of acute DVT (Table 31.13) should be considered for direct admission to an intermediate care facility for treatment. This will often follow an initial presentation in the office, urgent care, or emergency room. Those patients who are clinically unstable on presentation, or whose funding sources mandate a 3-day hospitalization prior to transfer (Medicare), may require a brief admission to the acute hospital to initiate therapy and monitor stability prior to transfer.

5 *Address pain management and mobility issues,* especially with the need for assistance with activities of daily living and adaptive aids.

Congestive heart failure

OVERVIEW

Congestive heart failure (CHF) is a significant public health problem in the USA affecting more than four million people. It is one of the most common medical problems in patients admitted to nursing homes and home care programs. It is the leading cause of hospitalization among older adults, and the rate of CHF admissions has been increasing over the past two decades. Most of this increase has occurred in adults aged 75 years and older. Patients with advanced CHF suffer major morbidity and mortality, and total costs approach $40 billion annually, including acute hospitalizations, emergency room visits, office visits, treatment modalities, home care and nursing home costs.[38,39]

The patient who presents in acute CHF has traditionally been managed in the acute hospital setting. Importantly, patients hospitalized for CHF are at increased risk for re-admission, with nearly 50 per cent re-admitted within 3–6 months of discharge. While CHF exacerbation was the most common cause for re-admission, a variety of diagnoses were responsible for repeated admissions, reflecting co-morbid diseases.[40–42] Although there is no 'low-risk group', certain correlates of early hospital readmission or 'high-risk' patients can be identified.[40,41,43,44] (Table 31.15). Advanced age and degree of functional disability are not independently associated with early re-admission. Upon discharge, 30 per cent of persons with heart failure receive post-hospital services (home care, nursing home, rehabilitation hospital). Heart failure is a major cause of functional decline in the elderly.[45]

Table 31.15 *Factors associated with early hospital readmission among patients hospitalized with congestive heart failure (CHF)*

Male gender
Single (unmarried or widowed)
Social isolation
Prior admissions within the preceding 6 months
Prior history of CHF
Diabetes mellitus
Presence of co-morbid conditions
Prolonged hospital stay (greater than 7 days)
Lower systolic blood pressure (<100 mm Hg)
Lower serum sodium (<132 meq/L)
Absence of new ST–T wave changes

HOME HEALTH CARE IN THE MANAGEMENT OF HEART FAILURE: THE NEW PARADIGM

Introduction

Current practice patterns in the management of heart failure have been insufficient in preventing hospital re-admissions and the associated social and functional declines.[46] Multiple factors often contribute to early re-admission, many of which are potentially remediable. It is estimated that up to 50 per cent of re-admissions are potentially preventable[47] (Table 31.16). Physicians underuse medications such as angiotensin-converting enzyme (ACE) inhibitors, and many patients either self-adjust or discontinue cardiac medications even when these medications are prescribed.[48] Poor adherence to dietary therapy is a common cause of re-admission, and patient's knowledge about heart failure and symptom identification is limited. Financial pressures impact on medication and dietary compliance.

Despite involvement with visiting nurse programs, many of these patients become a casualty of the systematic fragmentation of care, where the assessment arm (visiting nurse) is not closely enough tied to the treatment arm (primary care physician) to ensure comprehensive care and prompt, effective responses to symptoms. For example, a recent study showed that older adult patients with heart failure experience many

Table 31.16 *Potentially preventable factors contributing to early readmission among patients with congestive heart failure*

Suboptimal medication regimen
Medication non-adherence
Dietary non-adherence (salt, water)
Failure to seek medical help
Inadequate social support
Inadequate discharge planning and follow-up
Suboptimal management of co-morbid illness (depression,
    dementia)

of the symptoms of exacerbation for days before hospital admission.[49] Edema, cough, fatigue and weight gain are noted by patients for a week prior to admission. Progressive dyspnea and orthopnea are noted for 2–3 days, and patients with self-described 'acute' dyspnea are symptomatic at home for 12 hours before seeking assistance. This strongly suggests that there is a window of opportunity to intervene medically and avoid acute hospitalization.

These striking facts in a common diagnosis have attracted the attention of both clinicians and administrators seeking to improve the health of patients with heart failure and decrease costs. As noted, Rich and colleagues recently demonstrated that a multidisciplinary home intervention program, which was nurse-directed and included active physician participation, resulted in 44 per cent fewer hospital re-admissions than in the control group.[17] This prospective randomized trial resulted in improved quality of life and reduced hospital use and medical costs for elderly patients with heart failure. Although various other management programs have been advanced, they have in common a broad systems approach coordinating care through a strong physician/nurse alliance, emphasizing patient and family education, skilled assessment, and prompt, on-site treatment capabilities.

Recommendations for clinical management of CHF in a home health care program

Elderly patients with heart failure benefit from home health care programs. In most instances, a nurse case-manager coordinates the care, although some HHC teams are physician-led. The physician oversees medical care, and advises and supports the patient and family. A social worker, dietitian, rehabilitation therapist and pharmacist complete the core group. Comprehensive assessment and education, monitoring and treatment consistent with patient and family goals are critical components of a successful program. The HHC team often functions as the primary care provider, managing not only heart failure but the whole patient.

Typically the patient is visited at home by the nurse within 24–48 hours for initial comprehensive assessment. Follow-up visits are scheduled based upon clinical needs, but initially occur at least weekly. Frequent telephone contact supplements visits. The nurse completes a comprehensive assessment, including medical, cognitive, nutritional, and functional domains. The social worker addresses psychosocial (spiritual), and financial issues, transportation needs, and caregiver stress. The registered dietitian develops an individualized dietary assessment and provides instruction (Table 31.17).

The nurse begins intensive education about heart failure and its treatment, using written material to

Table 31.17 *Components of a multidisciplinary home intervention program for patients with congestive heart failure*

Nurse case-manager, physician, social worker, dietitian, rehabilitation therapist, pharmacist, and other team members are clearly identified

Primary care is provided, including treatment of co-morbid illness

24-hour clinical coverage is provided by the team

Communication lines between the patient, case-manager and physician are simplified

Integrated communication and medical information systems are available

Clinical practice guidelines are utilized to optimize medication therapy

Medication regimen is simplified and reinforced

Patients are educated about heart failure, medications, diet, and exercise

Recurrent symptoms amenable to treatment are identified

Patients receive environmental and functional home assessments to promote maximum independence and comfort

Social services provide psychosocial, spiritual and financial assistance, and address caregiver stress

Intensive home follow-up through home visits and telephone contact is provided, including physician home visits

Technology to provide comprehensive care at home is available, including diagnostic and therapeutic interventions

Advance directives and end-of-life issues are discussed

supplement teaching. The medication regimen is reviewed with the physician, optimized, and simplified to a twice- or thrice-daily schedule. Medication dispensing sets are distributed. The importance of recording daily weight is stressed, and scales may be provided. Environmental and functional adaptations maximize the patient's ability to remain independent, and ease the caregiver's role. Exercise for conditioning, and techniques for conservation of energy, improve the patient's ability to pursue meaningful activities. The patient is screened for depression and dementia, common illnesses in the homebound elderly, which interfere with compliance with behavioral interventions, and negatively impact on quality of life. Symptoms of heart failure are reviewed, and the patient is given individual guidelines and procedures for initiating contact with the home care team. The patient is prescribed an individualized home crisis medication kit for prompt treatment of CHF symptoms as instructed by the physician.

During routine visits and via telephone contact, the nurse reviews the educational program, and reinforces compliance with medications, diet, and exercise. New symptoms or signs of illness are rapidly assessed, reported to the physician, and treated. In 1999, a national quality improvement collaborative demonstrated that comprehensive home care teams can dramatically reduce emergency room visits and acute

hospitalizations for CHF, often providing care and services on site at home.[50]

Physician home visits are generally less frequent than visits from other team members, and the timing and frequency varies among patients. Typically the physician discusses with the patient the disease process and treatment options, the expected course of the illness, and the importance of compliance and monitoring, and early signs of instability. Discussion concerning advance directives and end-of-life issues is of paramount importance in developing a plan of care consistent with the patient's goals.

Home hospitalization As of yet, no clinical pathway is available to select those patients with exacerbation of CHF who may safely remain at home for treatment. Indeed, the American Heart Association guidelines for CHF note that 'with few exceptions, patients presenting with acute heart failure require hospital admission.'[51] Familiarity with known high-risk clinical conditions may identify the best candidates for triage to the hospital, such as hypotension, tachypnea, hyponatremia, or electrocardiographic changes of ischemia.[43] However, this information must be balanced against the known hazards of hospitalization in the elderly, the patient's goals and preferences, available family and caregiver support (financial, emotional, and physical), co-morbid illness, the patient's prognosis, and care and services available on site. These issues are especially important for patients with refractory or decompensated advanced systolic heart failure, when consideration is being made for chronic, intermittent intravenous inotropic therapy, or continuous intravenous diuretic therapy.

Although patients with advanced heart failure have high rates of re-admission to the hospital, nearly 50 per cent of these admissions are for reasons other than decompensated heart failure, such as acute pneumonia and myocardial infarction.[40] Therefore, the home care team will be called upon to assess and treat a variety of acute illnesses.

Home intravenous inotropic therapy Intermittent inotropic treatment has been recognized as an option in the treatment of patients with advanced systolic heart failure, either as palliative therapy or as a bridge to transplantation, when the oral regimen has been maximized. Studies of intermittent infusion therapy have demonstrated significant and sustained clinical benefits and reduced acute hospitalizations in selected patients.[52] Following an acute hospitalization to determine safety and efficacy, subsequent infusions can be done in outpatient clinics, subacute care units, or at home. Medicare guidelines require that the patient be dyspneic at rest with maximal therapy, and specify dosage ranges, and pre/post-cardiac index and pulmonary capillary wedge (CPW) parameters. The patient should report an increase in well-being, and receive ongoing, documented assessment, education, and management.[53,54]

Many studies of intermittent infusion therapy have demonstrated significant and sustained clinical benefits and reduced acute hospitalizations in selected patients.[52,54] However, the cost effectiveness of this therapy is still under evaluation despite these studies because of significant design flaws.

SUBACUTE CARE IN THE MANAGEMENT OF PATIENTS WITH CONGESTIVE HEART FAILURE

Subacute care units should be considered for the patient with CHF under certain clinical situations. Following acute hospitalization, the patient may require continued skilled nursing assessments and laboratory monitoring until stable. The hospitalized patient may also have developed progressive deconditioning, and benefit from transfer to a subacute unit for rehabilitation. Intensive education and comprehensive discharge planning can continue within this setting.

A patient with acute exacerbation may not have the required support at home to allow for home treatment. In this instance, if acute hospital admission is not required, a direct admission to a subacute care unit may be a management option. Similarly, a patient may require admission to a subacute care unit for continuation of intermittent inotropic therapy for refractory systolic heart failure.

FUTURE DIRECTIONS

Visiting nurse programs, subacute care units, and home health care offers many opportunities for cost-effective, high-quality care for patients with cardiovascular disease. Medical specialties and other professional groups will need to address these new paradigms of care from the educational, clinical, and research arenas.

Comprehensive curricula in home and subacute care need to be developed for medical schools and residency programs, supported through the introduction of established teaching sites and committed faculty. Specialty societies are encouraged to develop educational programs for practicing physicians, with the consideration of added qualification certification. Both sites will need to develop integrated communication and medical information systems to be effective sites for patient care, medical education, and research.

A requirement for all home care agencies to have a medical director is strongly encouraged. The statutory requirements for medical directors would be the same as for nursing homes and hospices. This would increase the direct physician involvement in home health care management and provide an opportunity to develop comprehensive, primary home health care teams within the home care agency.

Medical directors in subacute care units will need to expand their roles in quality improvement, staff educa-

tion, program development, and liaison with community physicians. Current Medicare barriers to direct patient admission to SCUs will need to be reviewed. SCUs will require stable professional staffing, equipment, and support systems to provide higher-acuity care.

Barriers to physician involvement in home care need to be modified, including reimbursement formulas and legal and regulatory restrictions, and a balance found to enable innovative programming while protecting against fraud and excess. New reimbursement formulas, in addition to providing adequate compensation for the work component of more complex home visits, should also address practice expense (e.g. travel time) in addition to time for patient/family education, counseling, and case coordination.

There are many opportunities for clinical research to answer the questions of cost and quality of these newly developing programs. The ethical issues raised by shifting the burden of care to the patient and family at home will be more difficult to resolve.

SUMMARY

- The demand for out-of-hospital care is growing rapidly, fueled by health care financing and enabled by medical technology, information systems, and patient preferences.
- Current regulatory and legal issues, though meant to limit fraud and abuse, complicate the ability of the physician to provide coordinated, comprehensive home care services.
- Visiting nurse programs are primarily used to provide long-term management of chronic disease, and a majority of visits are no longer linked to acute care needs.
- An emerging form of team care at home, termed 'Home Health Care' is characterized by the active involvement of the physician and expands on-site assessment and treatment capabilities, including home hospitalization.
- Subacute care units, based in nursing homes or hospitals, have expanded clinical care teams, laboratory and imaging services, to provide less costly sites of care than the acute hospital for selected patients.
- Many cardiovascular conditions, including endocarditis, cardiac rehabilitation, postoperative cardiac care, congestive heart failure, and acute thromboembolic disease, can be managed in the home or the subacute care unit.
- The management of patients with acute thromboembolic disease is changing because of the development and clinical acceptance of low-molecular-weight heparins.

- Elderly patients hospitalized for congestive heart failure have a high rate of re-admission (approximately 50 per cent within 6 months); nearly 50 per cent of these re-admissions are potentially avoidable with comprehensive home management.

REFERENCES AND RECOMMENDED READING

1. Goldberg AI. Physician participation in home care. *Home HealthCare Consult* 1996; **3**(4): 9–16.
2. Koren MJ. Home care – who cares? *N Engl J Med* 1986; **314**: 917–20.
3. Health and Public Policy Committee, American College of Physicians. Home health care. *Ann Intern Med* 1986; **105**: 454–60.
4. Welch HG, Wennberg DE, Welch WP. The use of medicare home health care services. *N Engl J Med* 1996; **335**: 324–9.
5. Boling PA. Improving economics of home care practice. *Home HealthCare Consult* 2001; **8**: 36–43.
6. Goldberg AI. Physician Participation in Home Care. *Am Acad Home Care Phys News* 1996; **3**: 1–6.
7. Hoyer TE. Letters of December 15, 1995 and February 29, 1996 policy interpretation. *Home Care News* 1996; June: 1–2.
8. National Association for Home Care. *NAHC Report* 1996; August 9: no. 673.
9. Keenan J. Update on physician reimbursement for home care. *Am Acad Home Care Phys News* 1994; **6**: 1–3.
10. Bayne CG. Home care, clinical laboratory improvement amendments (CLIA) and the portable lab. *Am Acad Home Care Phys News* 1996; **8**: 4–6.
♦11. Leff B, Burton JR. Acute medical care in the home. *J Am Geriatr Soc* 1996; **44**: 603–5.
♦12. American Medical Association Department of Geriatric Health. *Physicians and home care: guidelines for the medical management of the home care patient.* Chicago, IL, 1992.
13. American Medical Association. *Council on Scientific Affairs report: on-site physician home health care.* 1996; 9-I-96.
14. Zimmer JG, Groth-Juncker A, McCusker J. A randomized controlled study of a home health care team. *Am J Public Health* 1985; **75**: 134–41.
15. Creditor MC: Hazards of hospitalization of the elderly. *Ann Intern Med* 1993; **118**: 219–35.
16. Cummings JE, Hughes SL, Weaver FM, *et al.* Cost effectiveness of Veterans Administration hospital based home care. *Arch Intern Med* 1990; **150**: 1274–80.
♦17. Rich MW, Beckham V, Wittenberg C, *et al.* A multidisciplinary intervention to prevent the readmission of elderly patients with congestive heart failure. *N Engl J Med* 1995; **333**: 1190–5.
18. Kornowski R, Zeeli D, Averbuch M, *et al.* Intensive home-care surveillance prevents hospitalization and improves morbidity rates among elderly patients with severe congestive heart failure. *Am Heart J* 1995; **129**: 762–6.
19. Fanale JE, Markson L, Cooney L, Katz P. Role of the physician. In: Besdine RW, Rubenstein LZ, Snyder L, eds *Medical care of the nursing home resident.* Philadelphia: American College of Physicians, 1996; 3–15.
♦20. American Medical Association: *Guidelines for physician responsibilities in subacute care 1995*, Report 21-I-95.
21. Smith RL, Osterweil D. The medical director in hospital-based transitional care units. *Clinics Geriatr Med* 1995; **11**: 373–89.
22. Micheletti JA, Shlala TJ. Understanding and operationalizing subacute services. *Nursing Manag* 1995; **26**: 49–55.
23. Tokarski C. Riding the express: is your subacute strategy on track? *Hospitals Health Networks* 1995; July 5: 21–3.
24. Kane RL, Chen Q, Blewett LA, Sangl J. Do rehabilitative nursing homes improve the outcomes of care? *J Am Geriatr Soc* 1996; **44**: 545–54.
○25. Wenger NK. Alternate approaches to the delivery of cardiac rehabilitation services: home-based cardiac rehabilitation. *Home HealthCare Consult* 1996; **3**: 9–26.
26. DeBusk RF, Miller NH, Superko HR, *et al.* A case management system for coronary risk factor modification after acute myocardial infarction. *Ann Intern Med* 1994; **120**: 721–9.
27. Wilson WR, Karchmer AW, Dajani AS, *et al.* Antibiotic treatment of adults with infective endocarditis due to streptococci, enterococci, staphylococci, and HACEK microorganisms. American Heart Association. *JAMA* 1995; **274**: 1706–13.
28. Dunstan JL, Riddle MM. Rapid recovery management: the effects on the patient who has undergone heart surgery. *Heart Lung* 1997; **26**: 289–98.
29. Ginsberg JS. Management of venous thromboembolism. *N Engl J Med* 1996; **335**: 1816–28.
30. Hull RD, Raskob GE, Rosenbloom D, *et al.* Heparin for 5 days as compared with 10 days in the initial treatment of proximal venous thrombosis. *N Engl J Med* 1990; **322**: 1260–4.
31. Schafer AI. Low-molecular weight heparin – an opportunity for home treatment of venous thrombosis. *N Engl J Med* 1996; **334**: 724–5.
32. Lensing AWA, Prins MH, Davidson BL, Hirsh J. Treatment of deep venous thrombosis with low-molecular-weight heparins. *Arch Intern Med* 1995; **155**: 601–7.
33. Levine M, Gent M, Hirsh J, *et al.* A comparison of low-molecular-weight heparin administered primarily at

home with unfractionated heparin administered in the hospital for proximal deep-vein thrombosis. *N Engl J Med* 1996; **334**: 677–81.

34. Koopman MMW, Prandoni P, Piovella F, *et al.* Treatment of venous thrombosis with intravenous unfractionated heparin admininstered in the hospital as compared with subcutaneous low-molecular-weight heparin administered at home. *N Engl J Med* 1996; **334**: 682–7.

○35. Thomas DR. Advances in treatment of thromboembolic disease. *Home HealthCare Consult* (Suppl) 2000: 1–20.

36. Hull RD, Raskob GE, Rosenbloom D, *et al.* Treatment of proximal vein thrombosis with subcutaneous low-molecular-weight heparin vs intravenous heparin – an economic perspective. *Arch Intern Med* 1997; **157**: 289–94.

○37. Hull RD, Pineo GF. Economic aspects of deep vein thrombosis treatment and outpatient management. *Home HealthCare Consult* 2000; **7**: 22–9.

37a. Merli G, Spiro TE, Olsson C, *et al.* Subcutaneous enoxaparin once or twice daily compared with intravenous unfractionated heparin for treatment of venous thromboembolic disease. *Ann Intern Med* 2001; **134**: 191–202.

38. Croft JB, Giles WH, Pollard RA, *et al.* National trends in the initial hospitalization for heart failure. *J Am Geriatr Soc* 1997; **45**: 270–5.

39. Schocken DD, Arrieta MI, Leaverton PE, Ross EA. Prevalence and mortality rates of congestive heart failure in the United States. *J Am Coll Cardiol* 1992; **20**: 301–6.

40. Krumholz HM, Parent EM, Tu N, *et al.* Readmission after hospitalization for congestive heart failure among Medicare beneficiaries. *Arch Intern Med* 1997; **157**: 99–104.

41. Goldberg RJ. Advances and stagnations in heart failure. *Arch Intern Med* 1997; **157**: 17–19.

42. Wolinsky FD, Smith DM, Stump TE, *et al.* The sequelae of hospitalization for congestive heart failure among older adults. *J Am Geriatr Soc* 1997; **45**: 558–63.

43. Chin MH, Goldman L. Correlates of major complications or death in patients admitted to the hospital with congestive heart failure. *Arch Intern Med* 1996; **156**: 1814–20.

44. Chin MH, Goldman L. Correlates of early hospital readmission or death in patients with congestive heart failure. *Am J Cardiol* 1997; **79**: 1640–4.

45. Burns RB, McCarthy EP, Moskowitz MA, *et al.* Outcomes for older men and women with congestive heart failure. *J Am Geriatr Soc* 1997; **45**: 276–80.

46. Kerzner R, Rich MW. Does multidisciplinary management of chronic heart failure improve clinical outcomes? *J Clin Outcomes Manag* 2001; **8**: 41–9.

47. Vinson JM, Rich MW, Sperry JC, *et al.* Early readmission of elderly patients with congestive heart failure. *J Am Geriatr Soc* 1990; **38**: 1290–5.

48. West JA, Miller NH, Parker KM, *et al.* A comprehensive management system for heart failure improves clinical outcomes and reduces medical resource utilization. *Am J Cardiol* 1997; **79**: 58–63.

49. Friedman MM. Older adults' symptoms and their duration before hospitalization for heart failure. *Heart Lung* 1997; **26**: 169–76.

○50. Lynn J, Schall MW, Milne C, *et al.* Quality improvements in end of life care: insights from two collaboratives. *J Quality Improvement* 2000; **26**: 254–67.

51. ACC/AHA Task Force. Report on practice guidelines for evaluation and management of heart failure. *Circulation* 1995; September.

52. Marius-Nunez AL, Heaney L, Fernandez RN, *et al.* Intermittent inotropic therapy in an outpatient setting: a cost-effective therapeutic modality in patients with refractory heart failure. *Am Heart J* 1996; **132**: 805–8.

○53. Sherman A. Critical care management of the heart failure patient in the home. *Crit Care Nursing Quarterly* 1995; **18**: 77–87.

54. Boyer J. Infusion therapy with milrinone in the home care setting for patients who have advanced heart failure. *J Intravenous Nursing* 1997; **10**: 145–50.

32

Coordinated anticoagulation services and home management programs

JACK E ANSELL AND RICHARD C BECKER

The potential risk of poorly regulated oral anticoagulant therapy coupled with the labor intensity of routine monitoring impact treatment decisions and the clinical use of currently available agents among health care professionals. Coordinated anticoagulation programs and anticoagulation management services are designed to overcome existing barriers and have been shown to reduce thromboembolic and hemorrhagic event rates. Patient self-testing and self-management, representing an outgrowth of coordinated anticoagulation programs, are increasing worldwide and, in addition to providing safe, cost-effective and efficient care, offer the important dimension of patient empowerment.

INTRODUCTION

Oral anticoagulation is a time-tested and effective therapy for patients at risk for thromboembolism,[1] but patients may not receive the full benefits of therapy in situations where the risk of serious adverse events outweighs the benefits of preventing thrombotic episodes. Because of the perceived high risk–benefit ratio of oral anticoagulation, physicians are sometimes reluctant to initiate therapy even for well-established indications.[2,3] Furthermore, the management of oral anticoagulation is known to be labor intensive, and the degree of effort needed to achieve good clinical outcomes is an additional deterrence to the use of oral anticoagulation.[2,3] These factors can be minimized, and the benefits of oral anticoagulation maximized, by the implementation of an expert model of management that can be achieved with a coordinated and focused system of care known as an anticoagulation management service.[4]

The following chapter describes the elements of an anticoagulation management service and substantiates its benefits over traditional models of anticoagulation management. The authors also describe future approaches to management employing patient self-testing of prothrombin times and the potential for these management schemes to further enhance therapy.

HISTORIC LANDMARKS

Since dicoumarol's isolation and initial clinical use in 1941,[5,6] there have been several important developments toward establishing the benefits of oral anticoagulation, identifying the proper indications for treatment and improving its management (Table 32.1). Research in the last 15 years has validated the role of anticoagulation in a number of conditions by providing strong clinical evidence from randomized controlled trials; by improving the monitoring of oral anticoagulation through the use of the international normalized ratio (INR) and the promotion of sensitive thromboplastins for the prothrombin time (PT) test; and by identifying

Table 32.1 *Historical landmarks in the use and management of oral anticoagulation*

1940s	Discovery and first human use of oral anticoagulants
1950s–early 1960s	Initiation of therapy with loading dose. Clinical use in myocardial infarction and pulmonary embolism
Late 1960s–1970s	Loading dose eliminated. Mechanism of vitamin K and coumarin anticoagulants unraveled
Early 1980s	Variability of thromboplastin and inaccuracy of prothrombin times widely recognized. Low- and high-intensity therapy guidelines
Late 1980s	International normalized ratio (INR) promoted. Expanding indications based on randomized controlled trials. Refinement of low- and high-intensity therapy guidelines
1990s–2000s	Value of coordinated anticoagulation care recognized and programs promoted. Studies of patient self-testing and patient self-management initiated

both the potential pitfalls of traditional management and the benefits of a coordinated and focused approach achieved through an anticoagulation management service (AMS). The concept of an AMS, or anticoagulation clinic as it is often called, is not new. Programs focusing on the management of oral anticoagulation have existed in the USA for over 40 years, and several Scandinavian and other European countries are well known for their coordinated programs,[7] some of which oversee the care of all anticoagulated patients in their respective countries. In the USA, AMS programs are growing, spurred on by increasing evidence of improved clinical outcomes and cost effectiveness. The basic elements of an AMS include:

1 a manager or team leader (physician, pharmacist);
2 support staff (nurse practioner, pharmacist, or physician's assistant);
3 standardized record keeping;
4 a manual of operation and practice guidelines;
5 a formal mechanism for communicating with referring physicians and patients.

COORDINATED ANTICOAGULATION CARE

Most oral anticoagulation therapy in the USA is presently managed by a patient's personal physician (along with all the other patients in that physician's practice). In essence, the monitoring and dose titration of patients with thromboembolic disease represents a relatively small aspect of the physician's overall clinical practice. This approach can be characterized as traditional or 'routine medical care' (RMC). There may be no specialized system or guidelines in place to track patients or to assure their regular follow-up. An AMS employs a focused and coordinated approach to managing anticoagulation.[8] What constitutes an AMS may vary depending on the individuals involved and the health care system or practice setting, but in most cases, it is a specialized program of patient management focused predominantly, if not exclusively, on the management of anticoagulation. The program is often directed by a single physician who assumes no major responsibility for the primary care of the patients under management. The actual management is usually conducted by registered nurses, nurse practitioners, pharmacists, or physician assistants. In some settings, these individuals will manage a panel of patients with direction provided by different primary or referring physicians for individual patients. At a minimum, the goals of an AMS are to coordinate and optimize anticoagulation by:

- helping to determine the appropriateness of care;
- managing anticoagulation dosing;
- providing systematic monitoring and patient evaluation;
- providing ongoing education;
- communicating with other providers involved in the patient's care.

This approach to managing anticoagulation has grown considerably over the last decade, and substantial evidence has accumulated documenting its superiority over RMC.[8] Unfortunately, the clinical outcomes experienced under either of these two models of management have not been evaluated by randomized controlled studies. Most studies to date would be characterized predominantly as Level III, IV, or V evidence as defined by Cook *et al.*[9] Although the quality of the study designs is less than optimal, the weight of the evidence does suggest that the model of management is an important risk factor influencing the likelihood of an adverse event, and that coordinated care through an AMS leads to better outcomes.

Risk reduction with coordinated care

There are very few studies assessing clinical outcome when oral anticoagulation is managed under a model of routine medical care as defined above[10,11] (Table 32.2). Although the information is limited, the literature suggests that a major rate of hemorrhage of at least 7–8 per cent per patient year of therapy is expected. There is a similar rate of recurrent or *de novo* thromboembolism in these patients for an overall serious adverse event rate of between 15 and 20 per cent per patient year of therapy. Many studies indicate that the high adverse event rates are a consequence of poor therapeutic control with hemorrhage or thrombosis occurring as a

Table 32.2 *Frequency of major hemorrhage/thromboembolism in patients managed under a usual care model. (Adapted with permission from Ansell JE, Hughes R. Evolving models of warfarin management: anticoagulation clinics, patient self-monitoring, and patient self-management. Am Heart J 1996; 132: 1095–100)*

Study	Number of patients	Number of patient years	Years of data collection	New (N) or established (E) patients	Indications[a]	Target INR	Hemorrhage Major	Fatal[b]	Minor[c]	Recent TE[c]
Landefeld and Goldman[10]	565	876	1977–1983	N	Ven & Art	NA	7.4%	10	7.4%	NA
Gitter et al.[11]	261	221	1987–1989	E	Ven & Art	2.4 (Median achieved)	8.1%	1	14.5%	8.1%

[a]Ven & Art = mixed indications in the venous and arterial systems.
[b]Fatal bleeds included with major bleeds.
[c]Expressed as per cent per patient year of therapy.
INR = international normalized ratio; NA = not available; TE = thromboembolism.

consequence of excessive or subtherapeutic anticoagulation.

The observed outcomes from RMC can be contrasted to the rates identified in a large number of retrospective and some prospective studies of the outcomes experienced when care is delivered under the model of an AMS[12–22] (Table 32.3). Although the studies performed to date are mostly observational in design, they suggest at least a 50 per cent reduction in both major hemorrhagic and thrombotic events.

A summary of studies examining both models of management, where coordinated care is measured against a control group of routine medical care within each study[23–26] is presented in Table 32.4. These mostly non-randomized, retrospective analyses tend to assess the care provided to patients before and after enrollment in an AMS; despite a methodologic limitation, they do provide evidence for the benefit of coordinated care. The rates for major adverse events for RMS are remarkably similar to those found in Table 32.2, whereas the coordi-

Table 32.3 *Frequency of major hemorrhage/thromboembolism in patients managed under an anticoagulation management service. (Adapted with permission from Ansell JE, Hughes R. Evolving models of warfarin management: anticoagulation clinics, patient self-monitoring, and patient self-management. Am Heart J 1996; 132: 1095–100)*

Study	Number of patients	Number of patient years	Years of data collection	New (N) or established (E) patients	Indications[a]	Target[b] PTR/INR	Hemorrhage Major[c]	Fatal[d]	Minor[c]	Recent TE[c]
Forfar et al.[12]	541	1362	1970–1978	N & E	Ven & Art	1.8–2.6	4.2%	2	NA	NA
Errichetti et al.[13]	141	105	1978–1983	N & E	Ven & Art	1.3–2.0	6.6%	NA	24.7%	NA
Conte et al.[14]	140	153	1975–1984	N & E	Ven & Art	1.7–2.5	2.6%	NA	58%	8.4%
Petty et al.[15]	310	385	1977–1980	N & E	Ven & Art	NA	7.3%	3	NA	NA
Charney et al.[16]	73	77	1981–1984	N & E	Ven & Art	1.5–2.5	0	0	42%	5.0%
Bussey et al.[17]	82	199	1977–1986	N	Ven & Art	NA	2.0%	NA	15.5%	3.5%
Seabrook et al.[18]	93	158	1981–1988	N	Ven & Art	1.5–2.0	3.8%	0	6.9%	2.5%
Fihn et al.[19]	928	1950	NA	N	Ven & Art	1.3–1.5 1.5–1.8	1.7%	4	54.9%	7.5%
van der Meer et al.[20]	6814	6085	1988	N & E	Ven & Art	2.4–5.3 (INR)	3.3%	39	13.8%	NA
Cannegieter et al.[21]	1608	6475	1985–	N & E	Mech valves	3.6–4.8 (INR)	2.5%	22	NA	0.7%
Palareti et al.[22]	2745	2011	1993–1995	N	Ven & Art	2.0–3.0 2.5–4.5 (INR)	1.4%	5	6.2%	3.5%

[a]Ven & Art = mixed indications in the venous and arterial systems; Mech = mechanical.
[b]Target PTR = prothrombin time ratio unless INR indicated.
[c]Expressed as per cent per patient year of therapy.
[d]Fatal bleeds included with major bleeds.
NA = not available; TE = thromboembolism.

Table 32.4 *Frequency of major hemorrhage/thromboembolism in patients managed under usual care (UC) anticoagulation management service (AMS). (Adapted with permission from Ansell JE, Hughes R. Evolving models of warfarin management: anticoagulation clinics, patient self-monitoring, and patient self-management.* Am Heart J *1996; **132**: 1095–100)*

Study	Model of care	Number of patients	Number of patient years	Years of data collection	Indications[a]	Target[b] PTR/INR	Hemorrhage Major[c]	Fatal[d]	Minor[c]	Recent TE[c]
Garabedian-Ruffalo et al.[23]	UC	26	64.3	1977–1980	Ven & Art	1.5–2.5	12.4%	0	NA	6.2%
	AMS	26	41.9	1980–1983	Ven & Art	1.5–2.5 (PTR)	2.4%	0	NA	0
Cortelazzo et al.[24]	UC	271	677	1982–	Mech valves	25–35%[e]	4.7%	0	NA	6.6%
	AMS	271	669	1987–1990	Mech valves	3.0–4.5 (INR)	1.0%	0	NA	0.6%
Wilt et al.[25]	UC	44	28	1988–1993	Ven & Art	NA	17.8%	0	7.1%	42.8%
	AMS	68	60	1988–1993	Ven & Art	NA	0	0	3.3%	0
Chiquette et al.[26]	UC	142	102	1991–1992	Ven & Art	2.0–3.0	4.3%	1	55.0%	11.7%
	AMS	176	123	1992–1994	Ven & Art	2.5–3.5	0.9%	0	27.0%	3.6%

[a]Ven & Art = mixed indications in the venous and arterial systems.
[b]Target PTR = prothrombin time ratio unless INR indicated.
[c]Expressed as per cent per patient year of therapy.
[d]Fatal hemorrhagic events included with major hemorrhage.
[e]Prothrombin activity.
TE = thromboembolism; Mech = mechanical.

nated care group outcomes are further improved compared to the results in Table 32.3. Based on this evidence, it appears that coordinated care offers the possibility of improved clinical outcomes, presumably through maintenance of more effective therapeutic anticoagulation, patient education, and communication, resulting in a reduction in hemorrhage and thromboembolism.

The Agency for Health Care Policy and Research is currently supporting a study known as PORT (Patient Outcomes Research Team) MAST (Managing Anticoagulation Service Trial) that is designed to develop AMS programs in randomly selected clusters of practices within managed care organizations. The practice can then refer to the AMS, or not, as they choose (without the potential financial disincentive of paying for a referral). There will be five sites across the USA, each with two practice clusters including 2000–2500

patients with atrial fibrillation. The major outcome measures will include: (1) the proportion of patients receiving warfarin; (2) the quality of anticoagulation management (percentage of time the INR is within the target range); and (3) the cost effectiveness of anticoagulation.

Cost effectiveness of coordinated care

Although there is a relative paucity of information in the published literature addressing the issue of the cost effectiveness of AMS *vs* RMC, some studies do suggest a cost reduction with the former. The benefit is derived by a reduction in adverse clinical events and reduced utilization of hospital services. Table 32.5 summarizes the findings of several studies where the issue of cost effectiveness has been addressed.[25–28] Gray *et al.*[27] esti-

Table 32.5 *Cost savings due to reduced hospital and emergency department use by an anticoagulation management service*

Gray *et al.*[27]	0.48[a] *vs* 3.22[a] hospital days per patient year. $860/patient year of therapy.
Wilt *et al.*[25]	0 *vs* 21 hospital or emergency room (ER) visits. $4072/patient year of therapy.
Chiquette *et al.*[26]	11 *vs* 41 hospital or ER visits. $1320/patient year of therapy.
Lee and Schommer *et al.*[28]	3 *vs* 15 hospital admissions. $ savings not determined.

[a]Rates for coordinated care versus routine medical care.

mated a benefit–cost ratio of 6.5, or a savings of $860 per patient year of therapy due to a reduction in hospital days per patient year. Wilt et al.,[25] in a relatively small study, identified an extraordinary cost saving in favor of AMS reduction in hospital or emergency room visits. Chiquette et al.[26] reported their estimates of cost savings through a coordinated approach compared to routine care with 11 vs 41 hospital or emergency room visits for complications resulting in approximately $1320 per patient year of therapy. Lee and Schommer[28] also found a reduction in hospital admissions with coordinated care, but did not estimate the dollars saved.

The savings from coordinated care can also be estimated by comparing the rates of major bleeding and thromboembolism as presented in Table 32.4. If one excludes the report by Wilt et al.,[25] which had a disproportionately high complication rate for RMC, the reduction of major bleeding is roughly five events averted per 100 patient years by coordinated care. Eckman et al.[29] estimated the in-patient cost of major hemorrhage as being between $3000 and $12 000 depending on outcome. Thus, using a median value of $7500, the annual savings achieved by preventing five major events would be $33 750 for 100 patients, or $337 per patient year. Similarly, the decreased incidence of thromboembolism achieved by coordinated care is approximately five events per 100 patient years. Eckman et al.[29] estimated the in-patient hospital cost of a thromboembolism as between $5000 and $18 000 depending on outcome. Therefore, using a median cost of $11 500, the data would indicate an annual saving of $57 500 per 100 patient years or $575 per patient year. Based on these assumptions, neither of which take into account the long-term morbidity or costs of complications, the combined savings of coordinated care, by lowering the incidence of both major bleeding and thromboembolism, is approximately $912 per patient year. This number is very close to that reported by Gray et al.[27] and Chiquette et al.[26] Taken together, these estimates provide a relatively consistent picture of cost savings that can be achieved through prevention of major bleeding and thromboembolism via AMS care that nears $1000 per patient year. Therefore, the available data indicate that not only will coordinated care reduce the incidence of adverse outcomes, but will also reduce health care costs.

The availability of an AMS may also reduce cost by facilitating appropriate treatment of thromboembolic disease. Specifically, patients at risk for clinical events (e.g. atrial fibrillation) may be treated more often if a coordinated program is available with treatment; the rate of stroke would decline, thereby reducing hospital and rehabilitation cost. Needless to say, the greatest benefit will be to the patient. The PORT MAST Study will be evaluating the cost effectiveness of coordinated anticoagulation programs. The means to establish an AMS is beyond the scope of this chapter. The reader is referred to other sources that provide guidelines[8] and detailed operational and organizational policies and procedures.[30]

ADVANCES IN PROTHROMBIN TIME MEASUREMENT: PATIENT SELF-TESTING AND PATIENT SELF-MANAGEMENT

As a result of technological advances in prothrombin time measurement in the last few years, the potential of further simplifying and improving management is now possible. The major advance allows for the determination of a prothrombin time from a fingerstick sample of whole blood, and consequently, opens the possibility for patient self-testing. Portability of instrumentation means that prothrombin time measurements are no longer confined to the physician's office, a private laboratory, or a nearby hospital, but can be moved into the patient's home or even taken with the patient when traveling. Standardization of reagents and instruments, as well as reliance on the INR, will reduce the inaccuracies of multiple reagents and laboratories, and simplicity of the actual procedure further establishes the possibility of patient self-testing.

Since the late 1980s, a number of instruments have been introduced or are in development for point of care testing (Table 32.6).[31] In general, these instruments are based on a clot detection methodology that uses thromboplastin to initiate clot formation, but the end point of clot detection varies from instrument to instrument.

Clinical studies

In 1987, Lucas et al.[32] first reported on the precision and reliability of an instrument that measures a capillary whole blood prothrombin time from a fingerstick sample of blood using a standardized thromboplastin reagent. They extensively tested the system comparing capillary whole blood and standard plasma PTs in 858 paired samples and showed an excellent correlation between the two methods ($r = 0.96$). Using the same instrument other investigators have also shown good to excellent correlation between this new method and standard testing.[33–36] Yano et al.,[33] Weibert et al.[34] and White et al.[35] all compared capillary whole blood PTs to plasma PTs in different clinical settings and obtained excellent correlation coefficients of 0.95, 0.91, and 0.92, respectively. Anderson et al.[36] found agreement in 83–95 per cent of paired samples depending on two different sets of criteria. However, two groups of investigators have identified limits of comparability when the INR is used for comparative purposes. Jennings et al.[37] found discrepancies due to the high international sensitivity index (ISI) (i.e. low sensitivity) of one company's thromboplastin, as well as the inability to determine a true geometric mean normal prothrombin time for the instrument. Similarly,

Table 32.6 *Capillary whole blood (point-of-care) prothrombin time instruments. (Adapted with permission from Leaning KE, Ansell JE. Advances in the monitoring of oral anticoagulation: point-of-care testing, patient self-monitoring and patient self-management.* J Thromb Thrombolys *1996;* **3***: 377–83)*

Name of instrument	Methodology
Protime Monitor 1000[a] Coumatrak[a] Ciba Corning 512 Coagulation Monitor[a] CoaguCheck Plus[a]	Thromboplastin based Clot detection: cessation of blood flow
CoaguCheck Thrombolytic Assessment System	Thromboplastin based Clot detection: cessation of movement of iron particles
ProTIME Monitor	Thromboplastin based Clot detection: cessation of blood flow through capillary channel
AvoSure PT Monitor	Thromboplastin based. Clot detection: fluorescent thrombin substrate

[a]All instruments based on original Biotrack model and licensed under different names and now marketed as CoaguCheck Plus (some with added capabilities).

Tripodi et al.[38] found that back calculating the ISI of the instrument from a reference preparation produced a significantly higher ISI than stated by the manufacturer. Additional studies by McCurdy and White[39] indicated that the INR correlation was adequate within an INR range of 2.0–3.0 (the therapeutic range for most indications), but it began to lose its comparability as the INR increased to the 4.5 range. These limitations suggest that this particular system can be further improved to report accurate prothrombin times, but it does not negate the potential advantages of such a system. Although the appropriate studies have not been done, it is possible that this new system is significantly more reliable and consistent than the variable PT monitoring often employed in the usual care of a majority of patients on oral anticoagulants. These 'point-of-care' instruments have been tested in a number of different clinical settings and, in each case, although limitations are noted,[40] their accuracy and precision are considered to be more than adequate for the monitoring of oral anticoagulant therapy in both adults and children.[41–48] The variability between individual point-of-care instruments and between the instruments and standard laboratory INR measurements is directly influenced by the lack of whole blood and ISI calibration models.[49] Further work in this area will reduce method biases.

Patient self-testing is the next logical step in the application of this technology. A number of studies have demonstrated the ability of patients to perform self-testing and obtain an accurate result.[35,36,45,50] White et al.[35] showed the potential value of having patients perform their own PT monitoring following hospital discharge. In a randomized study, 23 patients instructed in the use of a fingerstick sampling method and a portable anticoagulation monitor were discharged and asked to perform their own testing, reporting the results to their physicians for dose adjustments. Compared to a standard treatment group, these patients spent a greater percentage of time within therapeutic range (87 per cent vs 68 per cent; P=0.003) and were significantly less likely to be in a subtherapeutic range during the follow-up period (6.3 per cent vs 23 per cent; P<0.001). In this small trial, the investigators failed to find significant differences in other parameters studied including above target range PTs, hemorrhagic or thrombolic complications. In a more recent trial of patient self-testing, Anderson et al.,[36] confirmed the feasibility of self anticoagulation monitoring in 40 patients over a period of 6–24 months and demonstrated a high degree of patient satisfaction as well. In a relatively large study, Byeth and Landefeld[51] followed 325 elderly patients, 163 of whom were managed by a single investigator based on INR results from home self-testing and compared outcomes with 162 patients managed by their private physicians. Over a 6-month period, the investigators recorded a rate of major hemorrhage of 12 per cent in the latter group and 5.7 per cent in the self-testing group. This finding was based on an intention to treat analysis; for those actually performing self-testing, there was only a 1.2 per cent incidence of major hemorrhage.

Home PT monitoring, in essence, is analogous to home glucose monitoring which raises the possibility of self-management as patients with diabetes have done for years. Although anticoagulation monitoring is not as intense as glucose monitoring for insulin therapy, relatively frequent assessment of its biological effect and regular dose adjustments are still required. The concept of self-management is not new. In a study by Erdman et al.[52] performed over 20 years ago, the investigators developed a protocol for patient self-adjustment of warfarin dosing based on physician-derived guidelines. The PTs were obtained on plasma samples by routine laboratory instrumentation. Overall, there was a greater proportion of patients within the target range of anticoagulation (98 per cent of 195 patients enrolled) compared with a retrospective survey of patients managed in a routine fashion (71 per cent success rate). Using a similar protocol, Schachner et al.[53] compared self-managed patients (n = 59) and standard care patients (n = 61). The self-management group experienced four episodes of thromboembolism compared to 24 episodes in the standard care group (P<0.0005). Similarly, the self-management group experienced fewer total hemorrhagic events (5.7 per cent/patient year) compared to the standard care group (7.5 per cent/patient-year; P<0.05).

Ansell and colleagues[50,54] updated the results of a pilot study of patient self-testing and self-management using point-of-care methodology in 20 patients followed for 7 years. Patients ranged in age from 3 to 87 years, had a wide variety of indications for anticoagulation, performed home testing, and adjusted their warfarin doses according to specified guidelines. The study group was compared to matched controls managed by an established anticoagulation service. Self-managed patients were found to be in the predetermined target range for 88.6 per cent of PT determinations versus 68 per cent of PT determinations in the controls (P<0.001). Fewer dose changes were required by study patients than by controls (10.7 per cent vs 28.2 per cent, P<0.001). Complication rates did not differ between the groups and study patients were satisfied with this mode of therapy (based on their responses to a survey questionnaire).

Bernardo[55] has published the experience from her work in Germany where patient self-management is widespread. A report based on 216 self-monitored and self-managed patients between the years of 1986 and 1992 concluded that a majority (83.1 per cent) of the PT results were within target range; perhaps even more impressive, there were no serious adverse events recorded during the observation period.

Horstkotte and colleagues[56] reported on the outcome from a randomized prospective study of 150 patients with prosthetic heart valves who managed their own warfarin therapy (n = 75) and were compared to a control group (n = 75) managed by their private physicians (usual case). The self-managed patients tested themselves approximately every 4 days and achieved the target INR 92 per cent of the time. The physician-managed patients were tested approximately every 19 days and only 59 per cent of INRs were found to be in the pre-specified range. They also experienced adverse clinical events more often than patients who were self-managed and an 11 per cent incidence of any type of bleeding.

The Early Self-Controlled Anticoagulation Trial (ESCAT), an investigation conducted between 1994 and 1997 in Bad Oeynhausen, Germany, has reported findings on 600 patients followed for 2 years. Patients with mechanical heart valve replacement randomized to self-management experienced fewer hemorrhagic and thromboembolic events than patients managed by their family practitioners.[57] Nearly 80 per cent of INR values were within the pre-specified target range (INR 2.5–4.5) with self-management compared to 62 per cent in routine care. Sawicki[58] performed a randomized, single-blind trial that included 179 patients to investigate the effect of self-management on accuracy of control and treatment-related quality of life. The control group received conventional care as provided by family physicians, including referral to specialists if necessary. Deviation from the target INR value was significantly less frequent in the self-management group at 3- and 6-month follow-up. Patient satisfaction was very high with self-management of anticoagulation.

Most recently, Watzke et al.[59] compared weekly INR patient self-management in 49 patients with management by an anticoagulation clinic in 53 patients. The self-management group was within therapeutic range a greater percentage of time and had a significantly smaller mean deviation from the target INR.

In a similar study employing a cross-over design, 50 patients on long-term oral anticoagulant treatment were self-managed or managed by an anticoagulation clinic for a period of 12 weeks. The odds ratio for better control of anticoagulation (defined as the period of time within the therapeutic target range) during self-management compared with anticoagulation clinic-guided management was 4.6.[60]

Based on the available information one could conclude that point-of-care coagulation monitoring offers the potential to: (1) lower the risk/benefit profile of warfarin therapy; (2) improve patient satisfaction and possibly patient compliance; and (3) by reducing the labor intensity of physician management facilitate the more widespread use of warfarin. The cost-effectiveness and the effect of self-monitoring and management on the incidence of thromboembolic or hemorrhagic complications can only be determined through large scale clinical trials.

Considerations for patient education

Patient education should initially begin with the determination of candidacy for self-monitoring or management. Clearly, not all patients will be able or willing to perform the test and keep the necessary records to ensure safe and accurate monitoring.

The first and perhaps most important consideration in the identification of a good candidate is incentive. Patients should not be expected to comply with testing unless there is an incentive to do so. Less frequent clinic visits may be a major incentive for some patients, particularly those who travel or have a difficult time reaching the clinic laboratory. Patients may have an aversion to phlebotomy, or have poor venous access, and therefore appreciate the ease of fingerstick sampling. Some patients enjoy the opportunity to learn more about their condition and take an active role in their treatment. Patients whose PT fluctuates, necessitating more frequent monitoring, may appreciate a less invasive sampling method and a means to increase the likelihood of achieving the desired target INR range. Although the incentives for home monitoring and management will differ, the key to safe and effective management is appropriate patient selection. Further considerations in identifying ideal candidates include: (1) adequate motor skills to perform the test; (2) sufficient cognitive capability; (3) adequate reading and writing capabilities; and (4) visual acuity (with or without glasses) to see the monitor screen. In the absence of one or more of these required attributes, a responsible family member or care giver may assume the responsibility of home testing or management.

Patients (and their family members) must understand their indication for warfarin, the importance of careful monitoring and the use of the monitor. The health care provider (typically a member of an experienced AMS) must convey the necessary information and train the patient, striving to simplify the process. Written instructions should also be provided, allowing the patient to continue their education at home. Instructions are usually provided by the instrument manufacturer as well.

After performing a test, each patient must record their results. A printed calendar to use both as a testing schedule and place for recording results should be provided. During the initial training session it is important to discuss on which days, the time of doses, and the place that the patient should perform the test, and to practice careful documentation (on the calendar). Adequate time should be allotted in the training session for patients and their family members to ask questions. It is also important to outline common problems that can arise and the best way to approach these. Needless to say, patients should be contacted at established intervals to provide continuous, high quality of care.

Finally, follow-up visits should be scheduled and recorded on the calendar. It may well take more than one visit to train a patient in all the aspects of home testing. Trainers should not assume their patients remember everything during the training session. Patients should know who, when, and what phone numbers to call for potential problems.

Instrumentation

The CoaguChek® (Roche Diagnostics), ProTime® Monitor (International Technidyne Corporation) and AvoSure® (Avoset Inc) are three instruments currently available for home use. Costs vary from approximately $600 to $1200 (US) and the testing cartridges (a new cartridge is required for each test) are approximately $5 to $7. Several instruments are currently in development and will create competition and ultimately lower prices. It is important to mention, however, that Medicare has not yet decided whether the cost of instruments and cartridges will be reimbursed. The managed care industry and third-party payers have not yet established a formal position.

The issue of liability with self-monitoring and management programs has been raised by health care professionals. Since the devices are FDA approved for home use, it is important for physicians to familiarize themselves with the technology and carefully manage warfarin dosing in response to results generated by patient self-testing. Self-management should be considered only for a highly selected group of patients with the intention of careful follow-up provided by an experienced AMS.

SUMMARY

- Anticoagulation management services and coordinated anticoagulation programs provide a focused approach for the management of patients with thromboembolic disease. In experienced hands, safe and effective anticoagulation can be achieved in a majority of patients thereby reducing complication rates and cost.
- Capillary whole blood prothrombin time measurement is available for use in patients with thromboembolic disease who require warfarin. The instrumentation is portable and the methodology is simple, allowing patient self-testing. The available technology also offers the potential for reduced variability of results, reduced costs of monitoring therapy, increased patient comfort and satisfaction, improved compliance, and possibly better overall outcomes.
- The full utilization of coordinated anticoagulation programs and point-of-care instruments for self-monitoring and management of anticoagulant therapy will require further investigation through large-scale clinical trials.

REFERENCES

1. Ansell JE. Oral anticoagulant therapy – 50 years later. *Arch Intern Med* 1993; **153**: 586–96.
2. Kutner M, Nixon G, Silverstone F. Physicians' attitudes toward oral anticoagulants and antiplatelet agents for stroke prevention in elderly patients with atrial fibrillation. *Arch Intern Med* 1991; **151**: 1950–3.

○3. McCrory DC, Matchar DB, Samsa G, Sanders LL, Pritchett ELC. Physician attitudes about anticoagulation for nonvalvular atrial fibrillation in the elderly. *Arch Intern Med* 1995; **155**: 277–81.

4. Ansell JE, Hughes R. Evolving models of warfarin management: anticoagulation clinics, patient self-monitoring, and patient self-management. *Am Heart J* 1996; **132**: 1095–100.

○5. Campbell HA, Link KP. Studies on the hemorrhagic sweet clover disease, IV: the isolation and crystallization of the hemorrhagic agent. *J Biol Chem* 1941; **138**: 21–33.

○6. Butt HR, Allen EV, Bollman JL. A preparation from spoiled sweet clover which prolongs coagulation and prothrombin time of the blood: preliminary reports of experimental and clinical studies. *Mayo Clin Proc* 1941; **16**: 388–95.

7. Loeliger EA, van Dijk-Wierda CA, van den Besselaar AMHP, Broekmans AW, Roos J. Anticoagulant control and the risk of bleeding. In: Meade TW, ed. *Anticoagulants and myocardial infarction: a reappraisal*. Chichester: John Wiley & Sons, Ltd, 1984: 135–77.

8. Ansell JE, Buttaro ML, Orsula Voltis T, Knowlton CH, and Anticoagulation Guidelines Task Force. Consensus guidelines for coordinated outpatient oral anticoagulation therapy management. *Ann Pharmacother* 1997; **31**: 604–15.

9. Cook DJ, Guyatt GH, Laupacis A, Sackett DL, Goldberg RJ. Clinical recommendations using levels of evidence for antithrombotic agents. *Chest* 1995; **108**(suppl): 227S–230S.

10. Landefeld CS, Goldman L. Major bleeding in outpatients treated with warfarin: incidence and prediction by factors known at the start of outpatient therapy. *Am J Med* 1989; **87**: 144–52.

11. Gitter MJ, Jaeger TM, Petterson TM, Gersh BJ, Silverstein MD. Bleeding and thromboembolism during anticoagulant therapy: a population-based study in Rochester, Minnesota. *Mayo Clin Proc* 1995; **70**: 725–33.

12. Forfar JC. A seven year analysis of haemorrhage in patients on long-term anticoagulant treatment. *Br Heart J* 1979; **42**: 128–32.

13. Errichetti AM, Holden A, Ansell J. Management of oral anticoagulant therapy: experience with an anticoagulation clinic. *Arch Intern Med* 1984; **144**: 1966–8.

14. Conte RR, Kehoe WA, Nielson N, Lodhia H. Nine-year experience with a pharmacist-managed anticoagulation clinic. *Am J Hosp Pharm* 1986; **43**: 2460–4.

15. Petty GW, Lennihan L, Mohr JP, *et al*. Complications of long-term anticoagulation. *Ann Neurol* 1988; **23**: 570–4.

16. Charney R, Leddomado E, Rose DN, Fuster V. Anticoagulation clinics and the monitoring of anticoagulant therapy. *Int J Cardiol* 1988; **18**: 197–206.

17. Bussey HI, Rospond RM, Quandt CM , Clark GM. The safety and effectiveness of long-term warfarin therapy in an anticoagulation clinic. *Pharmacother* 1989; **9**: 214–19.

18. Seabrook GR, Karp D, Schmitt DD, Bandyk DF. An outpatient anticoagulation protocol managed by a vascular nurse-clinician. *Am J of Surg* 1990; **160**: 501–4.

○19. Fihn SD, McDonell M, Martin D, *et al*. Risk factors for complications of chronic anticoagulation: a multicenter study. *Ann Intern Med* 1993; **118**: 511–20.

20. Van der Meer FJ, Rosendaal FR, Vandenbrouke JP, Briet E. Bleeding complications in oral anticoagulant therapy: an analysis of risk factors. *Arch Intern Med* 1993; **153**: 1557–62.

◆21. Cannegieter SC, Rosendaal FR, Wintzen AR, van der Meer FJM, Vandenbroucke JP, Briet E. Optimal oral anticoagulant therapy in patients with mechanical heart valves. *N Engl J Med* 1995; **33**: 11–17.

22. Palareti G, Leali N, Coccheri S, *et al*. Bleeding complications of oral anticoagulant treatment: an inception-cohort, prospective collaborative study (ISCOAT). *Lancet* 1996; **348**: 423–8.

23. Garabedian-Ruffalo SM, Gray DR, Sax MJ, *et al*. Retrospective evaluation of a pharmacist-managed warfarin anticoagulation clinic. *Am J Hosp Pharm* 1985; **42**: 304–8.

24. Cortelazzo S, Finazzi G, Viero P, *et al*. Thrombotic and hemorrhagic complications in patients with mechanical heart valve prostheses attending an anticoagulation clinic. *Thromb Haemostas* 1993; **69**: 316–20.

25. Wilt VM, Gums JG, Amhed OI, Moore LM. Outcome analysis of a pharmacist-managed anticoagulation service. *Pharmacotherapy* 1995; **15**: 732–9.

26. Chiquette E, Amato MG, Bussey HI. Comparison of an anticoagulation clinic and usual medical care: anticoagulation control, patient outcomes and health care costs. *Arch Intern Med* 1998; **158**: 1641–7.

27. Gray DR, Garabedian-Ruffalo SM, Chretien SD. Cost-justification of a clinical pharmacist-managed anticoagulation clinic. *Drug Intell Clin Pharm* 1985; **19**: 575–80.

28. Lee YP, Schommer JC. Effect of a pharmacist-managed anticoagulation clinic on warfarin-related hospital readmissions. *Am J Health Sys Pharm* 1996; **53**: 1580–3.

29. Eckman MH, Levine JH, Pauker SG. Making decisions about antithrombotic therapy in heart disease. *Chest* 1995; **108**(suppl): 457S–470S.

30. Ansell JE, Oertel LB, Wittkowsky AK, eds. *Managing oral anticoagulation: clinical and operational guidelines*. Gaithersburg, MD: Aspen Publishers, Inc., 1997.

○31. Leaning KE, Ansell JE. Advances in the monitoring of oral anticoagulation: point-of-care testing, patient self-monitoring and patient self-management. *J Thromb Thrombolys* 1996; **3**: 377–83.

♦32. Lucas FV, Duncan A, Jay R, *et al*. A novel whole blood capillary technique for measuring prothrombin time. *Am J Clin Pathol* 1987; **88**: 442–6.

33. Yano Y, Kambayashi J, Murata K, *et al*. Bedside monitoring of warfarin therapy by a whole blood capillary coagulation monitor. *Thromb Res* 1992; **66**: 583–90.

34. Weibert RT, Adler DS. Evaluation of a capillary whole blood prothrombin time measurement system. *Clin Pharm* 1989; **8**: 864–7.

35. White RH, McCurdy SA, von Marensdorff H, Woodruff DE, Leftgoff L. Home prothrombin time monitoring after initiation of warfarin therapy. *Ann Intern Med* 1989; **111**: 730–7.

♦36. Anderson D, Harrison L, Hirsh J. Evaluation of a portable prothrombin time monitor for home use by patients who require long-term oral anticoagulant therapy. *Arch Intern Med* 1993; **153**: 1441–7.

37. Jennings I, Luddington RJ, Baglin T. Evaluation of the Ciba Corning Biotrack 512 coagulation monitor for the control of oral anticoagulation. *J Clin Pathol* 1991; **44**: 950–3.

38. Tripodi A, Arbini A, Chantarangkul V, Bettega D, Mannucci PM. Are capillary whole blood coagulation monitors suitable for the control of oral anticoagulant treatment by the International Normalized Ratio? *Thromb Haemostas* 1993; **70**: 921–4.

39. McCurdy SA, White RH. Accuracy and precision of a portable anticoagulation monitor in a clinical setting. *Arch Intern Med* 1992; **152**: 589–92.

40. Kaatz AA, White RH, Hill J, et al. Accuracy of laboratory and portable monitor International Normalized Ratio determinations. *Arch Intern Med* 1995; **155**: 1861–7.

41. Oberhardt BJ, Dermott SC, Taylor M, Alkadi ZY, Abruzzini AF, Gresalfi NJ. Dry reagent technology for rapid, convenient measurements of blood coagulation and fibrinolysis. *Clin Chem* 1991; **37**: 520–6.

42. Rose VL, Dermott SC, Murray BF, *et al*. Decentralized testing for prothrombin time and activated partial thromboplastin time using a dry chemistry portable analyzer. *Arch Pathol Lab Med* 1993; **117**: 611–17.

43. Fabbrini N, Messmore H, Balbale S, *et al*. Pilot study to determine use of a TAS analyzer in an anticoagulation clinic setting. *Blood* 1995; **86**(suppl 1): 869a.

44. Kapiotis S, Quehenberger P, Speiser W. Evaluation of the new method Coaguchek for the determination of prothrombin time from capillary blood: comparison with Thrombotest on KC-1. *Thromb Res* 1995; **77**: 563–7.

45. Ansell J, Becker D, Andrew M, *et al*. Accurate and precise prothrombin time measurement in a multicenter anticoagulation trial employing patient self-testing. *Blood* 1995; **86**(suppl 1): 864a.

46. Andrew M, Marzinotto V, Adams M, Cimini C, Triplett D, LaDuca F. Monitoring of oral anticoagulant therapy in pediatric patients using a new microsample PT device. *Blood* 1995; **86**(suppl 1): 863a.

47. Zweig SE, Meyer BG, Sharma S, Min C, Krakower JM, Shohet SB. Membrane-based, dry-reagent prothrombin time tests. *Biomed Instrument Technol* 1996; **30**: 245–56.

48. van den Besselaar AMHP, Breddin K, Lutze G, *et al*. Multicenter evaluation of a new capillary blood prothrombin time monitoring system. *Blood Coag Fibrinolys* 1995; **6**: 726–32.

49. Gosselin R, Owings JT, White RH, *et al*. A comparison of point-of-care instruments designed for monitoring oral anticoagulation with standard laboratory methods. *Thromb Haemostas* 2000; **83**: 698–703.

♦50. Ansell J, Holden A, Knapic N. Patient self-management of oral anticoagulation guided by capillary fingerstick whole blood prothrombin times. *Arch Intern Med* 1989; **149**: 2509–11.

51. Byeth RJ, Landefeld CS. Prevention of major bleeding in older patients treated with warfarin: results of a randomized trial. *J Gen Intern Med* 1997; **12**: 66.

52. Erdman S, Vidne B, Levy MJ. A self-control method for long-term anticoagulation therapy. *J Cardiovasc Surg* 1974; **15**: 454–7.

53. Schachner A, Deviri E, Shabat S. Patient-regulated anticoagulation. In: Butchart EG, Bodnar E, eds. *Thrombosis embolism and bleeding*. London: ICR Publishers, 1992; 318–24.

♦54. Ansell J, Patel N, Ostrovsky D, Nozzolillo E, Peterson AM, Fish L. Long-term patient self-management of oral anticoagulation. *Arch Intern Med* 1995; **155**: 2185–9.

♦55. Bernardo A. Experience with patient self-management of oral anticoagulation. *J Thromb Thrombolysis* 1996; **2**: 321–5.

56. Horstkotte D, Piper C, Wiemer M, Schulte HD, Schultheiss H-P. Improvement of prognosis by home prothrombin estimation in patients with life-long anticoagulant therapy. *Eur Heart J* 1996; **17**(suppl): 230.

57. Koertke H, Minami K, Bairaktaris A, *et al*. INR self-management following mechanical heart valve replacement. *J Thromb Thrombolysis* 2000; **9**: 541–5.

♦58. Sawicki PT. A structured teaching and self-management program for patients receiving oral anticoagulation: a randomized controlled trial. *JAMA* 1999; **281**: 145–50.

59. Watzke HH, Forberg E, Svolba G, Jimenez-Boj E, Krinninger B. A prospective controlled trial comparing weekly self-testing and self-dosing with the standard management of patients on stable oral anticoagulation. *Thromb Haemost* 2000; **83**: 661–5.

♦60. Cromheecke ME, Levi M, Colly LP, *et al*. Oral anticoagulation self-management and management by a specialist anticoagulation clinic: a randomized cross over comparison. *Lancet* 2000; **356**: 97–102.

33

Establishing an out-patient (home) deep vein thrombosis treatment program using low-molecular-weight heparin therapy

WENDY A LEONG*

The development of low-molecular-weight heparin preparations with predictable pharmacokinetics and pharmacodynamics, coupled with their ability to be administered subcutaneously without routine coagulation monitoring, has paved the way for home deep vein thrombosis treatment programs. The key to a successful program lies within careful patient selection, follow-up and the coordinated efforts of physicians, nurses, pharmacists and other support staff.

INTRODUCTION

Low-molecular-weight heparin (LMWH) therapy has revolutionized the treatment of deep vein thrombosis (DVT).[1-10] Researchers and clinicians believe that the second generation of LMWH may replace intravenous unfractionated heparin (UH) therapy for most indications.[11,12]

The paradigm shift from traditional in-patient management to out-patient (ambulatory/home) care is a significant change in DVT treatment. In this chapter, the care of DVT patients will be discussed, with emphasis on practical tips for establishing out-patient treatment with LMWH therapy.

VENOUS THROMBOEMBOLISM

Pathophysiology

The underlying pathophysiology in thrombogenesis (clot formation) has been described as Virchow's triad with three major contributing variables:[13]

1 hypercoagulability, e.g. deficiency of protein C, protein S or antithrombin; estrogen, malignancy;
2 endothelial (vascular) damage, e.g. trauma, orthopedic surgery; and
3 hemostasis (sluggish blood flow), e.g. bed rest, immobility, venous obstruction.

*Disclaimer: I have participated in clinical research studies, pilot projects, professional presentations, seminars, advisory boards, journal publications and other projects involving the use of warfarin (Dupont Canada Inc.), dalteparin (Pharmacia Upjohn), enoxaparin (Aventis) and tinzaparin (Leo Laboratories Canada Inc.).

Venous thromboembolism is a clotting disorder with high potential for vascular occlusion. The thrombus (clot) usually begins in the deep veins of the legs as a DVT, and may progess to a life-threatening pulmonary embolism (PE) in the lungs. Figure 33.1 shows the two major types of DVT based on anatomical location:[14–19]

1 proximal DVT: femoral or popliteal veins; higher incidence of PE;
2 distal DVT: tibial veins; low risk of progressing to a proximal DVT or PE.

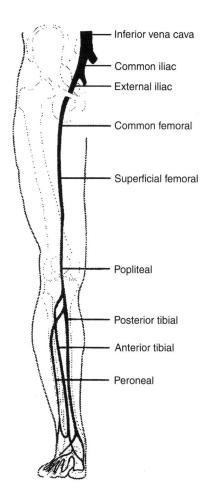

Inferior vena cava
Common iliac
External iliac
Common femoral
Superficial femoral
Popliteal
Posterior tibial
Anterior tibial
Peroneal

Figure 33.1 *Location of the deep vein thrombosis.*

Predisposing factors for DVT have been classified by level of risk by the American College of Chest Physicians' (ACCP) Sixth Consensus Conference on Antithrombotic Therapy.[20] The very high risk classification included major surgery in patients older than 40 years, plus previous venous thromboembolism or malignancy, or orthopedic surgery or hip fracture or stroke or spinal cord injury.[20]

Diagnosis and prognosis

Classic signs and symptoms of DVT such as calf pain or swelling have not been proven to be reliable, as only 20–30 per cent of patients with symptoms suggestive of a DVT have a positive diagnosis of DVT.[15,16] In Canada, the diagnosis of DVT is most commonly confirmed by non-invasive venous ultrasonography (Doppler ultrasound), while in the USA, invasive contrast venography (venogram) is preferred.

The location of the thrombus determines the prognosis and management of DVT. Proximal DVTs (thrombus in the femoral and/or popliteal veins) have a higher incidence of progressing to PE than distal DVTs (thrombus in the tibial veins) (Fig. 33.1). There is a lower risk of distal DVTs progressing to a proximal DVT or PE.[14,16] The diagnostic management of DVT and PE has been described in detail elsewhere.[14,16–18]

Undiagnosed or untreated DVT may increase morbidity (i.e. post-phlebitic syndrome, recurrent thromboembolism) and mortality (respiratory failure secondary to PE).[18] PE has been called a clinically silent disease with a mortality rate exceeding 50 per cent, owing to the rapid onset of respiratory failure and confirmed diagnosis on autopsy.[18]

Importance to clinical practice

DVT PROPHYLAXIS

A major area for improvement is the prevention of DVT. Fatal PE may be the most common preventable cause of death in hospitalized patients, yet DVT prophylaxis continues to be underutilized in up to 40 per cent of high-risk patients.[18,20,21]

A secondary diagnosis of DVT means that the patients were admitted for another medical condition (e.g. hip fracture, pneumonia) and developed a DVT as a complication of hospitalization.[19] The consequences would result in prolonged hospitalization, and increased risk of morbidity and mortality.[20,21] The ACCP has published clear consensus guidelines for DVT prophylaxis that needed to be incorporated into daily patient care;[20] for example, clinical protocols and pathways.

DVT TREATMENT

The paradigm shift from in-patient management with 5–10 days of intravenous (iv) UH to out-patient (ambulatory) care with LMWH is exciting. In Canada, there are an estimated 9000 patients admitted to hospitals annually with a primary diagnosis of DVT (i.e. reason for admission was DVT). Potentially 40 per cent of all uncomplicated DVT patients may avoid hospitalization.[9] In Canada, 40 per cent means 3600 patients per year could be treated safely on an out-patient basis and over 25 000 hospital days avoided per year. The literature strongly supports out-patient DVT treatment, but the barriers to establishing an out-patient DVT treatment program have restricted its widespread, routine use as standard care.[1–10]

TREATMENT OPTIONS AND PHARMACOTHERAPY

There are several factors to consider in the treatment of DVT such as the anatomical location of the DVT, primary versus secondary diagnosis of DVT, anticoagulation and non-drug measures.

Anatomical location and cause of DVT

The location of the DVT most often determines the treatment plan.[22] Proximal DVTs (in the femoral and/or popliteal vein) are routinely treated for a minimum of 3 months with anticoagulation due to the high risk of fatal PE and recurrent thromboembolism. Distal DVTs may not require any anticoagulation, and only follow-up with serial non-invasive venous ultrasonography (Doppler) for 10–14 days, to identify progression to proximal DVT.

The cause of the DVT may determine if the patient is eligible for out-patient treatment. For example, consider the two following categories.

- Primary diagnosis of DVT means that the reason for admission was a confirmed DVT.[19] For 40 per cent of all cases, out-patient treatment with LMWH therapy has been shown to be safe and effective.[1–10]
- Secondary diagnosis of DVT means that the patient developed a DVT during hospitalization after admission for another medical condition (e.g. hip fracture, congestive heart failure).[19] This group of patients may be less suitable for out-patient DVT treatment with LMWH due to their underlying medical condition.[19] The emphasis should be focused on improving DVT prophylaxis in this patient population.[20,21]

Anticoagulation and thrombolysis

UNFRACTIONATED INTRAVENOUS HEPARIN

Traditional management for DVT patients has been 5–10 days of hospitalization for the administration of a continuous iv infusion of unfractionated heparin (iv UH), aiming for a therapeutic prothrombin time (PTT) of 1.5–2.5 times control (e.g. 60–86 seconds), achieved by multiple daily blood tests (e.g. PTT every 6 hours) and iv UH dosage infusion adjustments up to four times daily.[22,23]

The minimum in-patient hospital stay would be 5 days: an average of 3 days to reach a therapeutic international normalized ratio (INR) of 2.0–3.0 with warfarin therapy, plus 2 more days for the overlap with iv UH to prevent heparin rebound.[22,23]

LOW-MOLECULAR-WEIGHT HEPARIN THERAPY

The purpose of the LMWH is to replace iv UH and to provide full anticoagulation until a therapeutic INR has been achieved for 2 consecutive days with warfarin therapy; a minimum of 5 days of LMWH.[1–10,22] A delay in reaching a therapeutic INR of 2.0–3.0 will result in prolonged LMWH usage.

LMWHs are the second generation of heparin therapy with a superior pharmacokinetic profile than iv UH.[12] LMWH may be described as a cleaner, filtered, smaller heparin molecule with more specific antifactor Xa activity.[12] Intravenous UH may become obsolete, to be replaced by LMWH for most indications.[11] For an excellent review of LMWH, please refer to Fareed et al.[12]

The constant half-life of LMWH allows for once or twice daily dosing (instead of a continous iv infusion). The excellent bioavailability of LMWH allows for subcutaneous dosing (no iv access necessary). PTT monitoring is not necessary for dosage adjustment (unlike iv UH). These combined advantages of LMWH allow for the treatment of DVT on an out-patient basis. There are studies supporting the use of dalteparin (Fragmin[R]), enoxaparin (Lovenox[R]), nadroparin (Fraxiparin[R]), and tinzaparin (Logiparin[R], Innohep[R]) for the treatment of DVT.[1–10,24] Each LMWH has been recognized as a distinct entity by the World Health Organization, and may not be interchanged at this time.[11]

Reported adverse drug reactions with LMWH therapy include hemorrhage, heparin-induced thrombocytopenia (HIT) and osteoporosis. The incidence of HIT may be lower with LMWH (0 per cent) compared to iv UH (2.7 per cent).[25] HIT has been defined as: (1) positive test for heparin-dependent immunoglobulin G (IgG) antibodies; and (2) a decrease in the platelet count to below 150 000 mm[3] after five days of heparin therapy.[25,26] Platelet monitoring is still required up to 2 weeks after discontinuation of LMWH or iv UH. HIT should be considered life-threatening due to the hypercoagulability and high risk of morbidity and mortality.[26]

WARFARIN

An out-patient DVT treatment program will fail if there is subtherapeutic warfarin dosing and poor follow-up. Warfarin does not act immediately.[22,27,28] There is often a 2-day delay to achieve a therapeutic INR of 2.0–3.0, which is why iv UH or LMWH must be used in the initial treatment of DVT. Although the emphasis has been on out-patient DVT treatment with LMWH therapy, more attention should be paid to the chronic warfarin management.[29] The literature suggests that up to 20 per cent of warfarin patients have subtherapeutic dosing.[27]

The duration of anticoagulation must be patient specific, depending on risk factors such as active malignancy or recurrent thromboembolism.[14,22] The LMWH therapy may only be used for 5 days initially, whereas the warfarin therapy will continue for a minimum of 3 months for the treatment of DVT. A delay in reaching a therapeutic INR of 2.0–3.0 will result in prolonged LMWH usage. A warfarin dosing service, anticoagulation clinic, or warfarin dosing protocol is highly recommended.[27,29]

THROMBOLYSIS

Fibrinolytic agents are not routinely recommended to treat DVT.[14,22]

Inferior vena cava (Greenfield) filter

Insertion of an inferior vena cava filter is an invasive procedure to prevent PE in patients with high risk or confirmed proximal DVT, and a contraindication to anticoagulation; or for patients with recurrent DVT or PE despite therapeutic doses of anticoagulation.[14]

FIVE MODELS FOR AN OUT-PATIENT DVT TREATMENT PROGRAM

The key to successfully establishing an out-patient DVT treatment program is the optimal use of each site's available resources and clinical expertise. Case management by a core group of clinicians is essential for continuity of care; even if it is only two people (e.g. one physician and one pharmacist).[29,30] DVT is a potentially life-threatening disease and requires careful screening, monitoring, and

follow-up. Table 33.1 shows five different clinical practice models:

1 anticoagulation clinic or thromboembolic service;
2 medical day care unit or ambulatory care clinic;
3 emergency department fast-track area;
4 one visit and self-injection only; and
5 physician office follow-up.[8,10,30–32]

Anticoagulation clinic or thromboembolic service

An existing anticoagulation clinic or thromboembolic service may be the easiest method of establishing out-patient treatment of DVT. The clinic could simply expand its services and accept referrals directly from the emergency department or physicians' offices after positive diagnosis. These types of resource may be more readily available at tertiary care centers with a multidisciplinary team, including hematology, pharmacy, nursing, research staff, etc. Case management by the clinic staff is necessary for continuity of care.[29,30] Patients could return to the clinic daily for nurse-administered subcutaneous (sc) injections, or they could be taught to self-inject at home. Warfarin dosing would be managed by the clinic, usually by telephone. The major disadvantage is that most sites do not have an anticoagulation clinic or a thromboembolic service.

Table 33.1 *Five models for an out-patient deep vein thrombosis treatment program*[8,10,30–32]

	Anticoagulation clinic or thromboembolic service	Ambulatory care clinic or medical day care unit	Emergency department fast track	One visit and self-injection	Physician office follow-up
Screening, enrolling, counseling	✓	✓	✓	✓	✓
sc injection given by					
Patient	✓ (or nurse)	✗	✗	✓	✓
Nurse	✓ (or patient)	✓	✓	✗	✗
Daily visits for sc injection	✓ (by nurse)	✓	✓	✗	✗
LMWH supply (reimbursement)					
Hospital, clinic	✓ (or patient)	✓	✓	✗	✗
Prescription for patient (i.e. third party)	✓	✗	✗	✓	✓
Warfarin dosing and INR monitoring					
At hospital, clinic	✓ (or phone)	✓ (or phone)	✓ (or phone)	✗	✗
By telephone	✓	✓	✓	✓	✓
Disadvantages					
High risk of sc non-compliance	✗	✗	✓	✓	✓
High risk of subtherapeutic warfarin dosing	✗	✗	✓	✓	✓

✓ = Yes; ✗ = no; sc = subcutaneous; INR = international normalized ratio.

Medical day care unit or ambulatory care clinic

An existing ambulatory care clinic could be modified to include out-patient DVT treatment. Some primary and secondary care centers already have a home parenteral antibiotic program, which has the same concept as an out-patient DVT treatment program, that is, patients either return to hospital once/twice daily for treatment, or a home care nurse administers daily treatment in the patient's home.

A core group of clinicians (e.g. physician, pharmacist, nurse), an examining room, access to a laboratory, and an office would be necessary for the ambulatory care clinic. Patients could return once or twice daily for nurse-administered sc injections and have their warfarin dosing managed for the first 5 days. The disadvantage of this model is that patients must have access to transportation or home care nurses must be readily available for home visits. This medical day care unit model will be described in more detail, based on our experiences at Burnaby Hospital.[30–32]

Emergency department fast-track area

Many emergency departments have a treatment area sometimes called *fast-track* for the *walking wounded*, including patients that may return once or twice a day for antibiotics. It may be an ideal setting for an out-patient DVT treatment program, as patients could return once or twice daily for nurse-administered sc LMWH injections. The major disadvantages are the lack of case management with rotating emergency physicians and nurses; a potentially long waiting time for the patient in high-volume sites; and a possible delay in reading therapeutic INR depending on the physician's expertise in warfarin dosing. A consistent person needs to track these DVT patients and monitor their medication compliance and warfarin therapy closely.[29] A clinical pharmacist in the emergency department would be an ideal person.[10,30]

One visit and self-injection only

Some sites may choose to see their DVT patients only once, at the time of diagnosis.[10] These patients may be taught to self-inject the sc LMWH at home and be followed up by telephone for warfarin dosing. It is imperative that these patients be monitored daily by a core group for medication compliance and for warfarin dosing. A prescription for LMWH would be filled at the patient's local pharmacy. Although this may be the ideal model, the disadvantages include: the patient's reluctance to self-inject; the patient's inability to self-inject with proper technique; non-compliance with sc injec-

tions and progression to PE. Unlike one missed intravenous antibiotic dose for cellulitis, one missed LMWH sc dose could mean the loss of its anticoagulation effect and increased risk of PE or respiratory failure.

Physician office follow-up

It is also possible for a physician to coordinate all the activities for outpatient management of DVT independently from his/her office, without the involvement of any clinics, hospital-based services or other health care team members. Once the diagnosis has been confirmed, the patient could have a prescription for LMWH filled at his/her local pharmacy. Sufficient time for counseling to self-inject is essential to ensure medication compliance. Warfarin dosing and laboratory monitoring could be coordinated by the physician. The major disadvantages to this model are: the physician's time; the high potential for medication non-compliance if there is no daily follow-up while on LMWH therapy; and the possible delay in reaching therapeutic INR with warfarin dosing, depending on the physician's expertise with oral anticoagulation dosing.

PROGRAM DEVELOPMENT

The remainder of this chapter will discuss the Burnaby Hospital Outpatient DVT Treatment Program that was implemented in May 1996, using the Medical Day Care Unit Model.[8,31,32] Practical recommendations have been included that may be useful for any of the five models described previously. Program development, implementation and step-by-step program instructions are provided as a template for those health care team members who are interested in establishing an outpatient DVT treatment program at their site using their existing resources.[31]

What is Burnaby Hospital? A Canadian primary and secondary care center

At the time of writing, Burnaby Hospital was a 515-bed, university-affiliated, primary and secondary care center with 60 000 emergency visits annually. Medical services included cardiology, critical care, general/orthopedic surgery, general medicine, geriatrics, neurology, oncology, palliative care and several ambulatory care programs. The hospital had limited resources with one hematologist, one cardiologist, two neurologists, five internal medicine specialists, nine clinical pharmacists, and over 200 family physicians with admitting privileges.

The Out-patient DVT Treatment Program was developed by a multidisciplinary Anticoagulation Working

Group, represented by hematology, pharmacy, nursing, laboratories, and cardiology. This group had been instrumental for the implementation of a standardized iv UH protocol (1994);[24] a pharmacy warfarin dosing service (1995);[27,29] a comprehensive evaluation of DVT prophylaxis (1995)[21] and DVT treatment (1995);[19] an out-patient DVT treatment program (1996);[8,30–32] and LMWH in unstable angina (1998, in progress). The hematologist, clinical pharmacist and program nurse were also investigators in thromboembolic research studies with LMWH since 1994.

How was the program justified?

In Canada, there are approximately 9000 patients admitted to hospitals annually with a primary diagnosis of DVT (i.e. reason for admission was DVT). Potentially 40 per cent of all uncomplicated DVT patients could avoid 5–10 days of hospitalization for continuous iv UH by using LMWH.[1–10,30–32] Forty per cent means that 3600 patients per year could be treated safely on an out-patient basis in Canada, avoiding over 25 000 hospital-days per year. (Accurate and verified statistics for the number of DVT patients admitted per year in the USA were not available to the writer at the time of this publication.)

In British Columbia, a Canadian western province, 40 per cent means 450 DVT patients could be treated without the traditional 5–10 days of hospitalization per patient; avoiding 2250–4500 hospital days per year. The literature strongly supports out-patient DVT treatment,[1–10,30–32] but the barriers to implementing an out-patient DVT treatment program have restricted its widespread routine use. There is no doubt that LMWH therapy has revolutionized the management of venous thromboembolism.

To prove that an out-patient DVT treatment program would be valuable at Burnaby Hospital, a continuous quality improvement project on DVT management was completed in 1995 by the Clinical Pharmacy Services. There were 75 patients with a primary diagnosis of DVT, an average of 8 days of hospitalization and an in-hospital gross mortality rate of 3 per cent.[19] The Anticoagulation Working Group received the report and recommended improving DVT prophylaxis in high-risk patients;[21] and implementing an out-patient DVT treatment program potentially to treat 40–50 patients per year and avoiding over 200 hospital-days per year.[19]

In addition, the pharmacy warfarin dosing service was well recognized and strongly supported for hospital-wide use since 1995. Clinical pharmacists were able to achieve a therapeutic INR of 2.0–3.0 in 86 per cent of patients by day 4 compared to physician dosing.[27] It was clear that the duration of hospital stay could be reduced with the warfarin dosing service for admitted DVT and PE patients.

PROGRAM IMPLEMENTATION

Establishing an out-patient DVT treatment program is not difficult and simply requires some strategic planning, in particular, trying to align this new program with existing resources. A 26-page Burnaby Hospital Outpatient Deep Vein Thrombosis Treatment Resource Guide was published in February 1997, upon demand, to provide practical information and useful standardized forms to any clinicians interested in implementing an out-patient DVT treatment program (Figs 33.2 and 33.3).[31]

Why was the medical day care unit selected and how does the program work?

For our site and its limited resources, the *medical day care unit* was the most feasible model, which is featured in the Outpatient DVT Treatment Resource Guide,[21] but this model was actually our third choice.[30,31]

There was no existing anticoagulation clinic or thromboembolic service at Burnaby Hospital, so our first choice was the *one visit and self-inject* model, but there was insufficient home care nursing resources available for the mandatory follow-up. We decided not to teach the patients how to self-inject at home, based on our experience of a high dropout rate with a previous LMWH sc self-injection research study. Our second choice was the *emergency department fast-track* model, but the high volume of 60 000 visits per year and a very busy fast-track area made this option unappealing to our emergency department staff who were already short-staffed.

Figure 33.4 is an overview of the Burnaby Hospital Outpatient DVT Treatment Program. Phase One was implemented in May 1996 using the Medical Day Care Unit to pilot the program. It was our intention to progress to Phase Two, the one visit and self-inject model by October 1997. Once again, owing to insufficient home care nursing resources at our site, Phase Two had not been implemented at the time of publication.

The Medical Day Care Unit was an open room with several chairs and two stretchers to accommodate nursing assessment, patient counseling, and out-patient treatment with iv antibiotics, blood transfusions, etc. Enrollment for the out-patient DVT treatment program was restricted from Monday to Friday, 0800–1600h, due to the availability of the hematologist and clinical pharmacist. On weekends, nights, and holidays, the patients were admitted overnight, then screened for out-patient treatment as soon as possible. Once patients were enrolled in the program, they received their first sc dose of LMWH (enoxaparin 1 mg/kg twice daily), usually in the emergency department. Patients were instructed to return to the hospital twice a day for 5 consecutive days (including weekends if necessary), as follows.

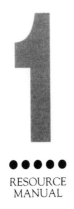

Purpose:
To provide practical
information and useful
standardized forms for
implementation of an
outpatient DVT
Treatment Program.

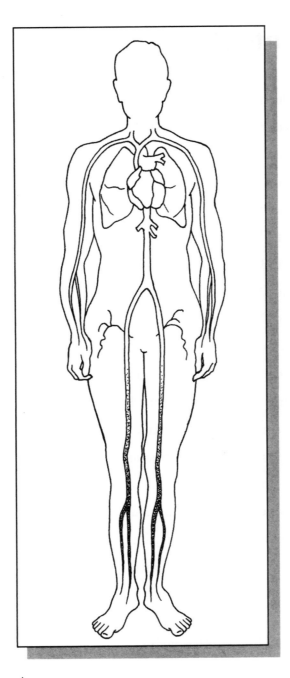

Resource Manual

- **Primary Diagnosis of DVT**

- **Low Molecular Weight Heparin Therapy**

- **Warfarin Dosing Service**

- **Patient Counselling**

Figure 33.2 *Resource manual.*

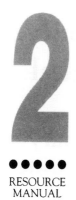

RESOURCE MANUAL

Contents

Figure 33.3 *Contents.*

Overview of Phase One and Two

PHASE ONE:
MEDICAL DAY CARE UNIT (MDCU)
(Implemented May 1996)

*The Outpatient DVT
Treatment Program
was implemented at
Burnaby Hospital in
two phases, due to
issues such as drug
reimbursement, patient
self-injection, optimal
oral anticoagulation,
and availability of
resources.*

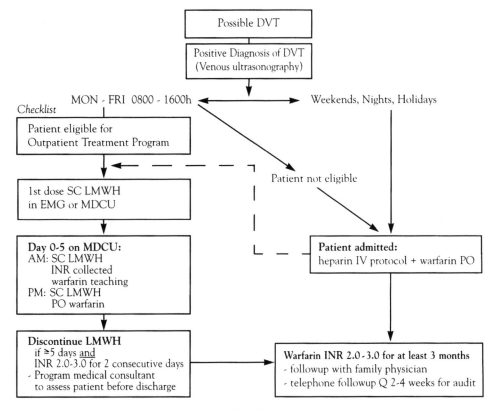

PHASE TWO:
HOME CARE
(Implementation scheduled for Fall 1997)

- Positive diagnosis of DVT (Venous ultrasonography)
- Screening / Enrollment
- Home Care & Patient Self-Injection

Figure 33.4 *Overview of phase one and two.*

- At 0800h: go to the hospital laboratory for an INR blood test, then go directly to the Medical Day Care Unit for the first daily, nurse-administered sc injection (enoxaparin 1 mg/kg).
- At 1700h: go to the Medical Day Care Unit for the second daily, nurse-administered sc injection (enoxaparin 1 mg/kg) and the daily oral warfarin dose (co-prescribed by the clinical pharmacist).

The LMWH may be discontinued after 5 days, once a therapeutic INR of 2.0–3.0 has been achieved with warfarin for two consecutive days.[1–10,30–32] The patient is then referred to his/her family physician who will assume responsibility for the chronic warfarin dosing.

Questions to consider before starting

A wise person once said that '*failing to plan is planning to fail*'! Therefore, it is important to consider the following questions when establishing an out-patient DVT treatment program at your site.

STATISTICS

Your medical records department may be able to provide these initial statistics.

1 How many patients were hospitalized per year with an admitting diagnosis of DVT?
- Only include patients with a primary diagnosis of DVT (i.e. their reason for admission was DVT).[19]
- Do not include patients with a secondary diagnosis of DVT (i.e. they developed a DVT as a complication of hospitalization, but were actually admitted for another medical condition such as pneumonia or total hip replacement).[19] DVT prophylaxis is the key for this patient population.[20,21]
2 What is the duration of hospitalization for these patients?
- Obtain the mean, median, and range for their length of stay (in days).
3 What are the patient demographics such as age, gender, history of DVT or PE, progression to PE, mortality rate and cause of death?
- Try to obtain as much information from your medical records department to save time. The basic required information is age, gender, mortality rate, and cause of death.
- For the patients' ages, obtain the mean, median, and range.
4 How many patients could potentially be treated on an out-patient basis?
- Use 40 per cent of the total number of primary diagnosis DVT patients as a guideline.[9,30] For example, 100 patients admitted per year, therefore 40 patients could be potentially treated on an out-patient basis.
5 What is the estimated number of hospital days avoided per year?
- For example, 400 hospital days per year (a mean or median of 8 days/DVT admission) × (50 DVT admissions/year)

RESOURCES

Using your existing resources and starting slowly means that an out-patient DVT treatment program could be established at most sites. Consider the five models described previously. Which model is best for your site?

1 Who will be the core group of clinicians that will assume ownership? What is their availability, defined roles, and responsibilities? When will patients be recruited?
- It is possible to have a core group of only two people (e.g. one physician and one clinical pharmacist), but someone must take ownership of the program. Continuity of care through case management is mandatory for a safe and effective out-patient DVT treatment program.[10,30]
- Design your new program around the core clinicians' availability, which may mean restricting the number of patients enrolled per week and restricting the recruitment hours. For example, if the hematologist and clinical pharmacist are only available 0800–1600h, Monday to Friday, then initially restrict patient enrollment to this time period only.
- Present this information to your site's administrators together with the DVT admission statistics. (If there is a desire to increase the recruitment to include all 40 per cent of your uncomplicated DVT patients and avoid 5–10 days of hospitalization per patient, then increased staffing may be required.)
2 Could an existing out-patient (ambulatory care) program be expanded to include out-patient DVT treatment?
- An anticoagulation clinic or thromboembolic service?[29]
- A medical day care unit or ambulatory care clinic?
- Also, a home parenteral (iv) antibiotic program?
3 Could the program be coordinated in the emergency department?
- For continuity of care, there needs to be one consistent person (e.g. a clinical pharmacist or a program nurse).[10,30]
4 Are home care nurses readily available?
- If so, try to organize the first home visit within 24 hours. Depending on the patient's degree of cooperation, home care nurses could teach the self-injection technique in the patient's home, or return once to twice daily to administer the sc doses.

5 Are there any protocols available to use as a template?
- Save time and avoid re-inventing the wheel by learning from other sites that have established a similar program.[10,30–32] The Burnaby Hospital Outpatient DVT Treatment Resource Guide may be useful as a starting point with pre-printed doctors' orders, letters for the patient, family physician, etc.[31]

6 How will the cost of the LMWH be reimbursed?
- Investigate all the alternatives available for your site, such as: (a) third-party reimbursement for the patient after the prescription has been filled at a local pharmacy; (b) LMWH cost incorporated into your site's annual drug budget; or (c) LMWH cost incorporated into an ambulatory care program's annual drug budget (which may be separate from your site's total annual drug budget).

7 Who will provide the warfarin dosing for these patients?
- It is best to have a trained person or group of clinicians responsible for the warfarin dosing.
- This tip is frequently overlooked and has significant consequences such as prolonged, subtherapeutic warfarin dosing, resulting in extended LMWH use greater than 5 days, and a higher risk of PE.
- A warfarin nomogram is highly recommended.[27,28]

8 What are some common mistakes?
- No continuity of care. There may be a higher risk of medication non-compliance, subtherapeutic warfarin dosing and, therefore, a higher risk of fatal PE.
- No time to build up to the 40 per cent of uncomplicated DVT patients. Instead of starting slowly (e.g. a maximum of two patients per week), testing the new program and measuring the impact on workload, some sites may become ambitious and quickly overwhelmed by accepting 5–10 patients in the first week with no additional staffing or resources.

STEP-BY-STEP PROGRAM INSTRUCTIONS

Please refer to the Burnaby Hospital Outpatient DVT Treatment Resource Guide for this section.[31] Step-by-step instructions are shown in Fig. 33.5.

It may require 1–1.5 hours *at bedside* to screen, enroll, counsel, coordinate the care plan with the physician, initiate a patient file, and activate the doctors' orders for each patient in the Outpatient DVT Treatment Program. Thereafter, daily follow-up care is minimal (approximately 10 minutes per visit).

Step 1: Screening and enrollment

- Patients may be screened by reviewing the daily results of venous ultrasonography (Doppler ultrasound) or invasive contrast venography (venogram); or by direct referrals from a physician, nurse, or pharmacist. At Burnaby Hospital, the emergency physicians initially contacted the clinical pharmacist to screen all patients with a positive diagnosis of DVT.
- An inclusion/exclusion checklist (Fig. 33.6) may be useful to determine which patients are suitable. Contraindicatons need to be considered on an individual basis (e.g. patients with recurrent DVT, or stable, submassive PE could be eligible).
- Enrollment must be confirmed with the most responsible physician.
- Standardized doctors' orders (Fig. 33.7), a warfarin dosing nomogram (Fig. 33.8) and a nursing documentation flow chart (Fig. 33.9) are convenient and will facilitate standardized patient care.
- Progress notes in the patient's medical chart are a medical–legal necessity and an effective method of communication.

Step 2: Patient counseling

- Teaching pamphlets may be given to the patient, but it is recommended that a health care team member review the literature with the patient and family members to optimize compliance and to address any concerns.
- Often the patients need to be reassured that their diagnosis of DVT is a serious condition but may be treated on an out-patient basis, safely and effectively. It is important to discuss DVT, the risk of PE, respiratory failure, signs and symptoms of PE.
- Counseling for warfarin, risk of hemorrhage, signs and symptoms of hemorrhage and INR monitoring may all be reinforced with a warfarin calendar and an anticoagulation pamphlet (Fig. 33.10). At Burnaby Hospital, we encourage our patients to *police* their INR results, by encouraging them to record their INR results. The patients are counselled to ask their physicians why their INR results are not between 2.0 and 3.0, if this happens while on warfarin therapy.
- It is essential to review the overall care plan with the patient and to answer all their questions (i.e. twice daily visits for 5 days, anticoagulation for at least 3 months, and morning laboratory work). If possible, reviewing the information with a family member may ensure compliance. The patient may need a pager number to call if there are any problems. At Burnaby Hospital, our patients have access to the clinical pharmacist's pager number.

Step-by-Step Program Instructions

This two-page document is a guideline with step-by-step instructions, from screening to discharge follow-up. It is completed by the clinical pharmacist and program nurse for each enrolled patient.

Screening And Enrollment (Monday-Friday, 0800-1600H)
(Check & Initial each box when completed)

1. Screen for patients daily: Doppler reports, EMG, and MD referral. ☐

2. Enter patient's information into the screening log. ☐

3. Complete Inclusion/Exclusion Checklist. ☐

4. Speak with the patient to determine if they are capable of entering the program. (i.e. transportation to hospital). If the patient is admitted in hospital, consult the ward staff. ☐

5. Notify Dr. Sparling and Wendy Leong. ☐

6. Ensure that the patient is admitted to 3B MDU (Medical Day Care Unit), and that the booking form is completed. If the EMG nurse is giving the first dose of Enoxaparin, then the patient can be admitted to 3B MDU for the next visit. If this is not feasible (i.e. 3B nurses to give first dose), then the patient needs to be taken to Admitting, paper work completed and forwarded to 3B. ☐

7. Enter the patient's weight on the preprinted outpatient DVT orders for medication dosage. Sign preprinted orders per Dr. Sparling, and yourself. Send the yellow copy to Pharmacy. ☐

8. Ensure the patient's blood work is completed. Make a photocopy of the orders for the Lab for five days (CBC/INR). Verify with the Lab the patient's prearranged visit times for outpatient blood work, and tests on each visit. ☐

9. Discuss the morning and evening dosing times with the patient. Give the teaching pamphlet on anticoagulation and introductory letter to the patient to reinforce the program expectations. ☐

10. Initiate baseline teaching. Review signs and symptoms of bleeding and pulmonary embolism. ☐

11. Make a note in the Progress Notes of the patient's chart. ☐

12. Contact the pharmacist for anticoagulation teaching. Diary will be given to the patient. ☐

(Page 1 of 2)

Step-by-Step Program Instructions

Screening And Enrollment (Monday-Friday, 0800-1600H)

(Check & Initial each box when completed)

13. Send e-mail to notify that a new patient is in the
outpatient DVT program (Lab, 3B Nursing, Pharmacy, Medicine)   ☐

14. Send 3 discharge letters to the ward with the patient. Write on
order to "Please call the Program Nurse or W. Leong prior to discharge."   ☐

15. Start a patient file for the program office (i.e. follow-up sheet), while the
patient is being treated on 3B MDCU. The Program Nurse will complete
the telephone follow-up forms, (i.e. verify phone and work numbers,
preferred time for us to call the patient, and if the patient consents to
be called at work).   ☐

DAILY FOLLOW-UP

1. Check the patient's chart daily, for any possible problems or
complications. Contact Wendy Leong or Dr. Sparling if necessary.   ☐

2. If dosing times coincide with schedule availability, try to meet with
the patient for an assessment.   ☐

3. Be available by pager Monday to Friday, from 0800-1600H, if
the 3B staff have any problems or concerns regarding the program.   ☐

DAY OF DISCHARGE

1. Dr. Sparling or designate will complete and sign the 3 letters to:
(1) the patient's family physician; (2) to the external (private) lab
and (3) the patient's discharge letter. These 3 letters will be given
to the patient prior to discharge. The patient will give the family
physician a letter at his first follow-up visit; and a letter to the lab
where the blood work will be collected.   ☐

2. Remind the patient that we will be calling on a weekly basis, and
write the date of the first telephone follow-up on the program
office's calendar.   ☐

(Page 2 of 2)

Figure 33.5 *Step-by-step program instructions.*

Inclusion & Exclusion Checklist

10

●●●●●
RESOURCE
MANUAL

The purpose of this Inclusion & Exclusion Checklist is to assist in the appropriate selection of patients for outpatient treatment, after initial diagnosis of DVT. The completed form is filed permanently in the patient's medical record.

INCLUSION/EXCLUSION CHECKLIST

(Nurse or Pharmacist may complete, but checklist must be verified and co-signed by a physician)

Inclusion Criteria	YES	NO
1. Positive diagnosis of DVT, confirmed by Doppler Ultrasound	☐	☐
2. No obvious signs or symptoms of pulmonary embolism (PE)	☐	☐

Relative Contraindications

	YES	NO
1. History of previous DVT and/or PE	☐	☐
2. History of CVA known to be hemorrhagic	☐	☐
3. Recent bleeding (e.g. PUD, hematuria)	☐	☐
4. Any bleeding and/or hematological disorder (*e.g. coagulopathy, Hb < 8.0, thrombocytopenia*)	☐	☐
5. Recent surgery within 2 weeks (i.e. potential for bleed)	☐	☐
6. Recent trauma (less than 2 weeks ago, potential for bleed)	☐	☐
7. Severe uncontrolled hypertension: SBP $\geq$ 180 or DBP $\geq$ 110	☐	☐
8. Renal failure (SCr > 200 umol/L) and/or hepatic failure	☐	☐
9. Potential for medication non-compliance (*e.g. mental confusion, inability to care for self, poor vision*)	☐	☐
10. Patient unable to complete 5 day course of SC injections as an outpatient (i.e. unable to return to hospital twice daily)	☐	☐

Dr. T. Sparling (Hematology, pager 650-2119) and Dr. W. Leong (Pharmacy, pager 680-4355) will be consulted for every patient to confirm eligibility. "Relative" contraindications means that the risks will be weighed against the benefits for every patient.

_____ _____ _____
Physician's Signature   Printed Name   Date
PHA - 101.96

Figure 33.6 *Inclusion and exclusion checklist.*

Standardized Doctor's Orders

The preprinted doctor's orders were developed to streamline patient care for the 5-day program.

LMWH
low molecular weight heparin

Warfarin
dosing protocol

Action Taken	Date & Time	List Directives:

		OUTPATIENT DVT TREATMENT PROGRAM
		(Enrolment Monday to Friday, 0800-1600h only)
		
		1. Diagnosis - Deep Vein Thrombosis (DVT)
		
		    1.1 Most Responsible Physician: Dr. T. Sparling
		    1.2 Family Physician: Dr. _____
		    1.3 Old chart to unit if available
		
		    1.4 Location of DVT (confirmed by Doppler ultrasound):
		
		         ☐ Proximal ☐ Left ☐ Unilateral
		         ☐ Distal ☐ Right ☐ Bilateral
		
		2. Screen for eligibility by completing the Outpatient DVT Treatment Program Checklist (PHA-101.96).
		
		    2.1 Contact Dr. T. Sparling, Hematology (pager 650-2119) and Dr. W. Leong (pager 680-4355) to confirm eligibility.
		
		    2.2 If patient is ineligible for the Outpatient DVT Treatment Program, admit under Family Physician and start Heparin IV Protocol (with warfarin).
		
		3. Baseline laboratory data:
		
		    3.1 CBC, INR, PTT
		    3.2 Electrolytes, blood glucose, SCr, BUN
		    3.3 AST, ALT, Alk phosph, TBil
		
		4. Daily CBC and INR every morning.
		
		5. Give enoxaparin SC 1st dose STAT, then
		
		    _____ (1 mg/kg) SC BID into abdomen X 5 days on 3BMDU
		
		    On day #5, reassess. Continue enoxaparin until warfarin INR 2-3 for 2 consecutive days.
		
		6. Give first dose of warfarin PO on day #1 of enoxaparin. Daily warfarin PO doses, as per pharmacy dosing service. Warfarin to be administered daily on 3BMDU after 1800h. Goal: INR 2-3 for 3 months.
		
		Physician's Signature: Printed Name: Date:
		
		_____ _____ _____

P&T Approval **APR 1996** **Revised:** **MAR 1996** **Contact:** **Hematology** **Pharmacy**		
PHA-102.96		White Copy for Chart, Yellow Copy for Pharmacy

Figure 33.7 *Standardized doctor's orders.*

Warfarin Dosing Protocol

This warfarin nomogram is used only as a guideline with the goal of achieving a therapeutic INR of 2.0 - 3.0 within 3-4 days.

Clinical judgement is required. For example, dosage reduction in elderly, low body weight (e.g. 40 kg) and warfarin sensitivity.

A Warfarin Dosing Service Starter Kit is available for purchase.

WARFARIN DOSING SERVICE
Burnaby Hospital

Action Taken	Warfarin Dosing Protocol Directives:
Date: _____ Time: _____ NURSING PLEASE CLARIFY	1. Discontinue all previous warfarin orders. 2. Baseline laboratory data: INR, CBC, Platelets. 3. Daily laboratory monitoring: INR, CBC. 4. No NSAIDs or ASA (unless specifically ordered by physician). 5. No IM injections. 6. At any sign of hemorrhage and/or INR > 6, call physician STAT. 7. Nursing: Please check - Is patient currently on heparin IV? ☐ Yes ☐ No 8. Nursing: Please check - Was patient taking warfarin on admission? ☐ Yes ☐ No If Yes, indicate dose: _____

WARFARIN THERAPY

PHYSICIAN PLEASE CLARIFY

9. Physician: Please check one of the following:

Indication for therapy	Target INR
___ Thromboembolism	2.0 - 3.0
___ Mechanical valve replacement	2.5 - 3.5
___ Other indication _____	_____

PHARMACY PLEASE CLARIFY

10. Start Warfarin Dosing Protocol. Daily Warfarin dosing to be adjusted and co-written by pharmacy based on the following nomogram (modifications may be necessary for patient-specific dosing titration):

	INR	WARFARIN DOSE (mg)
DAY 1	< 1.3	10
	1.3 - 1.5	5
	> 1.5	0
DAY 2	< 1.3	10
	1.3 - 1.5	5
	> 1.5	0
DAY 3	< 1.6	10
	1.6 - 1.8	7.5
	1.81 - 2.1	5
	2.11 - 2.4	2.5
	2.41 - 2.7	1.0
	> 2.7	0
DAY 4+	< 1.8	10
	1.8 - 2.1	7.5
	2.11 - 2.4	5
	2.41 - 2.5	2.5
	2.51 - 2.7	1.0
	> 2.7	0

11. Warfarin drug interactions: documentation by pharmacy.
12. Warfarin patient teaching: prior to discharge by pharmacy.

Physician's Signature and Code: _____

PHA-73-96	P&T Approval December 1994 - Revised May 1996	Yellow Copy - Pharmacy

Figure 33.8 *Warfarin dosing protocol.*

Nursing Documentation

15

•••••
RESOURCE
MANUAL

This patient log is used daily to chart dosage administration; assessment of DVT, PE and hemorrhage.

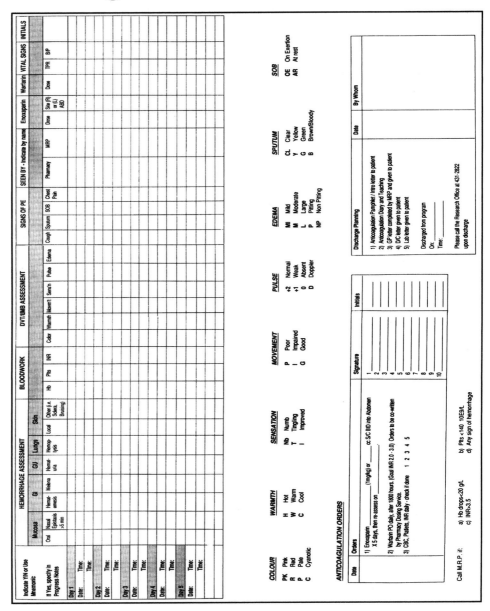

Figure 33.9 *Nursing documentation.*

Patient Counselling

Printed material provided by The Thrombosis Interest Group is distributed to the patient with one-on-one medication counselling by the clinical pharmacist or program nurse.

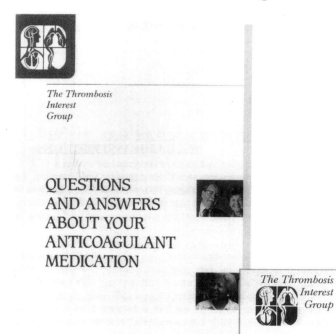

The Thrombosis
Interest
Group

QUESTIONS AND ANSWERS ABOUT YOUR ANTICOAGULANT MEDICATION

The Thrombosis
Interest
Group

DOSAGE CALENDAR

You are being treated with the anticoagulant crystalline warfarin sodium.

Circle appropriate tablet.

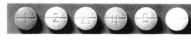

pink   lavender   green   blue   peach   white

Figure 33.10 *Patient counseling.*

Step 3: Warfarin dosing service

- A standardized warfarin dosing nomogram is recommended (Fig. 33.8).
- Training in warfarin dosing will ensure optimal, rapid therapeutic dosing.
- It is best to have a consistent person or trained group of clinicians to be responsible for the warfarin dosing, to ensure continuity of care (e.g. warfarin dosing service, anticoagulation clinic, thromboembolic service).[27]
- Clinical pharmacists may co-prescribe the daily warfarin orders and resolve any major warfarin drug interactions.
- A patient monitoring form is suggested for continuity of care.

Step 4: Discharge planning and counseling

- The last day of the out-patient DVT treatment program may be as important as the first day of the program, to maintain therapeutic anticoagulation.
- The patient must have clear written instructions for the next INR, the next warfarin dosage, and a follow-up appointment with his/her family physician (Fig. 33.11).
- A discharge letter for the family physician is often appreciated (Fig. 33.12).
- For data collection purposes only, we ask the patients to forward a letter to their local laboratory requesting that the INR results be faxed to the program office (Fig. 33.13).
- The most responsible physician needs to be contacted to confirm the discharge plan. Often a telephone call is sufficient. Some physicians prefer to see the patient on the last day of LMWH therapy.

Step 5: Post-discharge follow-up

- A telephone follow-up 3 months post-discharge may be useful in evaluating the out-patient DVT treatment program (Fig. 33.14). For a newly established program, it is recommended that the first ten patients be monitored for 3 months for quality assurance.
- The patient's local laboratory will send the INR results to your site upon request (Fig. 33.13). At Burnaby Hospital, we have not participated in the warfarin dosing after the patient has been discharged from the program, because there was no anticoagulation clinic available at the time of this publication. The INR results are collected for quality assurance. For example, if an out-patient DVT treatment patient developed PE within 3 months, we would check for subtherapeutic warfarin dosing first.

Step 6: Core group meetings

- The core group of clinicians who are most responsible for the out-patient program should meet on a regular basis to review any problems or concerns.
- Continuous quality improvement through program evaluation will ensure optimal patient care.

PROGRAM EVALUATION

The Burnaby Hospital Outpatient DVT Treatment Program won the 1996 Best Overall Acute Care Project Award for the Simon Fraser Health Region in British Columbia, Canada. Formal program evaluation is in progress but the interim evaluation has demonstrated overwhelming success. For example, we safely and effectively treated seven patients in a 2-week period, avoiding 35–70 hospital days or \$24 500–\$49 000; with no major bleeding and no recurrence of thromboembolism.

There is a demand to expand the program to 24 hours per day, 7 days per week, but further funding is required. Phase two with home care nursing visits had not been implemented owing to insufficient staffing at the time of this publication. The section below highlights the perspectives of the patient, the physician, the nurse, and the pharmacist.

What is the patient's point of view?

'Convenient', 'I can still go to work', 'Better for my kids', 'Thanks for all the TLC!', 'That's it?', 'Are you sure that I can go home?'

There was a 68-year-old woman with recurrent DVT (due to malignancy) who insisted on the out-patient program, refusing to be admitted. She had been hospitalized for 8 days 1 year ago and preferred to stay home. She had memories of the numerous blood tests and hematomas at the iv site during her last hospitalization. Warfarin had mistakenly been discontinued at 3 months instead of chronic therapy.

For the out-patient program, she was counselled by the pharmacist and given an introductory letter with full instructions for twice-daily visits, teaching pamphlets on DVT, and anticoagulation. The twice-daily visits to the Medical Day Care Unit were convenient for her family, as the total time per visit was only 15–20 minutes with no need to go to the Admitting Department.

On day 5, after two consecutive therapeutic INR results, the LMWH was discontinued. She was counselled by the pharmacist, given written instructions to see her family doctor the following day, and asked to deliver one discharge letter to her family doctor and one letter to her local laboratory. We informed her that our

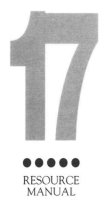

Discharge Letter To The Patient

This letter is discussed with the patient on the last day of the program (i.e. 2 day overlap of LMWH and therapeutic warfarin).

INFORMATION FOR THE PATIENT

Date:

Dear Patient:

RE: **DISCHARGE INSTRUCTIONS**

Thank you for your cooperation with the outpatient DVT program. For the past 5 days, you have been receiving injections of a blood thinner called enoxaparin, and an oral blood thinner called warfarin (Coumadin). For the next three months, it will be necessary for you to continue taking warfarin (Coumadin) to prevent the clot in your leg from getting larger or progressing to the lung.

Please see your family doctor on _____. It will be necessary to have blood tests done regularly for follow-up with your family doctor. In your medication calendar for warfarin, please record your dose of warfarin daily and any INR results that you get back from the lab. Please feel free to ask your doctor for your INR result, so that you can record it in the calendar. Remember that the target for the INR is between 2.0-3.0, which means that the blood is thin enough to prevent clotting, but not too "thin" as to increase your risk of bleeding.

Please remember that if you have any signs or symptoms of bleeding, such as vomiting blood, blood in the urine, black stool, or excessive bruising, you need to seek medical assistance immediately by going to the emergency department, by calling Dr. Sparling, or your family physician . We will be contacting you from the program office on a weekly basis to monitor your progress by telephone.

If you have any questions or concerns, please feel free to contact your family doctor, the program nurses at 431-2875, or Dr. Sparling at 650-2119.

Sincerely,

Program Nurse, on behalf of
Dr. T. Sparling, Hematology
Dr. W. Leong, Pharmacy

Figure 33.11 *Discharge letter to the patient.*

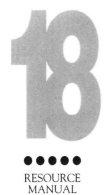

Discharge Letter to the Family Physician

This letter is completed and forwarded to the patient's family physician for follow-up care and warfarin dosing.

INFORMATION FOR FAMILY PHYSICIAN

Date:

Dear Dr.

Patient:

RE: <u>**OUT PATIENT DVT TREATMENT PROGRAM**</u>

This patient was admitted to Burnaby Hospital on _____ for a diagnosis of DVT. After careful screening and assessment, your patient was enrolled in the Outpatient DVT Treatment Program, which included:

1.   Enoxaparin (low molecular weight heparin) _____ mg SC BID for 5 days.
2.   Warfarin for _____ days, titrated to a therapeutic INR of 2.0-3.0
        by the Pharmacy Dosing Service.
3.   Last INR was drawn on _____.
        The last dose of warfarin was _____mg.

This patient has now been referred back to your care and therefore, we recommend the following:

1.   Warfarin therapy for 3 months, titrated to a therapeutic INR of 2.0-3.0.
2.   INR weekly for _____ weeks, then monthly.
3.   CBC weekly for _____ weeks, then monthly.

Thank you for allowing us to assist in the care of your patient. We are excited that the Burnaby Hospital Outpatient DVT Treatment has provided optimal patient care without the usual hospitalization of 5 to 10 days.

If there are any questions or concerns, please do not hesitate to contact Dr._____ at pager _____, or the program office at 431-2875.

Sincerely,

Program Nurse, on behalf of
Dr. T. Sparling, Hematology
Dr. W. Leong, Pharmacy

Figure 33.12 *Discharge letter to the family physician.*

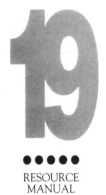

19

●●●●●
RESOURCE
MANUAL

The patient is asked to forward this letter to the outpatient laboratory that will be collecting their INRs (i.e. closest to the patient's home or workplace). INR results are collected for data analysis only, as the family physician will be primarily responsible for warfarin dosing.

Outpatient Laboratory Letter

INFORMATION FOR LAB STAFF

Date:

Patient:

RE: **OUTPATIENT DVT TREATMENT PROGRAM**

Please be advised that this patient was treated at Burnaby Hospital and discharged from our outpatient DVT treatment program on _____ . The last dose of warfarin was _____ mg. The last INR result was _____ . This patient will require continued INR monitoring.

The patient's family physician, Dr._____ , will be responsible for supervising all warfarin dosage adjustment, but we will continue to follow this patient for the duration of their treatment. For the purpose of data collection, we request that a copy of all bloodwork be faxed to us at 431-4770, attention W. Leong.

If there are any questions or concerns, please contact our program office at 431-2875 or page me at 680-4355.

Sincerely,

Dr. W. Leong,
Clinical Pharmacy Specialist

Figure 33.13 *Out-patient laboratory letter.*

program nurse would be telephoning for the next 3 months for data collection.

What is the physician's point of view?

'Great idea!', 'How is this possible?', 'LMWHs are that good?', 'Let's do it!'

The multidisciplinary Anticoagulation Working Group (AWG, mentioned previously) has earned a solid, reliable reputation in patient care since 1994. This new program was promoted as another AWG patient care project supported by the hospital's Pharmacy and Therapeutics Committee, and the Medical Advisory Committee.

The emergency physicians wholeheartedly supported the program and would like to see further progress such as: (1) enrollment 24 hours per day, 7 days per week; and (2) during evenings when venous ultrasonography is not available, the option of giving one dose of LMWH and having the patient return the next morning for follow-up, instead of admitting the patient overnight. At the time of this publication, these improvements were not possible due to insufficient resources at Burnaby Hospital.

Our specialists in hematology, internal medicine, and respirology have enrolled DVT and submassive PE patients in the program with no problems (enoxaparin 1 mg/kg sc twice daily). All out-patient DVT patients are discussed with our hematologist who is the program medical consultant. The family physicians were informed of the patient's care plan and were very supportive. Our hematologist also gave an educational session to the physician group prior to the program's initiation.

What is the nurse's point of view?

'Fantastic', 'What will they think of next?', 'Is it safe?', 'Can we send him home now please?'

Nurses in the emergency department have been enthusiastic, although there was some initial skepticism due to the significant change from in-patient management. There has been a noticeable decrease in bedside care with LMWH compared to establishing an iv access for a continuous infusion of UH and PTTs every 6 hours. No hospitalization has meant no chance of an overnight stay in the emergency department when the hospital has been full. Educational in-services by the clinical pharmacist were provided before the program was started.

Our program runs smoothly with the Medical Day Care Unit nurses and with a clinical pharmacist responsible for daily warfarin co-prescribing and patient counseling. Our program nurse played an important role in developing the documentation (e.g. a nursing documentation flow chart, Fig. 33.9), promoting the program,

recruiting patients, and collecting follow-up data. For clarification, our program nurse worked part-time in the emergency department, where she has been very active in patient enrollment, and part-time in research. Her availability for the out-patient DVT treatment program varied from 1–2 days per week.

What is the clinical pharmacist's point of view?

'Good timing with bed shortages becoming more frequent', 'Better for the patients'

There is ample opportunity for the clinical pharmacist to become involved in an out-patient DVT treatment program, from patient counseling to comprehensive case management. The goal is to optimize drug therapy and improve patient outcomes (i.e. pharmaceutical care).

At Burnaby Hospital, we restructured our department with no additional staffing, from one pharmacist on the wards per day in 1993, to six clinical pharmacists per day in 1995. A commitment to patient care has been the driving force. The Outpatient DVT Treatment Program was dependent on the clinical pharmacists at our hospital, from screening to discharge counseling (i.e. case management).[8,30]

What is the laboratory's point of view?

A laboratory technician and a pathologist have participated on the AWG projects since 1994. With LMWH, there is a significant decrease in PTTs required compared to iv UH. With the warfarin dosing service, our laboratory is aware that the INRs are ordered and followed appropriately, 7 days a week, by the clinical pharmacists. If there are any concerns with supratherapeutic INR results, a clinical pharmacist may be contacted to follow-up.

FUTURE DIRECTIONS

LMWH will replace iv UH for most indications.[11] In the future, out-patient treatment with LMWH will likely include:

- submassive, stable PE;[33,34]
- stable cardiac patients waiting for angioplasty or coronary artery bypass grafting;
- prolonged DVT prophylaxis after orthopedic surgery with early hospital discharge;
- patients with a contraindication or allergy to warfarin.

Prevention of thromboembolism must not be an option and must be incorporated into routine care, as per ACCP guidelines.[20] Other future directions in cardio-

23

●●●●●

RESOURCE
MANUAL

*For purposes of
continuous quality
improvement, data is
collected on every patient
for 3 months after
discharge from the
Outpatient DVT
Treatment Program.*

Data Collection Forms

Name: _____ **Lab results from:** _____

Phone Number: _____

Work Number: _____ **Ok to contact at work: Y/N** _____

Week # 1 Date: _____ | **Week # 2 Date:** _____

Bleeding:

Gums	Y/N	_____
GI	Y/N	_____
GU	Y/N	_____
Skin	Y/N	_____

Signs and Symptoms of P.E.:

Cough   Y/N _____
SOB   Y/N _____
Chest Pain   Y/N _____
Recurrence of
DVT symptoms Y/N _____
Last INR: _____
Next INR due: _____
Present dose of
Warfarin :   _____
Comments: _____
                 _____

Bleeding:

Gums   Y/N _____
GI   Y/N _____
GU   Y/N _____
Skin   Y/N _____

Signs and Symptoms of P.E.:

Cough   Y/N _____
SOB   Y/N _____
Chest Pain   Y/N _____
Recurrence of
DVT symptoms Y/N _____
Last INR: _____
Next INR due: _____
Present dose of
Warfarin :   _____
Comments: _____

Week # 3 Date: _____

Bleeding:

Gums   Y/N _____
GI   Y/N _____
GU   Y/N _____
Skin   Y/N _____

Signs and Symptoms of P.E.:

Cough   Y/N _____
SOB   Y/N _____
Chest Pain   Y/N _____
Recurrence of
DVT symptoms Y/N _____
Last INR: _____
Next INR due: _____
Present dose of
Warfarin :   _____
Comments: _____

Week # 4 Date: _____

Bleeding:

Gums   Y/N _____
GI   Y/N _____
GU   Y/N _____
Skin   Y/N _____

Signs and Symptoms of P.E.:

Cough   Y/N _____
SOB   Y/N _____
Chest Pain   Y/N _____
Recurrence of
DVT symptoms Y/N _____
Last INR: _____
Next INR due: _____
Present dose of
Warfarin :   _____
Comments: _____

(Page 1 of 2)

Data Collection Forms

Name: _____   Lab results from: _____

Phone Number: _____

Work Number: _____   Ok to contact at work: Y/N _____

Month 2 Date: _____

Bleeding:

Gums   Y/N _____

GI   Y/N _____

GU   Y/N _____

Skin   Y/N _____

Signs and Symptoms of P.E.:

Cough   Y/N _____

SOB   Y/N _____

Chest Pain   Y/N _____

Recurrence of

DVT symptoms Y/N _____

Last INR: _____

Next INR due: _____

Present dose of

Warfarin :   _____

Comments: _____

              _____

Month 3 Date: _____

Bleeding:

Gums   Y/N _____

GI   Y/N _____

GU   Y/N _____

Skin   Y/N _____

Signs and Symptoms of P.E.:

Cough   Y/N _____

SOB   Y/N _____

Chest Pain   Y/N _____

Recurrence of

DVT symptoms Y/N _____

Last INR: _____

Next INR due: _____

Present dose of

Warfarin :   _____

Comments: _____

              _____

Month 4 Date: _____

Bleeding:

Gums   Y/N _____

GI   Y/N _____

GU   Y/N _____

Skin   Y/N _____

Signs and Symptoms of P.E.:

Cough   Y/N _____

SOB   Y/N _____

Chest Pain   Y/N _____

Recurrence of

DVT symptoms Y/N _____

Last INR: _____

Next INR due: _____

Present dose of

Warfarin :   _____

Comments: _____

              _____

Overall Satisfaction With the Program: _____

_____

_____

_____

_____

_____

_____

_____

_____

_____

_____

_____

_____

(Page 2 of 2)

Figure 33.14 *Data collection forms.*

vascular management will likely include increased point-of-care testing for INR results with hand-held devices, similar to glucometers. More anticoagulation clinics will provide optimal patient care with minimal resources and facilitate further out-patient treatment.[29]

The development of a second-generation warfarin would be ideal. This oral agent would have a rapid onset of less than 1 hour, a fixed dosage without the need for INR monitoring, a low risk of hemorrhage, and no drug interactions. This ideal agent could potentially replace LMWH therapy!

CONCLUSION

The second generation of LMWH therapy may replace unfractionated iv heparin for most indications.[11] LMWH therapy has revolutionized the management of DVT from the traditional 5–10 days of in-patient care to out-patient management.[1–10,23,30–32] The literature has strongly supported the treatment of DVT with LMWH.[1–10,30–32] Potentially 40 per cent of all uncomplicated DVTs could be treated on an out-patient basis, which extrapolates to 3600 patients per year in Canada. The challenge for the health care team is to make out-patient treatment a standard practice in DVT.

SUMMARY

- Forty per cent of all uncomplicated deep vein thrombosis (DVT) patients may be treated safely and effectively on an out-patient basis using low-molecular-weight heparin (LMWH; the second generation of heparin therapy), which may be given as a fixed-dose, subcutaneous regimen with no prothrombin time monitoring required.
- Traditionally, these patients were hospitalized for 5–10 days for a continous intravenous infusion of unfractionated heparin, until oral warfarin therapy had reached a therapeutic international normalized ratio (INR) for 2 consecutive days.
- The paradigm shift from in-patient management to out-patient care of 3600 DVT patients could avoid over 25 000 hospital-days per year in Canada.
- Equally important and often overlooked is the therapeutic dosing of warfarin for a minimum of 3 months. Rapid titration and maintenance of a therapeutic INR of 2.0–3.0 is essential for a successful out-patient DVT treatment program. A delay in reaching a therapeutic INR of 2.0–3.0 will result in prolonged LMWH usage.

- Depending on each site's available resources, there are five models for establishing an out-patient (ambulatory/home) DVT treatment program: (1) anticoagulation clinic or thromboembolic service; (2) medical day care unit or ambulatory care clinic; (3) emergency department fast-track area; (4) one visit and self-injection only; and (5) physician office follow-up.

ACKNOWLEDGMENTS

Special thanks are due to two key people in the Burnaby Hospital Out-patient DVT Treatment Program: Dr Terence G. Sparling, Hematology/Oncology, Director of the Burnaby Hospital Regional Cancer Center; and Liz Brown, RN, Emergency Department/Research. We thank Rhone Poulenc Rorer for a restricted financial grant. I would also like to record my appreciation to the outstanding health care team at Burnaby Hospital including the Pharmacy Department (John Hope, Director), the Emergency Department and the Medical Day Care Unit (3B).

CONTACT ADDRESS

For a copy of the 26-page Burnaby Hospital Out-patient DVT Treatment Resource Guide, please send, fax or email your request to (while supplies last): Dr Wendy A. Leong, Burnaby Hospital Pharmacy Department, 3935 Kincaid Street, Burnaby, BC, Canada V5G 2X6. Telephone: (604) 431-2875; Fax: (604) 431-4770; Email: buh.wleong@sfhr.hnet.bc.ca.

REFERENCES

1. Hull RD, Raskob GE, Pineo GF, *et al*. Subcutaneous low molecular weight heparin compared with continuous intravenous heparin in the treatment of proximal vein thrombosis. *N Engl J Med* 1992; **326**: 975–82.
2. Leizorovicz A, Simonneau G, Decousus H, *et al*. Comparison of efficacy and safety of low molecular weight heparins and unfractionated heparin in initial treatment of deep venous thrombosis: a meta-analysis. *Br Med J* 1994; **309**: 299–304.
3. Lensing A, Prins M, Davidson B, *et al*. Treatment of deep vein thrombosis with low molecular weight heparins: a meta-analysis. *Arch Intern Med* 1995; **155**: 601–7.
4. Siragusa S, Cosmi B, Piovella F, *et al*. Low molecular weight heparins and unfractionated heparin in the treatment of patients with acute venous thromboembolism: results of a meta-analysis. *Am J Med* 1996; **100**: 269–77.

♦5. Levine M, Gent M, Hirsh J, *et al*. A comparison of low molecular weight heparin administered primarily at home with unfractionated heparin administered in the hospital for proximal deep vein thrombosis. *N Engl J Med* 1996; **334**: 677–81.

♦6. Koopman M, Prandoni P, Piovella F, *et al*. Treatment of venous thrombosis with intravenous unfractionated heparin administered in the hospital as compared with subcutaneous low molecular weight heparin administered at home. *N Engl J Med* 1996; **334**: 682–7.

7. Schafer A. Low molecular weight heparin – an opportunity for home treatment of venous thrombosis. *N Engl J Med* 1996; **334**: 724–5.

8. Brown L, Leong WA and Sparling TG. Outpatient DVT treatment program. *Canadian Nurse* 1996; **92**(10): 18.

9. Hull RD, Raskob GE, Rosenbloom D, *et al*. Treatment of proximal vein thrombosis with subcutaneous low molecular weight heparin versus intravenous heparin. *Arch Intern Med* 1997; **157**: 289–94.

10. Dedden P, Chang B, Nagel D. Pharmacy-managed program for home treatment of deep vein thrombosis with enoxaparin. *Am J Health Syst Pharm* 1997; **54**: 1968–72.

○11. Leong W, Fareed J. Unfractionated iv heparin may be replaced by low molecular weight heparin for most indications. *Int Angiol* 1997: **16**(suppl 1–3): 92.

12. Fareed J, Hoppensteadt D, Jeske W, *et al*. Low molecular weight heparins: a developmental perspective. *Exp Opin Invest Drugs* 1997; **6**: 705–33.

13. Cotran RS, Kumar V and Robbins SL. Fluid and hemodynamic derangements. In: Cotran RS, Kumar V and Robbins SL, eds *Robbins pathologic basis of disease*, 4th edn. Philadelphia: WB Saunders Co, 1989: 99–101.

○14. Ginsberg JS. Management of venous thromboembolism. *N Engl J Med* 1996; **335**: 1816–28.

15. Haeger K. Problems of acute deep vein thrombosis. The interpretation of signs or symptoms. *Angiology* 1969; **20**: 219–23.

16. Cranley JJ, Canos AJ, Sull WJ. The diagnosis of deep vein thrombosis: fallibility of clinical symptoms and signs. *Arch Surg* 1976; **111**: 34–6.

17. Haines ST, Bussey HI. Diagnosis of deep vein thrombosis. *Am J Health Syst Pharm* 1997; **54**: 66–74.

18. Morrell MT, Dunnill MS. The post-mortem incidence of pulmonary embolism in a hospital population. *Br J Surg* 1968; **55**: 347–52.

19. Leong W, Siu A, Sparling T. Evaluation of DVT and PE treatment at a primary and secondary care centre. In: Balas P, ed. *International Congress of Phlebology*, Bologna, Italy, 1996: 141–4.

20. Geerts WH, Heit JA, Clagett P, *et al*. Prevention of venous thromboembolism. *Chest* 2001; **119**: 312S–175S.

21. Leong W, Siu A, Sparling T. Evaluation of venous thromboembolism prophylaxis in high risk patients at a primary and secondary care centre. In: Balas P, ed. *International Congress of Phlebology*, Bologna, Italy, 1996: 303–7.

22. Hyers TM, Agnelli G, Hull RD, *et al*. Antithrombotic therapy for venous thromboembolic disease. *Chest* 2001; **119**: 176S–193S.

23. Hull R, Raskob G, Rosenbloom D, *et al*. Heparin for 5 days as compared with 10 days in the initial treatment of proximal venous thrombosis. *N Engl J Med* 1990; **322**: 1260–4.

24. Leong W, Sparling T. Implementation and evaluation of a standardized heparin protocol. Abstract presented at the *Canadian Society of Hospital Pharmacy Professional Practice Conference*, February 1995, Toronto, Ontario.

♦25. Warkentin T, Levine M, Hirsh J, *et al*. Heparin-induced thrombocytopenia in patients with low molecular weight heparin or unfractionated heparin. *N Engl J Med* 1995; **332**: 1330–5.

26. Green R. Treatment of heparin-induced thrombocytopenia and thrombosis. *Semin Vasc Surg* 1996; **9**: 292–5.

27. Andricevic M, Leong W. Patient-centred warfarin dosing service. Abstract presented at the *American College of Clinical Pharmacy Winter Practice and Research Forum*, February 1996, Monterrey, California.

28. Harrison L, Johnston M, Massicotte P, *et al*. Comparison of 5-mg and 10-mg loading doses in initiation of warfarin therapy. *Ann Intern Med* 1997; **126**: 133–6.

29. Ansell J, Hirsh J, Dalen J, *et al*. Managing oral anticoagulant therapy. *Chest* 2001; **119**: 22S–38S.

30. Leong W. Outpatient DVT treatment. *Hosp Pharm Practice* 1998; **6**: 1,24–31.

31. Leong W, Brown L, Sparling T. Outpatient deep vein thrombosis resource guide, February 1997, Vancouver, Canada. *Int Angiol* 1997; **16**(suppl 1–3): 83 (abstract).

32. Leong W. Burnaby Hospital. In: *Out-patient management of deep vein thrombosis, Canadian options and issues*. Toronto: Leo Laboratories Canada Inc., 1996.

33. Thery C, Simonneau G, Meyer G, *et al*. Randomized trial of subcutaneous low molecular weight heparin CY 216 (fraxiparine) compared with intravenous unfractionated heparin in the curative treatment of submassive pulmonary embolism: a dose-ranging study. *Circulation* 1992; **85**: 1380–9.

34. Simonneau G, Sors H, Charbonnier B, *et al*. A comparison of low molecular weight heparin with unfractionated heparin for acute pulmonary embolism. *N Engl J Med* 1997; **337**: 663–9.

PART 6

Medicolegal and ethical issues

34

Medicolegal and quality of care implications of consensus statements

KEVIN M McINTYRE

Consensus statements are designed to elevate the standard of care for patients and provide evidence-based guidelines for practising clinicians. Toward these important goals, consensus conferences must take several appropriate steps that include: (1) establishing objectives; (2) providing balanced and diverse views through carefully chosen participants; (3) meticulously reviewing the scientific evidence; and (4) following a consensus process that assures a comprehensive presentation of all relevant scientific information.

CONSENSUS STATEMENTS AND THE STANDARD OF CARE

In 1995, a new format was proposed by the *Journal of the American Medical Association* (JAMA) for the organization and implementation of consensus statements in the January 4, 1995, issue.[1] Emphasis was placed on a clear definition of the objective of the statement, the basis for the selection of the participants, the manner in which the evidence was reviewed and evaluated, the manner in which 'consensus' was developed, and the conclusions of the consensus conference. In the same issue of *JAMA*, Olson presented the rationale for the newly proposed format in an editorial in a clear and helpful manner and provides a useful framework within which to evaluate the quality of the consensus conference process according to the proposed new *JAMA* format.[2]

The most important responsibility of the consensus conference is to evaluate and prioritize the quality of the science in the subject areas of the conference and in so doing, lay the scientific groundwork for the 'standard of care' in these areas. This is particularly important when the conference product is likely to form the basis for the codification of clinical practice guidelines. While this product may reflect the standard of care in normative terms, application of that standard to a specific set of circumstances, as in a courtroom in a malpractice action, may be difficult since a number of other determinants enter into the equation, not the least of which being the relative strengths of the opposing expert witnesses. The primary value of practice guidelines, of course, is not their use in litigation but their use in *practice*: the extent to which they effectively elevate the quality of care is the measure of success. But, whether the work product of a consensus conference is used to improve care quality of the practitioner or as a measure of the adequacy of the defendant's care of a particular patient in a particular set of circumstances, the guidelines need to be both credible and usable. The new *JAMA* format appears to be an excellent model for use in planning a consensus conference since the key elements of credibility are elicited. 'Usability' perhaps is more a function of organization and style: it is impaired if the published guidelines are either overly specific or hopelessly general. In either case, the worth of the guidelines is diminished for both medical practitioners and litigants, be they plaintiff or defense attorneys. Ultimately, as Olson wrote in *JAMA*, 'Readers themselves must assess the quality and the validity of consensus statements as they do for all literature'.[2]

Objectives of the consensus statement

The consensus statement must define its objective clearly. While clearly expressing the immediate objective, e.g. to assist the practicing physician in proving better, safer care in the area under consideration, it is appropriate as well to underscore the important catalytic role of such conferences for the achievement of longer term objectives such as the development of perfections in the scientific data over time that may be expected to improve therapy in the future. The legal implication of such statements are also clear: all the answers are not in. Thus, there is likely room for the clinician to exercise his or her judgement with regard to a specific patient with a specific set of clinical characteristics. The guidelines then are intended to be just that – guidelines. If ideally developed and ideally packaged, these guidelines will be of the greatest use to the greatest number of practitioners in providing safe and effective therapy. As such, they will be optimal guides to the standard of care for the protection of the practitioner from committing malpractice, thus performing a legally beneficial role for the benefit of patient and practitioner alike. While guidelines to the standard of care, they are not the standard of care. It is not until the physician makes a judgment as to how a specific patient should be treated (or not treated) that the theory becomes actuality. It is the action or the inaction in a given set of circumstances that will be judged to fall within the standard of care or below the standard of care. The better the guidelines, the easier it will be for the physician to act properly in the best interests of his or her patient, and this result is clearly the most desirable from both a legal and a medical viewpoint.

Evidence has been provided to indicate that clinical guidelines may improve clinical practice when introduced in the context of rigorous evaluations.[3,4] Unfortunately, credible evaluations of the impact of clinical practice guidelines (CPGs) have to date been few and far between, a problem which we will consider below.

Participants

The critical currency of the consensus conference is credibility and the credibility of the recommendations of such a conference will depend on the degree to which legitimate differing views are presented and discussed openly. This is important not only for the purposes of comprehensive discussion, but from a legal viewpoint in that the law has recognized the opinions of 'respected' minorities, which may differ from the majority opinion. 'Consensus' should not be forced. If legitimate respected minority opinions exist, these should be put forward.

To assure that a comprehensive range of scientific and medical opinions will be presented and discussed as fully as necessary, the selection of participants is of paramount importance. There should be a balance in representation with regard to issues of content, particularly in controversial areas. There should also be balance on the issue of personality. A daunting figure on one pole of an argument should not be permitted the opportunity to intimidate a less confident presenter at the other pole.

Finally, the practice of bringing manuscripts to the conference so that publication deadlines can be met should be regulated carefully if such a policy is to be considered at all. Clearly all such manuscripts should be subject to prior review and open discussion and debate at the time of the conference.

Other ingredients that support credibility include the 'stature, expertise and intellectual integrity of the participants' and identification of sponsors and sources of financial support, as Olson points out.[2]

Evidence

When prior consensus conferences have been held and their recommendations published, each of the prior recommendations must be carefully reviewed and critiqued by experts who represent the extent range of opinions on the subject. Criteria for evaluating new scientific and medical data that may bear on the process of modification of prior recommendations and development of new recommendations have now been developed in advance in a number of cases based on suggested models.[4–6] Opinion, however expert, should clearly be subservient to credible data, particularly controlled clinical trials published in one or more respected peer-reviewed journals. Absent a credible scientific database, expert opinion based on clinical experience and open critical discussion may be the only available basis for recommending an appropriate approach to care until scientific data can be developed to answer the extent question definitively.

When contradictory opinions are present in respected medical journals, the work of the consensus conference becomes yet more important. A careful discussion of all credible information may lead to an impasse. If so, opposing views should be analyzed so that the best recommendations, i.e. safest and most likely to be effective, should be reported. A frank statement of the dilemma created by the insufficiency of scientific data should be one of the objectives of the consensus conference and should serve as a stimulus to the initiation of needed research in the area in question.

Consensus process

It is hardly avoidable that the process by which 'consensus' is developed will influence the final therapeutic recommendations that will ultimately appear in the form of clinical practice guidelines.[7] A number of approaches to the development of consensus have been identified, including the National Institutes of Health process that '. . . combines aspects of the judicial system [in which an impartial jury makes a decision based on the evidence presented], a scientific meeting [in which professional colleagues share their findings], and a town meeting [where any interested person can express an opinion].[2,7,8,9]

The central purpose in the consensus process, whatever format is chosen, is the following:

1   to assure a comprehensive presentation of all relevant scientific information, including minority opinions by respected experts who are dedicated to the objectives of the conference;
2   to assure a full and balanced discussion of this information among these experts, usually in small groups and in a manner in which the facts are emphasized and personal qualities of persuasion are minimized;
3   presentation of what has been agreed on and what has not been agreed on to the plenary session; and
4   faithful incorporation of the developed consensus and exceptions to consensus in the article for publication.

Role of professional organizations in the development of CPGs

In the area of cardiovascular medicine, the American College of Cardiology (ACC) and the American Heart Association (AHA), have maintained a propitious relationship in the development of CPGs as is witnessed by their co-sponsorship of virtually every set of CPGs in this area. Practice guidelines for the use of both diagnostic procedures and therapeutic interventions developed jointly by AHA and ACC include those for myocardial infarction, heart failure, electrocardiography, and cardiac catheterization, among many others. The purpose of these guidelines is to make clear to the practicing physician/cardiologist what experts in cardiovascular medicine consider to be the minimum acceptable performance standards in each of these areas. Such impartial guidelines should provide a clearer indication to physicians of what is expected of them by their peers. This, in turn, will tend to make the somewhat abstract 'standard-of-care' considerably more concrete for physicians, patients, lawyers, and judges. In terms of balance, this should work in favor of the conscientious practitioner both from a medical and from a legal point of view.

QUALITY OF CARE

Defining 'quality of care'

The Institute of Medicine has defined quality of medical care as 'the degree to which health services for individuals and populations increases the likelihood of desired health outcomes and are consistent with professional knowledge'.[10] More recently, quality of care has been viewed in three relatively distinct dimensions, i.e. effec-

tiveness of care, satisfaction with care, and access to care. All three of these parameters are unavoidably patient sensitive. An important and likely deliberate omission is cost. Over the past decade, the percentage of individuals in managed care has tripled while the rate of increase in health care spending has declined steadily. Clearly, the role of cost containment pressures on quality of care must be monitored carefully if quality of care under either definition is to be maintained.

In his review of the relationship between managed care and quality of care, Hellinger concluded that managed care had not decreased the overall effectiveness of care but may have adversely affected the health of some vulnerable subpopulations.[11] Further, satisfaction with care was lower in managed care plans and enrollees in such plans had more difficulty accessing specialty services. Young, wealthier, healthier persons were more satisfied with their plans than older, poorer, sicker persons. However, Hellinger points out that relatively little data on the effect of managed care on quality was reported from the 1990s and little was known about the newer types of HMOs. Further, the variability of HMOs made comparisons difficult.

If the ascendency of cost controls and profit motives have not negatively influenced the quality and availability of care, there is a widespread sense that the expanding power and influence of the market-oriented environment has, over the decade of the nineties, presided over the dissolution of the 'safety net' and has progressively excluded the indigent and diminished availability of care to the elderly, the disabled and those with chronic diseases.

Answering the question: what impact do HMOs have on quality of care?

Only a properly designed and controlled clinical study will answer this question and this would be expensive and difficult, if not impossible. One important reason for this is the fact that HMOs are changing so rapidly that any data developed in a given time window may no longer be applicable by the time the study was completed. The closest thing to an ideal study appears to be the Rand Corporation's Health Insurance Experiment, but a number of limitations to the results of this study have been cited and one of the most compelling must be the fact that it was carried out more than 15 years ago.[12]

Thus, it is quite likely that this important question will remain unanswered or incompletely answered for the foreseeable future.

MEDICAL PRACTICE GUIDELINES: SOME SUCCESSES, SOME FAILURES

'Practice guidelines', as defined in the Institutes of Medicine 1990 report, are 'systematically developed statements to assist practitioner and patient decisions about appropriate health care for specific clinical circumstances'.[10] Medical review criteria are 'systematically developed statements that can be used to assess the appropriateness of specific health care decisions, services and outcomes'. The latter publication included a section on the assessment of clinical practice guidelines which included a 'draft' instrument, reactions to which were described to be 'extremely varied'. For example, on the positive side, one comment was 'well written, concise' while on the negative side 'this instrument was very confusing, almost "impossible" ' and 'the instructions are verbose and redundant, almost legalistic. They are not user-friendly'.[13]

In the 1980s, CPGs were relative rarities. Perhaps the most notable example of widely accepted and used CPGs were those which formulated relatively uniform approaches to cardiopulmonary resuscitation (CPR) and emergency cardiac care (ECC). There is no doubt that the CPR and ECC guidelines have gone a long way toward standardizing practice in these important areas and have been used frequently in courts of law to support both the plaintiff's and the defendant's position. From the late 1980s to the present, there has been an explosion of CPGs as everyone, from organized medicine, peer review organizations, insurers, and state legislatures to the US Congress has become interested. By 1997, over 2500 CPGs had become available. Earlier CPGs were developed primarily through the use of peer review and consensus conferences. More recently, the trend has been to base the CPGs on a comprehensive evaluation and weighting of scientific evidence by panels of experts. And the enthusiasm for CPGs has not been limited to the USA. Evaluations of the impact of CPGs on the quality of care and outcomes has been distinctly less frequent than the emergence of new CPGs themselves. Of 59 evaluations of CPGs in Britain, most found some effect on the process of care delivery but only 11 of 59 looked at the impact of CPGs on the outcomes of clinical care. A Canadian review of the impact of CPGs on patient outcomes provided little support that CPGs improved patient outcomes at the primary care level but most studies looked at process rather than outcomes.[14] It has been suggested that the failure to demonstrate positive outcome impact may relate to the lack of methodologically sound studies, and it is not yet clear that evidence-based CPGs are any better than consensus-based CPGs.

Evidence of efficacy of CPGs

The lack of evidence for the efficacy of CPGs, despite what appears to be unbridled enthusiasm, may be due to the fact that they indeed may not positively affect clinical practice and outcomes. Alternatively, acceptance may be low, implementation inadequate or the evaluation process may so far be ineffective. However, the sheer weight of enthusiastic support is insufficient reason to disregard the fact that an innovation of such magnitude should not be permitted to go on unevaluated. For all the enthusiasm, there remains the possibility that CPGs could be having a negative impact on care, at some level, in some sector, on physician performance or on the physician–patient relationship, which appears to be under continuing attack by the forces of market-driven medical practice.

Since it is now clear that CPGs are the principal means by which evidence-based medicine is introduced into clinical practice, credible research on the impact of CPGs on the quality of care delivery and outcomes may be more valuable than the publication of more CPGs.

Market-driven medicine: impact on quality of care

The growth of CPGs has taken place during a period of vastly increased market-driven changes in medical care delivery, which have transformed the medical care delivery system and continue to do so in an ongoing manner. One of the many consequences of the intensive market competition that has resulted is an instability in the managed care system, which tends to impact negatively on continuity of care. Some employees may offer a single health plan that may or may not be able to provide care up to the CPG expectations.

Thus, while it is not yet clear whether CPGs have a positive impact on patient outcomes, it is quite clear that the number of CPGs which have been developed is greatly disproportionate to the paucity of evidence supporting the efficacy of CPGs.

Critical questions about CPGs

The ACC publication on CPGs states that 'Clinical practice guidelines are developed primarily to serve patient care needs'. As of the April 1998 ACC index of ACC/AHA Practice Guidelines, 13 have been published from 1989 through April 1998. The first, on ambulatory electrocardiography, was published in January 1989 and, since then, CPGs have ranged over the spectrum of diagnostic procedures and therapeutic interventions from cardiac catheterization through coronary artery by-pass graft surgery, etc., to pacemakers and anti-arrhythmic devices. To date, no comprehensive evidence that CPGs do indeed 'serve patient care needs' has been put forward. Most of us would attest to the value of disciplined codification of approaches to clinical practice, but we as yet do not know whether CPGs affect clinical practice in a positive manner. It is important to find out, for a number of reasons, not the least of which is that if CPGs have a strongly positive effect in a certain practice area, we should move to optimize these effects throughout that practice area. Are CPGs implemented more fully in managed care environments or in conventional insurance plans? Can this new technology be underused or misused in such a manner that appropriate care is withheld?

Absent critical evaluation, appropriate course corrections and enhancements cannot be implemented.

MEDICOLEGAL IMPLICATIONS OF CONSENSUS CONFERENCES AND CPGS

Malpractice liability

Codification of the product of a credible consensus conference into CPGs should make it easier for both the physician and the attorney to identify the appropriate 'standard' of practice in a given set of circumstances. Theoretically, then, the physician should be better informed as to minimal practice standards and thus less likely to act inappropriately. In addition, should a malpractice action be initiated, the physician should be better able to defend his or her position using the CPGs if *that physician acted in a manner consistent with the CPGs.* Alternatively, if the physician's action was inconsistent with the CPGs, the CPGs could become formidable evidence to persuade a jury that indeed the physician's performance fell below the standard of care. Further, if the physician failed to perform according to the CPGs, that failure could be either because he or she was aware of the CPGs and for some reason acted inconsistently with them, or because the physician was unaware of the CPGs. In the latter circumstance, a question likely to arise is whether implementation efforts were appropriate and this question may have broader implications, e.g. to the institutional setting in which the physician practiced.

PHYSICIAN JUDGMENT AND CPGS

One of the more serious legal dangers may be the use of CPGs to convince a jury of the liability of a practitioner when an apparent deviation from the CPGs was legitimately based on the physician's best judgment under the circumstances at the time. This, of course, is one of the risks of CPGs and another reason why credible information is needed to try to avoid unjust legal outcomes. The argument that the physician charged with malpractice deviated from the apparent applicable standard based on his or her judgment and experience is not new, and has sometimes been effective, and sometimes has failed. Whether CPGs become an inappropriately powerful weapon for the plaintiff's bar remains to be seen. There is no good data at the moment to determine whether CPGs are either helpful or harmful to the physician charged with malpractice.

INCONSISTENT GUIDELINES

Inconsistent guidelines could be problematic, of course, for both the plaintiff and the defendant in a malpractice case, and efforts to either reconcile inconsistencies or rationalize them in a coherent manner should be given a high priority, primarily because of the likely positive effect on practice and patient outcomes by reducing confusion as to proper procedures. Co-sponsorship by leading professional and public organizations in the same field such as the ongoing cooperative efforts by ACC and AHA are important steps toward reducing the problem of inconsistent guidelines.

Informed consent: an important process

SIGNING THE CONSENT FORM ALONE IS INADEQUATE

The widespread belief that the patient's signature on an 'informed consent' form is sufficient to meet the legal requirements for informed consent is in error. The purpose of informed consent is to protect patient autonomy. The legal requirement to show that the patient's autonomy has been protected is that the patient has sufficient understanding to choose whether or not to agree to a certain diagnostic procedure or to a certain form of therapy. To have a sufficient understanding, the patient needs to be able to understand the benefits and dangers of accepting and the consequences to him or her if the procedure or therapy is rejected. In addition, the patient must be informed about other tests and therapies that may represent reasonable alternatives, and the risks and benefits of each of these. The patient's questions need to be answered in a manner sufficient to satisfy the patient's concerns. There are unlikely to be any pre-printed 'consent forms' that can satisfy all of these requirements. Accordingly, a signed consent form may be no more than evidence that the patient signed the consent form and this is insufficient evidence to satisfy the legal requirements for informed consent. In addition to the signed consent form, it is highly desirable that a note be written in the record indicating the substance of the conversation with the patient, the specific concerns and questions raised by the patient, and the answers provided by the physician.

INFORMED CONSENT AS AN ENHANCEMENT TO THE PHYSICIAN–PATIENT RELATIONSHIP

The process of obtaining informed consent is often given short shrift. Such a practice may cause serious damage to the physician–patient relationship by diminishing patient trust and in so doing, increase the likelihood of legal action on the part of the patient should there be an adverse outcome. Rather, the process of obtaining informed consent should provide a basis for reinforcing the physician–patient relationship and enhancing patient trust and confidence.

One of the areas that has suffered in the revolution toward managed care is the physician–patient relationship. Since a meaningful discussion of all *material* risks to the patient required by the doctrine of informed consent is greatly facilitated by an atmosphere of trust, and an atmosphere of trust may be difficult to develop instantly between two individuals who may never have met before, informed consent may become a more difficult problem than ever. The absence of patient trust when the patient is being asked to consent to a potentially dangerous experience can be a strong stimulus to blame-placing, if an outcome is less than was anticipated by the patient. Care taken to gain the patient's confidence and trust is not only good medical practice but is a wise investment of time, especially now that most patients are well aware of the depersonalizing pressures imposed on the physician by managed care.

A sensitive approach to the informed consent process may have another intangible benefit that might be called 'emotional' informed consent, that is, not only has the patient been provided with the legal elements required for informed consent, but has been reassured that *this physician* has *this patient's* best interests at heart.

Achieving such a bonus as a result of the informed consent process can have appreciable positive benefits for patient, physician, and the liability risk.

SUMMARY

- The format for consensus statements proposed by the Journal of the American Medical Association in 1995 emphasized: objectives, selection of participants, methods of review and evaluation, manner of reaching a 'consensus' and overall conclusions.
- The primary value of consensus statements and clinical practice guidelines lies in their provision of a scientific groundwork for establishing a 'standard of care'.
- The impact of clinical practice guidelines on patient outcomes has not been rigorously tested.
- Consistency in practice guidelines is important and can be achieved through cooperative efforts involving leading professional and public organizations.

REFERENCES

1. Instructions for preparing structured abstracts. *JAMA* 1995; **273**: 28–30.
2. Olson CM. Consensus statements: applying structure. *JAMA* 1995; **273**: 72–3.
3. Grimshaw JM, Russell IT. Effect of clinical guidelines on medical practice: a systematic review of vigorous evaluations. *Lancet* 1993; **342**: 1317–22.
4. Weingarten SR, Riedinger MS, Conner L, *et al*. Practice guidelines and reminders to reduce duration of hospital stay for patients with chest pain. *Ann Intern Med* 1994; **120**: 257–63.
5. Squires BP. Statements from professional associations, specialty groups, and consensus conferences: what editors expect. *Can Med Assoc J* 1991; **145**: 297–98.
6. Woolf SH. Practice guidelines, a new reality in medicine: II. Methods of developing guidelines. *Arch Intern Med* 1992; **152**: 946–52.
7. Guidelines for cardiopulmonary resuscitation and emergency cardiac care. *JAMA* 1992; **268**: 1172.
8. Hillman BJ. The consensus of committees. *Invest Radiol* 1992; **27**: 1.
9. Tong R. The epistemology and ethics of consensus: uses and misuses of 'ethical' expertise. *J Med Philos* 1991; **16**: 409–26.
10. *Guidelines for clinical practice: from development to use*. Washington, DC: Institutes of Medicine, National Academy Press, 1992: 27.
11. Hellinger FJ. The effect of managed care on quality: a review of recent evidence. *Arch Intern Med* 1998; **158**: 833–41.
12. Manning WF, Leibowitz A, Goldberg GA, Rogers WH, Rogers JP. A controlled trial of the effects of a prepaid group practice on use of services. *N Engl J Med* 1984; **310**: 1505–10.
13. *Guidelines for clinical practice: from development to use*. Washington, DC: Institutes of Medicine, National Academy Press, 1992: 349.
14. Worrall G, Chaulk P, Freake D. The effects of clinical practice guidelines on patient outcomes in primary care: a systematic review. *Can Med J* 1997; **156**: 1705–12.

35

Ethical and legal issues in a managed medical care system

JAMES S FORRESTER AND SYLVAN LEE-WEINBERG

The transition from traditional fee-for-service medicine to managed care has created a new set of ethical questions, centered on the physician's role as patient advocate. This traditional medical tenet is put in conflict with a non-physician corporate interest, to provide profit for corporate shareholders. Consistent with this latter goal, effective reduction of patient care costs can be achieved by requiring physicians to obtain prior authorization for treatment from non-physicians, and by restricting access to specialty care. Ethical dilemmas are created when a decision to restrict care is not in the patient's best interest. Additional ethical conflicts are those placed directly upon the physicians by financial incentives to withhold care, and by contractual clauses that prohibit a physician from discussing therapeutic options not offered by the managed care organization. Ironically, issues of medical ethics, long the purview of the medical profession, are likely to be resolved by legislatures and by courts of law.

INTRODUCTION

> Whether the patient be a pauper or a millionaire, whether he be treated gratuitously or for reward, the physician owes him precisely the same measure of duty, and the same degree of skill and care.

Becker *vs* Janinski, 15 NYS 675, 1891[1]

So it was in New York in 1891. Does this ethical principle still hold today? The cost controls used in the practice of managed care medicine have created a new set of ethical dilemmas for physicians. Those who contract with managed care organizations have found themselves put in the role of 'double agents',[2] trying to balance the competing interests of their patients and their managed care employer. The most prominent managed care practices that raise ethical issues are prior approval of physician care by non-experts, restriction of access to specialty care, physician incentives to withhold care, and restriction of patient's access to medical and financial informa-

tion. In this chapter we will describe these ethical dilemmas, then analyze how they are being debated, clarified, and resolved.

HISTORICAL PERSPECTIVE

In 1973, Congress and states passed legislation that empowered the creation of health maintenance organizations (HMOs), by permitting selective contracting between doctors and hospitals. In the ensuing years, HMOs recruited clients who paid premiums for insured health care. Large companies who provided health care as part of their employee benefit packages found the lower premiums charged by HMOs particularly attractive compared to traditional private insurance. HMOs were able to deliver a large number of potential customers, so they then negotiated reduced charges for their medical services with both hospitals and doctors. The reduced revenue to hospitals and physicians precipitated both vigorous efforts at containment of health care costs, and concomitant huge profits for HMOs. Initially, these cost reductions could be accomplished by increased efficiencies, and later by reducing hospital profits and physician incomes. As competition among HMOs increased, however, the pressure for further cost reductions became intense. By the late 1980s it became apparent that the 'corporatization' of American medicine had created a new set of serious ethical and legal dilemmas centering around the conflict between the corporate mandate to reduce the cost of care and the medical mandate to maintain the quality of patient care. In simplified terms, the ethical and legal issue had become profits versus patients.

ETHICAL DILEMMAS

Prior authorization of appropriate care

In managed care, physicians are required to seek prior authorization for various medical and surgical interventions. HMOs deny in accordance with unilaterally established managed care criteria to which the physician has no access. In such cases a medical decision is made by an individual not directly involved in the patient's care, based on financial considerations. This external, financially motivated denial of care is often not made apparent to the patient. Consequently, the external review process raises the ethical issue as to whether a medical decision, potentially adverse to the patient's interest, can be made for financial reasons by a non-medical person, based on the financial interest of the insurer. Of profound additional importance, this practice undermines the ethical basis of medical professionalism,[3] since autonomy is one of the single most important elements that define a profession.[4]

Restriction of access to specialty care

An important factor in the rapid rise in the cost of medical care in the past two decades has been the emergence of specialty care. Consequently managed care organizations (MCOs) have sought to limit access to specialists and to restrain their use of expensive technology. One effective method is to prohibit referral of a patient to a physician not associated with the HMO. The practice that raises the most serious ethical questions, however, is use of a primary care 'gatekeeper' who must approve referral to a specialist. The issue has profound implications for patient outcomes. Recent studies have indicated that patient outcomes are less favorable when complex medical conditions are treated by non-specialists. For example, Jollis et al. examined mortality according to the specialty of the admitting physician among 8241 Medicare patients who were hospitalized

with myocardial infarction in four states.[5] At 1 year follow-up, patients who were admitted by a cardiologist were 12 per cent less likely to die than those admitted by a primary care physician. The ethical question raised by the gatekeeper concept is whether the restriction of a patient's access to a more qualified specialist violates the patient's reasonable expectation that the primary care physician is committed to providing the best possible care, an implied contract that is the foundation of the traditional doctor–patient relationship.

Physician incentives to withhold care

The American Medical Association's Council on Ethics and Judicial Affairs states that under no circumstances may physicians ethically place their own financial interests above the welfare of their patients. MCOs use financial incentives and disincentives extensively, in ways that seem designed to circumvent this ethical precept. The most common type of incentive is a periodic or year-end bonus to the physician for meeting a reduced cost of care target. Coercive disincentives, which effectively alter physician behavior are also used. These methods include termination of contracts with physicians who are identified as having an above average number of hospitalizations, mean length of hospital stay, referrals to specialists, or use of diagnostic and therapeutic technologies. These contract terminations have typically occurred without reference to the quality of care provided by the physician, and have not been subject to appeal. The potential for violation of the ethical mandate to place the patient's interest above all else is self-evident; detection of the abuse is extraordinarily difficult except when an ethical violation is flagrant.

Restriction of patients' access to information

Until recently most managed care contracts included 'gag clauses', which prohibit doctors from discussing forms of treatment not covered by the MCO, or revealing the existence of incentives for withholding care.[6] For example, typical language from one such contract states that 'physicians shall take no action or make any communication which undermines or could undermine the confidence of Enrollees, potential Enrollees, their employers, Plan Sponsors or the public in this organization or in the quality of care which this organization's Enrollees receive'. Other plans include phrases such as 'in no event shall Physician market or offer to enrollees services beyond those which are medically necessary or which are prescribed by the referring participating physician'. The ethical problem that is raised by these clauses is that information critical to a patient's decision about his/her best care may be withheld, in the best financial interest of the health care provider.

PRACTICAL IMPACT OF ETHICAL ISSUES

Physician behavior

Doctors subjected to such pressures over a protracted period of time tend to modify their medical decisions without realizing that they are no longer acting in the interest of their patients.[7] The impact of MCOs on physician behavior was documented in a Louis Harris survey, commissioned by the Commonwealth Fund.[8] Approximately 1700 randomly selected office-based physicians who spend at least half of their time in direct patient care were the subject of the study. Approximately 40 per cent of the physicians admitted that 'their ability to make decisions they think are right for their patients has declined during the past three years'. This view was held by a greater percentage of specialists than generalists. In addition, 41 per cent of the physicians reported the time they spent with their patients had decreased because of managed care, and 60 per cent of the respondents reported that external review limited their ability to make clinical decisions. Among physicians in discounted and capitated provider plans, 80 per cent reported they experienced limits on referrals to specialists and serious limitations on obtaining approval for admission of their patients to a hospital. Finally, a striking difference in satisfaction paralleled these changes: 40 per cent of physicians whose patients were in managed care plans were dissatisfied with their medical practice, compared to 18 per cent among those who had no managed care patients.

Potential disappearance of traditional medical ethical standards

Defenders of MCOs often point to the ethical abuses due to overutilization of services that have occurred in fee-for-service medicine. This kind of behavior, however, is condemned by the medical profession and clearly violates established ethical codes of organized medicine. In contrast, the new ethical questions, such as delaying and denying care, are part of an institutionalized management strategy in the MCO industry. As a consequence, a number of organizations, including the Group Health Association of America, the American Managed Care and Review Association, and the American Association of Health Plans have maintained that the MCO industry does not have a defined standard of ethics.[9]

A quarterly report on the health industry titled 'Health Care International'[10] observes that regulators who have long relied on physicians to guard the quality of medicine may no longer be able to do so because physicians who accept the legitimacy of managed care practices may no longer have the motivation to act as advocates for patients. The report notes that there is no ready system for monitoring the underutilization of medical care. While HMOs have set up their own professional body, the National Committee for Quality Assurance, to develop criteria with which to govern their members, this organization has not yet established a satisfactory method for measuring its effectiveness.[10,11]

CONFRONTING AND RESOLVING THE NEW ETHICAL ISSUES

Ironically it now appears that the resolution of these new ethical conflicts in medicine will not come from either thoughtful physicians or ethicists, but rather from the courts and from legislation. Although both legislation and case law is still evolving, there are already some remarkable legal decisions and pending legislation which deal with HMOs most controversial strategies – denial of billing authorization, physician incentives to withhold care, restriction on specialty referral, and gag rules.

Prior authorization and restriction of appropriate care

Courts have not been sympathetic to physicians caught in this particular version of the double-agent dilemma. A classic case is that of Lois Wickline, a 40-year-old woman who was approved for a 10-day hospitalization for placement of an abdominal vascular prosthesis.[12] In the postoperative period the graft occluded, necessitating additional surgery and prolongation of her hospitalization. Based on the postoperative complication, Ms Wickline's physicians filed a request for an 8-day extension. Her third-party payor, however, approved only 4 days of additional hospitalization. Consequently, her physicians discharged her early. Out of the hospital, Ms Wickline's graft again failed, leading to an above-knee amputation. In a subsequent lawsuit the court held Ms Wickline's physicians liable in unequivocal terms, creating a modern version of the century-old New York decision: 'The physician who complies without protest with the limitations imposed by a third party payor, when his medical judgment dictates otherwise, cannot avoid the ultimate responsibility for his patient's care. He cannot point to the healthcare payor as the liability scapegoat when the consequences of his own determinative medical decisions go sour'. This 'new' concept has not been seriously challenged in other analogous cases[13] and, further, the court's message is clearly consistent with a long history of American common law. We may reasonably conclude that the physician is required by common law precedent to be his/her patient's advocate, consistent with his/her medical judgment.

This principle, however, does not mean that the third-party payor always escapes responsibility. As an example, Howard Wilson was hospitalized for anorexia, severe depression, and drug dependency.[14] His physician concluded that based on the severity of his emotional problems, he required 4 weeks of in-patient care. Western Medical Review Organization, a utilization review corporation employed by Blue Cross, however, refused to authorize more than 10 days of hospitalization, and Mr Wilson was discharged. Less than 3 weeks later, he committed suicide. The court held that Blue Cross and its utilization review consultants were liable, because their refusal to provide coverage was a substantial factor in Mr Wilson's subsequent adverse outcome. In this and other analogous decisions,[14] the courts have typically assigned shared culpability. Thus we may also anticipate that, when both a third payor's prior restriction of coverage and the compliant physician's subsequent alteration of care leads to an adverse patient outcome, the law will find both parties accountable.

A special case of the profits vs patients conflict is the situation in which a physician assumes the responsibility of utilization review officer for an HMO, and then chooses to override another physician's best judgment. Lewis Hand, a 49-year-old hypertensive came to a Texas emergency room (ER) with a 3-day severe headache and nausea.[15] His father had died of an aneurysm. After observing Mr Hand's symptoms rise and fall with his blood pressure, ER physician Boyle told Mr Hand that he required hospitalization. Dr Boyle then discussed the case by telephone with Humana Healthcare Plan's on-call physician Dr Robert Tavera, who refused admission. Instead, Dr Tavera said that Mr Hand should be given medication to control his headache and blood pressure, and return for follow-up on the following morning to the Humana Out-patient Clinic. In the parking lot on his way home, Mr Hand suffered a paralyzing stroke. One might wonder which of four possible defendants – the hospital, ER physician Boyle, the third-party payor Humana, or Humana's on-call physician Tavera – might be liable. During a subsequent lawsuit, Dr Boyle was dropped from the case, and the hospital made a seven figure settlement. The on-call physician Dr Tavera claimed he could not be held responsible because he had not established a doctor–patient relationship with Mr Hand. Perhaps to many physician's surprise, the trial court accepted Dr Tavera's argument. The Texas Court of Appeals, however, reversed the decision based on review of the contractual language between Humana and Tavera's group: 'the Humana plan brought Hand and Tavera together just as surely as though they had met directly and entered the physician–patient relationship. Hand paid premiums to Humana to purchase medical care in advance of need, Humana met its obligation to Hand and its other enrollees by employing Tavera's group to treat them; and Tavera's medical group agreed to treat Humana enrollees in exchange for the fees received from Humana'. In this case, the court separated the responsibility of the physician who denied coverage from that of his HMO employer. From this decision, it becomes apparent that a physician who makes coverage

decisions for a HMO must exert extraordinary caution in countermanding the recommendation of an on-site physician. It is clearly possible to commit malpractice without ever seeing a patient.

A major impediment in implementing ethical reform: ERISA

Ironically a law that is not directly related to medical practice has had major impact on HMO malpractice case law. The Employee Retirement Income Security Act (ERISA), passed in 1974, was designed to safeguard employee benefits, including self-insured health care plans. ERISA includes a provision that, as a federal law, it pre-empts state laws that relate to employee benefit plans. Both state and federal courts have concluded that, when a company's HMO contract is part of an employee benefit plan, it is covered by ERISA. As a consequence an HMOs refusal to pre-certify payment for necessary medical services is defined as an insurance benefit decision. The remarkable outcome of this reasoning is that the liability of the HMO in an alleged malpractice action has been limited to payment of the cost of denied services, whereas the physician remains liable for both improper treatment and for additional punitive damages for willful disregard of the patient's interest. ERISA, therefore, creates a dichotomy in which the physician assumes the liability for a plan's decision with which he may not agree, while the plan's non-physician decision maker remains protected from liability.

Buddy Kuhl sustained a heart attack in a mid-western city.[16] After documenting inducible ventricular tachycardia, his cardiologist determined that he was at 'high risk for sudden death' and required electrophysiologically guided left ventricular aneurysmectomy. Because the area hospitals did not have equipment to perform this type of complex surgery, Mr Kuhl's cardiologist concluded that his best chance for survival lay in referral to Barnes Hospital in St Louis, which was outside the service area of Mr Kuhl's Lincoln National Health Plan. Arrangements were made for his surgery, but Lincoln National refused to pre-certify payment. After a second plan-retained cardiologist agreed with Mr Kuhl's physicians that he should be transferred to Barnes, the HMO informed Mr Kuhl that it would authorize the surgery. Owing to the HMOs delay in making this decision, however, the scheduled surgery had been canceled. When Mr Kuhl finally arrived at Barnes approximately 4 months after the original recommendation, his condition had further deteriorated, precluding the possibility of surgical repair. Buddy Kuhl died 3 months later while awaiting cardiac transplantation. In the subsequent malpractice suit, the court held that when Mr Kuhl's insurer canceled the proposed surgery in response to the physician's requested pre-certification review, it was not providing the patient with medical advice and therefore could not be held liable on the basis of medical malpractice. On the other hand, in response to the plaintiff's assertion that the HMO had interfered with medical practice, the court used the convoluted logic of the ERISA pre-emption to conclude that, since Mr Kuhl was a retirement benefit plan beneficiary, the plan was liable only for medical costs, not for the treatment outcome.

Physicians providing care to plan patients are clearly not covered by the ERISA pre-emption. In 1992, Glenn Nealy had been under treatment for cardiac disease with a personal physician for some time.[17] He enrolled in his employer's US Healthcare Plan after being told that he could continue treatment by his current physicians. The plan's administrators created considerable delay in approving this continuing relationship, and in addition provided incorrect information to his pharmacy. Consequently, during this time Mr Nealy was unable to see his personal cardiologist or to obtain needed medications. In the period during which he was without medication, Mr Nealy suffered a massive myocardial infarction and died. The plaintiffs brought suit against US Healthcare and the plan physician who did not approve Mr Nealy's request for referral to his non-plan physician. The court ruled that Mr Nealy's inability to obtain needed medications was not a basis for liability of US Healthcare, based on the ERISA exemption. On the other hand, the claims against US Healthcare's physician were remanded to state court, based on his potential malpractice liability arising from abuse of the doctor–patient relationship.

While courts have been quite consistent in protecting HMOs from liability based on ERISA legislation,[18–21] there are a few exceptions. These cases typically involve application of some other legal principle, which creates liability for the HMO. Carolyn Verzicco came to her physician complaining of chest pain, shortness of breath, and numbness in her shoulders of 20 minutes duration.[22] Her primary care found T-wave abnormalities on the electrocardiogram (ECG) and ordered a Holter monitor recording. US Healthcare denied payment for the Holter monitor recording. As a consequence, the recording was not reviewed. A few weeks later Ms Verzicco experienced severe chest pain radiating down her arm and up her neck. She went to the ER where she was found to have a blood pressure of 180/110 mm Hg and ECG evidence of anterior myocardial ischemia or infarction. She was sent home on medication and instructed to return if her condition worsened. The following day, while driving her car, Ms Verzicco again experienced severe chest pain, followed by syncope. She was again taken to the ER where prolonged resuscitation was performed. She sustained anoxic encephalopathy, from which she did not regain consciousness and entered a prolonged and persistent vegetative state. The court found that US Healthcare was liable for the actions of their physicians, because they had been selected and credentialed as a plan provider and had failed to diagnose the patient's

cardiac disease. Consistent with the ERISA principle, however, US Healthcare was not held liable for failing to approve an appropriate procedure to diagnose the patient's cardiac condition. Thus the Verzicco case stands as a exception to the many rejected claims of liability, which have been barred by the courts under ERISA. As a consequence of the questionable fairness and logic of these many ERISA-based decisions, ERISA has become one important target of proposed health care reform legislation.

In 1995, case law and legislation finally began to erode the ERISA pre-emption. In Dukes *vs* US Healthcare, a physician ordered blood tests on Mr Dukes, but the hospital laboratory refused to perform them, presumably because it did not have HMO authorization. Mr Dukes died soon thereafter. Mrs Dukes alleged that the failure to obtain these crucial blood tests led to her husband's death.[19] She accused US Healthcare of negligent administration of the health care plan, because it failed to use reasonable care in evaluating its medical contractors. The court ruled that ERISA did not pre-empt the malpractice claim: 'Patients enjoy the right to be free of medical malpractice whether or not their medical care is provided through an ERISA plan'. In the same year, an Oklahoma court ruled that an HMO was liable for the negligent care provided by one of its physician gatekeepers, because it bore responsibility for its physician–employee actions: 'Just as ERISA does not preempt a malpractice claim against the doctor, it should not preempt the vicarious liability claim against the HMO if the HMO has held out the doctor as its agent'.[23]

Physician incentives to withhold care

In the previously described cases, physicians withheld care because they deferred to a third-party recommendation that did not correspond to their own judgment. In physician incentive and capitation plans, however, the ethical problem is created when a physician appears to withhold care for personal financial gain. A physician who personally profits from limiting medical care when reasonable practice dictates otherwise is subject to litigation. The most widely publicized case involving physician incentive compensation began on August 14, 1992 in Southern California, when 35-year-old Joyce Ching presented to her primary care physician, Dr Elvin Gaines, with severe abdominal pain and rectal bleeding.[24] Dr Gaines diagnosed peptic ulcer, and for approximately 3 months, despite Mrs Ching's continuing severe pain, refused to do additional tests or refer her to a specialist. On October 30, 1992, after repeated requests from Mrs Ching and her family, Dr Gaines referred Ms Ching to a specialist. Three days later, she was found to have metastatic colon carcinoma. In the jury trial that followed her death, Joyce Ching's family argued that the MetLife HMO contract encouraged Dr Gaines' group to limit both referrals and diagnostic tests, and that Dr Gaines had failed to disclose these incentives. Dr Gaines conceded that reduction in referrals to medical specialists increased the income to his medical group. Nonetheless, the judge threw out the claims against Dr Gaines. The jury, however, brought back a $2.9 million judgment against MetLife. From the Ching case and a number of similar cases, it is apparent that the courts will not be sympathetic when a gatekeeper restricts a patient's access to specialty care in the mutual financial interest of the gatekeeper and HMO, if that decision violates reasonable standards of care, and results in an adverse patient outcome.

The attack on physician incentives to withhold care was extended to ERISA in 1997. A primary care physician whose HMO contract included a financial incentive to limit specialty referrals was sued when his refusal to refer a patient with severe heart failure to a cardiologist was followed a few months later by the patient's death.[25] The plaintiff alleged she and her deceased husband were victims of fraudulent misrepresentation because the physician and the HMO failed to inform them of the incentive plan. The court held that 'when the HMO's financial incentives discourage a treating doctor from providing essential health care referrals... the failure to do so is a breach of ERISA's fiduciary responsibility'.

Prohibitions on physician–patient communication: 'gag clauses'

Gag clauses became a national issue in 1996 following the widely publicized termination of Harvard University primary care physician David Himmelstein after his criticism of the gag clause and incentives to withhold care in his HMO contract on the Phil Donahue talk show.[26] Three days later, without accompanying explanation, he received a letter from US Healthcare dropping him from the network. The defense raised in this and similar cases is that these clauses protect proprietary information such as utilization review criteria, and encourage physicians to air their concerns about questionable HMO policies with the plan rather than with their patients. Because of the public response to the revelation of gag clauses, however, they are now being made illegal through both federal and state legislation.

FUTURE DIRECTIONS

Resolution of the ethical dilemmas raised by managed care practices

In the past year, a substantial segment of the American public has become aware of the risk–benefit dilemmas inherent in economically driven medical decisions. One might speculate that a majority will come to agree that

there are good and bad ways to reduce the costs of health care. Each of these ethically controversial methods – non-physician denial of care, restriction on the choice of physician and specialty referral, physician incentives to withhold care, and gag clauses – are now the subject of proposed legislation in state legislatures and in Congress. These initiatives seek to establish strict criteria for denial of care, prohibit the use of financial incentives to withhold care, provide for second opinions, establish appeal processes, and eliminate gag clauses. Thus it now seems likely that many of the ethical issues raised by managed care practices will be resolved not by thoughtful physicians and ethicists, but rather by legislatures, judges, and juries.[27]

SUMMARY

- Enabling legislation and the rising cost of employee health care benefits led to the emergence of managed care.
- An entirely new set of ethical dilemmas has been created by the 'corporatization' of medical care.
- Denial of care reduces costs but can lead to patient injury.
- Physician incentives to withhold care undermine the traditional basis of medical ethics.
- Restriction of patients' access to information creates new legal, as well as ethical, issues.
- Coercive practices effectively intimidate physicians and alter their behavior.
- Contracts with gag clauses are being eliminated by public demand rather than by litigation.
- Case law is being developed in response to the new ethical dilemmas raised by managed care practices.
- The future development of the ethics for medical care will be determined by legislatures and courts, not by ethicists and physicians.

REFERENCES

1. Becker v Janinski, 15 NYS 675,1891.
2. Angell M. The doctor as double agent. *Kennedy Inst Ethics J* 1993; **3**: 279–86.
3. Newcomer LN. Measures of trust in health care. *Health Affairs* 1997; **16**: 50–1.
4. Freidson E. *The profession of medicine: an essay in sociology of applied knowledge.* New York: Dodd Mead.
5. Jollis JG, DeLong ER, Peterson ED, *et al.* Outcome of acute myocardial infarction according to the specialty of the admitting physician. *N Engl J Med* 1996; **335**: 1880.
6. Smith J. Physician hold thy tongue. *LACMA Physician* 1996; 39–43.

○7. Kassirer JP. Managed care and the morality of the marketplace. *N Engl J Med* 1995; **333**: 50–2.

8. Scott Collins K, Schoen C, Sandman DR. *The Commonwealth fund survey of physician experiences with managed care*. New York: Commonwealth Fund, 1997: 1.

○9. Gray BH. Trust and trustworthy care in the managed care era. *Health Affairs* 1997; **16**: 34–49.

10. *Health Care International*, 1st quarter. London: The Economist Intelligence Unit, 1997.

11. Kassirer JP. The quality of care and quality of measuring it. *N Engl J Med* 1993; **329**: 1263.

12. Wickline *v* State of California 192 Cal. App. 3d 1630, 1986.

13. Boyd *v* Albert Einstein Medical Center, 377 Pa. Super. 609, 547 A.2d 1229, 1234–5, 1988.

14. Wilson *v* Blue Cross of Southern California 222 Cal. App. 3d 660, 1990.

15. Hand *v* Tavera, 864 S.W.2d 687 (Tex. App), 1993.

16. Kuhl *v* Lincoln Nat. Health Plan, 999 F.2d 298, 303 (8th Circuit), 1993.

17. Nealy *v* US Healthcare HMO, 844 F. Supp. 966, 973 (S.D.N.Y.), 1994.

18. Corcoran *v* United Healthcare, Inc., 965 F.2d 1321, 1332 (5th Circuit.), 1992.

19. Dukes *v* US Healthcare, Inc., 57 F.3d 350 (3d Circuit), 1995.

20. Holmes *v* Pacific Mutual Life Ins. Co., F. Supp 733 (C.D. Cal), 1989.

21. Marshall *v* Banker's Life & Casualty Co: 2 Cal 4th 1045, 1992.

22. Elsesser *v* Hospital of Philadelphia College, 802 F. Supp. 1286, 1291–2 (E. D. Pa.), 1992.

23. Pacificare of Oklahoma, Inc. *v* Burrage, 59 F.3d 151(10th Circuit),1995.

24. Azevedo D. Did an HMO doctor's greed kill Joyce Ching? *Med Econ* 1996; **73**: 43–4, 47–8, 50 passim.

25. Shea *v* Eisenstein, CA 8, No 95-4029 NM, 2/26/97.

26. Olmos DR, Roan S. HMO 'Gag clauses' on doctors spur protest. *Los Angeles Times* (*Home Edition Ed.*) 1996; A1.

27. Weinberg S. *Managing the excesses of managed care: the courts or the Congress in the golden age of medical science and the black age of health care delivery*. Philadelphia: Charles Pass Publishers, 2000: 76–8.

PART 7

Medical education

36

Clinical decision making and information management in the era of managed care

FARRELL J LLOYD AND VALERIE F REYNA

Current models of managed care impose significant administrative burdens, but their benefits for costs and quality have not been unambiguously demonstrated. We introduce an alternative approach that incorporates providers' decisions as the fundamental unit of analysis, as well as evidence-based practice guidelines, medical outcomes, and measures of efficiency that are tied to clinical indicators of quality of care. Information management can improve outcomes data, but outcomes cannot be interpreted in the absence of information about decision making. Realistic proposals to affect providers' decisions must incorporate research that provides insight into cognitive processes and how these processes affect health care delivery.

INTRODUCTION

The economic infrastructure of medical practice is undergoing rapid change. Recent developments include the emergence of managed care, and its spread from regional enclaves throughout the USA. These changes have subjected medicine to greater scrutiny, especially regarding health care costs and quality. In this chapter, we explore the implications of these economic developments for the practice of medicine. Although the chapter is directed primarily at practitioners, the framework we introduce should also be of practical benefit to health care administrators and policy makers.

We begin with a brief review of the problems that precipitated recent changes in health care. Then, we discuss the nature of these changes, such as the shift from a fee-for-service reimbursement system to capitation, and how they affect the day-to-day practice of medicine. Next, we analyze the assumptions behind these new approaches and introduce an alternative framework that addresses some of the same concerns (e.g. costs and quality of care) but that is without, we believe, some of the drawbacks of current models of managed care and quality improvement. As shall be seen,

this alternative framework highlights the importance of clinical information management and decision analysis in providing objective measures of performance for both health care systems and individual practitioners.

BACKGROUND

'Health care crisis' and rise of managed care

Although there is debate about the precise origins of the so-called 'health care crisis', most observers agree that rapidly increasing health care costs were the precipitating factor. Costs, in turn, were related to induced demand (e.g. increasing hospital beds), price inflation, employer-based insurance, rising numbers of uninsured, and government's expanding role in financing health care.[1] By introducing business efficiencies, it was thought that such costs could be contained. Managing care, then, consisted of implementing efficient business practices. A key assumption underlying managed care is that there is 'waste' in the health care system that can be eliminated without jeopardizing quality of care.[2]

Managed care uses a variety of methods to organize providers including preferred provider organizations (PPO), managed service organizations (MSO), provider hospital organizations (PHO), independent practice associations (IPA), group practice plans, and staff models. (Health maintenance organizations, HMOs, are businesses that use managed care and may employ providers in any one of these methods.) These methods can be distinguished according to the degree to which providers have autonomy. For example, physicians in PPOs may be in private practice (with a discounted fee schedule and contracted with HMOs), whereas physicians in staff model organizations typically are salaried employees.

Managed care also uses a variety of methods to control costs. The 'gatekeeper' model, in which primary care physicians constrain referral of patients to specialists, procedures, tests and evaluations, was designed to minimize unnecessary care in order to conserve economic resources (and, ostensibly, to protect patients from overtreatment).[3] In addition to gatekeeping, managed care uses clinical resource management methods, such as referral review, prior approval for admissions and procedures, restricted drug formularies, and case management to reduce length of hospital stays. Clinical resource management includes what is commonly referred to as utilization management (UM),[4] which most often pertains to out-patient referral authorization processes. Utilization review (UR) usually applies to a *post hoc* review of referrals (whereas UM involves a priori review).

Financial methods are also used that establish incentives to providers to reduce costs. These range from discounted fee-for-service to full capitated risk. In the latter, providers are paid a fixed amount per patient over a specified time, usually per month of a contracted period (i.e. per member per month). Thus, costs incurred treating patients are deducted from a provider's predetermined income. Utilization management, therefore, is used to keep providers' expenses within their predetermined budget.

Clinical resource management is defined relative to appropriate care. That is, costs should be reduced only to the extent that unnecessary or inappropriate care is eliminated. Quality assurance (QA) and, more recently, quality improvement (QI) are designed to address underutilization. Quality improvement as an industrial concept is increasingly accepted as a standard in health care delivery.[5] Some health care organizations report success in reducing inappropriate variability by employing industrial quality improvement methods.[6] An extensive description of these methods is beyond the scope of this chapter. The key points relating to health care include:

- concentrating on process rather than individuals;
- breaking down the process to standard data elements and performing statistical analysis to identify variability;
- instituting guidelines to reduce variability; and
- providing feedback to decision makers on their measured variability.[7]

The intent of these efforts is to reduce and ultimately eliminate inappropriate variability in the processes of health care with an assumption that this will lead to better patient outcomes.

Although reports of industrial methods of quality improvement are appearing in the medical literature,[8] most often, QA and QI amount to compliance with external standards such as the Health Employer Data Information Set (HEDIS)[9] established by the National Commission on Quality Assurance (NCQA)[10], and the Joint Commission for Accreditation of Health Care Organizations (JCAHO).[11] Quality improvement standards in health care take different forms depending on the way providers are organized.[12] For example, HEDIS was designed primarily for HMOs for accreditation purposes, and JCAHO is primarily used by hospitals for accreditation purposes but is evolving to include integrated out-patient and in-patient delivery systems. Other delivery systems (e.g. PPOs and IPAs) employ an array of standards that vary with the particulars of contracts and accrediting agencies. These methods of external evaluation tend to emphasize process outcomes (e.g. number of patients immunized) rather than clinical outcomes (e.g. mortality).

Role of protocols and guidelines

Improving clinical outcomes has been a motivating factor in the development of practice guidelines.[13] Guidelines can take the form of recommendations of professional organizations, such as the National Cholesterol Education Program.[14] As the industrial methods of quality improvement have gained favor, guidelines have been regarded as a possible solution to rising costs.[15] The assumption is that, if providers are given the appropriate guidelines, patient care will improve because patients will receive the necessary treatment without the risk of over- or undertreatment. This assumption was the impetus for the federal government's decision to sponsor the development of clinical practice guidelines.[16] The Agency for Health Care Policy and Research (AHCPR) developed a number of these guidelines that are also available on the World Wide Web (now called the Agency for Healthcare Research and Quality; AHRQ). Since 1999, clinical practice guidelines have been available through the National Guideline Clearinghouse (http://www.guideline.gov).

Effects of new demands on clinical practice

What impact, if any, AHCPR and other guidelines have made in actual clinical practice remains unclear.

Empirical evidence of their adoption is lacking.[17] One retrospective analysis indicated that adopting the guideline on the Diagnosis and Management of Unstable Angina would have little impact in actual clinical settings.[18] This conclusion was based on the finding that few low-risk patients were identified and, therefore, that there was little opportunity to decrease unnecessary admissions. However, these results underestimated the number of low-risk patients for whom significant reductions in admissions might have been made.[19]

The ability of physicians and delivery systems to incorporate these guidelines into clinical decision making is also untested. Once implemented, improving the guidelines and updating them is also problematic. Efforts to incorporate guidelines into computer-aided decision support systems are under way. Despite some success in a few health centers,[8] these methods are not routinely used. One problem is that the information systems requirements change as the delivery systems needs change. That is, as delivery systems undergo a transformation to managed care and its various processes, the information needs of the organization can change dramatically, placing new demands on the expectations of automated systems.

The shift from traditional fee-for-service to full-risk capitation reimbursement creates new administrative and clinical demands as well. Documentation and justification of treatment plans is usually required to a much greater extent. Drug formularies may change frequently and physicians are expected to stop therapeutic medication and order new medication on the formulary. The number of patients in a physician panel becomes a critical number because income is increased on a per member basis (not on the basis of services rendered). Increasing numbers in patient panels means that physicians have patients whom they have never seen demanding prescriptions and referrals. These patients are assigned to the provider but have not been seen (ABNS) and may be treated in emergency rooms with instructions to follow-up with their primary physician. Therefore, the primary care physician is responsible for large numbers of patients with whom they are unfamiliar.

As administrative barriers are erected as a result of managed care, patients' calls to medical offices multiply due to patient demands for non-formulary medications, emergency consultations, and referrals. Requested referrals for procedures, tests, and evaluations are usually scrutinized and may be denied after having been discussed as needed with patients. Often, this referral denial is not communicated until considerable time has elapsed from the original encounter. Patients may believe that the physician is the denying party, creating a perception that the physician is no longer an advocate for the patient. Adverse incentives, usually financial, that encourage underutilization of procedures, tests, and evaluations may further undermine the advocacy role of the physician. In practice, physicians are rarely provided

feedback by QA and QI about specific instances of underutilization, although feedback is occasionally given about overutilization through UM or UR.[4]

Assumptions of managed care

Although the assumption is that managed care reduces costs,[20] such reductions have not been rigorously demonstrated. For example, the point of diminishing returns, at which economic benefits no longer justify gatekeeping, is poorly defined in practice. Managed-care organizations typically do not perform empirical analyses of the trade-offs between complex approval processes for referrals and their economic returns. The observation that most referrals are approved in most systems does not necessarily imply that costs are not contained by these methods. The procedures, tests, and evaluations that are denied may be among the most expensive (although little evidence exists to support that conjecture). Also, the possibility of scrutiny has been shown to inhibit utilization.[21] However, specific efforts to reduce costs have not been directly linked to documented decreases in costs.

Another major assumption of managed care is that efforts to reduce costs will not adversely affect patient outcomes. Managed care contracts may turn over on a yearly or sooner basis, making long-term health benefits not especially relevant to short-term financial interests. As we have noted, QA and QI are assumed to counteract any tendency to underutilize. However, there is little conclusive evidence on this point. Arguments have been made that restricting access to specialists and advanced technology will deprive patients of timely care and ultimately lead to higher costs.[22] Research indicates, for example, that mortality rates for patients with acute coronary syndrome who are treated by cardiologists are lower than those treated by internists.[23,24] Hence, restricting access to cardiologists might be expected to lead to higher mortality for such patients. A direct comparison of managed care and fee-for-service patients with hypertension and diabetes mellitus found significantly lower subjective well-being for the former group (as measured by the Short Form 36 (SF-36)).[25] As these examples illustrate, however, there is a lack of research relating objective medical outcomes to different reimbursement structures. Thus, although anecdotes have been widely reported, conclusive evidence that managed care yields poor health outcomes is sparse.

Alternatively, the emphasis in some managed care organizations (e.g. many HMOs) on traditional preventive medicine (e.g. cancer screening, immunizations, coronary artery disease risk factor screening) may improve long-term outcomes (although the cost effectiveness of these efforts is in dispute). In addition, lack of access to specialty care in acute situations may offset any potential gains due to traditional prevention efforts. Despite the increased scrutiny of providers, neither traditional nor newer managed-care approaches currently offer objective measures of quality of outcomes. However, NCQA and JCAHO are beginning to incorporate outcomes management in their accreditation requirements.[11]

These and other assumptions of managed care are shown below:

- no adverse outcomes as a result of UM and UR;
- excess quality in the system;
- physicians are ethical and not influenced by money;
- primary is better than specialty care;
- less technology is better than more technology;
- primary care is better than urgent care, which is better than emergency care;
- specialists are more expensive than primary care physicians;
- adherence to explicit standards results in quality, i.e. ensures good outcomes;
- provide explicit standards and compliance will follow;
- good providers can be distinguished from bad providers in terms of utilization and quality;
- more utilization is bad and less is good;
- case mix can be safely ignored in setting capitation rates and in comparing providers or provider groups despite differences in severity of illness.

In summary, health care delivery is experiencing a comprehensive transition in methods of provider reimbursement and this has created administrative complexities for patients and their physicians. The primary impact occurs when the financing of care changes from fee-for-service to full risk capitation. Managed care attempts to provide appropriate care by instituting administrative processes to reduce overutilization (UM, UR) and processes to prevent underutilization (QA, QI). Organizations and individual physicians have experienced a dramatic change in incentives to see and treat patients based on reimbursement issues. Since the financial incentives to physicians are changing, the question as to whether patient outcomes are better, worse, or no different, based on whether a physician or physician group is paid per case or per member per month has been the subject of recent debate. The question has not been answered definitively. Surprisingly, we have little data concerning the a priori decision making of the physician and the linking of these decisions to patients' medical outcomes.

AN ALTERNATIVE FRAMEWORK

As our discussion indicates, there are obstacles to meeting patients' needs in delivery systems with capitated managed care. Administrators, physicians, and patients require data to navigate these new trends in health care delivery. Administrators need input to deliver cost-effective and efficient care in order to compete in managed care markets. Physicians need information to improve decision making and accountability. Patients need information to help them choose quality health plans and reassurance that their physician is their advocate. A framework that leads to appropriate operational research will facilitate efforts to meet these needs.

In the framework that we propose, clinical decisions that are associated with disease processes are assessed and ultimately linked to patient outcomes. Disease processes consist of a series of clinical events and decisions across related episodes of care, from which outcomes are derived[26] (see Fig. 36.1). Knowledge of those processes allows outcomes to be explained and predicted. The nature of the outcomes determines health care costs and quality.

The framework is designed to improve health care by analyzing the practice of medicine with the highest quality as the ideal. We define quality as the best medical decision and the best implementation of this decision.[27] The framework uses information management to relate clinical decisions to patient outcomes. Information management facilitates the measurement and interpretation of both clinical decision making (e.g. clinical assessments and plans) and administrative processes (e.g. UM and QI). The result is a description of the relationships among provider characteristics, patient characteristics, delivery-system characteristics, and patient outcomes (all of which bear on cost and quality). With this description, we can develop tools, such as computer software, to improve areas of deficiency in decisions and in their implementation. Therefore, our objectives include improved measurement, prediction, and intervention without the obtrusive administrative burden of current models of managed care.

Clinical decision making

The current emphasis on assessment of outcomes is a predictable consequence of the increasing scrutiny of medicine. Rising costs and putative 'overtreatment' have been used to justify oversight by business entities, as well as governmental, accrediting, and other regulatory agencies. Outcomes assessment addresses this desire for accountability. Theoretically, public and private expenditures can be rationally traded off against improvements in outcomes. The impact of changes in utilization management can be gauged so that underutilization is avoided. Thus, outcomes assessment can provide an empirical foundation for health care policies, both public and private.

In order to affect medical outcomes, however, it is necessary to understand how they are generated. Medical outcomes are the result of decisions made by patients and physicians in the context of available alternatives.

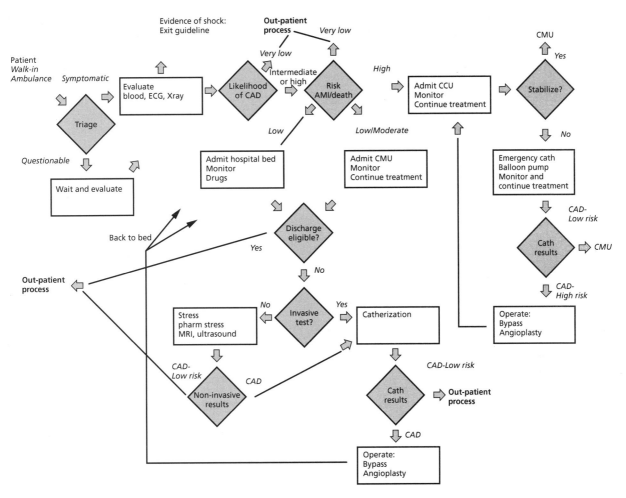

Figure 36.1 *In-patient chest pain process flow. AMI = acute myocardial infarction; CAD = coronary artery disease; Cath = catheterization; CCU = cardiovascular intensive care unit; CMU = cardiac monitoring unit (telemetry); ECG = electrocardiogram; MRI = magnetic resonance imaging; Pharm = pharmacological.*

One way to change medical outcomes, therefore, is to change the available alternatives, for instance, through advances in clinical research or reforms in government policy. The other way to change outcomes – the option that is of greater relevance in this chapter – is through changes in medical decision making.

Indeed, prior research has indicated that 'approximately 80% of health-care costs are associated with physician decision making'.[28] Of course, clinical outcomes are also directly influenced by physicians' decisions. Thus, physicians' decisions are a fundamental unit of analysis in evaluating costs and quality of care. Fortunately, an extensive and empirically grounded research literature exists regarding decision making.[29–32] That literature provides guidance about how the quality of decision making can be rigorously judged, and it contradicts some of the assumptions of the industrial model of quality control (as discussed later).

Moreover, medical outcomes cannot be interpreted in the absence of information about decision making. As is well known, good outcomes can be achieved in spite of

poor medicine, and vice versa. The science of decision analysis offers concepts and techniques, used for decades in other fields, that provide a principled basis for judgments about human performance. In general, decision analysis does not impose particular beliefs or values on decision makers, but it does allow them (and others) to judge whether their decisions are consistent with those beliefs and values and with the laws of logic and probability.

Decision analysis can, for example, help physicians select an appropriate diagnostic threshold for breast cancer screening, one that reflects the relative frequency of occurrence of breast cancer and the 'benefits and costs, respectively, of correct and incorrect decisions'.[32] If physicians believe that failing to detect breast cancer is worse than falsely detecting it, their threshold for screening should be low. A low threshold, or lenient criterion, means that more true positives would be detected (at the expense of more false positives). However, the base rate of the positive condition should also influence the screening threshold. When the condition is common, a low threshold will correctly yield many positive decisions. When the condition is relatively rare, as in the case of breast cancer among women in their 40s, a low threshold will yield many false positives. At the level of clinical decision making, matters are further complicated by the need to incorporate risk factors that alter a priori probabilities for individual patients. The precise implications of clinical decisions may not be fully appreciated without a formal analysis of their potential consequences.

On the other hand, such formal analysis would not be warranted if the benefits to clinical practice were minimal. However, research has amply demonstrated that actual medical decisions can deviate considerably from formal prescriptions.[27,31] A host of systematic biases in information processing have been demonstrated in physicians, including difficulties in incorporating the key base rates noted above into judgments of risk and probability. These findings do not imply that most medical decisions are biased. On the contrary, research has also indicated that human information-processing strategies are generally adaptive.[33–36] It does suggest, however, that when deviations occur, they are likely to be widespread among physicians and to occur automatically and unconsciously. Decision analysis can be used to make these biases explicit.[37]

Decision analysis, then, indicates what the parameters of ideal decision making should be, and it can be used to evaluate actual decision making. In this view, variability in decision making is expected. Surprisingly, some of that variability is principled and, thus, defensible. If, for example, two physicians disagree about the a priori probability of disease, and both probability estimates are consistent with the research literature (or the absence of research), as long as their decision processes are internally coherent, they should not be faulted. Box 36.1 provides a detailed presentation of such a case. As we have seen, however, other kinds of variability indicate biases and cannot be logically defended. Decision analysis makes it possible to discriminate good from bad variability.

The applicability of decision analysis to the development of health care policies and to the establishment of system-wide clinical protocols is, in principle, straightforward. Guidelines concerning the ordering of diagnostic or screening tests, for example, should reflect deliberate choices about tradeoffs among base rates and different kinds of decision errors. Multiple tests should be minimized on the basis of their informativeness, providing superior information to physicians while reducing costs. Utilization management and quality improvement should be consistent with rational constraints on decision making. If such guidelines and protocols were developed, health care systems could then focus on effectively implementing coherent policies. Although these changes are feasible at the system level, there are reasons to believe that the ideal of decision analysis is difficult to implement at the level of individual decision makers.

Consider our earlier analysis of breast cancer screening. Balancing the factors involved in a decision to order a screening mammogram in a 45-year-old woman is cognitively complex. As noted, that process is fraught with reasoning biases that have little to do with level of knowledge or training.[31,33] If we assumed that human information processing is analogous to machine computation, then we would design tools and interventions that helped physicians process more information more thoroughly and more quantitatively.[38] However, recent research indicates that human reasoning is primarily qualitative.[33–36] Qualitative reasoning has been shown to underlie judgment and decision making even in quantitatively sophisticated populations, such as statisticians.[31] In fact, increasing the detail and precision of thinking has been shown to increase human error.[39] Reasoning seems to compensate for weaknesses in verbatim memory and processing by relying on intuitive gist-like mental representations of information. Thus, it is impractical to assume that physicians will base day-to-day decisions on formal analysis, and errors might be exacerbated if they did.

Research also shows, however, that interventions can be designed that are compatible with humans' intuitive decision making and that improve performance. Thus, realistic proposals to affect physicians' decisions must include research that provides insight into the measurement and interpretation of cognitive processes, as well as into how these processes affect systemic aspects of health care delivery. Our framework is designed to capitalize on such research, especially about intuitive decision processes, and to translate it into recommendations for practice.

Some progress has been made without an awareness of the research in this area, however. Based on efforts to teach formal decision analysis, observers have concluded that this kind of analysis is time consuming and not likely to be readily embraced by physicians. Decision analysis techniques, which are based on Bayes' theorem and other probabilistic models, may predict patient outcomes acceptably but these techniques may not be incorporated into clinical decision making at the individual patient encounter because of predictable cognitive barriers. For example, empirical evidence exists that humans make systematic errors when information is presented in different, though equivalent, formats.[40,41] This leads to questions that are not addressed in decision analysis alone, but that concern those cognitive characteristics of decision makers that determine decisions and, therefore, patient outcomes.

Implications of the framework for managed care

Although biases are somewhat disturbing, cognitive research also has the potential to lead to important interventions that may improve patient outcomes by improving the decision making of providers. In addition, a framework that incorporates the important aspects of human decision making is likely to lead to better health care delivery systems. Unlike many industrial products like a computer chip, our patients' health care may never be standardized, even with ideal non-variable implementation processes, because of the relative unpredictable nature of biologic systems and the inherent and appropriate variability in human decision making.

In the industrial model of quality improvement, the process, not individuals, is the object of interest. The variability of outcomes is measured as a performance indicator. In our framework, in contrast, the decision processes of individuals must be taken into account and these are seen as a source of outcomes. As we have

discussed, diagnosis and management in many clinical scenarios results in practice variability. The industrial assumptions about variability may hold in, for example, well-defined surgical procedures and pre- and post-surgical management[8] but, in other areas, such as evaluating patients with chest pain, variability is likely to be refractory.

Using the industrial model, health care systems are attempting to measure practice variability, as well as physician productivity and patient outcomes. The example in Box 36.1 illustrates the difficulty of these tasks. If the administrators of an emergency room (ER) had a guideline which placed the patient in Box 36.1 at high/intermediate risk and the emergency physician discharged the patient to home, the hospital may believe the physician is in error. Conversely, if the guideline rated the patient as low/intermediate and the ER physi-

---

Box 36.1 *An example of decision making in clinical cardiology*

Clinical scenario
Two physicians are discussing a patient that was evaluated in the emergency room recently for a chief complaint of chest pain. Ms G. is a 49-year-old premenopausal female who reported sharp chest pain under her left breast and radiating to her left arm. The pain occurred while running the cash register at her business and has re-occurred on exertion and at rest. The pain resolved after taking her husband's nitroglycerin. On evaluation Ms G. has hypertension treated with a calcium-channel blocker, she smokes one pack of cigarettes per day and has for 20 years, her cholesterol is 180 mg/dL, her triglycerides are normal and high-density lipoprotein is 55. She has no history of diabetes. Her mother died at the age of 72 of an acute myocardial infarction. The emergency room physician, after noting that the electrocardiogram was normal and Ms G's physical examination was non-diagnostic, placed Ms G. on aspirin and a nitroglycerin patch, and sent her to the medicine out-patient clinic for further evaluation and management of possible unstable angina.

Clinical impressions of physician A and physician B
Physician A acknowledges there is some risk but believes it to be low. Physician B is concerned that Ms G. is at high risk for acute coronary syndrome. When asked to quantify their subjective probability estimates, physician A reports 30% or less and physician B reports 80% or more. Which physician is correct? What is the correct test to order: an exercise tolerance test (ETT), stress sestamibi or thallium, dipyridimole sestamibi, dobutamine echo, positron emission tomography scan, cardiac catheterization? An important point is that both physicians may be correct based on published data on prevalence of coronary artery disease.[47–50]

Diagnostic test ordered
The physicians agree that an ETT is the appropriate next step. Ms G. achieved 85% of expected heart rate and exercised for a total of 12 minutes with no ST or T-wave abnormalities noted. Physician A is satisfied but physician B is not, and is considering a nuclear stress test or possibly a cardiac catheterization. Which physician is correct?

Examination of positive and negative predictive values
Based on their a priori probability estimates, the negative predictive value of an ETT for physician A would be above 85%; however, for physician B it is below 45%. (Given a positive test the predictive values would be just the reverse: 46% for physician A and 89% for physician B.) When examining these numbers, we may begin to see that both physicians have evidence to support their point of view. The ETT was a good test for physician A because of the relatively high negative predictive value (given physician A's a priori probability). However, physician B is not so sure given the relatively low negative predictive value (given physician B's a priori probability). For this physician the correct initial test may have been a stress sestamibi, stress echo, or a cardiac catheterization. For example, the negative predictive value would approach 80% for the stress sestamibi, and if the test were negative, the physician may have more confidence in the result. This example is illustrative of the range in possible pretest probabilities given present clinical research.

Assumptions analyzed
This example illustrates physicians' use of probability calculations to order diagnostic tests, which is possible but not very probable. In fact, there may be systematic bias in the subjective estimates of pretest probabilities and there are likely to be systematic errors in interpretation of diagnostic tests. This has been demonstrated in cognitive research, and empirically confirmed in medical decision making, and may have profound effects on patient outcomes.

cian admitted the patient the physician would also be considered in error. The clinic physician who orders a stress sestamibi may be considered an overutilizer because he did not order the cheaper exercise tolerance test (ETT) when in fact the sestamibi may be the appropriate test given the physician's a priori risk estimate.[31] This expected and appropriate variability, if unaccounted for, could lead to administrative rules that produce systematically worse patient outcomes in terms of both cost and quality.

The example in Box 36.1 can also be used to illustrate the linking of physician decision making and utilization of clinical resources. Measuring appropriate utilization, then, depends not only on patient characteristics but on decision making characteristics.

There are three standard ways to evaluate decisions.[42] One is to compare the decision to some externally derived standard such as a guideline. Preferably the guideline has been validated empirically with at least a preponderance of strong evidence, such as medical outcomes, to support it. Another method would be to compare decision makers – that is, to compare one physician's decisions to that of the group (the so-called 'consensus' method or 'standard of care'). A third would be to evaluate the decision based on internal coherence, which is a minimal expectation that a decision maker agrees with his or her own estimations of risk.

Implementation of the decision

In our framework, quality of care includes decision making and the implementation of the decision. Implementation of a decision as part of a traditional quality improvement methodology involves improving performance of the delivery system's administration of services. This kind of industrial model is now commonly employed in health care delivery. Efficiency and effectiveness in terms of customer satisfaction have been the targets of NCQA and JCAHO, as well as numerous re-engineering efforts of health care delivery systems.[43] Important components of these efforts are that the health care organizations employing these methods must measure efficiency, effectiveness, and cost appropriately. Again, variability is the key to most quality improvement efforts with the assumption being that reducing variability will lead to higher quality.

Our framework also incorporates measures of efficiency and effectiveness, and of customer satisfaction. However, in our view, efficiency and effectiveness must be tied to clinical indicators of quality of care. Health care systems should be judged by the timeliness and accuracy with which they implement the best medical decisions. Those aspects of customer satisfaction that are more closely tied with good patient outcomes should

receive greater weight. Evaluations of administrative systems' delivery of services should be based on reliable data that is appropriately analyzed so that it accurately reflects cost and quality. For example, the evaluation of an electronic medical record should not depend solely on case histories from other institutions or on a site visit at which anecdotes about effectiveness are traded. Instead, performance should be assessed by such measures as the time taken for encounters before versus after adoption, or the availability of chart information and its effect on adherence to clinical guidelines. Thus, our framework includes measurement of the performance of providers and of the systemic aspects of health care delivery. To employ the framework, accurate indicators of cost and quality must be analyzed, such as patient outcomes. The framework takes into account patient outcomes and links these outcomes to patient and provider characteristics.

In summary, the framework allows analysis of the relationships between cost and quality. Specifically, the framework is designed to facilitate the ability of health care systems to:

1 provide measurably appropriate care to patients;
2 generate reliable estimates of costs and accurate measures of quality;
3 establish contracts that are outcomes-based, thereby shifting the emphasis from care at the lowest cost to the lowest-cost best care provided;
4 identify, collect, and analyze the data needed to provide information, ensuring (1), (2), and (3), above;
5 obtain the tools to perform (4) above, that will facilitate cost and quality improvements.

Application of the framework to clinical practice

Consider how points (1)–(5) are reflected in gatekeeping. Physicians, physician assistants, and nurse practitioners all see patients and are referred to as providers in managed care plans. As described above, in many instances the plans encourage a gatekeeper system. The primary care provider then is responsible for referring patients to specialists, and for special examinations such as magnetic resonance imaging, positron emission tomography, sestamibi, cardiac catheterization, physical therapy, etc. Several questions have been raised about this system including: is quality reduced, improved, or no different from standard fee-for-service; are primary care providers diagnosing and managing patients more efficiently; are fewer patients receiving high-technology care; does the physician reimbursement scheme influence ordering behavior; and are patient outcomes affected?

According to the framework, these questions could be addressed by studying providers as gatekeepers and comparing their decision making to non-gatekeeper providers. Disease processes could be mapped across episodes of care for different providers using information systems to track related episodes. After measuring the provider's decisions, the effect of decision making on outcomes can be assessed. To accomplish this, we must link disease-specific patient episodes of care and measure the clinical and cost outcomes.

As an illustration of how such a framework would apply in practice, consider a patient, Mr Jones, a 77-year-old member of a senior care HMO. He began experiencing substernal chest pressure that awoke him from sleep. It went away with three sublingual nitroglycerin spaced 5 minutes apart. The next morning Mr Jones called his primary care provider's (PCP) office. He was transferred to the triage nurse in the PCP's clinic who advised Mr Jones to go to the emergency room. Upon arrival at the emergency room, the physician evaluates Mr Jones and makes a determination of risk of coronary artery disease and of the possibility of acute myocardial infarction. She may decide to admit Mr Jones or discharge Mr Jones with out-patient follow-up. She also may decide to order diagnostic tests. If she admits Mr Jones, she may order a cardiac intensive care, telemetry, or regular ward bed.

Assume that she sent Mr Jones home with instructions to follow-up with his PCP. Mr Jones calls to get an appointment and is told that his PCP's next available appointment is in 2 months. He tells the scheduler that he needs an earlier appointment and is transferred to the clinic triage nurse who schedules a same-day or urgent-care visit with another doctor. (Mr Jones's doctor has no available slots.) When Mr Jones is seen in the clinic, his chart is unavailable but the physician assesses Mr Jones, who has had two similar episodes in the last 2 days. The physician decides to add a calcium-channel blocker and writes a referral for an ETT. He also tells Mr Jones to make an appointment with his PCP. Mr Jones leaves the clinic with instructions to call back 'in a few days' to see if the ETT is approved and to schedule the test. He is given an appointment with his PCP (to be seen in 2 months).

How can the framework help identify whether appropriate decisions were made? First, we identify all of the medical decision makers: the triage nurse, the emergency physician, the urgent-care physician (note that the PCP may or may not be aware of the situation). Were appropriate decisions made? Were the decisions implemented appropriately? What is the patient's expected outcome(s)? The patient may be at high, intermediate, or low risk of death or acute myocardial infarction, and he may have high, intermediate, or low likelihood of coronary artery disease. Clinical decision makers estimate these probabilities, if only implicitly. We can expect that if he is at high risk of acute myocardial infarction and he is not admitted to the hospital with unstable angina he is at increased risk of poor outcome(s).

In addition, an elderly person negotiating through this process may have difficulty complying with the requests for a 'call back in a few days'. Given that decisions were made without the benefit of a chart, did the patient's memory serve him well enough to recall medications or past work-ups?[44] Did the patient's providers have access to alternate forms of information, such as shadow charts or automated information? Did the providers caring for the patient page the PCP and discuss the case? Was the referral processed and approved efficiently? Was an appropriate appointment made for the ETT? Were the results conveyed to one of the patient's providers? Was the calcium-channel blocker on the HMO's formulary?

Databases and information management

The above example is meant to serve as 'grist for the mill' in forming hypotheses that the framework can test. The data gathering, analysis, and linkage, i.e. operational research, requires sophisticated information systems. The technical capability is present to perform these tasks but they have yet to be tested. With the framework in mind, two questions should be asked of any information system. Does the technology improve clinical decision making? Does it improve implementation of the decision? A database that was formed as a result of this operational research would be valuable in forming contracts. Because such a database would link episodes of care (e.g. from emergency room to out-patient clinic to the cardiac stress testing laboratory), it would contain the key information for predictions in terms of cost and quality.

For example, HMOs may be considering contracting with a multispecialty physician group and hospital for all chest pain service. A disease management strategy could be seen as a way to improve economic efficiency. In order to manage the contract well, the physician group should collect data on presentation to the emergency room that allows the prediction of cost and quality over the following year. The physician group then can negotiate from a much better position when determining whether the HMO's capitation rate is advantageous. The HMO will be interested in such data as well because this will quantify any cost-quality gaps that may be real or perceived, and could help improve the HMO's market share.

The electronic medical record is touted as having solutions to many of the problems we have discussed.[7,38] Unfortunately, empirical evidence of its utility is sparse. There are, however, reports of success with certain processes such as order entry and hospital management. A major issue is the shift in emphasis from hospital to out-patient care. Many of the out-patient systems are only months from initial testing in actual clinical environments. Order entry systems have been shown to improve physician compliance with minimal standards of quality.[28] These systems also may be helpful in the referral management process but this remains untested as well.

Information systems should be compatible with human information processing, which research shows is intuitive, i.e. qualitative and gist-based. Therefore, large amounts of precise detail should be eschewed in favor of information displays that do not create confusion or information overload. Thus, an information system in the era of managed care should have the following characteristics:

- referral management;
- documentation capabilities that comply with practice standards;
- ability to manage and display order entry, and results of procedures, tests and evaluations;
- clinical assistance, such as dealing with multiple formularies;
- tools such as e-mail and access to information sources, such as Medline;
- implementation issues, such as maintenance and security, are known upfront;
- technical capabilities are consistent with an open architecture to ensure accurate and reliable reporting capabilities.

FUTURE DIRECTIONS

Implications for physicians in the emerging medical market place

Physicians are being asked to serve in a number of new roles in the emerging medical market place. For example, physicians will be serving on committees to develop clinical guidelines, establish policies for utilization management, review provider decisions regarding procedures, tests and evaluations, implement NCQA and JCAHO requirements, manage new delivery systems, reduce costs and re-engineer clinics and hospitals, select electronic medical records, and advise/consent on negotiated contracts. Using the framework described above, physicians can generate critical questions that will address the cost and quality implications of proposed changes. These questions fall into two categories: those concerning the physician–patient relationship, and the system-level operations.

In dealing with patients, physicians should ask whether their decisions are consistent with high-quality practice guidelines, peer groups, and the laws of logic and probability. The best decisions, however, will lead to poor outcomes if they are ineffectively implemented.

Therefore, physicians should demand that operational infrastructure, including information systems, facilitate implementation of their clinical decisions. Information systems, such as electronic medical records, hold promise since disease processes could be mapped from decisions across episodes of care to outcomes. Therefore, physicians must inquire about the capability of systems to perform these important linkages.

Physicians' input to operations will often occur in the context of their service on utilization management and quality improvement committees. In reviewing other physicians' decisions, the usual assumption is that variability is undesirable. Given the same patient, two physicians should reach the same decision. As an abstract ideal, this assumption is correct. However, uncertainty in the clinical literature and differences in experience (e.g. with different patient populations) justify some variability in judgments. By analyzing decision processes for internal coherence, this kind of justifiable variability can be identified. Thus, most diagnostic decisions are inherently uncertain. Simply providing protocols or guidelines cannot eliminate this uncertainty. Guidelines can play a useful role, however, in reducing uncertainty when combined with information about decision processes and patient outcomes. This 'three-legged stool' of guidelines, decision processes, and patient outcomes provides a foundation to measure quality of care. Appropriate utilization, then, depends not only on patient characteristics but also on decision-making characteristics.

As delivery systems seek to comply with accreditation and re-engineering efforts, physicians will be asked to help implement clinical components, and they can expect audits by internal and external reviewers. Quality standards that focus on service requirements should be distinguished from standards that have direct implications for clinical outcomes. For example, NCQA's requirements on timely appointments may be considered a direct indicator of clinical efficiency but an indirect indicator of clinical quality. That is, new patients who are not given appointments within a few weeks of the request (efficiency) should be distinguished from patients with high risk of coronary artery disease or high risk of acute myocardial infarction who are not admitted to the coronary intensive care unit (quality).

Concerns about quality have arisen because, with capitation, organizations have financial incentives to withhold care. In fact, incentives in managed care are often the mirror image of those in fee-for-service reimbursement where there are financial incentives to overtreat. The difficulty lies in determining whether over- or undertreatment has occurred. According to our framework, adherence to evidence-based guidelines is one indicator of decision-making quality. For example, a guideline might indicate that a patient should be admitted to a hospital but the patient was actually discharged and vice versa. Undertreatment would correspond to failure to admit (when indicated by the guideline) and overtreatment to unnecessary admission. In a fee-for-service system, failure to admit leads to a loss in revenue and unnecessary admissions may increase revenue. In a capitated system, failure to admit prevents short-term revenue loss. Unnecessary admissions, of course, are a financial loss. Therefore, although treatment of patients incurs costs in both systems, reimbursement incentives are different.

The obvious financial loss associated with failure to admit in fee-for-service systems may also apply to capitated systems, however. The long-term costs of undertreatment may outweigh any short-term gain. For example, a high-risk patient for acute coronary syndrome who is discharged from the emergency room inappropriately may develop an acute myocardial infarction leading to cardiogenic shock with placement of a balloon pump after admission to the cardiovascular intensive care unit (CCU). If the patient had been admitted on first presentation and received a cardiac catheterization with resultant percutaneous transluminal coronary angioplasty, the CCU admission would likely have been prevented. The cost of the CCU admission is assessed against the capitated budget as are any out-patient evaluations. These costs are frequently overlooked in capitated systems and may not be fully recovered in fee-for-service systems.[45] Thus, short-term decision making, and resultant cost shifting, should be discouraged to reduce overall health care costs.

Regardless of the health care system or reimbursement mechanisms, over- and undertreatment are indicative of poor quality. Health care organizations and policy makers should measure the frequency of these errors.[46] Their interpretation, however, requires a decision analytic framework that incorporates clinical outcomes. Such a framework provides explicit definitions of quality and empirical measures of errors. A scientific approach to understanding the cost of quality health care will allow policymakers to focus on those issues that are likely to have the greatest impact on patients.

SUMMARY

- The shift from a fee-for-service reimbursement system to capitation is changing the day-to-day practice of medicine, subjecting physicians to greater administrative oversight.
- Utilization management is used to conserve resources within a capitated budget; quality improvement is an industrial concept used to ensure that care does not fall below an acceptable standard.
- Protocols and guidelines are being developed in an attempt to standardize processes of care.

- Fundamental assumptions of managed care have yet to be tested including the tradeoffs involved in gatekeeping.
- An alternative framework is necessary that incorporates clinical information management and decision analysis to provide objective measures of performance for health care systems and practitioners.
- Quality of health care can be defined as the best medical decision and its best implementation.
- Guidelines, patient outcomes, and provider's decisions form the basis of quality measurement; outcome data are ambiguous without decision analysis.
- Clinical information systems can be used to link episodes of care, to generate reliable estimates of costs and accurate measures of quality, and to provide technological interventions that improve decision making.

AUTHOR NOTE

Preparation of this manuscript was supported in part by grants to both authors from the Academic Medicine and Managed Care Forum and the National Science Foundation (SBR973-0143) and to the second author from the National Institutes of Health (NIH P50 AT00003), US Department of Health and Human Services (HRSA 1D34MB02077-O1), and the US Department of Commerce (04-60-98039).

REFERENCES

1. Feldstein, Paul J. *Health care economics*, New York: Delmar Publishers, Inc., 1993.
2. Iglehart JK. The American health care system: managed care. *N Engl J Med* 1992; **327**: 742–7.
3. Franks P. Sounding board. Gatekeeping revisited – protecting patients from overtreatment. *N Engl J Med* 1992; **327**: 424–9.
4. Bailit H, Sennett C. Utilization management as cost containment strategy. *Health Care Financing Rev Ann Suppl* 1991.
5. Berwick DM. Health services research and quality of care. Assignments for the 1990s. *Med Care* 1989; **27**: 763–71.
6. Kuperman G, James B, *et al*. Continuous quality improvement applied to medical care: experiences at LDS Hospital. *Med Decision Making* 1991; **11**(suppl): S60–5.
7. Elson RB, Faughnan JG, Connelly DP. An industrial process view of information delivery to support clinical decision making: implications for systems design and process measures. *JAMA* 1997; **4**: 266–78.

8. Evan RS, Classen DC, Pestonik SL, Lundsgaarde HP, Burke JP. Improving empiric antibiotic selection using computer decision support. *Arch Intern Med* 1994; **154**: 878–84.

9. Corrigan JM, Nielsen DM. *Toward the development of uniform reporting standards for managed care organizations: the Health Plan Employer Data and Information Set Joint Commission on Quality Improvement* (Version 2.0). 1993 (Dec); **19**(12): 566–75.

10. Corrigan JM, Griffith H. NCQA external reporting and monitoring activities for health plans: preventive services programs. *Am J Prev Med* 1995; **11**: 393–6.

11. Campion FX, Rosenthall MS. Quality assurance and medical outcomes in the era of cost containment. *Surg Clinics North Am* 1996; **76**: 139–59.

12. Hanchak NA. Managed care, accountability, and the physician. *Med Clinics North Am* 1996; **80**: 245–61.

13. Brook RH. Practice guidelines and practicing medicine. Are they compatible? *JAMA* 1989; **262**: 3027–30.

14. Summary of the Second Report of the National Cholesterol Education Program (NCEP) Expert Panel on Detection, Evaluation and Treatment of High Blood Cholesterol in Adults (Adult Treatment Panel 11). *JAMA* 1993; **269**: 3015–23.

15. Weingarten SR, Riedinger MS, Conner L, *et al*. Practice guidelines and reminders to reduce duration of hospital stay for patients with chest pain. *Ann Intern Med* 1994; **120**: 257–63.

16. Van Amringe M, Shannon TE. Awareness, assimilation, and adoption: the challenge, dissemination, and the first AHCPR-sponsored guidelines, *Qual Rev Bull* 1992; **18**: 397–404.

17. Weingarten S. Practice guidelines and prediction rules should be subject to careful clinical testing. *JAMA* 1997; **277**: 1977–8.

18. Katz D, Griffith J, Beshansky J, Selker H. The use of empiric clinical data in the evaluation of practice guidelines for unstable angina. *JAMA* 1996; **276**: 1568–74.

19. Lloyd FJ, Reyna VF, Liebowitz RL, Valenzuela TD. Letter to the editor: The AHCPR unstable angina algorithm in practice. *JAMA* 1997; **12**: 961.

20. Pretzer M. The managed-care juggernaut: explosive growth nationwide. *Med Econ – Pediat Ed* 1996; May: 20–6.

21. Rosenberg S, Allen D, Handte J, *et al*. Effect of utilization review in a fee-for-service health insurance plan. *N Eng J Med* 1995; **333**: 1326–30.

22. Ubel P, DeKay M, Baron J, Asch D. Cost-effectiveness analysis in a setting of budget constraints. *N Engl J Med* 1996; **334**: 1174–7.

23. Schreiber TL, Elkhatib A, Grines CL, O'Neill WW. Cardiologist versus internist management of patients with unstable angina: treatment patterns and outcomes. *J Am Coll Cardiol* 1995; **26**: 577–82.

24. Jollis JG, Delong AR, Peterson ED, Mulbaier LH, Fortin DF, Califf RM, Mark DB. Outcome of acute myocardial infarction according to the specialty of the admitting physician. *N Engl J Med* 1996; **335**: 1880–7.

25. Greenfield S, Rogers W, Mangotich M, Carney M, Tarlov A. Outcomes of patients with hypertension and non-insulin dependent diabetes mellitus treated by different systems and specialties. Results from the Medical Outcomes Study. *JAMA* 1995; **274**: 1436–44.

26. Braunwald E, Mark DB, Jones RH, *et al*. Unstable angina: diagnosis and management. Clinical Practice Guideline no. 10 (amended) AHCPR Publication No. 94-0602. Rockville, MD: Agency for Health Care Policy and Research and the National Heart Lung and Blood Institute, Public Health Service, US Department of Health and Human Services, May 1994.

27. Eddy DM. *Clinical decision making from theory to practice*. Boston: Jones and Bartlet Publishers, 1996.

28. Tierney W, Miller ME, Overhage JM, McDonald CJ. Physician inpatient order writing on microcomputer workstations. Effects on resources utilization. *JAMA* 1993; **269**: 379–83.

29. Dawes RM. *Rational choice in an uncertain world*. San Diego: Harcourt Brace Jovanovich, 1995.

30. Fischhoff B, Lichtenstein S, Slovic P, Derby S, Keeney R. *Acceptable risk*. New York: Cambridge University Press, 1981.

31. Kahneman D, Slovic P, Tversky A. *Judgment under uncertainty: heuristics and biases*. New York: Cambridge University Press, 1982.

32. Swets JA. The science of choosing the right decision threshold in high-stakes diagnostics. *Am Psychol* 1992; **47**: 522–32.

○33. Reyna VF, Brainerd CJ. Fuzzy-trace theory: an interim synthesis. *Learning Individ Diff* 1995; **7**: 1–75.

34. Reyna VF, Brainerd CJ. The origins of probability judgment: a review of data and theories. In: Wright G, Ayton P, eds *Subjective probability*. New York: Wiley, 1994: 239–72.

35. Reyna VF, Brainerd CJ. Fuzzy memory and mathematics in the classroom. In: Davies GM, Logie RH, eds *Memory in everyday life*. Amsterdam: North Holland Press, 1993: 91–119.

○36. Reyna VF. Class inclusion, the conjunction fallacy, and other cognitive illusions. *Dev Rev* 1991; **11**: 317–36.

37. van Miltenburg-van Zijl AJM, Bossuyt PMM, Nette RW, Simoons ML, Taylor TR. Cardiologists' use of clinical information for management decisions for patients with unstable angina. *Med Decision Making* 1997; **17**: 292–7.

38. Shortliffe EH, Perreault LE. *Medical informatics: computer applications in health care*. New York: Addison-Wesley Publishing, 1990.

39. Reyna VF. Interference effects in memory and reasoning: a fuzzy-trace theory analysis. In: Dempster FN, Brainerd CJ, eds *Interference and inhibition in cognition*. San Diego, CA: Academic Press, 1995: 29–59.

♦40. Reyna VF, Brainerd CJ. Fuzzy-trace theory and framing

effects in choice: gist extraction, truncation, and conversion. *J Behav Decision Making* 1991; **4**: 249–62.

41. Tversky A, Kahneman D. The framing of decisions and the psychology of choice. *Science* 1981; **211**: 453–8.

42. Liberman V, Tversky A. On the evaluation of probability judgments: calibration, resolution, and monotonicity. *Psychol Bull* 1993; **114**: 162–73.

43. Evans JH, Hwang Y, Nagarajan NJ. Cost reduction and process reengineering in hospitals. *J Cost Manag* 1997; May/June: 20–7.

44. Reyna VF, Lloyd FJ. Theories of false memory in children and adults. *Learning Individ Diff* 1997; **9**: 95–123.

45. Schroeder S, Cantor J. On squeezing balloons. Cost control fails again. *N Engl J Med* 1991; **325**: 1099–100.

○46. Kohn LT, Corrigan JM, Donaldson MS. *To err is human: building a safer health system*. Washington, DC: National Academy Press, 2000.

47. Wenger NK, Speroff l, Packard B. Cardiovascular health and disease in women. *N Engl J Med* 1993; **329**: 247–56.

48. Pagley PR, Goldberg RJ. Coronary artery disease in women. A population-based perspective. *Cardiology* 1995; **86**: 265–9.

49. Douglas P, Ginsburg GS. The evaluation of chest pain in women. *N Engl J Med* 1996; **334**: 1311–15.

50. Diamond GA, Forrester JS. Analysis of probability as an aid in the diagnosis of coronary artery disease. *N Engl J Med* 1979; **300**: 1350–8.

37

Use of continuous quality improvement to increase utilization of proven therapies for acute myocardial infarction

JEFFREY I LEAVITT

Despite advances in our understanding of heart disease, fibrinolytic therapy, aspirin and β-blockers are underutilized. Barriers to optimal physician practice patterns include gender and age bias, lack of awareness of clinical trial data, perceived contraindications and side effects of therapy, and resistance to change. Traditional continuing medical education (CME) methods have little sustained impact on practice patterns. The development of a continuous quality improvement approach by institutions and managed care organizations is ideal for addressing systematic barriers to quality of care. A variety of methods including new CME approaches, practice guidelines, critical pathways, outcomes reporting and computerized decision support systems may be used successfully to modify physician practice patterns.

MANAGEMENT OF ACUTE MYOCARDIAL INFARCTION: HISTORICAL LANDMARKS

Coronary heart disease (CHD) is the leading cause of death in the USA, accounting for approximately one-quarter of all deaths annually. Each year, acute myocardial infarction (AMI) strikes about 1.5 million people in the USA, of which 500 000 will die. The estimated annual economic cost due to AMI, including health care expenditures and loss of productivity, is approximately $70 billion.[1,2]

The CHD mortality rate has steadily declined over the past three decades, especially in the latter half of the 1980s, when age-adjusted mortality from AMI decreased by 25–35 per cent in the USA, Canada, and Europe.[3-7] A similar pattern has been described in the elderly.[8] Improvements in acute coronary care and primary and secondary prevention have all played a role in the decline in AMI mortality. Much of the decline, especially in recent years, is attributable to recognition of the importance of aspirin, thrombolytic therapy and β-blockade in the management of AMI.

The main goals of therapy for AMI are improved survival, prevention of complications, and improved symptoms and quality of life. In the acute phase, these goals are mediated in large part by limitation of infarct size. This is achieved by improving coronary blood supply to the infarct zone (addressed via fibrinolysis or angioplasty, aspirin, glycoprotein IIb/IIIa platelet receptor antagonists, and heparin) and reducing myocardial oxygen demand (using β-blockade, nitroglycerin, and angiotensin-converting enzyme inhibitors). In the recovery phase after AMI, therapy is guided toward secondary prevention of recurrent events.

The many large randomized trials of therapy for AMI conducted in the last two decades have provided a solid foundation upon which to practice evidence-based medicine. While use of appropriate agents has improved, however, proven therapies for AMI are still significantly underutilized. Greater use of these modalities would have a major impact on AMI mortality and its associated economic and social costs.

MANAGEMENT OF AMI: PHYSICIAN PRACTICE PATTERNS

Many studies have shown that usage of recommended therapy for AMI is increasing, but a significant segment of the AMI population are still not being treated appropriately. In this chapter, the available utilization data will be reviewed for certain key agents, with outcomes data when possible. Data regarding use of pharmacologic agents in AMI have been obtained from population-based studies, administrative databases, randomized trial registries, and prospective surveys of AMI admissions.

Fibrinolytic therapy

The first large randomized controlled trial documenting a survival benefit with the use of fibrinolytic therapy was published in 1986.[9] Understandably, utilization of thrombolysis was low at that time, ranging from 5 per cent of AMI patients in Canada[4] to 24 per cent in a European population-based study,[5] which focused on patients less than 65 years of age. By the early 1990s, thrombolytic usage increased to 26–45 per cent of all patients with AMI,[3–5,10–14] an important factor in the rapid decline in AMI mortality in this time period (as noted above). The utilization rate is now similar among most developed nations.

These figures indicate, however, that the majority of AMI patients are still not treated with fibrinolytic therapy. The proportion estimated to be eligible for treatment with fibrinolysis or primary angioplasty (i.e. those with symptoms for less than 12 hours, electrocardiographic (ECG) ST segment elevation or new bundle branch block, and no contraindications) ranges from 30 to 55 per cent.[13–15] The primary reasons for non-eligibility include delayed presentation and lack of ECG criteria; only 2–7 per cent of patients possess definite contraindications to therapy.[13,14] The 'shortfall' or proportion of untreated eligible patients without a clear reason for withholding treatment has been estimated to be 20 per cent of the AMI population, or 36 per cent of eligible patients.[13] Other studies report that 72–88 per cent of eligible patients appropriately received fibrinolytic therapy.[14–16] Importantly, among eligible patients, those receiving thrombolytic therapy have a significantly lower unadjusted mortality rate than untreated patients.[14,16]

The most important predictor of non-use of fibrin-olytics is advanced age;[13,15–17] other undertreated populations include women[13,16,17] and blacks.[17] Thrombolysis is of proven benefit in the elderly, and its use in this population is recommended by current guidelines.[18] In an effort to improve the quality of care provided to elderly patients with AMI, the Health Care Financing Administration (HCFA) developed the Cooperative Cardiovascular Project (CCP), which profiles patterns of medical care provided to Medicare beneficiaries. In the CCP pilot study, involving more than 16 000 patients, only 10 per cent of patients were considered eligible for fibrinolytic therapy, and 70 per cent of these patients were treated.[19] This study used overly strict exclusion criteria, however (e.g. symptoms greater than 6 hours). Using criteria more reflective of current guidelines, Krumholz et al. examined a subset of 3093 CCP patients and found that 24 per cent were eligible for fibrinolytic therapy, and only 44 per cent of eligible patients were treated.[20] These figures are far lower than those noted above for the overall myocardial infarction (MI) population. This pattern of underuse in the elderly is noted routinely in studies of fibrinolytic usage, although few studies have identified the proportion eligible for treatment. Again, eligible patients who received fibrinolytic therapy had a lower mortality rate than untreated eligible patients (14.7 per cent vs 20.5 per cent).[20] The First National Registry of Myocardial Infarction (NRMI-1), a prospective registry involving more than 1000 US hospitals and over 240 000 patients, found that age greater than 75 years was the reason cited for not administering fibrinolytic therapy in 20 per cent of subjects.[11]

Time to treatment with fibrinolytic therapy

The efficacy of fibrinolytic therapy in improving survival from AMI is closely linked to the delay between symptom onset and initiation of the fibrinolytic agent. This time period has been divided into two phases: the time from symptom onset to hospital arrival (pre-hospital phase) and the time from hospital arrival to initiation of thrombolysis ('door-to-needle time'). The greatest delay is routinely the pre-hospital phase. Among NRMI-1 subjects, the median pre-hospital time was 130 minutes; the median door-to-needle time was 57 minutes.[11] Reported pre-hospital time intervals are variable; a coronary care unit (CCU)-based US study[10] and the Canadian Global Utilization of Streptokinase and Tissue Plasminogen Activator for Occluded Coronary Arteries (GUSTO-1) investigators[21] reported shorter times, and a French intensive care unit survey[22] reported a median pre-hospital time of 250 minutes. In a prospective survey of CCUs in New Zealand, French et al. found that 14.4 per cent of AMI patients met ECG criteria for thrombolysis but presented greater than 12 hours after symptom onset.[14] Similarly, a European population-based study reported that 20 per cent of patients presented after 12 hours.[13] One reason for this delay is inadequate knowledge of heart attack symptoms, as shown in a recent population survey.[23] These findings are important in that they represent a possible avenue for improving access to fibrinolytic therapy. However, prior attempts at reducing the delay in hospital presentation have met with limited success.[24]

Hospitals have focused primarily on reducing door-to-needle time, over which they have more control. The median door-to-needle time in most studies is about 1 hour; hospitals have had some success in reducing this time, although limited published data are available.[25] The National Heart Attack Alert Program (NHAAP) has identified three critical time intervals, which together comprise door-to-needle time: 'door-to-data' (time interval from hospital arrival until first ECG is obtained), 'data-to-decision' (the time taken for physician to order thrombolysis after obtaining ECG), and 'decision-to-drug' (time from physician order to initiation of fibrinolytic infusion). The NHAAP has recommended that hospitals monitor their own door-to-needle time and use continuous quality improvement techniques to reduce them; the optimal door-to-needle time has been identified as less than 30 minutes.[26] Only 23 per cent of NRMI-1 subjects received fibrinolytic therapy within 30 minutes.[25]

The major predictors of delay in hospital presentation and door-to-needle time are female gender[10,21,25,27,28] and advanced age.[25] For unclear reasons, women present about 30 minutes later after symptom onset than do men.[27,28] An NRMI-1 report found that door-to-data, door-to-decision, and overall door-to-needle times were all significantly longer in women.[28] Of note, Rosamond et al. found an improvement in both pre-hospital delay (by 17 minutes) and door-to-needle time (by 20 minutes) in women from 1990–1991 to 1992–1993, achieving a time to treatment equivalent to that of men in 1992–1993.[10] The median door-to-needle time was 72 minutes in the elderly CCP subjects; only 11 per cent of patients given fibrinolytic agents received them within 30 minutes of hospital arrival.[19]

Aspirin

When administered within the first 24 hours of AMI, aspirin reduces short-term mortality by 23 per cent and non-fatal reinfarction by 49 per cent.[29] This agent is also highly effective in reducing late cardiac events. The use of aspirin in AMI is extremely cost effective, with cost estimates as low as $13 per life saved.[30] Despite its efficacy, low cost and excellent safety profile, however, usage rates in AMI are suboptimal. NRMI-1 data show that 70 per cent of AMI patients receive aspirin, with a higher rate (84 per cent) in patients receiving thrombolytic therapy.[11] Other studies have reported higher in-hospital aspirin usage, ranging from 81 to 89 per cent.[3–5,22] While

in-hospital administration rates may be reasonable, only 45 per cent of patients with AMI received aspirin in the emergency department (ED) in one report.[31] This may be clinically relevant given the importance of early treatment, the diagnostic uncertainty in a significant proportion of patients, and the efficacy of aspirin in reducing cardiac event rates in patients with unstable angina as well as AMI.

At least 70–80 per cent of patients are eligible for aspirin use in the acute phase, and only 4–5 per cent possess absolute contraindications to its use (active bleeding or allergy).[15,32] In the CCP population, only 58 per cent were said to be eligible for aspirin use upon hospital discharge, however.[19] Patients over 75 years of age who are otherwise eligible for aspirin treatment are 60 per cent less likely to be treated than are younger patients.[15] In another CCP report, Krumholz et al. found that 64 per cent of eligible elderly patients were treated within 48 hours of onset of AMI.[32] Treated patients had a mortality rate of 14 per cent, while untreated patients had a mortality rate of 24 per cent. After adjusting for multiple variables, aspirin use was associated with 22 per cent lower odds of 30-day mortality. The investigators estimated that giving aspirin to all eligible elderly patients with AMI would save more than 3000 lives each year in the USA.[32]

One reason for undertreatment is lack of awareness of the available data. Ayanian et al. reported that only about half of internists and three-fourths of cardiologists surveyed believed that aspirin definitely improves short- or long-term survival after AMI.[33] These results highlight the need for improved communication of the findings of clinical trials to community physicians so that they may incorporate these findings into practice.

β-Blockers

Long-term administration of oral β-blockers after AMI has clear benefits, reducing overall mortality by 22 per cent and reinfarction by 27 per cent.[34] Despite this evidence, which has been available since at least the mid-1980s, only about only 30–50 per cent of patients receive β-blockers post-MI.[3,4,11,17,35] Two major barriers to care are lack of awareness of clinical trial results, as noted above,[33] and the many perceived contraindications to these agents. Indeed, the proportion of patients reported to have potential contraindications to β-blockers ranges from 19 to 70 per cent depending on the exclusion criteria used.[15,35–37] The available data, however, do not support the contention that β-blockers should be avoided in many of these conditions (e.g. diabetes mellitus, peripheral vascular disease, and left ventricular dysfunction).[38,39] For instance, patients with AMI complicated by congestive heart failure derive a greater benefit from β-blockade than do those without heart failure.[40] Indeed, a report from the CCP database demonstrated that β-blockers reduce mortality to a similar degree in all patient subgroups, including those with perceived contraindications.[39]

Among eligible patients without any of the above perceived contraindications, only about 40–50 per cent receive β-blockade,[15,35] even when treated by a cardiologist.[36] As with aspirin and thrombolytic therapy, the populations undertreated with β-blockers include women and the elderly.[15,17] Soumerai et al. studied β-blocker usage in over 5000 New Jersey Medicare patients with prior AMI and found that only 21 per cent of eligible patients were treated with β-blockers in the 90-day period following AMI. Furthermore, after controlling for other predictors of mortality, treatment of eligible patients with β-blockers resulted in a 43 per cent lower mortality rate compared to untreated eligible patients.[37] A larger study from the CCP using somewhat different eligibility criteria reported that 50 per cent of eligible patients were discharged on β-blockers, with an adjusted 14 per cent lower risk of mortality at 1 year.[41] It has been estimated that increased usage of β-blockers in infarct survivors would save over 3000 lives per year in the USA.[42]

CONTINUOUS QUALITY IMPROVEMENT: THEORY AND PRACTICE

Up to this point, I have focused on potential areas for improvement in the care of the post-myocardial infarction patient (Table 37.1), providing evidence for improved outcomes if optimal practice patterns can be achieved. The remainder of this chapter will address how this improvement may be achieved.

Historical landmarks and development

Traditionally, perceived deficiencies in quality of care have been addressed by peer review organizations (PROs). PROs responded to complaints regarding care provided by an individual practitioner or institution, investigated the matter, and instituted sanctions as necessary. This model thus addressed problems retrospectively, on a case-by-case or 'hunt and peck' approach. In the late 1980s, HCFA and the state-based PROs that contracted with HCFA began to publicly report hospital- and diagnosis-specific mortality rates, with crude adjustments for co-morbid conditions. Historically, however, systematic evaluation of quality of care indicators, such as outcomes, processes of care (e.g. prescribing aspirin for AMI patients), and patient satisfaction was not undertaken. While the traditional PRO model may have succeeded in 'weeding out' a small number of incompetent providers, there is no evidence that it improved the overall quality of care.

In the early 1990s, HCFA announced the Health Care Quality Improvement Initiative, which was later developed into the Health Care Quality Improvement Program (HCQIP) in 1993, the pilot program of which was the CCP. This represented a radical shift in direction for HCFA and the PROs. This new paradigm follows the principles of continuous quality improvement (CQI), which had been adopted and used by commercial industry for many years. The CQI approach is founded upon prospective and systematic attention to the processes and outcomes of care. Rather than *reacting* to problems as they arise, the CQI approach involves *acting* to prevent problems before they arise. Through this initiative, PROs analyze and profile patterns of medical care, encourage hospitals to address problem areas by developing their own quality improvement initiatives, and provide non-punitive feedback to clinicians and institutions regarding their own performance in relation to national and regional benchmarks. The Joint Commission on Accreditation of Healthcare Organizations (JCAHO) is also shifting from a strictly punitive approach to one that encourages quality improvement efforts. Managed care organizations have followed these leads by profiling the practice patterns of their providers utilizing a variety of instruments. The National Committee on Quality Assurance (NCQA), a health maintenance organization (HMO) accreditation agency, has designed and proposed the Health Plan Employer Data and Information Set (HEDIS) as a standardized tool for reporting quality of care within managed care organizations.

Table 37.1 *Physician practice patterns in acute myocardial infarction*

Therapy	% of all patients treated	% of eligible patients treated	References
Thrombolysis	26–45	62–88	3,4,10–15,16,22
Aspirin – early[a]	88	81	4,15
Aspirin – late[b]	70–89	–	3,11,22
β-Blockers – early[a]	48	53	4,15
β-Blockers – late[b]	29–52	38–48	3,4,11,17,35,36

Includes studies without age limits. For studies reporting prescription rates over time, data from latest time period were used.
[a] Within 24 hours of admission.
[b] Treatment received in-hospital or upon discharge.

Developing a quality improvement program

The term continuous quality improvement refers to a systematic approach to improving the quality of care that employs a multidisciplinary team addressing a limited number of pre-specified goals, which are decided upon by consensus, based on initial data at the institution, and supported by literature documenting the benefits of improving such care. As the term implies, attention to such issues must be continuous; that is, even after a specific goal has been achieved, periodic data collection should be performed to ensure that this improvement is maintained (Fig. 37.1). Some of the key elements of this definition include the need for a *multidisciplinary* team approach, *data-* and *evidence-*based analysis, and *continuous* improvement.

Development of a quality improvement program at an institution requires a commitment and often a shift in mind-set by the hospital administration. While each member of the CQI team is important, real success cannot be achieved if institutional leaders have not 'bought in' to the key concepts of CQI. When a quality improvement program is initiated, there is generally a CQI executive committee that is composed of senior clinical and administrative leadership, with board representation. Participation of key physician leaders such as the department chiefs of medicine and surgery are a key to success. The executive committee will establish the overall mission of the component CQI teams, which is individualized according to the needs and biases of each institution. The mission may include goals, such as reducing the cost of care for given conditions, reducing length of stay, improvement in outcomes such as mortality, and improving the processes of care. The CQI executive committee selects the number and focus of the component CQI teams. Teams may be given a general focus such as 'improving the care of the cardiac patient' or very specific instructions, such as reducing door-to-needle time.

CQI teams

The optimal team size is 7–9 members. Representatives from multiple disciplines should be chosen on the basis of the issues addressed. For example, a CQI team focusing on reducing door-to-needle time should involve key players involved in the administration of thrombolytic therapy, such as an ED physician, a cardiologist, an ED nurse, an ECG technician, and a representative from pharmacy. Membership of such teams may be fluid, as goals shift. For instance, if in the analysis of thrombolysis administration it is determined that ED nurses rather than ECG technicians should obtain ECGs, and one component of delay is felt to be in the admission process, the team leaders may ask a representative from the admitting department to replace the ECG technician on the team. Other members of the team should include a facilitator and a data collector or quality advisor.

The team leader has a very important role in ensuring the success of the CQI team. Team leaders are generally physicians who have leadership roles in the institution. This is important to achieve 'buy-in' and better compliance from team members. Although it is important that every member of the team contribute, the leader must feel responsible for the success of the team. He/she should also be a good motivator. Another reason for choosing a senior physician is that they are more likely to be successful in negotiating with management for resources. Many teams employ co-leaders; in such cases, it is useful to have a nurse as one of the co-leaders. Again, this should generally be a nurse manager (or other nursing leadership position) to facilitate buy-in from the nursing staff.

The facilitator is generally an administrator who has experience with groups, has 'clout' with administration, and preferably, experience with the CQI process. The facilitator helps the team work through group dynamics issues and 'growing pains', which are a feature of any group. The facilitator will have special knowledge of problem-solving tools and techniques to help the group accomplish their goals. Finally, the facilitator acts as a liaison with management to help provide the necessary resources for the team.

Another important component of the team is the quality advisor, who is schooled in the CQI process and the use of CQI tools and techniques. The quality advisor helps educate the leaders and members about the CQI process, and guides the team through problem-solving by recommending the appropriate CQI tool(s) to address a problem. In addition, the quality advisor usually supervises data collection.

The team members should have a basic understanding of CQI principles and tools, which may be attained via

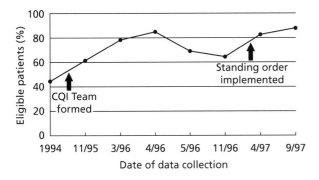

Figure 37.1 *Rate of administration of aspirin in the Memorial Hospital of Rhode Island emergency department to patients admitted for suspected acute myocardial infarction. Emergency department aspirin use steadily improved after initiation of an educational program, but declined over the next several months until a standing order for aspirin was instituted.*

handouts or workshops developed by the CQI facilitator or quality advisor. Members are expected to contribute actively to team discussions, assist in the design of the management plan, collect data when necessary, and devise and carry out interventions proposed by the team. In addition, they should be encouraged to network with their peers to promote the goals of the team. Team members should feel mutually accountable for achieving the goals of the CQI team.

Some of the issues that arise during the initial stages of CQI team growth include problems with group dynamics, inadequate communication of team goals, lack of support from administration or practicing physicians, difficulties with data collection, and lack of resources. The leader(s) and facilitator must pay attention to group dynamics and guide the team in the right direction; group rules may be established. It is vitally important to team success that there be clear communication. Roles and tasks should be well defined and team goals should be specific and concise, and understood by the team members. Adequate data collection must be ensured, as decisions should always be based on data. Furthermore, continuous or frequent data collection allows for necessary feedback to the team regarding their progress.

CQI process

Prior to the initial team meeting, leaders should select team members and design a preliminary management plan. When the team assembles, the management plan will be discussed and refined, and tasks should be assigned for completion prior to the next meeting. Initially, baseline data will be obtained on the process of care that is being addressed (e.g. door-to-needle time). After baseline data collection, the team gathers to analyze the components of the process, and brainstorms on the perceived causes of the problem and potential areas for improvement. This list is then narrowed down by team consensus and a few specific, measurable goals are selected. A plan for achieving these goals is developed and implemented. After a short period of time, data are then re-collected and re-analyzed by the group to determine if the interventions were successful, and a further course of action is planned. The specific elements of this process will be discussed in more detail below.

DATA COLLECTION

Collection of accurate data is the linchpin of the CQI process. Team goals should be measurable, and the process should be guided by the available data. Data collection is often labor intensive, thus only meaningful data related to the specific goals of the team should be collected. Preliminary goals are chosen based on feedback from managed care organizations employing HEDIS, from the CCP, NRMI, or other registries, as well as from the clinical experience of team members. Baseline data related to these goals are collected, often via retrospective chart reviews by team members. As the team progresses, more sophisticated data collection instruments may be used, including database software, prospective registries such as NRMI, or tools developed by the team such as critical pathways or care maps, which may be used to document certain critical elements. In addition, sophisticated hospital computer systems employing on-line order entry allow for automated data collection.

Data collection need not always be comprehensive; the group should decide on an adequate sample size for their purposes. In the example of door-to-needle time, however, the number of patients receiving thrombolytic therapy is low enough in most small- to medium-sized institutions that it is usually best to measure this indicator for all patients. Furthermore, complete data collection allows for identification of the range of door-to-needle time and of outliers. It is important that a physician oversee development of data collection tools (to ensure that they are clinically relevant) as well as initial efforts at data collection. Once a suitable and reliable tool has been developed, simple data elements may be collected by data abstractors with minimal supervision.

An institution committed to developing a quality improvement program should have a department of quality management. The members of this department are responsible for orchestrating data collection for the various CQI teams, assisting in data abstraction and analysis, and preparing reports. Data summaries and graphs are used to report results to the hospital board, CQI executive committee, other administrative committees, managed care organizations, and hospital employees. The quality management department should employ people with clinical experience (such as nurses) who are schooled in CQI methodology, as well as less highly trained individuals who function as data abstractors.

After initial data collection, it is important to view it in the context of 'benchmarks', data obtained by other institutions or reported in the literature. For instance, the literature on door-to-needle time would be reviewed to help determine a specific goal, which in this example would likely be a median time less than 30 minutes, as recommended by the NHAAP. Literature review is also used to learn methods employed by other institutions and investigators to improve processes of care in their institutions. In addition, national, regional, and peer (similar-sized hospitals with similar available facilities) data may be obtained through the NRMI, CCP, NCQA, or commercial databases.

DATA ANALYSIS

After baseline data have been collected, it should be presented to the team in an appropriate format decided upon by the quality advisor and team leader(s). Graphic representation of data is an effective form of communication. Types of graphs utilized include *run charts*, which display quantifiable data over time to show trends; *control charts*, which are essentially run charts with upper and/or lower control limits set according to statistical formulas (e.g. 1–2 standard deviations above and below the mean) to monitor the stability of data over time and easily identify outliers; *histograms* or bar graphs which segregate data according to categories or time intervals (Fig. 37.2); and *Pareto analysis*, which is a form of histogram, arranging data into separate categories and displaying them in a descending order of frequency. Pareto analysis allows a team to focus their attention on the largest problems by identifying, for instance, the major causes of delay in thrombolytic administration, or the most costly features of admission for AMI.

When a problem is identified and presented to the team, the team then dissects out the process into its component parts in order to identify features that are impeding quality of care. This exercise is facilitated by the use of CQI tools and techniques. Again, door-to-needle time is a useful example for this discussion, as the process is comprised of multiple steps involving many different disciplines, and is amenable to the CQI approach. While there is limited space for a comprehensive discussion, some of the more important CQI methodologies will be presented.

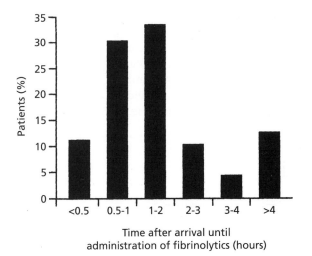

Figure 37.2 *Time from hospital arrival until initiation of fibrinolytic therapy (door-to-needle time) in the Cooperative Cardiovascular Project pilot study. Only 11 per cent of patients received treatment within 30 minutes, as recommended by the National Heart Attack Alert Program.[26] (Reproduced with permission from Ellerbeck EF, et al. Quality of care for Medicare patients with acute myocardial infarction: 4-state pilot study from the Cooperative Cardiovascular Project. JAMA 1995; 273: 1509–14.)*

'Brainstorming' is a technique that can be used at any phase in the quality improvement process. It is used to generate a large quantity of ideas in a short period of time. For instance, after baseline data demonstrating excessively long door-to-needle time are presented, the group is asked to brainstorm about the reasons for delay. The object of brainstorming is to solicit as many ideas as possible and not to criticize or edit these ideas. Exaggeration is welcomed and members are encouraged to build on others' ideas. Active participation by group members is essential. The benefits of brainstorming include its ability to generate ideas, spur creativity, and increase group involvement in the process. This technique frees up the group, allowing them to have fun while simultaneously stimulating creative ideas. During this exercise, the quality advisor or facilitator records all ideas on a flip chart or blackboard for the group to see.

Once a list of ideas is generated, group consensus is used to narrow it down to those ideas felt to be most important. A common technique used to narrow down a list is multivoting. Initially, team members review the original list and may ask for clarification of any of the ideas listed. Each team member then votes on the ideas that they feel are most appropriate. Those items getting the most votes are carried over into another round of voting and so on, until a handful of items are left, which presumably reflect group consensus.

Another technique used to organize the list of ideas generated by brainstorming is to create an affinity diagram. With this technique, it is helpful to record each idea on a separate index card. The entire team looks through the list and sorts the cards into similar groupings. Each group is then assigned a heading and broken down into subgroups as needed. The completed affinity diagram appears as a chart with the various headings that were created, and a list of related ideas under each heading.

Using the example of thrombolytic therapy administration, two useful CQI tools, the flow chart and cause and effect diagram, can be described. The flow chart is a graphic representation of the entire sequence of steps involved in the process of care under study. This tool is useful to help visualize the many components of a given process. Often, any one discipline is only really aware of the segments of the process in which they take part. Creating a flow chart allows the team to identify inefficiencies or rate-limiting steps easily, as well as potential areas for improvement. In order to create a flow chart, all of the disciplines involved in the process need to be present. First, the start and end points of the process are identified, e.g. arrival at the ED entrance and initiation of thrombolytic infusion. The team then reconstructs the entire process. Each component is identified; arrows show the direction of flow and diamonds indicate where a decision is to be made, e.g. whether to use thrombolytic therapy or not. The flow chart is not necessarily linear; it may branch out and there may be feedback loops involved. The NHAAP recommends that each institution create a flow chart outlining their process for thrombolytic therapy administration using the time intervals discussed earlier, i.e. door-to-data (ECG), data-to-decision (thrombolytic order), and decision-to-drug (initiating thrombolytic infusion). Potential causes of delay at each stage can then be identified. Table 37.2 lists a number of methods for eliminating this delay.

Table 37.2 *Methods for reducing door-to-needle time*

Data
- EMS screening for contraindications
- Pre-hospital 12-lead ECG
- Transmission of pre-hospital ECG
- Immediate triage
- Protocol for chest pain/MI patients including standing order for 12-lead ECG
- Nurses obtain ECG
- Hand-delivery of ECG to ED physician

Decision
- ED physician orders drug without consult
- When consult is necessary, easy access to consultants, including fax
- When ECG is non-diagnostic:
  - Repeat serial ECGs frequently
  - ST segment monitoring
  - Encourage posterior chest leads
  - Consider echocardiogram
- Guidelines for thrombolysis posted in ED and on 'pocket cards'
- Reference materials readily available

Drug
- Store drug in ED
- Train nurses to mix and administer drug
- Initiate treatment in ED

ECG = electrocardiogram; ED = emergency department;
EMS = emergency medical system; MI = myocardial infarction.

The cause and effect diagram, or 'fishbone', is used to display and categorize all of the possible root causes of a specific problem. The problem is displayed in a box on the right-hand side of the diagram with arrows pointing towards it. A list of contributing causes is generated, e.g. by brainstorming. These causes are then grouped into major categories, such as employees, equipment, methods, and materials. This format helps to graphically demonstrate the relationship between causes and effects in the process under study (Fig. 37.3).

PLANNING AND IMPLEMENTING CHANGE

The techniques and tools mentioned above highlight the major problem areas in the process being studied and suggest avenues for improvement. Upon review of the sample cause and effect diagram in Fig. 37.3, systematic impediments in the thrombolytic decision process are identified, and potential solutions become readily apparent: purchasing additional ECG machines, encouraging serial ECGs in patients with non-diagnostic changes and/or obtaining continuous ST segment monitoring capabilities (Fig. 37.4), improving access to prior ECGs, ongoing education of ED nurses and physicians, acquiring a system for receiving pre-hospital ECGs, and improving hospital interpreter services. Again, it is important to remember when entering the planning phase that a small number of specific well-defined goals should be agreed upon by the group, as well as a target date for achieving these goals. These goals should be well communicated, so that each of the members is able to voice them.

There are a whole host of intervention tools that may be utilized to bring about quality improvement (Table 37.3). These methodologies are used to educate providers, document care, and standardize processes and procedures. The use of standardized treatment protocols, pre-printed orders, and standing orders are effective tools for streamlining care (Fig. 37.5). They assist in

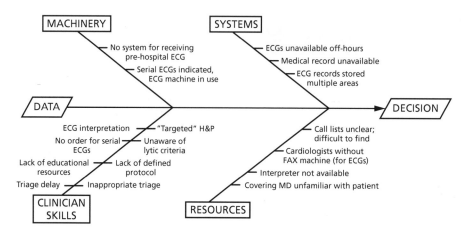

Figure 37.3 *Cause and effect diagram. This diagram lists and categorizes causes of delay in the decision to order fibrinolytic therapy in acute myocardial infarction. H & P = history and physical; ECG = electrocardiogram.*

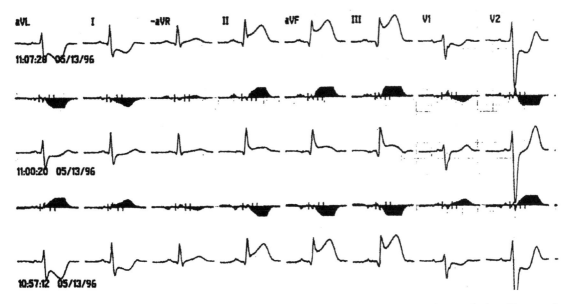

Figure 37.4 *ST segment monitoring in a patient with acute inferior wall myocardial infarction. Strips are displayed in ascending chronological order; time of each strip is displayed on left side, leads are displayed on top. Note the significant fluctuation in ST deviation from one strip to the next (over a 10-minute period of time). Intermittent 12-lead electrocardiograms would be less likely to show these dynamic changes, and may not capture significant ST deviation at all, e.g. if obtained at time of middle strip.*

Table 37.3 *Intervention tools for improving practice patterns*

- Educational tools – multimedia, interactive
- Peer education by local medical opinion leaders
- Guidelines
- Clinical prediction guides
- Critical pathways
- Care maps
- Pre-printed orders
- Standing orders
- Outcomes reporting (scorecards):
  - Institution-wide
  - Physician-specific
- Computerized decision support/ order entry:
  - Access to reference materials
  - Prompts for drug–drug, drug–laboratory interactions
  - Critical event monitors (abnormal laboratory results)
- Patient-specific 'reminders' to physicians
- Algorithms
- Case management

reducing delays such as door-to-needle time, and improving access to therapy, e.g. standing orders for aspirin in ED patients with suspected AMI. Some of the more commonly used intervention modalities will be discussed in further detail below.

COMPLETING THE LOOP

After an intervention plan is designed and implemented, an appropriate period of time is generally given to educate personnel to the change and allow them to incorporate it into their practice. The CQI team will have

already established a target goal, e.g. door-to-needle time of 30 minutes, aspirin administration to > 90 per cent of eligible patients with chest pain, etc. Data are then re-collected and brought back to the group. If the target has been achieved, the group may choose to address a new problem. If there has been limited or no improvement, the team should reassess the intervention that was implemented to see if the problem was due to non-compliance or due to the intervention itself. A new plan devised to improve compliance with the tool or to implement additional interventions is then carried out. In any event, data collection should be repeated periodically to monitor the process. It is not uncommon for an intervention to achieve initial success, only to have practice patterns regress to prior levels due to lack of compliance, or the 'out of sight, out of mind' phenomenon. This pattern seems to be especially common when the intervention is primarily educational, as the message delivered in, for example, a lecture, tends to fade over time. An example of this pattern is seen in Fig. 37.1, in which the rate of aspirin administration in the ED faded after an initial impressive response to an educational program. After standing orders for aspirin were implemented, the utilization rate improved again, and has thus far stabilized at this high rate (unpublished data). This highlights the need to standardize changes that have proven effective. Incorporating a desired process into a standardized protocol or pre-printed orders helps to ensure compliance with the desired process of care, in a sense by taking the 'human' element out of it. Of course, such standardized protocols must contain parameters as necessary to ensure safety, e.g. blood pressure parameters

EMERGENCY DEPARTMENT
CHEST PAIN

AUTHORIZATION IS GIVEN TO DISPENSE A GENERIC EQUIVALENT
UNLESS THE PHYSICIAN'S SIGNATURE APPEARS HERE:

_____ M.D./D.O.

ADDRESSOGRAPH

INSTRUCTIONS FOR USE: **USE BAL**
CHECK ALL APPLICABLE BOXES   *FAX* to Pharmacy

DATE/TIME	ORDERS

ALLERGIES:

Care Map   [   ]   **Chest Pain Care Map appropriate for use. Initiate CHEST PAIN PROTOCOL**

IV   [   ]   0.9% Sodium Chloride @ _____ mL / h

     [   ]   Saline Lock

Oxygen   [   ]   2 liters / min via nasal cannula

     [   ]   100% via non-rebreather mask

     [   ]   O2 at _____

Tests   [   ]   PA & Lateral Chest X-ray

Labs

     [   ]   PT *(Select if already on oral anticoagulants)*

     [   ]   aPTT *(Select if Heparin or Thrombolytics to be initiated)*

Meds   [   ]   Nitroglycerin 1/150 grs SL q 5 min X _____ for chest pain if SBP > 90

     [   ]   Nitroglycerin Ointment 1" applied to chest wall

     [   ]   Nitroglycerin IV 50 mg / 250 mL D5W. Start at 10 micrograms/min and titrate until pain free or maximum of 100 micrograms/min. Maintain SBP $\geq$ 90

     [   ]   Morphine Sulfate _____ mg IV

     [   ]   Repeat Morphine Sulfate _____ mg IV x 1 after _____ min if needed

HEPARIN   [   ]   Bolus with 5,000 units Heparin IV followed by a Heparin drip: 25,000 units / 500 mL 0.45% Sodium Chloride at 1,000 units / hour

     [   ]   aPTT 6 hours after Heparin bolus and 6 hours after any dosing change

BETA BLOCKERS   [   ]   Metoprolol 5 mg IV q 5 min X 3 doses if SBP > 90 and heart rate > 50

     [   ]   Metoprolol 50 mg po, 15 minutes after the last IV dose

THROMBOLYTIC THERAPY

     [   ]   *Start 2-3 peripheral IV's.*

     [   ]   *Alteplase (rt-PA) 15 mg IV bolus, then*
Give 0.75 mg/kg over 30 min (DO NOT EXCEED 50 mg)
Give 0.50 mg/kg over next 60 min (DO NOT EXCEED 35 mg)
       TOTAL DOSE NOT TO EXCEED 100 mg

     [   ]   *Streptokinase 1.5 million units in 100 cc of NS*
administered IV over 60 min.

     [   ]   *Reteplase 10 units IV bolus followed by additional 10 units*
IV bolus in 30 minutes

Additional Orders

Chest Pain Protocol includes in part:
Aspirin
EKG, Portable Chest X-ray
Lytes, BUN, Cr, Glucose, CBC
Cardiac enzymes
Pulse Oximetry
Evaluation of continued need for O2 @ 8 h
Diet advancement @ 4 h
Activity progression @ 4 h
(if chest pain free)

Thrombolytic Screening
INCLUSION CRITERIA
[   ] Anginal chest pain or equivalent < 12 h with
   [   ] ST elevations $\geq$ 0.1 mV (2 or more leads)
     [   ] II, III, aVF
     [   ] I, aVL
     [   ] 2 or more precordial leads
   [   ] ST depressions V1, V2, V3 (2 or more leads)
   [   ] New LBBB

EXCLUSION CRITERIA	YES	NO
1. Active internal bleeding / bleeding disorder		
2. CNS hemorrhage, neoplasm, or recent stroke		
3. Recent major trauma, surgery, or prolonged CPR		
4. Severe uncontrolled hypertension		
Comments		

ADMIT TO: _____ **M.D. DIAGNOSIS:** _____

DISPOSITION: _____ **TIME:** _____

Physician's signature _____ **M.D./D.O.**

7773-708.WK4 (Rev. 3-17-98)   **White - Chart Copy**   **Yellow - ED Registration**   **Pink - Business Office**

Figure 37.5 *Sample pre-printed orders for patients with suspected myocardial ischemia in the emergency department. Orders are activated when physician checks appropriate box. Note the order for chest pain protocol, which triggers an array of standardized orders, including aspirin administration.*

for administering nitroglycerin. Certain potentially high-risk interventions, such as thrombolytic therapy and β-blockade, require physician evaluation prior to their use. As noted above, continuous monitoring of indicators is essential to maintain results.

An important aspect of the quality improvement process is communication of achievements to hospital administrators, employees, third-party payors, and the public, if appropriate. Communication of success can enhance employee morale, hospital reputation in the community, and hospital compliance with JCAHO requirements. Furthermore, success stories engage interest in and acceptance of the CQI process, which will promote adherence to future CQI interventions.

USING CQI STRATEGIES TO IMPROVE PHYSICIAN PRACTICE PATTERNS

Physician beliefs and practices have been shown to lag behind definitive results provided by randomized controlled trials.[33,38,43] Some of the contributing factors to the gap between clinical research and clinical practice are listed in Table 37.4. First of all, practitioners may not be aware of the clinical trial findings supporting a given form of therapy. For instance, cardiologists are more aware of and thus more likely than generalists to prescribe drugs of proven benefit in AMI, including aspirin, β-blockers and thrombolytic therapy;[33,43a] they are less likely to prescribe drugs of unproven benefit, including diltiazem and prophylactic lidocaine.[33] This difference in practice pattern appears to translate into a lower mortality rate for patients admitted to cardiologists.[43a] Similarly, a recent CCP report demonstrated higher administration rates for aspirin, angiotensin-converting enzyme inhibitors and β-blockers in AMI patients admitted to teaching vs non-teaching hospitals. These differences led to a lower mortality rate in the teaching hospitals.[43b] This relative lack of awareness among generalists can be attributed to comparatively less experience with acute treatment of MI, the essentially impossible task of keeping up with all of the various subspecialties of internal medicine in face of the 'information explosion', and perhaps the tendency of subspecialists to address their findings to those within their own field.[33] Other causes of undertreatment

include perceived contraindications to therapy and fear of side effects of therapy. Some of these perceptions relate to later disproven lessons taught in clinical training; thus, physicians who are farther removed from training tend to be more likely to hold on to these beliefs. A classic example of this is the teaching that β-blockers are contraindicated in patients with heart failure, whereas recent research suggests that β-blockers are of particular value in post-MI patients with left ventricular (LV) dysfunction or heart failure,[38–42] and in fact appear independently to improve outcomes in patients with both ischemic and non-ischemic cardiomyopathy.[44] The fear of side effects is also an important impediment to prescription of appropriate agents. This ranges from perceived impacts on lifestyle (e.g. impotence in patients treated with β-blockers) to fear of life-threatening events (e.g. major bleeding in patients treated with thrombolytic therapy). Contributing to this behavior is the fact that adverse events may have a very tangible and lasting influence on a physician's practice (e.g. intracranial hemorrhage after thrombolysis), while the beneficial effects of various agents are less tangible and must be taken on faith from the results of randomized trials (e.g. treatment of hypertension). Relative experience with a given condition probably plays a role in the level of caution that physicians display in accepting data and changing their practice patterns.[33] Finally, it has been noted that aggressive marketing by pharmaceutical manufacturers may play a role in physician prescribing patterns.[38] Agents that have clear-cut benefits, but which are low in cost and/or have generic equivalents (aspirin, β-blockers) are less likely to be 'pushed' by pharmaceutical representatives, whereas agents with limited or no role in AMI (e.g. calcium-channel blockers) have been marketed aggressively, owing to their favorable profit margins.[38] With the proliferation of quality improvement programs at hospitals and managed care organizations, which are paying attention to measures such as prescription of β-blockers after AMI (a HEDIS measure), some of these barriers may be addressed. New continuing medical education (CME) strategies and CQI methods are currently being utilized to address the deficiencies in care documented earlier in this chapter. Some of these approaches will be discussed in further detail below.

Continuing medical education

Traditional CME relied almost exclusively on didactic techniques directed from the teacher to the learner, primarily in the written format, consisting of textbooks and journal review articles, and the oral format, consisting of 'Grand Rounds' and CME conferences. Recognition of the limitations of this approach[45] have led to changes in CME in recent years.[46] In brief, these changes consist of breaking the barriers of the rigid

Table 37.4 *Reasons for physician underutilization of proven therapies*

Lack of awareness of clinical trial findings
Perceived contraindications to use
Fear of side-effects
Caution in accepting data and changing practice
Influence of aggressive marketing

traditional format. This involves shifting from the unidirectional approach described above to a much more interactive process. Examples of methods that have been successful include outreach visits by physician-educators such as pharmacists, practice-enabling strategies (techniques to reinforce appropriate care, e.g. reminders or physician-specific feedback), patient-mediated educational strategies and materials, informal communication among peers, physician self-directed learning, and financial incentives and disincentives to guide appropriate care. One of the reasons that a traditional didactic approach is of limited value is its short half-life. Practice changes generally are not stimulated by isolated exposures to lectures or conferences and, if change is initiated, it may not be sustained.[46]

The proliferation of guidelines for a variety of medical conditions has occurred in response to the unwieldy explosion in medical information previously referred to, and to the efforts of managed care and medical specialty organizations to support standardized practice patterns, when appropriate. Other techniques used to provide ongoing education include computerized decision support and institutional- and physician-specific outcomes reporting, which encourage physicians, groups and institutions to examine their own practice strategies. These methods are described in further detail below. An important aspect of the new CME strategy is the recognition that a multifaceted approach is necessary to impact on physician practice patterns.[33,45] Therefore, a CQI team seeking to improve utilization of thrombolytic therapy may employ lectures, 'pocket cards' outlining thrombolytic guidelines, posters and other visual aids identifying guidelines, CD-ROM software, and interactive workshops for ED and primary care physicians. Furthermore, as the internet expands into medical education, the opportunities for rapid and widespread dissemination of medical knowledge are greatly enhanced. This includes the ability for the learner to interact with the educational environment and readily allows for problem-based learning and case-based scenarios, toward which medical school curricula have shifted.[47] While broad dissemination of clinical trial findings and guidelines has been advocated, limited resources dictate that targeted education may be most effective. For instance, when trying to improve door-to-needle time or access to thrombolytic therapy, an educational program directed primarily towards ED physicians may be most appropriate, as they are now the 'front line' of initial care for AMI.

Practice guidelines

The intent of practice guidelines is to improve quality of care by informing medical decisions on appropriate preventive, diagnostic, and treatment modalities. The aims are to improve clinical outcomes, decrease variations in care, and optimize resource utilization.[48,49] Guidelines have traditionally been used for educational purposes, but managed care organizations are increasingly using them as a basis for decisions on reimbursement; typically, non-physician personnel following decision algorithms based on published guidelines dictate 'appropriateness of care' and influence reimbursement of procedures and consultations. While guidelines have been shown to affect processes and outcomes of care positively, the degree of improvement has varied greatly.[50] It is apparent that published guidelines used in isolation are of limited value; when used with concurrent reminders or feedback, however, they may be of significant value.[50,51]

Some reasons for the limited impact of guidelines on physician practice patterns include:

1 faulty development resulting in guidelines that are ineffective, poorly transportable from one health care environment to another, too restrictive, i.e. not broadly applicable, or that have unintended secondary effects (e.g. reduction in length of stay leading to increased out-patient costs);

2 faulty dissemination, leading to limited awareness; and

3 physician resistance to guidelines. Physician resistance is prevalent; practice guidelines may be derided as 'cookbook medicine', and paid little mind.[49,52,53] Physicians tend to have adverse reactions to guidelines because they are viewed as tools of managed care, thus threatening physician autonomy.[52,53]

General principles for creating optimal practice guidelines are outlined in Table 37.5. The three phases of practice guideline creation are development, dissemination, and implementation. Guideline development must be rigorous and evidence based whenever possible. In the absence of randomized or observational trial data to answer a given question, expert consensus is used. If systematic reviews on a given topic are not available in the literature, the team creating the guidelines should conduct their own review. Indeed, it has been shown that internal, locally derived guidelines are more likely to

Table 37.5 *Principles for creating optimal practice guidelines*

Rigorous development based on systematic reviews and
  expert consensus
Internal development with physician involvement
Elicit input from clinicians
Keep guidelines simple, straightforward; use bounding rules
Validate prospectively prior to implementation
Multifaceted implementation with repeated clinical exposure
Non-punitive implementation strategy
Maintain/update content frequently

References in text.

overcome suspicion and increase acceptance, especially if physicians are involved in their development.[48,54] Guidelines should contain bounding rules, that is, the minimum acceptable standard of care for a condition (e.g. treatment of patients with heart failure and an ejection fraction of < 40 per cent with an angiotensin-converting enzyme inhibitor).[54] Following this practice helps maintain one of the most important principles of guideline development, the need for simplicity. If the guidelines are simple, straightforward, and well-defined, they are more likely to be read and utilized than complex, intricate guidelines.[52,54] Negative results in a study of implementation of practice guidelines for unstable angina led to the advice that guideline developers seek empiric input from clinicians prior to guideline dissemination.[55] Finally, and importantly, guidelines should be validated prospectively prior to implementation, similar to the latter phases of pharmaceutical development.[49,52,54]

Prior to disseminating practice guidelines, the focus audience must be determined; this will help to choose the appropriate publication site and guide the implementation strategy. Implementation refers to the method of dissemination used. An ineffective imple-

mentation strategy can render the most well-written guidelines useless. A multifaceted implementation strategy involving publication of the guidelines in print and on the World Wide Web, as well as incorporation of guideline principles into pocket cards and pamphlets, posters, patient educational materials, critical pathways, decision algorithms (Fig. 37.6),[56] and patient-specific reminders will greatly enhance the efficacy of guideline dissemination.[49–52,57] Involvement of local medical 'opinion leaders' to educate peers via small and large group discussions coupled with individual performance feedback has been shown to impact physician prescribing patterns positively.[58,59] Two recently reported studies randomized hospitals to one of two groups: (1) a control group given 'usual' guideline dissemination or performance feedback; or (2) an experimental group receiving this information via an intensive educational approach spearheaded by locally recruited respected physicians. In both studies, the more intensive approach was more successful in increasing usage of proven beneficial therapies.[58,59]

Practice guidelines may also take the form of clinical prediction guides, which basically streamline information from clinical trials into probabilistic algorithms that

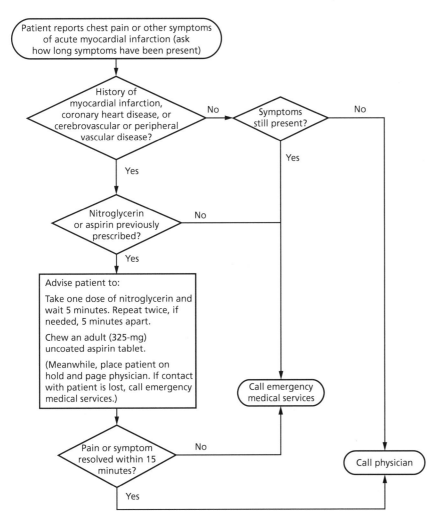

Figure 37.6 *Algorithm for triage of patients with chest pain by office clerical staff. This represents a typical algorithm, or decision tree. The flow of the process is shown by arrows; actions are displayed in boxes; decision points are displayed in diamonds; start point (input) and end points (output) are displayed in ovals. (Reproduced with permission from Dracup K, et al. The physician's role in minimizing prehospital delay in patients at high risk for acute myocardial infarction: recommendations from the National Heart Attack Alert Program. Ann Intern Med 1997;* **126***: 645–51.)*

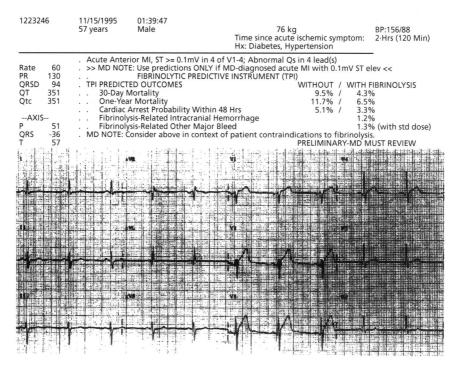

Figure 37.7 *The fibrinolytic predictive instrument, an example of a clinical prediction guide, used to assist in fibrinolytic decision-making. Based on patient-specific variables such as age, sex, blood pressure, and electrocardiographic findings, the instrument generates probabilities of clinical outcomes occurring with and without fibrinolytic therapy. In this patient with anterior ST segment elevation, the instrument predicts a significant benefit from fibrinolysis. (Reproduced with permission from Selker HP, et al. Patient-specific predictions of outcome in myocardial infarction for real-time emergency use: a thrombolytic predictive instrument.* Ann Intern Med *1997;* **127***: 538–56.)*

guide decision making (Fig. 37.7).[60] In order to achieve physician acceptance of guidelines, it is important to employ non-punitive methods of implementation. Above all, it should be made clear that the role of guidelines and related tools is to *support*, not *supplant* physician judgement.

Critical pathways

Critical pathways are schematic representations of diagnostic and treatment protocols for a given condition. While practice guidelines define goals of treatment and provide evidence to support such goals, critical pathways provide a step-by-step method for achieving such goals in an efficient manner (Table 37.6). Thus, critical pathways combine the goals of research-based guidelines with institution-specific processes of care to map the progression of care for all disciplines in one tool. These tools are designed to improve quality of care by highlighting standards of care, while encouraging the rational use of resources (Table 37.7). To achieve these goals, critical pathways promote a standardized approach to certain diagnoses and procedures in order to reduce unwanted and inefficient variations in care. The use of critical pathways has become widespread;

they are used in some form by the majority of health care facilities. A major impetus for critical pathway development and implementation has come from managed care organizations and third-party insurers in an effort to reduce costs and resource utilization. These tools are most effective in high-volume, predictable, relatively homogeneous conditions (Table 37.8). They are less useful in complex, chronic, or unstable health conditions. Procedures such as coronary angiography, angioplasty, or coronary artery bypass surgery are especially amenable to critical pathways, as the progression of care for multiple disciplines is readily mapped out.[61,62]

Concerns regarding the use of critical pathways are similar to those outlined above for practice guidelines. Most prominent are the concerns regarding 'cookbook medicine', as the sequence of care may be mapped out from prior to admission through hospitalization and into the out-patient setting. Given this prescribed approach, it has been suggested that critical pathways may inhibit independent thinking and decision-making by physicians-in-training. Finally, there is a perception that malpractice risks may be increased by highlighting variances of care by individual physicians.[61,62]

In response to these concerns, some of the advice used for practice guidelines can be applied to critical pathways. It is even more important that critical pathways are

Table 37.6 *Sample critical pathway for initial hospital management of ST elevation acute myocardial infarction*

	Critical pathway ST elevation or new BBB, chest pain ≤ 12 hours		
	Day 0 (ED)	Day 0 (CCU)	Day 1 (CCU)
Treatment	• Fibrinolysis if no contraindication[a] ☐ • If contraindicated → 1° PCI • Aspirin 160 mg chewed ☐ • IV heparin (optional with SK, low risk MI) • IV/ oral β-blocker if no contraindications ☐ • SL/ IV nitroglycerin if CHF, HTN, ongoing ischemia • Morphine prn • Oxygen per nasal cannula	• If persistent/recurrent pain, ECG changes or shock despite fibrinolysis → cath • Aspirin if not already given ☐ • Continue IV heparin, IV nitroglycerin as needed • Oral β-blocker • Consider oral ACE inhibitor if no contraindications • Stool softener, sedation prn • Continue oxygen	• Continue aspirin, IV heparin, β-blocker • Begin or continue ACE inhibitor, esp. if CHF, EF<40% ☐ • Coumadin if anterior MI, EF <40%, no cath planned • D/C nitroglycerin if no recurrent pain, CHF, HTN • D/C oxygen if sat >92%
Monitoring	• Vital signs • Continuous ECG monitoring • Oxygen saturation • ST segment monitoring • 2 peripheral IVs	• Vital signs q1-2 hrs • Continuous ECG monitoring • Oxygen saturation • ST segment monitoring • Admission weight • Stool occult blood	• Vital signs q2 hrs • Continuous ECG monitoring • Record weight
Tests	• CBC, electrolytes, Ca, Mg, P • PT/ PTT • Type and cross (with lysis) • ECG- repeat as needed; posterior, RV leads prn • Chest x-ray	• Serial CK, CK-MB, Troponin I • PTT at 6 hrs and 6 hrs after heparin dose change • ECG • Lipid profile ☐	• CBC, electrolytes • PTT • ECG • Echocardiogram
Activity	• Bedrest	• Bedrest with commode	• Ambulate in room tid
Diet	• NPO	• Low cholesterol, low fat, NAS	• Same
Education	• Instruct patient re: pain scale, reporting symptoms • Contact family, discuss dx	• Orient to CCU • Explain diagnosis, expected hospital course • Discuss treatments	• Explain tests and procedures • Discuss cardiac risk factors • Prepare for transfer from CCU
D/C planning	• Admit CCU		• If stable for 24–36 hours, may transfer to telemetry

[a] If fibrinolysis given, record times:
Symptom onset _____
ED arrival _____
Initial ECG _____
MD orders drug _____
Infusion begun _____

Shaded sections indicate critical intervention; check box if intervention done.
ACE = angiotensin-converting enzyme; BBB = bundle branch block; Cath = catheterization; CBC = complete blood count; CCU = coronary care unit; CHF = congestive heart failure; CK = creatine kinase; CK-MB = creatine kinase MB isoenzyme; D/C = discharge; dx = diagnosis; ED = emergency department; EF = ejection fraction; HTN = hypertension; IV = intravenous; NAS = no added salt; NPO = nil per os; PT/PTT = prothrombin time/partial thromboplastin time; PCI= percutaneous coronary intervention; RV = right ventricle; SK = streptokinase; SL = sublingual.

developed locally than it is for practice guidelines, as critical pathways must be adapted to each institution's processes of care. Again, clinicians must be involved in pathway development to increase clinical relevance and enhance acceptance. Staff roles and expectations should be clearly defined for each discipline before pathway implementation. With respect to their educational value,

critical pathways actually provide a unique opportunity to visualize the inter-relationship of different disciplines in the provision of care. By examining variances in care that are highlighted in critical pathways, insight may be gained into processes and potential solutions to improve efficiency. Furthermore, critical pathways may provide a tool for documentation and in certain cases may reduce

Table 37.7 *Benefits of critical pathways*

Improve quality of care by highlighting standards of care
Encourage provision of care in a timely fashion
Encourage standardized care when appropriate
Reduce hospital costs by eliminating unnecessary tests and
  procedures
Reduce hospital length of stay in low-risk patients
Improve patient education
Illustrate interrelationship of clinical processes and
  disciplines
Provide a tool for data collection

Table 37.8 *Clinical conditions best suited for critical pathway use*

High volume
High cost
Conditions with inappropriate variation in care
Procedures, e.g. coronary angioplasty, coronary artery bypass
  surgery
Medical conditions that lend themselves to homogeneous
  care plan

overall documentation, thus freeing up time for educational activities. By highlighting critical events (e.g. door-to-needle time, aspirin administration in AMI, etc.), data may be collected regarding these practices to provide important feedback to practitioners (Table 37.6). Finally, to counteract the claim of increased malpractice risk, it seems likely that the risk of malpractice may actually be decreased, as the intent of critical paths is to ensure that standards of care are maintained. By the nature of their design (e.g. by asking to document the reason that β-blockers are not used), these tools should improve documentation of practice variations, which is likely to reduce exposure to litigation. Of course, critical pathways are not intended to force patients into a course of action that may not be appropriate for that individual; they are no replacement for clinical judgement in individual cases. While the use of critical pathways appears promising, there are very few controlled trials available to establish their efficacy, although a recent trial reported a decrease in resource utilization associated with critical pathway usage, without impacting patient outcomes.[63] Research is needed to provide further evidence as well as to guide optimal critical pathway development.

Outcomes reporting

Use of outcomes reporting, or 'scorecards' is widespread among managed care organizations. HEDIS and other performance measures are used to monitor quality of care and benchmark with regional or national data.

Corporations and other health care purchasing groups are using these data to guide their choice of health plans. This practice achieved nationwide publicity when surgeon-specific mortality rates for coronary artery bypass surgery in New York State were published in 1990.[64] The basic philosophy behind outcomes reporting is that provision of institution-specific or physician-specific data benchmarked to peer institutions or providers will spur efforts to improve quality of care. Some positive aspects of this method include the greater emphasis placed on preventive care measures, which previously received little attention from health care organizations; its apparent success at stimulating quality improvement efforts with an attendant improvement in outcomes;[65-67] and its ability to identify 'outliers', e.g. low-volume interventional cardiologists with increased complication rates who merit closer scrutiny, further training, or perhaps withdrawal of privileges. Studies from New York[65] and northern New England[66] have reported improved outcomes coincident with published annual institution-specific reports of coronary artery bypass surgery mortality rates. The decline in mortality was felt to be due to the practice of outcomes reporting. However, Ghali *et al.* reported a similar improvement in cardiac surgery mortality in Massachusetts, which did not have a statewide quality improvement program in place at the time of data collection.[68] These data suggest that declining surgical mortality may simply reflect a nationwide trend due to factors other than outcomes reporting.[69] A recent review of the limited available evidence regarding the impact of public disclosure of hospital performance data revealed a modest improvement in health outcomes afforded by this practice.[67] Similarly, data regarding the impact of physician-specific outcomes reporting (or 'profiling') demonstrate only a very modest effect on physician practice patterns, including prescribing and test-ordering practices.[70] A more recent non-randomized study from the CCP, however, suggested that states receiving feedback of hospital-specific data regarding use of beneficial AMI therapy subsequently showed more appropriate use of such therapy than did states not receiving this feedback.[71] As noted earlier, the use of a strategy coupling performance feedback with an educational campaign utilizing local opinion leaders appears to provide optimal results.[58,59]

While scorecards appear to be here to stay, the main problem with this method is the need for accurate risk-adjustment, which is very difficult. Certainly, morbidity and mortality rates cannot be viewed in isolation; they must be adjusted for the disease severity and co-morbidities of the population at risk. Outcomes reporting is of no use if there is inadequate risk adjustment. Other problems with outcomes reporting are related to the attendant intense focus on numbers. Concerns have been raised that surgeons would avoid high-risk patient populations because of the impact on their surgical mortality rate. In addition, it becomes difficult for new proceduralists to get started because of the tendency towards a higher complication rate while they are on the 'learning curve'.[72] In order to prepare for such external scrutiny, Topol *et al.* recommend that cardiology divisions or groups maintain a database of all cardiac procedures and diagnoses, with relevant procedure- and diagnosis-specific outcome measures. They also recommend that all invasive and non-invasive cardiac laboratories develop written CQI plans with monitoring of volume, complication rates, credentialing, and staff development, as well as patient satisfaction.[72] Further research is indicated to determine how to use outcomes data optimally to improve quality of care.

Computerized decision support

It has been noted above that a multifaceted implementation approach to guideline dissemination and CME is most effective. 'Reminders', i.e. patient-specific messages to physicians regarding the use of laboratories, diagnostic tests, or medications are especially effective, as they provide timely feedback, which reinforces guideline content.[45,51,73] Such a system of reminders is expensive and labor intensive in the absence of an information system capable of providing immediate on-line feedback.[49] Systems such as these are said to provide 'decision support'. Sophisticated computerized decision support (CDS) systems interface with electronic medical records systems to provide:

1 access to guidelines and other references;
2 feedback regarding drug–drug, drug–laboratory, and drug–diagnosis interactions;
3 dosing guidelines;
4 adverse drug event detection and prevention; and
5 continuous data collection and on-line quality improvement.

The utility of such systems is optimized when combined with physician order entry, i.e. computerized orders. When order entry is used, the CD system can generate prompts to improve compliance with standards of care, reduce costs (by suggesting lower cost alternatives), and alert the physician when certain critical events, e.g. panic laboratory values occur. The alert may be in the form of a highlighted message or e-mail the next time the physician logs on, or may occur through an automated paging system. Interventions such as these cut down significantly on response times to abnormal laboratory values and medication errors,[74] and improve compliance with standards of care.[75]

Order entry and CDS systems have some drawbacks. The greatest impediment to initiating an order entry/CDS system is the high start-up and maintenance cost involved. Proponents argue, however, that the money saved by reducing adverse drug events, recommending lower cost medications, and suggesting more appropriate laboratory or diagnostic tests more than makes up for these expenses. A second drawback is that patient care becomes highly reliant on technology and thus vulnerable to the inevitable system 'crash'. While this potential exists, back-up systems are able to ease this burden. A third drawback is the steep learning curve associated with using these complex systems, which may require significant resources for training. In this era of ubiquitous computers, however, users are often fairly adept at picking up new systems. As more people learn the system, they may train colleagues, thus the training budget may decrease over time. Fourth, order entry takes more time to use in comparison to written orders, even for experienced users. The use of pre-designed templates for certain diagnoses and procedures help address this concern. Finally, the initial positive impact of a CDS system has been reported to diminish over time,[75] which again points to the limitations of relying on any one system to achieve sustained quality improvement.

FUTURE DIRECTIONS

The quality improvement 'movement' has become incorporated to some degree into all hospitals and managed care organizations (especially the latter). Two areas that deserve a great deal of attention and resources in the future are further research into CQI methods and ongoing development of computerized decision support systems.

Systematic reviews of randomized trials evaluating the independent effects of CME, guideline implementation strategies, physician profiling, and CDS on processes and outcomes of care have demonstrated modest benefits accruing to each of these approaches.[45,50,70,73,74] Studies have consistently shown that optimal quality improvement strategies employ a multifaceted approach using a combination of methods, including physician-specific feedback, patient-specific reminders, and other tools noted in this chapter.[45,50,51] Practitioners may become habituated to a particular stimulus (e.g. written length of stay reminders) over time and, if an intervention is withdrawn, practice change is generally not sustained. Repeated exposure of physicians to guideline recommendations from a variety of sources seems to be the most successful way to effect change. Recently, targeted educational approaches utilizing local opinion leaders have proven successful.[58,59] Guideline development must be rigorous and based on published research whenever possible. Similarly, implementation methods, such as prediction guides, critical paths, etc., should be subjected to the same rigorous methods and outcomes assessment as the processes themselves. This includes prospective validation against real patient cases prior to broad dissemination.[49,54] These tools should be developed or adapted by institutions for their own use with the input of clinicians using a CQI approach.

Another effective intervention strategy may be to target the implementation method used to the desired goal to be achieved; each method may have its 'niche'. Thus, clinical prediction guides are useful for triage and treatment decisions (Fig. 37.7), critical paths are effective for reducing length of stay, guidelines provide appropriateness criteria for procedures, and CDS systems are ideally suited for guiding use of ancillary tests.

It has been argued that in certain cases, 'guidelines' should become *standards* for which physicians are accountable.[53] These may be appropriate in scenarios where the process involved has significant benefit and cost effectiveness based on sound evidence. Leape has proposed creation of a National Medical Standards Board to oversee the development, dissemination, and monitoring of standards. Such overseeing is compared to the need for the Federal Aviation Administration to ensure that airlines and pilots meet certain safety standards.[53] Such a mechanism may prove effective and become necessary should CQI approaches show limited success.

It has been stressed that physicians must be involved in the quality improvement process and that implementation approaches can never replace clinical judgement. However, as stated by Leape, 'systems that depend on memory or on single individuals are doomed to fail. Instead, we need automatic fail-safe mechanisms to ensure that every patient who needs a required test receives it every time it is needed'.[53] This points to the need for CDS systems to interact with physicians and provide prompts for preventive tests, treatment standards, drug interactions, etc. The quality improvement method described in this chapter can be labor intensive, especially in the phases of data collection and implementation of interventions. CDS combined with order entry can perform ongoing data collection and employ CQI methods in an automated fashion.[49,53,54] Such an approach is promising, but it can only be achieved with ongoing attention and revisions guided by current clinical trials, research into optimal implementation methods, and the participation and acceptance of clinicians.

SUMMARY

- Coronary heart disease mortality has decreased by one-third in the last decade alone owing to improvements in acute coronary care and primary and secondary prevention.
- Fibrinolytic therapy, aspirin and β-blockers improve survival in acute myocardial infarction and yet they are underutilized, especially in the elderly and, to a lesser extent, in women.

- Continuous quality improvement (CQI) is founded upon prospective and systematic attention to the processes and outcomes of care, as guided by data.
- CQI teams are multidisciplinary and require active participation of all members.
- Based on preliminary data highlighting an unwanted variation from practice standards, the CQI team analyzes the components of the process and, utilizing CQI tools and techniques, designs and implements an improvement plan.
- After an intervention has been made, data are recollected to assess its impact; periodic or continuous data collection ensures that success is achieved and maintained.
- Contributing factors to the gap between research and clinical practice include lack of awareness of clinical trial results, perceived contraindications to therapy, resistance to change, and aggressive marketing of higher cost, less effective products to physicians.
- Continuing medical education is more effective when a multifaceted, interactive approach is employed.
- Clinical practice guidelines inform medical decisions on appropriate preventive, diagnostic and treatment modalities, and may be implemented in the form of clinical prediction rules, critical pathways, and patient-specific reminders using computerized decision support systems.
- The Health Care Financing Administration and managed care organizations are increasingly using outcomes reporting to give providers a risk-adjusted 'scorecard' in order to encourage quality improvement efforts.

REFERENCES

1. *American Heart Association heart and stroke facts: 1995 statistical supplement.* Dallas, TX: American Heart Association, 1995.
2. *Morbidity and mortality chartbook on cardiovascular, lung, and blood diseases.* Washington, DC: National Heart, Lung, and Blood Institute, 1994.
3. McGovern PG, Pankow JS, Shahar E, *et al.*, for the Minnesota Heart Survey Investigators. Recent trends in acute coronary heart disease: mortality, morbidity, medical care, and risk factors. *N Engl J Med* 1996; **334**: 884–90.
4. Le Feuvre CA, Connolly SJ, Cairns JA, Gent M, Roberts RS. Comparison of mortality from acute myocardial infarction between 1979 and 1992 in a geographically defined stable population. *Am J Cardiol* 1996; **78**: 1345–9.

5. Ferrieres J, Cambou JP, Ruidavets JB, Pous J. Trends in acute myocardial infarction prognosis and treatment in southwestern France between 1985 and 1990 (The MONICA Project-Toulouse). *Am J Cardiol* 1995; **75**:1202–5.

6. Salomaa V, Miettinen H, Kuulasmaa K, *et al*. Decline of coronary heart disease mortality in Finland during 1983 to 1992: roles of incidence, recurrence, and case-fatality. The FINMONICA MI Register Study. *Circulation* 1996; **94**: 3130–7.

7. Naylor CD, Chen E. Population-wide mortality trends among patients hospitalized for acute myocardial infarction: the Ontario experience, 1981 to 1991. *J Am Coll Cardiol* 1994; **24**: 1431–8.

8. Gottlieb S, Goldbourt U, Boyko V, *et al*., for the SPRINT and Thrombolytic Survey Groups. Improved outcome of elderly patients (≥ 75 years of age) with acute myocardial infarction from 1981–1983 to 1992–1994 in Israel. *Circulation* 1997; **95**: 342–50.

♦9. Gruppo Italiano per lo Studio della Streptochinasi Nell'infarto Miocardico (GISSI). Effectiveness of intravenous thrombolytic treatment in acute myocardial infarction. *Lancet* 1986; **1**: 397–402.

10. Rosamond WD, Shahar E, McGovern PG, Sides TL, Luepker RV. Trends in coronary thrombolytic therapy for acute myocardial infarction (The Minnesota Heart Survey Registry, 1990 to 1993). *Am J Cardiol* 1996; **78**: 271–7.

11. Rogers WJ, Bowlby LJ, Chandra NC, *et al*. Treatment of myocardial infarction in the United States (1990 to 1993): observations from the National Registry of Myocardial Infarction. *Circulation* 1994; **90**: 2103–14.

12. Maynard C, Weaver WD, Litwin PE, *et al*. Hospital mortality in acute myocardial infarction in the era of reperfusion therapy (the Myocardial Infarction Triage and Intervention project). *Am J Cardiol* 1993; **72**: 877–82.

13. European Secondary Prevention Study Group. Translation of clinical trials into practice: a European population-based study of the use of thrombolysis for acute myocardial infarction. *Lancet* 1996; **347**: 1203–7.

14. French JK, Williams BF, Hart HH, *et al*. Prospective evaluation of eligibility for thrombolytic therapy in acute myocardial infarction. *Br Med J* 1996; **312**: 1637–41.

15. McLaughlin TJ, Soumerai SB, Willison DJ, *et al*. Adherence to national guidelines for drug treatment of suspected acute myocardial infarction. *Arch Intern Med* 1996; **156**: 799–805.

♦16. Barron HF, Bowlby LJ, Breen T, *et al*., for the National Registry of Myocardial Infarction 2 Investigators. Use of reperfusion therapy for acute myocardial infarction in the United States. Data from the National Registry of Myocardial Infarction 2. *Circulation* 1998; **97**: 1150–6.

17. Pashos CL, Normand SLT, Garfinkle JB, Newhouse JP, Epstein AM, McNeil BJ. Trends in the use of drug therapies in patients with acute myocardial infarction: 1988 to 1992. *J Am Coll Cardiol* 1994; **23**: 1023–30.

○18. Ryan TJ, Antman EM, Brooks NH, *et al*. 1999 update: ACC/AHA guidelines for the management of patients with acute myocardial infarction: a report of the American College of Cardiology/American Heart Association Task Force on Practice Guidelines (Committee on Management of Acute Myocardial Infarction). *J Am Coll Cardiol* 1999; **34**: 890–911.

19. Ellerbeck EF, Jencks SF, Radford MJ, *et al*. Quality of care for Medicare patients with acute myocardial infarction: 4-state pilot study from the Cooperative Cardiovascular Project. *JAMA* 1995; **273**: 1509–14.

20. Krumholz HM, Murillo JE, Chen J, *et al*. Thrombolytic therapy for eligible elderly patients with acute myocardial infarction. *JAMA* 1997; **277**: 1683–8.

21. Cox JL, Lee E, Langer A, Armstrong PW, Naylor CD, for the Canadian GUSTO Investigators. Time to treatment with thrombolytic therapy: determinants and effect on short-term nonfatal outcomes of acute myocardial infarction. *Can Med Assoc J* 1997; **156**: 497–505.

22. Danchin N, Vaur L, Genes N, *et al*. Management of acute myocardial infarction in intensive care units in 1995: a nationwide French survey of practice and early hospital results. *J Am Coll Cardiol* 1997; **30**: 1598–605.

23. Goff DC, Sellers DE, McGovern PG, *et al*., for the REACT Study Group. Knowledge of heart attack symptoms in a population survey in the United States. The REACT Trial. *Arch Intern Med* 1998; **158**: 2329–38.

24. Moses HW, Engelking N, Taylor GJ, *et al*. Effect of a two-year public education campaign on reducing response time of patients with symptoms of acute myocardial infarction. *Am J Cardiol* 1991; **68**: 249–51.

25. Maynard C, Weaver WD, Lambrew C, Bowlby LJ, Rogers WJ, Rubison RM, for the Participants in the National Registry of Myocardial Infarction. Factors influencing the time to administration of thrombolytic therapy with recombinant tissue plasminogen activator (data from the National Registry of Myocardial Infarction). *Am J Cardiol* 1995; **76**: 548–52.

○26. National Heart Attack Alert Program Coordinating Committee, 60 Minutes to Treatment Working Group. Emergency department: rapid identification and treatment of patients with acute myocardial infarction. *Ann Emerg Med* 1994; **23**: 311–29.

27. Weaver WD, White HD, Wilcox RG, *et al*., for the GUSTO-1 Investigators. Comparisons of characteristics and outcomes among women and men with acute myocardial infarction treated with thrombolytic therapy. *JAMA* 1996; **275**: 777–82.

28. Lambrew CT, Bowlby LJ, Rogers WJ, Chandra NC, Weaver WD, for the Time to Thrombolysis Substudy of the National Registry of Myocardial Infarction-1. Factors influencing the time to thrombolysis in acute myocardial infarction. *Arch Intern Med* 1997; **157**: 2577–82.

29. ISIS-2 (Second International Study of Infarct Survival) Collaborative Group. Randomized trial of intravenous streptokinase, oral aspirin, both or neither among 17,187 cases of suspected acute myocardial infarction. *Lancet* 1988; **2**: 349–60.

30. Hennekens CH, Jonas MA, Buring JE. The benefits of aspirin in acute myocardial infarction. *Arch Intern Med* 1994; **154**: 37–9.

31. Saketkhou BB, Conte FJ, Noris M, *et al.* Emergency department use of aspirin in patients with possible acute myocardial infarction. *Ann Intern Med* 1997; **127**: 126–9.

32. Krumholz HM, Radford MJ, Ellerbeck EF, *et al.* Aspirin in the treatment of acute myocardial infarction in elderly medicare beneficiaries. *Circulation* 1995; **2**: 2841–7.

♦33. Ayanian JZ, Hauptman PJ, Guadagnoli E, Antman EM, Pashos CL, McNeil BJ. Knowledge and practices of generalist and specialist physicians regarding drug therapy for acute myocardial infarction. *N Engl J Med* 1994; **331**: 1136–42.

34. Yusuf S, Peto R, Lewis J, *et al.* Beta blockade during and after myocardial infarction: an overview of the randomized trials. *Prog Cardiovasc Dis* 1985; **27**: 335–71.

35. Sial SH, Malone M, Freeman JL, Battiola R, Nachodsky J, Goodwin JS. Beta blocker use in the treatment of community hospital patients discharged after myocardial infarction. *J Gen Intern Med* 1994; **9**: 599–605.

36. Brand DA, Newcomer LN, Freibruger A, Tian H. Cardiologists' practices compared with practice guidelines: use of beta-blockade after acute myocardial infarction. *J Am Coll Cardiol* 1995; **26**: 1432–6.

37. Soumerai SB, McLaughlin TJ, Spiegelman D, Hertzmark E, Thibault G, Goldman L. Adverse outcomes of under use of beta-blockers in elderly survivors of acute myocardial infarction. *JAMA* 1997; **277**: 115–21.

38. Kennedy HL, Rosenson RS. Physician use of beta-adrenergic blocking therapy: a changing perspective (editorial). *J Am Coll Cardiol* 1995: **26**: 547–52.

♦39. Gottlieb SS, McCarter RJ, Vogel RA. Effect of beta-blockade on mortality among high-risk and low-risk patients after myocardial infarction. *N Engl J Med* 1998; **339**: 489–97.

40. Chadda K, Goldstein S, Byington R, *et al.* Effect of propranolol after acute myocardial infarction in patients with congestive heart failure. *Circulation* 1986; **73**: 503–10.

41. Krumholz HM, Radford MJ, Wang Y, Chen J, Heiat A, Marciniak TA. National use and effectiveness of β-blockers for the treatment of elderly patients after acute myocardial infarction. National Cooperative Cardiovascular Project. *JAMA* 1998; **280**: 623–9.

42. Viskin S, Barron HV. Beta blockers prevent cardiac death following a myocardial infarction: so why are so many infarct survivors discharged without beta blockers? (editorial) *Am J Cardiol* 1996; **78**: 821–2.

43. Antman EM, Lau J, Kupelnick B, Mosteller F, Chalmers TC. A comparison of results of meta-analyses of randomized controlled trials and recommendations of clinical experts: treatments for myocardial infarction. *JAMA* 1992; **268**: 240–8.

43a. Jollis JG, DeLong ER, Peterson ED, *et al.* Outcome of acute myocardial infarction according to the specialty of the admitting physician. *N Engl J Med* 1996; **335**: 1880–7.

43b. Allison JJ, Kiefe CI, Weissman NW, *et al.* Relationship of hospital teaching status with quality of care and mortality for Medicare patients with acute MI. *JAMA* 2000; **284**: 1256–62.

44. Packer M, Bristow MR, Cohn JN, *et al.*, for the US Carvedilol Heart Failure Study Group. The effect of carvedilol on morbidity and mortality in patients with chronic heart failure. *N Engl J Med* 1996; **334**: 1349–55.

○45. Davis DA, Thomson MA, Oxman AD, Haynes RB. Changing physician performance: a systematic review of the effect of continuing medical education strategies. *JAMA* 1995; **274**: 700–5.

46. Felch WC, Scanlon DM. Bridging the gap between research and education: the role of continuing medical education (editorial). *JAMA* 1997; **277**: 155–6.

47. MacKenzie JD, Greenes RA. The World Wide Web: redefining medical education. *JAMA* 1997; **278**: 1785–6.

48. Cook DJ, Greengold NL, Ellrodt AG, Weingarten SR. The relation between systematic reviews and practice guidelines. *Ann Intern Med* 1997; **127**: 210–16.

49. Weingarten S. Practice guidelines and prediction rules should be subject to careful clinical testing (editorial). *JAMA* 1997; **277**: 1977–8.

○50. Grimshaw JM, Russell IT. Effect of clinical guidelines on medical practice: a systematic review of rigorous evaluations. *Lancet* 1993; **342**: 1317–22.

51. Weingarten SR, Riedinger MS, Conner L, *et al.* Practice guidelines and reminders to reduce duration of hospital stay for patients with chest pain: an interventional trial. *Ann Intern Med* 1994; **120**: 257–63.

52. Lee TH, Cooper HL. Translating good advice into better practice (editorial). *JAMA* 1997; **278**: 2108–9.

53. Leape LL. Translating medical science into medical practice: do we need a National Medical Standards Board (editorial)? *JAMA* 1995; **273**: 1534–7.

54. McDonald CJ, Overhage JM. Guidelines you can follow and can trust: an ideal and an example (editorial). *JAMA* 1994; **271**: 872–3.

55. Katz DA, Griffith JL, Beshansky JR, Selker HP. The use of empiric clinical data in the evaluation of practice guidelines for unstable angina. *JAMA* 1996; **276**: 1568–74.

56. Dracup K. Alonzo AA, Atkins JM, *et al*. The physician's role in minimizing prehospital delay in patients at high risk for acute myocardial infarction: recommendations from the National Heart Attack Alert Program. *Ann Intern Med* 1997; **126**: 645–51.

57. Stiell IG, McKnight RD, Greenberg GH, *et al*. Implementation of the Ottawa ankle rules. *JAMA* 1994; **271**: 827–32.

♦58. Soumerai SB, McLaughlin TJ, Gurwitz JH, *et al*. Effect of local medical opinion leaders on quality of care for acute myocardial infarction. A randomized controlled trial. *JAMA* 1998; **279**: 1358–63.

59. Leviton LC, Goldenberg RL, Baker CS, *et al*. Methods to encourage the use of antenatal corticosteroid therapy for fetal maturation. A randomized controlled trial. *JAMA* 1999; **281**: 46–52.

60. Selker HP, Griffith JL, Beshansky JR, *et al*. Patient-specific predictions of outcome in myocardial infarction for real-time emergency use: a thrombolytic predictive instrument. *Ann Intern Med* 1997; **127**: 538–56.

61. Pearson SD, Goulart-Fisher D, Lee TH. Critical pathways as a strategy for improving care: problems and potential. *Ann Intern Med* 1995; **123**: 941–8.

62. Every NR, Hochman J, Becker R, Kopecky S, Cannon CP, for the Committee on Acute Cardiac Care, Council on Clinical Cardiology, American Heart Association. Critical pathways: a review. *Circulation* 2000; **101**: 461–5.

63. Marrie TJ, Lau CY, Wheeler SL, Wong CJ, Vandervoort MK, Feagan BG, for the CAPITAL Study Investigators. A controlled trial of a critical pathway for treatment of community-acquired pneumonia. *JAMA* 2000; **283**: 749–55.

64. Zinman D. Ranking open heart surgery. *Newsday*, 1990; December 5: 4,33.

65. Hannan EL, Kilburn H, Racz M, Shields E, Chassin MR. Improving the outcomes of coronary artery bypass surgery in New York State. *JAMA* 1994; **271**: 761–6.

66. O'Connor GT, Plume SK, Olmstead EM, *et al*. A regional intervention to improve the hospital mortality associated with coronary artery bypass graft surgery. *JAMA* 1996; **275**: 841–6.

67. Marshall MN, Shekelle PG, Leatherman S, Brook RH. The public release of performance data: what do we expect to gain? A review of the evidence. *JAMA* 2000; **283**: 1866–74.

68. Ghali WA, Ash AS, Hall RE, Moskowitz MA. Statewide quality improvement initiatives and mortality after cardiac surgery. *JAMA* 1997; **277**: 379–82.

69. Jencks SF. Can large-scale interventions improve care? *JAMA* 1997; **277**: 419–20.

70. Balas EA, Boren SA, Brown GD, *et al*. Effect of physician profiling on utilization. Meta-analysis of randomized clinical trials. *J Gen Intern Med* 1996; **11**: 584–90.

♦71. Marciniak TA, Ellerbeck EF, Radford MJ, *et al*. Improving the quality of care for medicare patients with acute myocardial infarction. Results from the Cooperative Cardiovascular Project. *JAMA* 1998; **279**: 1351–7.

72. Topol EJ, Block PC, Holmes DR, Klinke WP, Brinker JA. Readiness for the scorecard era in cardiovascular medicine. *Am J Cardiol* 1995; **75**: 1170–3.

73. Szilagyi PG, Bordley C, Vann JC, *et al*. Effect of patient reminder/recall interventions on immunization rates: a review. *JAMA* 2000; **284**: 1820–7.

74. Johnston ME, Langton KB, Haynes RB, Mathieu A. Effects of computer-based clinical decision support systems on clinician performance and patient outcome: a critical appraisal of research. *Ann Intern Med* 1994; **120**: 135–42.

75. Demakis JG, Beauchamp C, Cull WL, *et al*., for the Department of Veterans Affairs Cooperative Study Group on Computer Reminders in Ambulatory Care. Improving residents' compliance with standards of ambulatory care: results from the VA Cooperative Study on Computerized Reminders. *JAMA* 2000; **284**: 1411–16.

38

A national certification program for anticoagulation therapy providers

LYNN B OERTEL*

The striking efficacy and safety of warfarin therapy are well documented, however, the monitoring and management aspects to achieve optimal therapy continues to challenge health care providers. Warfarin, with its relatively narrow therapeutic index, has potential catastrophic adverse outcomes, is often implicated in litigation cases, and has been under-utilized in some patient populations. This creates unnecessary costs to society. The purpose of a national certification process is to protect public health and well being by focusing efforts at the level of the direct care provider. This Certified Anticoagulation Care Provider (CACP) credential is the only multidisciplinary certification in the USA.

INTRODUCTION

Clinical research findings continue to stimulate interest to optimize oral anticoagulation therapy for patients. The primary focus of earlier research reports was to determine the safest, most appropriate therapeutic intensity level of oral anticoagulation for disease-specific conditions.[1–3] Once this was established, standardizing the approach to monitoring therapy by utilizing the most appropriate laboratory value, namely the international normalized ratio (INR), became the subject of numerous reports.[4–8] Additionally, results of randomized, clinical trials, such as the atrial fibrillation trials and prevention of complications in postmyocardial infarction, have expanded the clinical indications for therapeutic treatment using oral anticoagulants.[9–14] More recent reports describe the therapeutic outcomes achieved for specific populations.[15–17]

The importance of patient education and improved management strategies are frequently cited in these reports.

The approach to, or style of, care delivery is a key variable for achieving optimal anticoagulation outcomes in patients.

Indications of this can be found by comparing outcomes between traditional modes of patient management and organized anticoagulation clinic modes of care delivery.[16,18–20]

Furthermore, evidence is accumulating that demonstrates that health care costs are reduced and patient satisfaction levels are enhanced with this type of delivery mode.[18,21,22]

Already, over 2 million Americans are prescribed oral

*Lynn B Oertel representing the National Certification Board for Anticoagulation Providers: Richard C Becker, Stuart T Haines, Sally Loken, Mary Lynn McPherson, Geno Merli, Lynn B Oertel, William Rock, Gordon J Vanscoy, and Thomas H Wiser.

anticoagulants[23] and this number is expected to increase, along with the complexity and diversity of medical issues surrounding these patients. The challenge facing health care providers today is how to best provide optimal patient care with anticoagulation therapy.

Increasingly, efforts are focused upon determining the best model of care delivery to meet the demands of these ever larger numbers of patients. It is believed that an organized, systematic approach to care will achieve the best possible outcomes for patients, improve satisfaction and adherence to treatment plans and, ultimately, have a positive impact on the financial aspects of treatment. Anticoagulant therapy, specifically with warfarin sodium, encompasses a broad clinical spectrum with which health care providers must be knowledgeable and competent. However, what is not clear is how these health care providers will be prepared and educated; a key factor in optimizing patient care.

> A certification program is one mechanism to validate the advanced knowledge and skills necessary to optimize patient care and management with this challenging treatment modality.

Defining measurable competencies, specifically related to antithrombotic and anticoagulant therapies, will help standardize patient care across the country.

HISTORICAL LANDMARKS AND DEVELOPMENT

The number of patients treated with warfarin therapy is expected to grow; especially as the population in the USA continues to age. Recent developments, as a result of clinical research trials, have opened the door for increased use of warfarin as well as the potential for other types of antithrombotic or anticoagulant agents. Management and surveillance for many of the time-consuming aspects of anticoagulant therapy, previously undertaken by physicians, are now assumed by other health care professionals, such as pharmacists, nurses, advanced practice nurses, and physician's assistants. This transition allows physicians to devote more time and effort to other areas. Changes in health care delivery systems also play a role as non-physician providers assume more responsibility in monitoring and management of patients' anticoagulant therapy or in establishing anticoagulation management services. However, until recently, standards of care or clinical guidelines for coordinated out-patient anticoagulation therapy did not exist. A paper published by Ansell et al., provides consensus guidelines for coordinated out-patient oral anticoagulation therapy management.[24] These guidelines create a reproducible framework for the provision of services, suggest a structure and process for care delivery, and evaluate outcomes of coordinated out-patient anti-coagulation services. These guidelines, along with current Consensus Panel recommendations,[8] provide a strong theoretical base for developing competency-based guidelines for anticoagulation therapy providers.

Health issues pertaining to antithrombotic and anticoagulant therapies encompass a broad clinical spectrum. The health care professionals who assess, diagnose, and determine the management and educational needs for these patients have first-hand appreciation of the considerable time and effort needed to achieve success. The narrow therapeutic window of effectiveness of warfarin requires continual assessments of patients' risk–benefit ratio, persistent surveillance or monitoring, and in-depth patient education provided by skilled professionals.

In recent years, a national group, the Anticoagulation Forum, was established with a primary goal to pursue excellence in patient management through education, promotion of research, and professional dialogue. This group is comprised of physicians, nurses, pharmacists, and other health care professionals who have an interest in anticoagulation. The Anticoagulation Forum has sponsored five national conferences on a bi-annual schedule. Each conference has surpassed the previous in attendance and scope of the program scheduling. On a smaller scale, regional forums have been organized across the country that continue to offer educational and professional networking opportunities. Interest and attendance at courses and symposiums are growing and provide a valuable source of continuing education for clinicians.

While each of these opportunities fills a gap for knowledge, there are no standards addressing the scope, breadth, or achievement of minimal competencies in anticoagulation and antithrombotic therapies. To make a significant impact on patient care and ultimately clinical and financial outcomes of therapy at a national level, a national certification program must be developed to ensure that this can be achieved. Of note, there are several programs which offer a certificate course of study but, in general, these are limited to pharmacists, thus preventing clinicians from nursing and medicine to participate. For example, the American Society of Health System Pharmacists (ASHP) sponsors a certificate and training course in anticoagulant therapy; however, this course is limited to relatively few pharmacists each year. The Veterans Affairs Medical Center in Pittsburgh also has developed a program to certify anticoagulation providers,[25] but it, too, limits the number of participants.

The University of Southern Indiana has developed an internet-based continuing education course on anti-coagulation management. This course attracts clinicians with various disciplines from across the country. As a side note, the curriculum for this course of study is based upon the knowledge domains (or competency statements) developed by the National Certification Board for Anticoagulation Providers (NCBAP) for their national certification program which is described in more detail below.

Establishing a formal process for a national certification program was a logical step in defining minimum competencies for clinical practice for providers of anticoagulant therapy.

> By definition, a certification process will validate achievement of a specific set of knowledge-based competencies, thus promoting standards of care within a specific area. Credentialing or certification processes undertaken by a professional practice help assure the quality of care rendered to patients.

Relative to the history of the American Board of Internal Medicine, Benson[26] discusses certification in the context of achieving professional accountability. Styles and Gouley et al. have expressed similar views about the credentialing or certification process and its value to the profession and patient care from a nurse's and pharmacist's view, respectively.[27,28] The competitive managed care market, along with the demand for measurable quality outcomes, forces providers to offer high-quality programs. Certification in anticoagulation is timely as changes in the health care market continue and new roles are emerging. Health care services and providers who demonstrate advance levels of education and clinical competence may have a competitive edge in future health care settings.

DEVELOPMENTAL PROCESS TO CREATE A NATIONAL CERTIFICATION PROGRAM IN ANTITHROMBOTIC AND ANTICOAGULATION THERAPIES

A multidisciplinary group of clinicians was organized during the fall of 1996 with the belief that a certification process would demonstrate acquisition of specific knowledge and clinical competencies. The value of developing and implementing a provider competency program that included professionals from three distinct disciplines, namely medicine, nursing, and pharmacy, is an innovative collaboration. This collaborative effort mirrors what is often found in real-world practice sites and has the greatest potential to ensure the best clinical decision-making for patient care and management. Additionally, the results of a survey conducted by the Anticoagulation Forum during the winter of 1997 revealed strong support and belief in the need for a certification program.[29]

The grass roots effort of these clinicians began to take further definition by adopting the name Certified Anticoagulation Provider Working Group. However, in 1998, the name was officially changed to the National Certification Board of Anticoagulation Providers (NCBAP) to reflect the formal changes in the organizational structure of the entire certification process. Initially, the aim was to develop the objectives and process required to achieve the competencies for anticoagulation therapy providers, and to propose a framework for a national certification process that validates achievement of anticoagulation therapy providers' competencies.[25] After months of work, a framework emerged and efforts to clarify the clinical knowledge content was begun in earnest. A mission statement of the NCBAP evolved and reads: 'To develop, maintain and protect the Certified Anticoagulation Care Provider (CACP) credential and the certification process'.

Sharing a common goal of improving patient care, the collective knowledge, skills, and expertise this group represented helped to develop a high-quality interdisciplinary product. The group reviewed existing certifications programs such as the Certified Diabetes Educator model, and others, to aid in their efforts. The group determined that the level of professional care that would have the largest impact on the delivery of patient care was the anticoagulation provider; in other words, clinicians who spent a majority of time managing patients' anticoagulant therapy as opposed to medical directors overseeing clinic operations or generalists who occasionally are involved with patients' warfarin therapy.

A major element in this developmental process was to define the theoretical constructs of the certification process. Five content areas (or knowledge domains) were identified. Competency-based learning objectives were created for each domain to further augment the theoretical framework. Throughout the development of the domains, the group periodically solicited comments and opinions from experts and colleagues in the field. This was an important step in order to reflect the multidisciplinary approach that the group believed was extremely important. Some of the group members had first-hand experience in developing certificate courses with their affiliated academic institutions and this provided additional insight in the decision making.

An important event during this stage was the opportunity to present the 'work-in-progress' to colleagues and experts in the field. This opportunity took place during the Anticoagulation Forum's Fourth National Conference in May of 1997. At this time, the knowledge domains were presented and distributed to the attendees. Comments and feedback from this national forum meeting were incorporated into further revisions. Of note, the enthusiasm and interest generated as a result of this interaction reinforced the beliefs in the need for such a program. As a result of the efforts described above, these five content areas formulate the knowledge domains upon which this certification process is based:

I applied pathophysiology of thromboembolic disease
II patient assessment and management
III patient education
IV applied pharmacology of antithrombotic agents
V operational (administrative) procedures

Details of the current version of the knowledge domains are located in the Appendix to this chapter and a list of valuable resources and references is also included.

Determining the eligibility criteria was another challenge in the overall process. The Board requires current registration as a registered nurse, advance practice nurse, registered or licensed pharmacist, licensed physician or certified physician's assistant. This requirement is consistent with national trends for minimal entry-into-practice levels and imparts a broad enough scope of practice expected of a CACP. Additionally, candidates must hold a professional licence for a minimum of 18 months and provide evidence as anticoagulation therapy providers.

The final stage of this process was devoted to the creation of test items for use in the certification examination. The examination's content was derived from the clinical competency statements associated with each domain and measure one's knowledge and skills related to antithrombotic and anticoagulation therapy management. The Board made a deliberate decision to emphasize patient assessment, management, and education – the foundation for optimizing patient care. Thus, 50 per cent of the test items are derived from the second domain, patient assessment and management. The domain on patient education was deemed second most important; therefore 20 per cent of the test items were developed using this domain's theoretical content. The remainder of the examination content is equally divided among the three remaining domains (applied pathophysiology of thromboembolic disease, applied pharmacology of antithrombotic agents and operation (administrative) procedures) with 10 per cent of the test items derived from each domain's content.

An extensive amount of time and energy was spent to validate the bank of accumulated test items. This was accomplished by: (1) consulting with experts in the field; (2) conducting a pilot testing phase including experts and generalists, and (3) analyzing the results to discard or rewrite poor test items. The consequences of these procedures yielded a fair, yet decisive, examination. The certification examination is composed of 150 multiple-choice questions and a minimum score of 80 per cent is required to pass.

THE NATIONAL CERTIFICATION PROCESS

The Certified Anticoagulation Care Provider (CACP) credential is governed and awarded by the National Certification Board for Anticoagulation Providers. Clinicians who meet the eligibility requirements are welcome to participate in the CACP certification process. A candidate handbook for the application process is available which describes the eligibility criteria and procedures in further detail. The knowledge domains that describe the scope of knowledge from which the examination is based and a recommended reference list is also available. This national certification process requires evidence of clinical experience with direct patient management and is an important aspect of the application itself. Therefore, a minimum of 75 patient encounter forms must be submitted which serve to document these experiences. The entire application must be submitted 60 days prior to the test date one wishes to apply for. A board member of the NCBAP reviews the entire application packet and determines approval. If deficiencies are detected, the candidate is informed and an opportunity is provided for the candidate to make appropriate revisions and satisfy requirements. An application fee of $300 US is required.

The first certification examination was conducted in 1999, just two and a half years after the start of this process. Since then, five additional testing opportunities have occurred across the USA and the certification process continues. To date, there are nearly 90 CACPs with representation from almost 30 states. The majority of CACPs are pharmacists, followed by nurses, nurse practitioners (advance practice nurses), and one physician assistant.

Recently, the Board conducted a survey of all clinicians who pursued CACP credentials, regardless of performance in the examination. The results of the survey indicate three primary reasons for pursuing the CACP credential: (1) to improve one's clinical skills; (2) to increase marketability or patient referrals; and (3) to validate one's knowledge and level of expertise in the area of anticoagulation. The vast majority of clinicians would recommend this certification process to a colleague.

FUTURE DIRECTIONS

Although still in the infancy of its development, this national certification process continues to gain recognition and acceptance in the anticoagulation and antithrombotic arenas.

> Although continuing education courses and symposiums are available, there remains a need for advanced education and to validate the achievement of clinical expertise and competency in this specific area.

Continued research in the clinical arena may establish the need for organized, systematic approaches to patient care management along with the importance of having skilled, knowledgeable providers at the level of direct patient contact.

The process to develop a national certification program remains successful due to the collective talents and commitment of those involved. The National

Certification Board for Anticoagulation Providers is committed to establishing mechanisms for sustaining and strengthening this process. This credentialing process has been well received and work continues on various fronts. The Board is actively seeking ratification of organizational by-laws, rotating new members to the Board, and establishing sub-committees to address specific issues such as web-page development, test item writing, and so on. Increasing the accessibility for interested providers is key to the program's success. Therefore, opportunities for eligible candidates to sit for the certification examination are planned several times per calendar year in varying geographical locations throughout the USA. In the meanwhile, additional and up-to-date information can be obtained by visiting the following website: www.acforum.org.

SUMMARY

- The number of Americans who require warfarin and other antithrombotic drugs continues to increase and standardizing the approach to monitor and manage warfarin therapy will have a positive impact on their therapeutic outcomes.
- The National Certification Board for Anticoagulation Providers sponsors the only multidisciplinary certification process for anticoagulation therapy in the country.
- The certification process is designed and intended for practitioners whose primary role as an anticoagulation provider includes systematic, organized, and on-going patient education and therapeutic management.
- Five knowledge domains (or content areas), and their related clinical competency objectives, form the theoretical base of this certification process.
- The Certified Anticoagulation Care Provider (CACP) credential requires evidence of satisfactory clinical experience as well as achieving a passing score on the certification examination.
- Nearly 90 health care providers (pharmacists, advance practice nurses, nurses and a physician assistant) have earned the CACP credential, representing approximately 30 states in the USA.

REFERENCES

1. Hull RD, Hirsh J, Jay R, et al. Different intensities of oral anticoagulant therapy in the treatment of proximal-vein thrombosis. N Engl J Med 1982; **307**: 1676–81.
2. Saour JN, Sieck JO, Mamo LAR, et al. Trial of different intensities of anticoagulation in patients with prosthetic heart valves. N Engl J Med 1990; **322**: 428–32.
3. Turpie ACG, Hirsh J, Gunstensen J, et al. Randomised comparison of two intensities of oral anticoagulant therapy after tissue heart valve replacement. Lancet 1988; **1**: 1242–5.
4. Bussey HI, Force RW, Bianco TM, et al. Reliance on prothrombin time ratios causes significant errors in anticoagulation therapy. Arch Intern Med 1992; **152**: 278–82.
5. Hirsh J, Poller L. The international normalized ratio. Arch Intern Med 1994; **154**: 282–8.
6. Poller L. A simple nomogram for the derivation of international normalised ratios for the standardisation of prothrombin time. Thromb Haemost 1988; **60**: 18–20.
7. Hirsh J. Substandard monitoring of warfarin in North America: time for change. Arch Intern Med 1992; **153**: 257–8.
8. Hirsh J, Dalen JE, Deykin D, Anderson DR, Poller L, Bussey H, Ansell J. Oral anticoagulants: mechanism of action, clinical effectiveness, and optimal therapeutic range. Chest 1998; **114**(suppl): 445S–69S.
9. Stroke Prevention in Atrial Fibrillation Investigators. Stroke prevention in atrial fibrillation study: final results. Circulation 1991; **84**: 527–39.
10. The Boston Area Anticoagulation Trial for Atrial Fibrillation Investigators. The effect of low-dose warfarin on the risk of stroke in patients with nonrheumatic atrial fibrillation. N Engl J Med 1990; **323**: 1505–11.
11. Ezekowitz MD, Bridgers SL, James KE, et al. Warfarin in the prevention of stroke associated with non-rheumatic atrial fibrillation. N Engl J Med 1992; **327**: 1406–12.
12. Godtfredsen J, Boysen G, Anderson ED, Anderson B. Placebo-controlled, randomized trial of warfarin and aspirin for prevention of thromboembolic complications in chronic atrial fibrillation: the Copenhagen AFASAK Study. Lancet 1989; **1**: 175–7.
13. Connolly SJ, Laupacis A, Gent M, Roberts RS, Carins JA, Joyner C. Canadian atrial fibrillation anticoagulation (CAFA) study. J Am Coll Cardiol 1991; **18**: 349–55.
14. ASPECT Research Group. Effect of long-term oral anticoagulant treatment on mortality and cardiovascular morbidity after myocardial infarction. Lancet 1994; **434**: 499–503.
15. Cannegieter SC, Rosendaal FR, Wintzen AR, van der Meer FJM, Vandenbroucke JP, Briet E. Optimal oral anticoagulant therapy in patients with mechanical heart valves. N Engl J Med 1995; **333**: 11–17.
16. Cortelazzo S, Finazzi G, Viero P, et al. Thrombotic and hemorrhagic complications in patients with mechanical heart valve prosthesis attending an anticoagulation clinic. Thromb Haemost 1993; **69**: 316–20.
17. Van den Besselaar AM, van der Meer FJM, Gerrits-Drabbe CW. Therapeutic control of oral anticoagulant treatment in the Netherlands. Am J Clin Pathol 1988; **90**: 685–90.
18. Bussey HI, Chiquette E, Amato MG. Anticoagulation clinic care versus routine medical care: a review and interim report. J Thromb Thrombolys 1996; **2**: 315–19.
19. Garabedian-Ruffalo SM, Gray DR, Sax MJ, et al.

Retrospective evaluation of a pharmacist-managed warfarin anticoagulation clinic. *Am J Hosp Pharm* 1985; **42**: 304–8.

20. Cohen IA, Hutchison TA, Kirking DM, Shue ME. Evaluation of a pharmacist-managed anticoagulation clinic. *J Clin Hosp Pharm* 1985; **10**: 167–75.

21. Gray DR, Garabedian-Ruffalo SM, Chretien SD. Cost-justification of a clinical pharmacist-managed anticoagulation clinic. *Drug Intell Clin Pharm* 1985; **19**: 575–80.

22. Lee YP, Schommer JC. Effect of a pharmacist-managed anticoagulation clinic on warfarin-related readmissions. *Am J Health Sys Pharm* 1996; **53**: 1580–3.

23. Cypress BK. *Patterns of ambulatory care in internal medicine, The National Ambulatory Care Survey, United States, January 1980–December 1981*. Vital and Health Statistics, Public Health Service. US Government Printing Office, Washington, DC, 1984. DHHS publication No. (PHS) 84–1741.

♦24. Ansell JE, Buttaro ML, Voltis TO, Knowlton CH, and the Anticoagulation Guidelines Task Force. Consensus guidelines for coordinated outpatient oral anticoagulation therapy management. *Ann Pharmacother* 1997; **31**: 604–15.

25. Vancscoy GJ. Workshop: Credentialing of anticoagulation providers: a proposed model. *J Thromb Thrombolys* 1998; **5**: S53–S61.

26. Benson JA. Certification and recertification: one approach to professional accountability. *Ann Intern Med* 1991; **114**: 238–42.

27. Styles MM. Credentialing: pretensions and realities. *Credentialing News*, a publication of the American Nurses Credentialing Center, Washington, DC, Winter 1996–97: 1,6.

28. Gouley DR, Fitzgerald WL, Davis RL. Competency, board certification, credentialing, and specialization: who benefits: *Am J Managed Care* 1997; **3**: 795–801.

29. Anticoagulation Forum 1997 Winter Survey. Presented at *Anticoagulation Forum's 4th National Conference*, San Antonio, Texas, May, 1997.

APPENDIX: NATIONAL CERTIFICATION BOARD FOR ANTICOAGULATION PROVIDERS KNOWLEDGE DOMAINS (COMPETENCY STATEMENTS) FOR CERTIFIED ANTICOAGULATION CARE PROVIDERS (VERSION: 3/1/2000)

Domain I: Applied physiology and pathophysiology of thromboembolic disorders

GOAL

The Certified Anticoagulation Care Provider must have a working knowledge regarding the normal physiological processes of hemostasis and thrombosis. In addition, the Certified Anticoagulation Care Provider must be knowledgeable regarding the etiology, risk factors, and clinical manifestations of pathologic thrombus formation. To meet this goal, the Certified Anticoagulation Care Provider should be able to:

1 Describe the general process of hemostasis and thrombosis, including the role of the vascular endothelium, platelets, circulating clotting factors, endogenous anticoagulants, and thrombolytic proteins.

2 Describe the clotting cascade including the major functions of thrombin and fibrin. Identify the intrinsic (contact) pathway, extrinsic pathway, and the common pathway.

3 Explain how vitamin-K dependent coagulation proteins (including proteins C and S) are produced. State the role of vitamin K in their production. State the relative physiological half-life of vitamin-K dependent proteins.

4 Define the terms platelet adhesion, activation, and aggregation.

5 Compare and contrast the formation of a thrombus under conditions of high flow (arteries) and static flow (veins and cardiac chambers). State the relative contribution of the vascular subendothelium, platelets, and clotting factors in each.

6 Recognize the most frequent signs and symptoms of deep vein thrombosis.

7 Recognize the most frequent signs and symptoms of pulmonary embolism.

8 List the objective tests that may be employed to diagnose deep vein thrombosis and pulmonary embolism.

9 Recognize well-documented risk factors for venous thromboembolism.

10 List the most frequent signs and symptoms of the post-thrombotic (post-phlebitic) syndrome and state how the syndrome may be distinguished from acute deep vein thrombosis.

11 List the most frequent signs and symptoms of peripheral arterial disease and peripheral arterial ischemia/infarct.

12 List the most frequent signs and symptoms of coronary artery disease and cardiac ischemia/infarct.

13 List the most frequent signs and symptoms of cerebral vascular disease and cerebral ischemia/infarct.

14 List the major distinguishing characteristics of ischemic stroke, transient ischemic attacks (TIA's), and hemorrhagic stroke.

15 List the most frequent signs and symptoms of atrial fibrillation and atrial flutter.

16 List the most frequent signs and symptoms of heart failure.

17 Identify the types of cardiac replacement valves

commonly in use and rank the relative risk of thrombosis associated with each based on type and position.

18 List the diseases and risk factors associated with cardioembolic stroke.

19 Recognize, based on major clinical parameters, when an individual may have an inherited or acquired disorder of hypercoagulabilty including protein C deficiency, protein S deficiency, antithrombin III deficiency, activated protein resistance, antiphospholipid antibodies, and occult malignancy.

Domain II: Patient assessment and management

GOAL

The Certified Anticoagulation Care Provider must possess the knowledge, skills, and competencies to manage and monitor patients on anticoagulant therapy. This includes the ability to assess the efficacy and toxicity of the prescribed antithrombotic treatment, determine if the therapeutic goals have been achieved, and identify patient-related variables that effect therapy. The Certified Anticoagulation Care Provider should be able to:

1 List the appropriate indications for the use of antithrombotic agents including Food and Drug Administration (FDA)-approved indications as well as the grade A, B, and C recommendations published in American College of Chest Physicians (ACCP) Consensus Conference on Antithrombotic Therapy.

2 List the components of a problem-oriented anticoagulant therapy database. The database should include relevant subjective and objective findings necessary to appropriately monitor patients on antithrombotic therapy.

3 List the medical problems or clinical conditions that would preclude the use of antithrombotic agents or require alteration in dosing (e.g. peptic ulcer, thyroid disease, and congestive heart failure).

4 Given a specific patient history including co-morbid diseases, perform a benefit and risk analysis regarding the use of antithrombotic agents (warfarin, heparin, low-molecular-weight heparin, and antiplatelet medications).

5 Describe the potential adverse effects to a fetus or infant associated with the maternal use of antithrombotic agents (warfarin, heparin, low-molecular-weight heparin, and antiplatelet medications) during pregnancy and while breastfeeding.

6 Explain/describe the appropriate use of antithrombotic agents when used in special patient

groups (e.g. children, elderly, patients with warfarin resistance, hepatic cirrhosis, or seizures). State the most common adverse effects in these special population groups.

7 Describe/analyze the commonly used laboratory methods for monitoring antithrombotic therapy including prothrombin time (PT), prothrombin time ratio (PTR), international normalized ratio (INR), activated partial thromboplastin time (aPTT), anti-Xa activity, heparin concentration, hemoccult test, hematocrit, platelet count, and absolute neutrophil count. Provide a systematic plan for continuous monitoring of the appropriate test in a patient-specific manner.

8 Identify normal/therapeutic/toxic values and potential interpretation problems with the use of each of the following laboratory tests: prothrombin time (PT), prothrombin time ratio (PTR), international normalized ratio (INR), activated partial thromboplastin time (aPTT).

9 Make appropriate decisions when adjusting the dose of antithrombotic therapy to improve anticoagulation control (i.e. tailor dosage adjustments based on patient-related variables).

10 Develop a plan to detect, evaluate, and manage a hemorrhagic event in a patient who experiences bleeding while taking anticoagulant therapy.

11 Determine the appropriate action to detect, evaluate, and manage a non-hemorrhagic adverse event in a patient who is taking anticoagulation therapy (e.g. skin necrosis, thrombocytopenia, diarrhea).

12 List and state the relative effectiveness of commonly used non-pharmacological methods for the prevention and treatment of thromboembolism.

13 Describe and recommend an appropriate plan to initiate anticoagulant therapy including the concomitant use of multiple antithrombotic agents.

14 Develop a plan for systematic, continuous follow-up care (e.g. management and coordination) for patients on anticoagulation therapy.

15 Describe and implement appropriate plans for discontinuing antithrombotic therapy taking into account disease-related and patient-related variables (e.g. non-compliance, thromboembolic risk, development of new medical problems).

16 Identify illnesses and lifestyle behaviors that may alter anticoagulation response. Specifically, describe their likely impact (e.g. increased or diminished anticoagulant effect), clinical significance, and appropriate actions to take to avoid them.

17 Develop rational strategies to manage drug–drug and drug–food (including nutrient) interactions with antithrombotic therapy.

18 Identify and measure outcome criteria for patient satisfaction.

19 Identify risk factors for anticoagulation-induced

bleeding. Appropriately assess a patient at risk for bleeding, and describe appropriate situations when a patient should be referred to a physician for further evaluation.

20 Identify risk factors for the development of thromboembolism. Appropriately assess a patient at risk and recognize circumstances when a patient should be referred to a physician for further evaluation.

21 Develop a specific plan to manage a patient's anticoagulant therapy in situations requiring temporary discontinuation (e.g. dental procedures, surgery, colonoscopy).

22 Compare the potential advantages and disadvantages of point-of-care testing, patient self-testing, and patient self-management for monitoring antithrombotic therapies.

23 Describe the procedures to properly use capillary blood testing devices (e.g. Coumatrak, Coaguchek, ProTime).

24 Recognize and describe conditions that require emergency triage (e.g. acute shortness of breath, severe chest pain, loss of consciousness, or apnea).

25 Interact and communicate effectively with other health care professionals to facilitate the care of patients on anticoagulation therapy.

Domain III: Patient education

GOAL

The Certified Anticoagulation Care Provider must provide patient education that is tailored to patients' specific needs to promote safety, enhance adherence, and positively effect clinical outcomes. Anticoagulation providers must be able to perform an educational assessment, develop an educational plan, and document the educational activities in the patient's medical record. The Certified Anticoagulation Care Provider should be able to:

1 Identify and define at least four elements that should be evaluated in an educational assessment.

2 Identify the critical elements of a patient education plan.

3 List and compare learning and teaching styles.

4 Evaluate family/social supports and the potential impact on the educational process.

5 Describe the educational needs of special populations (e.g. children, elderly, mentally impaired, primary language is non-English).

6 Identify appropriate methods to determine a patient's knowledge, skill, and attitudes regarding anticoagulation therapy.

7 Identify appropriate educational materials and determine methods to obtain them.

8 Recognize behaviors that may be an indicator for non-adherence to antithrombotic therapy and develop appropriate educational interventions.

9 Identify community resources to reinforce/augment plan of care.

10 Develop a list of specific learning objectives regarding the use of antithrombotic drugs (regarding drug knowledge, potential interactions with therapy, safety issues, signs and symptoms of adverse affects).

11 Develop a list of specific learning objectives regarding the use of point-of-care testing devices.

Domain IV: Applied pharmacology of antithrombotic agents

GOAL

The Anticoagulation Therapy Care Provider must possess and maintain an in-depth knowledge regarding the pharmacological properties of antithrombotic drugs. To meet this goal the Anticoagulation Therapy Care Provider shall be able to:

1 List the brand name(s) and generic name of drugs currently approved by the FDA or frequently used in clinical practice for the prevention or treatment of thrombosis including warfarin, heparin, low-molecular-weight heparins, and antiplatelet agents.

2 List the currently available dosage forms, including strength(s) and administration route(s), of antithrombotic drugs.

3 Describe the mechanism of action (if known) of the following antithrombotic drugs: warfarin, heparin, low-molecular-weight heparins, and antiplatelet agents.

4 Summarize, by comparing and contrasting, the basic pharmacokinetic properties of each antithrombotic drug, including absorption, distribution, route(s) of elimination, half-life, and time to full antithrombotic effect.

5 List the most common side effects and major adverse effects associated with each antithrombotic drug.

6 List factors that increase the risk of adverse effects associated with antithrombotic drugs.

7 List the major potential adverse effects associated with each antithrombotic drug when used by pregnant or breastfeeding women.

8 Recognize clinically significant drug–drug and drug–food interactions documented to occur with antithrombotic drugs. Explain the likely mechanism of the interaction, time course to clinical effect, and the effect the interaction may produce (e.g. increased or decreased antithrombotic response or bleeding risk).

9 List the currently available dosage forms, including strength(s) and administration route(s), of drugs that may be used to reverse anticoagulation.

10 Describe the mechanism of action of vitamin K and protamine sulfate to reverse anticoagulation.

Domain V: Operational (administrative) procedures

GOAL

The Certified Anticoagulation Care Provider must possess the knowledge, skills, and competencies necessary to assist in the management of an anticoagulation service. This will include: (1) evaluating the need for anticoagulation services; (2) determining personnel requirements; (3) developing a proposal for an anticoagulation service; (4) developing effective communication strategies with the patient and other members of the health care team; (5) documenting patient care activities; (6) performing quality assurance and risk management activities; (7) complying with state and federal regulations governing patient care and laboratory services; and (8) seeking compensation for anticoagulation therapy services. The Certified Anticoagulation Care Provider should be able to:

1 Identify the population that will benefit most from anticoagulation monitoring services.
2 Identify appropriate criteria to define the role of each team member in the care of a patient taking antithrombotic therapy.
3 Identify goals for an anticoagulation management service.
4 Identify potential sources of compensation for the services provided by an anticoagulation service.
5 Identify key clinical outcomes indicators (e.g. bleeding and thromboembolic complications, INR performance measures) to evaluate the effectiveness of an anticoagulation service.
6 Justify the need and identify procedures for assuring continuing education for all members of an anticoagulation service.
7 Develop criteria and measure patient satisfaction.
8 Define full and complete patient care documentation, including patient education.
9 Identify the purpose(s) of International Classification Disease (ICD-9) and Current Procedural Terminology (CPT) coding.
10 List the entities that may govern the laboratory monitoring of antithrombotic therapy (e.g. Occupational Safety and Health Administration (OSHA), Clinical Laboratory Improvement Amendments (CLIA), Joint Commission on Accreditation of Healthcare Organizations (JCAHO), National Committee for Quality Assurance (NCQA), Health Plan Employer Data and Information Set (HEDIS)).
11 Describe the elements of collaborative practice agreements.

12 Identify the essential information regarding patients' anticoagulation status that should be communicated periodically to primary care providers.
13 Identify policies and procedures that enable an efficient method of ordering and obtaining laboratory parameters from laboratories affiliated with the anticoagulation service.

Resources and references

The National Certification Board for Anticoagulation Providers does not provide training to individuals who are seeking certification. Numerous training programs are available in the United States and Canada. The Board neither recommends nor endorses any specific training program or process of professional development. To prepare for the examination, candidates for certification should rely on the scientific evidence published in primary literature sources. Review articles and textbooks may also be helpful in preparation for the examination but candidates are responsible for the latest information regarding antithrombotic therapy. The Board expects candidates to be knowledgeable regarding all major scientific reports (except abstracts) that appear in peer-reviewed journals published six or more months prior to the examination. Conversely, scientific works that appear in the literature less than six months prior to the examination will NOT be included on the examination.

The Board considers the following sources of information as useful resources in preparation for the certification examination:

JOURNAL SUPPLEMENT

Fifth American College of Chest Physicians (ACCP) Consensus Conference on Antithrombotic Therapy. Dalen JE and Hirsh J, eds. *Chest* 1998; **114** (suppl).
[This supplemental issue to the journal Chest is published a few months after each ACCP Consensus Conference on Antithrombotic Therapy (conducted every 2-3 years). This volume is a comprehensive review of the literature and international experts evaluate the weight of the evidence to develop practice recommendations. This is undoubtedly the single most important reference for anticoagulation care providers.]

TEXTBOOKS

Ansell JE, Oertel LB, Whittkowsky A, eds. *Managing oral anticoagulation therapy: clinical and operational guidelines.* Gaithersburg, MD: Aspen Publishing Co., 1997, with annual supplements.
[Most comprehensive text available on all aspects of anticoagulation therapy management including clinical practice management, forms and flow sheets, basic physiology and pathophysiology, indications for treatment, technical

aspects of coagulation testing, and much more. This is an invaluable reference.]

Colman RW, Hirsh J, Marder VJ, Salzman EW, eds. *Hemostasis and thrombosis*, 3rd edn. Philadelphia: J.B. Lippincott Co., 1994.
[This textbook is without a doubt the most comprehensive and exhaustive volume ever written regarding the pathophysiology and treatment of thrombosis. Although some information is outdated, this is an excellent source to study background information about hemostasis and the pathophysiology of thrombosis-associated disorders.]

Bates B. *A guide to physical examination and history taking*, 6th edn. *Physical assessment. A guide for evaluating drug therapy.* Philadelphia: J.B. Lippincott Co., 1995.
[This textbook is a classic and is widely used by medicine, nursing, and pharmacy schools to teach students basic physical examination techniques. There are many excellent physical examination textbooks available. If you do not feel comfortable with your physical examination skills, you should consider taking a refresher course or reviewing a physical assessment text.]

Redman BK. *The practice of patient education*, 8th edn. St. Louis, Missouri: Mosby, Inc., 1997.
[Reviews theories and principles of adult education.]

Cross PA. *Adults as learners.* San Francisco: Posey-Bass Publishers, 1983.
[The last chapter is particularly helpful in discussing and comparing learning theories and characteristics of adult learners.]

Joint Commission on Accreditation of Healthcare Organizations. *Accreditation manual for hospitals*, Vol. 1: Standards. Oakbrook Terrace, Illinois: JCAHO, 1996.
[Defines current standards for health care delivery overall, specifically review sections pertaining to patient education.]

JOURNAL ARTICLES

Ansell JE, Buttaro ML, Voltis TO, Knowlton CH, and the Anticoagulation Guidelines Task Force. Consensus Guidelines for Coordinated Outpatient Oral Anticoagulation Therapy Management. *Ann Pharmacother* 1997; **31**: 604–15.
[Consider this article as mandatory reading. It describes guidelines for developing policies and procedures to ensure safe and effective anticoagulation therapy management.]

Ansell JE, Hughes R. Evolving models of warfarin management: anticoagulation clinics, patient self-monitoring, and patient self-management. *Am Heart J* 1996; **132**: 1095–100.
[One of many articles that examines the benefits of anticoagulation management services on therapeutic and economic outcomes.]

Basskin L. How to calculate the cost effectiveness of a specialty clinic. *Formulary* 1997; **32**: 527–37.
[Describes the processes involved in demonstrating the cost effectiveness and cost benefit of an anticoagulation clinic.]

Additional resources available for patient education materials from manufacturers

Barr Laboratories, Inc. (Tel: 888.WARFARIN)
[Patient educational materials on warfarin therapy.]

DuPont Pharmaceuticals (Tel: 800.COUMADIN)
[Patient educational materials on Coumadin therapy and management.]

International Technidyne Corporation
(Tel: 800.631.5945)
[Patient educational materials for Point-of-Care Testing device. (ProTime Microcoagulation System)]

Rhone-Poulenc Rorer Pharmaceuticals Inc.
(Tel: 800.340.7502)
[Drug information and video on enoxaparin sodium (Lovenox) available to providers.]

Roche Diagnostics (Tel: 800.852.8766)
[Patient educational materials for Point-of-Care Testing device and patient self-testing. (Coaguchek)]

Additional resources for patient education materials, therapeutic drugs, point-of-care devices are available from additional manufacturers.

39

Advanced medical education in the managed care era

PANG-YEN FAN

The rise of managed care has greatly affected graduate medical education. Financial pressures have shifted health care from the in-patient to out-patient setting, reduced federal and institutional funding, and decreased time and incentives for attending physician teaching. Academic institutions will need new methodology to determine educational costs and optimally allocate limited resources. Attending physicians should develop new strategies and techniques to optimize teaching in ambulatory clinic settings.

INTRODUCTION

Over the past decade, economic forces have dramatically altered the fundamental approach to health care in the USA. The evolution of a highly competitive health care market, epitomized by managed care, has resulted in a shift from hospital, specialist, and technology-based patient care toward an ambulatory clinic, primary care, outcome-based system. The financial pressures that have transformed clinical practice will similarly change medical research and education.

Preliminary data suggest that managed care and market competition may adversely affect research. For example, the rate of growth of federal research funding for medical schools appears inversely correlated with the level of managed care in the area.[1] Clinical researchers at institutions in highly competitive health care markets have fewer publications than colleagues in less competitive areas.[2] While managed care's impact on residency and fellowship training remains to be determined, health care reform clearly presents significant challenges to

academic institutions, teachers, and trainees, and necessitates the development of new approaches to graduate medical education.

HISTORICAL OVERVIEW

In 1765, the 'College of Philadelphia', which ultimately became the University of Pennsylvania, was founded as the first American medical school. However, apprenticeship remained the dominant form of medical education through the early nineteenth century, as many early medical schools were proprietary operations that delivered highly variable levels of training.[3] During this period, organizations such as the American Medical Association (1847) and Association of American Medical Colleges (1890) developed more stringent medical school accreditation and physician licensure criteria and procedures. As state medical boards began requiring internship for licensure in the early twentieth century, graduate medical education programs were established.[3]

Prior to World War II, internship and residency included a significant ambulatory care experience, since a large proportion of patient care was delivered in the out-patient setting.[4] However, as a result of increasing numbers and growing complexity of hospitalized patients, increased financing for hospital care, and wartime staffing shortages, house officer duties became concentrated almost exclusively on in-patient management. As federal clinical research funding increased, hospital staff became increasingly weighted toward specialists, and residency training became oriented toward specialty care. Not surprisingly, postresidency fellowship training became commonplace, if not expected. Given the perception of an overall physician shortage, many programs, particularly academic medical centers, emphasized and encouraged further specialty training without regard to societal physician needs.

As a result, the number of doctors, particularly specialists, has grown sharply over the past several decades. From 1960 to 1990, the ratio of physicians to population increased from approximately 140 per 100 000 to 240 per 100 000 population and the proportion of specialists rose from one-half to two-thirds of all doctors.[5] The total number of active physicians in the USA has increased to nearly 600 000 with an additional 100 000 currently in graduate medical training. At present, approximately 17 000 US medical graduates and nearly 7000 foreign medical graduates enter residency programs annually.[5]

In recent years, a number of studies have reported that the USA currently has or will develop a surfeit of specialists and possibly doctors in general.[6–8] These studies suggest that this surplus likely contributes to the spiraling medical costs observed in fee-for-service health care systems. These controversial reports have stimulated re-evaluation and revision of medical school curricula and graduate training programs to increase numbers of primary care physicians. In addition, including reductions in both undergraduate and graduate medical training positions are under active consideration. More extensive discussion of these difficult and complex issues is beyond the scope of this chapter.

OBSTACLES TO MEDICAL EDUCATION IN THE MANAGED CARE ERA

The sweeping changes wrought by managed care, particularly the shift from hospital to clinic-based patient care, have created a number of potential obstacles to graduate medical training at the level of the institution, attending physician, and trainee (Table 39.1). In addition, factors unrelated to economic pressures, including the tremendous proliferation of medical information and research, also pose challenges to the educational process.

Table 39.1 Obstacles to medical education

Institutional obstacles
Decreased state and federal funding
Decreased clinical revenue
Poor methodology to quantify educational costs
Limited methodology to evaluate and quantify educational effort

Disincentives for attending physician teaching
Limited time availability
Increased documentation requirements
Increased emphasis on cost
Lack of compensation for teaching
Limited methodology to evaluate and quantify teaching effort and quality
Unfamiliarity with clinical practice in managed care environment

Disincentives for trainee learning
Reduced autonomy/responsibility
Restricted access to diagnostic testing
Restricted choice of medications
Restricted access to specialty consultants

Non-economic obstacles
Information overload
Limited bedside teaching

Institutional obstacles to graduate medical education

Institutions face the daunting challenge of maintaining graduate medical training as clinical revenues and government funding decline. While educational expenditures are highly dependent on clinical revenue,[9] these expenses contribute to the higher costs that limit the ability of academic medical centers to contend in a competitive health care system. Inability to attract adequate patient volumes reduces clinical income and threatens the viability of training programs. This bleak financial quandary is exacerbated by reductions in state and federal funding. At present, the federal government provides over six billion dollars for graduate medical education.[10] However, the amount provided by academic medical centers appears likely to shrink as a result of an unfavorable allocation system and funding reductions. Institutional requests for governmental support of educational expenses are hampered by inadequate methodology for determining these costs. The true expenditures for teaching are extremely difficult to quantify due to elaborate networks of cross-subsidies.[9,11]

Academic institutions have traditionally rewarded scientific research to a much greater extent than clinical activity, teaching, or community service. This approach, coupled with the difficulty of documenting educational 'productivity' or scholarship, encourages attending physicians to redirect their efforts into more easily measured activities.

Disincentives for attending physician teaching

In order to maintain revenues and reduce costs, medical centers have required staff to increase productivity. Accordingly, many faculties have increased their clinical activity and therefore have less time available for teaching. These time constraints are worsened by new federal regulations necessitating increased attending physician presence and documentation.[10] In addition, emphasis on productivity encourages staff physicians to pursue activities that can be readily quantified. Unfortunately, as discussed above, teaching effort and effectiveness remain difficult to assess. In contrast, patient care can be measured by visit volumes, billings, or collections, and research by grants and publications.

Fiscal constraints can also limit attending physician teaching by necessitating increased attending control over patient management. This is a particular problem in systems where expenses generated by house staff for excess testing, expensive medications, or delayed discharge may result in financial penalties to the attending physician. However, these pressures are likely to increase with the implementation of managed care capitation and the transfer of financial risk for patient care from the insurer to the provider. Furthermore, many staff physicians, unaccustomed and possibly uncomfortable with incorporating the cost considerations in clinical decision making, are still learning to practice in the managed care setting and remain uncertain as to the most appropriate approach and material to teach in this setting.

Disincentives for trainee learning

The fiscal pressures of the current health care environment have significantly altered the nature of attending physician–house staff interactions and threaten to diminish the educational value of these exchanges. Most importantly, economic considerations virtually mandate increased attending physician supervision to avoid the inefficiencies associated with patient care by less experienced trainees. Efforts to streamline care have led to the development of data-based practice guidelines to standardize and hopefully optimize care for patients with common disorders. These developments have greatly decreased house staff autonomy. This reduction of responsibility and authority limits trainee growth by diminishing opportunities for independent analysis and action. House staff assume a passive role, simply carrying out staff physician instructions rather than formulating their own diagnostic and therapeutic approaches.

Other obstacles include trends to avoid testing for purely diagnostic or screening purposes. Fiscal restraints have prompted some physicians to order laboratory and radiological studies only if the results would affect management. While useful when appropriately applied by established clinicians, this approach increases the risk of inaccurate or missed diagnoses by inexperienced house staff. Economic considerations have also affected graduate medical education in medication selection. Many health insurers provide lists of preferred medications, which may be chosen principally by price rather than factors such as side effect profiles or dosing frequency. Finally, financial incentives to minimize costs may reduce consultation, decreasing exposure to specialist expertise and further reducing learning opportunities.

Non-economic obstacles to graduate medical education

Not all obstacles to graduate medical education are related to the current economics of the health care system. Problems resulting from the shift from hospital-based to clinic-based patient care are discussed below. In addition, the rapid pace of scientific research and technological advance has made it difficult for physicians to stay current with the expanding fund of medical knowledge. Information overload obligates physicians to learn information retrieval skills rather than simply absorb data.

House staff training has also suffered from the decline in bedside teaching. The use of this technique in attending rounds has decreased from 75 per cent during the 1960s to less than 16 per cent at present.[12] The loss of bedside teaching may impair development of trainee physical examination skills and increase reliance on technology-based means of patient assessment.

HOSPITAL-BASED MEDICAL EDUCATION

Despite being the central component of graduate medical training for many years, hospital-based teaching plays a greatly diminished role today. Although the medical center remains the site for training house staff in the care of acutely or critically ill patients, factors such as decreased admission rates and shortened length of stays have significantly reduced educational opportunities from in-patient care. Certainly, the frenetic pace of ward work minimizes time for meaningful contact between attending physician, house staff, and patient. Indeed, patients are frequently away for testing or treatment for much of the day, thus limiting availability for bedside teaching. Pressure to achieve brief lengths of stay, early discharge, and out-patient management may leave the trainee little time to observe or learn about the patient's illness. In fact, patients may be discharged prior to establishing a diagnosis or may leave with a diagnosis that is later proven to be incorrect. These problems are often exacerbated by the minimal or incomplete follow-up that trainees receive regarding the patient's course after discharge.

In a health care environment that stresses efficiency, the traditional ward structure of rounding physicians performing patient care and teaching attending physicians for educational purposes may be disadvantageous.[13] This separation of teaching and patient management is inefficient and may reduce the perceived importance of teaching rounds. In addition, the large number of attending physicians involved may limit interactions with house staff to brief, task-oriented encounters, which are unsatisfying and contribute to fragmented patient care.

CLINIC-BASED MEDICAL EDUCATION

As patient care shifts from the hospital to the clinic, graduate medical education in ambulatory care must increase. Unfortunately, current out-patient training experiences are characterized by a number of problems (Table 39.2), particularly limited attending physician–trainee interaction. Available data suggest that fewer than a third of clinic patients are presented to the staff physician and less than 20 per cent are examined by the attending physician.[14] Furthermore, the duration of discussion averages approximately 2 minutes. Not surprisingly, studies have documented minimal faculty observation of trainee–patient interaction, assessment of trainee fund of knowledge, or feedback to the trainee.[14] In addition, house staff rarely receive instruction or orientation regarding their role in the clinic environment. Finally, continuity of care is limited, particularly since ambulatory training is often scheduled as a block rotation due to logistical considerations. Lack of continuity combined with rushed, brief patient encounters further reduces the educational value of the clinic experience.

The conversion from in-patient to ambulatory care teaching poses a number of additional challenges. For example, many attending physicians are simply unfamiliar with teaching in this setting. In addition, the clinic environment presents far greater time constraints than the hospital ward, since the patient is available for a very brief and specific period of time. As patient volumes increase under managed care and requirements for preceptor presence tighten with new federal regulations, time pressures will further intensify.

STRATEGIES TO IMPROVE ADVANCED MEDICAL EDUCATION IN THE MANAGED CARE ERA

Just as clinical practice has changed, graduate medical education must also evolve in response to economics of managed care. This process will involve institutional restructuring and development of new strategies and approaches to both teaching and learning.

Institutional strategies (Table 39.3)

As clinical income and governmental funding dwindle, many institutions are considering administrative and fiscal reorganizations to protect funding for graduate medical education. An extensive discussion of these efforts is beyond the scope of this chapter. However, a number of academic medical centers have also sought to enhance and reward non-research-based scholarship through redefined promotion criteria and increased

Table 39.2 *Site-specific obstacles to graduate medical education*

Hospital
Decreased admissions
Reduced length of stay
Busy attending physician, trainee, and patient schedule
Incomplete patient evaluation
Lack of clinical follow-up after discharge
Traditional ward structure?

Clinic
Brief attending physician–trainee interaction
Rigid time schedule
High patient volume
Lack of continuity of care
Preceptor inexperience

Table 39.3 *Strategies to improve advanced medical education in the managed care era*

Institutional strategies
Administrative and fiscal reorganization
Faculty development
Redefined promotion criteria for teaching excellence
Estimate of educational expenditures

Hospital-based strategies
Reorganization of ward structure?
Increased bedside teaching

Clinic-based strategies
Structured teaching approach
Increased preceptor observation of trainee–patient interaction
Increased trainee observation of preceptor–patient interaction
Wave scheduling

Miscellaneous strategies
Improved information retrieval skills
Computer competency
Internet access
CD-ROM-based educational resources
Standardized patients

faculty development.[15] These efforts may induce faculty to resist growing financial pressure to abandon teaching for more lucrative endeavors. In addition, institutions have begun to evaluate training expenses more precisely. Well-documented estimates of graduate medical education costs are essential to any effort to establish governmental or even industry-based funding systems for teaching.

Hospital-based strategies

The hospital remains the ideal site for close and intense observation of seriously ill patients and will always maintain an important place in house staff training. However, the changes in clinical practice brought on by managed care have exposed inefficiencies of the traditional ward structure of separate teaching and patient care attendings.

> Therefore, consolidation of the teaching and rounding attending physician may improve hospital-based graduate medical education.

Available data suggest that this intervention increases the percentage of time devoted by house staff to educational activity, increases bedside teaching, improves the quality and educational value of the preceptor–trainee interactions, and may even reduce length of stay.[13] However, this system forces physicians to transfer care of their patients upon admission. As a result, poor communication between primary and ward attending physicians could potentially result in unnecessary testing and suboptimal care. In addition, this system may disadvantage physicians with high levels of out-patient activity by necessitating prolonged absences during ward rotations and may financially penalize clinics dependent on income generated by their physicians' in-patient rounding.[13]

Clinic-based strategies

> As attending physicians increase their teaching activities in the ambulatory care setting, a structured approach can facilitate the educational process (Table 39.4). One major element is preparation by both the preceptor and trainee as the time constraints of the ambulatory setting are so restrictive that any inefficiency will greatly reduce the value of the teaching encounter.

Preceptors should identify patients with communication skills and medical complexity appropriate for the participating house officer. The preceptor must also ensure that the trainee is exposed to a relevant and representa-

Table 39.4 *Structured ambulatory care clinic medical education. (Adapted from Kurth RJ, Irigoyen M, Schmidt HJ. A model to structure student learning in ambulatory care settings.* Acad Med *1997;* **72**: 601–6)

Preparation

Trainee	Reviews record, formulates tentative patient care agenda and educational agenda
	Presents to preceptor
Time:	5–15 minutes
Preceptor	Assess trainee presentation
	Give trainee brief orientation to major clinical issues, relevant physical examination
Time:	2–5 minutes

Patient encounter

Trainee	Interview and examine patient, formulate assessment and plan, present case
Time:	20–30 minutes
Preceptor	Assess trainee presentation, preferably at bedside
	Confirm trainee history and physical findings
Time:	5–10 minutes

Post-visit assessment

Trainee	Discuss case, formulate plan, and communicate with patient
	Complete charting
	Identify topics for further learning
Time:	10–15 minutes
Preceptor	Discuss case, formulate plan, and communicate with patient
	Assess trainee charting
	Identify topics for further teaching
Time:	5–10 minutes

tive mix of diseases. The house officer should review the patient charts and formulate a tentative plan to present to the attending physician prior to seeing the patient. The preceptor may then provide a brief orientation to the case including the most important issues that must be addressed and pertinent elements of the physical examination.[16]

> After the visit, the trainee presents to the preceptor, preferably in the presence of the patient. This process increases the attending contact with the patient and maximizes opportunities for house staff to observe the attending physician–patient interaction and receive bedside teaching.[16]

After leaving the examination room, the preceptor may discuss the case further and may offer feedback regarding the trainee's performance. Under this teaching system, time per visit is estimated at 40–70 minutes for house staff, 13–36 minutes for attending physicians, and 27–45 minutes for patients.[17]

Wave scheduling (Table 39.5) allows the attending physician to see patients independently while permitting the trainee adequate time to prepare for and evaluate the patient.

One disadvantage of this system is the need for increased clinic space when compared to a system where house staff simply accompany the attending physician.

Table 39.5 *Wave scheduling*

7.45–8.00 am	Trainee reviews records, formulates preliminary patient care agenda
8.00–8.20 am	Trainee sees Patient 1
	Preceptor sees Patient 2
8.20–8.40 am	Trainee and preceptor see Patient 1
8.40–9.00 am	Trainee charts on Patient 1 and prepares for Patient 4
	Preceptor sees Patient 3
9.00–9.20 am	Trainee and preceptor see Patient 4

Miscellaneous strategies

Other strategies may also improve graduate medical education (Table 39.3). In view of the exponential expansion of medical knowledge, instruction in data retrieval skills is essential preparation for a physician. Fortunately, computer advances have greatly facilitated this process. At present, a number of search programs allow users to perform rapid and highly specific literature searches. In addition, many educational resources, including many medical journals, are now available on the Internet. Various medical societies and academic institutions also offer on-line teaching material. Ironically, it appears that the proliferation of accessible medical information has been more rapidly utilized by patients than physicians.

Computer technology has also provided other benefits. The use of CD-ROMs to store vast quantities of data has led to computerized medical texts. Other media may also be stored, including images for histopathology and radiographs, video for echocardiograms or cardiac catheterization films, and audio for heart sounds.

Standardized patients offer another educational tool. While costly to establish and maintain, these programs allow assessment of house staff clinical skills[18] and provide valuable teaching exercises. Rigorously trained standardized patients present consistent case histories and simulate physical findings, and can generate reproducible evaluations of house staff. In addition, they can effectively provide feedback to trainees. In fact, standardized patients have been used successfully in a continuing medical education program in cardiology for practicing primary care physicians.[19] The use of a program by multiple institutions will mitigate cost considerations.

CLINICAL PERSPECTIVE

The economic forces epitomized by managed care have forced the US health care system to acknowledge and adjust to societal demands. These pressures have reshaped clinical practice and will similarly alter medical research and education. The difficult restructuring process provides a painful reminder that graduate medical education, along with the rest of the American medical system, must shape itself to address the nation's health care requirements.

As managed care's influence grows, both hospital and ambulatory care training must become more efficient. The strategies outlined in Table 39.3 may improve house staff training. Tables 39.4 and 39.5 will help structure the ambulatory teaching environment to allow for meaningful preceptor–trainee interaction while maintaining clinic efficiency.

FUTURE DIRECTIONS

The future direction of graduate medical education depends on a variety of forces. Techniques to assess societal requirements accurately are necessary to guide national decisions on the numbers and specialty mix of physician training positions. In addition, teaching institutions must develop more precise estimates of the cost of medical education. Armed with this information, academic centers can work with governmental and health care industry groups to establish reliable funding. Academic medical centers should establish improved methods for assessing, evaluating, and rewarding teaching excellence.

Structured approaches to both hospital and ambulatory care training will need to be refined as the health care environment changes. Research to develop methodology for evaluating teaching outcomes will greatly enhance this process.

Above all, graduate medical education must preserve the spirit of scientific inquiry that has led to so many medical advances. If we can impart this sense of curiosity and enjoyment of the practice of medicine to our future physicians during this time of economic constraints, we will have conquered the primary challenge of the managed care era.

SUMMARY

- Declining clinical revenues and federal funding have limited institutional support for graduate medical education.

- Increased emphasis on productivity creates a disincentive for attending physician participation in relatively poorly compensated activities such as teaching.
- Pressure to control costs has necessitated greater attending physician supervision of patient management and has reduced trainee autonomy.
- As health care shifts from the hospital wards to ambulatory clinics, a greater proportion of graduate medical education will occur in the out-patient setting. Attending physicians and trainees will face the challenges of increased time constraints and limited continuity of care.
- Academic institutions will need now methods for accurate assessment of educational expenses and determination of appropriate funding of teaching activities.
- Attending physicians should develop new strategies and techniques to improve teaching encounters in the clinic environment. Careful preparation and creative scheduling will help maximize the educational value of brief interactions between attending physicians and trainees.

REFERENCES

1. Moy E, Mazzaschi AJ, Levin RJ, Blake DA, Griner PF. Relationship between National Institutes of Health research awards to US medical schools and managed care market penetration. *JAMA* 1997; **278**: 217–21.

2. Campbell EG, Weissman JS, Blumenthal D. Relationship between market competition and the activities and attitudes of medical school faculty. *JAMA* 1997; **278**: 222–6.

○3. Council on Medical Education. History of accreditation of medical education programs. *JAMA* 1983; **250**: 1502–8.

4. Stoeckle JD, Leaf A, Grossman JH, Goroll AH. A case history of training outside the hospital and its future. *Am J Med* 1979; **66**: 1008–14.

5. Mullan F. Medical education in the USA: lessons from the health care reform era. *Med Educ* 1995; **29**(suppl 1): 57–60.

6. Council on Graduate Medical Education. *Third report: improving access to health care through physician workforce reform: directions for the 21st century.* Rockville, MD: US Department of Health and Human Services, 1992.

7. Council on Graduate Medical Education. *Fourth report: recommendations to improve access to health care through physician workforce reform.* Rockville, MD: US Department of Health and Human Services, 1994.

8. Billi JE, Wise CG, Bills EA, Mitchell RL. Potential effects of managed care on specialty practice at a university medical center. *N Engl J Med* 1996; **333**: 979–83.

9. Jones RF, Sanderson SC. Clinical revenues used to support the academic mission of medical schools, 1992–93. *Acad Med* 1996; **71**: 299–307.

10. Association of Professors of Medicine. 1997 ASP leadership conference: report on the status of subspecialty training. *Am J Med* 1997; **103**: 87–91.

11. Gold MR. Effects of the growth of managed care on academic medical centers and graduate medical education. *Acad Med* 1996; **71**: 828–38.

12. Lacombe MA. On bedside teaching. *Ann Intern Med* 1997; **126**: 217–20.

13. Ben-Menachem T, Estrada C, Young MJ, *et al.* Balancing service and education: improving internal medicine residencies in the managed care era. *Am J Med* 1996; **100**: 224–9.

14. Irby DM. Teaching and learning in ambulatory care settings: a thematic review of the literature. *Acad Med* 1995; **70**: 898–931.

15. Nieman LZ, Donoghue GD, Ross LL, Morahan PS. Implementing a comprehensive approach to managing faculty roles, rewards, and development in an era of change. *Acad Med* 1997; **72**: 496–504.

♦16. Ferenchick G, Simpson D, Blackman J, Darosa D, Dunnington G. Strategies for efficient and effective teaching in the ambulatory care setting. *Acad Med* 1997; **72**: 277–80.

♦17. Kurth RJ, Irigoyen M, Schmidt HJ. A model to structure student learning in ambulatory care settings. *Acad Med* 1997; **72**: 601–6.

18. Stillman PL, Swanson DB, Smee S, *et al.* Assessing the skills of residents with standardized patients. *Ann Intern Med* 1986; **105**: 762–71.

19. O'Brien MK, Feldman D, Alban T, *et al.* An innovative CME program in cardiology for primary care practitioners. *Acad Med* 1996; **71**: 894–7.

Appendices

Appendix A: Computer programs and on-line services

FREDERICK A SPENCER

CARDIOLOGY WEB SITES

Societies
- American College of Cardiology — www.acc.org
- American College of Chest Physicians — www.chestnet.org
- American Heart Association — www.amhrt.org
- American Society of Nuclear Cardiology — www.asnc.org
- American Society of Echocardiography — www.asecho.org
- European Society of Cardiology — www.escardio.org
- National Heart, Lung and Blood Institute — www.nhlbi.nih.gov
- North American Society of Pacing and Electrophysiology — www.naspe.org

Journals and publications
- *American Heart Journal* — www.mosby.com(ah)
- *American Journal of Cardiology* — www.elsevier.com/locate/umjcard
- *Annals of Thoracic Surgery* — www.sts.org/annals/
- *Canadian Journal of Cardiology* — www.pulsus.com/cardiol/
- *Circulation* — www.circulationaha.org
- *Clinical Cardiology* — www.clinical-cardiology.org/
- *Echocardiography Journal of University of Medicine and Dentistry of New Jersey (UMDNJ)* — www2.umdnj.edu/~shindler/echo.html
- *European Heart Journal* — www.hbuk.co.uk/wbs/ehj/
- *Heart Web* — www.heartweb.org/
- *Herz* — www.bnk.de/herz.htm
- *Internet Journal of Thoracic and Cardiovascular Surgery* — www.ispub.com/journals/ijtcus.htm
- *Journal of Thoracic and Cardiovascular Surgery* — www1.mosby.com/Mosby/Periodicals/Medical/JTCS/tctc1296.html
- *Journal of American Society of Echocardiography* — www.Mosby.com/echo

General cardiology
- 12-lead electrocardiogram library and related sites — homepages.enterprise.net/djenkins/ecgurls.html
www.heartinfo.org/physician/ecg/index.htm
- Ascultation Assistant — www.med.ucla.edu/wilkes/intro.html
- Cardiosource — www.cardiosource.com
- Cardiovascular Consultants Medical Group Recommended Links — www.dendrites.com/heartlinks.htm
- McGill University Virtual Stethoscope — sprojects.mmi.mcgill.ca/mus/MUSTETH.HTM

- Synapse Heart Sounds
- University of Florida ACLS Algorithms
- Web Doctor Section on Cardiology
- Practice Guidelines

www.medlib.com/spi/coolstuff2.htm
www.med.ufl.edu/medinfo/baseline/acsthms.html
www.gretmar.com/webdoctor/cardiology.html
www.cardiologycompass.com/guidelines.html

Cardiovascular pathology and images
- George Simon Radiology Collection
- University of Michigan Thoracic Radiology
- Computer Simulation and Visualization in the
  Cardiovascular System
- University of Utah Gross and Microscopic Images

www.sbu.ac.uk/~dirt/museum/gs-heart.html
www.med.umich.edu/lrc.radiology/radio.html
www.ncsa.uiuc.edu/SCMS/DigLib/text/biology/
  Cardiovascular-System-Clark.html
medstat.med.utah.edu/WebPath/CVHTML/

Cardiac catherterization and intervention
- Atlanta Cardiology Group – Complex Interventions
- Angioplasty/PTCA Home Page
- University of Tasmania – Hemodynamics Review

www.atlcard.com/complex.html
www.ptca.org
www.healthsci.utas.edu.au/physiol/tute1/hd.html

Echocardiography
- American Society of Echocardiography
- Columbia University – Adult Echocardiography
- *Echocardiography Journal of UMDNJ*
- University of Chicago Echo Laboratory

www.asecho.org
cpmcnet.columbia.edu/dept/ cardiology/echo
www2.umdnj.edu/~shindler.echo.html
card-mac.14bsd.uchicago.edu/levin/pages/
  echo-home/echo-home.html

Electrophysiology
- North American Society of Pacing and
  Electrophysiology (NASPE)
- *Heart Web – online journal of electrophysiology*
- Implantable Pacemaker and Defibrillator Index
- Intermedics Home Page
- Metronics Home Page
- Guide to Cardiac Pacemakers

www.naspe.org

www.heartweb.org
www.implantable.com
www.imed.com
www.medtronic.com
www2.interpath.net/devcomp/guide/bindexl.htm

Congenital heart disease
- Congenital Heart Disease – Radiologic Case Studies

- Canadian Adult Congenital Heart Network
- Pediatric Cardiology Almanac
- University of Kansas Pediatric Cardiology

www.tc.umn.edu/nlhome/m475/bjarn001/stuff/
  introscreen.html
www.cachnet.org
www.neosoft.com/~rlpierce/pc.htm
www.kumc.edu/instruction/medicine/pedcard/
  cardiology/chdefect.html

Patient education
- General Cardiology Education
- National Heart, Lung and Blood Institute (NHLBI)
  Patient Education Materials (Smoking)

home.hkstar.com/~shwan/Cardiology.html
gopher//lido.nhlbi.gov/oo/educprog/other/pubs/
  public/
    angina.txt
    arrhythm.txt
    hrtfail.txt
    hrtlung.txt

- University of California at Irvine (UCI) Heart Disease
  Prevention Program
- Franklin Institute – The Heart: a virtual exploration

www.heart.uci.edu

www.fi.edu/biosci/heart.html

Clinical trials
- Cardiovascular Clinical Trials Forum
- Center Watch Clinical Trials Listing Source

science-forum.com/cvct
www.centerwatch.com

Appendix B: Cardiovascular drugs – pharmacology, indications, and cost

PRITESH J GANDHI AND JILL AUGER

Cardiovascular agent	Pharmacology	Indication(s)	Cost[a,1]
Abciximab (ReoPro®)	Glycoprotein IIb/IIIa receptor antagonist resulting in the inhibition of platelets binding to fibrinogen[2]	• High-risk patients undergoing percutaneous coronary intervention (PCI)[3,4]	2 mg/mL, $ 540.02
Acebutolol (Sectral®)	Selective β_1-adrenergic receptor antagonist with membrane stabilizing and intrinsic sympathomimetic activity (ISA)	• Hypertension • Angina	200 mg, $0.80 400 mg, $1.07
Acetazolamide (Diamox®)	Non-competitive inhibition of carbonic anhydrase resulting in increased excretion of Na^+, K^+, HCO_3^- and water	• Metabolic alkalosis • Edematous states	250 mg po, $0.04 500 mg po, $1.20 500 mg iv, $31.20
Adenosine (Adenocard®)	Slows conduction through the AV node. In addition, it can slow conduction through reentry pathways[5]	• Paroxysmal supraventricular tachycardia (PSVT) due to AV node reentry and accessory pathways (including Wolff–Parkinson–White syndrome)	3 mg/mL (2 mL), $33.35
Alteplase (Activase®)	Activates plasminogen bound to fibrin ('fibrin selective') resulting in local fibrinolysis[6]	• Acute myocardial infarction[7] • Acute pulmonary embolism • Acute ischemic stroke	100 mg, $2750.00
Amiloride (Midamor®)	K^+ sparing diuretic that inhibits Na^+/H^+ exchange in the proximal tubule	• Hypertension • Edema	5 mg, $0.37
Amiodarone (Cordarone®)	Designated a Class III antiarrhythmic agent (K^+ channel-blocking properties); however, it also blocks the fast inward Na^+ current, it is a non-competitive β-blocker, and it has Ca^{2+} channel and α-blocking characteristics[8]	• Management of ventricular tachyarrhythmias in the acute setting • Prevention of paroxysmal supraventricular tachycardia (PSVT) and VT • Cardiopulmonary resuscitation[9]	200 mg po, $3.06 50 mg/mL iv, $84.03

Cardiovascular agent	Pharmacology	Indication(s)	Cost[a,1]
Amlodipine (Norvasc®)	Dihydropyridine slow Ca²⁺ channel blocker resulting in peripheral vasodilatation and inhibition of coronary vasospasm	• Hypertension • Angina (chronic stable or Prinzmetal's)	2.5 mg, $1.37 5 mg, $1.37 10 mg, $2.17
Amrinone (Inocor®)	Inhibits myocardial cyclic adenosine monophosphate (cAMP) phosphodiesterase III activity thereby augmenting cellular cAMP levels and increasing Ca²⁺ influx. In addition, amrinone possesses systemic and pulmonary vasodilator effects resulting in pre- and afterload reduction. Amrinone enhances AV nodal conduction	• Severe decompensated congestive heart failure • Pulmonary hypertension	5 mg/mL, $80.58
Anistreplase (Eminase®)	Activates the conversion of plasminogen to plasmin resulting in the degradation of fibrin, fibrinogen, and other procoagulant proteins into soluble fragments	• Management of acute myocardial infarction[10]	30 U, $2835.58
Aprotinin (Trasylol®)	Inhibits trypsin, chymotrypsin, cathepsin, plasmin and kallikrein. Overall, inhibition of these plasma and tissue polypeptide proteases results in antifibrinolytic effects[11]	• Used in conjunction with cardiopulmonary bypass surgery with extracorpeal circulation, to decrease intraoperative and postoperative bleeding[11]	10,000 kIU/mL (100 mL), $206.68 (200 mL), $413.35
Ardeparin (Normiflo®)	Low-molecular-weight heparin that inhibits Factor Xa to a greater extent than thrombin (Anti-Xa: Anti-IIa = 1.9)[12]	• Deep vein thrombosis (DVT) prophylaxis in patients undergoing orthopedic surgery	5000 U/0.5 mL, $15.98 10 000 U/0.5 mL, $25.33
Argatroban (Novastan®)	Direct antithrombin activity[13]	• Management of heparin-induced thrombocytopenia (HIT)	¶
Aspirin	Prevents the conversion of arachidonic acid by irreversibly inhibiting cyclooxygenase[14]	• Inhibition of platelet aggregation • Analgesia • Anti-inflammatory	81 mg, $0.04 325 mg, $0.02 325 mg (enteric coated), $0.04
Atenolol (Tenormin®)	Selectively inhibits β₁-adrenergic receptors. Selectivity is lost at higher doses	• HTN • Angina[15] • Peri- and post-myocardial infarction	25 mg po, $0.04 50 mg po, $0.04 100 mg po, $0.06 0.5 mg/mL (10 mL), $7.16
Atorvastatin (Lipitor®)	Competitively and selectively inhibits 3-hyroxyl-3-methylglutaryl coenzyme A (HMG-CoA), the rate-limiting enzyme that catalyzes the formation of mevalonic acid (a cholesterol precursor)[16]	• Adjunct to dietary and lifestyle modifications in hypercholesterolemia	10 mg, $1.97 20 mg, $3.05 40 mg, $3.50
Atropine	Antagonizes the actions of acetylcholine at parasympathetic sites	• Bradycardia • Asystole	0.4 mg/mL (1 mL), $1.12 0.5 mg/mL (1 mL), $1.33

Cardiovascular agent	Pharmacology	Indication(s)	Cost[a,1]
Azimilide (Stedicor®)	Class III antiarrhythmic agent with non-selective blockade of both the I_{Kr} (rapidly activating K^+ current) and I_{Ks} (slowly activating K^+ current) channels resulting in prolongation of the refractory period without slowing conduction velocity[17]	• Preventing recurrence of symptomatic atrial fibrillation. Pending FDA approval[17]	¶
Benazeparil (Lotensin®)	Competitive inhibitor of the angiotensin converting enzyme (ACE) resulting in lower levels of angiotensin II and reduction in aldosterone secretion[18]	• Hypertension	5 mg, $0.83 10 mg, $0.83 20 mg, $0.83 40 mg, $0.83
Bepridil (Vascor®)	Type 4 slow Ca^{2+} channel blocker producing coronary vasodilatation. In addition, bepridil inhibits fast Na^+ channels	• Chronic stable angina	200 mg, $3.45 300 mg, $3.82
Bisoprolol (Zebeta®)	Competitively and selectively blocks β_1- adrenergic receptors	• Hypertension	5 mg, $1.19 10 mg, $1.19
Bretylium (Bretylol®)	Class III antiarrhythmic agent that blocks K^+ channels resulting in prolonged refractoriness. In addition, it may cause hypotension due to α-blocking properties[8]	• Acute ventricular tachycardia • Acute ventricular fibrillation	50 mg/mL (10 mL), $2.99
Bumetanide (Bumex®)	Inhibits absorption of Na^+ and Cl^- in the ascending loop of Henle[19]	• Acute oliguria • Edematous states • Hypertension	0.5 mg po, $0.15 1 mg po, $0.17 2 mg po, $0.21 0.25 mg/mL (4 mL) iv, $1.90
Captopril (Capoten®)	Competitive inhibitor of the angiotensin converting enzyme (ACE) resulting in lower levels of angiotensin II and reduction in aldosterone secretion[18]	• Hypertension • Congestive heart failure[20,21] • Treatment of hemodynamically stable patients within 24-hours of an acute myocardial infarction[22] • Diabetic nephropathy	12.5 mg, $0.04 25 mg, $0.05 50 mg, $0.10 100 mg, $0.19
Carvedilol (Coreg®)	Non-selective β-adrenergic receptor blockade and vasodilatation due to α_1-adrenoceptor blockade[23]	• Mild to moderate congestive heart failure[24,25] • Hypertension	3.125 mg, $1.59 6.25 mg, $1.59 12.5 mg, $1.59 25 mg, $1.59
Cerivastatin (Baycol®)	Competitively and selectively inhibits 3-hyroxyl-3-methylglutaryl coenzyme A (HMG-CoA), the rate-limiting enzyme that catalyzes the formation of mevalonic acid (a cholesterol precursor)[26]	• Adjunct to dietary and lifestyle modifications for the treatment of elevated LDL-cholesterol in primary hypercholesterolemia and mixed dyslipidemia	0.2 mg, $1.42 0.3 mg, $1.42
Chlorothiazide (Diuril®)	Inhibits Na^+ reabsorption in the distal tubules causing excretion of water, Na^+, K^+, H^+, and Mg^{2+} [19]	• Hypertension • Edema	250 mg po, $0.05 500 mg po, $0.06 500 mg iv, $10.13
Cholestyramine (Questran®)	Exchanges Na^+ for bile acids resulting in an increase in bile acid synthesis from cholesterol[26]	• Adjunct to dietary and lifestyle modifications for the treatment of primary hyperlipidemia	4 g/packet, $0.95

Cardiovascular agent	Pharmacology	Indication(s)	Cost[a,1]
Clofibrate (Atromid-S®)	Mechanism of action is not clearly elucidated but it is thought to reduce cholesterol synthesis and hepatic-vascular transference[26]	• Adjunct to diet and lifestyle modifications in the management of hypertriglyceridemia	500 mg, $0.87
Clonidine (Catapres®)	Stimulates α_2-adrenerigic receptors centrally resulting in attenuated sympathetic outflow, decreased peripheral vascular resistance, and inhibition of renin and aldosterone secretion	• Hypertension • Withdrawal (opiates, nicotine, alcohol)	0.1 mg po, $0.06 0.2 mg po, $0.07 0.3 mg po, $0.10 0.3 mg/24 hours transdermal, $23.08
Clopidogrel (Plavix®)	Selectively inhibits adenosine diphosphate (ADP)-induced platelet aggregation[27]	• Reduces atherosclerotic events in patients with recent stoke, recent MI or established peripheral arterial disease[28]	75 mg, $3.22
Colestipol (Colestid®)	Exchanges Na^+ for bile acids resulting in an increase in bile acid synthesis from cholesterol[26]	• Adjunct to dietary and lifestyle modifications for the treatment of primary hyperlipidemia	1 g po, $0.38 5 g/packet, $1.66
Dalteparin (Fragmin®)	Low-molecular-weight heparin that inhibits Factor Xa to a greater extent than thrombin (Anti-Xa: Anti-IIa = 2.7)[12,29]	• Prophylaxis against deep vein thrombosis for patients undergoing hip replacement or abdominal surgery • Unstable angina or non-ST-segment elevation MI[30,31]	2500 IU/0.2 mL, $15.35 5000 IU/0.2 mL, $24.90
Danaparoid (Orgaran®)	Predominantly anti-Factor Xa activity[13]	• Prevention of postoperative deep vein thrombosis following elective hip replacement surgery. • Management of heparin-induced thrombocytopenia ('off label')	750 anti-Factor Xa U/0.6 mL, $123.24
Digoxin (Lanoxin®)	Inhibits the Na^+/K^+ ATPase pump causing an increased concentration of intracellular Ca^{2+} thereby resulting in an augmented cardiac output. In addition, digoxin prolongs refractoriness in the AV node secondary to its indirect vagotonic effects	• Supraventricular tachycardias (atrial fibrillation/flutter) • Congestive heart failure[32]	0.125 mg po, $0.09 0.25 mg po, $0.09 0.50 mg po, $0.15 0.25 mg/mL (1 mL), $2.48
Digoxin Immune Fab (Digibind®)	Binds with free digoxin and is excreted by the kidneys	• Severe digoxin intoxication manifested by life-threatening ventricular arrhythmias, hemodynamically significant bradyarrhythmias, acute digoxin intoxication (>10 mg in adults or >4 mg in children) and a serum $K^+ \geq 5$ mEq/L	10 mg/mL (4 mL), $558.36

Cardiovascular agent	Pharmacology	Indication(s)	Cost[a,1]
Diltiazem (Cardizem®, Dilacor®)	Blocks Ca^{2+} entry into cells through slow Ca^{2+} channels. Also depresses SA and AV nodal function resulting in a decreased cardiac output	• Ischemic heart disease • Hypertension • Rate control in atrial fibrillation/flutter, paroxysmal supraventricular tachycardia (*do not use in patients with accessory bypass tracts*)	30 mg po, $0.08 60 mg po, $0.14 90 mg po, $0.19 120 mg po, $0.24 60 mg po (extended release), $0.94 90 mg po (extended release), $1.07 120 mg po (extended release), $1.39 5 mg/mL (5 mL) iv, $14.30
Dipyridamole (Persantine®)	Interferes with platelet aggregation via inhibition of adenosine deaminase and phosphodiesterase. In addition, dipyridamole stimulates the release of prostacyclin or PGD_2 resulting in coronary vasodilatation[14]	• Prevention of thrombosis/ thromboembolism • As an alternative to exercise during thallium myocardial perfusion imaging for the evaluation of coronary artery disease	25 mg po, $0.03 50 mg po, $0.04 75 mg po, $0.06 5 mg/mL (2 mL) iv, $23.04
Disopyramide (Norpace®)	Class IA antiarrhythmic. Decreases myocardial excitability and conduction velocity. Other properties include: anticholinergic, peripheral vasoconstrictive and negative inotropic effects.	• Maintains normal sinus rhythm in patients converted from atrial fibrillation or atrial flutter	100 mg, $0.27 150 mg, $0.31 150 mg (extended release), $0.97
Dobutamine (Dobutrex®)	Stimulates β_1-adrenergic receptors resulting in an increased cardiac output and enhanced AV conduction	• Severe congestive heart failure • Mitral regurgitation	12.5 mg/mL (20 mL), $3.13
Dofetilide (Tikosyn®)	Antiarrhythmic agent with selective K^+ channel blocking properties	• Maintenance of and conversion to normal sinus rhythm in patients with highly symptomatic atrial fibrillation or atrial flutter	
Doxazosin (Cardura®)	Highly selective antagonist at postsynaptic α_1-adrenergic receptors	• Hypertension[33,34]	1 mg, $1.03 2 mg, $1.03 4 mg, $1.08 8 mg, $1.13
Enalapril (Vasotec®)	Competitive inhibitor of the angiotensin converting enzyme (ACE) resulting in lower levels of angiotensin II and reduction in aldosterone secretion[18]	• Hypertension[35] • Congestive heart failure[36,37] • Treatment of hemodynamically stable patients within 24-hours of an acute myocardial infarction[22] • Diabetic nephropathy	2.5 mg po, $0.86 5 mg po, $1.09 10 mg po, $1.15 20 mg po, $1.63 1.25 mg/mL (1 mL) iv, $15.30
Enoxaparin (Lovenox®)	Low-molecular-weight heparin that inhibits Factor Xa to a greater extent than thrombin (Anti-Xa: Anti-IIa = 3.8)[12]	• Prophylaxis against deep vein thrombosis (DVT) in patients undergoing hip or knee replacement surgery or patients with abdominal surgery • Unstable angina or non-ST-segment elevation MI[38] • In-patient/out-patient treatment of DVT[39]	30 mg/0.3 mL, $18.35 40 mg/0.4 mL, $24.46 60 mg/0.6 mL, $36.74 80 mg/0.8 mL, $48.98 100 mg/mL, $61.23

Cardiovascular agent	Pharmacology	Indication(s)	Cost[a,1]
Epinephrine	Stimulates α, β_1- and β_2-adrenergic receptors. The net result is augmented cardiac output, increased heart rate and blood pressure	• Cardiopulmonary resuscitation • Hypotension • Myocardial failure • Anaphylaxis • Severe asthma	0.1mg/mL (1 mL), $1.38 1 mg/mL (1 mL), $1.64
Epoprostenol (Flolan®)	Vasodilator of all vascular beds. In addition, it has the ability to inhibit platelet aggregation via increased concentration of cyclic adenosine monophosphate (cAMP) within the platelet	• Management of primary pulmonary hypertension associated with NYHA class III and iv patients, ARDS and cardiopulmonary bypass surgery	0.5 mg, $17.40 1.5 mg, $34.81
Eptifibatide (Integrilin®)	Glycoprotein IIb/IIIa receptor antagonist resulting in the inhibition of platelets binding to fibrinogen[40]	• Unstable angina or non-ST-segment elevation MI[41,42]	2 mg/mL (10 mL), $52.92 0.75 mg/mL (100 mL), $165.36
Esmolol (Brevibloc®)	Selective β_1-adrenergic blockade. Selectivity is lost at high doses	• Rate control in atrial fibrillation/flutter	10 mg/mL (10 mL), $18.03 250 mg/mL (10 mL), $85.21
Ethacrynic acid (Edecrin®)	Inhibits absorption of Na$^+$ and Cl$^-$ in the ascending loop of Henle	• Acute oliguria • Edematous states • Hypertension	25 mg po, $0.34 50 mg po, $0.49 50 mg iv, $21.84
Felodipine (Plendil®)	Dihydropyridine slow Ca^{2+}-channel blocker resulting in peripheral vasodilatation and relaxation of coronary vascular smooth muscle	• Hypertension • Angina (chronic stable or Prinzmetal's)	2.5 mg, $0.99 5 mg, $0.99 10 mg, $1.79
Fenoldopam (Corlopam®)	Selective postsynaptic dopamine (D$_1$-receptors) agonist resulting in decreased peripheral vascular resistance and increased renal blood flow and diuresis[43]	• Severe hypertension. May be particularly helpful in patients with renal compromise	10 mg/mL (1 mL), $240.00
Flecainide (Tambocor®)	Class IC antiarrhythmic. Blocks Na$^+$ current and delayed rectifier K$^+$ current resulting in a shortened action potential duration in Purkinje cells but prolonged action potential duration in ventricular cells	• Paroxysmal supraventricular tachycardia (PSVT) • Ventricular tachycardia/fibrillation without structural heart disease	50 mg, $1.49 100 mg, $2.40 150 mg, $3.30
Fluvastatin (Lescol®)	Competitively and selectively inhibits 3-hyroxyl-3-methylglutaryl coenzyme A (HMG-CoA), the rate-limiting enzyme that catalyzes the formation of mevalonic acid (a cholesterol precursor)[26]	• Adjunct to dietary and lifestyle modifications in primary hypercholesterolemia	20 mg, $1.33 40 mg, $1.33
Fosinopril (Monopril®)	Competitive inhibitor of the angiotensin-converting enzyme (ACE) resulting in lower levels of angiotensin II and reduction in aldosterone secretion[18]	• Hypertension[35] • Congestive heart failure[44]	10 mg, $0.90 20 mg, $0.90 40 mg, $0.90

Cardiovascular agent	Pharmacology	Indication(s)	Cost[a,1]
Furosemide (Lasix®)	Inhibits absorption of Na^+ and Cl^- in the ascending loop of Henle[19]	• Acute oliguria • Edematous states • Hypertension	20 mg po, $0.02 40 mg po, $0.03 80 mg po, $0.05 10 mg/mL (2 mL) iv, $1.24
Gemfibrozil (Lopid®)	Increases the effect of lipoprotein lipase, the enzyme responsible for the hydrolysis of triglycerides from VLDL and IDL particles[26]	• Adjunct to diet and lifestyle modifications in the management of hypertriglyceridemia	600 mg, $0.18
Guanabenz (Wytensin®)	Stimulates α_2-adrenergic receptors in the brainstem resulting in the attenuation of sympathetic outflow	• Hypertension	4 mg, $0.41 8 mg, $0.58
Guanfacine (Tenex®)	Stimulates α_2-adrenergic receptors in the brainstem resulting in the attenuation of sympathetic outflow	• Hypertension	1 mg, $0.63 2 mg, $0.88
Heparin	Accelerates the function of antithrombin III thereby inactivating thrombin, Factors IX, X, XI, XII and plasmin. Heparin prevents the conversion of fibrinogen to fibrin[13]	• Prophylaxis and treatment of thromboembolic disorders	1000 U/mL (1 mL), $1.10 5000 U/mL (1 mL), $1.44 2500 U/mL (0.25 mL), $1.06
Hydralazine (Apresoline®)	Causes direct relaxation of arteriolar smooth muscle	• Hypertension • Congestive heart failure (when used in combination with isosorbide dinitrate)[37]	10 mg po, $0.02 25 mg po, $0.04 50 mg po, $0.05 100 mg po, $0.09 20 mg/mL (1 mL), $8.75
Hydrochlorothiazide	Inhibits Na^+ reabsorption in the distal tubule causing excretion of water, Na^+, K^+, H^+, and Mg^{2+} [19]	• Hypertension[34] • Edema	25 mg, $0.02 50 mg, $0.03 100 mg, $0.06
Ibutilide (Corvert®)	Class III antiarrhythmic agent that increases activation of slow inward Na^+ ($I_{Na\text{-}S}$) current to prolong the action potential and thereby delays repolarization[45]	• Restoration of normal sinus rhythm in patients with atrial fibrillation or atrial flutter of recent onset	0.1 mg/mL (10 mL), $221.34
Indapamide (Lozol®)	Inhibits Na^+ reabsorption in the proximal portion of the distal tubule causing excretion of water, Na^+, K^+, H^+, and Mg^{2+}	• Hypertension • Edema	1.25 mg, $0.39 2.5 mg, $0.20
Irbesartan (Avapro®)	AT_1-angiotensin receptor antagonist resulting in the inhibition of the effects of angiotensin II and aldosterone	• Hypertension	75 mg, $1.19 150 mg, $1.25 300 mg, $2.51
Isoproterenol (Isuprel®)	Stimulates β_1- and β_2-adrenergic receptors resulting in increased heart rate, contractility and automaticity	• Bradycardia • AV block • Torsades de pointes	0.2 mg/mL (1 mL), $5.73
Isosorbide dinitrate (Isordil®)	Relaxes vascular smooth muscles via activation of guanylate cyclase and elevated concentration of cGMP	• Management of angina • Congestive heart failure (when used in combination with hydralazine)[37]	5 mg, $0.02 10 mg, $0.02 20 mg, $0.02 30 mg, $0.05

Cardiovascular agent	Pharmacology	Indication(s)	Cost[a,1]
Isosorbide mononitrate (Imdur®)	Relaxes vascular smooth muscles via activation of guanylate cyclase and elevated concentration of cGMP	• Management of angina	20 mg, $0.72 60 mg, $1.17
Isradipine (DynaCirc®)	Slow Ca^{2+}-channel blocker resulting in peripheral vasodilatation and relaxation of coronary vascular smooth muscle	• Hypertension	2.5 mg, $0.74 5 mg, $1.08 5 mg (extended release), $1.22 10 mg (extended release), $1.94
Labetalol (Normodyne®, Trandate®)	Selective α_1-adrenergic and non-selective β-adrenergic antagonist. Ratio of α-blockade to β-blockade is 1:3 to 1:7	• Hypertension • Management of pheochromocytoma	100 mg po, $0.48 200 mg po, $0.68 300 mg po, $0.91 5 mg/mL (20 mL) iv, $31.80
Lepirudin (Refludan®)	Antithrombin activity[13]	• Management of heparin-induced thrombocytopenia	50 mg, $126.00
Lidocaine	Class IB antiarrhythmic. Depresses conduction velocity (phase 0) and slope of phase 4 of the action potential[8]	• Ventricular tachycardia/ fibrillation • Cardiopulmonary resuscitation	0.5% 50 mL, $3.92 1% 2 mL, $1.83 1% 5 mL, $12.13 1% 20 mL, $2.72 2% 2 mL, $1.83 2% 5 mL, $2.17
Lisinopril (Prinivil®, Zestril®)	Competitive inhibitor of the angiotensin-converting enzyme (ACE) resulting in lower levels of angiotensin II and reduction in aldosterone secretion[18]	• Hypertension • Congestive heart failure[46] • Treatment of hemodynamically stable patients within 24 hours of an acute myocardial infarction[22] • Diabetic nephropathy	2.5 mg, $0.60 5 mg, $0.90 10 mg, $0.93 20 mg, $0.99 40 mg, $1.45
Losartan (Cozaar®)	AT_1-angiotensin receptor antagonist resulting in the inhibition of the effects of angiotensin II and aldosterone[47]	• Hypertension • May prolong survival in patients with congestive heart failure[48]	25 mg, $1.25 50 mg, $1.25 100 mg, $1.88
Lovastatin (Mevacor®)	Competitively and selectively inhibits 3-hyroxyl-3-methylglutaryl coenzyme A (HMG-CoA), the rate-limiting enzyme that catalyzes the formation of mevalonic acid (a cholesterol precursor)[26]	• Adjunct to dietary and lifestyle modifications in hypercholesterolemia	10 mg, $1.37 20 mg, $2.42 40 mg, $4.35
Mannitol (Osmitrol®)	Increases osmotic pressure of the glomerular filtrate, which facilitates excretion of water and inhibits reabsorption of Na^+ and Cl^-	• Cerebral edema • Acute oliguria	5% 1000 mL, $62.62 10% 1000 mL, $79.96 15% 500 mL, $76.69 20% 250 mL, $60.15 20% 500 mL, $60.15 25% 50 mL $6.13
Methyldopa (Aldomet®)	Stimulates central α_2-adrenergic receptors resulting in the attenuation of sympathetic outflow	• Hypertension	125 mg, $0.06 250 mg, $0.08 500 mg, $0.13
Metolazone (Zaroxolyn®, Mykrox®)	Inhibits Na^+ reabsorption in the distal tubule causing excretion of water, Na^+, K^+, H^+, and Mg^{2+}	• Hypertension • Edema • Cardiac and renal insufficiency	0.5 mg, $0.90 2.5 mg, $0.65 5 mg, $0.73 10 mg, $0.88

Cardiovascular agent	Pharmacology	Indication(s)	Cost[a,1]
Metoprolol (Lopressor®, Toprol XL®)	Selectively inhibits β_1-adrenergic receptors. Selectivity is lost at higher doses	• HTN[49] • Angina • Peri- and post-myocardial infarction • Congestive heart failure[50,51] • Supraventricular arrhythmias • Management of ventricular arrhythmias	50 mg po, $0.07 100 mg po, $0.09 50 mg po (extended release), $0.58 100 mg po (extended release), $0.88 1 mg/mL (5 mL) iv, $4.92
Mexiletine (Mexitil®)	Class IB antiarrhythmic. Depresses conduction velocity (phase 0) and slope of phase 4 of the action potential		150 mg, $0.82 200 mg, $0.98 250 mg, $1.14
Milrinone (Primacor®)	Inhibits myocardial cyclic adenosine monophosphate (cAMP) phosphodiesterase III activity thereby increasing cellular cAMP levels and increased Ca^{2+} influx. In addition to augmenting cardiac output, milrinone possesses systemic and pulmonary vasodilator effects resulting in pre- and afterload reduction	• Severe decompensated congestive heart failure. Long-term therapy with milrinone may be associated with increased morbidity and mortality in patients with severe heart failure[52]	Dextrose/Milrinone 5% 20 mg/100 mL, $134.19 20 mg/200 mL, $262.65 Milrinone Lactate 1 mg/mL (5 mL), $42.95 1 mg/mL (10 mL), $73.76 1 mg/mL (20 mL), $134.79 1 mg/mL (50 mL), $330.67
Minoxidil (Loniten®)	Minoxidil N-O sulfate, an active metabolite, relaxes vascular smooth muscle	• Hypertension	2.5 mg, $0.27 10 mg, $0.54
Moexipril (Univasc®)	Competitive inhibitor of the angiotensin-converting enzyme (ACE) resulting in lower levels of angiotensin II and reduction in aldosterone secretion[18]	• Hypertension	7.5 mg, $0.62 15 mg, $0.62
Moricizine (Ethmozine®)	Class IC antiarrhythmic agent. Depresses the Na^+ current and shortens repolarization resulting in decreased action potential duration and effective refractory period	• Management of ventricular arrhythmias in patients without organic heart damage	200 mg, $1.15 250 mg, $1.37 300 mg, $1.56
Nadolol (Corgard®)	Non-selective β-adrenergic antagonist	• Hypertension • Angina pectoris	20 mg, $0.47 40 mg, $0.51 80 mg, $0.66 120 mg, $1.77 160 mg, $1.96
Niacin	Reduces the conversion of VLDL to LDL, decreases the synthesis of triglycerides, and increases HDL concentrations[26]	• Hypertriglyceridemia or hypercholesterolemia	500 mg, $0.28 1000 mg, $0.93 500 mg (extended release), $0.54 750 mg (extended release), $0.69
Nicardipine (Cardene®)	Dihydropyridine slow Ca^{2+}-channel blocker resulting in peripheral vasodilatation	• Hypertension • Angina (chronic stable or Prinzmetal's)	20 mg po, $0.42 30 mg po, $0.68 2.5 mg/mL (10 mL) iv, $26.84
Nifedipine (Procardia®)	Dihydropyridine slow Ca^{2+}-channel blocker resulting in peripheral vasodilatation	• Hypertension • Angina (chronic stable or Prinzmetal's)	10 mg, $0.09 20 mg, $0.17 30 mg (extended release), $1.43 60 mg (extended release), $2.47 90 mg (extended release), $2.85

Cardiovascular agent	Pharmacology	Indication(s)	Cost[a,1]
Nimodipine (Nimotop®)	Dihydropyridine slow Ca^{2+}-channel blocker resulting in peripheral vasodilatation	• Hypertension • Angina (chronic stable or Prinzmetal's)	30 mg, $6.47
Nisoldipine (Sular®)	Dihydropyridine slow Ca^{2+}-channel blocker resulting in peripheral vasodilatation	• Hypertension • Angina (chronic stable or Prinzmetal's)	10 mg, $0.96 20 mg, $0.96 30 mg, $0.96 40 mg, $0.96
Nitroglycerin	Relaxes vascular smooth muscles via activation of guanylate cyclase and elevated concentration of cGMP. Decreases preload	• Acute coronary syndromes • Stable angina • Congestive heart failure • Systemic and pulmonary hypertension	0.3 mg po (sublingual), $0.07 0.4 mg po (sublingual), $0.07 0.6 mg po (sublingual), $0.07 0.4 mg spray, $31.23 2 mg buccal, $0.42 3 mg buccal, $0.46 0.1 mg/hour transdermal, $1.63 0.2 mg/hour transdermal, $1.65 0.4 mg/hour transdermal, $1.85 0.6 mg/hour transdermal, $2.01 2.5 mg po (extended release), $0.11 6.5 mg po (extended release), $0.12 9 mg po (extended release), $0.17 30 g (ointment 2%), $6.95 60 g (ointment 2%), $10.62 5%–10 mg/100 mL (250 mL) iv, $21.05
Nitroprusside (Nitropress®)	Decomposes to nitric oxide to activate guanylate cyclase. Guanylate cyclase converts GTP to cGMP which dilates arteriole and venous blood vessels	• Hypertensive crisis • Congestive heart failure	50 mg, $5.00
Norepinephrine (Levophed®)	Moderate effect on β_1-adrenergic receptors on the heart and a pronounced effect on α_1-receptors in the periphery. The net result is peripheral vasoconstriction, increase coronary blood flow and positive inotropic effect	• Cardiac arrest • Severe hypotension	1 mg/mL (4 mL), $16.63
n-PA (Lanotreplase®)	Deletion and point mutation of wild-type t-PA results in n-PA[6,53]	• Acute myocardial infarction[54]	[b]
Pindolol (Visken®)	Non-selective β_1- and β_2-adrenergic receptor antagonist with membrane stabilizing and intrinsic sympathomimetic activity (ISA)	• Management of angina	5 mg, $0.13 10 mg, $0.17
Pravastatin (Pravachol®)	Competitively and selectively inhibits 3-hyroxyl-3-methylglutaryl coenzyme A (HMG-CoA), the rate-limiting enzyme that catalyzes the formation of mevalonic acid (a cholesterol precursor)[26]	• Adjunct to dietary and lifestyle modifications in hypercholesterolemia • Primary prevention of myocardial infarction[55]	10 mg, $2.26 20 mg, $2.43 40 mg, $3.94

Cardiovascular agent	Pharmacology	Indication(s)	Cost[a,1]
Prazosin (Minipress®)	Highly selective antagonist at postsynaptic α_1-adrenergic receptors	• Hypertension	1 mg, $0.07 2 mg, $0.07 5 mg, $0.14
Procainamide (Pronestyl®)	Class IA antiarrhythmic; blocks Na^+ and multiple cardiac K^+ currents[8]	• Conversion of atrial fibrillation/atrial flutter • Paroxysmal supraventricular tachycardia • Wolff–Parkinson–White syndrome	250 mg po, $0.15 375 mg po, $0.18 500 mg po, $0.16 250 mg po (extended release), $0.18 500 mg po (extended release), $0.28 750 mg po (extended release), $0.45 1000 mg po (extended release), $0.48 100 mg/mL (10 mL) iv, $4.00 500 mg/mL (2 mL) iv, $4.00
Propafenone (Rythmol®)	Class IC antiarrhythmic. Blocks the Na^+ and delayed rectifier K^+ currents resulting in slow conduction in fast-response tissues. It prolongs the PR and QRS durations	• Paroxysmal supraventricular tachycardia • Ventricular/tachycardia/ fibrillation without structural heart disease	150 mg, $1.35 225 mg, $1.92 300 mg, $2.45
Propranolol (Inderal®)	Non-selective β-adrenergic antagonist with moderate membrane stabilizing activity thereby decreasing heart rate and contractility of the myocardium	• Hypertension • Angina pectoris • Supraventricular arrhythmias • Symptomatic premature ventricular contractions (PVCs) • Pheochromocytoma • Post-myocardial infarction	10 mg po, $0.02 20 mg po, $0.03 40 mg po, $0.03 60 mg po, $0.04 80 mg po, $0.04 120 mg po, $1.36 160 mg po, $1.78 1 mg/mL (1 mL) iv, $14.27
Quinapril (Accupril®)	Competitive inhibitor of the angiotensin-converting enzyme (ACE) resulting in lower levels of angiotensin II and reduction in aldosterone secretion[18]	• Hypertension • Congestive heart failure	5 mg, $0.98 10 mg, $0.98 20 mg, $0.98 40 mg, $0.98
Quinidine	Class IA antiarrhythmic. Increases the QT_c interval and widens the QRS complex. In addition, quinidine has vagolytic and α-adrenergic blocking properties[8,56]	• Paroxysmal supraventricular tachycardia	200 mg po, $0.10 300 mg po, $0.15 275 mg po, $1.35 324 mg po (extended release), $0.51 80 mg/mL (10 mL) iv, $16.98
Ramipril (Altace®)	Competitive inhibitor of the angiotensin-converting enzyme (ACE) resulting in lower levels of angiotensin II and reduction in aldosterone secretion	• Hypertension • Congestive heart failure[57]	1.25 mg, $0.78 2.5 mg, $0.92 5 mg, $1.00 10 mg, $1.18
Reserpine	Depletes catecholamine and 5-hydroxytryptophan in the CNS and peripheral adrenergic neurons thereby decreasing peripheral resistance and heart rate with a slight decrease in cardiac output	• Mild–moderate hypertension	0.25 mg, $0.03 0.1 mg, $0.04

Cardiovascular agent	Pharmacology	Indication(s)	Cost[a,1]
Reteplase (r-PA) (Retevase®)	Activates plasminogen bound to fibrin ('fibrin selective') resulting in local fibrinolysis. It has a prolonged half-life of 18 minutes[6,53]	• Acute myocardial infarction	10.8 U, $2750.00
Simvastatin (Zocor®)	Competitively and selectively inhibits 3-hyroxyl-3-methylglutaryl coenzyme A (HMG-CoA), the rate-limiting enzyme that catalyzes the formation of mevalonic acid (a cholesterol precursor)[26]	• Adjunct to dietary and lifestyle modifications in hypercholesterolemia • Improves survival and reduces the rate of coronary events[58]	5 mg, $1.78 10 mg, $2.18 20 mg, $3.81 40 mg, $3.81 80 mg, $3.81
Sotalol (Betapace®)	Class III antiarrhythmic. Non-selective β-adrenergic antagonist that prolongs the cardiac action potential and increases the refractory period[59]	• Paroxysmal supraventricular tachycardia • Prevention of ventricular tachycardia/fibrillation[60]	80 mg, $2.12 120 mg, $2.83 160 mg, $3.53 240 mg, $4.60
Spironolactone (Aldactone®)	Aldosterone inhibitor in the cortical collecting tubule, thereby increasing Na^+ excretion and decreasing K^+ excretion (K^+-sparing diuretic)[19]	• Hypertension • Edema • Congestive heart failure[61]	25 mg, $0.08
Streptokinase	Activates the fibrinolytic system by forming a complex with plasminogen. This results in the activation of plasminogen which is then converted to the active enzyme plasmin[53]	• Acute myocardial infarction[62]	250 000 IU, $121.73 750, 000 IU, $268.65 1.5 million IU, $537.34
Telmisartan (Micardis®)	AT_1-angiotensin receptor antagonist resulting in the inhibition of the effects of angiotensin II and aldosterone	• Hypertension	40 mg, $1.29 80 mg, $1.29
Terazosin (Hytrin®)	Highly selective antagonist at postsynaptic α_1-adrenergic receptors	• Hypertension	1 mg, $1.60 2 mg, $1.60 5 mg, $1.60 10 mg, $1.60
Ticlopidine (Tilclid®)	Selectively inhibits adenosine diphosphate (ADP)-induced platelet aggregation[27]	• Thrombotic stroke, transient cerebral ischemia, acute myocardial infarction (if patient is allergic to aspirin) • Inhibition of stent thrombosis[63]	250 mg, $1.92
Tirofiban (Aggrastat®)	Glycoprotein IIb/IIIa receptor antagonist resulting in the inhibition of platelets binding to fibrinogen[40]	• Unstable angina or non-ST-segment elevation MI[64]	0.25 mg/mL (50 mL vial), $420.00 Pre-mixed, $840.00
TNK-tPA	TNK-tPA has very high fibrin specificity and binding thus producing more rapid and complete thrombolysis[53]	• Acute myocardial infarction[65]	$2750.00
Tocainide (Tonocard®)	Class IB antiarrhythmic. Depresses conduction velocity (phase 0) and slope of phase 4 of the action potential	• Ventricular arrhythmias	400 mg, $0.88 600 mg, $1.13

Cardiovascular agent	Pharmacology	Indication(s)	Cost[a,1]
Torsemide (Demadex®)	Inhibits absorption of Na⁺ and Cl⁻ in the ascending loop of Henle[19]	• Acute oliguria • Edematous states • Hypertension	5 mg po, $0.49 10 mg po, $0.55 20 mg po, $0.64 100 mg po, $2.36 10 mg/mL (2 mL) iv, $3.99 10 mg/mL (5 mL) iv, $5.47
Trandolapril (Mavik®)	Competitive inhibitor of the angiotensin-converting enzyme (ACE) resulting in lower levels of angiotensin II and reduction in aldosterone secretion[18]	• Hypertension • Congestive heart failure[66]	1 mg, $0.72 2 mg, $0.72 4 mg, $0.72
Triamterene (Dyrenium®)	K⁺-sparing diuretic that inhibits Na⁺/H⁺ exchange in the proximal tubule	• Hypertension • Edema	50 mg, $0.87 100 mg, $1.59
Urokinase (Abbokinase®)	Activates plasminogen directly resulting in the formation of the active enzyme plasmin[53]	• Pulmonary embolism • Coronary artery thrombosis • Intravenous catheter clearance	5000 IU, $59.59 9000 IU, $103.91
Valsartan (Diovan®)	AT₁-angiotensin receptor antagonist resulting in the inhibition of the effects of angiotensin II and aldosterone	• Hypertension	80 mg, $1.25 160 mg, $1.34
Verapamil (Calan®, Isoptin®)	Phenylalkylamine slow Ca²⁺-channel blocker resulting in peripheral and coronary vasodilatation. In addition, verapamil possesses negative inotropic effects	• Hypertension • Angina (Prinzmetal's, chronic stable and unstable) • Rate control in atrial fibrillation/flutter	40 mg po, $0.15 80 mg po, $0.05 120 mg po, $0.33 120 mg po (extended release), $1.16 180 mg po (extended release), $0.29 240 mg po (extended release), $0.31 360 mg po (extended release), $2.10 2.5 mg/mL (2 mL) iv, $2.85 2.5 mg/mL (4 mL), $4.76
Warfarin (Coumadin®)	Competes with hepatic synthesis of vitamin K-dependent clotting Factors II, VII, IX and X[67]	• Prophylaxis and treatment of venous thrombosis • Treatment of pulmonary embolism • Prevention of systemic embolism in valve replacements, atrial fibrillation and myocardial infarction	1 mg po, $0.58 2 mg po, $0.60 2.5 mg po, $0.63 3 mg po, $0.63 4 mg po, $0.63 5 mg po, $0.64 6 mg po, $0.90 7.5 mg po, $0.93 10 mg po, $0.97 $19.31

[a] Costs to the pharmacist per unit dose based on the average wholesale price (AWP) listings in the 2000 *Red Book*.[1] USD = US dollars
[b] Current medication costs not available.
ARDS = acute respiratory distress syndrome; AT₁ = angiotensin 1; AV = atrioventricular; cGMP = cyclic guanidine monophosphate; CNS = central nervous system; FDA = Food and Drug Administration; HDL = high-density lipoprotein; HTN = hypertension; IDL = intermediate-density lipoprotein; iv = intravenous; LDL = low-density lipoprotein; MI = myocardial infarction; n-PA = lanotreplase; PGD₂ = prostaglandin D₂; po = per os; SA = sinoatrial; TNK-tPA = tenecteplase; VLDL = very-low-density lipoprotein; VT = ventricular tachycardia.

REFERENCES

1. Cardinale V, ed. *2000 Drug Topics® Red book®*. Montvale, NJ: Medical Economics Company, Inc., 2000.
2. Genetta TB, Mauro VF. Abciximab: a new antiaggregant used in angioplasty. *Ann Pharmacother* 1996; **30**: 251–7.
3. The EPIC Investigators. Use of monoclonal antibody directed against the platelet glycoprotein IIb/IIIa receptor in high-risk coronary angioplasty. *N Engl J Med* 1994; **330**: 956–61.
4. The EPILOG Investigators. Platelet glycoprotein IIb/IIIa receptor blockade and low dose heparin during percutaneous coronary revascularization. *N Engl J Med* 1997; **336**: 1689–96.
5. Camm AJ, Garratt CJ. Adenosine and supraventricular tachycardia. *N Engl J Med* 1991; **325**: 1621–9.
6. Smalling RW. A fresh look at the molecular pharmacology of plasminogen activators: from theory to test tube to clinical outcomes. *Am J Heath Syst Pharm* 1997; **54**(suppl 1): S17–22.
7. The GUSTO Investigators. An international randomized trial comparing four thrombolytic strategies for acute myocardial infarction. *N Engl J Med* 1993; **329**: 673–82.
8. Nolan PE. Pharmacokinetics and pharmacodynamics of intravenous agents for ventricular arrhythmias. *Pharmacotherapy* 1997; **17**(2 Pt 2): 65S–75S.
9. Kudenchuck PJ, Cobb LA, Copass MK, *et al*. Amiodarone for resuscitation after out-of-hospital cardiac arrest due to ventricular fibrillation. *N Engl J Med* 1999; **341**: 871–8.
10. AIMS Trial Study Group. Long-term effects of intravenous anistreplase in acute myocardial infarction: final report of the AIMS Study. *Lancet* 1990; **335**: 427–31.
11. Robert S, Wagner BKJ, Boulanger M, *et al*. Aprotinin. *Ann Pharmacother* 1996; **30**: 372–80.
12. Stringer KA. Emergence of low-molecular weight heparins in cardiology. *Pharmacotherapy* 1999; **19**(9 Pt 2): 141S–6S.
13. Hirsh J, Warkentin TE, Raschke R, *et al*. Heparin and low-molecular weight heparin. *Chest* 1998; **114**: 489S–510S.
14. Patrono C, Coller B, Dalen JE, *et al*. Platelet active drugs: the relationship among dose, effectiveness, and side effects. *Chest* 1998; **114**: 470S–88S.
15. Pepine CJ, Cohn PF, Deedwania PC, *et al*. Effects of treatment on outcome in mildly symptomatic patients with ischemia during daily life: the atenolol silent ischemia study (ASIST). *Circulation* 1994; **90**: 762–8.
16. Malinowski JM. Atorvastatin: a hydroxymethylglutaryl-coenzyme A reductase inhibitor. *Am J Health Syst Pharm* 1998; **55**: 2253–67.
17. Tsikouris JP, Kluger J. Azimilide: a nonselective class III antiarrhythmic agent for use in atrial fibrillation. *Formulary* 1999; **34**: 737–50.
18. Verme-Gibboney C. Oral angiotensin-converting-enzyme inhibitors. *Am J Health Syst Pharm* 1997; **54**: 2689–703.
19. Brater DC. Diuretic therapy. *N Engl J Med* 1998; **339**: 387–95.
20. Pfeffer MA, Braunwald E, Moye LA, *et al*. Effect of captopril on mortality and morbidity in patients with left ventricular dysfunction after myocardial infarction. Results of the survival and ventricular enlargement trial. *N Engl J Med* 1992; **327**: 669–77.
21. Van Gilst WH, Kingma H, Peels KH, *et al*. Which patient benefits from early angiotensin-converting enzyme inhibition? Results of one year serial echocardiographic follow-up from the captopril and thrombolysis study (CATS). *J Am Coll Cardiol* 1996; **28**: 114–21.
22. ACE Inhibitor Myocardial Infarction Collaborative Group. Indications for ACE inhibitors in the early treatment of acute myocardial infarction: systemic overview of individual data from 100 000 patients in randomized trials. *Circulation* 1998; **97**: 2202–12.
23. Bleske BE, Gilbert EM, Munger MA. Carvedilol: therapeutic application and practice guidelines. *Pharmacotherapy* 1998; **18**: 729–37.
24. Packer M, Bristow MR, Cohn JN, *et al*. The effect of carvedilol on morbidity and mortality in patients with chronic heart failure. *N Engl J Med* 1996; **334**: 1349–55.
25. Australia–New Zealand Heart Failure Research Collaborative Group. Randomized, placebo-controlled trial of carvedilol in patients with congestive heart failure due to ischaemic heart disease. *Lancet* 1997; **349**: 375–80.
26. Knopp RH. Drug treatment of lipid disorders. *N Engl J Med* 1999; **341**: 498–511.
27. Quinn MJ, Fitzgerald DJ. Ticlopidine and clopidogrel. *Circulation* 1999; **100**: 1667–72.
28. CAPRIE Steering Committee. A randomized, blinded, trial of clopidogrel vs aspirin in patients at risk of ischaemic events (CAPRIE). *Lancet* 1996; **348**: 1329–39.
29. Howard PA. Dalteparin: a low-molecular-weight heparin. *Ann Pharmacother* 1997; **31**: 192–203.
30. Fragmin during Instability in Coronary Artery Disease (FRISC) Study Group. Low molecular weight heparin during instability in coronary artery disease. *Lancet* 1996; **347**: 561–8.
31. Fragmin and Fast Revascularization during Instability in Coronary Artery Disease (FRISC II) Investigators. Invasive compared to non-invasive treatment in unstable coronary artery disease: FRISC II prospective randomized multicentre study. *Lancet* 1999; **354**: 708–15.
32. The Digitalis Investigation Group. The effect of digoxin on mortality and morbidity in patients with heart failure. *N Engl J Med* 1997; **336**: 525–33.
33. Langdon CG, Packard RS. Doxazosin in hypertension: results of a general practice study in 4809 patients. *Br J Clin Pract* 1994; **48**: 293–8.
34. Grimm RH Jr, Flack JM, Schoenberger JA, *et al*. Alpha-blockade and thiazide treatment of hypertension. A double blind randomized trial comparing doxazosin and hydrochlorothiazide. *Am J Hypertension* 1996; **9**: 445–54.
35. Hansson L, Forslund T, Hoglund C, *et al*. Fosinopril vs enalapril in the treatment of hypertension: a double

blind study in 195 patients. *J Cardiovasc Pharmacol* 1996; **28**: 1–5.

36. The SOLVD Investigators. Effect of enalapril on survival in patients with reduced left ventricular ejection fractions and congestive heart failure. *N Engl J Med* 1991; **325**: 293–302.

37. Cohn JN, Johnson G, Zeische S, *et al*. A comparison of enalapril with hydralazine–isosorbide dinitrate in the treatment of chronic congestive heart failure. *N Engl J Med* 1991; **325**: 303–10.

38. Cohen M, Demers C, Gurfinkel EP, *et al*. A comparison of low molecular weight heparin with unfractionated heparin for unstable coronary artery disease. *N Engl J Med* 1997; **337**: 447–52.

39. Levine M, Gent M, Hirsh J, *et al*. A comparison of low-molecular-weight heparin administered primarily at home with unfractionated heparin administered in the hospital for proximal deep-vein thrombosis. *N Engl J Med* 1996; **344**: 677–81.

40. Stringer KA. The evolving role of platelet glycoprotein IIb/IIIa inhibitors in the management of acute coronary syndromes. *Ann Pharmacother* 1999; **33**: 712–22.

41. The IMPACT-II Investigators. Randomized, placebo-controlled trial of effect of eptifibatide on complications of percutaneous coronary intervention: IMPACT-II. *Lancet* 1997; **349**: 1422–8.

42. The PURSUIT Trial Investigators. Inhibition of platelet glycoprotein IIb/IIIa with eptifibatide in patients with acute coronary syndromes. *N Engl J Med* 1998; **339**: 436–43.

43. Murphy MB, McCoy CE, Weber RR, *et al*. Augmentation of renal blood flow and sodium excretion in hypertensive patients during blood pressure reduction by intravenous administration of the dopamine, agonist fenoldopam. *Circulation* 1987; **76**: 1312–8.

44. *Monopril (fosinopril sodium) package insert*. Princeton, NJ: Bristol-Myers Squibb, 1995.

45. Granberry MC. Ibutilide: a new class III antiarrhythmic agent. *Am J Health Syst Pharm* 1998; **55**: 255–60.

46. Clark AL, Coats AJS. Severity of heart failure and dosage of angiotensin converting enzyme inhibitors. *Br Med J* 1995; **310**: 973–4.

47. Schaefer KL, Porter JA. Angiotensin II receptor antagonists: the prototype losartan. *Ann Pharmacother* 1996; **30**: 625–36.

48. Pitt B, Martinez FA, Meurers GG, *et al*. Randomized trial of losartan vs captopril in patients ≥ 65 with heart failure (Evaluation of losartan in the elderly study, ELITE). *Lancet* 1997; **349**: 747–52.

49. LaPalio L, Schork A, Glasser S, *et al*. Safety and efficacy of metoprolol in the treatment of hypertension in the elderly. *J Am Geriatr Soc* 1992; **40**: 354–8.

50. Persson H, Rythe'n-Alder E, Melcher A, *et al*. Effects of β receptor antagonists in patients with clinical evidence of heart failure after myocardial infarction: double blind comparison of metoprolol and xamoterol. *Br Heart J* 1995; **74**: 140–8.

51. Waagstein F, Bristow MR, Swedberg K, *et al*. Beneficial effects of metoprolol in idiopathic dilated cardiomyopathy. *Lancet* 1993; **342**: 1441–6.

52. Packer M, Carver JR, Rodeheffer RJ, *et al*. Effect of milrinone on mortality in severe chronic heart failure. *N Engl J Med* 1991; **325**: 1468–75.

53. Becker RC. New thrombolytic, anticoagulants, and platelet antagonists: the future of clinical practice. *J Thromb Thrombolysis* 1999; **7**: 195–220.

54. den Heijer P, Vermeer F, Ambrosioni E, *et al*., for the TIME investigators. Evaluation of a weight-adjusted single bolus plasminogen activator in patients with myocardial infarction. A double-blind, randomized angiographic trial of lanotreplase versus alteplase. *Circulation* 1998; **98**: 2117–25.

55. West of Scotland Coronary Prevention Study Group. Influence of pravastatin and plasma lipids on clinical events in the West of Scotland Coronary Prevention Study (WOCOPS). *Circulation* 1998; **97**: 1440–5.

56. Grace AA, Camm AJ. Quinidine. *N Engl J Med* 1998; **338**: 35–45.

57. The AIRE Study Investigators. Effect of ramipril on mortality and morbidity of survivors of acute myocardial infarction with clinical evidence of heart failure. *Lancet* 1993; **342**: 821–8.

58. Scandinavian Simvastatin Survival Study Group. Randomized trial of cholesterol lowering in 4444 patients with coronary heart disease: the Scandinavian Simvastatin Survival Study (4S). *Lancet* 1994; **344**: 1383–9.

59. Bauman JL. Class III antiarrhythmic agents: the next wave. *Pharmacotherapy* 1997; **17**(2 Pt 2): 76S–83S.

60. Haverkamp W, Martinez-Rubio A, Hief C, *et al*. Efficacy and safety of d,l-sotalol in patients with ventricular tachycardia and in survivors of cardiac arrest. *J Am Coll Cardiol* 1997; **30**: 487–95.

61. Pitt B, Zannad F, Remme WJ, *et al*., for the RALES Investigators. The effect of spironolactone on morbidity and mortality in patients with severe heart failure. *N Engl J Med* 1999; 341: 709–17.

62. ISIS-2 Collaborative Group. Randomized trial of intravenous streptokinase, oral aspirin, both, or neither among 17 187 cases of suspected acute myocardial infarction: ISIS-2. *Lancet* 1998; **II**: 349–60.

63. Leon M, Baim D, Popma J, *et al*. A clinical trial comparing three antithrombotic drug regimens after coronary artery stenting. *N Engl J Med* 1998; **339**: 1665–71.

64. Platelet Receptor Inhibition in Ischemic Syndrome Management in Patients Limited by Unstable Signs and Symptoms (PRISM-Plus) Study Investigators. Inhibition of the platelet glycoprotein IIb/IIIa receptor with tirofiban in unstable angina and non-Q-wave MI. *N Engl J Med* 1998; **338**: 1488–97.

65. Cannon CP, Gibson CM, McCabe CH, *et al*., for the TIMI 10b Investigators. TNK-tPA compared with front-loaded alteplase in acute myocardial infarction: results of the TIMI 10b trial. *Circulation* 1998; **98**: 2805–14.

66. Kober L, Torp-Pedersen C, Clarsen JE, *et al*. A clinical trial of the angiotensin-converting enzyme inhibitor trandolapril in patients with left ventricular dysfunction after myocardial infarction. *N Engl J Med* 1995; **333**: 1670–6.

67. Hirsh J, Dalen JE, Anderson DR, *et al*. Oral anticoagulants: mechanism of action, clinical effectiveness, and optimal therapeutic range. *Chest* 1998; **114**: 445S–69S.

Index

Note: page numbers in *italics* refer to figures and tables